T0265246

DISSEMINATION AND IMPLEMENTATION RESEARCH IN HEALTH

THIRD EDITION

DISSEMINATION AND IMPLEMENTATION RESEARCH IN HEALTH

Translating Science to Practice

EDITED BY

ROSS C. BROWNSON,
GRAHAM A. COLDITZ, AND
ENOLA K. PROCTOR

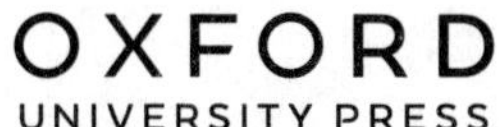

OXFORD
UNIVERSITY PRESS

Oxford University Press is a department of the University of Oxford. It furthers the University's objective of excellence in research, scholarship, and education by publishing worldwide. Oxford is a registered trade mark of Oxford University Press in the UK and certain other countries.

Published in the United States of America by Oxford University Press
198 Madison Avenue, New York, NY 10016, United States of America.

Library of Congress Cataloging-in-Publication Data
Names: Brownson, Ross C., editor. | Colditz, Graham A., editor. |
Proctor, Enola Knisley, editor.
Title: Dissemination and implementation research in health :
translating science to practice / edited by Ross C. Brownson,
Graham A. Colditz, Enola K. Proctor.
Description: 3. | New York, NY : Oxford University Press, [2023] |
Includes bibliographical references and index.
Identifiers: LCCN 2022051663 (print) | LCCN 2022051664 (ebook) |
ISBN 9780197660690 (hardback) | ISBN 9780197660713 (epub) |
ISBN 9780197660720
Subjects: MESH: Translational Research, Biomedical—methods |
Information Dissemination—methods | Implementation Science
Classification: LCC R852 (print) | LCC R852 (ebook) | NLM W 20.55.T7 |
DDC 610.72/4—dc23/eng/20230124
LC record available at https://lccn.loc.gov/2022051663
LC ebook record available at https://lccn.loc.gov/2022051664

DOI: 10.1093/oso/9780197660690.001.0001

Printed by Sheridan Books, Inc., United States of America

We dedicate this book to our spouses: Carol Brownson, Pat Cox, and Frank Proctor. We are grateful for their loving and life-long support, patience, and good humor.

CONTENTS

* New chapter for third edition.

FOREWORD

"10 Years Marked From the First of These"
—2017 Annual Dissemination and Implementation Science Conference Theme Song

YES AND . . .

The year 2021 marked the 20th (!) full year of my career at the National Institutes of Health (NIH), working to support the advancement of dissemination and implementation (D&I) research in health. I write with great appreciation for the efforts of so many, who have proposed and conducted influential studies; trained hundreds of aspiring scholars; convened thousands at workshops, webinars, and conferences; developed hundreds of conceptual advances; and harnessed methodological advances and created and validated new measures. We had followed a shift in thinking from "Why aren't our interventions implemented to the extent that they should be?" to "Can we get an intervention implemented?" to "What strategies can we use to support adoption, implementation, sustainment, and (where warranted) de-implementation?"

We saw a gradual shift from the linear pathway of research to recognition of reciprocal paths across stages of research and into an appreciation of dynamic evidence, interventions, and context.[1,2] Appreciation for the goals of D&I research was expressed across agencies, systems, and communities, and hundreds of trainees had developed study ideas that went from preliminary concept papers to full-fledged applications to research studies to outcomes papers.[3] D&I research has been prioritized nationally (e.g., National Cancer Institute's [NCI's] Cancer Moonshot, NIH's RADx-UP and Community Engagement Alliance [CEAL] initiatives) and globally (e.g., President's Emergency Fund for AIDS Relief [PEPFAR], household air pollution, Global Alliance for Chronic Diseases efforts)—so much to be grateful for.

At the close of this (literal) generation of work, we found ourselves with an even more daunting challenge that we continue to confront today—a global pandemic. We saw the manner in which work and society operated shift seismically; the need for public health, healthcare, and policy measures to be implemented vast; and a push for rapid, relevant, and robust studies to support a return to normalcy as the utmost priority. More than 2 years into this challenge, D&I research remains an opportunity to support community, population, and global health in the context of COVID and all areas of health.[4]

Reflecting on all of this in the presence of this third edited volume on the progress in D&I research, I have two words repeatedly echoing in my brain: "YES AND." This phrase was first explained to me by my brother-in-law, a former stand-up comedian and student of New York City's famed Upright Citizens Brigade as the first lesson of improv comedy. In that world, it's about acknowledging another's contribution and adding something to move the story along. It has implications for so many aspects of life, utilized in corporate and administrative retreats as a mantra for open and honest communication. And to me, it represents both progress and opportunity as the D&I research community continues to chart a more ambitious course for our collective future. YES AND says that we should celebrate the many successes, learn from myriad mistakes and limitations, and keep moving forward. It says that we can share in the conceptual and empirical gains in our D&I research knowledge base and listen intently to all who can shed light on what we have yet to uncover. As a framework, it calls out what we've written so far and sets us up for what could be even more impactful in the future.

A HANDFUL OF YES ANDS

YES, we've made great strides in building a large number of studies that test explicit implementation strategies hypothesized to drive uptake, implementation, and sustainment of individual evidence-based interventions. AND, we still need to expand our consideration of bundling both interventions and strategies. Indeed, many of our strategies are multicomponent, and yet we could do more to understand the mechanisms driving component and package to arrive at parsimonious bundles to improve implementation and sustainment.[5] On the intervention side, we can do more to test the implementation of interventions aggregated to encompass a broader care pathway (prevention, diagnosis, treatment, follow-up) or across multiple conditions (cancer, cardiovascular disease [CVD], depression, substance abuse, pain). YES, there are some nice examples of work in this area, AND much more that we can do together.

YES, we've seen significant contributions to the need for D&I to be equitable across all communities, systems, and populations. AND, we need to more extensively incorporate social determinants of health (e.g., education, transportation, social disorder); higher expectations for levels of uptake and sustainment; and recognition of the need for tailoring of interventions and strategies to improve scale-up for all.[6] In the past few years, many investigators and partners have raised awareness and advanced conceptual thinking of the interface between health equity and D&I research, as well as opportunities to address racism and discrimination.[7] There is still much more to do in our research designs, our collaborations, our engagement with partners, and our metrics for success.

YES, we've moved from the "kitchen sink" approach in developing and testing strategies to support D&I to a recognition that assessing hypothesized mechanisms is needed to determine how and why those strategies move D&I outcomes. AND, we need far more work to mechanistically understand the 73 (and counting) discrete strategies[8] and map how multiple strategies target specific influences individually and in tandem. This will enable more precision implementation approaches, efficiency in supporting key outcomes, and learnings that can generalize to a greater range of contexts and circumstances.

YES, we've developed a whole range of training materials, workshops, and institutes, building mentored and self-guided curricula that have supported hundreds of investigators in learning the basics of D&I research and how to apply them to specific study ideas, along with emerging courses and materials to support analogous learners in the policy and practice sphere.[9] AND, we need additional models to build multidisciplinary and multipartnered D&I research teams, twinning advances made in support for team science in concert with individual and community engagement.

YES, we have pursued and completed hundreds, if not thousands, of D&I studies across the globe, identifying facilitators and barriers to adoption and implementation; demonstrated improvements in key D&I outcomes; and supported tangible benefits to patients, clinicians, communities, and health systems. AND, we still need a larger concentration of studies looking at the long-term, dynamic outcomes of sustainment, adaptation (or evolution), and de-implementation.[10]

These YES ANDs represent a subset of the many markers of progress and the opportunities that lie ahead that provide such enthusiasm about the days to come. The past years have reinforced how important both dissemination and implementation processes are to address the largest challenges in healthcare and in society and the cost of not applying what we know and not learning what we do not.

ONE MORE YES AND FOR THE ROAD!

Finally, YES AND is about expressing gratitude for the people who have built a strong foundation for the next generation of studies and continually expanding the tent so that all who can influence population health, healthcare, and equity have a voice, an opportunity to share their expertise and experience, and keep us moving forward.

David A. Chambers, DPhil
Deputy Director for Implementation Science
Division of Cancer Control and
Population Sciences
National Cancer Institute
National Institutes of Health

REFERENCES

1. Chambers DA, Glasgow RE, Stange KC. The dynamic sustainability framework: addressing the paradox of sustainment amid ongoing change. *Implement Sci.* 2013 Oct 2;8:117. doi:10.1186/1748-5908-8-117
2. Aarons GA, Green AE, Palinkas LA, et al. Dynamic adaptation process to implement an evidence-based child maltreatment intervention. *Implement Sci.* 2012 Apr 18;7:32. doi:10.1186/1748-5908-7-32
3. Vinson CA, Clyne M, Cardoza N, Emmons KM. Building capacity: a cross-sectional evaluation of the US Training Institute for Dissemination and Implementation Research in Health. *Implement Sci.* 2019 Nov 21;14(1):97. doi:10.1186/s13012-019-0947-6
4. Chambers DA. Considering the intersection between implementation science and COVID-19. *Implement Res Pract.* January 2020;1(1). doi:10.1177/0020764020925994
5. Lewis CC, Boyd MR, Walsh-Bailey C, et al. A systematic review of empirical studies examining mechanisms of implementation in health. *Implement Sci.* 2020 Apr 16;15(1):21. doi:10.1186/s13012-020-00983-3
6. Brownson RC, Kumanyika SK, Kreuter MW, Haire-Joshu D. Implementation science should give higher priority to health equity. *Implement Sci.* 2021 Mar 19;16(1):28. doi:10.1186/s13012-021-01097-0
7. Shelton RC, Adsul P, Oh A, Moise N, Griffith DM. Application of an antiracism lens in the field of implementation science (IS): recommendations for reframing implementation research with a focus on justice and racial equity. *Implement Res Pract.* January 2021;2. doi:10.1177/26334895211049482
8. Powell BJ, Waltz TJ, Chinman MJ, et al. A refined compilation of implementation strategies: results from the Expert Recommendations for Implementing Change (ERIC) project. *Implement Sci.* 2015 Feb 12;10:21. doi:10.1186/s13012-015-0209-1
9. Proctor EK, Chambers DA. Training in dissemination and implementation research: a field-wide perspective. *Transl Behav Med.* 2017 Sep;7(3):624–635. doi:10.1007/s13142-016-0406-8
10. Norton WE, Chambers DA, Kramer BS. Conceptualizing de-implementation in cancer care delivery. *J Clin Oncol.* 2019 Jan 10;37(2):93–96. doi:10.1200/JCO.18.00589

PREFACE

To understand and fill the leaks in the pipeline between discovery of knowledge and application to improve population health and patient care, a distinct science has emerged. It goes by numerous titles, including translational research, knowledge translation, knowledge exchange, technology transfer, and dissemination and implementation (D&I) research. Although the terminology can be cumbersome and changing existing practices complex, the underlying rationale is simple: too often, discovery of new knowledge begets more discovery (the next study) with little attention on how to apply research advances in real-world public health, policy, social service, and health care settings. With early foundations in the work of Archie Cochrane in the 1970s showing that many medical treatments lacked scientific effectiveness, D&I research focuses on ways to increase the use of evidence-based interventions among practitioners, organizations, and systems. Research has shown that in efforts to disseminate practice guidelines using passive methods (e.g., publication of consensus statements, mass mailings), adoption has been relatively low, resulting in only small changes in the uptake of a new evidence-based practice. System change can be slower and more cumbersome. Thus, innovative and active approaches to D&I are needed, accounting for a wide array of contextual conditions.

As we began planning this new edition of our book, we realized how rapidly the science of D&I had grown since the second edition six years ago. Over this time period, we experienced the COVID-19 pandemic, which illustrated how a foundation in discovery research (e.g., developing a safe and effective vaccine) leads to a set of complex implementation challenges (e.g., scaling up strategies to promote vaccine uptake). COVID-19 also highlighted ongoing societal inequities, with substantially higher mortality among those living in poverty, and in some racial and minority groups, as well as in the elderly and chronically ill. This calls on us to redouble our efforts to address inequities and to do so with a sense of urgency.

These efforts require a return on investment—ensuring that the billions spent on basic and clinical research (discovery research) has proportional emphasis on translational research—moving discoveries into practice and policy. These efforts have been receiving much greater attention in mainline medical and public health journals. A growing set of journals are dedicated to D&I research, notably *Implementation Science* (begun in 2006), *Translational Behavioral Medicine* (begun in 2011), and *Implementation Research and Practice* (begun in 2020). In a PubMed search with the terms "implementation science" AND "methods" the number of articles increased from 2,542 in 2017 to 5,482 in 2021, a 116% increase. Similarly, in multiple countries, national agencies and foundations are beginning to support D&I research more fully.

The D&I gap has been shortened, perhaps best illustrated over the 20th century in the United States where life expectancy rose from 49 years in 1900 to 77 years in 2000. In large part, this increasing longevity was due to the application of discoveries on a population level (e.g., vaccinations, cleaner air and water). Yet for every victory, there is a parallel example of progress yet to be realized. For example, effective treatment for tuberculosis has been available since the 1950s yet globally, tuberculosis still accounts for 1.5 million annual deaths.

Despite a rich array of effective interventions and policies, tobacco use causes 7 million deaths per year. The chapters in this book draw on many successes and remaining challenges.

The rapid growth in our field, led to the need for several new or extensively revised chapters in this edition. In this third edition, 12 of 30 chapters are entirely new or extensively revised with mostly new material. In addition, all remaining chapters from the second edition have been updated.

This format of our book's new edition is organized to cover the major concepts for D&I researchers and practitioners. This edition draws on the talents of some of the top D&I scholars in the world—crossing many disciplines, health topics, and intervention settings. Our book has four sections. The first section provides a rationale for the book, highlights core issues needing attention, and describes the terminology for D&I research. In the second section, we highlight the theory and conceptual foundations of D&I research, including its historical roots, theories, core ethical issues. The third section focuses on a set of strategies and core methodologic concepts such as fidelity, adaptation, and organizational processes. In the next section, we cover design and measurement issues in depth, including concepts of external validity and mixed methods evaluation. The fifth section of the book focuses on settings and populations. Since D&I research occurs in places where people spend their lives (communities, schools, worksites) or receive care (health care, social service agencies), we devote chapters to specific settings. This section also recognizes the importance of policy influences on health, the science and practice of addressing health equity, and working in a global context. In the final section, we cover dissemination, the application of lessons from business and marketing, scale up, and capacity building.

The target audience for this text is broad and includes researchers and practitioners across many different disciplines including epidemiology, biostatistics, behavioral science, ethics, medicine, social work, psychology, and anthropology. It seeks to inform practitioners in health promotion, public health, health services, and health systems. We anticipate this book will be useful in academic institutions, state and local health agencies, federal agencies, and health care organizations. Although the volume is intended primarily for a North American audience, authors and examples are drawn from various parts of the world and we believe that much of the information covered is applicable in both developed and developing countries. The challenges of moving research to practice and policy appear to be universal, so future progress calls for collaborative partnerships and cross-country research.

Our book documents that in a time of substantial social and political changes resulting in increasing pressure on scientific and public resources, researchers must continue to meet the implied obligation to the public—that the billions of dollars invested in basic science will yield specific and tangible benefits to their health. Taxpayers have paid for a multitude of new discoveries—many of which are not being equitably translated into better patient care, public policy, and public health programs. We are confident that applying the principles in this volume will help to bridge the chasm between discovery and practice.

R. C. B.
G. A. C.
E. K. P.

ACKNOWLEDGMENTS

We are grateful to numerous individuals who contributed to the development of the third edition of this book. In particular, we are thankful to our extraordinary colleagues who contributed chapters. Their exceptional knowledge is reflected in the chapters, providing an up-to-date snapshot of dissemination and implementation science along with a peek into the future. We also appreciate the superb administrative assistance from Linda Dix.

Development of this book was supported in part by the National Institute of Diabetes and Digestive and Kidney Diseases (P30DK092950 and P30DK056341); the Centers for Disease Control and Prevention (U48DP006395); and the Foundation for Barnes-Jewish Hospital. This book was also supported by the Washington University Implementation Science Center for Cancer Control. The contents of this book are those of the authors and do not necessarily represent the official positions of the National Institutes of Health or the Centers for Disease Control and Prevention.

We acknowledge the remarkable leadership of Washington University's Brown School, Institute for Public Health, Alvin J. Siteman Cancer Center, Institute for Clinical and Translational Science, and Department of Surgery (Division of Public Health Sciences) for fostering an environment in which transdisciplinary and translational science are valued and encouraged. In particular, we are grateful to Tim Eberlein, Brad Evanoff, Eddie Lawlor, Andrew Martin, Mary McKay, Bill Powderly, Beverly Wendland, and Mark Wrighton. Finally, we are indebted to Sarah Humphreville and Emma Hodgdon, Oxford University Press, who provided valuable advice and support throughout the production of this new edition.

CONTRIBUTORS

Gregory A. Aarons, PhD
Department of Psychiatry
University of California
San Diego, CA, USA
UC San Diego Altman Clinical and Translational Research Institute, Dissemination and Implementation Science Center
University of California San Diego
La Jolla, CA, USA
Child and Adolescent Services Research Center
University of California, San Diego
La Jolla, CA, USA

Danielle R. Adams, PhD, MSW
Center for Mental Health Services Research, Brown School
Washington University in St. Louis
St. Louis, MO, USA

Prajakta Adsul, MBBS, MPH, PhD
Department of Internal Medicine, School of Medicine
University of New Mexico
Albuquerque, NM, USA
University of New Mexico Comprehensive Cancer Center
Albuquerque, NM, USA

Jennifer D. Allen, ScD, MPH
Department of Community Health
Tufts School of Arts and Sciences
Medford, MA, USA

Olakunle Alonge, MD, PhD, MPH
Bloomberg School of Public Health
Johns Hopkins University
Baltimore, MD, USA

Ana A. Baumann, PhD
Division of Public Health Sciences, Department of Surgery
Washington University in St. Louis
St. Louis, MO, USA

Jay M. Bernhardt, PhD, MPH
Moody College of Communication
University of Texas
Austin, TX, USA

Arleen Brown, MD
Division of General Internal Medicine, David Geffen School of Medicine
University of California Los Angeles
Los Angeles, CA, USA
Olive View UCLA Medical Center
Sylmar, CA, USA

C. Hendricks Brown, PhD
Department of Psychiatry and Behavioral Sciences
Northwestern University Feinberg School of Medicine
Chicago, IL, USA

Ross C. Brownson, PhD
Prevention Research Center in St. Louis, Brown School
Washington University in St. Louis
St. Louis, MO, USA
Division of Public Health Sciences and Alvin J. Siteman Cancer Center, Washington University School of Medicine
Washington University in St. Louis
St. Louis, MO, USA

Alicia C. Bunger, PhD
College of Social Work
The Ohio State University
Columbus, OH, USA

Leopoldo J. Cabassa, PhD
Brown School of Social Work
Washington University in St. Louis
St. Louis, MO, USA

David A. Chambers, DPhil
Division of Cancer Control and Population Sciences
National Cancer Institute, National Institutes of Health
Bethesda, MD, USA

Graham A. Colditz, MD, DrPH
Division of Public Health Sciences, Department of Surgery
Washington University School of Medicine
St. Louis, MO, USA

Todd B. Combs, PhD
Center for Public Health Systems Science, Brown School
Washington University in St. Louis
St. Louis, MO, USA

Erika L. Crable, PhD
Department of Psychiatry
University of California San Diego
San Diego, CA, USA

Gracelyn Cruden, PhD
Oregon Social Learning Center
Eugene, OR, USA

Geoffrey M. Curran, PhD
Departments of Pharmacy Practice and Psychiatry
University of Arkansas for Medical Sciences and Central Arkansas Veterans Healthcare System
Little Rock, AR, USA

Brittany Rhoades Cooper, PhD
Department of Human Development
Washington State University
Pullman, WA, USA

Melinda Davis, PhD, MCR
Oregon Rural Practice-Based Research Network, Department of Family Medicine, and School of Public Health
Oregon Health & Sciences University
Portland, OR, USA

Rachel Davis, PhD, MSc
Centre for Implementation Science, Health Services and Population Research Department
Kings College London
London, UK

James W. Dearing, PhD
Department of Communication
Michigan State University
East Lansing, MI, USA

S. Tiffany Donaldson, PhD
Department of Psychology and Honors College
University of Massachusetts Boston
Boston, MA, USA

Alex R. Dopp, PhD
RAND Corporation
Santa Monica, CA, USA

James M. DuBois, DSc, PhD
Department of Medicine
Washington University School of Medicine
St. Louis, MO, USA

O. Kenrik Duru, MD, MS
Division of General Internal Medicine/Health Services Research at the David Geffen School of Medicine
University of California Los Angeles
Los Angeles, CA, USA

Mark G. Ehrhart, PhD
Department of Psychology
University of Central Florida
Orlando, FL, USA

Andria B. Eisman, PhD
Community Health, Division of Kinesiology, Health and Sport Studies, College of Education
Wayne State University
Detroit, MI, USA
Center for Health and Community Impact
Wayne State University
Detroit, MI, USA

Karen M. Emmons, PhD
Department of Social and Behavioral Sciences
Harvard T. H. Chan School of Public Health
Boston, MA, USA

Maria E. Fernandez, PhD
Department of Health Promotion and Behavioral Science and Center for Health Promotion and Prevention Research
University of Texas Health Science Center at Houston
Houston, TX, USA

Stephanie L. Fitzpatrick, PhD
Kaiser Permanente Center for Health Research
Portland, OR, USA
Institute of Health System Science
Feinstein Institutes for Medical Research, Northwell Health
New York, NY, USA

Chandra L. Ford, PhD
Department of Community Health Sciences
University of California Los Angeles Fielding School of Public Health
Los Angeles, CA, USA

Meredith P. Fort, PhD, MPH
Department of Health Systems, Management and Policy; and Centers for American Indian and Alaska Native Health
Colorado School of Public Health
Aurora, CO, USA

Bridget Gaglio, PhD, MPH
Patient-Centered Research, Evidera
Bethesda, MD, USA

Elvin H. Geng, MD, MPH
Division of Infectious Diseases, Department of Medicine, School of Medicine, and Center for Dissemination and Implementation in the Institute for Public Health
Washington University
St. Louis, MO, USA

Russell E. Glasgow, PhD
Department of Family Medicine and Dissemination and Implementation Science Program of ACCORDS (Adult and Child Center for Health Outcomes Research and Delivery Science)
University of Colorado School of Medicine, Anschutz Medical Campus
Aurora, CO, USA

Beth A. Glenn, PhD
UCLA Kaiser Permanente Center for Health Equity, Department of Health Policy and Management
University of California Los Angeles Fielding School of Public Health
Los Angeles, CA, USA
Center for Cancer Prevention and Control Research, Jonsson Comprehensive Cancer Center
University of California Los Angeles
Los Angeles, CA, USA

Steven L. Gortmaker, PhD
Department of Social and Behavioral Sciences
Harvard T. H. Chan School of Public Health
Boston, MA, USA

Lawrence W. Green, DrPH**
Department of Epidemiology and Biostatistics, School of Medicine
University of California at San Francisco
San Francisco, CA, USA

Rebecca J. Guerin, PhD
Social Science and Translation Research Branch, Division of Science Integration, National Institute for Occupational Safety and Health
Centers for Disease Control and Prevention
Cincinnati, OH, USA

Alison B. Hamilton, PhD, MPH
VA HSR&D Center for the Study of Healthcare Innovation, Implementation & Policy
US Department of Veterans Affairs
Los Angeles, CA, USA
Department of Psychiatry and Biobehavioral Sciences, David Geffen School of Medicine
University of California Los Angeles
Los Angeles, CA, USA

Peggy A. Hannon, PhD, MPH
Health Promotion Research Center, Department of Health Systems and Population Health, School of Public Health
University of Washington
Seattle, WA, USA

Jeffrey R. Harris, MD, MPH, MBA
Health Promotion Research Center, Department of Health Systems and Population Health, School of Public Health
University of Washington
Seattle, WA, USA

Amy G. Huebschmann, MD, MSc**
Division of General Internal Medicine, Dissemination and Implementation Science Program of ACCORDS (Adult and Child Center for Health Outcomes Research and Delivery Science) and Ludeman Family Center for Women's Health Research
University of Colorado School of Medicine, Anschutz Medical Campus
Aurora, CO, USA

** Designates equal contributions to the authorship of this chapter.

Lisa A. Juckett, PhD
School of Health and Rehabilitation Science
The Ohio State University
Columbus, OH, USA

Christine M. Kava, PhD, MA
Health Promotion Research Center,
Department of Health Systems and Population Health, School of Public Health
University of Washington
Seattle, WA, USA

Kerk F. Kee, PhD
Department of Professional Communication
Texas Tech University
Lubbock, TX, USA

Bo Kim, PhD
Center for Healthcare Organization and Implementation Research
VA Boston Healthcare System
Boston, MA, USA
Department of Psychiatry
Harvard Medical School
Boston, MA, USA

JoAnn E. Kirchner, MD
VA Behavioral Health Quality Enhancement Research Initiative (QUERI)
Central Arkansas Veterans Healthcare System
North Little Rock, AR, USA
University of Arkansas for Medical Sciences
Little Rock, AR, USA

Harriet Koorts, PhD
Institute for Physical Activity and Nutrition,
School of Exercise and Nutrition Sciences
Deakin University
Geelong, Australia

Matthew W. Kreuter, PhD, MPH
Health Communication Research Laboratory,
Brown School
Washington University in St. Louis
St. Louis, MO, USA

Bethany M. Kwan, PhD
Department of Emergency Medicine and
Adult & Child Center for Outcomes Research and Delivery Science
University of Colorado School of Medicine,
Anschutz Medical Campus
Aurora, CO, USA

John Landsverk, PhD
Oregon Social Learning Center
Eugene, OR, USA

Matthew Lee, DrPH
Grossman School of Medicine
New York University
New York, NY, USA

Rebekka M. Lee, ScD, MS
Department of Social and Behavioral Sciences
Harvard T. H. Chan School of Public Health
Boston, MA, USA

Rebecca Lengnick-Hall, PhD
Brown School
Washington University in St. Louis
St. Louis, MO, USA

Jessenia De Leon, MSW
Suzanne Dworak-Peck School of Social Work
University of Southern California
Los Angeles, CA, USA

Cara C. Lewis, PhD
Kaiser Permanente Washington Health Research Institute
Seattle, WA, USA
Department of Psychiatry and Behavioral Sciences, Department of Health Systems and Population Health
University of Washington
Seattle, WA, USA

Laura A. Linnan, ScD
Department of Health Behavior
University of North Carolina Gillings School of Global Public Health
Chapel Hill, NC, USA

Douglas A. Luke, PhD
Center for Public Health Systems Science,
Brown School
Washington University in St. Louis
St. Louis, MO, USA

Sara Malone, PhD
Division of Public Health Sciences,
Department of Surgery
Washington University School of Medicine
St. Louis, MO, USA

Stephanie Mazzucca-Ragan, PhD
Prevention Research Center in St. Louis,
Brown School
Washington University in St. Louis
St. Louis, MO, USA

Collin McGovern
Department of Anthropology, School of Arts and Sciences
Washington University in St. Louis
St. Louis, MO, USA

Virginia R. McKay, PhD
Center for Public Health Systems Science, Brown School
Washington University in St. Louis
St. Louis, MO, USA

J. Curtis McMillen, PhD
The Crown Family School of Social Work, Policy, and Practice
The University of Chicago
Chicago, IL, USA

Demetria M. McNeal, PhD, MBA
Division of General Internal Medicine, and Dissemination and Implementation Science Program of ACCORDS (Adult and Child Center for Health Outcomes Research and Delivery Science)
University of Colorado School of Medicine, Anschutz Medical Campus
Aurora, CO, USA

Kayne Mettert, BA
Department of Psychology
University of Washington
Seattle, WA, USA
Kaiser Permanente Washington Health Research Institute
Seattle, WA, USA

Edward J. Miech, EdD
Center for Health Services Research
Regenstrief Institute
Indianapolis, IN, USA

Elecia Miller, BS
City of Lawrence Mayor's Health Task Force
Lawrence, MA, USA

Meredith Minkler, DrPH
Community Health Sciences, School of Public Health
University of California, Berkeley
Berkeley, CA, USA

Elaine H. Morrato, DrPH
Parkinson School of Health Sciences and Public Health
Loyola University Chicago
Maywood, IL, USA
Institute for Translational Medicine
Loyola University Chicago
Maywood, IL, USA

Alexandra B. Morshed, PhD, MS
Department of Behavioral, Social, and Health Education Sciences, Rollins School of Public Health
Emory University
Atlanta, GA, USA

Mosa Moshabela, MBChB, MMed, MSc, PhD
University of KwaZulu Natal
Durban, Republic of South Africa

Joanna C. Moullin, PhD
UC San Diego Altman Clinical and Translational Research Institute, Dissemination and Implementation Science Center
University of California San Diego
La Jolla, CA, USA
Curtin University, enAble Institute, Faculty of Health Sciences
Perth, Australia

Nicole Nathan, PhD
Hunter Medical Research Institute, Population Health Research Program
New Lambton Heights, Australia
National Centre of Implementation Science, Colleges of Health Medicine and Wellbeing
University of Newcastle
Callaghan, NSW, Australia
School of Medicine and Public Health
University of Newcastle
Callaghan, NSW, Australia

Per Nilsen, PhD
Division of Society and Health, Department of Health, Medicine and Caring Sciences
Linköping University
Linköping, Sweden

Daniel J. Niven, MD, PhD
Department of Critical Care Medicine, Cumming School of Medicine
University of Calgary and Alberta Health Services
Calgary, Canada

Lawrence A. Palinkas, PhD
Suzanne Dworak-Peck School of Social Work
University of Southern California
Los Angeles, CA, USA

Tai-Quan Peng, PhD
Department of Communication
Michigan State University
East Lansing, MI, USA

Byron J. Powell, PhD, LCSW
Center for Mental Health Services Research, Brown School
Washington University in St. Louis
St. Louis, MO, USA
Center for Dissemination & Implementation, Institute for Public Health
Washington University in St. Louis
St. Louis, MO, USA
Division of Infectious Diseases, John T. Milliken Department of Medicine, School of Medicine
Washington University in St. Louis
St. Louis, MO, USA

Enola K. Proctor, PhD
Brown School
Washington University in St. Louis
St. Louis, MO, USA

Beth Prusaczyk, MSW, PhD
Department of Medicine
Washington University School of Medicine
St. Louis, MO, USA

Jonathan Purtle, DrPH
School of Global Public Health
New York University
New York, NY, USA

Borsika A. Rabin, PhD, MPH, PharmD
Herbert Wertheim School of Public Health and Human Longevity Science
University of California, La Jolla, CA, USA
UC San Diego Altman Clinical and Translational Research Institute Dissemination and Implementation Science Center
University of California San Diego
La Jolla, CA, USA

Ramesh Raghavan, PhD
Silver School of Social Work
New York University
New York, NY, USA

Shoba Ramanadhan, ScD, MPH
Department of Social and Behavioral Sciences
Harvard T. H. Chan School of Public Health
Boston, MA, USA

Erika Salinas, MSW
Suzanne Dworak-Peck School of Social Work
University of Southern California
Los Angeles, CA, USA

Nick Sevdalis, PhD, MSc
Centre for Implementation Science, Health Services and Population Research Department
Kings College London
London, UK

Rachel C. Shelton, ScD, MPH
Department of Sociomedical Sciences
Columbia's Mailman School of Public Health
New York, NY, USA

Diana Silver, PhD
School of Global Public Health
New York University
New York, NY, USA

Michelle Silver, PhD, ScM
Division of Public Health Sciences, Department of Surgery
Washington University School of Medicine
St. Louis, MO, USA

Jeffrey L. Smith, BS
VA Behavioral Health Quality Enhancement Research Initiative (QUERI)
Central Arkansas Veterans Healthcare System
North Little Rock, AR, USA

Justin D. Smith, PhD
University of Utah Intermountain Healthcare Department of Population Health Sciences, Division of Health System Innovation and Research
Spencer Fox Eccles School of Medicine at the University of Utah
Salt Lake City, UT, USA

Joseph T. Steensma, EdD, MPH
Health Communication Research Laboratory, Brown School
Washington University in St. Louis
St. Louis, MO, USA

Rachel Sutherland
Hunter Medical Research Institute
Population Health Research Program
New Lambton Heights, Australia
National Centre of Implementation Science, Colleges of Health Medicine and Wellbeing
University of Newcastle
Callaghan, NSW, Australia
School of Medicine and Public Health
University of Newcastle
Callaghan, NSW, Australia
Hunter New-England Population Health
Hunter New England Local Health District
Wallsend, NSW, Australia

Rachel G. Tabak, PhD, RD
Prevention Research Center in St. Louis, Brown School
Washington University in St. Louis
St. Louis, MO, USA

Katy E. Trinkley, PharmD, PhD
Department of Family Medicine and Dissemination and Implementation Science Program of ACCORDS (Adult and Child Center for Health Outcomes Research and Delivery Science)
University of Colorado School of Medicine, Anschutz Medical Campus
Aurora, CO, USA

Niko Verdecias, DrPH, MPH
Health Communication Research Laboratory, Brown School
Washington University in St. Louis
St. Louis, MO, USA
Population Health, College of Health Solutions
Arizona State University
Phoenix, AZ, USA

Wouter Vermeer, PhD
Department of Psychiatry and Behavioral Science
Northwestern University Feinberg School of Medicine
Chicago, IL, USA

Clare Viglione, MPH, RD
Joint Doctoral Program at the Herbert Wertheim School of Public Health and Human Longevity Science at the University of California
San Diego and San Diego State University
La Jolla, CA, USA
UC San Diego Altman Clinical and Translational Research Institute Dissemination and Implementation Science Center
University of California San Diego
La Jolla, CA, USA

Cynthia A. Vinson, PhD, MPA
Division of Cancer Control and Population Sciences
National Cancer Institute
Bethesda, MD, USA

Simon Walker, MSc
Centre for Health Economics
University of York
York, UK

Callie Walsh-Bailey, MPH
Brown School
Washington University in St. Louis
St. Louis, MO, USA

Thomas J. Waltz, PhD, PhD
Eastern Michigan University
Department of Psychology
Ypsilanti, MI, USA

Eric M. Wiedenman, PhD
Division of Public Health Sciences, Department of Surgery
Washington University School of Medicine
St. Louis, MO, USA

Shannon Wiltsey Stirman, PhD
National Center for PTSD, Psychiatry and Behavioral Sciences
Stanford University
Palo Alto, CA, USA

Luke Wolfenden, PhD
Hunter Medical Research Institute, Population Health Research Program
New Lambton Heights, Australia
National Centre of Implementation Science, Colleges of Health Medicine and Wellbeing
University of Newcastle
Callaghan, NSW, Australia
School of Medicine and Public Health
University of Newcastle
Callaghan, NSW, Australia
Hunter New-England Population Health, Hunter New England Local Health District
Wallsend, NSW, Australia

Eva N. Woodward, PhD
VA Center for Mental Healthcare and Outcomes Research
Central Arkansas Veterans Healthcare System
North Little Rock, AR, USA
Department of Psychiatry
University of Arkansas for Medical Sciences
Little Rock, AR, USA

Sze Lin Yoong, PhD
Deakin University
Geelong, Australia
Global Centre for Preventive Health and Nutrition, Institute for Health Transformation, School of Health and Social Development, Faculty of Health
National Centre of Implementation Science, Colleges of Health Medicine and Wellbeing
University of Newcastle
Callaghan, NSW, Australia
Hunter New-England Population Health, Hunter New England Local Health District
Wallsend, NSW, Australia

SECTION 1

Background

1

The Promise and Challenges of Dissemination and Implementation Research

MICHELLE SILVER, GRAHAM A. COLDITZ, AND KAREN M. EMMONS

To him who devotes his life to science, nothing can give more happiness than increasing the number of discoveries, but his cup of joy is full when the results of his studies immediately find practical applications.

—Louis Pasteur

The ability of science to deliver on its promise of practical and timely solutions to the world's problems does not depend solely on research accomplishments but also on the receptivity of society to the implications of scientific discoveries.

—Agre and Leshner[1]

INTRODUCTION

Dissemination and implementation (D&I) of research findings into practice are necessary to achieve a return on investment in our research enterprise and to improve outcomes in the broader community. By not implementing prevention and treatment strategies equitably, we incur avoidable morbidity and mortality.[2] The translational challenge is an issue across the scientific continuum. At the level of molecular biology and pathogenesis of disease, we need more rapid translation from discovery of receptors or pathways to first-in-patient studies.[3] And once the benefit of a treatment or prevention strategy is demonstrated, it is in society's best interest to make it available to all. Thus, whether we are focusing on genomic discovery or evidence that treatment improves outcomes, moving from scientific discovery to broader application brings society the full return on our collective investment in research. Perhaps reflecting the historically low priority that has been placed on research related to implementation of scientifically proven approaches to care, in 2001 the Institute of Medicine noted a substantial gap between care that could be delivered if healthcare was informed by scientific knowledge and the care that is delivered in practice—defining this gap as a chasm.[4] More recently, the National Cancer Institute (NCI) Cancer Moonshot has placed emphasis on implementation science approaches to accelerate development, testing, and broader adoption of proven strategies to significantly reduce cancer risk and healthcare disparities in all populations, including medically underserved groups. It is precisely this gap between evidence and practice that D&I science is designed to address.

Implementation research is active inquiry that supports movement of evidence-based effective healthcare and prevention strategies or programs from the clinical or public health knowledge base into routine use (in some countries, the term *evidence informed* is used).[5] The Centers for Disease Control and Prevention (CDC) has defined implementation research as "the systematic study of how a specific set of activities and designated strategies are used to successfully integrate

Michelle Silver, Graham A. Colditz, and Karen M. Emmons, *The Promise and Challenges of Dissemination and Implementation Research* In: *Dissemination and Implementation Research in Health.* Edited by: Ross C. Brownson, Graham A. Colditz, and Enola K. Proctor, Oxford University Press. © Oxford University Press 2023. DOI: 10.1093/oso/9780197660690.003.0001 an evidence-based public health intervention within specific settings."[6(p6)] The NCI has defined implementation research as "the study of methods to promote the adoption and integration of evidence-based interventions, including practices and policies, into routine health care and community settings to improve health outcomes" (NCI Request For Applications CA21-056) (p. 3). The Canadian Institutes of Health Research (https://www.cihr-irsc.gc.ca/e/29418.html) uses the following definition for knowledge translation: "a dynamic and iterative process that includes synthesis, dissemination, exchange and ethically-sound application of knowledge to improve the health of Canadians, provide more effective services and products and strengthen the health care system." Despite this effort to clearly define the field, a 2004 survey of readers in *Nature Medicine* showed little agreement and understanding of translational research overall and D&I in particular.[7]

While government agencies frequently note the need to translate evidence-based interventions into practice to improve population health outcomes, the *process* for distribution of scientific findings, materials, and associated resources to support interventions is less developed. Dissemination is defined as "the targeted distribution of information and intervention materials to a specific public health or clinical practice audience."[8(p5)] Rabin et al. are more specific, calling for an active approach of spreading evidence-based interventions to the target audience via determined channels using planned strategies.[9] These definitions are similar to that of Lomas[10,11] but contrast to some extent with the approach of Curry,[12] who defined dissemination as a push-pull process. Those who adopt innovations must want them or be receptive (pull) while there is systematic effort to help adopters implement innovations (push). The intent of *dissemination research* is to spread knowledge and the associated interventions, building understanding of approaches to increased effectiveness of dissemination efforts. In understanding these approaches, numerous studies have shown that dissemination of evidence-based interventions using passive methods (e.g., publication of consensus statements in professional journals, mass mailings) has been ineffective, resulting in only small changes in the uptake of a new practice.[13] The intent of *implementation research* is to increase understanding of how to increase integration of evidence-based approaches into routine, real-world practices. Therefore, more targeted, active approaches to D&I are needed that take into account the many factors that influence uptake and integration, including the characteristics and needs of users, types of evidence needed, and organizational climate and culture. Greater stakeholder engagement across the D&I spectrum and systems approaches can increase the speed of change.[14] The definitions and other terms used in the field are described in more detail in chapter 2.

A review by Bowen and colleagues highlighted the impact that translation of discovery to applications could have for population health. In the past several years, implementation science has caught the attention of the translational research community, most notably through the engagement of implementation scientists in the nation's Clinical and Translational Science Award programs. A recent article noted several recommendations for integrating D&I science into clinical and translational research as a core component (see Box 1.1).[15] Notably, the recommendations specifically consider the importance of providing basic competencies related to D&I science to all investigators working on the translational continuum—even early stage translational researchers (see Table 1.1). By integrating D&I science more systematically throughout the substantial translational science infrastructure that has developed in the United States, we are more likely to speed the process by which implementation of the evidence base may have an impact on population health.

Through this book, we aim to lay out many options to help guide the field as it matures, thus speeding our progress toward improved health for all. This introductory chapter seeks to define D&I research and its significance, place it in context, and identify the challenges and opportunities moving forward.

BOX 1.1

RECOMMENDATIONS FOR EFFECTIVE INTEGRATION OF DISSEMINATION AND IMPLEMENTATION (D&I) SCIENCES IN CLINICAL AND TRANSLATIONAL SCIENCE AWARD (CTSA) PROGRAMS[a]

METHODS AND PROCESS

Develop standard expectations and processes for incorporating D&I expertise and perspectives in CTSA hub leadership and in key initiatives, methods, and processes.

Advance understanding of different models of D&I cores and other infrastructures for CTSAs and methods for collaboration and coordination across centers, including guidance from NCATS for incorporation into renewal proposals.

Increase involvement of D&I experts on cross-CTSA initiatives and working groups central to methods and processes, including topics from which they have traditionally been excluded, including clinical trial study design and the responsible conduct of research.

Identify methods by which D&I sciences can enhance sharing of best practices and programs between CTSA hubs to promote cross-hub adoption of CTSA innovations.

Support and track translation of a broader range of innovations into practice, for example, the spread and use of important innovations with high potential for health impact but low market potential.

EVALUATION

Develop a set of D&I competencies for early stage translational researchers.

Develop D&I sciences training curriculum for K-scholars, postdoctoral students in translational sciences, doctoral students, and master's level students.

Identify and catalogue novel methods to expand the workforce of D&I mentors, consultants, and collaborators.

Develop the set of core D&I competencies to assist partners to engage as scientists, stakeholders, and users of science.

EVALUATION

Develop novel measures and methods of assessing progress in D&I advancement and impact within CTSAs, including assessments of faculty D&I competency, training opportunities and quality, infrastructural and mentorship capacity, methodological alignment with D&I principles, and translational success.

Establish NCATS-coordinated effort to recruit and train D&I experts to evaluate CTSAs with the use of a standardized rubric and approach and a corresponding expectation that D&I experts should be systematically incorporated into eExternal advisory committees and funding review panels.

Identify standards for the evaluation of impact resulting from translation of research into practice.

Abbreviations: CTSA: Clinical and Translational Science Award; D&I: dissemination and implementation; NCATS: National Center for Advancing Translational Sciences.

[a]Adapted with permission from: Mehta TG, Mahoney J, Leppin AL, et al. Integrating dissemination and implementation sciences within Clinical and Translational Science Award programs to advance translational research: recommendations to national and local leaders. *J Clin Transl Sci.* 2021;5(1):e151.

TABLE 1.1 DISSEMINATION AND IMPLEMENTATION SCIENCE PRINCIPLES AND EXAMPLE COMPETENCIES APPLICABLE TO CLINICAL AND TRANSLATIONAL SCIENCE TRAINING[a]

Principle	Example Competencies to Maximize Design for Ultimate Translation
Context matters and is multilevel	Describe factors that influence research adoption, implementation, maintenance, and reach.
	Prioritize questions with high relevance to stakeholders.
It is not sufficient that evidence exists	Be familiar with user-centered design; making interventions useful, usable, and desirable (design for dissemination).
	Understand the stakeholders that should be engaged.
	Understand the value of early engagement of stakeholders.
	Understand the relevance of study design and choice of target group to external validity and ultimate translatability.
Change happens proactively	Understand the importance of value proposition, designing for dissemination, cost-effectiveness, and policy implications.
	Understand the value of type 1 hybrid design in all phases of clinical research.
	Understand the sources of error: fidelity/lapses in implementation as a source of reduced/heightened effect.
Both implementation practice and implementation science are team endeavors	Understand how to identify relevant nonacademic stakeholders in research and how and when to engage with them to aid in movement across research stages and translation into practice.
	Understand the benefit of communication and how to communicate with relevant stakeholders.
	Employ weighted evidence, cost-effectiveness, and translation into policy.

[a]Adapted with permission from: Mehta TG, Mahoney J, Leppin AL, et al. Integrating dissemination and implementation sciences within Clinical and Translational Science Award programs to advance transl ational research: recommendations to national and local leaders. *J Clin Transl Sci.* 2021;5(1):e151.

WHAT IS DISSEMINATION AND IMPLEMENTATION RESEARCH AND WHY DOES IT MATTER?

Given both the historic and current examples of D&I successes and failures, how do we conceptualize D&I research and classify it in relation to other systems or types of research? Growing emphasis on the pace of advances in medical systems leads to a number of approaches for classifying the continuum from discovery to delivery and the improvement of the health of the population. Classification of the research continuum from bench to bedside and use of population health metrics continues to evolve. Briefly, the language to describe these steps and procedures has evolved over the past decade (see chapter 2). Furthermore, the methods research to understand the limitations of research synthesis to gather information on effective interventions and inform next steps continues to provide caution in planning and evaluation of programs.[16,17] The Institute of Medicine has defined implementation research as an important component of the framework for clinical research, and Zerhouni called for reengineering the clinical research enterprise, but we are more broadly focused, including clinical research, health systems, and prevention.[18] The National Institutes of Health (NIH) roadmap[19] defines T1 as moving from basic science to clinical applications (translation to humans); T2 as clinical research (up to phase 3 trials) moving to broader clinical practice (translation to patients); and T3 as D&I research following development of guidelines for practice, moving research into public health and clinical practice through diffusion, dissemination, and delivery research (translation to practice) (see Figure 1.1). T4 research has now been added

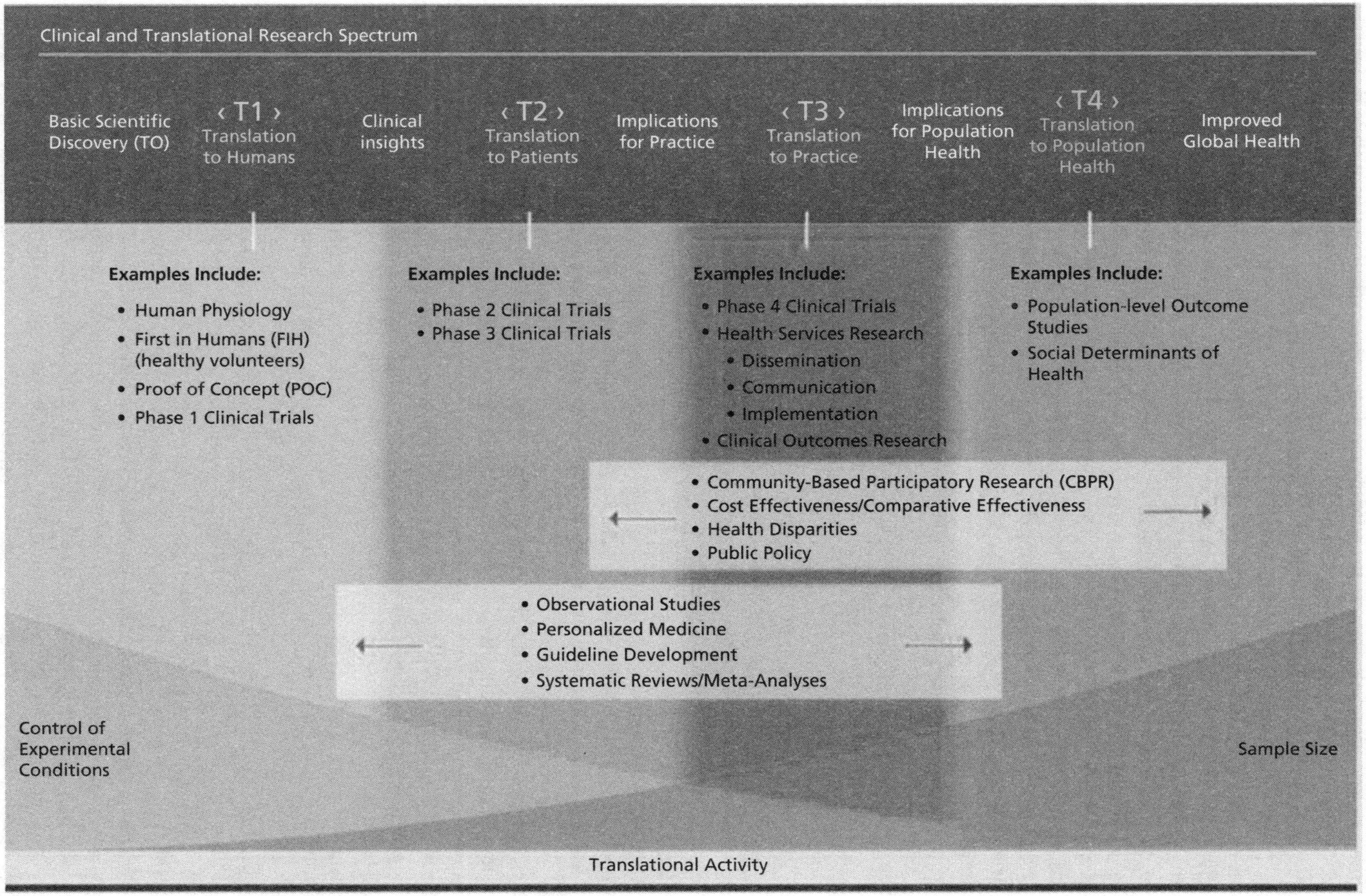

Clinical and Translational Research Spectrum

Basic Scientific Discovery (TO)
‹ T1 › Translation to Humans
Clinical insights
‹ T2 › Translation to Patients
Implications for Practice
‹ T3 › Translation to Practice
Implications for Population Health
‹ T4 › Translation to Population Health
Improved Global Health

Examples Include:

- Human Physiology
- First in Humans (FIH) (healthy volunteers)
- Proof of Concept (POC)
- Phase 1 Clinical Trials

Examples Include:

- Phase 2 Clinical Trials
- Phase 3 Clinical Trials

Examples Include:

- Phase 4 Clinical Trials
- Health Services Research
  - Dissemination
  - Communication
  - Implementation
- Clinical Outcomes Research

Examples Include:

- Population-level Outcome Studies
- Social Determinants of Health

- Community-Based Participatory Research (CBPR)
- Cost Effectiveness/Comparative Effectiveness
- Health Disparities
- Public Policy

- Observational Studies
- Personalized Medicine
- Guideline Development
- Systematic Reviews/Meta-Analyses

Control of Experimental Conditions

Sample Size

Translational Activity

FIGURE 1.1 The types of research across the translational research spectrum.

Reprinted with permission from Harvard Catalyst (Pathfinder—Harvard Catalyst).

to evaluate real-world outcomes from applying discoveries and bringing them to practice (translation to population). No doubt further subdivisions will be proposed in coming years. Public health approaches may broadly be defined as practice based (though health departments and social marketing strategies for health promotion may be beyond most people's vision for practice-based research).[20] Accordingly, our methods must be robust and adaptive to the situation where they are applied. In fact, the development and acceptance of a wide range of scientific methods as necessary for D&I research, beyond the randomized control trial, has helped to move the field significantly forward. These methods will be critical as new forms of discovery science proliferate, as some are anticipating for the field of precision medicine. Both the NIH Precision Medicine Initiative and the NCI's Cancer Moonshot Initiative are seeking to accelerate the pace and impact of genetic and genomic research on health. Chambers et al. noted the importance of implementation science as a mechanism for ensuring that precision medicine advances become integrated into healthcare delivery, which will ultimately be critical if the significant investment in these efforts is to be realized.[21]

A number of proposed models for D&I research are discussed in multiple chapters in this book. Some are "source based" (i.e., they view D&I from the lens of researchers pushing out science) (also see chapter 4). Others are community centered and focus on bringing research into practice settings. Systems approaches are also proposed to conceptualize the overall framework for D&I.[22] Underlying these approaches, the body of scientific evidence must be sufficient to justify moving from individual studies to broader practice (i.e., an evidence-based practice). How this is determined, through systematic synthesis, subgroup analysis, or other approaches continues to be debated. However, to move forward with an intervention one needs a strong scientific evidence base; political will to allocate resources to achieve the goal of implementation; and a social strategy that defines a plan of action to achieve the health goals.[23,24] We noted in our examples previously in the chapter that lack of political will may hinder the uptake of effective public health interventions, such as smallpox vaccination.

THE CHALLENGE IN TRANSLATING RESEARCH TO PRACTICE

There are a number of issues inherent in moving from discovery to application, which is essential if society is to fully benefit from our collective investment in research. Summarized below are some of the key issues that impact our ability to translate evidence-based programs into real-world practice.

Funding

Over the past 20 years, a relatively small proportion of the NIH budget, which is currently around $43 billion, has been expended on prevention research[25,26]—that is, the direct and immediate application of effective intervention strategies to benefit the public's health.[27(p93)] In 2019, primary and secondary prevention research represented 20.7% of NIH-funded projects and 27.4% of NIH research spending, but the funding for D&I research—that is how to integrate prevention into routine care was only a fraction of that. Across all funding sources through 2011—federal and foundations—spending on health services research, models of care, and service innovations, represented only 1/20th of biomedical research funding.[28] D&I research spans all areas from translating discoveries to bedside and broader clinical applications, to health services interventions to implement effective approaches to care. In global health it also spans from innovation in technology for extremely low-cost delivery systems to implementation in field settings.

Representation of D&I Science in the Scientific Literature

The past few years have witnessed an explosion of research in D&I across many diseases[29,30]; delivery settings; learning health systems[31]; and, to a lesser extent, policy,[32] reflecting changes in funding priorities and actions from funding agencies. Disease-focused infrastructure settings, such as NCI-designated cancer centers, are ideal settings in which to further D&I knowledge.[33] A recent study used the NIH Research Portfolio Online Reporting Tool (RePORTER) to examine the characteristics of NCI-funded D&I science grants in the nation's cancer centers to understand the nature, extent, and opportunity for this key type of translational work. There were 104 active

NCI-funded D&I research or training grants identified at the 64 clinical and comprehensive cancer centers; about 60% of cancer centers had at least one NCI-funded D&I grant. Two-thirds of awards were for research grants, and the remainder were for D&I-focused training grants. Although these findings indicate that D&I research is being conducted in our nation's cancer centers, it also illustrates that there is considerable room for further integration of D&I science into cancer center activities, which would further support NCI's translational mission.

What Are the Appropriate Outcomes for Progress in Dissemination and Implementation of Discoveries?

While the methods and issues used to advance population health through implementation science may appear to differ across fields of study, in this book we set forth principles and methods that should be applicable across settings. Like statistics, which has a long history of development in agriculture (the leading industry of the time—Cochran wrote on a meta-analysis of results from agriculture trial plots in 1937 and helped define modern approaches[34]), D&I research also grew from agriculture to guide thinking across many fields,[35] as discussed in a review of the history of D&I science in chapter 3. With healthcare expenditures consuming an ever-increasing portion of national and state budgets in the developed world, methods to maximize our societal benefit must be refined and accessible to end users—and will likely be developed and refined quickest in the context of health and wellness. In 2019, prior to the COVID-19 pandemic, expenditure was around 8.8% of the gross domestic product (GDP) in Organization for Economic Cooperation and Development (OECD) countries, unchanged since 2013, and in the United States it was 16.8% of the GDP.[36] There is no shortage of academic research, but how do we sift through studies and draw inference to disseminate and implement effective programs and policies more broadly? A recurring question as we approach D&I research is: Will the evidence and intervention be applicable to different settings?

Acceptance of Delays in Adoption

Delay in adoption of scientific discoveries is not a new phenomenon. We can look at Bayesian methods used in statistics in the 1960s to evaluate the authorship of the Federalist papers.[37] In the process, described in detail by Fred Mosteller in his autobiography, an empirical test of the Bayesian approach gave new insight to manuscript classification.[38] Mosteller also presented about using Bayesian approaches to combine means (Lake Junaluska, North Carolina, 1946; see pages 186–187 in Reference 38; also see 1948's "On Pooling Data"[39]).These statistical methods have only much more recently been adapted to widespread use, with modern computer technology supporting this application. So, advances in statistical methods development did not achieve widespread application for decades, perhaps in part due to not only the technical difficulty of implementing these approaches, but also reluctance on the part of investigators. Both individual and structural barriers impeded implementation, reflecting a complex interplay of barriers to implementation of innovations.

How can the principles and methods we see presented in this book help us move more quickly to build on research findings and apply them to improve health? Do we need new ways of thinking, conducting, and reporting research, or can we take our existing approaches and through consensus apply what is known more rapidly? The challenge of implementation extends along the continuum from discovery of biologic phenomena to clinical application in research settings and the broader application in the population at large. While a range of approaches to describing this continuum has been developed, perhaps more pertinent from the D&I perspective is the perspective summarized by Green and colleagues as a leaky pipeline from research to practice.[40] Across these approaches to defining stages of translation and application, some common themes emerged: (1) Discovery on its own does not lead to use of knowledge; (2) evidence of impact does not lead to uptake of new strategies; (3) organizations often do not support the culture of evidence-based practice; and (4) maintenance of change is often overlooked, leading to regression of system-level changes to a prior state. The focus of an intervention for implementation, whether at the implementer level or through system-level changes or policies, determines in part the breadth of change toward improved population outcomes. The lag from discovery to implementation of effective programs and practices may vary across disciplines. Examples from public health include the 50-year gap from perfecting the Papanicolaou (Pap) test in 1943 to the establishment of screening programs in all US states in 1995, and the 45-year delay from the 1964 surgeon general's report on smoking to effective statewide tobacco control programs and regulation of tobacco by the Food and Drug Administration (FDA) in 2009.[41] Of course, early applications will typically be in place to varying degrees before full widespread programs are implemented and sustained. As former NIH Director Francis Collins noted, many false starts or failures may be needed before successful translation of discoveries to human applications.[3] However, it is important to reduce the time lag from early adoption to comprehensive, widespread adoption, as this lag ultimately represents avoidable morbidity and mortality.

A frequently quoted statement about the total attrition in the funnel and the lapse between research and medical practice indicates that it takes 17 years to turn 14% of original research to the benefit of patient care and is attributed to Balas and Boren.[42] This evaluation lens has been applied in a more recent study of five cancer control evidence-based practices: The average time to implementation was still 15 years.[43] The leakage or loss of medical-clinical evidence from the pipeline at each stage from completed research through submission, publication, indexing, and systematic reviews that produce guidelines and textbook recommendations for best practices to the ultimate implementation of those practices in a health-care setting all contribute to these estimates. Changing technologies and priorities of publishing, bibliographic data management, and systematic reviews and disseminating evidence-based guidelines will lead to different estimates over time and in different fields. Green and colleagues depicted this flow of information as a leaky pipeline (Figure 1.2). In it, they identified many leakage points in the scientific process.[40]

Looked at from the other end, identifying major advances in engineering that have improved the quality of life in the 20th century, the National Academy of Engineering included electricity, electric motors, and imaging—each with a long line of scientific discovery and application before broader social impact was achieved.[44] Likewise, the lag from original discovery to formal recognition with Nobel Prizes grows exponentially.[45] A particular challenge in public health is that we are not producing a tangible product or commodity, as is the case with electricity and electric motors, but rather the intangible value of health and equity, which may be even more challenging. That said, the path from scientific discovery to social benefit from broad implementation has common challenges across many scientific disciplines.[46]

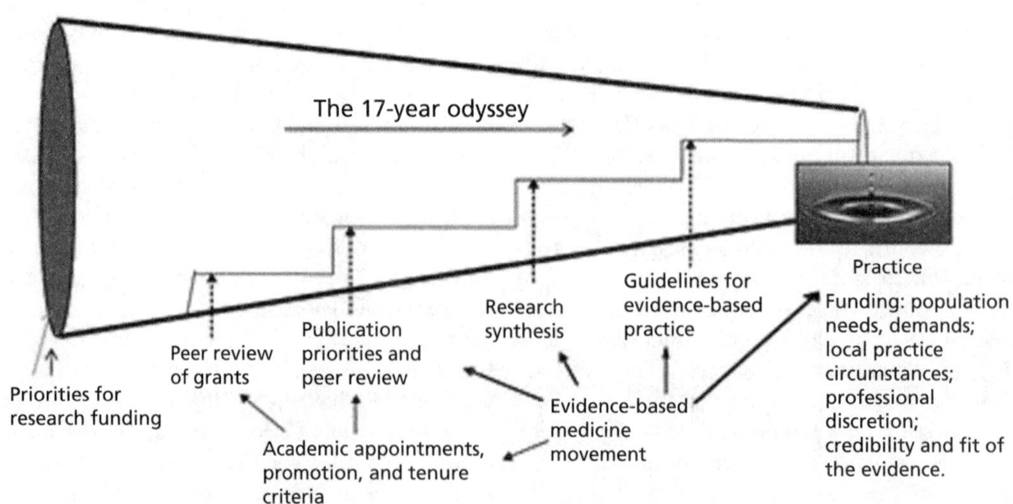

FIGURE 1.2 The funnel depicts loss in the pipeline from research to practice.

Reprinted with permission from: Green LW, Ottoson JM, Garcia C, Hiatt RA. Diffusion theory and knowledge dissemination, utilization, and integration in public health. *Annu Rev Public Health.* 2009;30:151–174).

CASE STUDIES: FROM BENCH TO BEDSIDE TO POPULATIONS

Several case studies can help illustrate the real-world challenges and successes in moving from research to practice. Of course, we learn both from successful translation of research to practice and from failures.

Insulin

Insulin offers an extreme example we do not see replicated today. Pancreas extract was evaluated in dogs in physiology laboratories in numerous medical centers in the early 1900s. After only 6 or so months of experimentation, Banting and Best moved from their physiology laboratory and animal studies in the Medical Building at the University of Toronto to the delivery to humans at Toronto General Hospital.[47] The clinical condition favored rapid translation to practice since patients routinely had a steady decline after onset of type 1 or insulin-dependent diabetes following therapies that were standard at the time, such as starvation, and ultimately dying from metabolic imbalances.[48] Rapid physiologic evidence of response to pancreatic extract in terms of blood sugar and urinary ketones led to demand for pancreas extract outstripping supply. Few medical discoveries have had such a huge effect that they move as quickly from bench to bedside and broader application in clinics across North America. In fact, the will of the patients and their providers outpaced the slower development of approaches to large-scale production. Eli Lilly had a major interest even before the discovery of the extraction methods in Toronto,[49] reinforcing the influence of market forces on implementation. More recent experience with HIV and the social forces brought to bear by AIDS activists, along with speed up of the drug approval process and marketing, led to faster developments, ranging from identification of a new disease condition to effective treatment.[50] This timeline spans from detection of AIDS cases in California and New York in 1981; to the viral cause identified in 1984; to AZT (azidovodine; azidothymidine) as the first drug for treating AIDS in 1987; to a US national education campaign in 1988; and to combination antiretroviral therapy that is highly effective against HIV in 1996. Like diabetes, the political will generated by an advocacy community garnered support for scientific advances at exceptional speed, with clear success making efforts in cancer and other chronic disease management pale in comparison. AIDS research and systems delivery leave open research questions such as optimal scaling up strategies to bring effective prevention and treatment to all.

Human Papillomavirus Vaccination

Human papillomavirus (HPV) vaccination provides a striking example of the differential impact of implementation strategies on outcomes. The vaccine, first approved in 2006, is highly effective at preventing cervical cancer and genital warts, as well as some vaginal, vulvar, anal, penile, and oropharyngeal cancers when administered prior to sexual activity and exposure to HPV and thus is best targeted towards 9- to 13-year-olds, though it is recommended through age 26. Australia became the first country to introduce a nationally funded school-based HPV vaccination program for girls in 2007 and expanded to include boys in 2013. The current program targets all students ages 12–13, and catch-up doses are available for free for everyone under 20 who is unvaccinated. This national school-based approach has resulted in very high HPV vaccine coverage, approaching 90% for initiation of the vaccine series and 80% for completion.[51] In contrast, rather than implementing a national vaccine program, the United States has left the decision up to each state, and to date, only three states (Hawaii, Rhode Island, and Virginia) and the District of Columbia have implemented an HPV vaccine requirement for school attendance. The lack of an organized national approach has led to much lower uptake than that seen in Australia, with around 75% initiating the HPV vaccine series, but less than 60% completing it.[52] Further, these national averages mask dramatic variation in uptake across the country and disparities in uptake across subgroups. The impact of these different implementation approaches can be seen in cervical cancer outcomes, as well as with rates in Australia below those in the United States. It is projected that Australia will be the first country to eliminate cervical cancer by 2035.[53]

COVID-19

The ongoing COVID-19 pandemic presents many learning opportunities about the need for and importance of D&I in public health. While rapid innovation and development occurred for testing and vaccination, there were many challenges in dissemination, implementation, and communication when rolling them out. Recommendations and guidelines were based on the best available data at a given time. However, with the rapid pace of discovery, frequent changes were made as new knowledge was gained. Updates were often presented without adequate context and explanation, perhaps complicated by the public's limited knowledge of the scientific process, leading some to question why scientists and policymakers were initially "wrong." These communication challenges, combined with readily available misinformation, resulted in slower uptake of testing, vaccination, and other prevention measures than anticipated and needed to manage the pandemic. To improve implementation and uptake of testing, particularly among traditionally underserved communities, NIH-funded initiatives such as the Rapid Acceleration of Diagnostics (RADx) and RADx-UP (underserved populations). RADx-UP is specifically designed to evaluate different implementation strategies for increasing testing among vulnerable groups, and while these studies are still underway, they should be very informative. We shouldn't forget that it has been a tremendous accomplishment to get the vaccine from development through testing and available to the population on such a short time frame, but at the same time we must learn from the challenges of getting those doses into actual arms to be better prepared for the next time.

These examples of translating discovery to widespread application in varying time frames demonstrate the enormous variation in implementation and some of the social and political factors that may facilitate implementing effective programs and practices. We must balance timely implementation with the caution that pervades the scientific process. Too rapid implementation of ineffective or even harmful technologies will have deleterious consequences for population health and for public confidence in science. Tempering such caution is evidence from public health, where use of lead in petroleum (gasoline) was opposed by Alice Hamilton as early as 1925 because of the expected adverse health effects, almost 50 years before the US Environmental Protection Agency began to restrict the lead content of gasoline in 1975, and 70 years before lead was phased out of gasoline entirely. Tobacco smoking continues to show just how slow we can be to implement effective prevention strategies when commercial interests oppose development of cohesive political will to advance population health. We contend, and the chapters in this book illustrate, that stronger methods for D&I research can help reduce this gap and bring population benefits. Chapter 24 focuses on policy D&I research in further detail.

Scientific Evidence Base

In moving forward with D&I research, we can start with the first of these three dimensions: the scientific evidence base. Here we see confusion in the field over when we have a sufficient scientific evidence base ready for broader implementation.[54] In chapter 16, Trinkley and colleagues highlight how the emphasis on internal validity in our research enterprise drives us to restricted populations and narrowly defined interventions. Do these interventions work? Will they work in a different setting? Will results from trials hold up with further evaluation?[17] The tension of priority on internal validity against external validity and the associated evidence to support broader applications of scientific findings continues within the scientific process.[55] Much of the evidence synthesis "industry" focuses on narrowing evidence to specific finite questions. In medicine and public health, this began by meta-analysis even excluding nonrandomized trials from study.[56] In an early application of research synthesis and meta-analysis to observational public health data, Berlin and Colditz evaluated quality of exposure measure and used regression methods to predict future health benefits from increases in physical activity.[57] Can stronger use of existing approaches to prediction (e.g., meta-regression and network meta-analysis) help us understand when interventions will work and how large a benefit we might ultimately see? What range of benefits will fit within the distribution of findings to date?

The scope of synthesis has broadened over time—from consensus and review articles[58] to rigorous panel (systematic review) methods such as those used by the US and Canadian Preventive Services[59] and the CDC community guide. The Grading of Recommendations, Assessment, Development and Evaluations (GRADE) system has been developed to more explicitly guide panel decision-making.[60–62] Despite these more formal approaches, a review of World Health Organization (WHO) guidelines shows that they systematically omit guidance on active implementation strategies.[63]

While reporting standards have focused on the internal validity of clinical trials and observational studies,[64] new approaches to make features of study design most relevant to effectiveness have been proposed (PRagmatic Explanatory Continuum Indicator Summary: PRECIS and PRECIS-2).[65,66] By making explicit a number of dimensions (e.g., flexibility of the comparison condition and experimental intervention; practitioner expertise; eligibility criteria participant compliance, etc.), approaches such as meta-regression[67] may be implemented to draw on these contextual factors to better understand if results can be applied in different settings. Furthermore, regression can then be used to predict what level of benefit may be seen in future applications (as has been done in the meta-analysis of BCG vaccine for prevention of tuberculosis).[68,69] While one often thinks of meta-analysis as driving for a common single answer to a clinical or public health problem, regression approaches and using meta-analysis to understand sources of heterogeneity highlight the many potentially untapped ways in which data can be synthesized to better inform policy and clinical decision-making.[70] Importantly, implementation science should study how to translate findings to be contextually relevant—and while regression and synthesis offer traditional quantitative approaches, broader system and contextual measures are likely needed to fully capture translation to practice.[71]

Bero has studied the delay in implementation of clinical practices—guidelines are typically published and sit on a bookshelf.[13] Practice does not change. She reviews effectiveness for a range of approaches that are commonly used. Importantly, while the field of healthcare has moved substantially to accepting a role for research synthesis over the past quarter century, the study of how to implement the effective approaches to health and public health practice has been far less rigorous. Approaches to synthesis of strategies that work[72] could strengthen the field. In addition, there is a set of contextual factors that influence dissemination to various audiences (Table 1.2).[73]

As in any field, a thorough review of evidence may provide a summary of where the field is or identify gaps that require further research.[74] Reviewing evidence in service organizations, Greenhalgh and colleagues[75]

TABLE 1.2 FACTORS INFLUENCING DISSEMINATION AMONG HEALTH ADMINISTRATORS, POLICYMAKERS, AND THE GENERAL PUBLIC[a]

Category	Influential Factor
Information	• Sound scientific basis, including knowledge of causality
	• Source (e.g., professional organization, government, mass media, friends)
Clarity of contents	• Formatting and framing
	• Perceived validity
	• Perceived relevance
	• Cost of intervention
	• Strength of the message (i.e., vividness)
Perceived values, preferences, beliefs	• Role of the decision maker
	• Economic background
	• Previous education
	• Personal experience or involvement
	• Political affiliation
	• Willingness to adopt innovations
	• Willingness to accept uncertainty
	• Willingness to accept risk
	• Ethical aspect of the decision
Context	• Culture
	• Politics
	• Timing
	• Media attention
	• Financial or political constraints

[a]Adapted with permission from Bero and Jadad.[73]

provided a model for diffusion of innovations in health service organizations, summarized methodology for review of evidence in this setting, and identified gaps for research focus. They argued that research on diffusion of innovations should be theory driven; process rather than package oriented; ecological; collaborative; multidisciplinary; detailed; and participatory. They distinguished between "letting it happen," "helping it happen," and "making it happen" as related to diffusion and dissemination. Letting or helping it happen relies on the providers or consumers to work out how to use the science, in contrast with "making it happen," which places accountability for implementation on teams of individuals who may coach, support, or guide the implementation. Ramanadhan and colleagues describe the value of participatory research in speeding implementation of research findings (see chapter 10).

POLICY IMPLEMENTATION SCIENCE

In the past two decades, implementation science has helped to create a strong focus on improving evidence-based practice at the clinical, community, organizational, and health system levels. There has been less success, however, in the translation of evidence into policy, especially outside healthcare. Given that policy sets the context for the delivery of preventive care and for mechanisms outside the healthcare system that influence health risk and outcomes, this is of particular concern. It is also clear that policy can eradicate or reinforce systemic structures that lead to health inequalities. The field has begun to recognize the importance of policy, and there are efforts underway to identify the resources needed to push policy implementation science forward. There has been an effort to identify the ways in which our current conceptual frameworks apply to policy implementation (Bullock), as well as to identify frameworks from other fields that would be useful, most notably from political science (Nilsen).[32] Emmons, Chambers, and Abazeed outlined four ways in which a greater understanding of political science could inform policy implementation science, including (1) deepening our understanding of the policymaking process, which reflects conceptualization of the problem and possible policy solutions, the political context, and the implementation process; (2) placing an emphasis on the outer context, such as the policy and political environment, which is often ignored or minimized in implementation science (IS) research; (3) identifying the range of policy instruments that can be used to translate evidence into policy; and (4) an appreciation of the long and complex time trajectory of policymaking and the interdependency between the many factors that influence the policy process.

A key gap has been the availability of valid measures that can enable us to disentangle the differential impacts of policy implementation determinants and outcomes. A recent systematic review by Allen et al. identified 15 "mostly transferable" measures from studies of health policy implementation, including measures of fidelity and adaptation, organizational culture and climate, implementation costs, acceptability, and readiness for implementation. However, it was rare for these constructs to be defined, and few data on measure validity and reliability were available. Without more emphasis on the development of precise and rigorous policy-relevant measures, it will be difficult for the field to move forward.

The COVID pandemic has illustrated the intersection between policy and politics, particularly when it pertains to scientific evidence. For policy translation to occur in the context of the current polarized political situation in the United States, it will be important to establish broad coalitions of support, as strong scientific evidence may be necessary but ever more so insufficient for policy enactment. It is also important to recognize that integration of science into policy is often incremental and requires a long time horizon, as noted above.

The framework of Kingdon[76] is useful in illustrating the policymaking process and its impact on D&I research. Kingdon argued that policies move forward when elements of three "streams" come together. The first of these is the definition of the problem (e.g., a high cancer rate or synthesis of the scientific knowledge base). The second is the development of potential policies to solve that problem (e.g., identification of policy measures to achieve an effective cancer control strategy). Finally, there is the role of politics, political will, and public opinion (e.g., interest groups supporting or opposing the policy). Policy change occurs when a "window of opportunity" opens and the three streams push policy change through.

The time frame for benefits of knowledge translation—D&I research—is in the future and runs counter to public policy and planning, conflicting with pressure to deliver services today.[77] In contrast with disease (e.g., breast cancer) and exposure advocacy groups (e.g., those focusing on environmental contaminants; or unions and related occupational exposures), prevention does not have a voice from those who benefit. Despite the apparent priority of tobacco control efforts since the 1964 surgeon general's report, we have only halved the rate of smoking in the United States. While this reduction in smoking may have prevented more cancer deaths than all adult cancer therapy advances over the same time frame, it leaves us with an enormous lack of accomplishment when the full burden of smoking is summed up. Where are all those who quit smoking or never started and are not suffering or dying prematurely from lung cancer and many other chronic diseases? A lack of voice leads to limited political will and lack of resource allocation to achieve the benefits of translating research to practice. Sometimes governments do step in and do the right thing—as illustrated by the significant progress in tobacco control during the Obama presidency.[78] Based on the significant foundation of evidence about the health impacts of tobacco and strategies for effective tobacco control, the Obama administration implemented FDA regulation of tobacco (Family Smoking Prevention and Control Act enacted by Congress and signed by President Obama in 2009); improved coverage of tobacco cessation services by health plans via the 2010 Affordable Care Act; funded the first national media campaign, designed to highlight the real human costs of smoking; expanded Medicare coverage for older smokers and expanded Medicaid coverage for pregnant smokers; and provided protection from exposure to secondhand tobacco smoke in public housing.

Social Strategy

In launching the first health goals for the nation, Richmond defined social strategy in the context of health—guiding both the landmark Healthy People 1980 and the first nutrition guidelines for the United States.[23] He proposed changes to promote health through healthcare providers, through regulations, and through community (individual and organizational changes). The Healthy People initiative has represented an ambitious yet achievable health promotion and disease prevention agenda for over four decades, but only recently has this effort fully embraced a comprehensive social determinants perspective. Koh and colleagues noted the importance of integrating social determinants of health into Healthy People 2020.[78] Healthy People 2020 included a new overarching goal to "create social and physical environments that promote good health for all" by accepting shared social responsibility for change. Healthy People 2030 expands on this by including an added emphasis on health equity and incorporating it into all five of its overarching goals.[79,80]

Now we may expand this concept to incorporate the D&I elements—the innovation; the communication channel; the time; and the social system.[81] Proctor[82] proposed a model of implementation research that defines the intervention (from the evidence base); the implementation strategy (systems environment; organizational; group/learning; supervision; and individual providers/consumers) (see Figure 1.3).

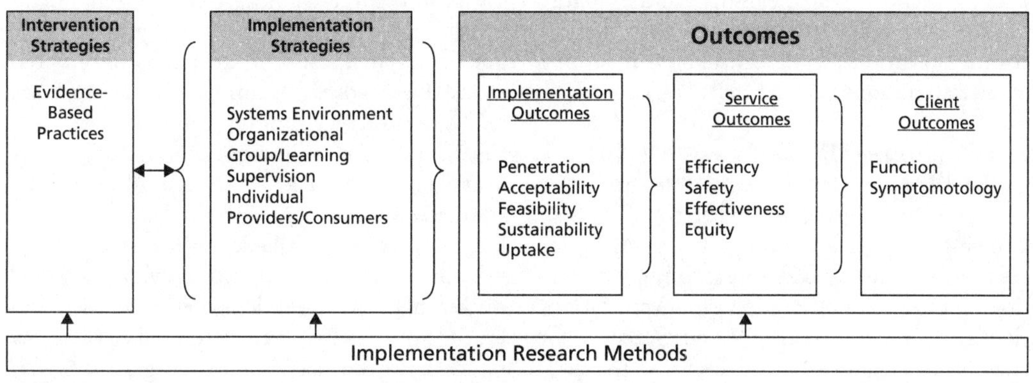

FIGURE 1.3 Conceptual model of implementation research.

Reprinted with permission from: Proctor E, Silmere H, Raghavan R, et al. Outcomes for implementation research: conceptual distinctions, measurement challenges, and research agenda. Research Support, N.I.H., Extramural. *Adm Policy Ment Health.* Mar 2011;38(2):65–76.

Here Proctor specifically defined the levels of change that an intervention is addressing: the larger system or environment; the organization; a group or team; or the individual. This is not unlike Richmond, who focused on changes to promote health at the policy level, provider level, and individual and community levels.[23] One can ask: Is there a parallel model for dissemination research addressing all these levels?

WHAT IS MISSING—OUR SOCIAL CONTEXT FOR TRANSLATING RESEARCH INTO PRACTICE

Expansion of D&I approaches to address issues in global health embraces many of the same issues as outlined in chapters throughout this book. Low-resource settings require rethinking delivery approaches and implementation outcomes,[83] as well as adaptation of interventions to fit the local setting, with a goal of achieving equity remaining paramount (see chapter 25). A systems thinking approach, including a focus on developing local capacity and thinking more broadly about context and strengthening health systems, can be an important approach to increasing equity globally.[84] Other examples include resource-stratified guidelines and stronger engagement of stakeholders for breast cancer programs.[85]

To place the growing emphasis on D&I in the context of current funding, manpower needs, and academic environments, we summarize a number of opportunities. We note the recent publication of Standards for Reporting Implementation Studies (StaRI)[86] and expect that the adoption of these standards over the coming years will further improve the quality of D&I research. Furthermore, topics such as scaling up and de-implementation are gaining greater attention and are briefly introduced.

Funding—NIH, CDC, Agency for Healthcare Quality and Research, and Canadian Priorities

Growing emphasis through funding adds credibility to the area of research implementation and evaluation. Requests for Applications (RFAs) from NIH, CDC, and Agency for Healthcare Quality and Research (AHRQ) attest to the growing commitment of resources in the United States. The NIH also has a study section, the Science of Implementation in Health and Healthcare (SIHH) to specifically review grants that "identify, develop, and evaluate dissemination and implementation theories, strategies and methods designed to integrate evidence-based health interventions into public health, clinical, and community settings." However, SIHH expects applications to have "a major methods, strategy, or theoretical development component,"[87] so researchers must find the delicate balance between applied implementation science and advancing the science of implementation. The Canadian Institutes of Health Research have also increased emphasis on funding of D&I, or knowledge translation. Priority for methods development and application is included in these funding opportunities and for many institutions provides the building block on which junior faculty members are themselves promoted (holding grants in addition to scientific productivity are often key components of promotion criteria). Many healthcare organizations are also beginning to recognize the importance of implementing evidence-based practices, which creates opportunities for research partnerships that can help to speed translation.[88]

Education and Training

A 2020 systematic review of capacity building in D&I identified the need to expand capacity-building initiatives by increasing training opportunities and expanding their reach to a broader audience to keep pace with the growing field of D&I. Challenges to capacity-building initiatives identified in the review included demand for training greatly outpacing the available slots and an emphasis on postdoctoral training, with few opportunities for predoctoral trainees, practitioners, and policymakers. The review also emphasized the need for training multidisciplinary teams, delivering training in low-resource settings, and increasing dissemination of widely available, often free, resources online. Shared resources of D&I teaching materials and toolkits are readily available online (see https://www.pcori.org/impact/putting-evidence-work/dissemination-and-implementation-framework-and-toolkit; https://cancercontrol.cancer.gov/is/training-education/training-in-cancer/TIDIRC-open-access) and expanding awareness and access to these tools will help support the training endeavors and make systematic training in D& I science more accessible and widely available.

There have been evaluations published of nationally focused D&I science training programs. Vinson et al. evaluated the first 5 years of the NCI's Training in Dissemination and Implementation Research in Health (TIDIRH) program,[89] which provided an in-person, week-long training to 197 investigators who were new to the D&I field. Trainees were compared to 125 unselected applicants (UAs) whose application score was within one standard deviation of the mean for all trainees' scores for the same application year. A portfolio analysis combining grant mechanisms showed that overall, TIDIRH trainees submitted more peer-reviewed NIH grants per person than UA and had significantly better funding outcomes (25% vs. 19% funded, respectively). The greatest difference was for large research projects, program/center, and cooperative agreement grant mechanisms. Other indicators suggested that the training program was effective at creating a network of scholars across institutions. An evaluation of the 2-year mentored Implementation Research Institute (IRI), which focuses on mental health, found that selected applicants' odds of publishing in implementation science were higher for earlier alumni, starting at 12% at 1 year out and increasing to 94% for those who were 4 years out from starting training.[90] Chances for nonselected applicants remained relatively stable, starting at 47% at 1 year and going to 33% at 4 years, controlling for demographic characteristics. Evaluations of other 2-year mentored programs suggested the strength of this model.[91,92]

Academic Rewards

Priority has historically been placed on novel contributions to science—that is, discovery. Even at the Nobel Prize level of recognition, debate was substantial regarding the role of Florey in moving from discovery of penicillin to the refinement of methods for mass production. From the point of view of impact, it was clearly the application of methods leading to broad use that saved lives during World War II, not the discovery years earlier that lay dormant in a journal article. So, how do we change our academic reward system to acknowledge that application of knowledge or translation to practice is an essential component of effective and affordable health and welfare services? Accountability given the high levels of government funding for research in the United States and many other countries does not on its own shift the reward system. In fact, Moses and Martin called for sweeping changes in the way we conduct research in academic medical centers and reward scientists to more efficiently translate research to practice,[93] yet 12 years later these same changes are still being called for. We need models that are implemented and evaluated within our major academic centers to show that the translation of science to practice is an academic discipline with methods and outcomes that can be evaluated like any other discipline. However, if junior investigators do not have options for a career path in these disciplines, then again the growth of this area will be limited. As an example, academic primary care has supported leading researchers at Dartmouth and Case Western to develop strategies for increased use of evidence-based preventive services, testing subsequent widespread implementation.[94–97] Broader recognition across health sciences disciplines will support methods development and applications to improve population health.

Innovation Versus Replication (Delivery of Effective Programs)

Again, the criteria for funding of grants and the promotion of faculty often hinge on innovation and discovery. Moving a discovery from bench to clinical application or from one health department to a statewide intervention may not appear to be as innovative as a more focused basic science contribution. We might argue it is, however, far more complex and less likely to succeed! Can we refine metrics that will help us estimate lives saved or improvement in quality-adjusted life years to summarize the public health impact of D&I research? How can we convey that the novelty or innovation lies not necessarily in the intervention itself, as by definition it has already proven to be effective, but in how we can implement it to increase its uptake and therefore impact? One recently developed framework, the translational science benefits model considers the impact of health research beyond the individual level and assesses impacts across four domains: (1) clinical and medical benefits; (2) community and public health benefits; (3) economic benefits; and (4) policy and legislative benefits.[98] Still, additional questions persist, such as how we should quantify the contextual factors that moderate the effectiveness of implementation. As Titler asked,[99]: Can we become consistent in approaches to circumstances and setting in which implementation or translation to practice is effective, and define mechanisms for effective interventions?

Scaling Up

As a field we frequently describe the need to take evidence-based interventions to scale and deliver them to all population groups equitably so that we can achieve population health benefits. However, a common and consistent definition of scaling up is not yet evident in the literature. Why aren't we studying large-scale implementation more routinely? How does scaling up differ from other implementation—if at all? Questions arise, such as the ability to deliver the intervention at low cost, the approaches to monitoring consistency or integrity of the intervention delivery, and outcomes across levels of health system (provider or health department), setting, and individuals. Will additional technical assistance be needed for broader implementation? How is this developed, delivered, and sustained? How flexible can and must the intervention be?[100] What are the measures of organizational success and of overall outcome? How important is the original intervention design for delivery at scale? One guide for scaling up interventions sets out a step-by-step process.[101] Scale-up, while an important goal for implementation, cannot alone be the end goal. While planning for scale-up, considerations of maintenance and sustainability must also be factored into the equation. A widespread program that requires continued inputs may not survive once training, temporary staffing, or initial funding ends. For more on this topic, see chapter 29.

De-implementation

There is growing interesting in de-implementation (see NIH funding opportunity announcements: PAR-22-042 and NOT-CA-20-021) or reduction of the use of strategies and interventions that are not evidence based.[8] NOT-CA-20-021 defines de-implementation research as "the scientific study of factors, processes, and strategies for reducing, replacing, or stopping the use of ineffective or low-value clinical practices in healthcare delivery settings" (p. 1), specifying that NCI "special interest in research on the de-implementation of ineffective or low-value clinical practices, programs, treatments, or interventions ('practices') along the cancer care continuum from detection to end-of-life." De-implementation is critically important because about 30% of all medical spending in the United States is unnecessary and doesn't add value. There has been a clinical focus on this over the last few years, largely as a result of the Choosing Wisely campaigns that target reduction/elimination of low-value care. Research in this area had been relatively limited, but is increasing in prevalence as of late.

There is a wide range of terms that are used to describe de-implementation, including de-adoption, exnovation, and de-innovation.[102,103] Some authors use the term *mis-implementation* to include both practices that end effective, evidence-based programs or continue non-evidence-based or ineffective ones.[104] Regardless of the terminology, it is important to understand that this area actually represents three different types of problems: (1) ending harmful practices, such as eliminating use of harmful drugs; (2) reducing use of ineffective practices, or those that offer no benefit over less invasive practices; and (3) reducing use of one practice while increasing the use of another.

Niven et al.[102] completed the first knowledge synthesis in the area of de-implementation in 2015. They concluded that most de-implementation that occurs is the result of scientific evidence, is focused on market withdrawal of harmful drugs, and results from active interventions. It was also noted that de-implementation studies were largely observational, and little systematic or rigorous work in this area had been conducted. A recently published systematic review examining studies from the last 30 years noted a similar lack of research in this area, identifying only a dozen studies with interventions to de-implement low-value care in cancer care delivery settings,[105] yet at the same time, a scoping review recently identified 27 frameworks and models for studying de-implementation.[106]

With all these available resources, the time is ripe for conducting rigorous research into how to reduce mis-implementation and de-implement low-value care. There are many critical questions to be answered related to de-implementation, including whether the processes are similar across the three different types of de-implementation problems and whether different people are needed to effectively address these different problems. There is also a real need to consider how to sustain de-implementation over time, especially when considering interventions other than drugs that are not driven by the market or regulatory factors.

There is also a critical need to understand the factors responsible for rapid and unplanned de-implementation, such as reduced use of hormone replacement therapy in the United States. Developing nimble mechanisms to allow for the study of population-level de-implementation as it is occurring may be particularly useful. For example, ongoing changes in practice, such as elimination of PAP smears in Australia's national cervical screening program, from January 2017, and replacement with 5-year HPV testing, offer opportunities to consider the perspectives, facilitators, and barriers to de-implementation from the patient, provider, testing laboratory, and insurance perspectives. De-implementation will likely not be the inverse of implementation and dissemination uptakes.[107] Further, there are likely very different social factors at work in the implementation versus de-implementation context. For example, women have been told for decades that they must have yearly mammograms and may have many friends who had breast cancer detected via routine mammography. Asking them now to have fewer mammograms or at older ages to stop completely may test their confidence in their provider and the healthcare system and go against deeply rooted beliefs about taking care of themselves. On the other hand, for women who have yet to establish lifelong routine screening regimens, recommendations to eliminate inefficient screening at younger ages have been more readily adapted.[108] Where to begin to remove inefficient or unnecessary practices remains an area of study, as does identifying the characteristics of the people who will lead or resist de-implementation and how they may differ from those who lead implementation.[109] For example, the Choosing Wisely campaign launched in 2012 in the United States aims to encourage abandoning care that wastes resources or delivers no benefit in specific health areas, such as management of blood sugar and diabetes and cancer screening. The approach to studying de-implementation mechanisms examines variation among systems, providers, patients, and the actual implementation strategies that may modify the success of the program.[110] See chapter 12 for more on de-implementation and mis-implementation.

Systems to Quantify Benefits of Effective Programs (Outcomes)

How do we sum up the benefits of implementation and effective programs being delivered to broad sectors of the population? Ginexi and Hilton proposed that focusing on evidence-based best practices may help bridge the gap from research to practice.[111] They argued that best and worst practice can inform practice improvement. How we quantify program fidelity and implementation remains at the core of the challenge. Proctor and colleagues[82] now propose a taxonomy of eight conceptually distinct implementation outcomes—acceptability, adoption, appropriateness, feasibility, fidelity, implementation cost, penetration, and sustainability—along with their nominal definitions. Further, they propose using a two-pronged agenda for research on implementation outcomes. Conceptualizing and measuring implementation outcomes (or process evaluation measures in the European framework) will advance understanding of implementation processes, enhance efficiency in implementation research, and pave the way for studies of the comparative effectiveness of implementation strategies. As we note in this book, several novel approaches are proposed, but coming to agreement on when these measures are most helpful will require further study.

New methods are needed and consistency across programs will add to the overall advance of the field. The magnitude of benefit, the proportion of the population reached, and the degree to which a program is sustained all impact the long-term population benefit. Proctor defined steps in the model of implementation, noting that conceptualizing and measuring implementation outcomes will advance understanding of implementation processes, enhance efficiency in implementation research, and pave the way for studies of the comparative effectiveness of implementation strategies.[82] Refinement to better incorporate ethical, legal, and social considerations through stakeholder engagement will further advance this model. Further, identifying implementation outcomes that are important to our stakeholders/

implementation partners is a critical aspect that deserves increased consideration. For example, the ways in which the RE-AIM (Reach, Effectiveness, Adoption, Implementation, and Maintenance) framework can inform evaluation are summarized in chapter 17. Other approaches that apply across settings will make for a more robust area of inquiry.

SUMMARY

Given the growing emphasis on D&I as a means to increase the effectiveness and efficiency of the research enterprise, public policy, and the services with which we work, refining methods that will facilitate translation and implementation are imperative. Cultural changes within the academy and in linking researchers and practitioners will be necessary adjuncts to effective progress. Bringing the D&I research community to common understanding of answers to our overarching questions will be a necessary step. Then we can more consistently answer the questions: How will we gather this information on effective interventions to form the evidence base? Will interventions be applicable to our setting? What methods should we use to decide what to disseminate or implement? Which implementation strategies will give us the greatest impact on population health? What outcomes should be tracked to know if we are making progress? How long will it take to show progress, or when will it be observed? The methods and examples outlined in this book will help answer these and other important questions.

SUGGESTED READINGS AND WEBSITES

Readings

Glasgow RE, Vinson C, Chambers D, Khoury MJ, Kaplan RM, Hunter C. National Institutes of Health approaches to dissemination and implementation science: current and future directions. *Am J Public Health*. 2012;102:1274–1281.

Addressing the gap between knowledge and practice, this article reviews core values necessary to advance implementation science. These include rigor and relevance, efficiency, collaboration, improved collaboration, and cumulative knowledge.

Glasziou P, Chalmers I, Altman DG, et al. Taking healthcare interventions from trial to practice. *BMJ*. 2010;341:c3852.

Improved reporting of details of trials will enable use of results in practice. An example of this is illusrated and a call for increased reporting of intervention details to improve replication and use in practice.

Green LW, Ottoson JM, Garcia C, Hiatt RA. Diffusion theory and knowledge dissemination, utilization, and integration in public health. Annu Rev Public *Health*. Apr 29 2009;30:151–174.

Rigorous review of public health implications of diffusion, dissemination, and implementation to improve public health practice and guide design of future research.

Ioannidis JP, Karassa FB. The need to consider the wider agenda in systematic reviews and meta-analyses: breadth, timing, and depth of the evidence. *BMJ*. 2010;341:c4875.

Thoughtful critique of limitations of meta-analysis of clinical interventions, the narrow scope of practice they cover, and the potential to draw misleading conclusions from systematic reviews and meta-analysis.

Lobb R, Colditz G. Implementation science and its application to population health. *Annu* Rev Public *Health*. 2013;34:235–253.

Thoughtful review of the role that stakeholder engagement and more rigorous study of barriers to implementation can help identify how systems can implement effective innovations in healthcare delivery.

Proctor E, Silmere H, Raghavan R, et al. Outcomes for implementation research: conceptual distinctions, measurement challenges, and research agenda. Adm Policy Ment *Health*. 2010;38:65–76.

Groundbreaking summary of issues in design and evaluation of implementation research setting out a model that defines steps in the process and discusses a model for quantifying benefits of program implementation.

Weiner BJ, Sherr K, Lewis CC, Eds. *Practical Implementation Science: Moving Evidence Into Action*. Springer Publishing; 2022.

This useful textbook describes how to implement evidence-based practices effectively through use of relevant theories, frameworks, models, tools, and research findings. It includes real-world case studies across a range of settings and topics.

Woolf SH. The meaning of translational research and why it matters. *JAMA*. 2008;299(2):211–213.

An important contribution defining stages of research and the importance of translation from bench to bedside and from reseach clinic to population-wide applications. Also calls for research funding to be directed to improving population health outcomes.

Selected Websites and Tools

National Cancer Institute Implementation Science Research and Practice Tools: https://cancercontrol.cancer.gov/is/tools

The Research and Practice tools acts a portal to provide access to data and resources for dissemination and implementation in both research and practice.

Dissemination and Implementation Research Core at the Institute for Clinical and Translational Science, Washington University in St Louis, Ana Baumann and Elvin Geng, co-directors. http://icts.wustl.edu/icts-researchers/icts-cores/find-services/by-core-name/dissemination-implementation-research-core

The Dissemination and Implementation Research Core (DIRC) provides methodological expertise to advance translational (T3 and T4) research to inform and move efficacious health practices from clinical knowledge into routine, real-world use. The DIRC works with scientists to move forward scientific agenda and grant writing related to D&I of healthcare discoveries. Furthermore, DIRC develops tools and methods for studying D&I.

Implementation Science Exchange (IMPSCIX), a public service of the North Carolina Translational and Clinical Sciences Institute (NC TRACS), UNC Chapel Hill. https://impsci.tracs.unc.edu/

This free online resource offers help to design, to get funded, and to execute implementation science research projects.

Task Force on Community Preventive Services. https://www.thecommunityguide.org

The Community Guide provides a repository of the more than 200 systematic reviews conducted by the Task Force on Community Preventive Services, an independent, interdisciplinary group with staff support by the CDC. Each review gives attention to the "applicability" of the conclusions beyond the study populations and settings in which the original studies were conducted.

Cochrane. https://www.cochrane.org/

Cochrane prepares Cochrane Reviews and aims to update them regularly with the latest scientific evidence. Members of the organization (mostly volunteers) work together to assess evidence to help people make decisions about healthcare practices and policies. Some people read the healthcare literature to find reports of randomized control trials; others find such reports by searching electronic databases; others prepare and update Cochrane Reviews based on the evidence found in these trials; others work to improve the methods used in Cochrane Reviews; and others provide a vitally important consumer perspective.

RE-AIM. https://www.RE-AIM.org

The acronym refers to Reach, Effectiveness, Adoption, Implementation, and Maintenance, all important dimensions in the consideration of D&I research and in the external validity or applicability of research results in original studies for the alternative settings and circumstances in which they might be applied. These were applied in the development of a set of guidelines for assessing and reporting external validity in Reference 29 below.

D-Cubed. http://www.uq.edu.au/evaluationstedi/Dissemination/?q=dissemination/

A review of dissemination strategies used by projects funded by the Australian Learning and Teaching Council promotes dissemination strategies that have facilitated effective dissemination. A useful framework for dissemination and guide for use is provided.

REFERENCES

1. Agre P, Leshner AI. Bridging science and society. Editorial. *Science.* Feb 19 2010;327(5968):921. doi:10.1126/science.1188231
2. Emmons KM, Colditz GA. Realizing the Potential of Cancer Prevention—The Role of Implementation Science. *N Engl J Med.* 2017 Mar 9;376(10):986–990. doi:10.1056/NEJMsb1609101. PMID: 28273020; PMCID: PMC5473684.
3. Collins FS. Reengineering translational science: the time is right. *Sci Transl Med.* Jul 6 2011;3(90):90cm17. doi:10.1126/scitranslmed.3002747
4. Institute of Medicine. *Crossing the Quality Chasm: A New Health System for the 21st Century.* National Academy Press; 2001.
5. Rubenstein LV, Pugh J. Strategies for promoting organizational and practice change by advancing implementation research. *J Gen Intern Med.* Feb 2006;21(suppl 2):S58–S64. doi:10.1111/j.1525-1497.2006.00364.x
6. United States Department of Health and Human Services. *Improving Public Health Practice Through Translational Research.* 2007. Accessed July 17, 2011. http://grants.nih.gov/grants/guide/rfa-files/rfa-cd-07-005.html
7. Lost in clinical translation. *Nat Med.* Sep 2004;10(9):879. doi:10.1038/nm0904-879
8. Department of Health and Human Services. Dissemination and Implementation Research in Health, PAR-16-238. NIH. Accessed September 4, 2016. https://grants.nih.gov/grants/guide/pa-files/PAR-16-238.html
9. Rabin BA, Brownson RC, Haire-Joshu D, Kreuter MW, Weaver NL. A glossary for dissemination and implementation research in health. *J Public Health Manag Pract.* Mar–Apr 2008;14(2):117–123. doi:10.1097/01.PHH.0000311888.06252.bb

10. Lomas J. Diffusion, dissemination, and implementation: who should do what? *Ann N Y Acad Sci.* Dec 31 1993;703:226–235; discussion 235–237.
11. Lomas J, Sisk JE, Stocking B. From evidence to practice in the United States, the United Kingdom, and Canada. *Milbank Q.* 1993;71(3):405–410.
12. Curry SJ. Organizational interventions to encourage guideline implementation. *Chest.* Aug 2000;118(2)(suppl):40S–46S.
13. Bero L, Grillr R, Grimshaw J, Harvey E, Oxman AD, Thompson M. Closing the gap between research and practice: an overview of systematic reviews of interventions to promote the implementation of research findings. *BMJ.* 1998;317:465–468.
14. Lobb R, Colditz GA. Implementation science and its application to population health. *Annu Rev Public Health.* 2013;34:235–251. doi:10.1146/annurev-publhealth-031912-114444
15. Mehta TG, Mahoney J, Leppin AL, et al. Integrating dissemination and implementation sciences within Clinical and Translational Science Award programs to advance translational research: recommendations to national and local leaders. *J Clin Transl Sci.* 2021;5(1):e151. doi:10.1017/cts.2021.815
16. Glasziou P, Chalmers I, Altman DG, et al. Taking healthcare interventions from trial to practice. *BMJ.* 2010;341:c3852. doi:10.1136/bmj.c3852
17. Ioannidis JP, Karassa FB. The need to consider the wider agenda in systematic reviews and meta-analyses: breadth, timing, and depth of the evidence. *BMJ.* 2010;341:c4875. doi:10.1136/bmj.c4875
18. Zerhouni E. Medicine. The NIH roadmap. *Science.* Oct 3 2003;302(5642):63–72. doi:10.1126/science.1091867
19. Westfall JM, Mold J, Fagnan L. Practice-based research—"Blue Highways" on the NIH roadmap. *JAMA.* Jan 24 2007;297(4):403–406. https://jamanetwork.com/journals/jama/article-abstract/205216
20. Frieden TR. A framework for public health action: the health impact pyramid. *Am J Public Health.* Apr 2010;100(4):590–595. doi:10.2105/AJPH.2009.185652
21. Chambers DA, Feero WG, Khoury MJ. Convergence of implementation science, precision medicine, and the learning health care system: a new model for biomedical research. *JAMA.* May 10 2016;315(18):1941–1942. doi:10.1001/jama.2016.3867
22. Wandersman A, Duffy J, Flaspohler P, et al. Bridging the gap between prevention research and practice: the interactive systems framework for dissemination and implementation. *Am J commun Psychol.* Jun 2008;41(3-4):171–181. doi:10.1007/s10464-008-9174-z
23. Richmond J, Kotelchuck M. Coordination and development of strategies and policy for public health promotion in the United States. In: Holland W, Detel R, Know G, eds. *Oxford Textbook of Public Health.* Oxford University Press; 1991:441–454.
24. Atwood K, Colditz GA, Kawachi I. From public health science to prevention policy: placing science in its social and political contexts. *Am J Public Health.* Oct 1997;87(10):1603–1606.
25. Farquhar JW. The case for dissemination research in health promotion and disease prevention. *Can J Public Health.* Nov–Dec 1996;87(suppl 2):S44–S49.
26. Harlan WR. Prevention research at the National Institutes of Health. *Am J Prev Med.* May 1998;14(4):302–307. doi:10.1016/s0749-3797(98)00005-1
27. Institute of Medicine. *Linking Research to Public Health Practice. A Review of the CDC's Program of Centers for Research and Demonstration of Health Promotion and Disease Prevention.* National Academy Press; 1997.
28. Moses H 3rd, Matheson DH, Cairns-Smith S, George BP, Palisch C, Dorsey ER. The anatomy of medical research: US and international comparisons. *JAMA.* Jan 13 2015;313(2):174–189. doi:10.1001/jama.2014.15939
29. Foraker RE, Benziger CP, DeBarmore BM, et al. Achieving optimal population cardiovascular health requires an interdisciplinary team and a learning healthcare system: a scientific statement from the American Heart Association. *Circulation.* Jan 12 2021;143(2):e9–e18. doi:10.1161/CIR.0000000000000913
30. Feofanova EV, Zhang GQ, Lhatoo S, Metcalf GA, Boerwinkle E, Venner E. The Implementation Science for Genomic Health Translation (INSIGHT) study in epilepsy: protocol for a learning health care system. *JMIR Res Protoc.* Mar 26 2021;10(3):e25576. doi:10.2196/25576
31. Braganza MZ, Pearson E, Avila CJ, Zlowe D, Ovretveit J, Kilbourne AM. Aligning quality improvement efforts and policy goals in a national integrated health system. *Health Serv Res.* Jun 2022;57 Suppl 1(Suppl 1):9–19. doi:10.1111/1475-6773.13944
32. Emmons KM, Chambers D, Abazeed A. Embracing policy implementation science to ensure translation of evidence to cancer control policy. *Transl Behav Med.* Nov 30 2021;11(11):1972–1979. doi:10.1093/tbm/ibab147

33. Mueller NM, Hsieh A, Ramanadhan S, Lee RM, Emmons KM. The prevalence of dissemination and implementation research and training grants at National Cancer Institute-Designated Cancer Centers. *JNCI Cancer Spectr.* 2021 Dec 15;6(1):pkab092.
34. Cochran W. Problems arising in the analysis of a series of similar experiments. *J R Stat Soc Suppl.* 1937;4:102–118.
35. Rogers E. *Diffusion of Innovations.* 3rd ed. Free Press; 1993.
36. OECD. Health at a Glance *2021.* OECD *Indicators.* OECD Publishing; 2021. doi:10.1787/ae3016b9-en
37. Mosteller F, Wallace D. *Inference and Disputed Authorship: The Federalist.* Addison-Wesley Publishing Company; 1964.
38. Mosteller F. *The Pleasures of Statistics. The Autobiography of Frederick Mosteller.* Springer; 2010.
39. Mosteller F. On pooling data. *J Am Stat Assoc.* 1948;43:231–242.
40. Green LW, Ottoson JM, Garcia C, Hiatt RA. Diffusion theory and knowledge dissemination, utilization, and integration in public health. *Annu Rev Public Health.* Apr 29 2009;30:151–174.
41. Brownson RC, Bright FS. Chronic disease control in public health practice: looking back and moving forward. *Public Health Rep.* May–Jun 2004;119(3):230–238. doi:10.1016/j.phr.2004.04.001
42. Balas EA, Boren SA. Managing clinical knowledge for health care improvement. In: Bemmel J, McCray A, eds. *Yearbook of Medical Informatics 2000: Patient-Centered Systems.* Schattauer Verlagsgesellschaft mbH; 2000:65–70.
43. Khan S, Chambers D, Neta G. Revisiting time to translation: implementation of evidence-based practices (EBPs) in cancer control. *Cancer Causes Control.* Mar 2021;32(3):221–230. doi:10.1007/s10552-020-01376-z
44. Goodwin I. Engineers proclaim top achievements of 20th century, but neglect attributing feats to roots in physics. *Physics Today.* 2000;53:48–49.
45. Fortunato S. Prizes: growing time lag threatens Nobels. *Nature.* Apr 10 2014;508(7495):186. doi:10.1038/508186a
46. Dzau VJ, Balatbat CA, Ellaissi WF. Revisiting academic health sciences systems a decade later: discovery to health to population to society. *Lancet.* Dec 18 2021;398(10318):2300–2304. doi:10.1016/S0140-6736(21)01752-9
47. Banting FG, Best CH. The internal secretion of the pancreas. 1922. *Indian J Med Res.* Mar 2007;125(3):251–266.
48. Banting FG, Best CH, Collip JB, Campbell WR, Fletcher AA. Pancreatic extracts in the treatment of diabetes mellitus. *CMAJ.* Mar 1922;12(3):141–146.
49. Bliss M. *The Discovery of Insulin.* 25th anniversary ed. University of Chicago Press; 2007.
50. US Department of Health and Human Services. A timeline of HIV/AIDS. Accessed February 22, 2017. https://www.aids.gov/hiv-aids-basics/hiv-aids-101/aids-timeline/
51. Department of Health. Historical data from the National HPV Vaccination Program Register. Immunizaton data up to 31 December 2018. Department of Health, Commonwealth of Australia. Updated January 7, 2020. Accessed April 3, 2022. https://www.health.gov.au/resources/collections/historical-data-from-the-national-hpv-vaccination-program-register#collection-description
52. Pingali C, Yankey D, Elam-Evans LD, et al. National, regional, state, and selected local area vaccination coverage among adolescents aged 13–17 years—United States, 2020. *MMWR Morb Mortal Wkly Rep.* Sep 3 2021;70(35):1183–1190. doi:10.15585/mmwr.mm7035a1
53. Hall MT, Simms KT, Lew JB, et al. The projected timeframe until cervical cancer elimination in Australia: a modelling study. *Lancet Public Health.* Jan 2019;4(1):e19–e27. doi:10.1016/S2468-2667(18)30183-X
54. Petticrew M, Tugwell P, Welch V, et al. Better evidence about wicked issues in tackling health inequities. Research Support, Non-U.S. Gov't. *J Public health.* Sep 2009;31(3):453–456. doi:10.1093/pubmed/fdp076
55. Lavis J, Davies H, Oxman A, Denis JL, Golden-Biddle K, Ferlie E. Towards systematic reviews that inform health care management and policy-making. Research Support, Non-U.S. Gov't. *J Health Serv Res Policy.* Jul 2005;10(suppl 1):35–48. doi:10.1258/1355819054308549
56. Sacks H, Berrier J, Reitman D, Ancona-Berk V, Chalmers T. Meta-analysis of randomized controlled studies. *N Engl J Med.* 1987;316:450–455.
57. Berlin J, Colditz G. A meta-analysis of physical activity in the prevention of coronary heart disease. *Am J Epidemiol.* 1990;132:612–628.
58. Bastian H, Glasziou P, Chalmers I. Seventy-five trials and eleven systematic reviews a day: how will we ever keep up? *PLoS Med.* 2010;7(9):e1000326. doi:10.1371/journal.pmed.1000326
59. Preventive Services Task Force. *Guide to Clinical Preventive Services.* 2nd ed. Williams and Wilkins; 1996.
60. Schunemann HJ, Oxman AD, Brozek J, et al. GRADE: assessing the quality of evidence

for diagnostic recommendations. *Evid Based Med.* Dec 2008;13(6):162–163. doi:10.1136/ebm.13.6.162-a

61. Jaeschke R, Guyatt GH, Dellinger P, et al. Use of GRADE grid to reach decisions on clinical practice guidelines when consensus is elusive. *BMJ.* 2008;337:a744. doi:10.1136/bmj.a744
62. Guyatt GH, Oxman AD, Vist GE, et al. GRADE: an emerging consensus on rating quality of evidence and strength of recommendations. *BMJ.* Apr 26 2008;336(7650):924–926. doi:10.1136/bmj.39489.470347.AD
63. Wang Z, Norris SL, Bero L. Implementation plans included in World Health Organisation guidelines. *Implement Sci.* May 20 2016;11(1):76. doi:10.1186/s13012-016-0440-4
64. Moher D, Schulz KF, Altman DG. The CONSORT statement: revised recommendations for improving the quality of reports of parallel-group randomized trials. *Ann Intern Med.* Apr 17 2001;134(8):657–662.
65. Thorpe KE, Zwarenstein M, Oxman AD, et al. A pragmatic-explanatory continuum indicator summary (PRECIS): a tool to help trial designers. *CMAJ.* May 12 2009;180(10):E47–E57. doi:10.1503/cmaj.090523
66. Loudon K, Treweek S, Sullivan F, Donnan P, Thorpe KE, Zwarenstein M. The PRECIS-2 tool: designing trials that are fit for purpose. *BMJ.* May 08 2015;350:h2147. doi:10.1136/bmj.h2147
67. Berkey CS, Hoaglin D, Mosteller F, Colditz GA. A random-effects regression model for meta-analysis. *Stat Med.* 1995;14:395–411.
68. Colditz GA, Brewer TF, Berkey CS, et al. Efficacy of BCG vaccine in the prevention of tuberculosis. Meta-analysis of the published literature. *JAMA.* Mar 2 1994;271(9):698–702.
69. Colditz GA, Berkey CS, Mosteller F, et al. The efficacy of bacillus Calmette-Guerin vaccination of newborns and infants in the prevention of tuberculosis: meta-analyses of the published literature. *Pediatrics.* Jul 1995;96(1 Pt 1):29–35.
70. Colditz G, Burdick E, Mosteller F. Heterogeneity in meta-analysis of data from epidemiologic studies: a commentary. *Am J Epidemiol.* 1995;142:371–382.
71. Glasgow RE, Chambers D. Developing robust, sustainable, implementation systems using rigorous, rapid and relevant science. *Clin Transl Sci.* Feb 2012;5(1):48–55. doi:10.1111/j.1752-8062.2011.00383.x
72. Proctor EK, Landsverk J, Aarons G, Chambers D, Glisson C, Mittman B. Implementation research in mental health services: an emerging science with conceptual, methodological, and training challenges. *Adm Policy Ment Health.* Jan 2009;36(1):24–34. doi:10.1007/s10488-008-0197-4
73. Bero LA, Jadad AR. How consumers and policy-makers can use systematic reviews for decision making. *Ann Intern Med.* 1997;127:37–42.
74. Mosteller F, Colditz G. Understanding research synthesis (meta-analysis). *Ann Rev Public Health.* 1996;17:1–32.
75. Greenhalgh T, Robert G, Macfarlane F, Bate P, Kyriakidou O. Diffusion of innovations in service organizations: systematic review and recommendations. *Milbank Q.* 2004;82(4):581–629. doi:10.1111/j.0887-378X.2004.00325.x
76. Kingdon JW. *Agendas, Alternatives, and Public Policies.* Addison-Wesley Educational Publishers, Inc.; 2003.
77. Hemenway D. Why we don't spend enough on public health. *N Engl J Med.* May 6 2010;362(18):1657–1658. doi:10.1056/NEJMp1001784
78. Koh HK, Piotrowski JJ, Kumanyika S, Fielding JE. Healthy People: a 2020 vision for the social determinants approach. *Health Educ Behav.* Dec 2011;38(6):551–557. doi:10.1177/1090198111428646
79. Levine RL. Healthy People 2030: a beacon for addressing health disparities and health equity. *J Public Health Manag Pract.* Nov–Dec 01 2021;27(suppl 6):S220–S221. doi:10.1097/PHH.0000000000001409
80. Gomez CA, Kleinman DV, Pronk N, et al. Addressing health equity and social determinants of health through Healthy People 2030. *J Public Health Manag Pract.* Nov–Dec 01 2021;27(suppl 6):S249–S257. doi:10.1097/PHH.0000000000001297
81. Bowen DJ, Sorensen G, Weiner BJ, Campbell M, Emmons K, Melvin C. Dissemination research in cancer control: where are we and where should we go? *Cancer Causes Control.* May 2009;20(4):473–485. doi:10.1007/s10552-009-9308-0
82. Proctor E, Silmere H, Raghavan R, et al. Outcomes for implementation research: conceptual distinctions, measurement challenges, and research agenda. Research Support, NIH, Extramural. *Adm Policy Ment Health.* Mar 2011;38(2):65–76. doi:10.1007/s10488-010-0319-7
83. Rivera AS, Hernandez R, Mag-Usara R, et al. Implementation outcomes of HIV self-testing in low- and middle-income countries: a scoping review. *PLoS One.* 2021;16(5):e0250434. doi:10.1371/journal.pone.0250434
84. Gravitt PE, Silver MI, Hussey HM, et al. Achieving equity in cervical cancer screening in low- and middle-income countries (LMICs): strengthening health systems using a systems thinking

approach. *Prev Med.* Mar 2021;144:106322. doi:10.1016/j.ypmed.2020.106322
85. Rositch AF, Unger-Saldana K, DeBoer RJ, Ng'ang'a A, Weiner BJ. The role of dissemination and implementation science in global breast cancer control programs: frameworks, methods, and examples. *Cancer.* May 15 2020;126(suppl 10):2394–2404. doi:10.1002/cncr.32877
86. Pinnock H, Barwick M, Carpenter CR, et al. Standards for Reporting Implementation Studies (StaRI): explanation and elaboration document. *BMJ Open.* Apr 03 2017;7(4):e013318. doi:10.1136/bmjopen-2016-013318
87. Wang W. Science of Implementation in Health and Healthcare—SIHH. National Institutes of Health, Center for Scientific Review. Updated January 17, 2022. Accessed April 3, 2022. https://public.csr.nih.gov/StudySections/DABP/HDM/SIHH
88. Gopalan A, Grant RW. Research to change health delivery systems: on the outside looking in? *J Gen Intern Med.* Oct 2018;33(10):1592–1593. doi:10.1007/s11606-018-4586-4
89. Vinson CA, Clyne M, Cardoza N, Emmons KM. Building capacity: a cross-sectional evaluation of the US Training Institute for Dissemination and Implementation Research in Health. *Implement Sci.* Nov 21 2019;14(1):97. doi:10.1186/s13012-019-0947-6
90. Baumann AA, Carothers BJ, Landsverk J, et al. Evaluation of the Implementation Research Institute: trainees' publications and grant productivity. *Adm Policy Ment Health.* Mar 2020;47(2):254–264. doi:10.1007/s10488-019-00977-4
91. Brownson RC, Jacob RR, Carothers BJ, et al. Building the Next Generation of Researchers: Mentored Training in Dissemination and Implementation Science. *Acad Med.* Jan 1 2021;96(1):86–92. doi:10.1097/ACM.0000000000003750
92. Padek M, Mir N, Jacob RR, et al. Training scholars in dissemination and implementation research for cancer prevention and control: a mentored approach. *Implement Sci.* Jan 22 2018;13(1):18. doi:10.1186/s13012-018-0711-3
93. Moses H 3rd, Martin JB. Biomedical research and health advances. *N Engl J Med.* Feb 10 2011;364(6):567–571. doi:10.1056/NEJMsb1007634
94. Dietrich A, Carney P, Winchell C, et al. An office systems approach to cancer prevention in primary care. *Cancer Pract.* 1997;5:375–381.
95. Dietrich AJ, Tobin JN, Cassells A, et al. Telephone care management to improve cancer screening among low-income women: a randomized, controlled trial. *Ann Intern Med.* Apr 18 2006;144(8):563–571. doi:144/8/563 [pii]. https://www.ncbi.nlm.nih.gov/pmc/articles/PMC3841972/
96. Dietrich AJ, Tobin JN, Cassells A, et al. Translation of an efficacious cancer-screening intervention to women enrolled in a Medicaid managed care organization. *Ann Fam Med.* Jul–Aug 2007;5(4):320–327. doi:10.1370/afm.701
97. Stewart EE, Nutting PA, Crabtree BF, Stange KC, Miller WL, Jaen CR. Implementing the patient-centered medical home: observation and description of the national demonstration project. *Ann Fam Med.* 2010;8(suppl 1):S21–S32; S92. doi:8/Suppl_1/S21 [pii] 10.1370/afm.1111
98. Luke DA, Sarli CC, Suiter AM, et al. The translational science benefits model: a new framework for assessing the health and societal benefits of clinical and translational sciences. *Clin Transl Sci.* Jan 2018;11(1):77–84. doi:10.1111/cts.12495
99. Titler MG. Translation science and context. *Res Theory Nurs Pract.* 2010;24(1):35–55.
100. Gopalan G, Franco LM, Dean-Assael K, McGuire-Schwartz M, Chacko A, McKay M. Statewide implementation of the 4 Rs and 2 Ss for strengthening families. *J Evid Based Soc Work.* 2014;11(1–2):84–96. doi:10.1080/15433714.2013.842440
101. Milat AJ, Newson R, King L, et al. A guide to scaling up population health interventions. *Public Health Res Pract.* Jan 28 2016;26(1):e2611604. doi:10.17061/phrp2611604
102. Niven DJ, Mrklas KJ, Holodinsky JK, et al. Towards understanding the de-adoption of low-value clinical practices: a scoping review. *BMC Med.* Oct 06 2015;13:255. doi:10.1186/s12916-015-0488-z
103. Gnjidic D, Elshaug AG. De-adoption and its 43 related terms: harmonizing low-value care terminology. *BMC Med.* Oct 20 2015;13:273. doi:10.1186/s12916-015-0511-4
104. Brownson RC, Allen P, Jacob RR, et al. Understanding mis-implementation in public health practice. *Am J Prev Med.* May 2015;48(5):543–551. doi:10.1016/j.amepre.2014.11.015
105. Alishahi Tabriz A, Turner K, Clary A, et al. De-implementing low-value care in cancer care delivery: a systematic review. *Implement Sci.* Mar 12 2022;17(1):24. doi:10.1186/s13012-022-01197-5
106. Walsh-Bailey C, Tsai E, Tabak RG, et al. A scoping review of de-implementation frameworks and models. *Implement Sci.* Nov 24 2021;16(1):100. doi:10.1186/s13012-021-01173-5
107. Davidoff F. On the undiffusion of established practices. *JAMA Intern Med.* May 2015;175(5):809–811. doi:10.1001/jamainternmed.2015.0167

108. Silver MI, Anderson ML, Beaber EF, et al. De-implementation of cervical cancer screening before age 21. *Prev Med.* Dec 2021;153:106815. doi:10.1016/j.ypmed.2021.106815

109. van Bodegom-Vos L, Davidoff F, Marang-van de Mheen PJ. Implementation and de-implementation: two sides of the same coin? *BMJ Qual Saf.* Aug 10 2016;26(6):495–501. doi:10.1136/bmjqs-2016-005473

110. Aron DC, Lowery J, Tseng CL, Conlin P, Kahwati L. De-implementation of inappropriately tight control (of hypoglycemia) for health: protocol with an example of a research grant application. *Implement Sci.* May 19 2014;9:58. doi:10.1186/1748-5908-9-58

111. Ginexi EM, Hilton TF. What's next for translation research? *Eval Health Prof.* Sep 2006;29(3):334–347. doi:10.1177/0163278706290409

2

Terminology for Dissemination and Implementation Research

BORSIKA A. RABIN, CLARE VIGLIONE, AND ROSS C. BROWNSON

BACKGROUND

Dissemination and implementation (D&I) research has become an established field in health sciences and public health and continues to be a growing priority for major health-related funding agencies.[1–3] While over the past decade progress has been made in harmonizing terminology for D&I research, there continues to be a need for further refinements to definitions and how they are used across different geographical areas, subfields, and professions.[4,5] As noted by Ciliska and colleagues: "Closing the gap from knowledge generation to use in decision-making for practice and policy is conceptually and theoretically hampered by diverse terms and inconsistent definitions of terms."[6(p2)] A survey conducted by *Nature Medicine* on how their readers defined the term "translational research" found substantial variation in interpretation by respondents. Some definitions were consistent with the National Institutes of Health (NIH) definition ("the process of applying ideas, insights and discoveries generated through basic scientific inquiry to the treatment or prevention of human disease" [7(p879)]), others believed that only research that leads to direct clinical application should be defined as translational research, and only a small group emphasized the bidirectional nature of the process (i.e., bench to bedside and back).[7] This phenomenon can be partly explained by the relatively new appearance of D&I research on the health research agenda and by the great diversity of disciplines that made noteworthy contributions to the understanding of D&I research.[8–10] Some of the most important contributions originate from the nonhealth fields of agriculture, education, marketing, communication, and management.[11] Diverse health-related areas contribute to D&I research, including health services research, HIV prevention, school health, mental health, nursing, cancer prevention and control, violence prevention, and disability and rehabilitation.[12] Further complexity is injected by the variation in terminology and classification of terms across countries. This book uses the term "dissemination and implementation research" to denote the newly emerging field in the United States; however, other countries and international organizations (e.g., the United Kingdom, Canada, the World Health Organization [WHO]) commonly use the terms "knowledge translation and integration," "population health intervention research," or "scaling up" to define this area of research.[13–16] Furthermore, Graham and colleagues identified 29 distinct terms referring to the some aspect of the D&I (or knowledge translation) process when they looked at the terminology used by 33 applied research funding agencies in nine countries,[16] and McKibbon and colleagues identified 100 terms that described knowledge translation or KT research.[17]

This chapter builds on the previous two editions as well as a published article that used an expert discussion to select definitions to be included from a list of 106 definitions. In this third edition, we expanded on the glossary to include updates to the original terms and definitions based on newer D&I publications published since the previous edition in 2018. We formalized our approach to identifying and revising glossary terms by systematically

Borsika A. Rabin, Clare Viglione, and Ross C. Brownson, *Terminology for Dissemination and Implementation Research* In: *Dissemination and Implementation Research in Health.* Edited by: Ross C. Brownson, Graham A. Colditz, and Enola K. Proctor, Oxford University Press.
 DOI: 10.1093/oso/9780197660690.003.0002

reviewing (1) publications that have been cited at least 50 times from prominent D&I journals, including *Implementation Science* and *Translational Behavioral Medicine*; (2) articles tagged as "most accessed" in *Implementation Science Communications*; (3) publications recommended by D&I experts, prioritizing those covering new areas or trends within D&I science; (4) the current list of terms in the Index; and (5) all chapters within this book.

Terms and definitions are organized in this chapter by the sections and subsections of the textbook. The first section (**Background**) provides definitions for the most commonly used terms in D&I research as well as identifies stages of the research process continuum. In section 2 (**Theory and Conceptual Foundations**), the most commonly used models and frameworks that can inform planning and evaluation activities in D&I research are discussed. Section 3 (**Strategies and Methods**) provides an overview of key D&I strategies along with concepts of adaptation and fidelity, organizational processes and participatory approaches associated with D&I science, system science, and factors associated with the success, speed, and extent of D&I. Section 4 (**Design and Measurement**) summarizes important concepts of study design and measurement that should be considered when evaluating D&I research. Section 5 (**Setting- and Population-Specific D&I**) includes critical concepts of policy and health equity. Finally, Section 6 (**Dissemination and Scale-up**) comprises terms relevant to designing for dissemination and sustainment, marketing and distribution systems, sustainability and scale-up, and training and capacity building for D&I. Because the list of terms is lengthy, we present a condensed list of key definitions in this chapter, and a longer version with all terms is available online (see https://doi.org/10.1093/oso/9780197660690.003.0002).

SECTION 1: BACKGROUND

Innovation

The term *innovation* can refer to "an idea, practice, or object that is perceived as new by an individual or other unit of adoption."[11(p12)] More specifically in the context of research, innovation refers to research evidence that is being implemented in a new setting. Some authors use this term interchangeably with the term *evidence-based intervention* (EBI).

Intervention

Interventions are the focus of D&I efforts (the thing).[18] Most interventions in D&I research are multifaceted with many interacting components and can be conceptualized as having "core components" (the elements of the intervention responsible for its effectiveness) and "adaptable components."[19–21] Interventions within D&I research are defined broadly and may include programs, practices, principles, procedures, products, pills, and policies.[22]

Evidence-Based Intervention

In D&I research, interventions are most often expected to have a certain level of evidence of efficacy or effectiveness (EBIs) to be deemed ready for D&I.[23–26]

The type and extent of evidence indicating action might differ depending on the context in which D&I occurs.[27]

Complex Intervention

In D&I research, we commonly work with complex interventions. Complexity can emerge from the properties of the intervention as well as the interaction between the intervention and context.[28,29] Key considerations for the complexity of the intervention include the number, diversity, and interaction of core components; target behaviors; expertise and skills needed for the delivery and receipt of the intervention; target groups, settings, and socioecological levels; and the level of flexibility allowed for the delivery of the intervention.[30] Further guidance about developing, implementing, and evaluating complex interventions is provided by Hawe and colleagues and Skivington et al.[30,31]

Evidence-Informed Practice or Interventions

The term *evidence-informed practice or interventions* expands the traditional EBI terminology and intends to emphasize that healthcare and population health should always be context sensitive and use a person- or client-focused (stakeholder) perspective and not be limited to the mere synthesis and application of scientific evidence.[32] In part, the "evidence-informed" framing seeks to emphasize that health-related decisions are not based only on research (particularly considering political and organizational factors).[33,34] This perspective highlights the importance of making health decisions using evidence-based methods (information based on the synthesis of scientific evidence) in conjunction with clinician and practitioner expertise and knowledge and information about the values, preferences, and circumstances of the target patient or population. Consequently, real-world experience suggests that the evidence should not be limited to quantitative evidence from highly controlled research trials but should also consider the use of many different levels and types of evidence, including qualitative studies, case reports, and expert opinion.[35] Despite the initial distinction in meaning between evidence-based and evidence-informed practice, the terms are commonly used interchangeably in the literature. Additional terms denoting the subject of D&I activities include best practices, evidence-based processes, and evidence-based healthcare.[36,37]

D&I Competencies

Competencies refer to a range of learning objectives, knowledge, and skills required to be successful and efficient as a D&I researcher.[38] Padek and colleagues developed and organized D&I strategies by levels of expertise as beginner, intermediate, and advanced. Additional D&I competencies are categorized then into four domains: (1) background and rationale (e.g., identifying gaps in D&I research); (2) theory and approaches (e.g., identifying appropriate conceptual models); (3) design and analysis (e.g., describing core components of external validity); and (4) practice-based considerations (e.g., considering the perspectives of different stakeholders).[38] More details about D&I competencies are provided in chapter 30.

Types of Evidence

The types of evidence available for decision-making in health can be classified as type 1, type 2, and type 3 evidence.[27,39] These evidence types differ in their characteristics, scope, and quality.

Type 1 Evidence

Type 1 evidence is concerned with etiology and burden and defines the cause of a particular outcome (e.g., health condition). This type of evidence includes factors such as magnitude and severity of the outcome (i.e., number, incidence, prevalence) and the actionability of the cause (i.e., preventability or changeability) and often leads to the conclusion that "*something* should be done."[27,39]

Type 2 Evidence

Type 2 evidence focuses on the relative impact of a specific intervention to address a particular outcome (e.g., health condition). This type of evidence includes information on the effectiveness or cost-effectiveness of a strategy compared to others and points to the conclusion that "*specifically, this* should be done."[25] Type 2 evidence (interventions) can be classified based on the source of the evidence (i.e., study design) as evidence-based, efficacious, promising, and emerging interventions.[27,39]

Type 3 Evidence

Type 3 evidence is concerned with the type of information that is needed for the adaptation and implementation of an EBI.[23]This type of evidence includes information on how and under which contextual conditions interventions were implemented and how they were received and addressed the issue of "*how* something should be done." Type 3 is the type of evidence we have the least of and derives from the context of an intervention, particularly concepts of external validity.[27,39]

Knowledge for Action

The terms **knowledge translation**, **knowledge transfer**, **knowledge exchange**, **and knowledge integration** are commonly used, especially outside of the United States, to refer to the entire or some aspects of the D&I process. This chapter uses definitions coined by the Canadian Institutes of Health Research (CIHR) and KT Canada, Graham and colleagues, Best and colleagues, and McKibbon and colleagues to define these terms.[15–17,40]As Best and colleagues suggested, these terms can be classified as linear (knowledge translation and transfer), relationship (knowledge exchange), or systems (knowledge integration) models of D&I.[40] Additional terms can be found in McKibbon and colleagues' platform for knowledge translation terms and definitions.[41]

Knowledge Translation

Knowledge translation is the term used by the CIHR to denote "a dynamic and iterative process that includes synthesis, dissemination, exchange and ethically sound application of knowledge." Knowledge translation occurs within a complex social system of interactions between researchers and knowledge users and with the purpose of improving population health, providing more effective health services and products, and strengthening the healthcare system.[16,42,43]

Knowledge Transfer

Knowledge transfer is a commonly used term both within and outside of the healthcare sector and is defined as the process of getting (research) knowledge from producers to potential users (i.e., stakeholders).[16,44] This term is often criticized for its linear (unidirectional) notion and its lack of concern with the implementation of transferred knowledge.[16]

Knowledge Exchange

Knowledge exchange is the term used by the Canadian Health Services Research Foundation and describes the interactive and iterative process of imparting meaningful knowledge between knowledge users (i.e., stakeholders) and producers, such that knowledge users (i.e., stakeholders) receive relevant and easily usable information and producers receive information about users' research needs.[16,40] This term was introduced, in contrast to the terms knowledge translation and knowledge transfer, to highlight the bi- or multidirectional nature of the knowledge transmission process (relationship model).[16,40,45]

Research Utilization

Research utilization is a form of knowledge utilization, and it has long traditions in the nursing literature. It refers to "the process by which specific research-based knowledge (science) is implemented in practice."[46,47(pp4–5)] Research utilization, similarly to knowledge translation and knowledge transfer, follows a linear model and is primarily concerned with moving research knowledge into action.[16]

Processes for D&I Science

Spread

Spread is the process of replicating an initiative or intervention within a new health system or community setting.[48,49]

Diffusion

Diffusion is the passive, untargeted, unplanned, and uncontrolled spread of new interventions. Rogers defined diffusion as the process by which an innovation is communicated through certain channels over time among the members of a social system.[11] Diffusion is part of the diffusion-dissemination-implementation continuum, and it is the least focused and intense approach.[50,51]

Dissemination

Dissemination is an active approach of spreading interventions to the target audience via determined channels using planned strategies.[50]

Implementation

Implementation is the actively planned process of putting evidence to use or integrating new interventions within a specific setting.[52] Implementation can also be conceptualized as the process through which interventions are operationalized in an organization or community setting. The process may involve multiple approaches used by change agents in a multistage, iterative, and dynamic process; it does not usually occur in a linear fashion and can involve a combination of planned implementation steps and unplanned, iterative corrections, refinements, or expansions.[53]

Types of Research

Translational Research

Translational research encompasses research with the explicit goal to produce more meaningful, applicable, and relevant research results and to speed the real-world application of scientific evidence.[54,55] It can be defined as research steps to take discoveries "from the bench to the beside and back again."[56] Translational research has been classified across five phases (T0 through T4).[57,58]

Translation

Translation is the process of applying scientific evidence to real-world practice.[59]

Efficacy Research

Efficacy research evaluates the initial impact of an intervention (whether it does more good than harm among the individuals in the target population) when it is delivered under optimal or laboratory conditions (or in an ideal setting). Efficacy trials typically use random allocation of participants and/or units and ensure highly controlled conditions for implementation. This type of study focuses on internal validity or establishing a causal relationship between exposure to an intervention and an outcome.[60,61]

Effectiveness Research

Effectiveness research determines the impact of an intervention with demonstrated efficacy when it is delivered under "real-world" conditions. As a result, effectiveness trials often must use methodological designs that are better suited for large and/or less controlled research environments with a major purpose to obtain more externally valid (generalizable) results.[60,61]

Dissemination Research

Dissemination research is the systematic study of processes and factors that lead to widespread use of an EBI by the target population. Its focus is to identify the best methods that enhance the uptake and utilization of the intervention.[10,60] Refer to chapter 3 for more on dissemination research.

Implementation Research

Implementation research seeks to understand the processes and factors that are associated with successful integration of EBIs within a particular setting (e.g., a worksite or school).[62,63] Implementation research assesses whether the core components of the original intervention were faithfully transported to the real-world setting (i.e., the degree of fidelity of the disseminated and implemented intervention with the original study) and also concerned with the adaptation of the implemented intervention to the local context).[63(p10-040)] Another, often overlooked but essential component of implementation research involves the enhancement of readiness through the creation of effective climate and culture in an organization or community.[19,64]

Finally, a broader interpretation of implementation research also includes the study of discontinuation of interventions and practices that do not work. See also mis-implementation and de-implementation in this chapter.[65] Refer to chapter 3, implementation science.

Quality Improvement

Quality improvement (QI) is defined as the concerted and ongoing activities that are undertaken systematically by diverse stakeholders to improve care. In the optimal case, this includes all relevant healthcare providers, organizational leaders, evaluators, and patients and their caregivers. QI efforts can address improving patient outcomes, healthcare services and system performance, and/or professional development (i.e., learning healthcare system) in the context of healthcare.[66–68] While QI and D&I science approach healthcare improvement from different paradigms and use different frameworks and methods, they share the ultimate goal of improving patient health outcomes.

The main differences between QI and D&I science involve their scope, starting point, and speed of action. QI is generally initiated at the local level to address a specific issue for a clinic or healthcare system, while D&I science often starts with an EBI or practice and explores how it can be spread and implemented at the health system or clinic level.[69] Usually QI efforts focus on or at least begin with very small "tests," even within a single healthcare team, using simple measures, often developed by local teams for rapid feedback (i.e., Plan-Do-Study-Act [PDSA] cycle). QI is also, by definition, iterative, whereas D&I is usually seen as slower, larger in scope, and more likely to use explicit theoretical or conceptual models and well-validated measures. Recent reviews and thought pieces suggested that if we are to make relevant, significant, and sustainable impact on health outcomes, D&I science should consider adopting some of the methods used by QI, such as the iterative, rapid testing, and adaptation of interventions and implementation strategies.[70] A proposal for the combination of QI and D&I science methods was described by Balasubramanian et al. in terms of learning evaluation.[71]

Improvement Science

Improvement science is considered a subtype of implementation science and refers to systems-level work to improve the quality, safety, and value of healthcare with an emphasis on creating generalizable knowledge.[72–75]

Learning Healthcare System

A learning healthcare system is defined by the Institute of Medicine (IOM), as a system in which "science, informatics, incentives, and culture are aligned for continuous improvement and innovation, with best practices seamlessly embedded in the delivery process and new knowledge captured as an integral by-product of the delivery experience."[76] As suggested by Chambers, Feero, and Khoury, D&I science has a critical role to play in creating and sustaining learning healthcare systems through providing evidence-based strategies, frameworks, and measures to support ongoing learning and integration of evidence into practice.[77–79]

Precision Medicine

Precision medicine merges information on genomic, biological, behavioral, environmental, and other data on individuals in order to identify factors that can support individualized treatment.[78,80] While to date most of the work in precision medicine has focused on the genomic and biological components, there is great need and opportunity in expanding our work to data elements related to the social and behavioral determinants of health, as well as patient values and preferences relevant for shared decision-making. These last factors are especially important when we consider the contextual and pragmatic issues involved in moving precision medicine activities from research into practice and policy. Chambers and colleagues suggested that the key potential of D&I science in precision medicine is to support the integration of various precision medicine interventions into learning healthcare systems.[78]

Precision Public Health

Precision public health involves the collection of more accurate population- and individual-level data on genes, exposures, behaviors, and other social/economic health determinants to enhance public health action and reduce health disparities in the population by using more precision data for action.[81]

Evidence Synthesis Approaches

In addition to more traditional evidence synthesis approaches of systematic reviews and meta-analysis, a number of more novel techniques are especially appropriate to use to summarize existing knowledge about D&I research and practice. These methods allow for a more relevant, real-world perspective on studies through a more inclusive, context-sensitive approach. For this chapter, three techniques were selected and are discussed below. For further guidance on review types, Right Review, a web-based interactive tool can support selection of the appropriate review methodology.[82]

Realist Review

Realist review (also known as realist evaluation) is a method for reviewing and synthesizing information about complex, real-world interventions using an explanatory approach and focusing on "what works for whom, in what circumstances, in what respects and how."[83(p21)] Instead of determining if a certain intervention will work, realist reviews provide rich, contextual, and practical information regarding the mechanisms by which the intervention or program works under certain circumstances. This information can support implementation of programs at different levels. Realist review considers interventions as complex systems that function within systems and will be limited in terms of scope (how much can be looked at), the availability of information (the need for an array of primary sources for information), and the nature of effectiveness information (lack fast truth about effectiveness).[83–85]

Scoping Review

Scoping reviews map key concepts underpinning a research area and the main sources and types of evidence available and can be efficiently used to explore complex areas or areas that have not been reviewed before.[86(p194)] The most important differences between a systematic review and a scoping review include level of specificity of the research question it is based on and the types of studies they draw on. Systematic reviews generally start off with well-defined research questions and are most frequently based on a narrow range of quality-assessed studies. Scoping reviews intend to explore broader topics and include more diverse study designs and are not concerned with quality assessment of included studies.[87,88] When undertaken as a stand-alone activity rather than in preparation of a systematic review, scoping reviews can be used to summarize and disseminate information about interventions to policymakers, practitioners, and consumers.[89–91]

SECTION 2: THEORIES AND CONCEPTUAL FOUNDATIONS

Theories, Models, and Frameworks

There are a large number of theories, models, and frameworks (TMFs) that shape the way that we think about D&I research and guide our planning, implementation, and evaluation activities.[92,93] Tabak and colleagues identified 63 distinct D&I models through their original review,[94] and a more recent review indicated more than 150 knowledge translation frameworks.[95,96] A web-based interactive tool, the D&I Models Webtool (https://dissemination-implementation.org) can help researchers and practitioners to select the D&I model that best fits their research question or practice problem, adapt the model to the study or practice context, fully integrate the model into the research or practice process, and find existing measurement instruments for the model constructs.[97] In this chapter, we discuss a few commonly used and influential TMFs, including (1) the diffusion of innovations theory[11,98]; the Consolidated Framework for Implementation Research (CFIR)[21]; the exploration, preparation, implementation, sustainment model[99,100]; the RE-AIM (Reach, Effectiveness, Adoption, Implementation, and Maintenance) framework[101,102]; the practical, robust implementation and sustainability model (PRISM),[103]; and the Promoting Action on Research Implementation in Health Services (PARIHS) framework.[104,105] More comprehensive discussion of D&I TMFs is provided in chapter 4.

Theory

Theories in D&I research attempt to explain the causal pathways of implementation processes and provide an overarching explanation of how and why relationships between variables lead to specific events. A theory in the D&I field implies some predictive capacity and attempts to explain the causal mechanisms of implementation. Theories are widely used in implementation science, and it is important to be explicit about the selection and use of specific theories in designing implementation research.[106]

Model

Models involve a deliberate simplification of a phenomenon or a specific aspect of a phenomenon.[107] and often demonstrate how different events are linked. Models can be described as theories with a more narrowly defined scope of explanation; a model is descriptive, whereas a theory is explanatory as well as descriptive.[13] Models in the D&I field are commonly used to describe and/or guide the process of translating research into practice.

Framework

Frameworks convey an overarching structure, outline of a system, or plan consisting of various interacting descriptive elements and categories.[107] Frameworks do not typically provide explanations; they describe empirical phenomena by fitting them into a set of categories.[108,109] There are several types of frameworks commonly used in implementations science, including determinant frameworks, causal frameworks, and explanatory frameworks. See chapter 4 for more information.

Determinant Frameworks

Determinant frameworks have a specific purpose to characterize factors that might influence implementation outcomes. They do not specify the mechanisms of change and typically operate like checklists of determinants at multiple levels.[110] Determinant frameworks are useful in defining both dependent and independent variables influencing implementation outcomes. They can draw links between dependent variables and can highlight barriers between variables that hinder interdependence and therefore have an impact on implementation.

Logic Model

A logic model is a diagram that describes in detail how a program or intervention operationally works to achieve benefits and captures the logical flow and linkages that exist within the program or intervention and its proximal and distal outcomes. It is the "if-then" sequence of changes that the program intends to set in motion through inputs, activities, and outputs.[111] Even in cases where the theory of a program has never been made explicit, the logic model approach can help to uncover, articulate, present, and examine theory.[112] A logic model specific to D&I science, the implementation research logic model, was developed by Smith and colleagues to specify conceptual linkages between the core elements of a D&I research project and enhance the rigor and transparency of processes of enhancing the uptake, implementation, and sustained use of interventions.[113]

SECTION 3: STRATEGIES AND METHODS

Dissemination and Implementation Strategies

Strategies for D&I

The D&I strategies promote and integrate evidence-based practice into real-world settings and are central to D&I science, which seeks to evaluate the effectiveness of strategies to integrate EBIs into specific settings.[114,115] D&I strategies can also be referred to as implementation interventions.[69]

Dissemination Strategy

Dissemination strategies describe mechanisms and approaches used to communicate and spread information about interventions to targeted users.[52] Dissemination strategies are concerned with the packaging of the information about the intervention and the communication channels to reach potential adopters and target audience. Passive dissemination strategies include mass mailings, publication of information that includes practice guidelines, and untargeted presentations to heterogeneous groups.[116] Active dissemination strategies include hands-on technical assistance, replication guides, point-of-decision prompts for use, and mass media campaigns.[116] It is consistently stated in the literature that dissemination strategies are necessary but not sufficient to ensure widespread use of an intervention.[117,118]

Implementation Strategy

Implementation strategies refer to the systematic processes or methods, techniques, activities, and resources that support the adoption, integration, and sustainment of EBIs into usual settings.[119–121] Fixsen and colleagues referred to implementation strategies as core implementation components or implementation drivers and list staff selection, preservice and in-service training, ongoing consultation and coaching, staff and program evaluation, facilitative administrative support, and systems interventions as components.[20,118] Powell and colleagues differentiated discrete (i.e., individual implementation actions, e.g., reminders, educational meetings), multifaceted (i.e., combination of two or more discrete strategies, e.g., training with technical assistance), and blended (i.e., implementation strategies). They used a review and expert consensus approach to create a consolidated compilation of 73 discrete implementation strategies and respective definitions.[120,122] Chapter 6 discusses these strategies in more detail.[120–122]

Expert Recommendations for Implementing Change Strategies

Expert Recommendations for Implementing Change (ERIC) refers to a compilation of implementation strategies developed to support systematic reporting of implementation strategies both prospectively and retrospectively. The ERIC compilation has 73 discrete strategies organized in 9 categories: (1) using evaluative and iterative strategies; (2) providing interactive assistance; (3) adapting and tailoring to context; (4) developing stakeholder interrelationships; (5) training and educating stakeholders; (6) supporting clinicians; (7) engaging consumers; (8) utilizing financial strategies; and (9) changing infrastructure.[122] These strategies can be viewed as the building blocks of multifaceted strategies used to address the potential determinants of implementation for a specific EBI.[122]

Dissemination Field Agent

Dissemination field agents work to generate awareness, provide training, and support use of evidence-based, practice-ready programs by adopters.[123] These specialists have extensive knowledge of EBIs and expertise in how to adapt and implement the interventions in different settings and for different populations. They would work closely and proactively with customers to help them understand and choose from available strategies. See chapter 28 for more details on dissemination field agents.

Knowledge Broker

A knowledge broker is an intermediary (individual or organization) who facilitates and fosters the interactive process between producers (i.e., researchers) and users (i.e., practitioners, policymakers) of knowledge through a broad range of activities (see information about knowledge brokering in References 124 and 125). More broadly, knowledge brokers assist in organizational problem-solving process through drawing analogic links between solutions learned from resolving past problems often in diverse domains and demands of the current project. Knowledge brokers also help "make the right knowledge available to the right people at the right time."[125(p67)]

A more detailed discussion of knowledge brokering and knowledge brokers was provided by Hargadon.[125]

Boundary Spanners

Boundary spanners are institutions, groups, or individuals that span the divide between researchers and users, enable communication between these two groups, and are accountable in some fashion to both groups.[126,127]

Intermediary and Purveyor Organizations

Intermediary and purveyor organizations (IPOs) develop, implement, disseminate, and support best practice programs or services. IPOs support implementation by engaging in consultation activities, training, QI, outcome evaluation, and policy development.[128–130]

Fidelity and Adaptations

Understanding the nature and origin of changes made to the EBIs and implementation strategies during the implementation process and assessing how these modifications might have impacted outcomes as well as using this information to inform future implementation efforts are critical topics for D&I research. In this section we define terms related to fidelity, adaptations, and core components.

Fidelity

Fidelity is the extent to which the core intervention elements (or implementation strategies) are successfully delivered as intended within a setting[131,132] and conceptualized as the continuation of elements found to be necessary for intervention effectiveness.[133] Fidelity is commonly measured by comparing the original EBI and the disseminated and implemented intervention in terms of (1) adherence to the program protocol, (2) dose or amount of program delivered, (3) quality of program delivery, and (4) participant reaction and acceptance.[134] A more comprehensive discussion of fidelity measurement of complex interventions is found in chapter 7.

Adaptation

For the success of D&I, interventions in most cases need to be adapted to fit the local context (i.e., needs and realities).[13,135] Adaptation is defined as the degree to which an EBI or implementation strategy is changed or modified by a user before, during, and after adoption and implementation to suit the needs of the setting or to improve the fit to local conditions.[11] Ideally, adaptation will lead to at least equal intervention effects as shown in the original efficacy or effectiveness trial. Furthermore, while modifications might facilitate implementation and sustainability by improving the fit between the intervention and the population or the facility, program fidelity and outcomes of interest may be affected. To reconcile the tension between fidelity and adaptation, it is suggested that the **core components** or **core functions** (see definitions in this section) must be identified and preserved during the adaptation process.[134] Frameworks have been developed to assist with systematically documenting adaptations to the EBI, such as the expanded Framework for Reporting Adaptations and Modifications,[136,137] or to the implementation strategies (Framework for Reporting Adaptations and Modifications to Evidence-Based Implementation Strategies [FRAME-IS]).[138] In addition the distinction of form and function by Jolles-Perez et al. is increasingly used to guide adaptations.[139] For a more comprehensive discussion of adaptations, see chapter 8 and a number of seminal papers on the topic.[134,140–143]

Cultural Adaptation

Cultural adaptation is considered a critical and distinct type of adaptation, defined as changes to an intervention in order to increase an intervention's cultural relevance and appropriateness. These could be changes to any aspects of the intervention, including but not limited to language, communication methods, imagery, materials, or delivery modality.[144,145] There is a need in early program stages to make planned "fidelity-consistent" adaptations that reflect diverse settings, cultures, and populations in which they are delivered.[137,146,147] Failing to make planned cultural or contextual adaptations may have an adverse impact on effectiveness and, ultimately, perpetuate health inequities.[134,147] Refer to chapter 8 for more on cultural adaptation.

Replication

Replication is the process of reproducing key aspects of a well-defined innovation with the intent of achieving the desired outcomes and building the evidence for that innovation.[148]

Core Components

Core components are defined as the active ingredients of the intervention that are essential to achieving the desired outcomes of the intervention.[20] Identification of core components is not always straightforward and can be facilitated by the use of theoretical frameworks and may "depend upon careful research and well-evaluated experiential learning from a number of attempted replications."[20(p26)] Core components can also refer to the drivers of the implementation process that are indispensable for the successful implementation of an intervention.[20,149] Refer to chapters 7 and 8 for more on core components.

Adaptable/Discretionary Components

The adaptable/discretionary components are intervention features that are not essential for the target user and are not supported by evidence or theory and thus are assumed to be modifiable without major impact on intervention effectiveness (e.g., provision of an additional class as part of a parenting intervention addressing trauma related to natural disasters).[150] Alternative terms are optional components or intervention's surface structure. Adapting evidence-informed complex population health interventions for new contexts is a systematic review of guidance.[135,151,152]

Organizational Processes in D&I Research

Organizational Culture

Organizational culture has been identified as a key element of EBI adoption, implementation, and sustainment[153,154] and is defined as the organizational norms and expectations regarding how people behave and how things are done in an organization.[155,156] This includes implicit norms, values, shared behavioral expectations, and assumptions that guide the behaviors of members of a work unit.[157–159] Organizational culture refers to the core values of an organization, its services or products, and how individuals and groups within the organization treat and interact with each other. Schein defined it as "the pattern of shared basic assumptions that was learned by a group as it solved its problems of external adaptation and internal integration, and that has worked well enough to be considered valid and, therefore, to be taught to new members as the correct way to perceive, think, and feel in relation to those problems."[160(p17)] Another way to characterize organizational culture is by layers or levels. Refer to chapter 9 for more information.

Organizational Climate

Organizational climate refers to the employees' perceptions of and reaction to the characteristics of the work environment.[158,161,162] There is a key distinction that emerged early in the history of the climate literature between molar (or generic) climate and focused (or strategic) climate. In contrast to molar climate, which attempts to capture the general "feel" of the organization (which overlaps more with organizational culture), the focused or strategic climate approach attempts to understand the extent to which employees perceive that management emphasizes a specific criterion of interest.[163,164] Please refer to chapter 9 for more information.

Organizational Readiness

Organizational readiness for change is defined as the extent to which organizational members are psychologically and behaviorally prepared to implement a new intervention.[165] Organizational readiness is widely regarded as an essential antecedent to successful implementation of change in healthcare and social service organizations.[166–168] Factors that are associated with organizational readiness for change include (1) change valence (i.e., the employees' perception of the personal benefit of implemented change); (2) change efficacy (i.e., the perception of their capability of implementing the change); (3) discrepancy (i.e., the employees' belief in the necessity of change to bridge the gap between the organization's current and desired state); and (4) principal support (i.e., the employees' perception of the commitment of the formal organizational leaders and opinion leaders to support successful implementation of change) and are discussed in more detail in chapter 9.[169–171]

Implementation Leadership

Implementation leadership refers to a set of behaviors, attitudes, and practices within the umbrella of general leadership focused on specific strategic imperatives related to the adoption and use of EBP.[158,172,173] Implementation leadership is posited to influence employee attitudes and behavior regarding the imperative and makes it more likely that an EBP will be adopted and sustained.[174] There are two types of leadership important in D&I. *Transformational* leadership includes those behaviors in which a leader attends to and develops followers to higher levels of performance and potential (individualized consideration), and *transactional* leadership involves exchanges between leaders and followers in which leaders reinforce or reward followers for engaging in certain behaviors and meeting practical and/or aspirational goals (contingent reward) as well as monitoring and correcting performance (passive or active management by exception).[175] Refer to chapter 9 for more information on leadership.

Participatory Approaches in D&I Research

Community-Based Participatory Research

Community-based participatory research (CBPR) is a collaborative approach to research that equitably involves all partners throughout the life cycle of the research process.[176–178] The principles of CBPR highlight trust among team members, respect for each person's expertise and contributions, mutual benefit for all community partners, and community-driven partnership with equitable and shared decision-making.[179] CBPR can maximize the economic and health benefits of interventions by increasing both the rigor and relevance of the research.[180] See chapter 22 for more on CBPR.

Community Engagement

Community engagement involves including and engaging with members and stakeholders from target communities that experience suboptimal health or undesirable health outcomes.[181] Community engagement in research necessitates community leadership in the direction of research priorities, intervention design, and implementation.[182] Community engagement can help identify the research questions of primary relevance to the community, potentially improving external validity and providing scientific evidence that is more likely to lead to improved health outcomes in those communities.[181]

Community Permission

Community permission is the critical process of seeking consent from members of a community using a variety of means, such as holding town hall style discussions or community voting.[183–185]

Stakeholder Engagement

Stakeholder engagement involves the deliberate inclusion and meaningful interaction and engagement with stakeholders (e.g., clinicians, patients, funders, community members) during the research process. Stakeholder engagement is especially critical when organizations face competing demands and scarce resources, such as opportunity costs for front line staff engaging in implementation efforts in lieu of billable patient care.[180]

Participatory Implementation Science

Participatory implementation science (PIS) is an iterative process alongside a variety of stakeholders to coproduce knowledge and create system-level change in order to integrate evidence into real-world and community settings.[186] PIS approaches improve the successful execution of research while increasing the utility and impact of the findings both locally and for the field broadly.[187] See chapter 10 for more on PIS.

Human-Centered Design

Human-centered design (HCD) is also known as user-centered design and is focused on developing compelling and intuitive products, grounded in knowledge about the people and contexts where an innovation will be deployed.[188] Although the application of HCD methods has typically been limited to digital technologies, their potential for broader applications in healthcare is increasingly recognized.[189] Using an HCD approach to the development of EBIs and implementation strategies will substantially increase their successful uptake, implementation, and sustained use.[190] Dopp and colleagues provided a glossary for HCD terms and strategies for implementation science experts.[191]

Economic Evaluation in D&I Research

Implementation Cost

Gold and colleagues defined implementation cost as "cost related to the development and execution of the implementation strategy that targets one or more specific evidence-based interventions."[192] Saldana and colleagues indicated that implementation costs emerge from activities associated with the building of an infrastructure that can support program development, stakeholder engagement, intervention delivery, and sustainment.[180,193]

Economic Evaluation

Economic evaluations in D&I address the question: How can organizations and systems invest in the D&I of evidence-based practices to maximize the value produced? The basic calculation of the economic evaluation in D&I is

$$\text{Economic Impact of Implementation} = \frac{(\text{Cost}_{\text{Implementation Strategy A}} + \text{Cost}_{\text{EBP}} |A) - (\text{Cost}_{\text{Implementation Strategy B}} + \text{Cost}_{\text{EBP}} |B)}{\text{Outcome}_{\text{Implementation Strategy A}} - \text{Outcome}_{\text{Implementation Strategy B}}}$$

Within healthcare specifically, the purpose of economic evaluation is to maximize outcomes related to health that are subject to a set of constraints.[194–196] The direction of the economic evaluation depends on many things, including the primary objective, the clinical or community context, and relevant decision makers and stakeholders who will utilize the information.[180] Refer to chapter 11 for more information on economic evaluation as well as a new collection of articles compiled on this topic in implementation science and implementation science communications.[195]

Mis-implementation and De-implementation

Mis-implementation

Mis-implementation refers to ending effective programs and policies prematurely or continuing ineffective ones.[197,198]

De-implementation

De-implementation is defined as stopping or abandoning practices that are not proved to be effective and are possibly harmful.[199–201] De-implementation is believed to be an effective approach for improving patient outcomes and to achieve cost saving. Early evidence indicates that similarly to D&I efforts, de-implementation also requires active approaches and local champions for success. Factors associated with successful de-implementation efforts are still being studied. Norton and colleagues provided an overview of multilevel factors that influence de-implementation, including characteristics of (1) the inappropriate intervention to be de-implemented; (2) the individual who receives the intervention; (3) the individual who delivers the intervention; and (4) the organization or setting where the intervention is delivered.[202] Walsh-Bailey and colleagues identified 27 unique frameworks and models to help conceptualize and guide de-implementation.[203] Chapter 12 provides an in-depth discussion of the concept of de-implementation.

Low-Value Care

Low-value care refers to services and clinical practices that provide little to no clinical benefit.[204] Low-value care can be defined in terms of net benefit for an individual or group and is assessed relative to alternatives, including no treatment.[200,205]

System Science Methods in D&I Research

Systems Thinking

Systems thinking is the process of understanding how things influence one another other within a whole and is based on the premise that societal problems are complex and that the response to these complex problems is only possible by intervening at multiple levels and with the engagement of stakeholders and settings across the different levels, including the home, school, workplace, community, region, and country.[206,207] Systems thinking is concerned with not only applying multiple strategies at multiple levels but also focusing on the interrelationships within and across levels and how interventions need to take these relationships into account in their design and implementation.[206,207] System science approaches to study design include the system dynamics method, agent-based modeling, social network analysis, system engineering, intelligent data analysis, and decision analysis with microsimulation modeling. Chapter 13 provides a detailed discussion of the concept of systems thinking for D&I.

System Dynamics Modeling

System dynamics modeling is a problem-oriented modeling approach originally developed for business but with wide-ranging applicability from public health to economics. System dynamics involves causal mapping and computer simulation to understand real-world system interactions and behavior. Policy and large-scale intervention scenarios are then iteratively tested to answer "what if" questions.[208,209] This process of decision experimentation creates a learning environment in which researchers gain an understanding of how the system will respond to decisions and potential unintended consequences. System dynamics modeling is increasingly used within implementation science and public health to understand larger healthcare systems level changes and policy behavior.

Participatory System Dynamics

Participatory system dynamics (PSD) builds on the rich theoretical and methodological foundation of group model building, but emphasizes embedded, participatory action research principles and processes.[210] PSD aims to facilitate community partner and researcher learning and empower those responsible for implementation decisions—especially those who have previously been left out of key implementation decisions that impact their daily workflow. Refer to chapter 13 for more on PSD.

Complexity

In complexity, the behavior embedded in highly complex systems or models with large numbers of interacting components (e.g., agents, artifacts and groups) and the ongoing, repeated interactions create local rules and rich, collective behaviors.[211]

Agent-Based Modeling

Agent-based modeling utilizes computer simulations to examine how elements of a system behave as a function of their interactions with each other and their environment.[212]

Social Network Analysis

Social network analysis is the process of systematically investigating social networks and the relationships and flows among social actors. Social network analysis characterizes social actors in terms of *nodes* (things within the network, e.g., people or organizations) and the relationships and links between them.[213,214]

Factors Associated With the Speed and Extent of D&I

Several factors (i.e., moderators) influence the extent to which D&I of EBIs occur in various settings.[11] Moderators are factors that alter the causal effect of an independent variable on a dependent variable.[215] In this case, organizational capacity can moderate the effect of an intervention on a desired outcome. These factors can be classified as the characteristics of the intervention, characteristics of the adopter (organizational and individual), and contextual factors. The adoption rate will be influenced by the interaction among the attributes of the innovation, characteristics of the intended adopters, and the given context.[19]

Characteristics of the Intervention

Characteristics of the intervention include important facets that impact decision-making related to the initial uptake, implementation, and sustained use of the innovation. Rogers identified five perceived attributes of an innovation that are likely to influence the speed and extent of its adoption: (1) relative advantage (effectiveness and cost efficiency relative to alternatives); (2) compatibility (the fit of the innovation to the established ways of accomplishing the same goal); (3) observability (the extent to which the outcomes can be seen); (4) trialability (the extent to which the adopter must commit to full adoption); and (5) complexity (how simple the innovation is to understand).[11,140] Relative advantage and compatibility are particularly important in influencing adoption rates.[11] Additional characteristics of the intervention, such as acceptability, appropriateness, and feasibility, have been highlighted in recent literature. Refer to chapters 7 and 22 for more on characteristics of the intervention.

Determinants

Determinants are factors that influence the effectiveness and implementation of an intervention, such as barriers (e.g., time and resource costs) or facilitators (e.g., skilled personnel and financial incentives).[110] See chapter 22 for more information on determinants.

Predictors

Predictors are constructs that act as precursors to implementation and dissemination of interventions.[216]

Mediating Variables/Mediators

Mediating variables or mediators are variables that reside in a causal pathway between the independent and dependent variables. Mediators cause variation in the dependent variable and are influenced by the independent variable.[215,217] In behavioral or public health interventions, mediators are often proximal behavioral variables, such as motivation or self-efficacy, which then lead to health behavior changes.

Moderating Variables/Moderators

Moderators or moderating variables, synonymous with "effect modifiers," refer to variation in the magnitude of an outcome across levels of another variable (i.e., moderator).[215,217,218] In behavioral interventions, dose or adherence to the intervention protocol are examples of moderating variables.

Mechanisms

Mechanisms explain how or why interventions create change. They are the underlying processes and drivers of change.[106] In the context of D&I, Lewis and colleagues indicated that in the context of D&I science, "mechanisms explain *how* an implementation strategy has an effect by describing the actions that lead from the administration of the strategy to the implementation outcomes."[219(p4)]

Context

Movsisyan and colleagues defined context as "a set of characteristics and circumstances that consist of active and unique factors within which the implementation of an intervention is embedded. Intervention effects are generated through interaction of new ways of working with existing contexts."[135(p2)] Implementation context is most often multilevel and dynamic (i.e., changes over time).[220] Considering the context can support or hinder the uptake, implementation, and sustained use of an intervention is essential for the success of the D&I.[221] Furthermore, when findings from D&I studies are considered with context taken into account, greater understanding around the mechanisms leading to said results might emerge more readily.[222] A number of D&I theories, models, and frameworks include some aspect of context.[97] Ones that are most useful conceptualize context at multiple levels and from the perspective of multiple stakeholders (e.g., CFIR; exploration, preparation, implementation, sustainment [EPIS] model; PRISM). Furthermore, while it is acknowledged as a critical area of influence for D&I, systematic documentation of context is still rarely reported on.[222] Context is best assessed using mixed-methods approaches, which requires the collection of rich qualitative data in addition to more traditional quantitative data collection efforts (see chapter 18). To explore more about context, see chapters 8 and 17.

SECTION 4: DESIGN AND MEASUREMENT

Study Designs in D&I Research

Traditional randomized controlled trials (RCTs) are not always desirable or feasible for the evaluation of D&I programs. To achieve a greater understanding of external validity, a variety of study designs that take into account contextual factors should be considered for the evaluation of D&I efforts.[223,224] In this section, we provide definitions for a number of innovative design options relevant to D&I science. For a more detailed discussion of designs for D&I, see chapter 14 and work by Brown and colleagues.[22]

Pragmatic or Practical Clinical Trial

Pragmatic or practical clinical trials (PCTs) are clinical trials that are concerned with producing answers to questions faced by decision makers.[225] Tunis and colleagues defined PCTs as studies that "(1) select clinically relevant alternative interventions to compare, (2) include a diverse population of study participants, (3) recruit participants from heterogeneous settings, and (4) collect data on a broad range of health outcomes."[225] PCTs prioritize external validity using methods more closely aligned with real-world settings[4] and take into rather than "take out of" (i.e., control for) consideration the large number of mediators and moderators that influence the D&I process. PCTs are ultimately more likely to produce practice-based evidence than their highly controlled counterparts.[4,223]

Observational Implementation Study

Observational implementation studies are studies of naturally occurring policy- and practice-led implementation processes. Observational implementation studies maximize external validity and offer opportunities to develop insights into barriers, facilitators, and key influences on routine implementation processes and success. Strong research designs are needed to achieve adequate internal validity. See chapter 21 for more information.

Interventional Implementation Study

Interventional implementation studies include (1) phase 1 pilot studies of implementation to develop initial evidence on the feasibility, acceptability, and potential effectiveness of implementation strategies; (2) phase 2 efficacy-oriented, small-scale studies of implementation programs; (3) effectiveness-oriented large trials of implementation programs; and (4) "post-marketing" studies of implementation initiatives. See chapter 21 for more information.

Effectiveness Trial

Effectiveness trials are typically embedded in the community and/or organizational system where such a clinical/preventive intervention would ultimately be delivered. Effectiveness trials often have clinicians, other practitioners, or trained individuals from the community deliver the intervention with supervision by researchers.[22]

Hybrid Effectiveness-Implementation Designs

Hybrid study designs or effectiveness-implementation hybrid designs blend the design characteristics of effectiveness and implementation studies to generate more timely uptake of desirable interventions, more effective implementation strategies, and more relevant information for future scale-up activities. Curran and colleagues identified three types of hybrid designs. Hybrid type 1 includes a primary focus on testing the effectiveness of an intervention while implementation-relevant data are also collected as a secondary outcome. Hybrid type 2 involves the parallel testing of intervention and implementation strategy effectiveness. Hybrid type 3 primarily focuses on testing of the effectiveness of an implementation strategy while gathering information on the intervention's impact on relevant secondary intervention effectiveness outcomes.[226–229]

Multiphase Optimization Strategy Implementation Trials

Testing all combinations in a single design is not feasible, but the multiphase optimization strategy implementation trials (MOST) design can be used to identify and test an optimized intervention. MOST has three phases. The first phase, preparation, involves selection and pilot testing components with a clear optimization criterion (e.g., most effective components subject to a maximum cost). In the second phase, optimization, a fully powered randomized experiment is conducted to assess the effectiveness of each intervention component. The number of distinct implementation strategies is minimized using a balanced, fractional factorial experiment. Fractional designs can make examination of multiple components feasible, even when cluster randomization is necessary.[227,230,231] The set of components that best meets the optimization criterion is identified based on the trial's results. In the third phase, evaluation, a standard randomized implementation trial is conducted comparing the optimized intervention against an appropriate comparison condition.[22]

Sequential, Multiple Assignment, Randomized Trial design

Sequential, multiple assignment, randomized trials (SMART) can be used to develop adaptive interventions and adaptive implementation strategies and involve multiple intervention stages, each indicating a decision point in the development of the adaptive intervention.[232–234] Adaptive interventions and adaptive implementation strategies allow using individual (e.g., preference, severity of condition) or setting level (e.g., local processes and resources) variables to adapt an intervention or implementation strategy and individual (e.g., treatment response, adherence) or setting level (e.g., uptake by providers, screening rates at clinic) outcomes to further readapt or refine the intervention or implementation strategy during implementation. These modifications can be important to address changes in circumstances, to reduce burden and cost, and to increase success as well as align with the more iterative approach to intervention and implementation strategy development.[230,233,235]

Stepped-Wedge Design

A stepped-wedge design uses a sequential rollout of the intervention to target sites or individuals in a manner that all sites or participants will receive the intervention by the end of the trial but the order in which they receive is determined randomly. Data collection happens at the end of each time segment or wedge. Stepped-wedge design is especially favorable to more traditional randomized trial designs when rollout of the intervention is not practical or feasible at once and when the intervention is believed to do more benefit than harm.[236] The use of the stepped-wedge design increased over the past decade and is especially suitable for multisite scale-up studies as it aligns with the realities of real-world settings.[237]

Learn as You Go Designs

Learn as you go (LAGO) designs can design and undergo adaptation and modification based on information gained during the conduct of the study.[238] The first stage of a LAGO study identifies the optimal strategy or strategy bundle, which is refined over time as information emerges from the implementation effort. Thus, the strategy or multifaceted strategy bundle can be considered a random variable that is informed by previous outcomes. While only emerging as a design in implementation science, LAGO studies hold the promise for real-time adaptations that can ultimately increase the rate at which implementation science knowledge is identified and spread.[239]

Measurement Issues in D&I Research

Measurement Considerations

In the context of measures of the D&I process, three main components should be considered: moderators (i.e., factors associated with the speed and extent of D&I), mediators (i.e., process variables), and outcomes. Moderators and mediators are defined in a previous section of this chapter. The measurement of moderators and mediators can help to identify the factors and processes that lead to the success or failure of an EBI to achieve certain outcomes. To reflect the complexity of interventions and diversity in the interest of potential stakeholders (i.e., policymakers, practitioners, clinicians), in D&I research we commonly measure multiple moderators, mediators, and outcomes and assess their relationship.[240] Chapters 15, 16, and 17 provide a more detailed overview of measurement and evaluation concepts for D&I.

Outcome Variables

Outcome variables, the end results of EBIs, in D&I research are often different from those in traditional health research and have to be defined broadly, including short- and long-term outcomes, individual- and organizational- or population-level outcomes, impacts on quality of life, adverse consequences, and economic evaluation.[116] Although individual-level variables can also be important (e.g., behavior change variables like smoking or physical activity), outcome measures in D&I research are typically measured at organizational, community, or policy level (e.g., organizational change, community readiness for change).

Implementation Outcomes

Implementation outcomes are distinct from system outcomes (e.g., organizational-level measures) and individual-level behavior and health outcomes and are defined as "the effects of deliberate and purposive actions to implement new treatments, practices, and services."[132(p65)] Implementation outcomes are measures of implementation success, proximal indicators of implementation processes, and key intermediate outcomes of effectiveness and quality of care. The main value of implementation outcomes is to distinguish intervention failure (i.e., when an intervention is ineffective in a new context) from implementation failure (i.e., when the incorrect deployment of a good intervention causes lack of previously documented desirable outcomes).[132] Proctor and colleagues proposed the following implementation outcomes: acceptability, adoption, appropriateness, costs, feasibility, fidelity, penetration, and sustainability.[132] The RE-AIM framework also proposes a set of implementation outcomes in the form of reach, adoption, implementation, and maintenance.[101] More recently, the CFIR 2.0 also specified anticipated and actual implementation outcomes (adoptability, implementability, sustainability and adoption, implementation, and sustainment).[241] A cross-walk of the Proctor Implementation Outcomes Framework and the RE-AIM framework was provided by Reilly et al.[216]

Dissemination Outcomes

Dissemination outcomes are defined as the effects of dissemination or the outcomes of targeted distribution of information related to an innovation, intervention, or best practice to a specific public health or clinical practice audience.[242]

Pragmatic Measures

Pragmatic measures were proposed by Glasgow and Riley as a set of criteria that should apply to instruments used in real-world studies, including studies of D&I. In addition to the traditional criteria of validity and reliability, the key characteristics of ideal pragmatic measures include (1) measure outcomes important to a diverse set of stakeholders (i.e., practitioners, patients, researchers); (2) low burden from both a data collection and analysis perspective (i.e., brief, user friendly, low cost); (3) broad applicability (i.e., works across populations, settings, languages, and cultures); (4) sensitivity to change (i.e., able to track change over time); (5) ability to yield information that enhances patient engagement; (6) actionability (i.e., based on information realistic action can be taken); (7) public health relevance; and (8) causing no harm (e.g., interferes with relationships, has unintended negative consequences).[243,244]

Reach

Reach refers to the ability of a program to engage its ultimate target audience in terms of both quantity (number/percentage of participants) and quality (representativeness of participants).[216] The reach of a program can greatly influence the level of public health impact the program can achieve.[101]

Adoption

Adoption is the decision of an organization or community to commit to and initiate an EBI.[11,60,245]

External Validity and D&I Research

Rapid, Responsive, Relevant Research

The concept of rapid, responsive, relevant (R3) research was coined by Riley and colleagues to provide a framework and set of strategies for a rapid learning health research approach and address limitations of traditional health research. Key criticisms of traditional health research include its slow pace, high cost and resource nature, and most importantly its lack of relevance to stakeholders that use the information for decision-making. Proposed strategies to achieve R3 research include greater and more meaningful stakeholder engagement; use of innovative, rapid, and flexible designs; streamlining of the review process; and creation and better use of research infrastructure, rapid learning systems, and other health information technologies.[246]

External Validity

External validity is the degree to which findings from a study (or set of studies) can be generalizable to and relevant for populations, settings, and times other than those in which the original studies were conducted.[247,248] Standardized and detailed reporting on factors that influence external validity (e.g., those recommended in the RE-AIM framework) can contribute to more successful D&I efforts.[101,247,249] Key threats to external validity include (1) unrealistic resource expectations and selection bias of settings; (2) low priority or externally imposed topics; (3) unrepresentative participants/selection bias of participants; (4) interventions too tightly controlled; and (5) Hawthorne effect. Chapter 16 provides a detailed description of each of these threats and key strategies to avoid them. In addition, Green and Glasgow have proposed rating criteria for external validity.[247] The concept of external validity is discussed in detail in chapter 18.

Implementability

Implementability is the extent to which an intervention, policy, or practice is easily implementable in a new setting.[250]

Pragmatic–Explanatory Continuum Indicator Summary

The Pragmatic–Explanatory Continuum Indicator Summary (PRECIS-2) is a tool to support researchers in deciding where their research study falls on the pragmatic–explanatory continuum for different aspects of the study design. PRECIS-2 is represented in the form of a nine-spoked wheel based on the nine domains of design decisions: (1) eligibility criteria; (2) recruitment); (3) setting; (4) organization; (5) flexibility delivery; (6) flexibility adherence; (7) follow-up; (8) primary outcome; and (9) primary analysis measured on a scale of 1 (very explanatory) through 5 (very pragmatic). More information about the PRECIS-2 is available on their website (https://www.precis-2.org/) and in Loudon et al.[251,252]

Standards for Reporting Implementation Studies

Standards for Reporting Implementation Studies (StaRI). StaRI offers authors and publishers guidelines for reporting context, adoption and adaptation strategies, and evaluation methods for both the intervention and the implementation strategy.[29,253,254] The authors posited that the use of StaRI guidelines might reduce the diffusion gap between evidence creation and common practice, raise the volume of publications, and improve the clarity and utility of implementation research narratives.[255]

The StaRI checklist encompasses 27 items and provides guidelines for implementation studies on reporting transparently, accurately, and consistently on various aspects of their work. The guidelines were developed using findings from a systematic review, a consensus-building e-Delphi exercise, and input from an international group of experts.[65]

Template for Intervention Description and Replication Checklist

The Template for Intervention Description and Replication (TIDieR) checklist prompts authors to describe interventions in sufficient detail to allow their replication. The checklist contains the minimum recommended items for describing an intervention.[256] TIDieR includes 12 items that are applicable across diverse types of simple and complex interventions and include consideration for (1) the intervention name; (2) why (rationale); (3) what (materials); (4) what (procedure); (5) who provided; (6) how (delivery mode); (7) where (locations); (8) when and how much (dose); (9) tailoring or planned adaptation; (10) unplanned modifications; (11) how well (planned fidelity); and (12) how well (actual fidelity).[256]

Qualitative, Quantitative, and Mixed Methods in D&I Research

Qualitative Methods

Qualitative methods (alone or in combination with quantitative methods) are critical in identifying factors that facilitate or hinder the implementation of EBIs in diverse settings and explain why implementation efforts succeed or fail.[257] The Qualitative Research in Implementation Science (QUALRIS) report[258] identified five needs for advancing the use of qualitative methods in D&I science: (1) bring greater transparency to and documentation of team-based analysis; (2) continue to strengthen tools and techniques for conducting rapid qualitative assessment and analysis; (3) explore methods of qualitative data collection and analysis not commonly used in implementation research; (4) contribute to the development of a common language while remaining "true" to a qualitative approach; and (5) develop meaningful approaches for cross-context comparison and synthesis of qualitative data.[259,260]

Rapid Qualitative Assessment

Rapid research is described as "research designed to address the need for cost-effective and timely results in rapidly changing situations."[261(p3)] Rapid qualitative assessment often involves the use of visual displays (e.g., matrices) to synthesize and share data in a succinct manner to guide decision-making. Rapid qualitative assessment using a matrix approach has been broadly used in D&I research to generate rigorous yet actionable information for implementers.[257,262,263]

Quantitative Methods

Quantitative methods focus on the quantity of phenomena being studied, mostly through the analysis of numeric data to determine statistical significance of the associations between constructs or the differences across groups. Quantitative methods in D&I research can be used for multiple purposes: (1) to quantify or characterize stages and processes of implementation specified in D& models and frameworks; (2) to test hypotheses related to predictors of successful implementation and to quantify implementation barriers and facilitators; (3) to test theoretically based assertions about how different aspects of implementation lead to intervention outcomes; (4) to determine the impact implementation strategies have on measurable implementation (e.g., adoption, fidelity, sustainability) and intervention outcomes (e.g., participant health outcomes); and (5) to summarize quantitative findings across multiple studies in systematic reviews and meta-analyses. Quantitative methods in isolation cannot achieve all the goals set out by D&I research (e.g., understanding why and how implementation success or failure occurs, etc.), which can be addressed using qualitative methods and mixed methods. Chapter 18 provides a more detailed description of quantitative methods in D&I research along with case examples.[132,264]

Mixed Methods

Mixed-methods designs involve the collection and analysis of multiple, both quantitative and qualitative, data in a single study to answer research questions using a parallel (quantitative and qualitative data collected and analyzed concurrently), sequential (one type of data informs the collection of the other type), or converted (data are converted—qualitized or quantitized—and reanalyzed) approach. The central premise of mixed-methods designs is that the use of quantitative and qualitative approaches in combination provides a better understanding of research issues than either approach alone.[265,266]

In mixed-method designs, qualitative methods are used to explore and obtain depth of understanding regarding the reasons for success or failure to implement an evidence-based practice or to identify strategies for facilitating implementation, while quantitative methods are used to test and confirm hypotheses based on a conceptual model and obtain breadth of understanding of predictors of successful implementation.[265,266] Mixed methods are often used to simultaneously answer confirmatory and exploratory research questions and therefore verify and generate theory in the same study.[267] The mixed-methods research design can generate rich data from multiple levels and a number of stakeholders and hence is appropriate to answer complex research questions (also see the Systems Thinking definition in this chapter).[268,269]

Configurational Comparative Methods

Configurational comparative methods (CCMs) involve a set of innovative techniques that integrate the strengths of both qualitative and quantitative approaches. It is a relatively new approach within implementation science that is a dynamic and systematic way to account for both complexity and context, allowing implementation scientists to identify deep patterns within their data, linking conditions with outcomes that might otherwise go undetected.[270] A broadly used CCM technique is qualitative comparative analysis (QCA).

Qualitative Comparative Analysis

Qualitative comparative analysis[271] is a form of CCM that can be used to examine complex combinations of explanatory factors associated with implementation outcomes when traditional statistical methods are not possible because of the limited number of cases. It can also be used to systematically combine quantitative and qualitative data.[272]

SECTION 5: SETTING- AND POPULATION-SPECIFIC DISSEMINATION AND IMPLEMENTATION

Policy Dissemination and Implementation

Small p Policy

"Small p" policies are localized, small-scale policies, including organizational changes, administrative or institutional policies, or non-governmental professional guidelines.[273]

Big P Policy

"Big P" policies are formal governmental policies, including laws, administrative rules, and regulations.[273]

Policy Implementation Research

Policy implementation research seeks to understand the complexities of the policy process and increase the likelihood that evidence reaches policymakers and influences their decisions so that the population health benefits of scientific progress are maximized.[274] A key objective of policy implementation is the enactment, enforcement, and evaluation of evidence-based policies, seeking to (1) understand approaches to enhance the likelihood of policy adoption (process); (2) identify specific policy elements that are likely to be effective (content); and (3) document the potential impact of policy (outcomes).[27,275] The two types of policy implementation research studies include policy process implementation and policy impact implementation. Policy process implementation studies describe the process through which a policy was implemented. Such studies can document what actions were performed by which stakeholders to execute policy implementation. Policy impact implementation studies use experimental or quasi-experimental designs to assess the main effect of a policy on implementation outcomes, the moderating effect of policy implementation outcomes on policy effectiveness outcomes, or the main effect of policy implementation strategies on policy implementation and/or effectiveness outcomes. Chapter 24 provides a more detailed overview of policy implementation research.

Policy Dissemination Research

Policy dissemination research seeks to understand how research evidence can be most effectively communicated to policymakers and integrated into policymaking processes.[276]

Dissemination Effectiveness Studies

Dissemination effectiveness studies involve the prospective randomization of policymakers to experimental conditions, deploying dissemination strategies, and assessing outcomes. The purpose of these studies is to determine which dissemination strategies are most effective.[277–279] See chapter 24 for more details.

Policy Diffusion Studies

A complement to studies focused on the uses of research evidence at the policymaker level, policy diffusion studies seek to understand how policy adoption (i.e., the enactment of a specific policy) spreads across geopolitical units (e.g., states).[280,281]

Formative Audience Research

Formative audience research seeks to describe the characteristics of policymakers with the goal of informing the design and distribution of dissemination materials.[282] Survey and interview methods are used in these studies. A formative audience research study may assess the sources that policymakers turn to for research evidence, such as the knowledge brokers and intermediary organizations with which policymakers have relationships.

Multiple-Streams Model

The multiple-streams model of public policymaking identifies three independent streams that flow through the policy system: politics, problems, and policy. The politics stream contains factors creating an environment conducive to agenda change; the problems stream contains concerns that come to the attention of policymakers; and the policy stream is where ideas are formulated.[283]

Health Equity

Broadly, equity is an ongoing process of assessing needs, correcting historical inequities, and creating conditions for optimal outcomes by members of all social identity groups (APA, 2021b).[284] Health equity is also the absence of avoidable, unfair, or remediable differences among groups of people, whether those groups are defined socially, economically, demographically, or geographically.[285] Equity implies everyone should have a fair opportunity (and not necessarily equivalent opportunities) to attain their fullest health potential and that no one should be disadvantaged from achieving this potential.[285,286] Specific opportunities to advance health equity within D&I science have been proposed by Brownson and colleagues and include (1) providing a key link between social determinants of health and health outcomes; (2) building equity into all policies; (3) using equity-relevant metrics; (4) studying what is already happening; (5) integrating equity into models; (6) designing and tailoring implementation strategies; (7) connecting systems and sectors outside of health; (8) engaging organizations (including community-based organizations) internally and externally; (9) building capacity for equity; and (10) focusing on equity in dissemination efforts. Chapter 25 provides more details and case examples about the use of a health equity lens in D&I research. Chapter 16 provides a framework on the relevance of health equity at different stages of research and its connection with external validity.

Health Equity Lens

The health equity lens has been defined by Kumanyika as "a set of field glasses that allows one to see both overt and subtle injustices at work, including the historical, social, political, and environmental contexts that may interfere with or facilitate a person being able to reach their full health potential."[287(p1354)] To do this means going beyond language translation to culturally adapt existing interventions for use in new settings and populations; identifying strategies to equitably disseminate, implement, and sustain interventions or emerging technologies that have the potential to be equally effective across diverse populations; and considering the various contextual systems and policies at the community and health system levels that may perpetuate or exacerbate inequities.[273]

Equity-Oriented Implementation

Equity-oriented implementation was defined by Loper and colleagues as the "explicit attention to the culture, history, values, assets, and needs of the community—integrated into the principles, strategies, frameworks, and tools of implementation science, and EBIs that promote equity and address inequities and their root causes are routinely implemented in settings serving historically marginalized communities."[288]

Racism

Racism is a hierarchical structure of oppression that operates at multiple levels and across systems (e.g., housing, education, employment, credit, healthcare, criminal justice) to create, reinforce, and maintain inequities based on racial characteristics.[289–291]

SECTION 6: DISSEMINATION AND SCALE-UP

Designing for Dissemination, Implementation, and Sustainability

Designing for Dissemination and Sustainment

Designing for dissemination and sustainability (D4DS) refers to principles and methods for enhancing the fit between a health program, policy, or practice and the context in which it is intended to be adopted. In this chapter, we first summarize the historical context of D4DS and justify the need to shift traditional health research and dissemination practices[292] D4DS allows researchers to better account for the needs, assets, priorities, and time frames of potential adopters and anticipates dissemination products by developing a dissemination plan that takes into account these audience differences, product messaging, channels, and packaging.[27,242,292,293] A key principle in D4DS is *beginning with the end in mind*, meaning plan for future dissemination and sustainability at the outset.[294] Another D4DS principle—*product-context fit*—occurs when the products of research match the needs, resources, workflows, and characteristics of the target setting. Chapter 27 provides a more detailed overview of D4DS.

Marketing and Distribution Systems

Marketing and distribution systems bring products and services from their point of development to their point of use. This occurs through interconnected organizations and intermediaries who work to identify users, promote products, and distribute through local channels.[295] Chapter 28 provides a detailed overview of marketing and distribution systems.

Audience Segmentation

Audience segmentation is the process of distinguishing between different subgroups of users and creating targeted marketing and distribution strategies for each subgroup. Dearing and Kreuter suggested that "segmentation of intended audience members on the basis of demographic, psychographic, situational, and behavioral commonalities" allows for the design of products and messages that are perceived more relevant by the intended target audience.[117(ps102)] Audience segmentation studies seek to understand how dissemination materials might be tailored for different types of policymakers.[278] Segments of policymakers may vary in terms of preferences for types of materials or attitudes about a health issue.[282] See chapter 24 for more information about audience segmentation.

Scale-Up and Sustainment

Sustainability

Sustainability describes the extent to which an EBI can deliver its intended benefits over an extended period of time after external support from the donor agency is terminated.[133,296] A number of models and instruments are available to conceptualize and measure sustainability.[297,298] Most often, sustainability is measured through the continued use of intervention components; however, Scheirer and Dearing suggested that measures for sustainability should also include considerations of maintained community- or organizational-level partnerships; maintenance of organizational or community practices, procedures, and policies that were initiated during the implementation of the intervention; sustained organizational or community attention to the issue that the intervention is designed to address; and efforts for program diffusion and replication in other sites.[299] Other terms that are commonly used in the literature to refer to program continuation include sustainment, incorporation, integration, local or community ownership, confirmation, durability, stabilization, and sustained use.[64]

Operational indicators of sustainability can be: (1) *maintenance* of a program's initial health benefits, (2) *institutionalization* of the program in a setting or community, (3) *capacity building* in the recipient setting or community, and (4) *sustainability capacity*.[297]

Maintenance

Maintenance refers to the ability of the recipient setting or community to continuously deliver the health benefits achieved when the intervention was first implemented.[297]

Institutionalization

Institutionalization assesses the extent to which the EBI is integrated within the culture of the recipient setting or community through policies and practice.[297,300,301] Three stages that determine the extent of institutionalization are (1) *passage* (i.e., a single event that involves a significant change in the organization's structure or procedures, such as transition from temporary to permanent funding); (2) *cycle or routine* (i.e., repetitive reinforcement of the importance of the EBI through including it into organizational or community procedures and behaviors, such as the annual budget and evaluation criteria); and (3) *niche saturation* (the extent to which an EBI is integrated into all subsystems of an organization).[44,297,302] Niche saturation is also referred to as *penetration* in the literature as described by Lewis and colleagues in chapter 14 of this book.[132]

Capacity Building

Capacity building in D&I usually refers to activities (e.g., training or facilitation) that build resources within the target setting to enable the continued delivery of an intervention after external support is terminated.[44,297,303] Leeman and colleagues identified six strategies for capacity building: training, tools, technical assistance, assessment and feedback, peer networking, and incentives.[304]

Sustainment

Sustainment is an outcome of interest in an implementation science study indicating an intervention continues to be implemented over time.[133]

Planning for Sustainability

Planning for sustainability involves addressing systems, resource needs, and cost-benefit trade-offs to support continued use of the intervention or product. Sustainability planning necessitates engagement of policy decision makers and funders to encourage continued financing.[305]

Scale Up

The term *scale up* is commonly used in the international health and development literature and refers to "deliberate efforts to increase the impact of health service innovations successfully tested in pilot or experimental projects so as to benefit more people and to foster policy and programme development on a lasting basis."[306–308] Scaling up most commonly refers to expanding the coverage of successful interventions; however, it can also be concerned with the financial, human, and capital resources necessary for the expansion.[6,82] It is suggested that sustainable scale up requires a combination of horizontal (e.g., replication and expansion) and vertical (institutional, policy, political, legal) scaling up efforts that benefit from different D&I strategies (i.e., training, technical assistance hands-on support vs. networking, policy dialogue, advocacy).[7] Furthermore, some researchers suggested that scale up has a broader reach and scope than D&I and expands to national and international levels.[83] The National Implementation Research Network uses the term going to scale when an EBI reaches 60% of the target population that could benefit from it.[84] Barker and colleagues identified three key components of scale up: (1) using a clear sequence of activities needed to take interventions to scale; (2) articulating the context and environmental factors that will foster scale up of best practices; and (3) describing the infrastructure that is required to support scale up.[309]

Scale Out

Scaling out refers to broadening an innovation to a setting or target population that is different from previous implementations.[148] There are three types of scaling out; the first variant, type I (population fixed, different delivery system) involves targeting the same population as previously tested, but through a different delivery system. The second type of scaling out, type II (delivery system fixed, different population) involves targeting a different population than previously tested, but through the same delivery system; and the final type of scaling out, type III (different population and delivery system) involves targeting a different population through a different delivery system as compared to the original EBI trial.[310,311]

Voltage Drop

Interventions are expected to yield lower benefits as they move toward sustainability due to the added complexity of heterogeneous beneficiaries, implementers, and settings.[69,235,312]

Team Science

Team science involves research collaboration among investigators from different disciplines who work interdependently to share leadership and responsibility to address a scientific challenge.

SUMMARY AND CONCLUSION

In order for a field to prosper and thrive, a common language is essential. As is often the case when many disciplines and numerous organizations converge in development of a field, D&I research is still characterized by inconsistent terminology. The lack of agreed-on language for D&I research impedes the systematic analysis and summary of existing evidence in the field and the communication across different stakeholders (i.e., researchers, practitioners, policymakers).[11,192] The purpose of this chapter is not to advocate or argue the superiority of one term or classification scheme over another, but to facilitate communication by beginning to define commonly used terms in D&I research for researchers,

TABLE 2.1 GLOSSARY

SECTION 1: BACKGROUND

INNOVATION

- Innovation
- Intervention
- Evidence-based intervention
    - The 7Ps[a]
    - Complex intervention
    - Empirically supported treatment[a]
- Evidence-informed practice or interventions
- Promising/emerging intervention[a]

D&I COMPETENCIES

TYPES OF EVIDENCE

- Type 1 evidence
- Type 2 evidence
- Type 3 evidence

KNOWLEDGE FOR ACTION

- Knowledge translation
- Knowledge transfer
- Technology transfer[a]
- Knowledge exchange
- Knowledge integration[a]
- Knowledge utilization[a]
- Research utilization

PROCESSES FOR D&I SCIENCE

- Spread
- Diffusion
- Dissemination
- Implementation

TYPES OF RESEARCH

- Translational research
- Translational science[a]
- Translation
- T0 research[a]
- T1 research[a]
- T2 research[a]
- Efficacy research
- Effectiveness research
- T3 research[a]
- Dissemination research
- Implementation research
- T4 research[a]
- Population Health Intervention[a]/Research[a]
- Quality improvement science[a]
- Quality improvement
- Improvement science
- Plan-Do-Study-Act cycles[a]
- Learning system
- Learning evaluation[a]
- Precision medicine
- Precision health[a]
- Precision public health

EVIDENCE SYNTHESIS APPROACHES

- Realist review
- Scoping review
- Rapid scoping review[a]

SECTION 2: THEORIES

THEORIES, MODELS, AND FRAMEOWORKS

- Theory
- Model
- Framework
- Determinant frameworks
- Select Theories, models, and frameworks[a]
    - Diffusion of innovations[a]
    - CFIR[a]
    - EPIS[a]
    - RE-AIM[a]
    - PRISM[a]
    - PARiHS[a]
- Logic model
- Theory of change[a]

SECTION 3: METHODS

D&I STRATEGIES

- Strategies for D&I
- Dissemination strategy
- Implementation strategy
- ERIC strategies[a]
- Needs assessment[a]
- Intervention mapping[a]
- Implementation mapping[a]
- Group model building[a]
- Financing Strategies[a]
- Behavioral economics[a]
- Opinion leaders[a]
- Change agent[a]
- Implementation agent[a]
- Dissemination field agent
- Knowledge brokering[a]
- Knowledge broker
- Boundary spanners
- Purveyor of change[a]
- Intermediary and purveyor organization[a]

FIDELITY & ADAPTATIONS

- Fidelity
    - Implementation fidelity[a]
    - Intervention fidelity[a]
- Adaptation
    - Fidelity-consistent adaptations[a]
    - Fidelity-inconsistent adaptations[a]
    - Cultural adaptation
- Adaptive interventions[a]
- Replication
- Core components
- Adaptable/discretionary components
- Adaptability[a]
- Function[a]
- Form[a]
- Fit[a]
- Dose[a]
- Participant responsiveness[a]
- Program drift[a]
- Evolvability[a]
- Transferability[a]
- Transferability failure[a]

ORGANIZATIONAL PROCESSES

- Organizational implementation context[a]
- Organizational culture
- Organizational climate
- Implementation climate[a]
- Organizational readiness
- Implementation leadership

PARTICIPATORY APPROACHES IN D&I

- CBPR
- Community engagement
- Community permission
- Stakeholder engagement
- Co-creation[a]
- Co-learning[a]
- Patient-centered outcomes research[a]
- Patient centered[a]
- Participatory Implementation science
- Integrated knowledge translation[a]
- Participatory team science[a]
- Transcreation[a]
- Human-centered design

ECONOMIC EVALUATION IN D&I

- Implementation cost
- Replication costs[a]
- Economic evaluation
- Activity-based costing methods[a]
- Cost-effectiveness[a]
- Cost-utility analysis[a]
- Cost-benefit analysis[a]
- Action period costs[a]

(continued)

TABLE 2.1 CONTINUED

DE-IMPLEMENTATION/ MISIMPLEMENTATION
Mis-implementation
De-implementation
De-prescribing[a]
Disinvestment[a]
Low-value care

SYSTEM SCIENCE METHODS IN D&I
Systems thinking
System dynamics modeling
Systems engineering[a]
Participatory system dynamics
Community-based system dynamics[a]
Complexity theory[a]
Complexity
Complex system[a]
Complexity science[a]
Agents[a]
Agent-based modeling
Social network analysis
Rapid cycle systems Modeling (RCSM)[a]

FACTORS ASSOCIATED WITH THE SPEED & EXTENT OF D&I
Characteristics of the intervention
- Relative advantage[a]
- Compatibility[a]
- Acceptability[a]
- Appropriateness[a]
- Feasibility[a]

Implementer characteristics[a]
Determinants
Predictors
Mediators
Moderators
Mechanisms
Equifinality[a]
Context
- Setting[a]
- Inner setting[a]
- Outer setting[a]

Service delivery system[a]
Nonclinical settings for D&I[a]
Social service settings[a]
D&I for workplace health promotion[a]
D&I in the global context[a]
- Health systems building blocks framework[a]

SECTION 4: DESIGNS
STUDY DESIGNS IN D&I
Pragmatic clinical trial
Observational implementation study
Interventional implementation study
Effectiveness trial
Within-site design[a]
Between-site design[a]
Within- and between-site comparison designs[a]
Roll-out Implementation Optimization (ROIO) design[a]
Hybrid designs
- Type 1 hybrid design[a]
- Type 2 hybrid design[a]
- Type 3 hybrid design[a]

Pre-post studies[a]
Controlled before- and after-study design[a]
Multiple baseline time-series design[a]
Interrupted time series[a]
New versus implementation as usual (IAU) design[a]
Head-to-head trial[a]
Factorial designs[a]
Adaptive design[a]
MOST design
SMART design
Stepped-wedge design
Just-in-time (JIT) adaptive interventions[a]
LAGO design
Regression-discontinuity design[a]
Dynamic wait-listed control trial[a]
Pairwise-enrollment rollout designs[a]
N-of-1 design[a]

MEASUREMENT ISSUES
Measure considerations
Outcome variables
Implementation outcomes
Dissemination outcomes
Implementation outcomes framework[a]
Pragmatic measures
Psychometric and Pragmatic Evidence Rating (PAPERS)[a]
Harmonized measures[a]
Patient-reported measures[a]
Reach
Adoption
Uptake[a]
Unintended consequences[a]

EXTERNAL VALIDITY AND D&I RESEARCH
Rapid, responsive, relevant research
External validity
Representativeness[a]
Implementability
Transportability theory[a]
Evaluability assessment[a]
Wicked problems[a]
PRECIS-2
StaRI
TIDier

QUALITATIVE, QUANTITATIVE, & MIXED METHODS
Qualitative methods
Rapid qualitative assessment
Ethnographic approaches[a]
Rapid Assessment Procedure Informed Clinical Ethnography (RAPICE)[a]
Periodic reflections[a]
Quantitative methods
Conjoint analysis[a]
Structural equation modeling[a]
Mixed methods
Configurational comparative methods
- Qualitative comparative analysis
- Coincidence analysis[a]

Matrixed multiple-case study[a]
Process evaluation[a]
Intelligent data analysis[a]

SECTION 5: SETTING AND POPULATION D&I
POLICY D&I
Small p policy
Big p policy
Policy implementation research
Policy dissemination research
Dissemination effectiveness studies
Policy diffusion studies[a]
Policymaker[a]
Research evidence in policymaking[a]
Narrative communication[a]

TABLE 2.1 CONTINUED

Formative audience research
Multiple-streams model

HEALTH EQUITY
Health[a]
Health equity
  Health equity lens[a]
Equity-oriented implementation
Health disparities[a]
Racism
Antiracism[a]
Structural racism[a]
Reciprocal dialogues[a]

SECTION 6: DISSEMINATION & SCALE-UP
Designing for dissemination and sustainability
  Planning for active dissemination[a]
Context and situation analysis[a]
Fit to context framework[a]
Marketing and distribution systems
Marketing and distribution teams[a]
Audience segmentation
7 Ps framework for stakeholder identification[a]

SCALE-UP AND SUSTAINMENT
Sustainability
Maintenance
Institutionalization
Capacity building
Sustainability capacity[a]
Sustainment
Planning for sustainability
Scale up
  Horizontal scale-up[a]
  Vertical scale-up[a]
Scale out
Scalability[a]
Scalable unit[a]
Voltage drop
Penetration[a]

TEAM SCIENCE

[a]Indicates term and definition are only available in online version of this chapter.

practitioners, policymakers, and funding agencies. A common language should help accelerate the scientific progress in D&I research by facilitating comparison of methods and findings, as well as identifying gaps in dissemination knowledge.

When compiling this chapter, we encountered a number of challenges. Our research was limited to English language documents, so we may have missed important information from non-English-speaking countries. Another challenge was the lack of consensus on the overall classification of terms in the literature that may lead to apparent contradictions. For example, this chapter defines the different stages (dissemination, adoption, implementation, and sustainability) of the process under the umbrella term "D&I research." Other stage models may discuss adoption and sustainability as a distinct stage.[138] Finally, it is important to note that we organized this chapter by the general structure of the book to make it easier for readers to cross-reference sections. Table 2.1 provides an overview of this structure. Some terms could have arguably been classified in multiple sections. At the end of this book, the index provides an alphabetized list of terms with respective page numbers to facilitate the search for definitions and the fuller context for each term.

While the "state of the art" might still not be advanced enough to resolve all of the existing inconsistencies in terminology, this chapter represents the tremendous amount of development that happened since the last edition of this book to create platforms and approaches for a more consistent, agreed-on language for D&I research across topic areas, stakeholder groups, and geographical areas. As the D&I field makes progress toward a shared terminology, we can expect to see higher quality D&I research and greater contribution of D&I science to improving public health and clinical practice.

ACKNOWLEDGMENTS

We are thankful to Drs. Melinda Davis, Jonathan Purtle, Shari Rogal, Nicole Vaughn, and Russell Glasgow for their valuable input on the organizing structure and approaches used in earlier versions of this chapter and to Ms. Shannon Keating for her assistance in preparing the first version of this chapter. An early version of this chapter was published in the *Journal of Public Health Management and Practice* in 2008 and was coauthored by Drs. Debra Haire-Joshu, Matthew Kreuter, and Nancy Weaver. We sincerely appreciate the dedication and contributions from Ms. Olivia Fang for organizing the formatting and references for the full version of this glossary.

REFERENCES

1. Patient-Centered Outcomes Research Institute. PCORI dissemination and implementation funding initiatives. 2022. Accessed May 14, 2022. https://www.pcori.org/impact/putting-evidence-work/pcori-dissemination-and-implementation-funding-initiatives
2. Oh A, Vinson CA, Chambers DA. Future directions for implementation science at the National Cancer Institute: implementation science centers in cancer control. *Transl Behav Med.* 2021;11(2):669–675. doi:10.1093/tbm/ibaa018
3. National Institutes of Health. PAR-22-105: Dissemination and Implementation Research in Health (R01 clinical trial optional). 2022. Accessed May 14, 2022. https://grants.nih.gov/grants/guide/pa-files/PAR-22-105.html
4. Wolfenden L, Foy R, Presseau J, et al. Designing and undertaking randomised implementation trials: guide for researchers. *BMJ.* 2021;372:m3721. doi:10.1136/bmj.m3721
5. Glasgow RE, Vinson C, Chambers D, Khoury MJ, Kaplan RM, Hunter C. National Institutes of Health approaches to dissemination and implementation science: current and future directions. *Am J Public Health.* 2012;102(7):1274–1281. doi:10.2105/AJPH.2012.300755
6. Ciliska D, Robinson P, Armour T, et al. Diffusion and dissemination of evidence-based dietary strategies for the prevention of cancer. *Nutr J.* 2005;4(1):13. doi:10.1186/1475-2891-4-13
7. Lost in clinical translation. *Nat Med.* 2004;10(9):879. doi:10.1038/nm0904-879
8. Dobbins M. *Is Scientific Research Evidence Being Translated Into New Public Health Practice?* Central East Health Information Partnership; 1999.
9. Mayer JP, Davidson WS. Dissemination of innovation as social change. In: Rappaport J, Seidman E, eds. *Handbook of Community Psychology.* Plenum Publishers; 2000:421–438. doi:10.1007/978-1-4615-4193-6_18
10. Green LW, Johnson JL. Dissemination and utilization of health promotion and disease prevention knowledge: theory, research and experience. *Can J Public Health.* 1996;87(suppl 2):S11–S17.
11. Rogers EM. *Diffusion of Innovations.* 5th ed. Free Press; 2003.
12. Kilbourne AM, Glasgow RE, Chambers DA. What can implementation science do for you? Key success stories from the field. *J Gen Intern Med.* 2020;35(suppl 2):783–787. doi:10.1007/s11606-020-06174-6
13. World Health Organization. Regional Office for Africa. *Practical Guidance for Scaling Up Health Service Innovations.* WHO; 2009. Accessed April 15, 2022. https://apps.who.int/iris/handle/10665/254748
14. Hawe P, Potvin L. What is population health intervention research? *Can J Public Health.* 2009;100(suppl I8–I14). doi:10.1007/BF03405503
15. Tetro J. Knowledge translation at the Canadian Institutes of Health Research: a primer. National Center for the Dissemination of Disability Research; 2007. Accessed April 15, 2022. https://ktdrr.org/ktlibrary/articles_pubs/ncddrwork/focus/focus18/
16. Graham ID, Logan J, Harrison MB, et al. Lost in knowledge translation: time for a map? *J Contin Educ Health Prof.* 2006;26:13–24. doi:10.1002/chp.47
17. McKibbon KA, Lokker C, Wilczynski NL, et al. A cross-sectional study of the number and frequency of terms used to refer to knowledge translation in a body of health literature in 2006: a Tower of Babel? *Implement Sci.* 2010;5:16. doi:10.1186/1748-5908-5-16
18. Curran GM. Implementation science made too simple: a teaching tool. *Implement Sci Commun.* 2020;1:27. doi:10.1186/s43058-020-00001-z
19. Greenhalgh T, Robert G, Macfarlane F, Bate P, Kyriakidou O. Diffusion of innovations in service organizations: systematic review and recommendations. *Milbank Q.* 2004;82(4):581–629. doi:10.1111/j.0887-378X.2004.00325.x
20. Fixsen D, Naoom S, Blase K, Friedman R, Wallace F. Implementation Research: A Synthesis of the Literature. National Implementation Research Network, University of South Florida; 2005. Accessed April 15, 2022. https://nirn.fpg.unc.edu/resources/implementation-research-synthesis-literature
21. Damschroder LJ, Aron DC, Keith RE, Kirsh SR, Alexander JA, Lowery JC. Fostering implementation of health services research findings into practice: a consolidated framework for advancing implementation science. *Implement Sci.* 2009;4:50. doi:10.1186/1748-5908-4-50
22. Brown CH, Curran G, Palinkas LA, et al. An overview of research and evaluation designs for dissemination and implementation. *Annu Rev Public Health.* 2017;38:1–22. doi:10.1146/annurev-publhealth-031816-044215
23. Rychetnik L, Hawe P, Waters E, Barratt A, Frommer M. A glossary for evidence based public health. *J Epidemiol Community Health.* 2004;58(7):538–545. doi:10.1136/jech.2003.011585
24. Sackett DL, Rosenberg WMC, Gray JAM, Haynes RB, Richardson WS. Evidence based medicine: what it is and what it isn't. *BMJ.* 1996;312(7023):71–72. doi:10.1136/bmj.312.7023.71

25. Brownson RC, Baker EA, Deshpande AD, Gillespie KN. *Evidence-Based Public Health*. Oxford University Press; 2003.
26. Jenicek M. Epidemiology, evidenced-based medicine, and evidence-based public health. *J Epidemiol*. 1997;7(4):187–197. doi:10.2188/jea.7.187
27. Brownson RC, Shelton RC, Geng EH, Glasgow RE. Revisiting concepts of evidence in implementation science. *Implement Sci*. 2022;17:26. doi:10.1186/s13012-022-01201-y
28. Dissemination & implementation models in health research & practice interactive webtool Accessed on January 11, 2023. Available at: https://dissemination-implementation.org/constructDetails.aspx?id=27
29. Pfadenhauer LM, Gerhardus A, Mozygemba K, et al. Making sense of complexity in context and implementation: the Context and Implementation of Complex Interventions (CICI) framework. *Implement Sci*. 2017;12:21. doi:10.1186/s13012-017-0552-5
30. Skivington K, Matthews L, Simpson SA, et al. A new framework for developing and evaluating complex interventions: update of Medical Research Council guidance. *BMJ*. 2021;374:n2061. doi:10.1136/bmj.n2061
31. Hawe P, Shiell A, Riley T. Complex interventions: how "out of control" can a randomised controlled trial be? *BMJ*. 2004;328(7455):1561–1563. doi:10.1136/bmj.328.7455.1561
32. Miles A, Loughlin M. Models in the balance: evidence-based medicine versus evidence-informed individualized care. *J Eval Clin Pract*. 2011;17(4):531–536. doi:10.1111/j.1365-2753.2011.01713.x
33. Armstrong R, Pettman TL, Waters E. Shifting sands—from descriptions to solutions. *Public Health*. 2014;128(6):525–532. doi:10.1016/j.puhe.2014.03.013
34. Yost J, Dobbins M, Traynor R, DeCorby K, Workentine S, Greco L. Tools to support evidence-informed public health decision making. *BMC Public Health*. 2014;14:728. doi:10.1186/1471-2458-14-728
35. Woodbury M, Kuhnke J. Research 101: evidence-based practice vs. evidence-informed practice: what's the difference? *Wound Care Canada*. 2014;12(1):26–29. Accessed April 15, 2022. https://www.woundscanada.ca/docman/public/wound-care-canada-magazine/2014-vol-12-no-1/510-wcc-spring-2014-v12n1-research-101/file
36. Borkovec TD, Costonguay LG. What is the scientific meaning of empirically supported therapy? *J Consult Clin Psychol*. 1998;66(1):136–142. doi:10.1037/0022-006X.66.1.136
37. Gambrill E. Evidence-based practice: implications for knowledge development and use in social work. In: Rosen A, Proctor EK, eds. *Developing Practice Guidelines for Social Work Intervention: Issues, Methods, and Research Agenda*. Columbia University Press; 2003:37–58.
38. Padek M, Colditz G, Dobbins M, et al. Developing educational competencies for dissemination and implementation research training programs: an exploratory analysis using card sorts. *Implement Sci*. 2015;10:114. doi:10.1186/s13012-015-0304-3
39. Brownson RC, Fielding JE, Maylahn CM. Evidence-based public health: a fundamental concept for public health practice. *Annu Rev Public Health*. 2009;30:175–201. doi:10.1146/annurev.publhealth.031308.100134
40. Best A, Hiatt RA, Norman CD, National Cancer Institute of Canada Joint Working Group on Translational Research and Knowledge Integration of the Advisory Committee for Research and the Joint Advisory Committee for Cancer Control. Knowledge integration: conceptualizing communications in cancer control systems. *Patient Educ Couns*. 2008;71(3):319–327. doi:10.1016/j.pec.2008.02.013
41. McKibbon KA, Lokker C, Keepanasseril A, Colquhoun H, Haynes RB, Wilczynski NL. WhatisKT wiki: a case study of a platform for knowledge translation terms and definitions—descriptive analysis. *Implement Sci*. 2013;8:13. doi:10.1186/1748-5908-8-13
42. Canadian Institutes of Health Research. Knowledge translation at CIHR. 2022. Accessed April 15, 2022. https://cihr-irsc.gc.ca/e/29529.html
43. Straus SE, Tetroe J, Graham I. Defining knowledge translation. *CMAJ*. 2009;181(3–4):165–168. doi:10.1503/cmaj.081229
44. Pluye P, Potvin L, Denis JL. Making public health programs last: conceptualizing sustainability. *Eval Program Plann*. 2004;27(2):121–133. doi:10.1016/j.evalprogplan.2004.01.001
45. Mitton C, Adair CE, McKenzie E, Patten SB, Waye Perry B. Knowledge transfer and exchange: review and synthesis of the literature. *Milbank Q*. 2007;85(4):729–768. doi:10.1111/j.1468-0009.2007.00506.x
46. Estabrooks CA. The conceptual structure of research utilization. *Res Nurs Health*. 1999;22(3):203–216. doi:10.1002/(sici)1098-240x(199906)22:3<203::aid-nur3>3.0.co;2-9

47. Estabrooks C, Wallin L, Milner M. Measuring knowledge utilization in health care. Int J Policy Eval Manage. 2003;1:3–36.
48. Nelson EC, Batalden PB, Huber TP, et al. Microsystems in health care: part 1. Learning from high-performing front-line clinical units. *Jt Comm J Qual Improv.* 2002;28(9):472–493. doi:10.1016/s1070-3241(02)28051-7
49. Massoud MR, Donohue KL, McCannon CJ. *Options for Large-Scale Spread of Simple, High-Impact Interventions.* University Research Co. LLC (URC); 2010.
50. Lomas J. Diffusion, dissemination, and implementation: who should do what? *Ann N Y Acad Sci.* 1993;703:226–235; discussion 235–237. doi:10.1111/j.1749-6632.1993.tb26351.x
51. MacLean DR. Positioning dissemination in public health policy. *Can J Public Health.* 1996;87(suppl 2):S40–S43.
52. National Institutes of Health. PAR-10-038: dissemination and implementation research in health (R01). 2010. Accessed April 15, 2022. https://grants.nih.gov/grants/guide/pa-files/par-10-038.html
53. May C. Towards a general theory of implementation. *Implement Sci.* 2013;8:18. doi:10.1186/1748-5908-8-18
54. De Maria Marchiano R, Di Sante G, Piro G, et al. Translational research in the era of precision medicine: where we are and where we will go. *J Pers Med.* 2021;11(3):216. doi:10.3390/jpm11030216
55. Ledford H. Translational research: the full cycle. *Nature.* 2008;453(7197):843–845. doi:10.1038/453843a
56. Fort DG, Herr TM, Shaw PL, Gutzman KE, Starren JB. Mapping the evolving definitions of translational research. *J Clin Transl Sci.* 2017;1(1):60–66. doi:10.1017/cts.2016.10
57. Woolf SH. The meaning of translational research and why it matters. *JAMA.* 2008;299(2):211–213. doi:10.1001/jama.2007.26
58. Szilagyi PG. Translational research and pediatrics. *Acad Pediatr.* 2009;9(2):71–80. doi:10.1016/j.acap.2008.11.002
59. Tansella M, Thornicroft G. Implementation science: understanding the translation of evidence into practice. *Br J Psychiatry.* 2009;195(4):283–285. doi:10.1192/bjp.bp.109.065565
60. Sussman S, Valente TW, Rohrbach LA, Skara S, Pentz MA. Translation in the health professions: converting science into action. *Eval Health Prof.* 2006;29(1):7–32. doi:10.1177/0163278705284441
61. Glasgow RE, Lichtenstein E, Marcus AC. Why don't we see more translation of health promotion research to practice? Rethinking the efficacy-to-effectiveness transition. *Am J Public Health.* 2003;93(8):1261–1267. doi:10.2105/ajph.93.8.1261
62. Leppin AL, Mahoney JE, Stevens KR, et al. Situating dissemination and implementation sciences within and across the translational research spectrum. *J Clin Transl Sci.* 2020;4(3):152–158. doi:10.1017/cts.2019.392
63. National Institutes of Health. PAR-10-040: dissemination and implementation research in health (R21). 2010. Accessed April 15, 2022. https://grants.nih.gov/grants/guide/pa-files/par-10-040.html
64. Center for Mental Health in Schools at UCLA. Systemic change and empirically-supported practices: the implementation problem. 2006. Accessed April 15, 2022. http://smhp.psych.ucla.edu/dbsimple2.php?primary=1401&number=9917
65. Pinnock H, Barwick M, Carpenter CR, et al. Standards for Reporting Implementation Studies (StaRI) statement. *BMJ.* 2017;356:i6795. doi:10.1136/bmj.i6795
66. Batalden PB, Davidoff F. What is "quality improvement" and how can it transform healthcare? *Qual Saf Health Care.* 2007;16(1):2–3. doi:10.1136/qshc.2006.022046
67. Health Center Resources & Services Administration. Clinical Quality Improvement; August 5, 2016. Accessed April 15, 2022. https://bphc.hrsa.gov/qualityimprovement/index.html
68. Kao L. Implementation science and quality improvement. In: Dimick JB, Greenberg CC, eds. *Success in Academic Surgery: Health Services Research.* Springer; 2014:85–100.
69. Bauer MS, Damschroder L, Hagedorn H, Smith J, Kilbourne AM. An introduction to implementation science for the non-specialist. *BMC Psychol.* 2015;3:32. doi:10.1186/s40359-015-0089-9
70. Rosin R. Keynote address: the innovation conundrum. Presented at: Ninth Annual Conference on the Science of Dissemination and Implementation in Health; December 14–15, 2016; Washington, DC. Accessed April 15, 2022. https://academyhealth.confex.com/academyhealth/2016di/meetingapp.cgi/ModuleSessionsByDay/0
71. Balasubramanian BA, Cohen DJ, Davis MM, et al. Learning evaluation: blending quality improvement and implementation research methods to study healthcare innovations. *Implement Sci.* 2015;10:31. doi:10.1186/s13012-015-0219-z
72. Mitchell SA, Chambers DA. Leveraging implementation science to improve cancer care delivery and patient outcomes. *J Oncol Pract.* 2017;13(8):523–529. doi:10.1200/JOP.2017.024729

73. Davidoff F, Dixon-Woods M, Leviton L, Michie S. Demystifying theory and its use in improvement. *BMJ Qual Saf.* 2015;24(3):228–238. doi:10.1136/bmjqs-2014-003627
74. Koczwara B, Stover AM, Davies L, et al. Harnessing the synergy between improvement science and implementation science in cancer: a call to action. *J Oncol Pract.* 2018;14(6):335–340. doi:10.1200/JOP.17.00083
75. Adesoye T, Greenberg CC, Neuman HB. Optimizing cancer care delivery through implementation science. *Front Oncol.* 2016;6:1. doi:10.3389/fonc.2016.00001
76. Institute of Medicine (US) Roundtable on Evidence-Based Medicine; Olsen L, Aisner D, McGinnis JM, eds. *The Learning Healthcare System: Workshop Summary.* National Academies Press; 2007. Accessed April 15, 2022. http://www.ncbi.nlm.nih.gov/books/NBK53494/
77. Platt JE, Raj M, Wienroth M. An analysis of the learning health system in its first decade in practice: scoping review. *J Med Internet Res.* 2020;22(3):e17026. doi:10.2196/17026
78. Chambers DA, Feero WG, Khoury MJ. Convergence of implementation science, precision medicine, and the learning health care system: a new model for biomedical research. *JAMA.* 2016;315(18):1941–1942. doi:10.1001/jama.2016.3867
79. Greenhalgh T, Papoutsi C. Spreading and scaling up innovation and improvement. *BMJ.* 2019;365:l2068. doi:10.1136/bmj.l2068
80. National Cancer Institute. National Cancer Moonshot Initiative. February 1, 2016. Accessed March 25, 2017. https://www.cancer.gov/research/key-initiatives/moonshot-cancer-initiative
81. Khoury MJ, Bowen MS, Clyne M, et al. From public health genomics to precision public health: a 20-year journey. *Genet Med.* 2018;20(6):574–582. doi:10.1038/gim.2017.211
82. Knowledge Translation Program. Right Review. 2023. Accessed April 15, 2022. https://rightreview.knowledgetranslation.net/
83. Pawson R. *Evidence-Based Policy: A Realist Perspective.* Sage; 2006. https://uk.sagepub.com/en-gb/eur/evidence-based-policy/book227875
84. Pawson R, Greenhalgh T, Harvey G, Walshe K. Realist review—a new method of systematic review designed for complex policy interventions. *J Health Serv Res Policy.* 2005;10(suppl 1):21–34. doi:10.1258/1355819054308530
85. Rycroft-Malone J, McCormack B, Hutchinson AM, et al. Realist synthesis: illustrating the method for implementation research. *Implement Sci.* 2012;7:33. doi:10.1186/1748-5908-7-33
86. Mays N, Roberts E, Popay J. Synthesising research evidence. In: Allen P, Allen P, Black N, Clarke A, Fulop N, Anderson S, eds. *Studying the Organisation and Delivery of Health Services: Research Methods.* Routledge; 2001:188–219. doi:10.4324/9780203481981
87. Arksey H, O'Malley L. Scoping studies: towards a methodological framework. *Int J Soc Res Methodol.* 2005;8(1):19–32. doi:10.1080/1364557032000119616
88. Munn Z, Peters MDJ, Stern C, Tufanaru C, McArthur A, Aromataris E. Systematic review or scoping review? Guidance for authors when choosing between a systematic or scoping review approach. *BMC Med Res Methodol.* 2018;18(1):143. doi:10.1186/s12874-018-0611-x
89. Dijkers M. What is a scoping review? *KT Update.* 2015;4(1). https://ktdrr.org/products/update/v4n1/dijkers_ktupdate_v4n1_12-15.pdf
90. Dopp AR, Narcisse MR, Mundey P, et al. A scoping review of strategies for financing the implementation of evidence-based practices in behavioral health systems: state of the literature and future directions. *Implement Res Prac.* 2020;1. https://doi.org/10.1177/2633489520939980
91. Colquhoun HL, Levac D, O'Brien KK, et al. Scoping reviews: time for clarity in definition, methods, and reporting. *J Clin Epidemiol.* 2014;67(12):1291–1294. doi:10.1016/j.jclinepi.2014.03.013
92. Crosswaite C, Curtice L. Disseminating research results—the challenge of bridging the gap between health research and health action. *Health Promot Int.* 1994;9(4):289–296. doi:10.1093/heapro/9.4.289
93. Johnson JL, Green LW, Frankish CJ, MacLean DR, Stachenko S. A dissemination research agenda to strengthen health promotion and disease prevention. *Can J Public Health.* 1996;87(suppl 2):S5–S10.
94. Tabak RG, Khoong EC, Chambers DA, Brownson RC. Bridging research and practice: models for dissemination and implementation research. *Am J Prev Med.* 2012;43(3):337–350. doi:10.1016/j.amepre.2012.05.024
95. Strifler L, Cardoso R, McGowan J, et al. Scoping review identifies significant number of knowledge translation theories, models, and frameworks with limited use. *J Clin Epidemiol.* 2018;100:92–102. doi:10.1016/j.jclinepi.2018.04.008
96. Esmail R, Hanson HM, Holroyd-Leduc J, et al. A scoping review of full-spectrum knowledge translation theories, models, and frameworks. *Implement Sci.* 2020;15:11. doi:10.1186/s13012-020-0964-5

97. Dissemination & Implementation Models in Heath Research & Practice. Helping navigate dissemination and implementation models. 2015 Accessed January 11, 2023. https://dissemination-implementation.org/
98. Oldenburg B, Glanz K. Diffusion of innovation. In: Glanz K, Rimer BK, Viswanath K, eds. *Health Behavior and Health Education: Theory, Research, and Practice.* 4th ed. Jossey-Bass; 2008:313–334.
99. EPIS Framework. The EPIS implementation framework. Accessed January 11, 2023. https://episframework.com
100. Moullin JC, Dickson KS, Stadnick NA, Rabin B, Aarons GA. Systematic review of the exploration, preparation, implementation, sustainment (EPIS) framework. *Implement Sci.* 2019;14:1. doi:10.1186/s13012-018-0842-6
101. Glasgow RE, Vogt TM, Boles SM. Evaluating the public health impact of health promotion interventions: the RE-AIM framework. *Am J Public Health.* 1999;89(9):1322–1327. doi:10.2105/ajph.89.9.1322
102. Glasgow RE, Harden SM, Gaglio B, et al. RE-AIM planning and evaluation framework: Adapting to new science and practice with a 20-year review. *Front Public Health.* 2019;7:64. doi:10.3389/fpubh.2019.00064
103. Feldstein AC, Glasgow RE. A practical, robust implementation and sustainability model (PRISM) for integrating research findings into practice. *Jt Comm J Qual Patient Saf.* 2008;34(4):228–243. doi:10.1016/s1553-7250(08)34030-6
104. Kitson A, Harvey G, McCormack B. Enabling the implementation of evidence based practice: a conceptual framework. *Qual Health Care.* 1998;7(3):149–158. doi:10.1136/qshc.7.3.149
105. Rycroft-Malone J, Kitson A, Harvey G, et al. Ingredients for change: revisiting a conceptual framework. *Qual Saf Health Care.* 2002;11(2):174–180. doi:10.1136/qhc.11.2.174
106. Moullin JC, Dickson KS, Stadnick NA, et al. Ten recommendations for using implementation frameworks in research and practice. *Implement Sci Commun.* 2020;1:42. doi:10.1186/s43058-020-00023-7
107. Nilsen P, Birken SA, eds. Handbook on Implementation Science. Edward Elgar Publishing; 2020. Accessed April 15, 2022. https://econpapers.repec.org/bookchap/elgeebook/18688.htm
108. Frankfort-Nachmias C, Nachmias D. *Research Methods in the Social Sciences.* St. Martin's Press; 1996.
109. Sabatier PA. *Theories of the Policy Process.* Westview Press; 1999.
110. Nilsen P, Bernhardsson S. Context matters in implementation science: a scoping review of determinant frameworks that describe contextual determinants for implementation outcomes. *BMC Health Serv Res.* 2019;19:189. doi:10.1186/s12913-019-4015-3
111. United Way of America. *Measuring Program Outcomes: A Practical Approach.* University of Nebraska Omaha; 1996:38. Accessed April 22, 2022. https://digitalcommons.unomaha.edu/slceeval/47
112. Savaya R, Waysman M. The logic model. *Adm Soc Work.* 2005;29(2):85–103. doi:10.1300/J147v29n02_06
113. Smith JD, Li DH, Rafferty MR. The implementation research logic model: a method for planning, executing, reporting, and synthesizing implementation projects. *Implement Sci.* 2020;15(1):84. doi:10.1186/s13012-020-01041-8
114. Leeman J, Birken SA, Powell BJ, Rohweder C, Shea CM. Beyond "implementation strategies": classifying the full range of strategies used in implementation science and practice. *Implement Sci.* 2017;12:125. doi:10.1186/s13012-017-0657-x
115. National Cancer Institute. Division of Cancer Control and Population Sciences (DCCPS). About implementation science. August 19, 2021. https://cancercontrol.cancer.gov/is/about
116. Rabin BA, Brownson RC, Kerner JF, Glasgow RE. Methodologic challenges in disseminating evidence-based interventions to promote physical activity. *Am J Prev Med.* 2006;31(4)(suppl):24–34. doi:10.1016/j.amepre.2006.06.009
117. Dearing JW, Kreuter MW. Designing for diffusion: how can we increase uptake of cancer communication innovations? *Patient Educ Couns.* 2010;81(suppl):S100–S110. doi:10.1016/j.pec.2010.10.013
118. Blase K, Fixsen D, Duda M, Metz A, Naoom S, Van Dyke A. Implementing and sustaining evidence-based programs: have we got a sporting chance? Presented at: Blueprints Conference; April 8, 2010; University of North Carolina, Chapel Hill. https://www.blueprintsprograms.org/conference/presentations/2010/keynote_kb.pdf
119. National Institutes of Health. PA-08-166: Dissemination, Implementation, and Operational Research for HIV Prevention Interventions (R01). 2009. Accessed April 20, 2022. https://grants.nih.gov/grants/guide/pa-files/pa-08-166.html
120. Powell BJ, McMillen JC, Proctor EK, et al. A compilation of strategies for implementing

clinical innovations in health and mental health. *Med Care Res Rev.* 2012;69(2):123–157. Doi:10.1177/1077558711430690

121. Proctor EK, Powell BJ, McMillen JC. Implementation strategies: recommendations for specifying and reporting. *Implement Sci.* 2013;8:139. Doi:10.1186/1748-5908-8-139
122. Powell BJ, Waltz TJ, Chinman MJ, et al. A refined compilation of implementation strategies: results from the Expert Recommendations for Implementing Change (ERIC) project. *Implement Sci.* 2015;10:21. Doi:10.1186/s13012-015-0209-1
123. Kreuter MW, Wang ML. From evidence to impact: recommendations for a dissemination support system. *New Dir Child Adolesc Dev.* 2015;2015(149):11–23. Doi:10.1002/cad.20110
124. Ward VL, House AO, Hamer S. Knowledge brokering: exploring the process of transferring knowledge into action. *BMC Health Serv Res.* 2009;9(1):12. Doi:10.1186/1472-6963-9-12
125. Hargadon A. Brokering knowledge: linking learning and innovation. *Research in Organizational Behavior.* 2002;24:41–85. Doi:10.1016/S0191-3085(02)24003-4
126. Tushman ML. Special boundary roles in the innovation process. *Adm Sci Q.* 1977;22(4):587–605. Doi:10.2307/2392402
127. Parker J, Crona B. On being all things to all people: boundary organizations and the contemporary research university. *Soc Stud Sci.* 2012;42(2):262–289. Doi:10.1177/0306312711435833
128. Franks RP, Bory CT. Who supports the successful implementation and sustainability of evidence-based practices? Defining and understanding the roles of intermediary and purveyor organizations. *New Dir Child Adolesc Dev.* 2015;2015(149):41–56. Doi:10.1002/cad.20112
129. Corcoran T, Rowling L, Wise M. The potential contribution of intermediary organizations for implementation of school mental health. *Adv School Mental Health Promot.* 2015;8(2):57–70. Doi:10.1080/1754730X.2015.1019688
130. Frank R. Role of the intermediary organization in promoting and disseminating best practices for children and youth: the Connecticut center for effective practice. *Emotional Behav Disord Youth.* 2010;10(4):87–93.
131. Proctor EK, Landsverk J, Aarons G, Chambers D, Glisson C, Mittman B. Implementation research in mental health services: an emerging science with conceptual, methodological, and training challenges. *Adm Policy Ment Health.* 2009;36(1):24–34. Doi:10.1007/s10488-008-0197-4
132. Proctor E, Silmere H, Raghavan R, et al. Outcomes for implementation research: conceptual distinctions, measurement challenges, and research agenda. *Adm Policy Ment Health.* 2011;38(2):65–76. Doi:10.1007/s10488-010-0319-7
133. Shelton RC, Cooper BR, Stirman SW. The sustainability of evidence-based interventions and practices in public health and health care. *Annu Rev Public Health.* 2018;39:55–76. Doi:10.1146/annurev-publhealth-040617-014731
134. Castro FG, Barrera M, Martinez CR. The cultural adaptation of prevention interventions: resolving tensions between fidelity and fit. *Prev Sci.* 2004;5(1):41–45. Doi:10.1023/b:prev.0000013980.12412.cd
135. Movsisyan A, Arnold L, Evans R, et al. Adapting evidence-informed complex population health interventions for new contexts: a systematic review of guidance. *Implement Sci.* 2019;14:105. Doi:10.1186/s13012-019-0956-5
136. Stirman SW, Miller CJ, Toder K, Calloway A. Development of a framework and coding system for modifications and adaptations of evidence-based interventions. *Implement Sci.* 2013;8:65. Doi:10.1186/1748-5908-8-65
137. Wiltsey Stirman S, Baumann AA, Miller CJ. The FRAME: an expanded framework for reporting adaptations and modifications to evidence-based interventions. *Implement Sci.* 2019;14(1):58. Doi:10.1186/s13012-019-0898-y
138. Miller CJ, Barnett ML, Baumann AA, Gutner CA, Wiltsey-Stirman S. The FRAME-IS: a framework for documenting modifications to implementation strategies in healthcare. *Implementation Sci.* 2021;16(1):36. Doi:10.1186/s13012-021-01105-3
139. Perez Jolles M, Lengnick-Hall R, Mittman BS. Core functions and forms of complex health interventions: a patient-centered medical home illustration. *J Gen Intern Med.* 2019;34(6):1032–1038. Doi:10.1007/s11606-018-4818-7
140. Dearing JW. Evolution of diffusion and dissemination theory. *J Public Health Manag Pract.* 2008;14(2):99–108. Doi:10.1097/01.PHH.0000311886.98627.b7
141. Bopp M, Saunders RP, Lattimore D. The tug-of-war: fidelity versus adaptation throughout the health promotion program life cycle. *J Prim Prev.* 2013;34(3):193–207. Doi:10.1007/s10935-013-0299-y
142. Carvalho ML, Honeycutt S, Escoffery C, Glanz K, Sabbs D, Kegler MC. Balancing fidelity and adaptation: implementing evidence-based chronic disease prevention programs. *J Public*

Health Manag Pract. 2013;19(4):348–356. Doi:10.1097/PHH.0b013e31826d80eb
143. Cohen DJ, Crabtree BF, Etz RS, et al. Fidelity versus flexibility: translating evidence-based research into practice. *Am J Prev Med.* 2008;35(5)(suppl):S381–S389. Doi:10.1016/j.amepre.2008.08.005
144. Bernal G, Domenech Rodríguez MM. Cultural adaptation in context: psychotherapy as a historical account of adaptations. In: Bernal G, Domenech Rodríguez MM, eds. *Cultural Adaptations: Tools for Evidence-Based Practice With Diverse Populations.* American Psychological Association; 2012:3–22. Doi:10.1037/13752-001
145. Cabassa LJ, Baumann AA. A two-way street: Bridging implementation science and cultural adaptations of mental health treatments. *Implement Sci.* 2013;8:90. Doi:10.1186/1748-5908-8-90
146. Shelton RC, Chambers DA, Glasgow RE. An extension of RE-AIM to enhance sustainability: addressing dynamic context and promoting health equity over time. *Front Public Health.* 2020;8:134. Doi:10.3389/fpubh.2020.00134
147. Baumann AA, Cabassa LJ, Stirman SW. Adaptation in dissemination and implementation science. In: Brownson RC, Colditz GA, Proctor EK, eds. *Dissemination and Implementation Research in Health: Translating Science to Practice.* 2nd ed. Oxford University Press; 2017:286–300.
148. Livet M, Haines ST, Curran GM, et al. Implementation science to advance care delivery: a primer for pharmacists and other health professionals. *Pharmacotherapy.* 2018;38(5):490–502. Doi:10.1002/phar.2114
149. Blase K, Fixsen D. *Core Intervention Components: Identifying and Operationalizing What Makes Programs Work.* Department of Health and Human Services; 2013. Accessed April 15, 2022. https://aspe.hhs.gov/reports/core-intervention-components-identifying-operationalizing-what-makes-programs-work-0
150. Dusenbury L, Brannigan R, Falco M, Hansen WB. A review of research on fidelity of implementation: implications for drug abuse prevention in school settings. *Health Educ Res.* 2003;18(2):237–256. Doi:10.1093/her/18.2.237
151. McKleroy VS, Galbraith JS, Cummings B, et al. Adapting evidence-based behavioral interventions for new settings and target populations. *AIDS Educ Prev.* 2006;18(4)(suppl A):59–73. Doi:10.1521/aeap.2006.18.supp.59
152. Wingood GM, DiClemente RJ. The ADAPT-ITT model: a novel method of adapting evidence-based HIV Interventions. *J Acquir Immune Defic Syndr.* 2008;47(suppl 1): S40–S46. Doi:10.1097/QAI.0b013e3181605df1
153. Aarons GA, Hurlburt M, Horwitz SM. Advancing a conceptual model of evidence-based practice implementation in public service sectors. *Adm Policy Ment Health.* 2011;38(1):4–23. Doi:10.1007/s10488-010-0327-7
154. Jacobs R, Mannion R, Davies HTO, Harrison S, Konteh F, Walshe K. The relationship between organizational culture and performance in acute hospitals. *Soc Sci Med.* 2013;76(1):115–125. Doi:10.1016/j.socscimed.2012.10.014
155. Gilson L, Schneider H. Commentary: managing scaling up: what are the key issues? *Health Policy Plann.* 2010;25(2):97–98. Doi:10.1093/heapol/czp067
156. Verbeke W, Volgering M, Hessels M. Exploring the conceptual expansion within the field of organizational behaviour: organizational climate and organizational culture. *J Manage Stud.* 1998;35(3):303–329. Doi:10.1111/1467-6486.00095
157. Cooke RA, Rousseau DM. Behavioral norms and expectations: a quantitative approach to the assessment of organizational culture. *Group Organ Stud.* 1988;13(3):245–273. Doi:10.1177/105960118801300302
158. Williams NJ, Beidas RS. Annual research review: the state of implementation science in child psychology and psychiatry: a review and suggestions to advance the field. *J Child Psychol Psychiatry.* 2019;60(4):430–450. Doi:10.1111/jcpp.12960
159. Schneider, B, González-Romá, V, Ostroff, C, West, MA. Organizational climate and culture: reflections on the history of the constructs in the *Journal of Applied Psychology. J Appl Psychol.* 2017;102(3):468–482.
160. Schein EH. *Organizational Culture and Leadership.* 3rd ed. Jossey-Bass; 2004. Accessed April 15, 2022. http://www.untag-smd.ac.id/files/Perpustakaan_Digital_2/ORGANIZATIONAL%20CULTURE%20Organizational%20Culture%20and%20Leadership,%203rd%20Edition.pdf
161. Hellriegel D, Slocum JW. Organizational climate: measures, research and contingencies. *Acad Manage J.* 1974;17(2):255–280. Doi:10.5465/254979
162. Reichers A, Schneider B. Climate and culture: an evolution of constructs. In: Schneider B, ed. *Organizational Climate and Culture.* Jossey-Bass; 1990:5–39.
163. Powell BJ, Mettert KD, Dorsey CN, et al. Measures of organizational culture, organizational climate, and implementation climate in behavioral

health: a systematic review. *Implement Res Pract.* 2021;2. Doi:10.1177/26334895211018862

164. Ehrhart, MG, Schneider, B, Macey, WH. *Organizational Climate and Culture: An Introduction to Theory, Research, and Practice.* Routledge; 2014. Accessed April 15, 2022. https://www.routledge.com/Organizational-Climate-and-Culture-An-Introduction-to-Theory-Research/Ehrhart-Schneider-Macey/p/book/9781848725287
165. Scaccia JP, Cook BS, Lamont A, et al. A practical implementation science heuristic for organizational readiness: R = MC2. *J Community Psychol.* 2015;43(4):484–501. Doi:10.1002/jcop.21698
166. Lehman WEK, Greener JM, Simpson DD. Assessing organizational readiness for change. *J Subst Abuse Treat.* 2002;22(4):197–209. Doi:10.1016/s0740-5472(02)00233-7
167. Weiner BJ. A theory of organizational readiness for change. *Implement Sci.* 2009;4:67. Doi:10.1186/1748-5908-4-67
168. Weiner BJ, Amick H, Lee SYD. Review: conceptualization and measurement of organizational readiness for change: a review of the literature in health services research and other fields. *Med Care Res Rev.* 2008;65(4):379–436. Doi:10.1177/1077558708317802
169. Brooke-Sumner C, Petersen-Williams P, Wagener E, Sorsdahl K, Aarons GA, Myers B. Adaptation of the Texas Christian University Organisational Readiness for Change Short Form (TCU-ORC-SF) for use in primary health facilities in South Africa. *BMJ Open.* 2021;11(12):e047320. Doi:10.1136/bmjopen-2020-047320
170. Shea CM, Jacobs SR, Esserman DA, Bruce K, Weiner BJ. Organizational readiness for implementing change: a psychometric assessment of a new measure. *Implement Sci.* 2014;9:7. Doi:10.1186/1748-5908-9-7
171. Nickel NC, Taylor EC, Labbok MH, Weiner BJ, Williamson NE. Applying organization theory to understand barriers and facilitators to the implementation of baby-friendly: a multisite qualitative study. *Midwifery.* 2013;29(8):956–964. Doi:10.1016/j.midw.2012.12.001
172. Avolio BJ, Bass BM, Jung DI. Re-examining the components of transformational and transactional leadership using the Multifactor Leadership Questionnaire. *J Occup Organ Psychol.* 1999;72(4):441–462. http://dx.doi.org/10.1348/096317999166789
173. Jung D, Sosik J. Who are the spellbinders? Identifying personal attributes of charismatic leaders. *J Leadersh Stud.* 2010;12(4):1071–7919.
174. Aarons GA, Ehrhart MG, Farahnak LR. The Implementation Leadership Scale (ILS): development of a brief measure of unit level implementation leadership. *Implement Sci.* 2014;9(1):45. Doi:10.1186/1748-5908-9-45
175. Bass B, Avolio B. *The Multifactor Leadership Questionnaire.* Consulting Psychologists Press; 1989.
176. Jull J, Giles A, Graham ID. Community-based participatory research and integrated knowledge translation: advancing the co-creation of knowledge. *Implement Sci.* 2017;12:150. Doi:10.1186/s13012-017-0696-3
177. Leung MW, Yen IH, Minkler M. Community based participatory research: a promising approach for increasing epidemiology's relevance in the 21st century. *Int J Epidemiol.* 2004;33(3):499–506. Doi:10.1093/ije/dyh010
178. Israel BA, Schulz AJ, Parker EA, Becker AB. Review of community-based research: assessing partnership approaches to improve public health. *Annu Rev Public Health.* 1998;19:173–202. Doi:10.1146/annurev.publhealth.19.1.173
179. Goodman MS, Sanders Thompson VL. The science of stakeholder engagement in research: classification, implementation, and evaluation. *Transl Behav Med.* 2017;7(3):486–491. Doi:10.1007/s13142-017-0495-z
180. Eisman AB, Quanbeck A, Bounthavong M, Panattoni L, Glasgow RE. Implementation science issues in understanding, collecting, and using cost estimates: a multi-stakeholder perspective. *Implement Sci.* 2021;16:75. Doi:10.1186/s13012-021-01143-x
181. Windle M, Lee HD, Cherng ST, et al. From epidemiologic knowledge to improved health: a vision for translational epidemiology. *Am J Epidemiol.* 2019;188(12):2049–2060. Doi:10.1093/aje/kwz085
182. Chen EK, Reid MC, Parker SJ, Pillemer K. Tailoring evidence-based interventions for new populations: a method for program adaptation through community engagement. *Eval Health Prof.* 2013;36(1):73–92. Doi:10.1177/0163278712442536
183. Dubois JM, Bailey-Burch B, Bustillos D, et al. Ethical issues in mental health research: the case for community engagement. *Curr Opin Psychiatry.* 2011;24(3):208–214. Doi:10.1097/YCO.0b013e3283459422
184. Quinn SC. Ethics in public health research: protecting human subjects: the role of community advisory boards. *Am J Public Health.* 2004;94(6):918–922. Doi:10.2105/ajph.94.6.918

185. Ross LF, Loup A, Nelson RM, et al. The challenges of collaboration for academic and community partners in a research partnership: points to consider. *J Empir Res Hum Res Ethics.* 2010;5(1):19–31. Doi:10.1525/jer.2010.5.1.19
186. Ramanadhan S, Davis MM, Armstrong R, et al. Participatory implementation science to increase the impact of evidence-based cancer prevention and control. *Cancer Causes Control.* 2018;29(3):363–369. Doi:10.1007/s10552-018-1008-1
187. National Research Council; Committee on the Science of Team Science; Cooke NJ, Hilton ML, eds. Board on Behavioral, Cognitive, and Sensory Sciences, Division of Behavioral and Social Sciences and Education. *Enhancing the Effectiveness of Team Science.* National Academies Press; 2015. Doi:10.17226/19007
188. Courage C, Baxter K. *Understanding Your Users: A Practical Guide to User Requirements Methods, Tools, and Techniques.* Gulf Professional Publishing; 2005.
189. Roberts JP, Fisher TR, Trowbridge MJ, Bent C. A design thinking framework for healthcare management and innovation. *Healthcare.* 2016;4(1):11–14. Doi:10.1016/j.hjdsi.2015.12.002
190. Dopp AR, Parisi KE, Munson SA, Lyon AR. Aligning implementation and user-centered design strategies to enhance the impact of health services: results from a concept mapping study. *Implement Sci Commun.* 2020;1:17. Doi:10.1186/s43058-020-00020-w
191. Dopp AR, Parisi KE, Munson SA, Lyon AR. A glossary of user-centered design strategies for implementation experts. *Transl Behav Med.* 2019;9(6):1057–1064. Doi:10.1093/tbm/iby119
192. Gold HT, McDermott C, Hoomans T, Wagner TH. Cost data in implementation science: categories and approaches to costing. *Implement Sci.* 2022;17:11. Doi:10.1186/s13012-021-01172-6
193. Saldana L, Ritzwoller DP, Campbell M, Block EP. Using economic evaluations in implementation science to increase transparency in costs and outcomes for organizational decision-makers. *Implement Sci Commun.* 2022;3:40. Doi:10.1186/s43058-022-00295-1
194. Neumann PJ, Ganiats TG, Russell LB, Sanders GD, Siegel JE, eds. *Cost-Effectiveness in Health and Medicine.* 2nd ed. Oxford University Press; 2016. Doi:10.1093/acprof:oso/9780190492939.001.0001
195. BioMed Central Ltd. Economic evaluation in implementation science. 2022. Accessed May 15, 2022. https://www.biomedcentral.com/collections/EconomicEvaluation
196. Clemmer B, Haddix A. Cost-benefit analysis. In: Haddix AC, Shaffer PA, Duñet DO, eds. *Prevention Effectiveness: A Guide to Decision Analysis and Economic Evaluation.* Oxford University Press; 1996:85–102.
197. Padek MM, Mazzucca S, Allen P, et al. Patterns and correlates of mis-implementation in state chronic disease public health practice in the United States. *BMC Public Health.* 2021;21:101. doi:10.1186/s12889-020-10101-z
198. Brownson RC, Allen P, Jacob RR, et al. Understanding mis-implementation in public health practice. *Am J Prev Med.* 2015;48(5):543–551. doi:10.1016/j.amepre.2014.11.015
199. Prasad V, Ioannidis JP. Evidence-based de-implementation for contradicted, unproven, and aspiring healthcare practices. *Implement Sci.* 2014;9:1. doi:10.1186/1748-5908-9-1
200. Norton WE, Kennedy AE, Chambers DA. Studying de-implementation in health: an analysis of funded research grants. *Implement Sci.* 2017;12(1):144. doi:10.1186/s13012-017-0655-z
201. Holtrop JS, Rabin BA, Glasgow RE. Dissemination and implementation science in primary care research and practice: contributions and opportunities. *J Am Board Fam Med.* 2018;31(3):466–478. doi:10.3122/jabfm.2018.03.170259
202. Norton WE, Chambers DA. Unpacking the complexities of de-implementing inappropriate health interventions. *Implement Sci.* 2020;15:2. doi:10.1186/s13012-019-0960-9
203. Walsh-Bailey C, Tsai E, Tabak RG, et al. A scoping review of de-implementation frameworks and models. *Implement Sci.* 2021;16:100. doi:10.1186/s13012-021-01173-5
204. Schwartz AL, Landon BE, Elshaug AG, Chernew ME, McWilliams JM. Measuring low-value care in Medicare. *JAMA Intern Med.* 2014;174(7):1067–1076. doi:10.1001/jamainternmed.2014.1541
205. Colla CH. Swimming against the current—what might work to reduce low-value care? *N Engl J Med.* 2014;371(14):1280–1283. doi:10.1056/NEJMp1404503
206. Trochim WM, Cabrera DA, Milstein B, Gallagher RS, Leischow SJ. Practical challenges of systems thinking and modeling in public health. *Am J Public Health.* 2006;96(3):538–546. doi:10.2105/AJPH.2005.066001
207. Leischow SJ, Best A, Trochim WM, et al. Systems thinking to improve the public's health. *Am J Prev Med.* 2008;35(2)(suppl):S196–S203. doi:10.1016/j.amepre.2008.05.014
208. Homer JB, Hirsch GB. System dynamics modeling for public health: Background

and opportunities. *Am J Public Health.* 2006;96(3):452–458. doi:10.2105/AJPH.2005.062059

209. Currie DJ, Smith C, Jagals P. The application of system dynamics modelling to environmental health decision-making and policy—a scoping review. *BMC Public Health.* 2018;18:402. doi:10.1186/s12889-018-5318-8
210. Zimmerman L, Lounsbury DW, Rosen CS, Kimerling R, Trafton JA, Lindley SE. Participatory system dynamics modeling: increasing stakeholder engagement and precision to improve implementation planning in systems. *Adm Policy Ment Health.* 2016;43(6):834–849. doi:10.1007/s10488-016-0754-1
211. Braithwaite J, Churruca K, Long JC, Ellis LA, Herkes J. When complexity science meets implementation science: a theoretical and empirical analysis of systems change. *BMC Med.* 2018;16:63. doi:10.1186/s12916-018-1057-z
212. Lewis E, Baumann A, Gerke D, et al. Dissemination and implementation research designs toolkits. July 2017. Accessed May 15, 2022. https://cpb-us-w2.wpmucdn.com/sites.wustl.edu/dist/6/786/files/2017/07/DIRC-designs-toolkit_7-27-17-2ir4zjl.pdf
213. Luke DA, Stamatakis KA. Systems science methods in public health: dynamics, networks, and agents. *Annu Rev Public Health.* 2012;33:357–376. doi:10.1146/annurev-publhealth-031210-101222
214. Otte E, Rousseau R. Social network analysis: a powerful strategy, also for the information sciences. *J Inf Sci.* 2022;28(6):441–453. doi:10.1177/016555150202800601
215. Last J. *A Dictionary of Epidemiology.* 4th ed. Oxford University Press; 2001.
216. Reilly KL, Kennedy S, Porter G, Estabrooks P. Comparing, contrasting, and integrating dissemination and implementation outcomes included in the RE-AIM and implementation outcomes frameworks. *Front Public Health.* 2020;8:430.
217. Kraemer HC, Stice E, Kazdin A, Offord D, Kupfer D. How do risk factors work together? Mediators, moderators, and independent, overlapping, and proxy risk factors. *An J Psychiatry.* 2001;158(6):848–856. doi:10.1176/appi.ajp.158.6.848
218. Rothman KJ, Greenland S. *Modern Epidemiology.* 2nd ed. Lippincott Williams & Wilkins; 1998.
219. Lewis CC, Klasnja P, Powell BJ, et al. From classification to causality: advancing understanding of mechanisms of change in implementation science. *Front Public Health.* 2018;6:136. doi:10.3389/fpubh.2018.00136
220. Hering JG. Implementation science for the environment. *Environ Sci Technol.* 2018;52(10):5555–5560. doi:10.1021/acs.est.8b00874
221. Bauman LJ, Stein RE, Ireys HT. Reinventing fidelity: the transfer of social technology among settings. *Am J Community Psychol.* 1991;19(4):619–639. doi:10.1007/BF00937995
222. Balasubramanian BA, Heurtin-Roberts S, Krasny S, et al. Contextual factors related to implementation and reach of a pragmatic multisite trial—the My Own Health Report (MOHR) study. *J Am Board Fam Med.* 2017;30(3):337–349. doi:10.3122/jabfm.2017.03.160151
223. Rabin BA, Glasgow RE, Kerner JF, Klump MP, Brownson RC. Dissemination and implementation research on community-based cancer prevention: a systematic review. *Am J Prev Med.* 2010;38(4):443–456. doi:10.1016/j.amepre.2009.12.035
224. Victora CG, Habicht JP, Bryce J. Evidence-based public health: moving beyond randomized trials. *Am J Public Health.* 2004;94(3):400–405. doi:10.2105/ajph.94.3.400
225. Tunis SR, Stryer DB, Clancy CM. Practical clinical trials: increasing the value of clinical research for decision making in clinical and health policy. *JAMA.* 2003;290(12):1624–1632. doi:10.1001/jama.290.12.1624
226. Landes SJ, McBain SA, Curran GM. An introduction to effectiveness-implementation hybrid designs. *Psychiatry Res.* 2019;280:112513. doi:10.1016/j.psychres.2019.112513
227. Curran GM, Bauer M, Mittman B, Pyne JM, Stetler C. Effectiveness-implementation hybrid designs: combining elements of clinical effectiveness and implementation research to enhance public health impact. *Med Care.* 2012;50(3):217–226. doi:10.1097/MLR.0b013e3182408812
228. Swindle T, Curran GM, Johnson SL. Implementation science and nutrition education and behavior: opportunities for integration. *J Nutr Educ Behav.* 2019;51(6):763–774.e1. doi:10.1016/j.jneb.2019.03.001
229. Landes SJ, McBain SA, Curran GM. Reprint of: an introduction to effectiveness-implementation hybrid designs. *Psychiatry Res.* 2020;283:112630. doi:10.1016/j.psychres.2019.112630
230. Collins LM, Murphy SA, Bierman KL. A conceptual framework for adaptive preventive interventions. *Prev Sci.* 2004;5(3):185–196. doi:10.1023/B:PREV.0000037641.26017.00
231. Collins LM, Baker TB, Mermelstein RJ, et al. The multiphase optimization strategy for engineering effective tobacco use interventions. *Ann*

Behav Med. 2011;41(2):208–226. doi:10.1007/s12160-010-9253-x
232. Collins LM, Nahum-Shani I, Almirall D. Optimization of behavioral dynamic treatment regimens based on the Sequential, Multiple Assignment, Randomized Trial (SMART). *Clin Trials.* 2014;11(4):426–434. doi:10.1177/1740774514536795
233. Lei H, Nahum-Shani I, Lynch K, Oslin D, Murphy SA. A "SMART" design for building individualized treatment sequences. *Annu Rev Clin Psychol.* 2012;8:21–48. doi:10.1146/annurev-clinpsy-032511-143152
234. Nahum-Shani I, Qian M, Adams D, et al. Experimental design and primary data analysis methods for comparing adaptive interventions. *Psychol Methods.* 2012;17(4):457–477. doi:10.1037/a0029372
235. Kilbourne AM, Neumann MS, Pincus HA, Bauer MS, Stall R. Implementing evidence-based interventions in health care: application of the replicating effective programs framework. *Implement Sci.* 2007;2:42. doi:10.1186/1748-5908-2-42
236. Brown CA, Lilford RJ. The stepped wedge trial design: a systematic review. *BMC Med Res Methodol.* 2006;6:54. doi:10.1186/1471-2288-6-54
237. Beard E, Lewis JJ, Copas A, et al. Stepped wedge randomised controlled trials: systematic review of studies published between 2010 and 2014. *Trials.* 2015;16:353. doi:10.1186/s13063-015-0839-2
238. Selby JV, Beal AC, Frank L. The Patient-Centered Outcomes Research Institute (PCORI) national priorities for research and initial research agenda. *JAMA.* 2012;307(15):1583–1584. doi:10.1001/jama.2012.500
239. Nevo D, Lok JJ, Spiegelman D. Analysis of "learn-as-you-go" (LAGO) studies. *Ann Stat.* 2021;49(2):793–819. doi:10.1214/20-AOS1978
240. Glasgow R. What outcomes are the most important in translational research? Presented at: From Clinical Science to Community: The Science of Translating Diabetes and Obesity Research Conference; 2004; Bethesda, MA.
241. Damschroder LJ, Reardon CM, Opra Widerquist MA, Lowery J. Conceptualizing outcomes for use with the Consolidated Framework for Implementation Research (CFIR): the CFIR outcomes addendum. *Implement Sci.* 2022;17:7. doi:10.1186/s13012-021-01181-5
242. Brownson RC, Jacobs JA, Tabak RG, Hoehner CM, Stamatakis KA. Designing for dissemination among public health researchers: findings from a national survey in the United States. *Am J Public Health.* 2013;103(9):1693–1699. doi:10.2105/AJPH.2012.301165
243. Glasgow RE, Riley WT. Pragmatic measures: what they are and why we need them. *Am J Prev Med.* 2013;45(2):237–243. doi:10.1016/j.amepre.2013.03.010
244. Rabin BA, Purcell P, Naveed S, et al. Advancing the application, quality and harmonization of implementation science measures. *Implement Sci.* 2012;7:119. doi:10.1186/1748-5908-7-119
245. Rapport F, Clay-Williams R, Churruca K, Shih P, Hogden A, Braithwaite J. The struggle of translating science into action: foundational concepts of implementation science. *J Eval Clin Pract.* 2018;24(1):117–126. doi:10.1111/jep.12741
246. Riley WT, Glasgow RE, Etheredge L, Abernethy AP. Rapid, responsive, relevant (R3) research: a call for a rapid learning health research enterprise. *Clin Transl Med.* 2013;2(1):10. doi:10.1186/2001-1326-2-10
247. Green LW, Glasgow RE. Evaluating the relevance, generalization, and applicability of research: issues in external validation and translation methodology. *Eval Health Prof.* 2006;29(1):126–153. doi:10.1177/0163278705284445
248. Huebschmann AG, Leavitt IM, Glasgow RE. Making health research matter: a call to increase attention to external validity. *Annu Rev Public Health.* 2019;40:45–63. doi:10.1146/annurev-publhealth-040218-043945
249. Rothwell PM. External validity of randomised controlled trials: "To whom do the results of this trial apply?" *Lancet.* 2005;365(9453):82–93. doi:10.1016/S0140-6736(04)17670-8
250. Klaic M, Kapp S, Hudson P, et al. Implementability of healthcare interventions: an overview of reviews and development of a conceptual framework. *Implement Sci.* 2022;17:10. doi:10.1186/s13012-021-01171-7
251. PRECIS-2. Home page. Accessed April 15, 2022. https://www.precis-2.org/
252. Loudon K, Treweek S, Sullivan F, Donnan P, Thorpe KE, Zwarenstein M. The PRECIS-2 tool: designing trials that are fit for purpose. *BMJ.* 2015;350:h2147. doi:10.1136/bmj.h2147
253. Möhler R, Köpke S, Meyer G. Criteria for Reporting the Development and Evaluation of Complex Interventions in healthcare: revised guideline (CReDECI 2). *Trials.* 2015;16:204. doi:10.1186/s13063-015-0709-y
254. Benchimol EI, Smeeth L, Guttmann A, et al. The REporting of studies Conducted using Observational Routinely-collected health Data (RECORD) statement. *PLoS Med.* 2015;12(10):e1001885. doi:10.1371/journal.pmed.1001885

255. Bazemore A, Neale AV, Lupo P, Seehusen D. Advancing the science of implementation in primary health care. *J Am Board Fam Med.* 2018;31(3):307–311. doi:10.3122/jabfm.2018.03.180091
256. Hoffmann TC, Glasziou PP, Boutron I, et al. Better reporting of interventions: Template for Intervention Description and Replication (TIDieR) checklist and guide. *BMJ.* 2014;348:g1687. doi:10.1136/bmj.g1687
257. Nevedal AL, Reardon CM, Opra Widerquist MA, et al. Rapid versus traditional qualitative analysis using the Consolidated Framework for Implementation Research (CFIR). *Implement Sci.* 2021;16:67. doi:10.1186/s13012-021-01111-5
258. Qualitative Research in Implementation Science (QualRIS) Group. Qualitative methods in implementation science. NIH National Cancer Institute Division of Cancer Control & Population Sciences; 2018:31. Accessed April 15, 2022. https://cancercontrol.cancer.gov/sites/default/files/2020-09/nci-dccps-implementationscience-whitepaper.pdf
259. Kozica SL, Lombard CB, Harrison CL, Teede HJ. Evaluation of a large healthy lifestyle program: informing program implementation and scale-up in the prevention of obesity. *Implement Sci.* 2016;11:151. doi:10.1186/s13012-016-0521-4
260. Colón-Emeric C, Toles M, Cary MP, et al. Sustaining complex interventions in long-term care: a qualitative study of direct care staff and managers. *Implement Sci.* 2016;11:94. doi:10.1186/s13012-016-0454-y
261. Beebe J. *Rapid qualitative inquiry: a field guide to team-based assessment.* Rowman & Littlefield; 2014 Oct 23.
262. Beebe J. Basic concepts and techniques of rapid appraisal. *Hum Organ.* 1995;54(1):42–51.
263. Hamilton AB, Finley EP. Qualitative methods in implementation research: an introduction. *Psychiatry Res.* 2019;280:112516. doi:10.1016/j.psychres.2019.112516
264. Chinman M, Goldberg R, Daniels K, et al. Implementation of peer specialist services in VA primary care: a cluster randomized trial on the impact of external facilitation. *Implement Sci.* 2021;16:60. doi:10.1186/s13012-021-01130-2
265. Creswell JW, Clark VLP. *Designing and Conducting Mixed Methods Research.* 3rd ed. Sage; 2018. Accessed April 15, 2022. https://us.sagepub.com/en-us/nam/designing-and-conducting-mixed-methods-research/book241842
266. Tashakkori AM, Johnson RB, Teddlie CB. *Foundations of Mixed Methods Research: Integrating Quantitative and Qualitative Approaches in the Social and Behavioral Sciences.* 2nd ed. Sage Publications, Inc; 2021.
267. Teddlie C, Tashakkori A. Major issues and controversies in the use of mixed methods in the social and behavioral sciences. In: Tashakkori A, Teddlie C, eds. *Handbook of Mixed Methods in the Social and Behavioral Sciences.* Sage; 2003:3–50.
268. Johnson RB, Onwuegbuzie AJ. Mixed methods research: a research paradigm whose time has come. *Educ Res.* 2004;33(7):14–26. doi:10.3102/0013189X033007014
269. Tashakkori A, Teddlie C. *SAGE Handbook of Mixed Methods in Social & Behavioral Research.* 2nd ed. Sage Publications, Inc.; 2010. doi:10.4135/9781506335193
270. Whitaker RG, Sperber N, Baumgartner M, et al. Coincidence analysis: a new method for causal inference in implementation science. *Implement Sci.* 2020;15(1):108. doi:10.1186/s13012-020-01070-3
271. Ragin CC. *Redesigning Social Inquiry: Fuzzy Sets and Beyond.* University of Chicago Press; 2009. Accessed April 15, 2022. https://press.uchicago.edu/ucp/books/book/chicago/R/bo5973952.html
272. Kane H, Lewis MA, Williams PA, Kahwati LC. Using qualitative comparative analysis to understand and quantify translation and implementation. *Transl Behav Med.* 2014;4(2):201–208. doi:10.1007/s13142-014-0251-6
273. Brownson RC, Kumanyika SK, Kreuter MW, Haire-Joshu D. Implementation science should give higher priority to health equity. *Implement Sci.* 2021;16(1):28. doi:10.1186/s13012-021-01097-0
274. McGinty EE, Tormohlen KN, Barry CL, Bicket MC, Rutkow L, Stuart EA. Protocol: mixed-methods study of how implementation of US state medical cannabis laws affects treatment of chronic non-cancer pain and adverse opioid outcomes. *Implement Sci.* 2021;16(1):2. doi:10.1186/s13012-020-01071-2
275. Dopp AR. *Comparing Two Federal Financing Strategies on Treatment Penetration and Sustainment (R01DA051545).* RAND Corporation; 2022.
276. Purtle J, Peters R, Brownson RC. A review of policy dissemination and implementation research funded by the National Institutes of Health, 2007–2014. *Implement Sci.* 2016;11:1. doi:10.1186/s13012-015-0367-1
277. Brownson RC, Dodson EA, Stamatakis KA, et al. Communicating evidence-based information on cancer prevention to state-level policy

makers. *J Natl Cancer Inst.* 2011;103(4):306–316. doi:10.1093/jnci/djq529

278. Purtle J, Lê-Scherban F, Wang X, Shattuck PT, Proctor EK, Brownson RC. Audience segmentation to disseminate behavioral health evidence to legislators: an empirical clustering analysis. *Implement Sci.* 2018;13:121. doi:10.1186/s13012-018-0816-8
279. Long EC, Pugel J, Scott JT, et al. Rapid-cycle experimentation with state and federal policymakers for optimizing the reach of racial equity research. *Am J Public Health.* 2021;111(10):1768–1771. doi:10.2105/AJPH.2021.306404
280. Volden C, Ting MM, Carpenter DP. A formal model of learning and policy diffusion. *Am Polit Sci Rev.* 2008;102(3):319–332.
281. Grossback LJ, Nicholson-Crotty S, Peterson DAM. Ideology and learning in policy diffusion. *Am Politics Res.* 2004;32(5):521–545. doi:10.1177/1532673X04263801
282. Slater MD. Theory and method in health audience segmentation. *J Health Commun.* 1996;1(3):267–283. doi:10.1080/108107396128059
283. Ackrill R, Kay A. Multiple streams in EU policy-making: the case of the 2005 sugar reform. *J Eur Public Policy.* 2011;18(1):72–89. doi:10.1080/13501763.2011.520879
284. American Psychological Association. *Equity, Diversity, and Inclusion Framework.* APA; 2021. Accessed April 15, 2022. https://www.apa.org/about/apa/equity-diversity-inclusion/equity-division-inclusion-framework.pdf
285. Sterling MR, Echeverría SE, Commodore-Mensah Y, Breland JY, Nunez-Smith M. Health equity and implementation science in heart, lung, blood, and sleep-related research: emerging themes from the 2018 Saunders-Watkins leadership workshop. *Circ Cardiovasc Qual Outcomes.* 2019;12(10):e005586. doi:10.1161/CIRCOUTCOMES.119.005586
286. Woodward EN, Matthieu MM, Uchendu US, Rogal S, Kirchner JE. The health equity implementation framework: proposal and preliminary study of hepatitis C virus treatment. *Implement Sci.* 2019;14:26. doi:10.1186/s13012-019-0861-y
287. Kumanyika SK. A framework for increasing equity impact in obesity prevention. *Am J Public Health.* 2019;109(10):1350–1357. doi:10.2105/AJPH.2019.305221
288. Annie E. Casey Foundation, National Implementation Research Network. Bringing equity to implementation: incorporating community experience to improve outcomes. 2021. Accessed April 15, 2022. https://ssir.org/supplement/bringing_equity_to_implementation
289. Shelton RC, Adsul P, Oh A, Moise N, Griffith DM. Application of an antiracism lens in the field of implementation science (IS): recommendations for reframing implementation research with a focus on justice and racial equity. *Implement Res Pract.* 2021;2:26334895211049480. doi:10.1177/26334895211049482
290. Reskin B. The race discrimination system. *Annu Rev Sociol.* 2012;38:17–35. doi:10.1146/annurev-soc-071811-145508
291. Bailey ZD, Krieger N, Agénor M, Graves J, Linos N, Bassett MT. Structural racism and health inequities in the USA: evidence and interventions. *Lancet.* 2017;389(10077):1453–1463. doi:10.1016/S0140-6736(17)30569-X
292. Kwan BM, Brownson RC, Glasgow RE, Morrato EH, Luke DA. Designing for dissemination and sustainability to promote equitable impacts on health. *Annu Rev Public Health.* 2022;43:331–353. doi:10.1146/annurev-publhealth-052220-112457
293. Knoepke CE, Ingle MP, Matlock DD, Brownson RC, Glasgow RE. Dissemination and stakeholder engagement practices among dissemination & implementation scientists: results from an online survey. *PLoS One.* 2019;14(11):e0216971. doi:10.1371/journal.pone.0216971
294. Balis LE, Strayer TE, Ramalingam N, Harden SM. Beginning with the end in mind: contextual considerations for scaling-out a community-based intervention. *Front Public Health.* 2018;6. doi:10.3389/fpubh.2018.00357
295. Kotler P, Keller K. *Marketing Management.* 15th ed. Pearson; 2014.
296. Moore JE, Mascarenhas A, Bain J, Straus SE. Developing a comprehensive definition of sustainability. *Implement Sci.* 2017;12:110. doi:10.1186/s13012-017-0637-
297. Shediac-Rizkallah MC, Bone LR. Planning for the sustainability of community-based health programs: conceptual frameworks and future directions for research, practice and policy. *Health Educ Res.* 1998;13(1):87–108. doi:10.1093/her/13.1.87
298. Luke DA, Calhoun A, Robichaux CB, Elliott MB, Moreland-Russell S. The Program Sustainability Assessment Tool: a new instrument for public health programs. *Prev Chronic Dis.* 2014;11:130184. doi:10.5888/pcd11.130184
299. Scheirer M, Dearing J. An agenda for research on the sustainability of public health programs. *Am J Public Health.* 2011;101:2059–2067. doi:10.2105/AJPH.2011.300193
300. Hoelscher DM, Kelder SH, Murray N, Cribb PW, Conroy J, Parcel GS. Dissemination and adoption of the Child and Adolescent Trial for

Cardiovascular Health (CATCH): a case study in Texas. *J Public Health Manag Pract*. 2001;7(2):90–100. doi:10.1097/00124784-200107020-00012

301. Goodman RM, Steckler A. A model for the institutionalization of health promotion programs. *Fam Community Health*. 1989;11(4):63–78.
302. Johnson K, Hays C, Center H, Daley C. Building capacity and sustainable prevention innovations: a sustainability planning model. *Eval Program Plann*. 2004;27(2):135–149. doi:10.1016/j.evalprogplan.2004.01.002
303. Kislov R, Waterman H, Harvey G, Boaden R. Rethinking capacity building for knowledge mobilisation: developing multilevel capabilities in healthcare organisations. *Implement Sci*. 2014;9:166. doi:10.1186/s13012-014-0166-0
304. Leeman J, Calancie L, Hartman MA, et al. What strategies are used to build practitioners' capacity to implement community-based interventions and are they effective? A systematic review. *Implement Sci*. 2015;10(1):80. doi:10.1186/s13012-015-0272-7
305. Brownson RC, Chriqui JF, Stamatakis KA. Understanding evidence-based public health policy. *Am J Public Health*. 2009;99(9):1576–1583. doi:10.2105/AJPH.2008.156224
306. Mangham LJ, Hanson K. Scaling up in international health: what are the key issues? *Health Policy Plan*. 2010;25(2):85–96. doi:10.1093/heapol/czp066
307. Milat AJ, King L, Bauman AE, Redman S. The concept of scalability: increasing the scale and potential adoption of health promotion interventions into policy and practice. *Health Promot Int*. 2013;28(3):285–298. doi:10.1093/heapro/dar097
308. Johns B, Torres TT, WHO-CHOICE. Costs of scaling up health interventions: a systematic review. *Health Policy Plan*. 2005;20(1):1–13. doi:10.1093/heapol/czi001
309. Barker PM, Reid A, Schall MW. A framework for scaling up health interventions: lessons from large-scale improvement initiatives in Africa. *Implement Sci*. 2016;11:12. doi:10.1186/s13012-016-0374-x
310. Aarons GA, Sklar M, Mustanski B, Benbow N, Brown CH. "Scaling-out" evidence-based interventions to new populations or new health care delivery systems. *Implement Sci*. 2017;12:111. doi:10.1186/s13012-017-0640-6
311. Mclaughlin M, Duff J, Sutherland R, Campbell E, Wolfenden L, Wiggers J. Protocol for a mixed methods process evaluation of a hybrid implementation-effectiveness trial of a scaled-up whole-school physical activity program for adolescents: Physical Activity 4 Everyone (PA4E1). *Trials*. 2020;21:268. doi:10.1186/s13063-020-4187-5
312. Chambers DA, Glasgow RE, Stange KC. The dynamic sustainability framework: addressing the paradox of sustainment amid ongoing change. *Implement Sci*. 2013;8:117. doi:10.1186/1748-5908-8-117

SECTION 2

Theory and Conceptual Foundations

3

Historical Roots of Dissemination and Implementation Science

JAMES W. DEARING, KERK F. KEE, AND TAI-QUAN PENG

INTRODUCTION

The science of dissemination and implementation (D&I) has been driven by new media, the interests of philanthropies and the needs of government agencies, and the persistent and growing applied problems that have been addressed but not solved by basic scientists in disciplines such as psychology, sociology, and political science. D&I science is being shaped by researchers in the professional and applied fields of study, including public health, health services, communication, marketing, education, criminal justice, and social work.

Research about D&I is a response to a general acknowledgment that successful, effective practices, programs, policies, and technologies resulting from clinical and community trials, demonstration projects, and community-based research as conducted by researchers very often do not affect the services that clinical staff, community service providers, and other practitioners fashion and provide to residents, clients, patients, and populations at risk. In any one sector or occupation (populated, e.g., by oncologists, or public health department directors or city-level parks and recreation planners), the state of the science (what researchers collectively know) and the state of the art (what practitioners collectively do) often coexist autonomously, each realm of activity having little effect on the other.

Dissemination science is the study of how evidence-based practices, programs, policies, and technologies (evidence-based interventions, EBIs) can best be communicated or spread to potential adopters and implementers to produce adoption and effective and sustained use. A *potential adopter* is someone targeted by a change agency to make a decision about whether to try a practice, program, policy, or technology that they perceive to be new (i.e., an *innovation*). While some dissemination activity is directed at individuals who are themselves at risk of disease or injury, such as people who ingest the synthetic opioid fentanyl knowingly or unknowingly, many dissemination efforts carried out by change agencies are aimed at intermediaries who serve people at risk, such as social workers, nurses, radiologists, and elementary schoolteachers. And in some dissemination efforts, adoption decisions and implementation activity are needed at multiple levels—that of the service provider(s) and of the person at risk—for an intervention to function effectively. The science of dissemination is the science of a special type of communication in which messages concern interventions that have been designed to improve conditions and for which there is reason to believe that those interventions are both internally valid (they work) and externally valid (they work well enough across settings, populations, and times).

The idea of *implementation science* has evolved to represent a study of the uptake and integration of EBIs within a particular setting (e.g., a school or worksite). Unlike dissemination science, which sometimes focuses solely on individuals at risk in order to inform and persuade them, implementation science concerns organizations, frequently complex organizations with countervailing agendas and interests, sophisticated stakeholder relations, imperfect coordination across divisions and

James W. Dearing, Kerk F. Kee, and Tai-Quan Peng, *Historical Roots of Dissemination and Implementation Science* In: *Dissemination and Implementation Research in Health*. Edited by: Ross C. Brownson, Graham A. Colditz, and Enola K. Proctor, Oxford University Press. © Oxford University Press 2023.
DOI: 10.1093/oso/9780197660690.003.0003

offices, constant employee churn, and evolution after evolution of information technology such as we experience in medical centers as researchers and—sometimes—as patients. For many of us, this is the trick: how to design an intervention that will achieve our objectives for it as an EBI and then somehow survive with an acceptable degree of robustness across multiple organizations of a type, in settings where it is implemented and subjected to the reality of everyday practice conditions (e.g., precious little time, competing demands, reduced budgets, imperfect information, and most importantly, patients in need). While some implementation scientists train their sights on this external validity objective, a smaller proportion of implementation researchers concern themselves with postimplementation behavior among practitioners, years after the vast majority of grants have ended.

An *implementer* is someone who will change his or her behavior to use an innovation in practice. In organizations, the people who make the decision to adopt an innovation are often not the users of innovations. The extent and quality of implementation and client or constituent responses to it have become dependent variables of study that are more important than initial adoption. Implementation researchers are increasingly studying sustainability, which may be even more important than implementation.

So, D&I science is a broad and colorful palette with which public health and health services researchers and practitioners can conceptualize research by posing rather different but perhaps equally fascinating questions, such as

- For a given innovation, does the change agency target organizations that serve people at greatest risk/highest need? Is equity a central determinant of which intermediaries receive the most technical assistance, or does the change agency simply target convenient or familiar organizations with which they've collaborated before?
- Does the change agency develop messages about the new program based on systematic formative evaluation?
- To what extent does the change agency strategically consider *when* to introduce the new program or do they just disseminate information as it becomes available?
- What is the competition for attention from the proponents of other similar programs, and how does this change over time?
- What proportion of organizations targeted with dissemination messages respond by contacting the change agency for more information?
- How many try the new program (which might qualify them as adopters) of all those targeted (a measure of *reach*)?
- Was the program truly new conceptually to decision makers in the adopting organizations, or were they already experimenting with similar programs?
- Do some organizations invest resources in adoption (taking the time to learn about the program, pay licensing fees, attend trainings, order booklets and train-the-trainer materials, become certified as coaches, etc.) but then never implement the program? And why?
- What proportion of adopting organizations actually offer the program but then discontinue it? And why?
- How many organizations stay in a holding pattern of adopting/not implementing/not discontinuing? And why?
- What proportion of implementers offer the program as its designers intended with the same content, same number of modules, same behavior stimuli, same support, and checks on enrollee or client performance?
- What types of adaptations to the program are made by implementers? Do they offer all of the program's core components? Are they true to the program's theory of behavior change? Do they drop some components, customize others, and/or create their own to better suit their organization and their clients? Does the design/research team pay attention to adaptations by implementers for the purpose of reinventing future iterations of the program on the basis of expert practitioner input?
- Does the implementing organization change in ways unanticipated by the program designers? Does learning the one program serve as a trigger or

precipitating event for organizational decision makers to adopt other consonant or complementary public health programs?
- Do implementers think they are offering the program as the designers intended but, in practice, do something quite different?
- Can a less expensive version of an EBI provide nearly as much benefit but to a wider range of beneficiaries than a version with all the bells and whistles?
- What is the client or enrollee yield? How many individuals sign up? How many complete all modules or classes? How many people actually do the variety of behavior changes—wearing pedometers, meeting in groups, writing in diaries, coming to class, completing their workbook, monitoring their progress—as suggested (and tested in efficacy trials) by the program designers?
- Is the public health program sustained by the organization? Do clients or enrollees also continue their participation? Is fidelity or adaptation a better predictor of sustainability?
- What are the individual outcomes (weight loss, muscle tone, etc.) and public health impacts (e.g., proportion of obese people in intervention communities)?
- How can implementers identify opinion leaders who are looked to by others for advice and as an example for practice improvement?
- How can cutting-edge computational approaches help health researchers understand public attention and emotion toward health issues and EBIs?

Dissemination and implementation science merges the objective of system-wide or sector-wide improvement with the study of complex organizations. For example, public health researchers or practitioners can encourage many county public health departments to adopt a new disease prevention program (a dissemination study objective) while preparing to support and assess what is done with the program in a random sample of all adopting departments (an implementation study objective). And cascades of adoptions, clustered together in time, can beget whole systems change in healthcare and public health.[1] A key, we suggest, is the stimulation of or tapping into intrinsic motivation of the staff in public health, healthcare, and other types of organizations and among their clients and program enrollees in communities. Certain innovations are met with enthusiasm, open arms, and eager learners who go on to champion new programs and advocate them to others. Innovations spread rapidly when people want and can access them and can then implement them to good effect.

Where does the emphasis on D&I science come from? How are new media altering the spread of new practices, programs, and beliefs? We turn to the diffusion of innovations paradigm to address these questions. In the health domain, a diffusionist lens blends the imperative of translation with the social attractiveness of imitative behavior and that which is fashionably new.[2]

THE CLASSICAL DIFFUSION PARADIGM

Diffusion is the process through which an innovation is communicated through certain channels over time among the members of a social system.[3] Health services and public health researchers are actively applying diffusion concepts to understand and affect the spread of EBIs[4] through structured efforts at improvement, by accounting for and explaining adaptations at implementing sites, by emphasizing user rationalities, or a combination of these logics.[5] For example, Munro and colleagues,[6] through semistructured interviews, showed how the attributes of innovations, system readiness, and the relationships among adopters affected the uptake of mifepristone, an abortion pill, by Canadian pharmacists in the context of an integrated knowledge translation effort that emphasized engagement and feedback. As a social process that may occur among the members of a system such as a professional association, a community of practice, an organization, or a neighborhood, diffusion is a potential product of organized and intentional D&I support activity: We disseminate EBIs hoping to trigger a diffusion effect among actual and potential adopters and implementers.

Diffusion studies have demonstrated a mathematically consistent sigmoid pattern (the S-shaped curve) of adoption over time for innovations that are perceived to be

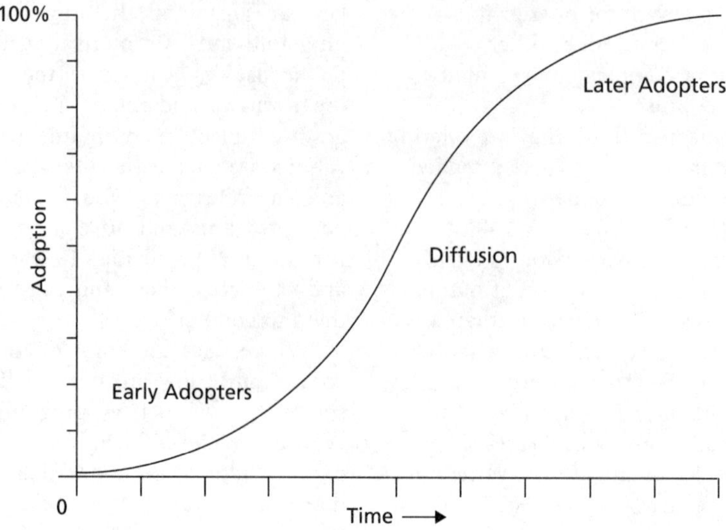

FIGURE 3.1 The generalized cumulative curve that describes the curvilinear process of the diffusion of innovations.

consequential by potential adopters, when the decisions to adopt are voluntary as opposed to them being compulsory, and with attendant logically related propositions, qualifying this literature as a theory of social change.[7] The "S" shape is due to the engagement of informal opinion leaders in talking about and modeling the innovation for others to hear about and see in action (Figure 3.1). For any given consequential innovation, the rate of adoption tends to begin slowly, accelerate because of the activation of positive word of mouth communication and social modeling by the 5% to 8% of social system members who are sources of advice (i.e., opinion leaders) for subsequent other adopters, and then slow as system potential is approached. Box 3.1 provides a summary of the evolving opinion leader research for D&I interventions.

Key components of diffusion theory are as follows:

1. Key components of diffusion theory are the *innovation* and especially potential adopter perceptions of its *attributes* of cost, effectiveness, compatibility, simplicity, observability, and trialability (see Table 3.1);
2. The *adopter*, especially each adopter's degree of *innovativeness* (earliness relative to others in adopting the innovation);
3. The *social system*, such as a geographic community, a distributed network of collaborators, a professional association, or a province or state, especially in terms of the *structure* of the system, its informal *opinion leaders*, and potential adopter perception of *social pressure* to adopt;
4. The *individual adoption process*, a stage-ordered model of awareness, persuasion, decision, implementation, and continuation[25];
5. The *diffusion system*, especially an external *change agency* and its paid *change agents*, who, if well trained, correctly seek out and intervene with the client system's opinion leaders and paraprofessional aides and support the enthusiasm of unpaid emergent innovation champions.

Diffusion occurs through a combination of (1) the need for individuals to reduce personal uncertainty when presented with information about an innovation, (2) the need for individuals to respond to their perceptions of what specific credible others are thinking and doing, and (3) the general felt social pressure to do as others have done. Uncertainty in response to an innovation typically leads to a search for information and, if the potential adopter believes the innovation to be interesting and with the potential for

BOX 3.1

EVOLVING OPINION LEADER

RESEARCH FOR D&I INTERVENTIONS

Opinion leaders are individuals who exert a disproportionate amount of influence on the decisions of others[8] within a social system. They can play important roles in the diffusion of creative ideas, innovative products, and new practices. Although the conceptualization of opinion leaders is rather clear, the empirical identification of opinion leaders has proven nontrivial.[9] In the past, self-reported individual attributes, such as education degree, social-economic status, and trustworthiness, were employed to measure individuals' opinion leadership. However, such attribute-based measurement does not fully capture the influence-susceptible relationship between opinion leaders and followers, which is central to Rogers and Cartano's conceptualization of opinion leaders.[10] Advances in network science can be combined with marketing approaches to help D&I researchers identify and intervene with opinion leaders for health.[11]

Individual persons or groups in a social system are considered network nodes that can be connected with one another via multiple types of links based on their similarities, social relations, interactions, or flows.[12] Such networks can be examined at the macro level to discover statistical regularities, at the meso level to reveal structural organizations, and at the micro level to uncover the positions occupied by individuals in a social system.[13] Micro-level analysis can allow researchers or practitioners to identify who is better connected in a social system and who is less so. Individuals in better connected positions have greater influence than those in poorly connected positions,[14] as the latter is dependent on the former for valued resources (e.g., knowledge, evaluation, and investment). Network science provides an array of centrality metrics to quantify the "better connected" positions, including degree centrality, closeness centrality, betweenness centrality, and eigenvector centrality.[15–17] More on network science is found in chapter 13.

These four network metrics have been used separately or in combination to identify opinion leaders for various health issues (e.g., obesity, HIV/AIDS, and smoking) among the general public,[18,19] medical professionals,[20] and specific groups of patients.[21] Albalawi and Sixsmith[18] employed the degree centrality of Twitter users to identify which users have the potential to raise awareness of health issues and advocate for health in Saudi Arabia. They identified 100 accounts with the greatest potential to influence, including religious men/women, traditional media, commercial companies, sports-related accounts, politically related accounts, and health accounts. Holliday et al.[19] developed a peer support network among high school students in the United Kingdom and employed the degree, closeness, and betweenness centrality metrics to identify and engage opinion leaders.

In addition to these four centrality metrics, network scientists have developed more sophisticated algorithms to identify opinion leaders in social networks, such as the stability-sensitivity method,[22] the path-counting method,[23] and VoteRank.[24] These metrics and algorithms can be applied in D&I science to help researchers and practitioners better understand, detect, and engage opinion leaders, which can facilitate the diffusion of ideas and practices among certain populations.

benefits, a search for evaluative judgments of trusted and respected others (informal opinion leaders). This advice-seeking behavior is a heuristic that allows the decision maker to avoid comprehensive information seeking, reflecting Herbert Simon's seminal insight about the importance of everyday constraints in "bounding" the rationality of our decision-making.[26]

TABLE 3.1 CLASSIC INNOVATION ATTRIBUTES, THEIR DEFINITIONS, AND APPLICATION TO THE CONTEXT OF PUBLIC HEALTH AND HEALTHCARE DELIVERY[a]

Innovation Attributes	Definitions	Application to Public Health and Healthcare Delivery
Cost	Perceived cost of adopting and implementing an innovation	How much time and effort are required to learn to use the innovation and routinize its use? How long does recouping of costs take?
Effectiveness	The extent to which the innovation works better than that which it will displace	Does a gain in performance outweigh the downsides of cost? Do different stakeholders agree on the superiority of the innovation?
Simplicity	How simple the innovation is to understand	How easy is an evidence-based program for adopters/implementers to understand and/or if it requires a steep learning curve and much training before actual implementation?
Compatibility	The fit of the innovation to established ways of accomplishing the same goal	How much/little would an evidence-based program disrupt the existing routine and/or workflow of the adopting/implementing organization?
Observability	The extent to which outcomes can be seen	How much and/or how quickly will the results of an evidence-based program become visible to an implementing organization, its clients, funders, and peer organizations?
Trialability	The extent to which the adopter must commit to full adoption	If an evidence-based program can be implemented as a pilot project without much investment and be abandoned without incurring much sunk cost?

[a]Application of diffusion principles to policy D&I is covered in chapter 24.

Needs or motivations differ among people according to their degree of innovativeness (earliness in adoption relative to others): The first 2.5% to adopt (*innovators*) tend to do so because of novelty and having little to lose; the next 13.5% to adopt (*early adopters*, including the subset of about 5% to 7% informal opinion leaders) do so because of an appraisal of the innovation's attributes; the subsequent 34% of early majority adopters and 34% of late majority adopters do so because others have done so. They come to believe that adoption is the right thing to do (an imitative effect rather than a carefully reasoned rational judgment). The last 16% to adopt do so grudgingly with reservations. Their recalcitrance is sometimes later proved to be well justified since new programs can have undesirable consequences.

One's orientation to an innovation and time of adoption are related to and can be predicted by each adopter's structural position in the network of relations that tie a social system such as a school, community, or even a far-flung professional network together. When viewed sociometrically (especially who-seeks-advice-from-whom within a social network) in two-dimensional space, the pattern of diffusion begins on the periphery of a network as the first to try the innovation then experiment with it; central members of the network—informal opinion leaders who are a special subset of early adopters—then adopt if they judge the innovation to have important advantages over current practices; the many others then follow, who pay attention to what these sociometrically central and highly connected network members do and advise.[27] This outside-inside-outward progression of adoption, when graphed as the cumulative number of adoptions over time, reflects an S-shaped diffusion curve (Figure 3.1).

Forefathers of the Diffusion Model

The French judge cum sociologist Gabriel Tarde explained diffusion as a societal-level phenomenon of social change in his 1902 book, *The Laws of Imitation*, including the identification of an S-shaped curve in cumulative adoptions over time, the role of conversation in producing mimicry, and the importance of informal opinion leaders in jumpstarting the S-shaped curve. As a judge, Tarde had taken note of the way people coming before the bench used new slang and wore new clothing fashions as if on cue. In Germany at the same time, Georg Simmel, a political philosopher, was writing about how individual thought and action were structured by the set of interpersonal relations to which a person was subject. Tarde's perspective was the forerunner for the macro, social system perspective on diffusion as the means by which cultures and societies changed and progressed. Simmel's contribution, explicated in his book, *Conflict: The Web of Group Affiliations*, was the forerunner for understanding how social network position affects what individuals do in reaction to innovations and when. Together, these perspectives provided an explanation for how system-level effects pressured the individual to adopt new things and how individuals can effect change through their relationships in social networks.

Following Tarde and Simmel, European anthropologists seized on diffusion as a means to explain the continental drift of people, ideas, means of social organization, and primitive technologies. American anthropologists such as Alfred Kroeber in the 1920s also conducted historical studies, but they confined their analyses—for the first time called *diffusion* study—to more discrete innovations in smaller social systems, such as a community or a region of the country. Anthropologists studying diffusion focused on not only spread of innovations but also how cultures in turn shaped those innovations[28] by giving them new purposes and by adapting them to suit local needs—the beginnings of what we now call implementation science. The studies of these early diffusion researchers encouraged sociologists to take up diffusion work in contemporary 1920s and 1930s society, focusing on informal communication in friendship or social support networks as an explanation for the city-to-rural spread of innovations, the importance of jurisdictions as barriers to diffusion, and the importance of proximity to the spread of ideas.[28] And diffusion was not only understood as a one-way process: The American sociologist Pitirim Sorokin saw diffusion as inherently recursive. More developed countries extract raw materials from developing countries and sent back finished goods; classical music composers, for example, absorbed ideas from folk tunes into the creation of symphonies.[29] Public health and healthcare can also be interpreted recursively: Epidemiologic data about communities and practice-based research results are "diffused" to researchers, who develop new public health and healthcare interventions and seek to disseminate them back to those same practitioner systems and communities.[30]

A landmark event for diffusion science occurred in 1943 with a report on the diffusion of hybrid seed corn in two Iowa communities.[31] This seminal article set the paradigm for many hundreds of future diffusion studies by emphasizing individuals as the locus of decision, adoption as the key dependent variable, a centralized innovation change agency that employed change agents, and the importance of different communication channels for different purposes at different times in the individual innovation-decision process. The Ryan and Gross article propelled diffusion study to center stage among rural sociologists. It also made the application of diffusion concepts a key set of tools in the work of agricultural extension agents. Rural sociologists were closely wedded to the extension services for funding and for providing the distribution system by which diffusion study ideas could be tested. The academics were practice oriented. From 1954 to 1969, key faculty in the Iowa State University Department of Sociology gave an estimated 600 presentations about the diffusion process, many to extension service groups. In 1958 alone, there were 35 publications reporting diffusion data collected in the United States by rural sociologists. Six years later, rural sociology publications about diffusion in less developed countries reached a peak of 20.[32] Diffusion studies by rural sociologists began to wane in 1969, but by that time scholars in sociology, medical sociology, education, communication, and public health had begun diffusion research, such as Coleman, Katz, and Menzel's classic study of physician's drug-prescribing behavior as a result of social network ties.[33]

Synthesizing the Diffusion Paradigm

The diffusion of innovations paradigm began to synthesize its approaches, central challenges, and lessons learned beginning in the 1960s. Internationally, an "invisible college" of rural sociologists based in the American Midwest had formed, drawn together both by intellectual questions and funding opportunities for research into a coauthorship, collaborative, and competitive network.[34] As these questions were answered by rural sociologists, diffusion research became fashionable to scholars in other disciplines and fields, who conceptualized somewhat different problems, especially concerning policymakers as adopters and the conditions of innovation and spread in complex organizations. Yet diversification did not limit the centrality of diffusion scholarship as it importantly related to the growing paradigms of knowledge utilization and technology transfer studies and then to the evidence-based medicine movement.[35]

Everett M. Rogers, trained as a rural sociologist at Iowa State University, defended his dissertation in 1957 after growing up poor on an Iowa farm.[36,37] While the dissertation was ostensibly about the diffusion of 2-4-D weed spray among farmers, Rogers's real interest was in drawing generalizations that he believed were warranted on the basis of commonalities he had discovered by reading diffusion studies being published in different fields. The authors of the studies were not aware that other researchers were studying diffusion in fields different from theirs. Rogers expanded his literature review into the 1962 seminal book, *Diffusion of Innovations*, synthesizing what was known about diffusion in general terms. His modeling of diffusion as an over-time social process and, at the individual level, as a series of stages that a person passes through in relation to an innovation would soon come to be recognized across fields of study as the diffusion of innovations paradigm. Though Rogers[38] would remain for decades the single most recognizable name associated with the diffusion of innovations, many other scholars were studying diffusion. And many diffusion scholars took a slightly different approach than Rogers. Many of these scholars were former students and colleagues of his; their contributions continue to push the paradigm forward and outward. In particular, some working in the paradigm took a macro structural perspective on diffusion, especially those in population planning, demography, economics, and international relations. Anthropologists studying the spread of culture and linguists studying the spread of language also preferred a structural perspective on diffusion, which conceptualized waves of innovations washing over societies. To these structuralists, the study of diffusion was the study of social change writ large. For them, units of adoption are countries or cultures.

This macro orientation to diffusion was highly enticing to scholars because of its deductive and parsimonious potential based in a simple mathematical law of nature that describes a logistic (S-shaped or exponential) growth curve. Marketing scientists, epidemiologists, demographers, and political scientists instantly appreciated the predictive potential and eloquence of the population perspective on diffusion. Mathematical modeling formed the basis of this work, most of which continues today in fields such as family planning apart from more qualitatively informed micro-level studies of diffusion.[39]

A major part of Rogers's contribution was in persuasively showing how macro-level processes of system change could be linked to micro-level behavior. These ideas harkened back to Simmel and Tarde: Individuals were influenced by system norms, and system structure and rules were the cumulative results of individual actions. Diffusion was one of the very few social theories that persuasively linked macro- with micro-level phenomena.

KNOWLEDGE UTILIZATION AND TECHNOLOGY TRANSFER

The agricultural extension model, with its basis in the training of social change concepts to full-time staff who were experts in areas such as cherry blight, zebra mussel eradication, and pine beetle control, was critical to the popularity of the diffusion of innovations paradigm. It was also important in the genesis of two closely related bodies of research. *Knowledge utilization* has been a robust paradigm for 50 years; its central problem was not how a new practice came to be voluntarily adopted by many people, but rather how knowledge in the form of prior results of a social program (the effectiveness of school busing, of curbside recycling, or of business enterprise zones in cities) affected the subsequent decisions of elected representatives and policy staff in government. This is another route to social change, one that relies more on policy action by formal authorities followed by the compulsory adoptions of others than the traditional diffusion attention to informal influence. Were ineffective programs phased out by policymakers while effective programs were replicated and expanded? Did the social and education programs that managed to spread across the American states deserve to spread? The key intellectual contributor to this paradigm was the education policy scholar, Carol H. Weiss.[40] Weiss's studies of policy decision-making showed that rational expectations between evidence and program continuation/expansion were not supported by social science study. And beyond the expectation of a rational outcomes-to-funding relationship, Weiss and other knowledge utilization researchers of the policymaking process showed that any direct program evaluation-to-policy decision link was rare; rather, policymaking was inherently political.[41] Many more factors besides evidence of program effectiveness factored into decision-making.[42] When program evidence did affect subsequent decisions by policymakers, it did so through circuitous cumulative learning by policymakers and staff as they became "enlightened" over time in terms of general programming lessons. In a gradual, accretionary way, indirect and partial knowledge diffusion did occur.

From the perspective of knowledge utilization, Blake and Ottoson[43] maintained that dissemination is the process of moving information from one source to another (as from program evaluators to policymakers), and the ultimate purpose of dissemination should be utilization by users. When utilization by users is achieved, information/knowledge has impact. This perspective has evolved with the field of knowledge utilization studies, through "waves" of research from the empirical studies in the 1940s by rural sociologists to studies of international development and family planning in the 1970s, to research in the 1990s about how research could improve human services in health and education.[44,45]

Researchers studying *technology transfer* identified a different problem. Beginning with Mansfield in the 1960s, scholars such as Leonard-Barton and von Hippel focused on the firm, especially complex organizations such as multinational corporations that partly by virtue of their size exhibited problems of coordination, knowledge sharing, and even knowing what was going on across its many divisions let alone having a managerial system for knowing which practices were more effective than others.[46] Whereas diffusion was about innovations that usually began with a single source and then spread broadly, technology transfer was one to one or "point to point." How can an innovative workflow redesign or unit-based team approach to scheduling that produces huge productivity gains in Argentina be applied to improve the same company's productivity in Canada? What sorts of adaptation might be necessary?[47]

Contrary to the technology transfer label, Dunn, Holzener, and Zaltman[48(p120)] argued that: "Knowledge use is transactive. Although one may use the analogy of 'transfer,' knowledge is never truly marketed, transferred or exchanged. Knowledge is really negotiated between the parties involved." Similarly, Estabrooks and colleagues[49(p28)] clarified that the Canadian Institutes of Health Research defines knowledge translation as the "exchange, synthesis and ethically sound application of knowledge—within a complex system of interactions among researchers and users." In other words, the notions of transaction, negotiation, interactions, and synthesis are key to the conceptualization of transfer (and dissemination/diffusion) of information/knowledge from producers to users. In health research and organizational technology transfer, one needs to understand what is being transferred, by whom, to which targets, through what process, and with what outcomes.[50] So, effective transfer has knowledge utilization at its core.[42]

EVIDENCE-BASED MEDICINE AND EVIDENCE-BASED PUBLIC HEALTH

Literatures about diffusion of innovations, knowledge utilization, and technology transfer have found new application and expansion in the fields of medicine and public health. *Evidence-based medicine* is the conscientious, explicit, and judicious use of current best evidence in making decisions about the care of individual patients. The practice of evidence-based medicine means integrating individual clinical expertise with the best available external clinical evidence from systematic research.[51]

Evidence-based medicine is an approach to medical practice that emphasizes the role of research literature (new information, latest knowledge), usually in the form of clinical practice or medical guidelines (increasingly based on comparative effectiveness research) over prior training and clinical experiences such that each becomes an input in decision-making about each particular patient's health. Although evidence-based medicine has been controversial among some medical professionals[52] and somewhat misunderstood as a movement to displace traditional practices in medicine, advocates[53] argue for augmentation rather than displacement. Clinical epidemiology, for example, has become infused with evidence-based knowledge generation, rapid critical appraisal of evidence, efficient storage and retrieval, and evidence synthesis.[54] When all four components are effectively practiced, the quality of patient care increases.

The desire for valid and generalizable evidence to inform decisions also has been applied to the domain of public health. Brownson and colleagues[55] proposed the following attributes as key to defining evidence-based public health: (1) Decisions are guided by best available peer-reviewed evidence and literature from a range of methodologies; (2) evidence-based public health approaches systematically make use of data and information systems; (3) its practice frameworks for program planning come from theories rooted in behavioral science; (4) the community of users are involved in processes of decision-making and assessment; (5) evidence-based public health approaches carry out sound evaluation of programs; and (6) lessons learned are shared with stakeholder groups and decision makers. Simmons, Fajans, and Ghiron[56] additionally emphasized contextual factors as key in matching practice refinements to local conditions.

During the dissemination of evidence-based practices, we believe that it is useful to consider the interplay between the technical rationalities of knowledge producers or change agencies and users' narrative rationalities, whether those users are patients and community members or healthcare providers and public health professionals. Technical rationalities are based on logics that are predictive, instructive, and technocratic, while narrative rationalities are stories of experiences that are interpretive, contextual, and dynamic.[56] Narratives can be illuminating to program planners as well as inform ongoing attempts to improve care and public health practice.[57,58] Collectively, these two perspectives represent the state of the science (what researchers collectively know) and the state of the art (what practitioners and policymakers collectively do). New media and emerging technologies can facilitate the access to and use of both technical rationalities (guideline content) and narrative rationalities (e.g., clinical practitioners' perspectives about how they have implemented such guidance given the realities of their practices).

NEW (AND NEWER) MEDIA

What are the effects of new information and communication technologies on dissemination activities by change agencies, the social diffusion processes that may result as potential adopters consider an innovation, and how implementation in organizations unfolds?

Collective knowledge of the diffusion of innovations paradigm has given way to a focus on those paradigmatic concepts that can be operationalized in purposive tests of how to best disseminate and implement evidence-based health practices, programs, and policies.[59] This has long been an objective in trying to spread effective innovations for improved global health as well as for domestic healthcare and public health.[60,61] New media, in the ways in which they affect the dissemination of information by change agencies, the subsequent diffusion process among targeted adopters, and the resultant critical stage of implementation of evidence-based practices in organizations, are iteratively changing how we work and how targeted adopters respond to change initiatives. D&I researchers and practitioners are well advised to be agile.

The traditional notion of an innovation as predesigned by centralized change agents is increasingly inaccurate. Increasingly, innovations are malleable and coproduced by researchers, practitioners, and those persons who adopt them, whether the researchers in question have this intention or not. Such a perspective on change has the advantage of enabling learning from those persons who are best positioned to make insightful and applicable real-time improvements to an innovation: users themselves.[62] This shift in emphasis to utilization by users would wed source perspectives on change with those of innovation users-as-creators. Utilization properly involves both the logics of innovation producers and the experiential expertise of users who are sensitized to issues of context and the everyday reality of compatibility.

Technologies can facilitate information access and knowledge creation in the context of dissemination. In terms of information access, it is clear that information technologies and certain new media accelerate our ability to disseminate information worldwide.[63] Do they also accelerate diffusion (i.e., resultant decision-making) among those healthcare and public health practitioners whom we sometimes try to reach and affect?[64] Technologies increase the dissemination of knowledge about innovations and expand reach in terms of health promotion,[65] disease prevention,[66] health compliance, telehealth,[67,68] and cybermedicine.[69] Technologies allow easy access to new information and latest knowledge via specialized knowledge management systems (e.g., medical literature databases), which healthcare providers can use to inform their medical practice, and general knowledge management systems (e.g., public web-based search engines) to help patients make better health-related choices in life.[70]

Furthermore, technologies may intensify the diffusion process among connected adopters whom change agents may target for change,[71] including tapping their weak ties and strong ties,[72] and designing strategic messages to drive views, comments, and shares on social media.[73] Traditionally and still today, diffusion is facilitated by mass media and interpersonal networks among people. In today's wired societies and more specifically in our networked market segments that are organized by common interests and professions, new media create new online social communities that are critical to the facilitation of information knowledge dissemination beyond geographically/temporally bound communities of the past. Technologies intensify the dissemination process by elevating social media platforms and their amateur broadcasters as well as new networks among people who do not know each other except through online communities[74] to an emerging position of intermediary, thus giving information/knowledge another push for dissemination throughout social systems.[75]

In terms of knowledge creation, technologies are enabling new and expanded professional networks among healthcare providers and public health professionals, leading to interorganizational sharing and cross-fertilization of information and knowledge about common challenges.[76] New media make coproduction of knowledge between producers and users easier to achieve because of the low cost and high speed for feedback and ongoing communication.[77] Technologies support automatic and cumulative data acquisition (including electronic medical records in healthcare organizations and online data mining) for computations and analyses that, in turn, can produce more knowledge. In this way, the use of technologies demonstrates Sorokin's view that diffusion is inherently recursive. We surmise that if potential adopters of innovations feel that they have been involved in the creation of or refinement of an innovation, their adoption and implementation is more likely. If new media lead to the experience of broader participation in knowledge creation, then those media will stimulate not only dissemination but also diffusion among adopters. Box 3.2 provides a summary of applications of computational social science to D&I research in health.

BOX 3.2

APPLICATIONS OF COMPUTATIONAL SOCIAL SCIENCE TO D&I RESEARCH IN HEALTH

Computational social science (CSS) has penetrated health research due to widely available massive ("BIG") data sets and increasingly sophisticated computational methods.[78] The computational paradigm has triggered the creativity of researchers from different disciplines (e.g., computer science, physics, communication and epidemiology) to examine health phenomena at an unprecedented scale. These CSS methods can identify targets for D&I strategies and aid in evaluation of such efforts.

Among the most visible application of CSS in public health is the forecasting of disease outbreaks with search query data. Ginsberg et al.[78] tracked the search volumes of 45 influenza-related queries at Google and found that the searching trends of these queries could alert the general public to flu pandemics earlier than could government statistics from the Centers for Disease Control and Prevention in the United States. Although recent studies found that Google search trends would overestimate the epidemic degree of influenza in the United States,[79,80] this study has prompted scholars to apply query data to monitor the trends of various diseases, such as dengue,[81] stroke,[82] tuberculosis,[83] and COVID-19 pandemic.[84,85] Researchers were also inspired to employ data from other social media platforms (e.g., Twitter) for influenza surveillance.[86] Such surveillance and forecasting of specific diseases is of great significance for public health professionals who can send timely alerts to the public and prepare adequate resources to address outbreaks.

Another notable application of CSS in health is the mining of voluminous textual information on the Internet to understand and monitor how the public thinks about and feels toward health issues. By combining manual content analysis and automatic text-mining algorithms, researchers analyzed information collected from various online sources (e.g., Twitter, blogs, and news) to understand public confidence toward vaccination,[87] discover major themes underlying public discussion about measles[88] and Zika,[89] and examine public sentiment toward depression and anxiety disorder.[90] User-generated content on Twitter has been employed to capture a pulse of mental health in communities throughout the COVID-19 pandemic, which led to considerable stress and anxiety among the public over a very extended period of time.[91]

The "always-on, always-on-you" quality of mobile technologies[92] has brought significant transformations to many practices in public health, which has resulted in the emergence of mobile health as an EBI.[93] Individuals, regardless of their individual characteristics, have adopted mobile health applications to seek health information, track daily workouts, manage chronic health conditions, and make medical appointments.[94] The real-time geographical information captured by mobile devices has played a significant role in tracking the origin and spread of the COVID-19 pandemic[95,96] and in evaluating the effectiveness and consequences of lockdown measures during the COVID-19 pandemic.[97,98]

A fourth application of CSS in public health is to investigate how offline and online social connections among individuals may lead to the diffusion of health behaviors. By creatively utilizing several large-scale longitudinal data sets, Nicholas Christakis, James Fowler, and their colleagues[99–102] conducted a series of studies to investigate how a specific health phenomenon (e.g., obesity, smoking, alcohol consumption, drug use, and depression) can spread across network ties. Researchers have designed experiments on social media platforms (e.g., Facebook and Twitter) to examine how individuals' online connections may lead to changes in health behavior in various domains, such as fitness,[103,104] sexual health,[105] and smoking.[106]

With the increasing availability of data sets from more platforms and the rapid development of computational algorithms, the CSS paradigm will contribute more theoretical insights and methodological options for D&I research in health.

SUMMARY

We have described the evolution of diffusion of innovations theory and how concepts from that paradigm as well as knowledge utilization and technology transfer research have contributed to the evidence-based medicine and evidence-based public health emphases in D&I. We suggest that D&I researchers and practitioners will continue to find relevance and applicability in these former research traditions as they seek ways to study and apply new information and communication technologies to the challenges of dissemination activity by innovation proponents, diffusion responses by adopters, and then subsequent implementation and sustained use.

SUGGESTED READINGS AND WEBSITES

Readings

Dearing JW, Cox JG. Diffusion of innovations theory, principles, and practice. *Health Aff.* 2018;37(2):183–190.

The authors review the tenets of diffusion theory and highlight new directions in diffusion research. The article emphasizes well-established concepts from the diffusion literature that can be operationalized as parts of a dissemination strategy to trigger adoptions and successful implementations.

Estabrooks C, Derksen L, Winther C, et al. The intellectual structure and substance of the knowledge utilization field: a longitudinal author co-citation analysis, 1945 to 2004. *Implement Sci.* 2008;3(1):49.

This article is a bibliographic analysis of the knowledge utilization field between World War II and the present and how it has evolved in that time. The authors cite the emergence of evidence-based medicine during this time period, a major advance with significant influences on models of evidence-based practice in other fields, including public health.

Green LW, Ottoson JM, Garcia C, Hiatt RA. Diffusion theory and knowledge dissemination, utilization, and integration in public health. *Annu Rev Public Health.* 2009;30:151–174.

Green et al. provide a rigorous review of the public health implications of diffusion, dissemination, and implementation to improve public health practice and guide the design of future research. The article suggests a decentralized approach to D&I, as well as ways diffusion may be combined with other theories.

Rogers EM. *Diffusion of Innovations.* 5th ed. Free Press; 2003.

Rogers's classic text describes on how ideas and opinions diffuse over time through various communication channels and networks. Because many new ideas involve taking a risk, people seek out others who have already adopted it. As a result, the new idea is spread through social networks over a period of weeks, months, or years.

Selected Websites and Tools

Chung M, Dekker D, Gridley-Smith C, Dearing JW. An emergent network for the diffusion of innovations among local health departments at the onset of the COVID-19 pandemic. *Prev Chronic Dis.* 2021;18:200536. http://dx.doi.org/10.5888/pcd18.200536

This article shows how simple sociometric questions posed to leaders of the same type of organization can reveal the informal structure of advice-seeking behavior among them, suggesting a social influence route to accelerating the adoption of innovations.

Zhang Y, Cao B, Wang Y, Peng T-Q, Wang X. When public health research meets social media: knowledge mapping from 2000 to 2018. *J Med Internet Res.* 2020;22:e17582. https://www.jmir.org/2020/8/e17582/

By reviewing more than 3,400 articles published from 2000 to 2018, this article provides a summary of how social media has altered the foci and methods in public health research.

It concludes that social media enables scholars to study new phenomena and propose new research questions in public health research. Meanwhile, the methodological potential of social media in public health research needs to be further explored.

Effective interventions. Centers for Disease Control and Prevention. Last reviewed March 7, 2022. Accessed November 27, 2020. https://www.cdc.gov/hiv/effective-interventions/index.html

This website is an excellent example of how diffusion concepts can be operationalized to accelerate the adoption of evidence-based programs. Building on the CDC's Diffusion of Evidence-Based Interventions (DEBI) initiative for HIV prevention, the above website models multiple EBPs for diagnosing HIV, treating patients with HIV, preventing HIV, and responding to HIV outbreaks by using well-designed content, graphics and tools for each program, as well as examples of how localities have successfully implemented each program.

REFERENCES

1. Berta W, Virani T, Bajnok I, Edwards N, Rowan M. Understanding whole systems change in health care: insights into system level diffusion from

nursing service delivery innovations—a multiple case study. *Evid. Policy.* 2014;10(3):313–336.

2. Czarniawska B, Sevon G. Translation is a vehicle, imitation its motor, and fashion sits at the wheel. In: Czarniawska B, Sevon G, eds. *Global Ideas: How Ideas, Objects and Practices Travel in the Global Economy.* Liber & Copenhagen Business School Press; 2005:7–12.
3. Bonacich P. Power and centrality: a family of measures. *Am J Sociol.* 1987;92(5):1170–1182.
4. Dearing JW, Cox JG. Diffusion of innovations theory, principles, and practice. *Health Aff.* 2018;37(2):183–190.
5. Greenhalgh T, Papoutsi C. Spreading and scaling up innovation and improvement. *BMJ.* 2019;365:12068.
6. Munro S, Wahl K, Soon JA, et al. Pharmacist dispensing of the abortion pill in Canada: diffusion of innovation meets integrated knowledge translation. *Implement Sci.* 2021;16:76.
7. Green LW, Gottlieb NH, Parcel GS. Diffusion theory extended and applied. *Adv Health Educ Promot.* 1991;3:91–117.
8. Rogers EM, Cartano DG. Methods of measuring opinion leadership. *Public Opin Q.* 1921;26(3):435–441.
9. Kim DK, Dearing JW, eds. *Health Communication Research Measures.* 2nd ed. Peter Lang Inc.; 2016.
10. Flynn LR, Goldsmith RE, Eastman JK. Opinion leaders and opinion seekers: two new measurement scales. *J Acad Market Sci.* 1996;24(2):137.
11. Dearing JW. Social marketing and the diffusion of innovations. In: Stewart DW, ed. *Handbook of Persuasion and Social Marketing.* Praeger; 2014:35–66.
12. Borgatti SP, Mehra A, Brass DJ, Labianca G. Network analysis in the social sciences. *Science.* 2009;323(5916):892–895.
13. Lu L, Chen D, Ren X-L, Zhang Q-M, Zhang Y-C, Zhou T. Vital nodes identification in complex networks. *Phys Rep.* 2016;650:1–63.
14. Burt RS. The network structure of social capital. *Res Organ Behav.* 2000;22:345–423.
15. Bavelas A. Communication patterns in task-oriented groups. *J Acoust Soc Am.* 1950;22:725–730.
16. Bonacich P. Power and centrality: a family of measures. *Am J Sociol.* 1987;92(5):1170–1182.
17. Freeman LC. Centrality in social networks: conceptual clarification. *Soc Networks.* 1979;1(3):215–239.
18. Albalawi Y, Sixsmith J. Identifying Twitter influencer profiles for health promotion in Saudi Arabia. *Health Promot Int.* 2015;32(3):456–463.
19. Holliday J, Audrey S, Campbell R, Moore L. Identifying well-connected opinion leaders for informal health promotion: the example of the ASSIST smoking prevention program. *Health Commun.* 2016;31(8):946–953.
20. Jonnalagadda S, Peeler R, Topham P. Discovering opinion leaders for medical topics using news articles. *J Biomed Semantics.* 2012;3:article 2.
21. Wang X, Shi J, Chen L, Peng T-Q. An examination of users' influence in online HIV/AIDS communities. *Cyberpsych Behav Soc Netw.* 2016;19(5):314–320.
22. Dangalchev C. Residual closeness in networks. *Physica A: Stat Mech Appl.* 2006;365(2):556–564.
23. Klemm K, Serrano MÁ, Eguíluz VM, Miguel MS. A measure of individual role in collective dynamics. *Sci Rep.* 2012;2:292.
24. Zhang J-X, Chen D-B, Dong Q, Zhao Z-D. Identifying a set of influential spreaders in complex networks. *Sci Rep.* 2016;6:27823.
25. Brownson RC, Ballew P, Brown KL, et al. The effect of disseminating evidence-based interventions that promote physical activity to health departments. *Am J Public* Health. 2007;97(10):1900–1907.
26. Gigerenzer G, Reinhard S. *Bounded Rationality. The Adaptive Toolbox.* MIT Press; 2001.
27. Kerckhoff AC, Back KW, Miller N. Sociometric patterns in hysterical contagion. *Sociometry.* 1965;28(1):2–15.
28. Katz E. Theorizing diffusion: Tarde and Sorokin revisited. *Ann Am Acad Pol Soc Sc.* 1999;566:144–155.
29. Katz E, Levin ML, Hamilton H. Traditions of research on the diffusion of innovation. *Am Sociol Rev.* 1963;28(2):237–252.
30. Orleans CT. Increasing the demand for and use of effective smoking-cessation treatments reaping the full health benefits of tobacco-control science and policy gains--in our lifetime. *Am J Prev Med.* 2007;33(6)(suppl):S340–S348.
31. Ryan B, Gross NC. The diffusion of hybrid seed corn in two Iowa communities. *Rural Sociol.* 1943;8(1):15–24.
32. Valente TW, Rogers EM. The origins and development of the diffusion of innovations paradigm as an example of scientific growth. *Sci Commun.* 1995;16(3):242–273.
33. Coleman JS, Katz E, Menzel H. The diffusion of an innovation among physicians. *Sociometry.* 1957;20:253–270.
34. Crane D. *Invisible Colleges: Diffusion of Knowledge in Scientific Communities.* University of Chicago Press; 1972.
35. Estabrooks CA, Derksen L, Winther C, et al. The intellectual structure and substance of the knowledge utilization field: a longitudinal author co-citation analysis, 1945 to 2004. *Implement Sci.* 2008;3:49.

36. Rogers EM. *A Conceptual Variable Analysis of Technological Change*. PhD dissertation. Iowa State University; 1957.
37. Rogers EM. *The Fourteenth Paw: Growing Up on an Iowa Farm in the 1930s*. Asian Media Information and Communication Centre; 2008.
38. Singhal A, Dearing JW. *Communication of Innovations: A Journey With Ev Rogers*. Sage Publications, Inc.; 2006.
39. Montgomery MR, Casteline JB. The diffusion of fertility control in Taiwan; evidence from pooled cross-section time series models. *Pop Stud.* 1993;47(3):457–479.
40. Weiss CH, Bucuvalas MJ. *Social Science Research and Decision-Making.* Columbia University Press; 1980.
41. Kingdon JW. *Agendas, Alternatives, and Public Policies*. Longman; 2003.
42. Anderson LM, Brownson RC, Fullilove MT, et al. Evidence-based public health policy and practice: promises and limits. *Am J Prev Med.* 2005;28(5)(suppl):226–230.
43. Blake SC, Ottoson JM. Knowledge utilization: implications of evaluation. *New Dir Eval.* 2009;124:21–34.
44. Backer TE. Knowledge utilization: the third wave. *Knowledge: Creation, Diffusion, Utilization.* 1991;12(3):225–240.
45. Green LW, Ottoson JM, Garcia C, Hiatt RA. Diffusion theory and knowledge dissemination, utilization, and integration in public health. *Annu Rev Public Health.* 2009;30:151–174.
46. O'Dell C, Grayson CJ. If only we knew what we know: identification and transfer of internal best practices. *Calif Manage Rev.* 1998;40(3): 154–174.
47. Leonard-Barton D. Implementation as mutual adaptation of technology and organization. *Res Policy.* 1988;17(5):251–267.
48. Dunn W, Holzener B, Zaltman G. Knowledge utilization. In: Husen T, Postlethwaite TN, eds. *The International Encyclopedia of Education.* Vol 1. Pergamon Press; 1985:2831–2839.
49. Estabrooks CA, Thompson DS, Lovely JJE, Hofmeyer A. A guide to knowledge translation theory. *J Contin Educ Health Prof.* 2006;26(1):25–36.
50. Lavis JN, Robertson D, Woodside J, McLeod CB, Abelson J. How can research organizations more effectively transfer research knowledge to decision makers. *Milbank Q.* 2003;81(2): 221–248.
51. Sackett DL, Rosenberg WMC, Gray JAM, Haynes RB, Richardson WS. Evidence based medicine: what it is and what it isn't. *Br Med J.* 1996;312:71–72.
52. Mykhalovskiy E, Weir L. The problem of evidence-based medicine: directions for social science. *Soc Sci Med.* 2004;59(5):1059–1069.
53. Haynes RB. What kind of evidence is it that evidence-based medicine advocates want health care providers and consumers to pay attention to? *BMC Health Serv Res.* 2002;2(1):3.
54. Sackett DL. Clinical epidemiology. What, who, and whither. *J Clin Epidemiol.* 2002;55(12):1161–1166.
55. Brownson RC, Fielding JE, Maylahn CM. Evidence-based public health: a fundamental concept for public health practice. *Annu Rev Public Health.* 2009;30:175–201.
56. Simmons R, Fajans P, Ghiron L. *Scaling Up Health Service Delivery From Pilot Innovations to Policies and Programmes.* Department of Reproductive Health and Research World Health Organization; 2007.
57. Greene JD. Communication of results and utilization in participatory program evaluation. *Eval Program Plann.* 1988;11(4):341–351.
58. Doolin B. Narratives of change: discourse, technology and organization. Organization. 2003;10(4):751–770.
59. Dearing JW. Evolution of diffusion and dissemination theory. *J Public Health Manag.* 2008;14(2):99–108.
60. Rogers EM. *Communication Strategies for Family Planning.* Free Press; 1973.
61. Office of Behavioral and Social Sciences Research. *Putting Evidence Into Practice: The OBSSR Report of the Working Group on the Integration of Effective Behavioral Treatments Into Clinical Care.* Office of Behavioral and Social Sciences Research; 1997.
62. von Hippel E. *Democratizing Innovation.* MIT Press; 2005.
63. Edejer TT. Disseminating health information in developing countries: the role of the internet. *BMJ.* 2000;321(7264):797–800.
64. Dearing JW, Maibach E, Buller DB. A convergent diffusion and social marketing approach for disseminating proven approaches to physical activity promotion. *Am J Prev Med.* 2006;;31(4S):S11–S23.
65. Korp P. Health on the Internet: implications for health promotion. *Health Educ* Res. 2006;21(1):78–86.
66. Atherton H, Huckvale C, Car J. Communicating health promotion and disease prevention information to patients via email: a review. *J Telemed* Telecare. 2010;16(4):172–175.
67. Tuerk PW, Fortney J, Bosworth HB, et al. Toward the development of national telehealth services: the role of Veterans Health Administration

and future directions for research. *Telemed J E* Health. 2010;16(1):115–117.

68. Dellifraine JL, Dansky KH. Home-based telehealth: a review and meta-analysis. *J Telemed* Telecare. 2008;14(2):62–66.
69. Eysenbach G, Sa ER, Diepgen TL. Shopping around the internet today and tomorrow: towards the millennium of cybermedicine. *Br Med J.* 1999;319(7220):1294.
70. Jadad AR, Haynes RB, Hunt D, Browman GP. The internet and evidence-based decision-making: a needed synergy for efficient knowledge management in health care. *CMAJ.* 2000;162(3):362–365.
71. Dearing JW, Kreuter MW. Designing for diffusion: how can we increase uptake of cancer communication innovations? *Patient Educ Couns.* 2010;81S:100–110.
72. Kee KF, Sparks L, Struppa DC et al. Information diffusion, Facebook clusters, and the simplicial model of social aggregation: a computational simulation of simplicial diffusers for community health interventions. *Health Commun.* 2016;31(4):385–399.
73. Liang YJ, Kee KF. Developing and validating the A-B-C framework of information diffusion on social media. *New Media Soc.* 2018;20(1):272–292.
74. Hawn C. Take two aspirin and tweet me in the morning: how Twitter, Facebook, and other social media are reshaping health care. *Health Aff (Millwood).* 2009;28(2):361–368.
75. Shirky C. *Here Comes Everybody: The Power of Organizing Without Organizations.* Penguin Press; 2009.
76. Eysenbach G. Medicine 2.0: social networking, collaboration, participation, apomediation, and openness. *J Med Internet Res.* 2008;10(3):e22.
77. Griffiths F, Lindenmeyer A, Powell J, Lowe P, Thorogood M. Why are health care interventions delivered over the internet? A systematic review of the published literature. *J Med Internet Res.* 2006;8(2):e10.
78. Ginsberg J, Mohebbi MH, Patel RS, Brammer L, Smolinski MS, Brilliant L. Detecting influenza epidemics using search engine query data. *Nature.* 2009;457(7232):U1012–U1014.
79. Butler D. When Google got flu wrong. *Nature.* 2013;494(7436):155–156.
80. Lazer D, Kennedy R, King G, Vespignani A. The parable of Google flu: traps in big data analysis. *Science.* 2014;343(6176):1203–1205.
81. Althouse BM, Ng YY, Cummings DAT. Prediction of dengue incidence using search query surveillance. *PLoS Negl Trop Dis.* 2011;5(8):1–7.
82. Walcott BP, Nahed BV, Kahle KT, Redjal N, Coumans J-V. Determination of geographic variance in stroke prevalence using internet search engine analytics. *Neurosurg Focus.* 2011;30(6):E19.
83. Zhou X, Ye J, Feng Y. Tuberculosis surveillance by analyzing Google trends. *IEEE Trans Biomed Eng.* 2011;58(8):2247–2254.
84. Rovetta A. Reliability of Google trends: analysis of the limits and potential of web infoveillance during COVID-19 pandemic and for future research. *Frontiers in Research Metrics and Analytics.* 2021;6:670226. doi:10.3389/frma.2021.670226
85. Mavragani A, Gkillas K. COVID-19 predictability in the United States using Google trends time series. *Sci Rep.* 2020;10(1):20693. doi:10.1038/s41598-020-77275-9
86. Broniatowski DA, Paul MJ, Dredze M. National and local influenza surveillance through Twitter: an analysis of the 2012–2013 influenza epidemic. *PLoS One.* 2013;8(12):e83672.
87. Larson HJ, Smith DMD, Paterson P, et al. Measuring vaccine confidence: analysis of data obtained by a media surveillance system used to analyse public concerns about vaccines. *Lancet Infect Dis.* 2013;13(7):606–613.
88. Mollema L, Harmsen IA, Broekhuizen E, et al. Disease detection or public opinion reflection? Content analysis of Tweets, other social media, and online newspapers during the measles outbreak in the Netherlands in 2013. *J Med Internet Res.* 2015;17(5):e128.
89. Fu K-W, Liang H, Saroha N, Tse ZTH, Ip P, Fung IC-H. How people react to Zika virus outbreaks on Twitter? A computational content analysis. *Am J Infect Control.* 2016;44(12):1700–1702.
90. Ji X, Chun SA, Wei Z, Geller J. Twitter sentiment classification for measuring public health concerns. *Soc Netw Anal Min.* 2015;5(1):13.
91. Guntuku SC, Sherman G, Stokes DC, et al. Tracking mental health and symptom mentions on Twitter during COVID-19. *J Gen Intern Med.* 2020;35(9):2798–2800. doi:10.1007/s11606-020-05988-8
92. Turkle S. Always-on/always-on-you: the tethered self. In Katz JE, ed. *Handbook of Mobile Communication Studies*: MIT Press; 2008:121–138.
93. Steinhubl SR, Muse ED, Topol EJ. The emerging field of mobile health. *Sci Transl Med.* 2015;7(283):283rv3. doi:10.1126/scitranslmed.aaa3487
94. Guan L, Peng TQ, Zhu JJ. Who is tracking health on mobile devices: behavioral logfile analysis in Hong Kong. *JMIR Mhealth Uhealth.* 2019;7(5):e13679. doi:10.2196/13679
95. Kraemer MU, Yang CH, Gutierrez B, et al. The effect of human mobility and control measures on the COVID-19 epidemic in China. *Science.* 2020;368(6490):493–497.

96. Xiong C, Hu S, Yang M, Luo W, Zhang L. Mobile device data reveal the dynamics in a positive relationship between human mobility and COVID-19 infections. *Proc Natl Acad Sci U S A.* 2020;117(44):27087–27089.
97. Bonaccorsi G, Pierri F, Cinelli M, et al. Economic and social consequences of human mobility restrictions under COVID-19. *Proc Natl Acad Sci U S A.* 2020;117(27):15530–15535.
98. Galeazzi A, Cinelli M, Bonaccorsi G, et al. Human mobility in response to COVID-19 in France, Italy and UK. *Sci Rep.* 2021;11(1):1–10.
99. Christakis NA, Fowler JH. The spread of obesity in a large social network over 32 Years. *N Engl J Med.* 2007;357(4):370–379.
100. Christakis NA, Fowler JH. The collective dynamics of smoking in a large social network. *N Engl J Med.* 2008;358(21):2249–2258.
101. Rosenquist JN, Fowler JH, Christakis NA. Social network determinants of depression. *Mol Psychiatry.* 2011;16(3):273–281.
102. Rosenquist JN, Murabito J, Fowler JH, Christakis NA. The spread of alcohol consumption behavior in a large social network. *Ann Intern Med.* 2010;152(7):W426–W141.
103. Centola D. An experimental study of homophily in the adoption of health behavior. *Science.* 2011;334(6060):1269.
104. Turner-McGrievy G, Tate D. Tweets, apps, and pods: results of the 6-month Mobile Pounds Off Digitally (Mobile POD) randomized weight-loss intervention among adults. *J Med Internet Res.* 2011;13(4):e120.
105. Bull SS, Levine DK, Black SR, Schmiege SJ, Santelli J. Social media–delivered sexual health intervention: a cluster randomized controlled trial. *Am J Prev Med.* 2012;43(5):467–474.
106. Graham AL, Cobb NK, Papandonatos GD, et al. A randomized trial of internet and telephone treatment for smoking cessation. *Arch Intern Med.* 2011;171(1):46–53.

4

The Conceptual Basis for Dissemination and Implementation Research

Lessons From Existing Theories, Models, and Frameworks

RACHEL G. TABAK, PER NILSEN, EVA N. WOODWARD, AND DAVID A. CHAMBERS

INTRODUCTION

Dissemination and implementation (D&I) research can be dynamic and complex. Studies lacking adequate underpinning from a theory, model, or framework (TMF; often referred to as theoretical or theory-based approaches) may miss key information related to system-wide processes, organizational factors, and measures required for D&I and may have a more limited contribution to the D&I research literature.[1,2] Evidence from other fields, such as public health, have found that interventions using health behavior theories are more effective than those lacking theoretical underpinning, as the theory can provide a way to tailor the intervention on components relevant to achieve the process of behavior change.[3] Similarly, as D&I research advances, evidence is building to show that the interpretability of study findings is improved by use of TMFs because the study can be better organized and strategies can more successfully intervene on and measure the components essential to a successful D&I outcome.[1,3]

There are a number of ways in which a TMF can improve a D&I study.[4] Theoretical approaches provide a systematic structure for the development, management, and evaluation of D&I efforts, linking study aims, design, measures, and analytic approaches.[5] D&I TMFs can help narrow the scope of a study by assisting with the focus of the research question and guiding the selection of constructs to measure. Using a D&I TMF provides a basis for explaining how and why a D&I strategy works or does not work since TMFs make assumptions explicit. Empirical findings from theory-based studies contribute to contextual understanding across studies, provide evidence to support understanding the mechanisms for D&I strategies, and move D&I research forward.[2,4,6] In this way, TMFs can help on the front end to organize and understand context and on the back end to understand why and how D&I strategies succeed or fail. This is particularly true if the field is to progress to the point when people conducting D&I studies regularly use TMFs to account for a different combination of factors affecting local implementation, and in this way can help to better tailor implementation strategies to an individual setting. Further, this understanding is important as there are a number of pathways through which a D&I strategy may operate.

The purpose of this chapter is to introduce TMFs to inform D&I research. The chapter begins with an overview of terminology. Subsequent sections provide guidance on and tools for (1) selecting a TMF and (2) adapting, combining, and applying TMFs. Case examples then demonstrate these processes in D&I research.

TERMINOLOGY

Dissemination and implementation research uses many TMFs, which are three related, yet distinct, concepts often used interchangeably in the

Rachel G. Tabak, Per Nilsen, Eva N. Woodward, and David A. Chambers, *The Conceptual Basis for Dissemination and Implementation Research*
In: *Dissemination and Implementation Research in Health.* Edited by: Ross C. Brownson, Graham A. Colditz, and Enola K. Proctor,
Oxford University Press. © Oxford University Press 2023. DOI: 10.1093/oso/9780197660690.003.0004

field. In general, a theory may be defined as a set of analytical principles or statements designed to structure our observation, understanding, and explanation of the world[7] and indicates relationships between constructs and concepts. Theories can be described on an abstraction continuum. High abstraction level theories (general or grand theories) have an almost unlimited scope, middle abstraction level theories explain limited sets of phenomena, and lower-level abstraction theories are empirical generalizations of limited scope and application.[8] A theory in the D&I field typically implies some predictive capacity and attempts to explain the causal mechanisms of implementation or factors serving as key components for change (e.g., an understanding of how an implementation strategy like training in a new evidence-based intervention works to improve practice through improving provider knowledge and skill, which builds their confidence and self-efficacy, thus making them more likely to integrate and use the intervention as part of their practice).[9]

Models typically involve deliberate simplifications of a phenomenon or a specific aspect of a phenomenon. Models need not be completely accurate representations of reality to have value.[10] Models can be described as theories with a more narrowly defined scope of explanation; a model is descriptive, whereas a theory is explanatory as well as descriptive.[7] Models in D&I research are commonly used to describe and/or guide the process of translating research into practice. For example, there is the Implementation Research Logic Model (see Figure 4.1), which is a visual depiction linking key elements in an implementation practice and/or research effort to make explicit what barriers and facilitators exist (determinants), how changes might be made (strategies, mechanisms), and what it is hoped will change (outcomes).[6] Although the implementation research logic model uses determinants of the Consolidated Framework for Implementation Research (CFIR) in its template, any determinant framework could replace it, and any evaluation framework could dictate outcomes of interest. The implementation research logic model is a tool to make clear some of the theoretical underpinnings in one specific project and improve planning and communication across teams.

A framework is usually a structure, overview, outline, system, or plan consisting of various descriptive categories and the relations between them that are presumed to account for a phenomenon.[11] Frameworks do not provide explanations; they only describe empirical phenomena by fitting them into a set of categories.[7] D&I frameworks often have a descriptive purpose by pointing to factors believed or found to influence implementation outcomes. Neither frameworks nor models specify the mechanisms of change; they are typically more like checklists of factors relevant to various aspects of D&I.

In explaining the conceptual underpinnings of D&I research, we recognize five categories of theoretical approaches:

- Process models
- Determinant frameworks
- Classic theories
- D&I theories
- Evaluation frameworks

The first category, process models, focuses on describing and/or guiding the process of translating research into practice. Process models incorporate the temporal sequence of implementation as well as the importance of barriers and facilitators to D&I efforts, but do not aim to identify or systematically structure what makes D&I efforts successful. Frameworks and theories in the categories of determinant frameworks, classic theories, and D&I theories are used to guide research aimed at understanding and/or explaining the factors that influence the outcomes of D&I efforts. Determinant frameworks usually describe four types (or domains) of determinants, which together influence the outcome(s): characteristics of the implementation object, the users/adopters, the context, and the implementation strategy. Theories from D&I research (D&I theories) or other fields (classic theories) are needed for research aimed at enhancing the understanding of relationships and change mechanisms or to predict outcomes. The last category, evaluation frameworks, can guide D&I research by identifying specific aspects of the D&I effort to evaluate to determine success.

It should be noted that the terminology for each TMF in D&I research is not always consistent with this taxonomy. Thus, a determinant framework might be called a model. For example, the Conceptual *Model* by Greenhalgh et al. (2005) is a determinant framework,[12]

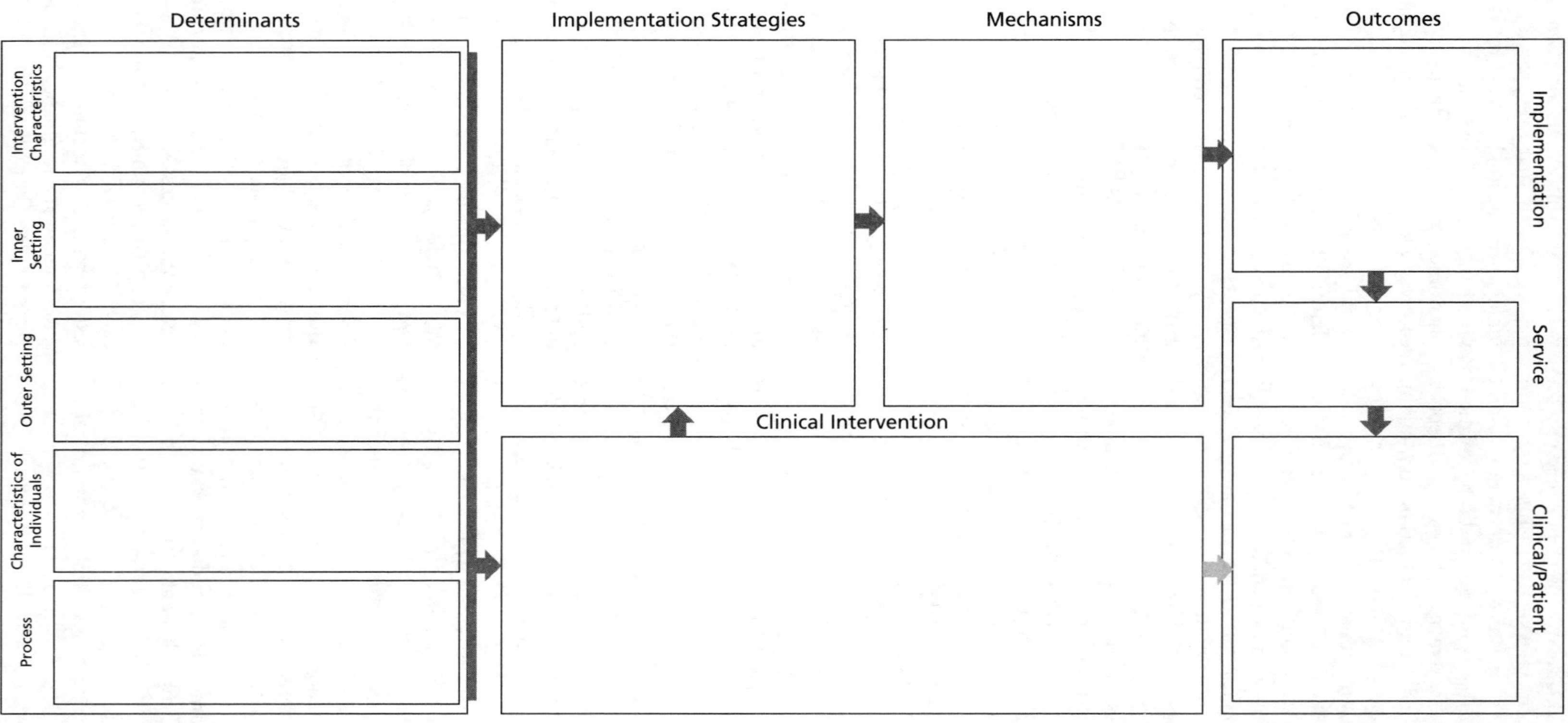

FIGURE 4.1 Implementation research logic model example.

whereas the Quality Implementation *Framework* by Meyers et al. (2012) is a process model. Some theoretical approaches also combine aspects of determinant frameworks *and* process models. For example, the EPIS (Exploration, Preparation, Implementation, Sustainment) framework identifies four phases of the implementation process (i.e., a process model feature) and four types of determinants that impact this process (i.e., a determinant framework feature).[13] In addition, these categories are not rigid, particularly as TMFs are adapted to include additional constructs, such as the evolution of the Promoting Action on Research Implementation in Health Services (PARIHS) to the integrated Promoting Action on Research Implementation in Health Services (i-PARIHS)[14]. Similarly, the CFIR has been updated based on user feedback[15] and additional guidance is available to support incorporating the Practical, Robust, Implementation, and Sustainability Model (PRISM) constructs, relevant to implementation determinants, with the Reach, Effectiveness, Adoption, Implementation, and Maintenance (RE-AIM) framework outcomes.[16] Thus, it is important for investigators to clearly communicate how they are using a TMF to guide their work, when they adapt one and why, and strive to use consistent terminology.

There has been an evolution of TMFs in fields outside healthcare, which can be applied within D&I research. For example, in the field of business/management, scholars incorporated a number of different ways to think about change, including change as rational action[17] and change as adaptation to environment, which included theories such as Contingency Theory,[18] Ecology Theory,[19] and Institutional Theory.[20] A theory familiar to many D&I health researchers, Rogers's Diffusion of Innovations,[21] became part of this literature as change was conceptualized as innovation; a further conceptualization was cultural change.[22] D&I research in health has learned a great deal from fields beyond health about the value of TMFs and can continue to look to these fields (e.g., business, engineering, political science) to develop and adapt new applications.[17,18]

SELECTING A THEORY, MODEL, OR FRAMEWORK

Researchers embarking on D&I research may wonder: How do I select an appropriate TMF to guide my work? Several efforts to collect, organize, and synthesize the many TMFs to guide D&I research are available.

Of particular relevance to this process include the review by Nilsen described above[23] and guidance provided by Lynch et al. on selecting a TMF.[24] In another review, TMFs were organized based on three continua: construct flexibility, dissemination and/or implementation (D/I), and the socioecological levels the framework addressed.[5] At one end of the construct flexibility spectrum are broad TMFs, those with more loosely defined or outlined constructs, and at the other end, operational TMFs offer more detailed step-by-step actions for organizing a D&I study. Because of the greater flexibility afforded by broad TMFs, more responsibility is placed on the researchers to operationalize, implement, and use the TMF; however, operational TMFs, because of their specificity, tend to be more clearly defined for a particular context and activity. Dissemination and/or implementation refers to whether the TMF is focused on using active efforts to spread evidence-based interventions to the target audience via determined channels using planned strategies (dissemination) or is focused on integrating an intervention within a setting (implementation); definitions for D&I have been provided in chapter 2. The socioecological framework includes these levels: individual, organization, community, and system. It describes that a TMF can operate at one or more of these; they can also include a policy component. It is also important to consider whether the constructs in the TMF are relevant to the research questions; as an example, Pinto et al. explored the presence of constructs related to community engagement across a sample of TMFs.[25]

Chambers laid out a set of questions that can be asked about a D&I effort to inform the choice of a model; these questions have been adapted and are summarized in Table 4.1.[26]

In a review of 61 TMFs,[5] at least four fell into each of the five categories for the construct flexibility and D/I scales. The approaches were spread across the socioecological framework levels, and every TMF operated at more than one level. The majority of approaches included community and/or organizational levels. Only eight touched on policy. Additional information about these TMFs is also provided, including the field in which the TMF was developed

TABLE 4.1 QUESTIONS TO CONSIDER WHEN SELECTING A THEORY, MODEL, OR FRAMEWORK (TMF)[a]

Question	Considerations
What is/are the research question(s) I am seeking to answer?	1. Reviewing D&I literature to identify and utilize essential concepts and established definitions[27] will enhance the overall generalizability of the effort. 2. Articulating a research question and aims can narrow the scope of which TMFs might fit the study well. 3. Beginning with a research question allows the researcher to determine what evidence is needed to answer that question.
What is the scope of the study?	1. Explanatory investigations certainly benefit from TMFs. 2. Earlier stage research such as measurement development or pilot work may not need to fully flesh the study out in terms of a TMF and might instead frame the study under the idea of a TMF.
What is the purpose of the TMF in the context of the study?[23]	Nilsen proposed[23] five categories and functions a TMF can have in guiding a study—you might need more than one TMF for a study: 1. Process models "describe and/or guide the process of translating research into practice." 2. Determinant frameworks help explain/understand influences on implementation outcomes by specifying determinants (barriers and facilitators). 3. Classical theories, which emerge from fields such as organizational theory, psychology, and sociology, can be applied to explain/understand implementation efforts. 4. Implementation theories, developed by implementation researchers, help understand/explain implementation. 5. Evaluation frameworks "specify aspects of implementation that could be evaluated to determine implementation success."
What socioecological level(s) of change am I seeking to explain?	1. Specifying the socioecological level in which the change will occur allows for selection of a TMF that corresponds to the types of change under investigation (e.g., individual, organizational, community, system). 2. When thinking about policy, it is important to consider that policy exists at two levels: "big P" policy (formal laws, rules, regulations enacted by elected officials) and "small p" policy (organizational guidelines, internal agency decisions/memoranda, social norms).[28]
What characteristics of context are relevant to the research questions?	1. Identifying aspects of the context that may be important to the D&I outcome is an important step.
What is the time frame?	1. There is variability between TMFs in terms of how many phases of the D&I process are included (e.g., exploration of an evidence-based intervention to be adopted, evidence-based intervention implementation, and sustainment of the practice). 2. A study may focus on some or all phases of the D&I process depending on the research question and scope of the study. 3. For studies covering multiple phases, multistage frameworks (Reach Effectiveness Adoption Implementation Maintenance [RE-AIM][29] and exploration, preparation, implementation, and sustainment [EPIS] framework)[30] can help organize studies in addition to providing context specific for those stages. 4. Other TMFs may focus on one specific phase of the D&I process.

TABLE 4.1 CONTINUED

Question	Considerations
Are measures available?	1. Measures are one of the important ways in which a TMF and its constructs are operationalized and are a way to tie the TMF to the research question. 2. Resources to help researchers identify measures for the constructs in their selected TMFs, including the availability/absence of psychometric properties for the measures, are available,[31] but considerable work is still needed.
Does the study need to be related to a single TMF, and how strict does the use of the model need to be?	1. Given the complexity of D&I research, it is possible that a single TMF may be inadequate or underspecified to fully inform a research study. 2. TMFs may be combined to complement their purpose (e.g., those laid out by Nilsen such as process models, implementation theories, or evaluation frameworks),[23] based on the level of context, and/or based on the phase of the D&I process under study.
Are resources, guidance, and/or examples available to support using the TMF?	1. Looking to the literature when considering a TMF, it may be possible to identify resources specific to using the TMF (e.g., for RE-AIM,[32] the Theoretical Domains Framework,[33] the health equity implementation framework,[34] CFIR,[35] PARIHS[36]). 2. Searching the references citing a TMF may help identify example studies that have used the TMF.
Does the TMF need to be adapted to fit the goal, setting, population, or other context?[5]	1. TMFs often need to be adapted to fit the study; theoretical and/or empirical adaptations can contribute to advancing D&I research. 2. Caution must be taken when adapting a TMF to provide evidence that supports the change without compromising the core elements.[5]

[a]Adapted with permission from Chambers 2016.[26]

as well as citations with examples where it was used empirically.

To provide an additional tool to identify TMFs and narrow the search, theoretical approaches from several reviews (i.e., Tabak et al.,[5] Mitchell et al.,[3] and Strifler et al.[37]) and newer TMFs from the literature have been collected and organized in a searchable website (https://dissemination-implementation.org/). A sample of highly cited, representative TMFs are displayed in Table 4.2 to demonstrate how these pieces of information about each TMF might be used. Within this sample are TMFs representing all categories in terms of dissemination to implementation and construct flexibility and all levels of the socioecological framework. From the table it is possible to narrow down the list of available TMFs to those that might best fit the intended study. Once the search has been narrowed to a small number of TMFs, the T-CAST (Theory Comparison and Selection Tool) can be a useful tool for comparing TMFs.[38]

It is important to consider the variety of theoretical approaches available for use in D&I research and to recognize the benefits of selecting an existing TMF from those already available, which includes an opportunity to advance the field by providing empirical evidence for the TMF in question. Applying an existing TMF can be a source of innovation for a study, especially if it is a TMF not previously used in the field. While there are many TMFs available, not all are well operationalized, and it may, therefore, require more effort to apply them in a study. The decision to attempt to develop a new TMF should be taken with caution, as this is a large undertaking, and there are many TMFs with similar and overlapping constructs that currently exist in the literature. However, there is no comprehensive TMF that will perfectly fit every study, so it may be necessary to adapt a TMF and/or to combine multiple TMFs to inform a study.

TABLE 4.2 CATEGORIZATIONS OF SELECTED THEORIES, MODELS, AND FRAMEWORKS (TMFS) BASED ON KEY CHARACTERISTICS

Theory, Model, or Framework	Dissemination and/or Implementation	Construct Flexibility: Broad (1) to Operational (5)	Socioecological Framework Level					Field of Origin	Selected Studies (by Reference Number) That Use the Model
			System	Community	Organization	Individual	Policy		
Diffusion of innovation[21]	D only	1		x	x	x		Agriculture	39–43
Streams of policy process[44,45]	D only	2	x	x	x		x	Political Science	46, 47
Greenhalgh Diffusion of Innovations in Service Organizations[12]	D > I	4		x	x			Health Services	48, 49
Framework for Dissemination of Evidence-Based Policy[28]	D > I	5		x	x	x	x	Public Health	50
Interactive Systems Framework[51]	D = I	2	x	x	x	x		Violence Prevention	52–54
The RE-AIM framework[16,55]	D = I	4		x	x	x		Public Health	56–58
Active Implementation Framework[59,60]	I only	3		x	x	x		Any Domain	61, 62
Implementation effectiveness model[63,64]	I only	3			x	x		Management	65–68
Exploration, preparation, implementation, sustainment (EPIS) model (conceptual model of evidence-based practice implementation in public service sectors)[13,30]	I only	4	x	x	x	x	x	Public sector services	69, 70
Theoretical Domains Framework[33,71,72]	I only	4		x	x	x		Health Psychology	73, 74
Consolidated Framework for Implementation Research (CFIR)[15,75]	I only	4		x	x			Health Services	76, 77

GUIDANCE ON ADAPTING, COMBINING, AND APPLYING THEORIES, MODELS, AND FRAMEWORKS

Adapt

In the process of adapting, combining, and using TMFs, investigators can consider them as living documents, or works in progress, rather than static entities (see examples above of TMFs, which have been updated: i-PARIHS,[14] RE-AIM,[16,55] CFIR[15,75]). The decision to adapt a TMF may be guided by several factors, including aligning the constructs of the TMF with the setting, population, or topic in which the study will take place (e.g., tailoring the name of a construct to align with the context); providing more specificity in constructs (e.g., providing examples of the construct or identifying subconstructs more specific to the study); incorporating additional constructs (e.g., those related to health equity) and/or emphasizing/de-emphasizing constructs based on their relevance to the study; and highlighting relationships between constructs. One example of this is an adaptation of the RE-AIM framework to advance sustainability and equity.[78] This can support the field by allowing researchers to build on previous findings by enhancing generalizability of the TMF and our understanding of how to operationalize its constructs and by testing modifications to existing TMFs. There is reason for caution, as drastic changes to a TMF can become a weakness of a study. Therefore, it is important to consider both the overall fit of the TMF to the study and to track, document, and monitor adaptations so these can be reported and incorporated into the literature (see Case Study 4.1 as an excellent example).

Combine

Many studies may be better supported by combining multiple TMFs. Reasons for this may include the following: The study may need TMFs from multiple categories of theoretical approaches in D&I research.[6,23] There may be a need for multiple frameworks for multiple functions. An example is the use of the CFIR as the determinant framework to better understand the outcomes informed by the RE-AIM framework. An example can be seen in Figure 4.2, which outlines how RE-AIM and CFIR, together, guided the study by Simione et al. (2021).[79]

Of note, RE-AIM has expanded the focus on determinants and the updated CFIR guides incorporation of implementation outcomes from additional TMFs.[15,16] Another reason to

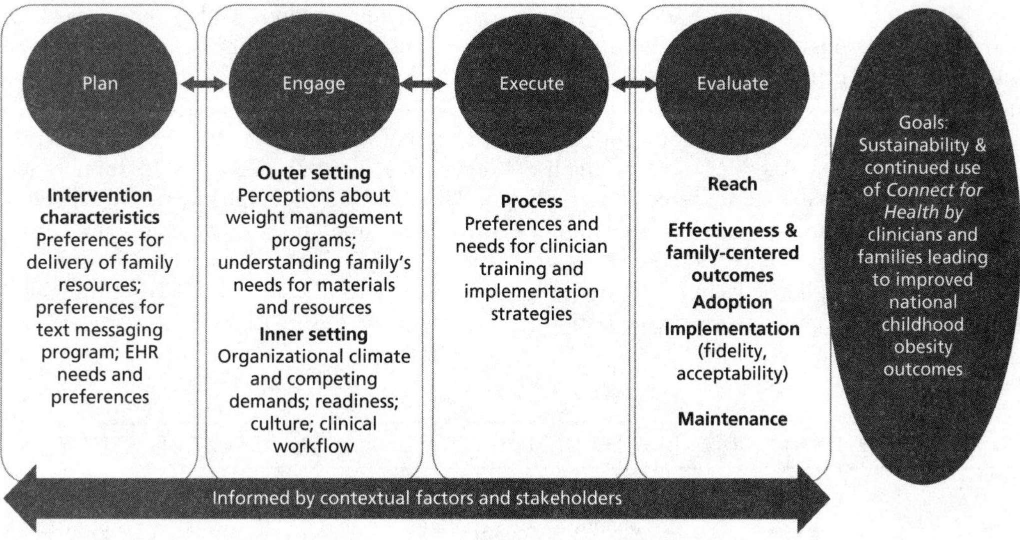

FIGURE 4.2 Summary of the implementation and evaluation approach for Connect for Health, a primary care-based pediatric weight management program. In the figure, the authors show how CFIR is used to consider determinants in the plan, engage, and execute phases, and RE-AIM is used to determine evaluation metrics in the evaluate phase.

Reprinted with permission from: Simione M, Farrar-Muir H, Mini FN, et al. Implementation of the Connect for Health pediatric weight management program: study protocol and baseline characteristics. *J Comp Eff Res*. Aug 2021;10(11):881–892.

combine theoretical approaches is the need to expand the depth of one TMF. For example, one might provide a broad, multilevel description of an issue or phenomenon and another help focus on an in-depth manner on one specific level of this issue (e.g., provider-level determinants), where another may allow for expansion of constructs in another broader, less specialized TMF. A widely used example is the combined use of the CFIR with the Theoretical Domains Framework (TDF), examples of which can be found in a review of the combined use of the TMFs.[80] Similarly, one TMF might help operationalize a construct from a larger TMF. Also, TMFs may be used in a temporal fashion, with some of the constructs playing key roles earlier (e.g., understanding determinants of implementation) and others at later phases (e.g., evaluation of implementation outcomes). It may also be helpful to combine a TMF from D&I research with a more specialized TMF from another discipline (e.g., health equity).

Apply

Theories, models, and frameworks can be used in all phases of the research process, from early development of D&I research questions through the analyses and dissemination of research findings and can help researchers interpret findings and contribute to the science.[2] In describing a research study, the TMF can be apparent in the aims, design, study activities, selections of measures, evaluation, analyses, and the interpretation and dissemination of findings (among others). Moullin et al. identified 10 recommendations for using TMFs from D&I research.[81] (1) First on the list is selecting a suitable TMF (covered above), (2) followed by continuous engagement of community stakeholders and partnerships. (3) Next, they suggested the TMF be used to frame a study, including shaping the research questions, specific aims, study hypotheses, and/or objectives and (4) conceptualize the activities and relationships that might be important in the study, for example, informing a logic model such as the one depicted in Figure 4.1. (5) The TMF can also inform study methods and measures of evaluation as well as (6) understanding implementation determinants.

An important part of operationalizing a TMF is to tie measures (qualitative and/or quantitative) to the TMF's constructs, which enables conceptualizing and evaluating/quantifying dependent and independent variables as well as mediators and moderators, as suggested in the TMF. A mediator is an "intervening variable that may account for the relationship between the implementation strategy and the implementation outcome" and a moderator is a "factor that increase or decrease the level of influence of an implementation strategy."[9] One example of how to connect TMFs to elements of a research study is shown in Table 4.3, which may help communicate this to readers.

Continuing the list of 10 recommendations, according to Moullin et al.,[81] the TMF can also guide (7) selection and tailoring of implementation strategies. For example, there have been efforts to use determinants identified with CFIR to match specific implementation strategies.[35] (8) Next, TMFs can guide specification of relevant implementation outcomes and (9) tailor implementation at the micro level. Of importance to the specific research effort and a contribution to the field is (10) incorporating the TMF in communicating about the study (e.g., grant proposal, manuscript, report, presentation). There are resources to support use of TMFs, including empirical studies applying the TMFs, and links to measures and guidance for use.[32,33,35,36,82] It is helpful to continually return to the selected TMF throughout the study to ensure that measures and data

TABLE 4.3 EXAMPLE TABLE TO DEMONSTRATE TMF IN RESEARCH STUDY

Construct	Description/ Definition	Level	Assessment Method	Data Source/ Reporter	Assessment Tool	No. of Items	Psychometric Properties

collection procedures align with the TMF and its key constructs. The case studies below outline examples of using a TMF.

CASE STUDY 4.1: HEALTH EQUITY IMPLEMENTATION FRAMEWORK

Background

Adaptation and development of the Health Equity Implementation Framework responded to a need for an implementation theory that could prospectively address health disparities in complex healthcare delivery systems, identified in a preliminary study in 2016.[83]

The specific driver for the framework's construction was the United States Food and Drug Administration's (FDA's) 2015 approval of a class of revolutionary new treatments for chronic hepatitis C virus (HCV) infection, a chronic blood-borne infection affecting 4 million people in the United States that had become the most common cause of liver failure and liver cancer in the country. Previous HCV treatments (i.e., interferon injections and daily oral ribavirin) were ineffective in the majority of patients, and extremely toxic, with many patients simply refusing treatment because of intolerable and potentially life-threatening side effects.

In contrast, the new HCV drugs, known as direct-acting antivirals, cured over 90% of HCV patients and generally had very few side effects and only required taking a single tablet daily by mouth for 8 to 12 weeks.[84] Thus, this pharmaceutical innovation was a dramatic therapeutic advance over the older interferon-based treatments. However, the extremely high cost and inadequate insurance coverage of the direct-acting antivirals quickly emerged as a major barrier to access, given that a 3-month treatment course could cost up to $84,000 in the United States.[85,86]

The Veterans Health Administration (VHA), the single largest provider of HCV care in the United States, was able to surmount cost and related barriers to direct-acting antiviral access. Congress appropriated directed funding to the VHA to cover costs; at the same time, VHA used statutory authorities to negotiate lower prices for the new drugs.[87] These actions allowed VHA to lift clinical restrictions on direct-acting antiviral treatment of HCV, as well as exempt most HCV patients in VHA care from virtually all copayment requirements. Removing cost as a barrier to access and uptake of direct-acting antivirals was particularly important for this population since veterans in VHA care were known to be much more likely than civilians to be diagnosed with HCV.[88]

However, nonfinancial barriers remained significant impediments to direct-acting antiviral uptake, in both the United States and the VHA. For subgroups based on race in the general US population, after adjustment for age, the prevalence of HCV among Black individuals was significantly higher than for White individuals.[88,89] Prior to FDA approval of direct-acting antivirals, there were significant racial disparities in HCV treatment in the United States and within the VHA, with Black patients 18% less likely to receive interferon-based treatment than White patients in the United States as a whole, and 62% less likely in the VHA.[90,91] Although lower response rates to interferon-based therapy among Black HCV patients were advanced as a basis for these disparities,[92] the finding that Black HCV patients in the VHA were also less likely to receive complete laboratory evaluation and viral genotype testing underscored the inadequacy of this explanation. As the authors of the VHA study noted: "Further investigation is warranted to help understand whether patient preference or provider bias may explain why HCV-infected Blacks were less likely to receive medical care than Whites."[90]

A retrospective cohort study published in 2016, early in the VHA's rollout of direct-acting antivirals, demonstrated evidence of a significantly lower odds ratio for treatment with the new drugs among Black HCV patients in the VHA compared to non-Black patients.[92,93] Although the retrospective nature of the analysis prevented drawing definitive conclusions, the size of the study sample and the magnitude of the differences between racial subgroups, combined with the previously demonstrated racial disparities in HCV treatment with interferon, made it clear that racial disparities in access to direct-acting antiviral treatment should be assumed until proven otherwise.

In 2016, the VHA's Office of Health Equity funded a research team to investigate Black and African American VHA patient perspectives on barriers and facilitators to uptake of the new drugs. The research team examined several existing implementation TMFs and decided to use i-PARIHS, a determinant and process framework, but noted there was little attention to factors with known associations with healthcare disparities in any existing implementation TMF, which was of direct importance to this study. They needed to adapt i-PARIHS to integrate key factors related to healthcare disparities, such as patients' prior experience with racial discrimination, provider racial bias, and poor patient-provider interactions.

Selecting and Adapting the Framework

The research team decided to add three health equity domains to the existing implementation-determinant framework (i-PARIHS), although not to the process element of i-PARIHS: culturally relevant factors of recipients, the clinical encounter, and societal context. To determine those three health equity domains, the lead researcher reviewed seminal, published texts on health and healthcare disparities, such as Kilbourne's framework[94] and LaVeist's textbook.[95] She extracted common factors theorized or documented to explain some variance in subpar healthcare or healthcare disparities across populations (e.g., Black individuals; lesbian, gay, bisexual, and queer individuals; individuals who were overweight). Ultimately, she selected Kilbourne's framework to add to i-PARIHS, specifically domains of the clinical encounter and "patient and provider factors" renamed "cultural factors of recipients." Then, she consulted with various D&I scientists and made iterations or clarified definitions. Then, she consulted with health disparities scientists and others at annual D&I research meetings, who suggested broader societal impacts, including structural violence and social determinants of health,[96–98] which were subsumed under the umbrella term "societal influences." Finally, she met with one of the creators of i-PARIHS and they reviewed iterations together. She returned to the literature to assess whether the final list of factors had prior research evidence that explained some variability in health or healthcare disparities.[99–101] If they did, she integrated them as determinants into those three broad health equity domains. Through revisions with blinded peer reviewers in two manuscript submissions, the three domains evolved to be "clinical encounter, culturally relevant factors of recipients, and societal context."

Context

The Health Equity Implementation Framework proposes several determinants important to assess and address in an implementation effort *and* a process by which implementation would occur (facilitation); see Figure 4.3. Therefore, it is a determinant and process framework. Three health equity domains are directly combined with typical implementation domains (e.g., innovation, inner and outer context). Assessing domains and their determinants would logically prompt one to then address those identified as barriers in the implementation process through strategies (e.g., facilitation). The framework is not yet adapted for how the process would change to address equity, as that science and work is emerging. So, the primary adaptation currently is the health equity focus on assessing and understanding determinants.

One domain is the characteristics of the innovation itself (e.g., pill, practice, policy). A second domain is recipients, the people who will have to do something differently for the innovation to be implemented: providers, staff, and patients. One important set of determinants is culturally relevant factors of those recipients, such as their attitudes toward a certain health problem or population, health literacy, and beliefs based on lived experiences. Another domain is the clinical encounter (patient-provider interaction), during which a staff person or provider might or might not offer the innovation to a patient, who has an opportunity to agree, decline, or question. The contextual domains are the inner, outer, and societal context. Inner and outer contexts are local wards, clinics, or services, whereas outer contexts are typically larger systems encompassing those units, such as parent facilities or regional hospital networks.

Although there are no explicit equity determinants in the organizational context, we should consider an equity lens to clinics and organizations and their prior experience with addressing disparities. Societal context involves influences that are upstream and may have a direct or indirect impact on the organizational context, recipients, or even the innovation, such as racial housing discrimination or restrictive immigration laws (sociopolitical forces), how healthcare is exchanged (economies), and the built environment patients navigate to access healthcare (physical structures). There are thorough descriptions of this framework[83] with

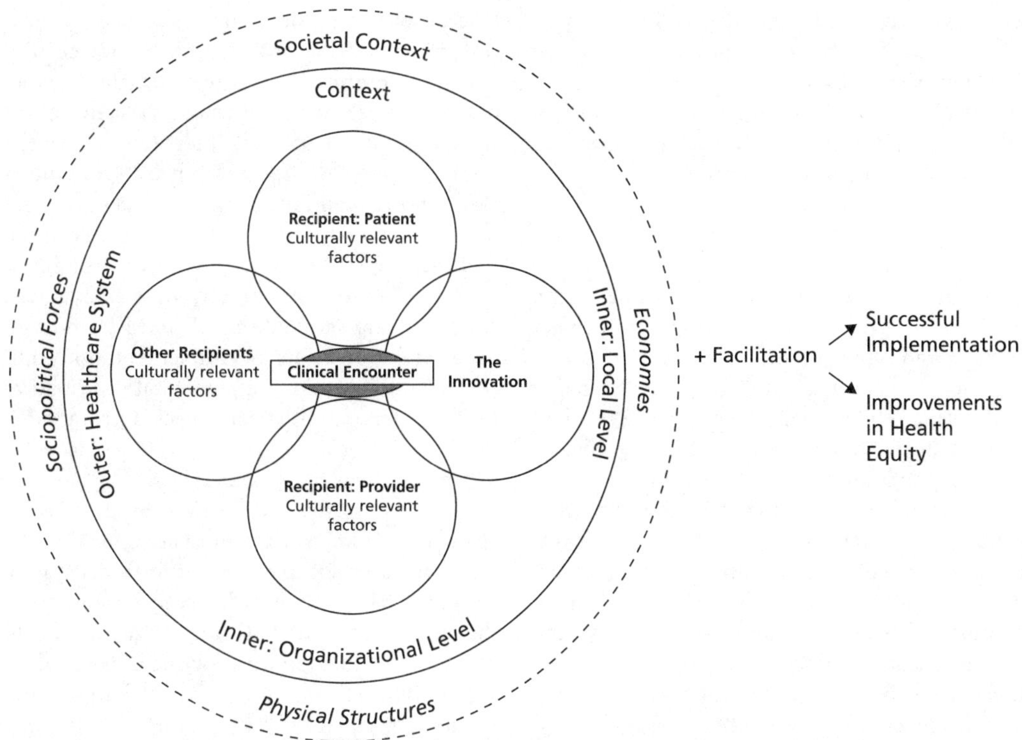

FIGURE 4.3 The Health Equity Implementation Framework, which showcases three equity domains (clinical encounter, culturally relevant factors of recipients, and societal context) adapted to an existing determinant and process framework, the integrated Promoting Action on Research Implementation in Health Services (i-PARIHS).

Reprinted with permission from: Woodward EN, Matthieu MM, Uchendu US, Rogal S, Kirchner JE. The health equity implementation framework: proposal and preliminary study of hepatitis C virus treatment. *Implement Sci.* Mar 12 2019;14(1):26.

practical guidance on possible measures and examples.[34]

Regarding disparate receipt of direct-acting antivirals between Black and White VHA patients, the research team assessed patient perspectives about barriers and facilitators to using the innovation (the new medicine). They created a qualitative interview guide asking about all domains of the Health Equity Implementation Framework, piloting questions about the three health equity domains. After analyzing data from the qualitative interviews, they identified several barriers typical in other implementation efforts, such as lack of connection to treatment after testing positive for HCV. They also identified strengths or facilitators, such as patient desires to try the new medicine. By asking specifically about clinical encounters in the past, culturally relevant factors of patients, and societal context, the research team also learned that prior racial discrimination experienced by themselves or their peers made them less inclined to initiate or attend healthcare appointments. Stigma about how they acquired HCV also made them less likely to share their condition with others and forgo or delay treatment to maintain privacy. Physical structural barriers like long commutes and limited physical transit to rural clinics occasionally created insurmountable barriers for patients to access healthcare.

In this case, the VHA deployed several research teams like this one to investigate different aspects of this problem, and all contributed knowledge back to clinical and operational leaders. Supported by a national operational office,[102] the VHA used a VHA-wide learning collaborative focused on HCV quality improvement, comprising clinicians from different disciplines, system redesign specialists, and clinic managers, with regional teams using Lean methods to affect critical changes in microsystems at individual facilities, as well as other strategies to plan, pilot, study, and use new approaches. Eventually, these efforts led to elimination of HCV among more than 95% of all VHA patients in care, equitably distributed across racial and ethnic subgroups.[103]

Lessons Learned

One lesson is that frameworks change over time, just as the Health Equity Implementation Framework evolved with consultation, peer review, and pilot testing. This is also documented well in the shift from PARIHS to i-PARIHS. Follow emerging science, adapt TMFs as needed, and allow TMFs to evolve as more information becomes known.

A second lesson is that adapting a framework and adding domains takes more time, requires thoughtfulness, and adds complexity to design of data collection, recruitment, training of data collectors, data analysis, and interpretation. The result is worth this extra investment, but it is important to plan for the extra time, training, or financial resources.

A final lesson is specific to scientists and practitioners who aim to understand factors driving inequities or disparities: Plan to assess *and address* factors related to inequities or they will likely be under detected and misunderstood. To do this in an implementation effort, individuals can (1) use the entire Health Equity Implementation Framework; (2) use only the three health equity domains added to another implementation determinant framework; or (3) find other domains or determinants relevant to health equity to add on to an existing framework. There is benefit to the field of making clear what was adapted and why, as evidenced in the case study.

CASE STUDY 4.2: RE-AIM (REACH, EFFECTIVENESS, ADOPTION, IMPLEMENTATION, AND MAINTENANCE) FRAMEWORK

Background

Project HEAL (Health Through Early Awareness and Learning) used a community-based, cluster-randomized trial in African American churches to compare a web-based technology to traditional classroom didactic methods for training community health advisors to implement an evidence-based cancer (breast, prostate, and colorectal cancer) educational intervention.[104] Reaching outside clinical and into community settings (e.g., faith-based organizations) with culturally targeted cancer screening interventions is important. Given the difficulty determining why projects to implement an intervention in a new setting are more or less successful (i.e., was the intervention ineffective in the new setting or was the intervention deployed incorrectly or weakly?), the research team selected the RE-AIM framework to guide evaluation of implementation outcomes (e.g., adoption, implementation) in addition to intervention effectiveness outcomes.

Context

In this case study,[104] RE-AIM was used as an evaluation framework, and over more than 20 years, it has been used to guide thousands of studies.[16] RE-AIM was developed to improve the speed and impact of translating science to practice and to support a focus on external, as well as internal, validity in study planning and evaluation. RE-AIM guides "an explicit focus on issues, dimensions, and steps in the design, dissemination, and implementation process that can either facilitate or impede success in achieving broad and equitable population-based impact."

RE-AIM informed the measures and evaluation for Project HEAL, guiding metrics for adoption; reach; implementation (i.e., adherence, does, quality); efficacy; and sustainability across multiple levels (e.g., individual participant, individual community health advisor, organization/church), with the outcomes reported over several manuscripts. This evaluation explored the potential for technology-based training by assessing adoption, reach, and implementation among community health advisors trained in this method versus those trained using traditional classroom methods.

Lessons Learned

Project HEAL evaluated all domains of RE-AIM and provided valuable information on the potential for training community health advisors using web-based technology or traditional classroom methods. Regarding adoption of the intervention, 41% of churches (organizations) approached agreed to participate, and reach was marginally greater among community health advisors trained traditionally, but church members attended a greater number of workshops from community health advisors trained using web-based technology.

Use of the RE-AIM framework in Project HEAL provided a broader picture of intervention and implementation effectiveness, especially as a clinical intervention was being spread into the community. The application of a TMF, in this case, RE-AIM, more deeply connects the findings to a broader D&I research literature and allows for more generalizable findings regarding implementation in community settings.

FUTURE DIRECTIONS

Given the plethora of TMFs to guide D&I studies and projects and the importance of using theory-based approaches to support these projects, it is essential to consider how D&I scientists facilitate the selection, adaptation, combination, and application of TMFs. While several options for categorization of existing TMFs have been described,[5,23] further categorizing TMFs by (1) type of intervention, (2) type of provider, (3) type of setting, (4) study aim, and (5) implications for health equity, as well as utility for implementing multiple evidence-based interventions simultaneously, could be beneficial to those selecting a TMF approach. There is much to be gained from employing TMFs, including contributions to empirical testing and understanding mechanisms for change in D&I studies, which can be facilitated by enabling more researchers to select from and employ existing TMFs.

As described above, there are many TMFs that have never been tested,[5,23] so their empirical use has potential to advance the field. Aside from TMFs existing within D&I research and health, TMFs for D&I may be adapted from fields outside of health, such as education, business, and engineering. There is room for additional work in specialty topics of D&I research to describe the TMFs used, though there has been advancement in important areas (e.g., health equity,[83] adaptation,[105–107] sustainment,[78,108] and de-implementation[109,110]).

While efforts to sort TMFs have been described, further synthesis of existing TMFs, including exploring the many common constructs across theoretical approaches, could help extend the existing TMFs to address key questions in D&I research. A better connection between various TMFs and the measures to assess their constructs is required for continuing to advance D&I research.

SUMMARY

Applying a TMF is important in all stages of research, from designing the study to interpreting the findings. There are tangible benefits to the use of TMFs to inform D&I research. However, D&I scientists may find it difficult to select, adapt, combine, and apply a specific TMF to their work. Guidance was provided on how to select a TMF, as answering several questions (e.g., the research question, scope of the study) can aid a research team in selecting a TMF. A case study example of adapting a TMF to better address health equity was also included, as for nearly all studies the selected TMF will need adaptation. Given the large number of TMFs available and the amount of work required to develop a new TMF, a researcher likely does not need to create a new TMF. An alternative might be to look outside the field of health (e.g., economics, political science, engineering) to identify other TMFs that could inform research, as reviews have identified gaps in availability of TMFs for certain types of D&I research (e.g., economics,[111] health equity,[83] sustainability[112]). The application and ongoing testing of theory-based approaches will increase our ability to ensure essential concepts are considered, enhance interpretability, support evaluation of outcome variations, and move the science forward.

SUGGESTED READINGS AND WEBSITES

Readings

Moullin JC, Dickson KS, Stadnick NA, et al. Ten recommendations for using implementation frameworks in research and practice. *Implement Sci Commun.* 2020;1:42.

This article provides 10 recommendations to improve the use of D&I frameworks and support work that advances generalizable knowledge for implementation science and practice.

Nilsen P. Making sense of implementation theories, models and frameworks. *Implement Sci* 2015;10:53.

In this article, Nilsen presents a strategy to categorize models to assist in model selection based on study aim. This review identified five categories of models and associated each with one of three common aims for D&I research (describing and/or guiding the process of translating research into practice, understanding and/or explaining what influences implementation outcomes, and evaluating implementation): process models, determinant frameworks, classic theories, implementation theories, and evaluation frameworks.

Nilsen P, Potthoff S, Birken SA. Conceptualising four categories of behaviours: implications for implementation strategies to achieve behaviour change. Hypothesis and theory. *Front Health Serv.* January 11, 2022. doi:10.3389/frhs.2021.795144

The authors explore concepts, theories, and empirical findings from different disciplines to categorize different types of influences on behaviors. They described four types of influences and provided a 2 × 2 conceptual map. The paper discusses the nature of the behaviors that need to be changed, thus providing guidance on the type of theory or framework that might be most relevant for understanding and facilitating behavior change.

Smith JD, Li DH, Rafferty MR. The implementation research logic model: a method for planning, executing, reporting, and synthesizing implementation projects. *Implement Sci.* 2020;15(1):84.

This article provides a description of the IRLM and its development as well as a guide to using the tool to improve the "specification, rigor, reproducibility, and testable causal pathways involved in implementation research projects." Blank models as well as examples are provided.

Strifler L, Cardoso R, McGowan J, et al. Scoping review identifies significant number of knowledge translation theories, models, and frameworks with limited use. *J Clin Epidemiol.* 2018;100:92–102.

This scoping review identified 159 TMFs. For the TMFs, the authors identified studies in which they were used, classified their use (e.g., planning/design, sustainability/scalability), and determined the level (e.g., individual, organizational) at which behavior change was targeted.

Tabak RG, Khoong EC, Chambers DA, Brownson RC. Bridging research and practice: models for dissemination and implementation research. *Am J Prev Med.* 2012;43(3):337–350.

This narrative review identified 61 models used in D&I research and organized them according to several continua (construct flexibility, dissemination and/or implementation [D/I], and the levels of the socio-ecological framework) in order to assist with model selection. Additional information about each model including the field in which it originated, examples of studies (where available) that use the model, and the number of times the model was cited. Case studies demonstrating model use are also included.

Selected Websites and Tools

Dissemination& Implementation Models in Health Web tool. https://dissemination-implementation.org/

This website provides a searchable database of models included in previous review papers and more recent TMFs. Search categories include dissemination to implementation, levels of the socioecological framework, *and included constructs. The database includes information about each model's categorization as well as citations for the model, and where possible, examples of its use. Resources on adapting and integrating the model are also provided.*

CFIR Technical Assistance Website. http://www.cfirguide.org/

This website has considerable information for those interested in the Consolidated Framework for Implementation Research (CFIR). This includes an overview of the framework, its domains and constructs, and a library of citations using CFIR. Other features of the site are tools and templates for data collection and analysis, which includes an interview guide tool designed to help researchers build interview guides based on CFIR.

RE-AIM Website. http://re-aim.org/

The RE-AIM website provides a number of resources related to the RE-AIM framework and external validity. Information on the overall framework and its application is provided, as well as information on RE-AIM's components—Reach, Effectiveness, Adoption, Implementation, and Maintenance—with examples of use. The website also includes many resources and tools, including guides on how to calculate the components of RE-AIM, and checklists and tools for intervention planning and assessing RE-AIM application

Theory, Model, and Framework Comparison and Selection Tool (T-CaST).https://impsci.tracs.unc.edu/tcast/

This site helps implementation researchers assess one or more TMF for a particular project and can help users consider what characteristics of a TMF are most important for the specific project, evaluate how each TMF meets those needs, compare TMFs, and identify how TMFs can be combined.

REFERENCES

1. Sales A, Smith J, Curran G, Kochevar L. Models, strategies, and tools. Theory in implementing evidence-based findings into health care practice. *J Gen Intern Med.* Feb 2006;21(suppl 2):S43–S49.
2. Davis M, Beidas RS. Refining contextual inquiry to maximize generalizability and accelerate the implementation process. *Implement Res Pract.*

January 2021;2. https://doi.org/10.1177/2633489521994941
3. Mitchell SA, Fisher CA, Hastings CE, Silverman LB, Wallen GR. A thematic analysis of theoretical models for translational science in nursing: mapping the field. *Nurs Outlook*. Nov–Dec 2010;58(6):287–300.
4. Damschroder LJ. Clarity out of chaos: use of theory in implementation research. *Psychiatry Res*. Jan 2020;283:112461.
5. Tabak RG, Khoong EC, Chambers DA, Brownson RC. Bridging research and practice: models for dissemination and implementation research. *Am J Prev Med*. Sep 2012;43(3):337–350.
6. Smith JD, Li DH, Rafferty MR. The implementation research logic model: a method for planning, executing, reporting, and synthesizing implementation projects. *Implement Sci*. Sep 25 2020;15(1):84.
7. Frankfort-Nachmias C, Nachmias D. *Research Methods in the Social Sciences*. Arnold; 1996.
8. Wacker J. A definition of theory: research guidelines for different theory-building research methods in operations management. *J Operat Manag*. 1998;16:361–385.
9. Lewis CC, Klasnja P, Powell BJ, et al. From classification to causality: advancing understanding of mechanisms of change in implementation science. *Front Public Health*. 2018;6:136. doi:10.3389/fpubh.2018.00136
10. Carpiano RM, Daley DM. A guide and glossary on postpositivist theory building for population health. *J EpidemiolCommunity Health*. 2006;60(7):564–570.
11. Sabatier PA. *Theories of the Policy Process*. Westview Press; 1999.
12. Greenhalgh T, Robert G, Macfarlane F, Bate P, Kyriakidou O. Diffusion of innovations in service organizations: systematic review and recommendations. *Milbank Q*. 2004;82(4):581–629.
13. Moullin JC, Dickson KS, Stadnick NA, Rabin B, Aarons GA. Systematic review of the exploration, preparation, implementation, sustainment (EPIS) framework. *Implement Sci*. Jan 5 2019;14(1):1.
14. Harvey G, Kitson A. PARIHS revisited: from heuristic to integrated framework for the successful implementation of knowledge into practice. *Implement Sci*. 2015;11(1):1–13.
15. Damschroder LJ, Reardon CM, Widerquist MAO, et al. The updated Consolidated Framework for Implementation Research based on user feedback. *Implement Sci*. 2022;17:75. https://doi.org/10.1186/s13012-022-01245-0.
16. Glasgow RE, Harden SM, Gaglio B, et al. RE-AIM planning and evaluation framework: adapting to new science and practice with a 20-year review. *Front Public Health*. 2019;7:64.
17. Delbecq AL, Van de Ven AH. A group process model for problem identification and program planning. *J Appl Behav Sci*. 1971;7(4):466–492.
18. Hage J, Aiken M. *Social change in complex organizations*. Vol. 43. Random House; 1970.
19. Hannan MT, Freeman J. Structural inertia and organizational change. *Am Sociol Rev*. 1984;49(2):149–164.
20. Dimaggio P, Powell W. The iron cage revisited: institutional isomorphism and collective rationality in organizational fields. *Am Sociol Rev*. 1983;48(2):147–160.
21. Rogers EM. *Diffusion of Innovations*. 5th ed. Free Press; 2003.
22. Schein E. *Organizational Culture and Leadership: A Dynamic View*. Joint publication in the Jossey-Bass management series and the Jossey-Bass social and behavioral science series; 1985.
23. Nilsen P. Making sense of implementation theories, models and frameworks. *Implement Sci*. 2015;10:53.
24. Lynch EA, Mudge A, Knowles S, Kitson AL, Hunter SC, Harvey G. "There is nothing so practical as a good theory": a pragmatic guide for selecting theoretical approaches for implementation projects. *BMC Health Serv Res*. Nov 14 2018;18(1):857.
25. Pinto RM, Park S, Miles R, Ong PN. Community engagement in dissemination and implementation models: a narrative review. *Implement Res Pract*. January 2021;2. https://doi.org/10.1177/2633489520985305
26. Chambers DA. Guiding theory for dissemination and implementation research: a reflection on models used in research and practice. In: Beidas RS, Kendall PC, eds. *Dissemination and Implementation of Evidence-Based Practices in Child and Adolescent Mental Health*. Oxford University Press; 2014:chap 2.
27. Baumann AA, Cabassa LJ, Wiltsey Stirman S. Adaptation in dissemination and implementation science. In: Brownson R, Colditz G, Proctor E, eds. *Dissemination and Implementation Research in Health: Translating Science to Practice*. 2nd ed. Oxford University Press; 2018:chap 17.
28. Dodson E, Brownson R, Weiss S. Policy dissemination research. In: Brownson R, Colditz G, Proctor E, eds. *Dissemination and Implementation Research in Health: Translating Science to Practice*. Oxford University Press; 2012:437–458.
29. Glasgow RE, McKay HG, Piette JD, Reynolds KD. The RE-AIM framework for evaluating interventions: what can it tell us about approaches

to chronic illness management? *Patient Educ Couns.* Aug 2001;44(2):119–127.

30. Aarons GA, Hurlburt M, Horwitz SM. Advancing a conceptual model of evidence-based practice implementation in public service sectors. *Adm Policy Ment Health.* Jan 2011;38(1):4–23.
31. Systematic reviews of methods to measure implementation constructs. Accessed January 22, 2022. https://journals.sagepub.com/topic/collections-irp/irp-1-systematic_reviews_of_methods_to_measure_implementation_constructs/irp
32. Glasgow RE, Harden SM, Gaglio B, et al. Use of the RE-AIM framework: translating research to practice with novel applications and emerging directions. *Front Public Health.* Updated December 18, 2021. Accessed January 7, 2023. doi:10.3389/978-2-88971-181-9. https://www.frontiersin.org/research-topics/10170/use-of-the-re-aim-framework-translating-research-to-practice-with-novel-applications-and-emerging-di#articles
33. Atkins L, Francis J, Islam R, et al. A guide to using the Theoretical Domains Framework of behaviour change to investigate implementation problems. *Implement Sci.* Jun 21 2017;12(1):77.
34. Woodward EN, Singh RS, Ndebele-Ngwenya P, Melgar Castillo A, Dickson KS, Kirchner JE. A more practical guide to incorporating health equity domains in implementation determinant frameworks. *Implement Sci Commun.* Jun 5 2021;2(1):61.
35. CFIR Research Team. Consolidated Framework for Implementation Research (CFIR). Accessed January 7, 2023. http://cfirguide.org/
36. Bergstrom A, Ehrenberg A, Eldh AC, et al. The use of the PARIHS framework in implementation research and practice—a citation analysis of the literature. *Implement Sci.* Aug 27 2020;15(1):68.
37. Strifler L, Cardoso R, McGowan J, et al. Scoping review identifies significant number of knowledge translation theories, models, and frameworks with limited use. *J Clin Epidemiol.* 2018;100:92–102.
38. Birken SA, Rohweder CL, Powell BJ, et al. T-CaST: an implementation theory comparison and selection tool. *Implement Sci.* Nov 22 2018;13(1):143.
39. Dingfelder HE, Mandell DS. Bridging the research-to-practice gap in autism intervention: an application of diffusion of innovation theory. *J Autism Dev Disord.* May 2011;41(5):597–609.
40. Glanz K, Steffen A, Elliott T, O'Riordan D. Diffusion of an effective skin cancer prevention program: design, theoretical foundations, and first-year implementation. *Health Psychol.* Sep 2005;24(5):477–487.
41. Shively M, Riegel B, Waterhouse D, Burns D, Templin K, Thomason T. Testing a community level research utilization intervention. *Appl Nurs Res.* Aug 1997;10(3):121–127.
42. Wiecha JL, El Ayadi AM, Fuemmeler BF, et al. Diffusion of an integrated health education program in an urban school system: planet health. *J Pediatr Psychol.* Sep 2004;29(6):467–474.
43. Al-Ghaith WA, Sanzogni L, Sandhu K. Factors influencing the adoption and usage of online services in Saudi Arabia. *Electronic J Inform Syst Dev Countries.* 2010;40(1):1–32.
44. Kingdon JW. *Agendas, Alternatives, and Public Policies.* Little, Brown; 1984:xi.
45. Kingdon JW. *Agendas, Alternatives, and Public Policies.* Updated 2nd ed. Longman; 2010:xx.
46. Craig RL, Felix HC, Walker JF, Phillips MM. Public health professionals as policy entrepreneurs: Arkansas's childhood obesity policy experience. *Am J Public Health.* Nov 2010;100(11):2047–2052.
47. D'Abbs P. Alignment of the policy planets: behind the implementation of the Northern Territory (Australia) Living With Alcohol programme. *Drug Alcohol Rev.* Mar 2004;23(1):55–66.
48. Deschesnes M, Trudeau F, Kebe M. Factors influencing the adoption of a Health Promoting School approach in the province of Quebec, Canada. *Health Educ Res.* 2010;25(3):438–450.
49. Hanbury A, Thompson C, Wilson PM, et al. Translating research into practice in Leeds and Bradford (TRiPLaB): a protocol for a programme of research. *Implement Sci.* 2010;5:37.
50. Hook ML. Using implementation theory to evaluate the impact of technology on nurses' knowledge and use of best practices in acute care. Presented at the 9th Annual Conference of the Science of Dissemination and Implementation, co-hosted by the National Institutes of Health and AcademyHealth; December 2016; Washington, DC.
51. Wandersman A, Duffy J, Flaspohler P, et al. Bridging the gap between prevention research and practice: the interactive systems framework for dissemination and implementation. *Am J Community Psychol.* Jun 2008;41(3–4):171–181.
52. Lee SJ, Altschul I, Mowbray CT. Using planned adaptation to implement evidence-based programs with new populations. *Am J Community Psychol.* Jun 2008;41(3–4):290–303.
53. Lesesne CA, Lewis KM, White CP, Green DC, Duffy JL, Wandersman A. Promoting science-based approaches to teen pregnancy prevention: proactively engaging the three systems of the interactive systems framework. *Am J Community Psychol.* Jun 2008;41(3–4):379–392.

54. Ozer EJ, Cantor JP, Cruz GW, Fox B, Hubbard E, Moret L. The diffusion of youth-led participatory research in urban schools: the role of the prevention support system in implementation and sustainability. *Am J Community Psychol.* 2008;41(3):278–289.
55. Glasgow RE, Vogt TM, Boles SM. Evaluating the public health impact of health promotion interventions: the RE-AIM framework. *Am J Public Health.* Sep 1999;89(9):1322–1327.
56. De Meij JSB, Chinapaw MJM, Kremers SPJ, Van der Wal MF, Jurg ME, Van Mechelen W. Promoting physical activity in children: the stepwise development of the primary school-based JUMP-in intervention applying the RE-AIM evaluation framework. *Br J Sports Med.* Sep 2010;44(12):879–887.
57. Glasgow RE, Nelson CC, Strycker LA, King DK. Using RE-AIM metrics to evaluate diabetes self-management support interventions. *Am J Prev Med.* Jan 2006;30(1):67–73.
58. Van Acker R, De Bourdeaudhuij I, De Cocker K, Klesges L, Cardon G. The impact of disseminating the whole-community project "10,000 Steps": a RE-AIM analysis. *BMC Public Health.* 2011;11(1):3.
59. Fixsen D, Naoom S, Blase K, Friedman R, Wallace F. *Implementation Research: A Synthesis of the Literature.* Tamps, FL: University of South Florida, Louis de la Parte Florida Mental Health Institute, National Implementation Research Network (FMHI Publicatino #231); 2005.
60. UNC Frank Porter Graham Child Development Institute, National Implementation Research Network. Active implementation hub. Accessed January 7, 2023. https://nirn.fpg.unc.edu/ai-hub
61. Casado BL, Quijano LM, Stanley MA, Cully JA, Steinberg EH, Wilson NL. Healthy IDEAS: implementation of a depression program through community-based case management. *Gerontologist.* 2008;48(6):828.
62. Graff CA, Springer P, Bitar GW, Gee R, Arredondo R. A purveyor team's experience: lessons learned from implementing a behavioral health care program in primary care settings. *Fam Syst Health.* 2010;28(4):356.
63. Klein KJ, Conn AB, Sorra JS. Implementing computerized technology: an organizational analysis. *J Appl Psychol.* 2001;86(5):811.
64. Klein KJ, Sorra JS. The challenge of innovation implementation. *Acad Manage Rev.* Oct 1996;21(4):1055–1080.
65. Dong L, Neufeld DJ, Higgins C. Testing Klein and Sorra's innovation implementation model: an empirical examination. *J Eng Technol Manag.* 2008;25(4):237–255.
66. Holahan PJ, Aronson ZH, Jurkat MP, Schoorman FD. Implementing computer technology: a multiorganizational test of Klein and Sorra's model. *J Eng Technol Manag.* 2004;21(1–2):31–50.
67. Robertson J, Sorbello T, Unsworth K. Innovation implementation: the role of technology diffusion agencies. *J Technol Manag Innov.* 2008;3(3):1–10.
68. Sawang S. Innovation implementation effectiveness: a multiorganizational test of Klein Conn and Sorra's model (Doctoral dissertation, Queensland University of Technology). 2008.
69. Brookman-Frazee L, Chlebowski C, Suhrheinrich J, et al. Characterizing shared and unique implementation influences in two community services systems for autism: applying the EPIS framework to two large-scale autism intervention community effectiveness trials. *Adm Policy Ment Health.* Mar 2020;47(2):176–187.
70. Aarons GA, Fettes DL, Sommerfeld DH, Palinkas LA. Mixed methods for implementation research: application to evidence-based practice implementation and staff turnover in community-based organizations providing child welfare services. *Child Maltreat.* Feb 2012;17(1):67–79.
71. Cane J, O'Connor D, Michie S. Validation of the theoretical domains framework for use in behaviour change and implementation research. *Implement Sci.* Apr 24 2012;7:37.
72. French SD, Green SE, O'Connor DA, et al. Developing theory-informed behaviour change interventions to implement evidence into practice: a systematic approach using the Theoretical Domains Framework. *Implement Sci.* Apr 24 2012;7:38.
73. Birken SA, Presseau J, Ellis SD, Gerstel AA, Mayer DK. Potential determinants of health-care professionals' use of survivorship care plans: a qualitative study using the Theoretical Domains Framework. *Implement Sci.* Nov 15 2014;9:167.
74. Curran JA, Brehaut J, Patey AM, Osmond M, Stiell I, Grimshaw JM. Understanding the Canadian adult CT head rule trial: use of the theoretical domains framework for process evaluation. *Implement Sci.* Feb 21 2013;8:25.
75. Damschroder LJ, Aron DC, Keith RE, Kirsh SR, Alexander JA, Lowery JC. Fostering implementation of health services research findings into practice: a consolidated framework for advancing implementation science. *Implement Sci.* 2009;4:50.
76. Lash SJ, Timko C, Curran GM, McKay JR, Burden JL. Implementation of evidence-based substance use disorder continuing care interventions. *Psychol Addict Behav.* Jun 2011;25(2):238–251.
77. Hartzler B, Lash SJ, Roll JM. Contingency management in substance abuse treatment: a

structured review of the evidence for its transportability. *Drug Alcohol Depend.* 2012;122.1-2:1–10. https://doi.org/10.1016/j.drugalcdep.2011.11.011

78. Shelton RC, Chambers DA, Glasgow RE. An extension of RE-AIM to enhance sustainability: addressing dynamic context and promoting health equity over time. *Front Public Health.* 2020;8:134.
79. Simione M, Farrar-Muir H, Mini FN, et al. Implementation of the Connect for Health pediatric weight management program: study protocol and baseline characteristics. *J Comp Eff Res.* Aug 2021;10(11):881–892.
80. Birken SA, Powell BJ, Presseau J, et al. Combined use of the Consolidated Framework for Implementation Research (CFIR) and the Theoretical Domains Framework (TDF): a systematic review. *Implement Sci.* Jan 5 2017;12(1):2.
81. Moullin JC, Dickson KS, Stadnick NA, et al. Ten recommendations for using implementation frameworks in research and practice. *Implement Sci Commun.* 2020;1:42.
82. Kirk MA, Kelley C, Yankey N, Birken SA, Abadie B, Damschroder L. A systematic review of the use of the consolidated framework for implementation research. *Implement Sci.* 2015;11(1):1–13.
83. Woodward EN, Matthieu MM, Uchendu US, Rogal S, Kirchner JE. The health equity implementation framework: proposal and preliminary study of hepatitis C virus treatment. *Implement Sci.* Mar 12 2019;14(1):26.
84. Kowdley KV, Gordon SC, Reddy KR, et al. Ledipasvir and sofosbuvir for 8 or 12 weeks for chronic HCV without cirrhosis. *N Engl J Med.* May 15 2014;370(20):1879–1888. doi:10.1056/NEJMoa1402355
85. *Hepatitis C and Veterans: Hearing before the U.S. Comm on Veterans Affairs,* 113th Cong. 1 (2014) (Statement of Sen. Bernie Sanders, Chair, S. Comm. on Veterans Affairs).
86. Lo Re V 3rd, Gowda C, Urick PN, et al. Disparities in absolute denial of modern hepatitis C therapy by type of insurance. *Clin Gastroenterol Hepatol.* Jul 2016;14(7):1035–1043. doi:10.1016/j.cgh.2016.03.040
87. Moon AM, Green PK, Berry K, Ioannou GN. Transformation of hepatitis C antiviral treatment in a national healthcare system following the introduction of direct antiviral agents. *Aliment Pharmacol Ther.* May 2017;45(9):1201–1212. doi:10.1111/apt.14021
88. Dominitz JA, Boyko EJ, Koepsell TD, et al. Elevated prevalence of hepatitis C infection in users of United States veterans medical centers. *Hepatology.* Jan 2005;41(1):88–96.
89. Armstrong GL, Wasley A, Simard EP, McQuillan GM, Kuhnert WL, Alter MJ. The prevalence of hepatitis C virus infection in the United States, 1999 through 2002. *Ann Intern Med.* May 16 2006;144(10):705–714.
90. Rousseau CM, Ioannou GN, Todd-Stenberg JA, et al. Racial differences in the evaluation and treatment of hepatitis C among veterans: a retrospective cohort study. *Am J Public Health.* May 2008;98(5):846–852.
91. Vutien P, Hoang J, Brooks L Jr, Nguyen NH, Nguyen MH. Racial disparities in treatment rates for chronic hepatitis C: analysis of a population-based cohort of 73,665 patients in the United States. *Medicine (Baltimore).* May 2016;95(22):e3719.
92. Reddy KR, Hoofnagle JH, Tong MJ, et al. Racial differences in responses to therapy with interferon in chronic hepatitis C. Consensus Interferon Study Group. *Hepatology.* Sep 1999;30(3):787–793. doi:10.1002/hep.510300319
93. Kanwal F, Kramer JR, El-Serag HB, et al. Race and gender differences in the use of direct acting antiviral agents for hepatitis C virus. *Clin Infect Dis.* Aug 1 2016;63(3):291–299.
94. Kilbourne AM, Switzer G, Hyman K, Crowley-Matoka M, Fine MJ. Advancing health disparities research within the health care system: a conceptual framework. *Am J Public Health.* Dec 2006;96(12):2113–2121.
95. LaVeist TA. *Minority Populations and Health: An Introduction to Health Disparities in the United States.* Jossey-Bass; 2005.
96. Page-Reeves J, Niforatos J, Mishra S, Regino L, Gingrich A, Bulten R. Health disparity and structural violence: how fear undermines health among immigrants at risk for diabetes. *J Health Dispar Res Pract.* 2013;6(2):30–47.
97. Thomas SB, Quinn SC, Butler J, Fryer CS, Garza MA. Toward a fourth generation of disparities research to achieve health equity. *Annu Rev Public Health.* 2011;32:399–416.
98. Marmot M. Social determinants of health inequalities. *Lancet.* Mar 19–25 2005;365(9464):1099–1104. doi:10.1016/S0140-6736(05)71146-6
99. Cooper LA, Roter DL, Carson KA, et al. The associations of clinicians' implicit attitudes about race with medical visit communication and patient ratings of interpersonal care. *Am J Public Health.* May 2012;102(5):979–987.
100. Blair IV, Steiner JF, Fairclough DL, et al. Clinicians' implicit ethnic/racial bias and perceptions of care among Black and Latino patients. *Ann Fam Med.* Jan–Feb 2013;11(1):43–52.

101. Sabin JA, Marini M, Nosek BA. Implicit and explicit anti-fat bias among a large sample of medical doctors by BMI, race/ethnicity and gender. *PLoS One*. 2012;7(11):e48448.
102. Belperio PS, Chartier M, Ross DB, Alaigh P, Shulkin D. Curing hepatitis C virus infection: best practices from the U.S. Department of Veterans Affairs. *Ann Intern Med*. Oct 3 2017;167(7):499–504.
103. Belperio PSK, Korshak L, Moy E. Hepatitis C treatment in minority veterans. 2020. Accessed January 22, 2022. https://www.va.gov/HEALTHEQUITY/Hepatitis_C_Treatment_in_Minority_Veterans.asp#:~:text=The%20Office%20of%20Health%20Equity%20%28OHE%29%20champions%20the,common%20in%20Veterans%20than%20the%20general%20U.S.%20population
104. Santos SL, Tagai EK, Scheirer MA, et al. Adoption, reach, and implementation of a cancer education intervention in African American churches. *Implement Sci*. Mar 14 2017;12(1):36.
105. Miller CJ, Barnett ML, Baumann AA, Gutner CA, Wiltsey-Stirman S. The FRAME-IS: a framework for documenting modifications to implementation strategies in healthcare. *Implement Sci*. 2021;16(1):1–12.
106. Stirman SW, Baumann AA, Miller CJ. The FRAME: an expanded framework for reporting adaptations and modifications to evidence-based interventions. *Implement Sci*. 2019;14(1):1–10.
107. Moore G, Campbell M, Copeland L, et al. Adapting interventions to new contexts—the ADAPT guidance. *BMJ*. Aug 3 2021;374:n1679.
108. Chambers DA, Glasgow RE, Stange KC. The dynamic sustainability framework: addressing the paradox of sustainment amid ongoing change. *Implement Sci*. Oct 2 2013;8:117.
109. Nilsen P, Ingvarsson S, Hasson H, von Thiele Schwarz U, Augustsson H. Theories, models, and frameworks for de-implementation of low-value care: a scoping review of the literature. *Implement Res Pract*. 2020;1:2633489520953762.
110. Walsh-Bailey C, Tsai E, Tabak RG, et al. A scoping review of de-implementation frameworks and models. *Implement Sci*. Nov 24 2021;16(1):100.
111. Brown V, Tran H, Blake M, Laws R, Moodie M. Correction to: a narrative review of economic constructs in commonly used implementation and scale-up theories, frameworks and models. *Health Res Policy Syst*. Oct 28 2020;18(1):124.
112. Shelton RC, Cooper BR, Stirman SW. The sustainability of evidence-based interventions and practices in public health and health care. *Annu Rev Public Health*. Apr 1 2018;39:55–76.

5

Ethical Issues in Dissemination and Implementation Research

JAMES M. DUBOIS AND BETH PRUSACZYK

INTRODUCTION

In contrast to theoretical ethics, which focuses on areas such as understanding the nature of ethical reasoning and ethical language, professional ethics are specific to a particular activity, such as practicing medicine, investment banking, or doing research. Professional ethics are frequently a concoction of norms stemming from diverse sources, including federal and state laws and regulations, the codes of professional associations, institutional policies, general ethical principles, scientific standards, and the decisions of oversight boards or stakeholder committees. Within the domain of research ethics, the content of these norms is also highly varied. In the broadest sense, the responsible conduct of research (RCR) involves protection of human subjects as well as standards for ensuring data integrity, good mentoring, authorship, peer review, and the social value of research.[1] This chapter focuses primarily on the protection of human participants in dissemination and implementation (D&I) studies. It begins by reviewing the Belmont principles that undergird US research regulations and considering the ethical case for D&I research, including emerging areas such as de-implementation. It then proceeds to examine some ethical issues that might arise during a public health, D&I research agenda in middle schools.

Moving beyond the content of the ethics of a profession, one may also focus on fostering ethical behavior. This can be accomplished by not only teaching rules but also increasing sensitivity to how ethical issues arise in specific contexts, fostering good ethical decision-making skills, creating an ethical climate in which leaders model good behavior and clearly state expectations, and providing oversight.[2–4] After examining how D&I raises special challenges in determining which rules and regulations apply to a study (increasing ethical sensitivity), we consider a series of decision-making strategies that can guide behavior in challenging situations that arise in D&I research, for example, when disagreement exists regarding which rules apply to a study or stakeholders seek competing goals. We conclude by exploring how D&I provides tools for implementing ethical policies or practices.

THE BELMONT PRINCIPLES

The Belmont Report: Ethical Principles and Guidelines for the Protection of Human Subjects of Research describes three general principles that are widely recognized in society and have implications for the ethical conduct of human subjects research.[5] The principle of *respect for persons* requires that insofar as human beings are capable of reasoning and self-determination, we should provide them with information about research studies and solicit their voluntary, informed consent. When human beings lack the cognitive capacity to provide informed consent (e.g., due to young age or cognitive impairments) or when voluntariness might be compromised (e.g., by being institutionalized or in a subordinate relationship to the researchers or sponsors of a project), then they are vulnerable and deserve additional protections. The *principle of beneficence* reminds us that research should pursue benefits that are proportionate to the risks involved, and that risks

James M. DuBois and Beth Prusaczyk, *Ethical Issues in Dissemination and Implementation Research* In: *Dissemination and Implementation Research in Health*. Edited by: Ross C. Brownson, Graham A. Colditz, and Enola K. Proctor, Oxford University Press.
 DOI: 10.1093/oso/9780197660690.003.0005

TABLE 5.1 BELMONT PRINCIPLES FOR THE PROTECTION OF HUMAN SUBJECTS APPLIED TO D&I RESEARCH

Belmont Principle	General Requirements	Application Questions in D&I Research
Respect for persons	• Obtain informed consent • Provide additional protections when participants are incapable of providing informed consent	• Who needs to provide informed consent when implementation is studied? • How can the voluntariness of participation be ensured when participants are students or employees?
Beneficence	• Minimize risk of harms, establish appropriate protections • Ensure anticipated benefits justify risks	• Must implementation trials have equipoise? • When interventions are effective, how can benefits be provided to control groups?
Justice	• The populations that undertake risks in research should also be beneficiaries of research • Vulnerable populations should not be targeted due to convenience	• How can community partners be engaged to address concerns about social justice within D&I studies? • When is there an obligation to engage in D&I research in order to justify the investment in efficacy research?

should be minimized and managed throughout studies. The *principle of justice* requires that, in general, those who are likely to benefit from a research study are the ones who should undertake the risks of research participation. Participants should not be recruited simply because it is convenient to access them (e.g., due to institutionalization).

When the Belmont Report was produced in the 1970s, the emphasis was on avoiding the exploitation of vulnerable groups of individuals as occurred in Nazi experimentations on human subjects held in concentration camps and in the Public Health Service study of syphilis at Tuskegee. Today, we additionally recognize that justice requires that research serves people in need without regard to their sex, sexual preferences, or financial means. Ironically, the desire to protect vulnerable populations—for example, those living with often-stigmatized diseases such as HIV or prisoners—may prevent them from benefiting from research participation and may slow advances in the treatment or prevention of diseases that disproportionately affect them.[6,7]

While the Belmont Report focused primarily on the treatment of research participants, which has led some to question its suitability for public health research,[8] each of its principles may be adapted to communities from which participants are drawn.[9] For example, while only individuals can provide informed consent in the traditional sense, community permission may be sought through a variety of means, such as holding town hall meetings, surveying community members, establishing community advisory boards, or including community members as full research partners using action research or community-based participatory research designs.[8,10,11] Engaging communities may serve to increase transparency, provide researchers with valuable guidance, facilitate recruitment by fostering buy-in, and provide the permission of representatives from the community.[11–14] Similarly, risks may be considered to not only individuals, but also communities, including the risk of breaching trust or stigmatizing groups. Within some public health circles, the need to adapt general ethical principles to the special features of communities has led to recognition of a fourth principle, *respect for communities*.[15,16]

Table 5.1 presents the Belmont principles and illustrates how they relate to current questions about ethics in D&I research.

THE ETHICAL CASE FOR D&I RESEARCH

Many have argued that funders and researchers have an ethical duty to disseminate and implement knowledge and evidence from efficacy trials so their full benefits can be realized.[17–19]

Only through implementation science can "our nation's investment in research in the life sciences yield the pay-off that patients and the public deserve."[19(p32)] The Public Health Leadership Society published *Principles of the Ethical Practice of Public Health*, which includes principles on the D&I of information, policies, and programs.[18] One of the underlying values and beliefs of the principles states that information is not gathered for "idle interest" but that: "Public health should seek to translate available information into timely action." The society continued by saying that people have a *responsibility* to act on the basis of what they know.

Mann offered several reasons why researchers have an ethical obligation to disseminate research findings, including the need for providing social value, facilitating production of credible and relevant systematic reviews and meta-analyses, honoring the altruistic motivation of study participants and participants' right to know the results of studies they were enrolled in, and complying with codes of ethical conduct that require sharing new knowledge with colleagues and the public.[20] Mann believed it is the responsibility of research ethics committees (e.g., institutional review boards [IRBs] in the United States) to ensure dissemination occurs; we believe the responsibility is shared with investigators as well.

As described in numerous chapters in this book, we know that some strategies for D&I are significantly more effective in achieving the goals of knowledge transfer, research utilization or adoption, and diffusion within communities, including utilizing audit and feedback, learning collaboratives, facilitation, and local needs assessments.[21] Thus, there is an imperative to engage in not only D&I, but also research on D&I aimed at making D&I more effective in achieving their goals.

Furthermore, experts have recently highlighted the ethical case for engaging in the emerging field of de-implementation research, specifically for advancing health equity.[22–24] De-implementation is defined as the removal or replacement of practices that are not supported by the best available evidence and/or are unnecessary, costly, or harmful or do not improve health outcomes (see chapter 12).[25] In some cases, racial and ethnic minority patients are more likely to receive low-value care than White patients,[26] which means de-implementation efforts have the potential to reduce this disparity and further health equity. However, there are important ethical challenges to consider when conducting de-implementation research, such as understanding the cultural and historical context of the practice targeted for de-implementation and ensuring there are adequate replacements (to not further disparities).[22–24]

COMMON ETHICAL CHALLENGES IN D&I RESEARCH

Several authors have argued that researchers and review boards must think about the ethical challenges of clinical efficacy studies differently from those of D&I research, a point that has also been made by others.[19,27–31] This chapter considers four questions that arise in D&I research more frequently than in common research activities such as drug trials:

1. Is it human subjects research?
2. Who are your research participants, and who should provide informed consent?
3. Is equipoise necessary?
4. How can scientific rigor be protected in a real-world setting (e.g., when participation cannot be blinded or participants are not interested in D&I research)?

A Focal Case

In order to illustrate how these questions arise when conducting D&I research, we build on a case presented in chapter 22, Health Dissemination and Implementation Within Schools. Lee and colleagues describe Planet Health, an obesity prevention program in middle schools. The Planet Health program aims to prevent obesity by "increasing physical activity, decreasing television viewing, improving diet through increased fruit and vegetable intake, and moderating fat intake."[32(p468)] The program is built around self-assessment and lessons delivered by social studies, language arts, math, and science teachers and micro units delivered by physical educators. The Planet Health field trial aimed not only to study the efficacy of the program, but also how the program was implemented and disseminated within the real-world context of schools. The project used a group- or cluster-randomized trial (CRT) design. Initially, 10 schools that were matched on key characteristics were randomized to receive the Planet Health intervention or nothing (until the end of the project period).

In what follows, we consider diverse projects—both real and fictitious—related to the Planet Health project, as well as ethical challenges and potential ethical solutions, again both real and fictitious.

Is It Human Subjects Research?

US Federal Regulations define research as "a systematic investigation, including research development, testing and evaluation, designed to develop or contribute to generalizable knowledge" (45CFR46.102(d)).

Dissemination and implementation are systematic activities. As defined in chapter 2, dissemination involves spreading evidence-based practices to a target group using planned strategies. Implementation involves using evidence-based practices within a real-world setting. Understood in this manner, D&I activities do not contribute to generalizable knowledge and do not constitute research. Accordingly, many aspects of research ethics such as review by an IRB, informed consent of participants, and privacy protections may not pertain to D&I activities.

In contrast to dissemination activities, D&I research aims to study the effects of interventions and diverse variables on outcomes such as uptake of evidence-based practices. Chapter 21, which focuses on healthcare settings, describes 11 different research activities commonly performed across the life of an implementation research program, ranging from preimplementation studies through four phases of implementation studies.

Whether human subjects protections and review by an IRB are required is primarily determined by the purpose of a study and whether human subjects or identifiable information about individuals are involved. If the purpose of an implementation project is strictly to improve outcomes at a hospital or the health of children at a school, then the activity may be treated as a quality improvement project. However, even when federal regulations do not apply to quality improvement projects, institutions or community organizations may nevertheless require some level of review and oversight.[33] Similarly, if a study does not examine outcomes at the level of individuals but only at the level of clusters or groups, it may not meet the definition of human subjects research and may not be addressed by research regulations. However, if determining the outcomes of a group involves examining identifiable, individual information, the regulations and IRB review do apply.[15]

Who Are Your Research Participants? Who Should Provide Consent?

D&I studies can be complicated because they may collect data on diverse outcomes, particularly in hybrid effectiveness-implementation designs.[34] For example, in the Planet Health study, investigators may be concerned with effectiveness—whether middle school children who receive the intervention have lower rates of obesity than children who do not receive the intervention. If the effectiveness outcome involves gathering data through interaction with the children or in some other manner that involves the collection of individually identifiable data, then the children are research subjects. Depending on the risk level of the intervention and the feasibility of obtaining consent, an IRB might (a) waive elements of consent (e.g., permit an opt-out approach); (b) require written, signed parental permission; and (c) require the verbal or written signed assent of the children. In several studies by the Planet Health principal investigator, the authors stated that they obtained both the written consent (permission) of parents and the consent (assent) of the children.[35,36] Requiring consent to establish the effectiveness of a hybrid D&I intervention can present a significant burden in school settings; it may mean excluding from participation students who might benefit from the program, and it might be finding alternative classroom space and meaningful activities for nonparticipating children. In other cases, however, a participating school may have the authority to make participation in a project's educational activities required or at least routine, and consent and assent are sought only for the collection of individual data.[35]

In other legs of the Planet Health project, the outcomes were all related to implementation, rather than effectiveness: "dose, acceptability, feasibility, and intent to continue use." All of these outcomes could be measured by engaging teachers as subjects; student participation was not necessary.[32] A common challenge investigators face when conducting D&I research relates to the collection of data from employees or providers in organizations whose supervisors or administrative leaders may have access to or request access to the data. Employees or providers may worry that their participation in the study or their feedback on the intervention or implementation strategies could impact their job security or standing in the organization. Investigators should anticipate this prior to beginning the study and map out strategies to ensure the privacy of employees or providers is protected.

Is Equipoise Necessary?

Within the world of efficacy trials such as randomized, controlled trials of pharmaceuticals, it is common to speak of clinical equipoise as a requirement[37] (though even in this domain the concept is somewhat controversial, and the term is not used in the Common Rule, 45CFR46).[38] Clinical equipoise is "a state of genuine uncertainty on the part of the clinical investigator regarding the comparative therapeutic merits of each arm in a trial."[37(141)] For example, in a study with three arms that compares a new drug to a standard of care drug and to placebo, equipoise would require uncertainty about the comparative merits of each arm. If one embraces clinical equipoise as an ethical requirement for clinical trials, then the use of placebo cannot always be justified. For example, if a serious medical condition urgently requires some form of treatment (e.g., lung cancer), then a placebo must be administered alongside a known effective treatment. However, if all available medications have serious side effects (while placebo rarely does) and a positive placebo effect has been observed in a clinical population (as is often the case in patients with depression), then the use of placebo might be justified.[39]

Implementation trials rarely occur in the absence of prior trials demonstrating efficacy. However, the point of implementation trials such as Planet Health is to establish effectiveness in real-world settings (as well as to examine factors that affect implementation outcomes) (see chapter 22). That is to say, the fact that a strategy for preventing obesity in children has been proven efficacious in a controlled setting does not mean it will be effective in the real-world setting of a middle school, which requires effective training of teachers, buy-in from administrators and teachers, and resources to sustain the program on a larger scale. So, uncertainty does exist regarding the comparative merits of being in the intervention arm versus a control arm.

Moreover, it is unclear whether the notion of equipoise—which arose from within the patient-physician relationship, in which patients present with health needs in the context of a fiduciary relationship[40]—should be extrapolated to public health settings. Some argue that the notion could be grounded in the relationship of trust that exists between the state and research subjects (or by analogy, a school and its students), and it remains useful as IRBs evaluate studies.[41] However, the Ottawa Statement on the Ethical Design and Conduct of Cluster Randomized Trials states that:

> Researchers must adequately justify the choice of the control condition. When the control arm is usual practice or no treatment, individuals in the control arm must not be deprived of effective care or programs *to which they would have access, were there no trial.*[15(p7)] [emphasis added]

That is, in a nontherapeutic trial—a trial in which no patient-physician relationship preexists to treat or prevent an illness or disease—one should focus on not harming, but there is no strict obligation to provide benefits to which one ordinarily would not have access. Nevertheless, when prior trials lead study teams and community members to believe an intervention will improve the lives of participants, the question of justice cannot be avoided. Community input may be particularly important when it is not feasible (e.g., due to limited funding) to provide everyone with a known effective intervention.[42] However, when it is feasible—except for reasons of scientific design (specifically the need for a control group)—then it is possible to provide control groups with the intervention following the conclusion of the study if the intervention proves effective.[35] This approach is often defensible because until the conclusion of the implementation study, genuine uncertainty exists whether it will have its intended effect in a real-world setting. In fact this approach is possible in D&I through the increasing use of the stepped-wedge research design, in which the intervention is rolled out to all participants over time.[43] This design is adaptive, and as the intervention and strategies are rolled out data are collected and analyzed then used to adapt the rollout for the next group of participants. This ongoing data collection and adaptation does present potential challenges with IRBs, who may request ongoing review and approval in tandem with the ongoing study procedures.

How Can Scientific Rigor Be Protected in Real-World Settings?

Emanuel, Wendler, and Grady reviewed international codes of research ethics to answer the question: What makes research with human subjects ethical?[44] *Scientific validity* was among the seven requirements that they identified. Research that lacks scientific merit exposes participants to risks for no purpose and wastes scarce research resources.

Threats to scientific validity in real-world settings are manifold. First, in real-world settings, it is difficult to identify all the factors that might mediate, moderate, or confound effects of interventions. Randomization may help establish that an intervention was effective, but implementation science aims to understand why and when it is effective in complex settings such as hospitals and schools. This may require not only statistical expertise, but also very large sample sizes, which in turn requires tremendous resources and buy-in from stakeholder groups.

In 2007, the research team that implemented the Planet Health and other health promotion programs in public schools published a "lessons learned" paper. Although the paper discussed few specific challenges that arose within these studies, focusing rather on positive lessons (above all, the need for early and ongoing stakeholder engagement, liaisons between research teams and schools, and project champions), it offered the following general observation:

> Creating public health partnerships with schools is challenging for many reasons, including the numerous academic and nonacademic demands placed on schools. In addition, school programs often lack sufficient funds, are subject to political vicissitudes, exist in complex bureaucracies that foster fragmentation, and vary across localities.[45(p2)]

The authors of an article on the importance of community engagement for ensuring the ethical design and conduct of research added caveats throughout. In particular, they offered two observations. First, communities are never fully engaged; they may lack organization, leaders, or spokespeople; they may be heterogeneous and speak with competing voices rather than one voice; and individuals may not want to engage researchers. Second, while community engagement may improve the conduct of research in many ways, it can also compromise scientific rigor when done poorly or when goals are not shared.[11]

How can one protect the rigor of a research study when problems arise, for example, when gatekeepers or IRBs resist the use of a control group, when parental consent is required and parents are not heavily engaged in their children's school activities, or when a commitment to co-design of a study[28] requires that the design be adaptive to emerging stakeholder concerns? The following sections offer strategies for addressing these and other concerns that may arise in D&I research.

STRATEGIES FOR ETHICAL DECISION-MAKING

A recent root cause analysis of why researchers were referred for remediation of research compliance and integrity violations found that researchers are at risk when they are overextended, rules and expectations are ambiguous (e.g., when moving into new areas of research or working in an unfamiliar culture), or relationships or communication are poor.[46] Engaging stakeholders well is time consuming (though often time saving in the long run), which is challenging for busy researchers; each institution has its own culture; and communication is difficult in studies that involve multiple sites or that gather data at several levels (e.g., schools, teachers, and students). Rules are often ambiguous in implementation trials because they include elements that do not exist in the standard clinical trials that IRBs routinely review. Relationships can be strained when diverse stakeholders have competing goals for a project.

What follows offers a series of evidence-informed professional decision-making strategies that can serve researchers well as they navigate the challenges that may arise in D&I research.[47,48] As observed repeatedly throughout this chapter, stakeholder engagement is often key to navigating ethical and scientific issues in D&I research.[16,28,45] Each of these strategies can be applied by individual investigators or adapted for application by research teams.

Seek Help

Uncertainty can arise at all stages of research regarding logistical, scientific, ethical, or regulatory matters. Seeking help—the input of stakeholders, compliance officers, research ethicists, or more experienced colleagues—may provide new information, identify new options, or establish new relationships that can enable projects to move forward positively. Given the novelty of many D&I designs or interventions, seeking help from investigators who have previously conducted D&I research on the ethical issues they encountered and how they solved them may prove especially beneficial.

Manage Emotions

As research moves from experimental settings to real-world settings, projects become more politically charged, a greater number of competing voices must be heard, and accordingly, tensions can run high.[11,45] Managing emotions is a key component to successful professional decision-making and relationship development.[49,50] Strategies for managing emotions can include reappraising a situation, engaging in stress management practices such as relaxation or mindfulness, or simply taking a timeout.[49,51,52]

Anticipate Consequences

In research and many other endeavors, we often focus on information that confirms what we expect.[53,54] Yet, deliberations about risks, benefits, fair outcomes, and protection of the trust of stakeholder groups requires consideration of possible short-term and long-term and positive and negative consequences of a project for different stakeholders.[55] Anticipating consequences is often best done in conjunction with many of the other strategies listed here, including seeking help, managing emotions, and testing assumptions.

Recognize Rules and Context

Recognizing rules sounds like a straightforward task. However, D&I research frequently spans the worlds of academic institutions and service organizations (e.g., hospitals, public health agencies, schools), which may have different rules and procedures. Moreover, research regulations require interpretation as they are applied to specific research protocols; for better or worse, the interpretation of rules offered by IRBs carries more authority than the interpretation of investigators. Additionally, community organizations may have unwritten rules that guide their interactions with researchers, rules that must be satisfied before partnership agreements can be established or executed successfully. Again, other strategies may assist in the execution of this strategy—particularly seeking help (e.g., calling the IRB or engaging communities through focus groups) and testing assumptions. Last, as with all human subjects research, there may be additional rules and regulations surrounding D&I research with some communities and populations such as prisoners, American Indians or Alaskan Natives, or pregnant women.

Test Assumptions and Motives

Researchers make a lot of assumptions, for example, assumptions about the value of a project, the needs of communities, the best design to test a hypothesis, the feasibility of recruiting participants, and the risks of a study to individuals or communities. Problems can arise when these assumptions are either mistaken or are not shared by other stakeholders. Good communication with others is an excellent way of testing assumptions. Sharing our thought processes with others enables correction of bias and reappraisal of situations, which in turn may reduce anxiety and facilitate constructive problem-solving.[56]

Researchers may also assume that IRBs have all the information they need to make effective decisions. However, particularly with complex and unfamiliar study designs, this may not be the case. D&I researchers may benefit significantly from serving on IRBs or writing protocols with detailed engagement of ethical issues.

IMPLEMENTING ETHICS

It is insufficient to identify ethical practices or develop ethical policies: To have a positive impact on the world, they must be implemented. A recent article presented an implementation science framework for implementing ethical policies and practices.[57] The practices of engaging stakeholders, identifying barriers and facilitators, and considering dissemination at the outset of an endeavor may help with the refinement and implementation of ethical policies and practices. Thus, it is best to see ethics in D&I as a two-way relationship: Ethics should guide our D&I activities, and the tools of D&I may assist us in achieving ethical goals such as reducing racial health disparities.[58,59]

SUMMARY

While the use of ethical decision-making strategies and practices such as stakeholder engagement may be beneficial to all researchers, we believe they are of particular value to D&I researchers because the nature of their work—context specific, complex, and unfamiliar to many peers, collaborators, and reviewers—means they will deal with uncertainty and conflict on a regular basis, and solutions to the problems they face will rarely be found through simple reference principles, rules, or regulations.

SUGGESTED READINGS AND WEBSITES

Readings

DuBois JM, Bailey-Burch B, Bustillos D, et al. Ethical issues in mental health research: the case for community engagement. *Curr Opin Psychiatry.* 2011;24(3):208–214.

This article makes the case for community engagement in research and illustrates diverse approaches to community engagement suitable for a wide range of study designs. This article tries to move beyond the all-or-nothing (or community-based participatory research-or-nothing) approach to community engagement in research.

Gopichandran V, Luyckx VA, Biller-Andorno N, et al. Developing the ethics of implementation research in health. *Implement Sci.* 2016;11(1):161.

This is a comprehensive overview of ethical issues in implementation research with case studies.

Helfrich CD, Hartmann CW, Parikh TJ, Au DH. Promoting health equity through de-implementation research. *Ethnicity & Disease,* 2019;29(suppl 1):93.

This article describes how de-implementation is critical for advancing health equity within the domains of healthcare overuse, highlighting a number of ethical issues.

Macklin R. Ethical challenges in implementation research. *Public Health Ethics.* 2014;7(1):86–93.

The article provides an excellent overview of ethical issues that arise in implementation research by a leading ethicist.

Weijer C, Grimshaw JM, Eccles MP, et al. The Ottawa Statement on the Ethical Design and Conduct of Cluster Randomized Trials. *PLoS Med.* 2012;9(11):e1001346.

A thoughtful consensus statement on the ethical design of cluster randomized trials, a study design commonly used in clinical effectiveness research. This resource may be particularly useful in engaging institutional research ethics committees or IRBs.

Selected Websites and Tools

The Belmont Report. https://www.hhs.gov/ohrp/regulations-and-policy/belmont-report/

This website provides the full text of the Belmont Report, which describes the principles of respect for persons, beneficence, and justice and applies them to the context of human research. This framework has been particularly influential in the United States, where specific rules and regulations are supposed to be based on these principles.

Public Health Ethics Resources hosted by the Centers for Disease Control and Prevention (CDC). https://www.cdc.gov/od/science/integrity/phethics/resources.htm

This website collects a variety of useful materials in the area of public health ethics, many of which are open access.

Public Health Ethics Training Materials from the CDC. https://www.cdc.gov/od/science/integrity/phethics/trainingmaterials.htm

This website provides access to training materials developed by the CDC, as well as other open access training materials in the area of public health ethics.

REFERENCES

1. Shamoo AE, Resnik DB. *Responsible Conduct of Research.* 3rd ed. Oxford University Press; 2015.
2. Antes AL, DuBois JM. Aligning objectives and assessment in responsible conduct of research instruction. *J Microbiol Biol Educ.* 2014;15(2): 108–116. doi:10.1128/jmbe.v15i2.852
3. Rest JR, Narvez D, Bebeau MJ, Thoma SJ. *Postconventional Moral Thinking: A Neo-Kohlbergian Approach.* Lawrence Erlbaum Associates, Inc.; 1999:ix.
4. Mulhearn TJ, Steele LM, Watts LL, Medeiros KE, Mumford MD, Connelly S. Review of instructional approaches in ethics education. *Sci Eng Ethics.* 2017;23(3):883–912.
5. National Commission. *The Belmont Report: Ethical Principles and Guidelines for the Protection of Human Subjects of Research.* Department of Health, Education, and Welfare. National Commission, for the Protection of Human Subjects of Biomedical and Behavioral Research; 1979.

6. King PA. Justice beyond Belmont. In: Childress JF, Meslin EM, Shapiro HT, eds. *Belmont Revisited: Ethical Principles for Research With Human Subjects*. Georgetown University Press; 2005:136–147.
7. DuBois JM, Beskow L, Campbell J, et al. Restoring balance: a consensus statement on the protection of vulnerable research participants. *Am J Public Health*. 2012;102(12):2220–2225. doi:10.2105/AJPH.2012.300757
8. Quinn S. Ethics in public health research: protecting human subjects: the role of community advisory boards. *Am J Public Health*. 2004;94(6):918–922.
9. Gostin L. Ethical principles for the conduct of human subject research: population-based research and ethics. *Law Med Health Care*. Fall-Winter 1991;19(3–4):191–201.
10. Ross LF, Loup A, Nelson RM, et al. The challenges of collaboration for academic and community partners in a research partnership: points to consider. *J Empir Res Hum Res Ethics*. Mar 2010;5(1):19–31. doi:10.1525/jer.2010.5.1.19
11. DuBois JM, Bailey-Burch B, Bustillos D, et al. Ethical issues in mental health research: the case for community engagement. *Current Opin Psychiatry*. May 2011;24(3):208–214. doi:10.1097/YCO.0b013e3283459422
12. Frerichs L, Kim M, Dave G, et al. Stakeholder perspectives on creating and maintaining trust in community-academic research partnerships. *Health Educ Behav*. 2016:1–10. doi:10.1177/1090198116648291
13. Ross LF, Loup A, Nelson RM, et al. Human subjects protections in community-engaged research: a research ethics framework. *J Empir Res Hum Res Ethics*. Mar 2010;5(1):5–17. doi:10.1525/jer.2010.5.1.5
14. Ross LF, Loup A, Nelson RM, et al. Nine key functions for a human subjects protection program for community-engaged research: points to consider. *J Empir Res Hum Res Ethics*. Mar 2010;5(1):33–47. doi:10.1525/jer.2010.5.1.33
15. Weijer C, Grimshaw JM, Eccles MP, et al. The Ottawa Statement on the Ethical Design and Conduct of Cluster Randomized Trials. *PLoS Med*. 2012;9(11):e1001346. doi:10.1371/journal.pmed.1001346
16. Weijer C. Protecting communities in research: philosophical and pragmatic challenges. *Cambridge Q Healthc Ethics*. Fall 1999;8(4):501–513. doi:10.1017/s0963180199004120
17. Woolf SH. The meaning of translational research and why it matters. *JAMA*. 2008;299(2):211–213. doi:10.1001/jama.2007.26
18. Public Health Leadership Society, Centers for Disease Control and Prevention. *Principles of the Ethical Practice of Public Health*. 2002. http://www.apha.org/~/media/files/pdf/membergroups/ethics_brochure.ashx
19. Solomon MZ. The ethical urgency of advancing implementation science. *Am J Bioeth*. Aug 2010;10(8):31–32. doi:10.1080/15265161.2010.494230
20. Mann H. Research ethics committees and public dissemination of clinical trial results. *Lancet*. 2002;360(9330):406–408. doi:10.1016/s0140-6736(02)09613-7
21. Brownson RC, Colditz GA, Proctor EK. *Dissemination and Implementation Research in Health: Translating Science to Practice*. 2nd ed. Oxford University Press; 2018:xxiii.
22. Helfrich CD, Hartmann CW, Parikh TJ, Au DH. Promoting health equity through de-implementation research. *Ethn Dis*. 2019;29(suppl 1):93–96. https://doi.org/10.18865/ed.29.S1.93
23. Walsh-Bailey C, Tsai E, Tabak RG, et al. A scoping review of de-implementation frameworks and models. *Implement Sci*. 2021;16(1):100. https://doi.org/10.1186/s13012-021-01173-5
24. Prusaczyk B, Swindle T, Curran G. Defining and conceptualizing outcomes for de-implementation: key distinctions from implementation outcomes. *Implement Sci Commun*. 2020;1:article 1. doi:10.1186/s43058-020-00035-3
25. Shelton RC, Brotzman LE, Johnson D, Erwin D. Trust and mistrust in shaping adaptation and de-implementation in the context of changing screening guidelines. *Ethn Dis*. 2021;31(1):119–132. doi:.org/10.18865/ED.31.1.119
26. Schpero WL, Morden NE, Sequist TD, Rosenthal MB, Gottlieb DJ, Colla CH. Datawatch: for selected services, Blacks and Hispanics more likely to receive low-value care than whites. *Health Aff*. 2017;36(6):1065–1069. doi:10.1377/hlthaff.2016.1416. PMID: 28583965; PMCID: PMC5568010.
27. Eccles MP, Weijer C, Mittman B. Requirements for ethics committee review for studies submitted to implementation science. *Implement Sci*. 2011;6(32):1–4.
28. Goodyear-Smith F, Jackson C, Greenhalgh T. Co-design and implementation research: challenges and solutions for ethics committees. *BMC Med Ethics*. Nov 16 2015;16:78. doi:10.1186/s12910-015-0072-2
29. Gopichandran V, Luyckx VA, Biller-Andorno N, et al. Developing the ethics of implementation research in health. *Implement Sci*. Dec 09 2016;11(1):161. doi:10.1186/s13012-016-0527-y

30. Hutton JL, Eccles MP, Grimshaw JM. Ethical issues in implementation research: a discussion of the problems in achieving informed consent. *Implement Sci.* 2008;3:52. doi:10.1186/1748-5908-3-52
31. Macklin R. Ethical challenges in implementation research. *Public Health Ethics.* 2014;7(1):86–93. doi:10.1093/phe/phu003
32. Wiecha JL, El Ayadi AM, Fuemmeler BF, et al. Diffusion of an integrated health education program in an urban school system: Planet Health. *J Pediatr Psychol.* 2004;29(6):467–474. doi:10.1093/jpepsy/jsh050
33. Bellin E, Dubler NN. The quality improvement-research divide and the need for external oversight. *Am J Public Health.* Sep 2001;91(9):1512–1517. doi:10.2105/ajph.91.9.1512
34. Curran GM, Bauer M, Mittman B, Pyne J, Stetler C. Effectiveness-implementation hybrid designs: combining elements of clinical effectiveness and implementation research to enhance public health impact. *Ann HSR.* March 2012;50(3):217–226.
35. Gortmaker SL, Cheung LW, Peterson KE, et al. Impact of a school-based interdisciplinary intervention on diet and physical activity among urban primary school children: eat well and keep moving. *Arch Pediatr Adolesc Med.* 1999;153(9):975–983. doi:10.1001/archpedi.153.9.975
36. Gortmaker SL, Lee RM, Mozaffarian RS, et al. Effect of an after-school intervention on increases in children's physical activity. *Med Sci Sports Exerc.* 2012;44(3):450–457. doi:10.1249/MSS.0b013e3182300128
37. Freedman B. Equipoise and the ethics of clinical research. *N Engl J Med.* Jul 16 1987;317(3):141–145. doi:10.1056/NEJM198707163170304
38. Castro M. Placebo versus best-available-therapy control group in clinical trials for pharmacologic therapies: which is better? *Proc Am Thorac Soc.* Oct 01 2007;4(7):570–573. doi:10.1513/pats.200706-073JK
39. Khan A, Warner HA, Brown WA. Symptom reduction and suicide risk in patients treated with placebo in antidepressant clinical trials: an analysis of the Food and Drug Administration database. *Arch Gen Psychiatry.* Apr 2000;57(4):311–317. doi:10.1001/archpsyc.57.4.311
40. Miller PB, Weijer C. Rehabilitating equipoise. *Kennedy Inst Ethics J.* Jun 2003;13(2):93–118. doi:10.1353/ken.2003.0014
41. Binik A, Weijer C, McRae AD, et al. Does clinical equipoise apply to cluster randomized trials in health research? *Trials.* 2011;12:118. doi:10.1186/1745-6215-12-118
42. Valdiserri RO, Tama GM, Ho M. The role of community advisory committees in clinical trials of anti-HIV agents. *IRB: Ethics Hum Res.* Jul-Aug 1988;10(4):5–7. doi:10.2307/3564624
43. Brown CA, Lilford RJ. The stepped wedge trial design: a systematic review. *BMC Med Res Methodol.* 2006;6(1):54. doi:10.1186/1471-2288-6-54
44. Emanuel EJ, Wendler D, Grady C. What makes clinical research ethical? *JAMA.* May 24–31 2000;283(20):2701–2711. doi:jsc90374 [pii]
45. Franks A, Kelder S, Dino G, et al. School-based programs: lessons learned from CATCH, Planet Health, and Not-On-Tobacco. *Prev Chronic Dis.* 2007;4(2):1–9.
46. DuBois JM, Chibnall JT, Tait RC, Vander Wal JS. Lessons from researcher rehab. *Nature.* 9 June 2016;534:173–175.
47. DuBois JC, Chibnall JT, Tait RC, et al. Professional decision-making in research (PDR): the validity of a new measure. *Sci Eng Ethics.* 2016;22(2):391416.
48. Mecca JT, Medeiros KE, Giorgini V, et al. The influence of compensatory strategies on ethical decision making. *Ethics Behav.* Jan 2 2014;24(1):73–89. doi:10.1080/10508422.2013.821389
49. Thiel CE, Connelly S, Griffith JA. Leadership and emotion management for complex tasks: different emotions, different strategies. *Leadership Q.* Jun 2012;23(3):517–533. doi:10.1016/j.leaqua.2011.12.005
50. Angie AD, Connelly S, Waples EP, Kligyte V. The influence of discrete emotions on judgement and decision-making: a meta-analytic review. *Cogn Emot.* 2011;25(8):1393–1422. doi:10.1080/02699931.2010.550751
51. Barrett LF, Gross J, Christensen TC, Benvenuto M. Knowing what you're feeling and knowing what to do about it: mapping the relation between emotion differentiation and emotion regulation. *Cogn Emot.* Nov 2001;15(6):713–724.
52. Roche M, Haar JM, Luthans F. The role of mindfulness and psychological capital on the well-being of leaders. *J Occup Health Psychol.* 2014;19(4):476–489.
53. Bazerman MH, Moore DA. *Judgment in Managerial Decision Making.* 8th ed. Wiley; 2013:vii.
54. Nickerson RS. Confirmation bias: a ubiquitous phenomenon in many guises. *Rev Gen Psychol.* 1998;2(2):175–220.
55. Stenmark CK, Antes AL, Thiel CE, Caughron JJ, Wang XQ, Mumford MD. Consequences identification in forecasting and ethical decision-making. *J Empir Res Hum Res Ethics.* Mar 2011;6(1):25–32. doi:10.1525/jer.2011.6.1.25

56. DuBois JM, Kraus E, Mikulec A, Cruz S, Bakanas E. A humble task: restoring virtue in medicine in an age of conflicted interests. *Acad Med.* 2013;88(7):924–928.
57. Sisk BA, Mozersky J, Antes AL, DuBois JM. The "ought-is" problem: an implementation science framework for translating ethical norms into practice. *Am J Bioeth.* 2020;20(4):62–70. doi:10.1080/15265161.2020.1730483
58. Nobis N, Sodeke S. Making ethics happen: addressing injustice in health inequalities. *Am J Bioeth.* May 2020;20(4):100–101. doi:10.1080/15265161.2020.1730498
59. Lavery JV. "Wicked problems," community engagement and the need for an implementation science for research ethics. *J Med Ethics.* Mar 2018;44(3):163–164. doi:10.1136/medethics-2016-103573

SECTION 3

Strategies and Methods

6

Implementation Strategies

JOANN E. KIRCHNER, THOMAS J. WALTZ, BYRON J. POWELL, EVA N. WOODWARD, JEFFREY L. SMITH, AND ENOLA K. PROCTOR

INTRODUCTION

The development, understanding, and application of strategies that enhance the uptake of evidence-based and evidence-informed practices are central to the science and practice of implementation. Implementation strategies are the methods or the "how to" approaches intended to support the uptake of innovations whether this occurs in a clinical, educational, or community setting. We use the term *innovation* inclusively. In a clinical setting, this may be a new clinical intervention or screening procedure. In a public health setting, it may be a prevention program or policy, or in a community setting, a new model of service. Our discussion focuses on strategies for implementation, but we note that these may overlap considerably with strategies for dissemination and de-implementation. Chapter 12 of this book addresses de-implementation specifically.

We define implementation strategies as methods to enhance the adoption, implementation, sustainment, and scale-up of an innovation.[1] Based on prior work by this team and others, we further differentiate discrete and multifaceted implementation strategies.[2,3] Discrete implementation strategies involve one action or process, such as educational meetings, reminders, or audit and feedback. The challenges of effective implementation often call for the use of multifaceted implementation strategies, which comprise multiple discrete strategies interwoven and packaged as protocolized or branded strategies. For example, the **W**orking with **HIV** clinics to adopt **A**ddiction **T**reatment using **I**mplementation **F**acilitation (WHAT-IF?) study identifies a set of strategies to promote adoption of addiction treatments in clinics that serve populations living with HIV, including but not limited to conduct of a formative evaluation, stakeholder engagement, education and academic detailing, and establishment of a learning collaborative.[4] Multifaceted implementation strategies can, but do not necessarily, reflect a logical analysis of how interrelationships among discrete strategies address determinants of implementation at multiple levels.[4–6]

This chapter presents methods to classify discrete implementation strategies; recommendations for how to adapt strategies to projects; processes through which one can identify, develop, or tailor an implementation strategy; recommendations on how to document an implementation strategy for replication; guidance for checking fidelity of strategy use; enhanced designs for assessing strategy outcomes; and examples of how to disseminate an effective implementation strategy using the WHAT-IF? Study.[4] We conclude with recommendations for future research.

CLASSIFYING IMPLEMENTATION STRATEGIES

Numerous taxonomies of implementation strategies have been developed, primarily based on scoping reviews of the literature.[2,7,8] Scoping reviews aim to rapidly map the key concepts underpinning a research area and the main sources and types of evidence available; they can be undertaken as stand-alone projects in their own right, especially where an area is complex or has not previously been reviewed comprehensively.[9] While scoping reviews are a

JoAnn E. Kirchner, Thomas J. Waltz, Byron J. Powell, Eva N. Woodward, Jeffrey L. Smith, and Enola K. Proctor, *Implementation Strategies* In: *Dissemination and Implementation Research in Health.* Edited by: Ross C. Brownson, Graham A. Colditz, and Enola K. Proctor, Oxford University Press.
 DOI: 10.1093/oso/9780197660690.003.0006

foundation, comprehensive, state-of-art compilations of discrete implementation strategies must reflect the experience and judgment of both researchers and practitioners who use these strategies under a variety of circumstances. The Expert Recommendations for Implementing Change (ERIC) project mobilized 71 of these stakeholders and utilized rigorous mixed-methods procedures to characterize expert consensus on an updated compilation of implementation strategies.[10]

Beginning with a compilation of 68 discrete implementation strategies from Powell and colleagues, an interactive three-round process engaged participants in providing feedback on the strategy labels, specifying synonyms for the strategies, editing the definitions, proposing alternate definitions, and proposing new strategies (with definitions) to be added to the compilation.[2] This resulted in a final compilation of 73 discrete implementation strategies.[3] *Additional File 6* for this compilation includes ancillary materials for most strategies reflecting resources and additional considerations for the strategy suggested by the panel. Table 6.1 provides an overview of the ERIC discrete implementation strategies and their definitions and includes two additional strategies (in italics) identified by Perry and colleagues,[11] further described in the Applying and Conceptualizing the ERIC Compilation section below.

The large number of discrete implementation strategies included in any compilation necessitates breaking them into superordinate categories, however tentative, to support their meaningful consideration. Ideally, a categorization scheme supports considering strategies that are similar in their action, function, or targets proximally to one another; otherwise, potential similarities among strategies may be obscured in a large compilation. The ERIC project took a stakeholder participatory approach (i.e., concept mapping) to implementation strategy categorization. For details for developing the cluster labels for the strategies reported in Table 6.1, see Waltz et al.[13]

Applying and Conceptualizing the ERIC Compilation

How applicable is the ERIC compilation across practice settings, implementation initiatives, implementation actors, and innovations to be implemented? Perry and colleagues[11] applied the ERIC compilation in a review of the implementation of cardiovascular preventive care in over 200 primary care practices. Based on this review, the team elaborated on several strategies and their ancillary materials they applied to the project. While this review was completed post hoc, adapted elaborations of implementation strategies to fit the specific actors, contexts, and outcomes of a particular project (as described below) should be considered routine practice. The working glossary for the implementation strategies used within a project may involve highly adapted language, but published reports of implementation activities should report strategy labels from the ERIC compilation (or another established taxonomy) to facilitate meta-analytic efforts in the field of implementation science (e.g., those of Jones et al.).[14]

When and How Might Such Applications Reveal New Strategies That Are Not Included in ERIC?

While researchers should expect new strategies to emerge, language harmony and consistency are critical to replicating and developing a knowledge base. Rebranding strategies as new when instead they are but offshoots of extant strategies may thwart capturing knowledge about established strategies in literature reviews or meta-analyses. To determine whether a strategy as operationalized for a project is conceptually unique from existing ERIC strategies, investigators should consider the operationalized strategy's fit to the superordinate categories (i.e., clusters) in established compilations, such as ERIC, asking: Is the operationalized strategy conceptually unique from strategies in the existing cluster? This can minimize the risk of treating operationalized elements of a strategy (e.g., different actors or settings) as justification for considering the effort a "new" discrete implementation strategy.

Perry and colleagues[11] identified two additional discrete implementation strategies: *assess and redesign workflow* (a conceptual fit with the *use evaluative and iterative strategies* superordinate cluster) and *engage community resources* (a conceptual fit with the *develop stakeholder interrelationships* superordinate cluster). See Table 6.1 for definitions. A third strategy, *create online learning communities*, was proposed, but this addition is not distinct from the existing *create a learning collaborative* strategy. Perry's work illustrates the importance of considering

TABLE 6.1 ERIC IMPLEMENTATION STRATEGY COMPILATION[a]

Strategy	Cluster/Definition
	Use evaluative and iterative strategies
Assess and redesign workflow	*Observe and map current work processes and plan for desired work processes, identifying changes necessary to accommodate, encourage, or incentivize use of the clinical innovation as designed*[12i]
Assess for readiness and identify barriers and facilitators	Assess various aspects of an organization to determine its degree of readiness to implement, barriers that may impede implementation, and strengths that can be used in the implementation effort.
Audit and provide feedback	Collect and summarize clinical performance data over a specified time period and give it to clinicians and administrators to monitor, evaluate, and modify provider behavior.
Conduct cyclical small tests of change	Implement changes in a cyclical fashion using small tests of change before taking changes system-wide. Tests of change benefit from systematic measurement, and results of the tests of change are studied for insights on how to do better. This process continues serially over time, and refinement is added with each cycle.
Conduct local needs assessment	Collect and analyze data related to the need for the innovation.
Develop a formal implementation blueprint	Develop a formal implementation blueprint that includes all goals and strategies. The blueprint should include the following: (1) aim/purpose of the implementation; (2) scope of the change (e.g., what organizational units are affected); (3) time frame and milestones; and (4) appropriate performance/progress measures. Use and update this plan to guide the implementation effort over time.
Develop and implement tools for quality monitoring	Develop, test, and introduce into quality-monitoring systems the right input—the appropriate language, protocols, algorithms, standards, and measures (of processes, patient/consumer outcomes, and implementation outcomes), which are often specific to the innovation being implemented.
Develop and organize quality monitoring systems	Develop and organize systems and procedures that monitor clinical processes and/or outcomes for the purpose of quality assurance and improvement.
Obtain and use patients/consumers and family feedback	Develop strategies to increase patient/consumer and family feedback on the implementation effort.
Purposefully reexamine the implementation	Monitor progress and adjust clinical practices and implementation strategies to continuously improve the quality of care.
Stage implementation scale up	Phase implementation efforts by starting with small pilots or demonstration projects and gradually move to a system-wide rollout.
	Provide interactive assistance
Centralize technical assistance	Develop and use a centralized system to deliver technical assistance focused on implementation issues.
Facilitation	Use a process of interactive problem-solving and support that occurs in a context of a recognized need for improvement and a supportive interpersonal relationship.
Provide clinical supervision	Provide clinicians with ongoing supervision focusing on the innovation. Provide training for clinical supervisors who will supervise clinicians who provide the innovation.

(continued)

TABLE 6.1 CONTINUED

Strategy	Cluster/Definition
Provide local technical assistance	Develop and use a system to deliver technical assistance focused on implementation issues using local personnel.
	Adapt and tailor to context
Promote adaptability	Identify the ways a clinical innovation can be tailored to meet local needs and clarify which elements of the innovation must be maintained to preserve fidelity.
Tailor strategies	Tailor the implementation strategies to address barriers and leverage facilitators that were identified through earlier data collection.
Use data experts	Involve, hire, and/or consult experts to inform management on the use of data generated by implementation efforts.
Use data warehousing techniques	Integrate clinical records across facilities and organizations to facilitate implementation across systems.
	Develop stakeholder interrelationships
Build a coalition	Recruit and cultivate relationships with partners in the implementation effort.
Capture and share local knowledge	Capture local knowledge from implementation sites on how implementers and clinicians made something work in their setting and then share it with other sites.
Conduct local consensus discussions	Include local providers and other stakeholders in discussions that address whether the chosen problem is important and whether the clinical innovation to address it is appropriate.
Develop academic partnerships	Partner with a university or academic unit for the purposes of shared training and bringing research skills to an implementation project.
Develop an implementation glossary	Develop and distribute a list of terms describing the innovation, implementation, and stakeholders in the organizational change.
Engage community resources	*Connect practices and their patients to community resources outside the practice.*
Identify and prepare champions	Identify and prepare individuals who dedicate themselves to supporting, marketing, and driving through an implementation, overcoming indifference or resistance that the intervention may provoke in an organization.
Identify early adopters	Identify early adopters at the local site to learn from their experiences with the practice innovation.
Inform local opinion leaders	Inform providers identified by colleagues as opinion leaders or "educationally influential" about the clinical innovation in the hopes that they will influence colleagues to adopt it.
Involve executive boards	Involve existing governing structures (e.g., boards of directors, medical staff boards of governance) in the implementation effort, including the review of data on implementation processes.
Model and simulate change	Model or simulate the change that will be implemented prior to implementation.
Obtain formal commitments	Obtain written commitments from key partners that state what they will do to implement the innovation.
Organize clinician implementation team meetings	Develop and support teams of clinicians who are implementing the innovation and give them protected time to reflect on the implementation effort, share lessons learned, and support one another's learning.
Promote network weaving	Identify and build on existing high-quality working relationships and networks within and outside the organization, organizational units, teams, and so on to promote information sharing, collaborative problem-solving, and a shared vision/goal related to implementing the innovation.

TABLE 6.1 CONTINUED

Strategy	Cluster/Definition
Recruit, designate, and train for leadership	Recruit, designate, and train leaders for the change effort.
Use advisory boards and workgroups	Create and engage a formal group of multiple kinds of stakeholders to provide input and advice on implementation efforts and to elicit recommendations for improvements.
Use an implementation advisor	Seek guidance from experts in implementation.
Visit other sites	Visit sites where a similar implementation effort has been considered successful.
	Train and educate stakeholders
Conduct educational meetings	Hold meetings targeted toward different stakeholder groups (e.g., providers, administrators, other organizational stakeholders, and community, patient/consumer, and family stakeholders) to teach them about the clinical innovation.
Conduct educational outreach visits	Have a trained person meet with providers in their practice settings to educate providers about the clinical innovation with the intent of changing the provider's practice.
Conduct ongoing training	Plan for and conduct training in the clinical innovation in an ongoing way.
Create a learning collaborative	Facilitate the formation of groups of providers or provider organizations and foster a collaborative learning environment to improve implementation of the clinical innovation.
Develop educational materials	Develop and format manuals, toolkits, and other supporting materials in ways that make it easier for stakeholders to learn about the innovation and for clinicians to learn how to deliver the clinical innovation.
Distribute educational materials	Distribute educational materials (including guidelines, manuals, and toolkits) in person, by mail, and/or electronically.
Make training dynamic	Vary the information delivery methods to cater to different learning styles and work contexts and shape the training in the innovation to be interactive.
Provide ongoing consultation	Provide ongoing consultation with one or more experts in the strategies used to support implementing the innovation.
Shadow other experts	Provide ways for key individuals to directly observe experienced people engage with or use the targeted practice change/innovation.
Use train-the-trainer strategies	Train designated clinicians or organizations to train others in the clinical innovation.
Work with educational institutions	Encourage educational institutions to train clinicians in the innovation.
	Support clinicians
Create new clinical teams	Change who serves on the clinical team, adding different disciplines and different skills to make it more likely that the clinical innovation is delivered (or is more successfully delivered).
Develop resource-sharing agreements	Develop partnerships with organizations that have resources needed to implement the innovation
Facilitate relay of clinical data to providers	Provide as close to real-time data as possible about key measures of process/outcomes using integrated modes/channels of communication in a way that promotes use of the targeted innovation.
Remind clinicians	Develop reminder systems designed to help clinicians to recall information and/or prompt them to use the clinical innovation.
Revise professional roles	Shift and revise roles among professionals who provide care, and redesign job characteristics

(*continued*)

TABLE 6.1 CONTINUED

Strategy	Cluster/Definition
	Engage consumers
Increase demand	Attempt to influence the market for the clinical innovation to increase competition intensity and to increase the maturity of the market for the clinical innovation.
Intervene with patients/consumers to enhance uptake and adherence	Develop strategies with patients to encourage and problem solve around adherence.
Involve patients/consumers and family members	Engage or include patients/consumers and families in the implementation effort.
Prepare patients/consumers to be active participants	Prepare patients/consumers to be active in their care, to ask questions, and specifically to inquire about care guidelines, the evidence behind clinical decisions, or available evidence-supported treatments.
Use mass media	Use media to reach large numbers of people to spread the word about the clinical innovation.
	Utilize financial strategies
Access new funding	Access new or existing money to facilitate the implementation.
Alter incentive/allowance structures	Work to incentivize the adoption and implementation of the clinical innovation
Alter patient/consumer fees	Create fee structures where patients/consumers pay less for preferred treatments (the clinical innovation) and more for less-preferred treatments.
Develop disincentives	Provide financial disincentives for failure to implement or use the clinical innovations.
Fund and contract for the clinical innovation	Governments and other payers of services issue requests for proposals to deliver the innovation, use contracting processes to motivate providers to deliver the clinical innovation, and develop new funding formulas that make it more likely that providers will deliver the innovation.
Make billing easier	Make it easier to bill for the clinical innovation.
Place innovation on fee-for-service lists/formularies	Work to place the clinical innovation on lists of actions for which providers can be reimbursed (e.g., a drug is placed on a formulary, a procedure is now reimbursable).
Use capitated payments	Pay providers or care systems a set amount per patient/consumer for delivering clinical care.
Use other payment schemes	Introduce payment approaches (in a catch-all category).
	Change infrastructure
Change accreditation or membership requirements	Strive to alter accreditation standards so that they require or encourage use of the clinical innovation. Work to alter membership organization requirements so that those who want to affiliate with the organization are encouraged or required to use the clinical innovation.
Change liability laws	Participate in liability reform efforts that make clinicians more willing to deliver the clinical innovation.
Change physical structure and equipment	Evaluate current configurations and adapt, as needed, the physical structure and/or equipment (e.g., changing the layout of a room, adding equipment) to best accommodate the targeted innovation.
Change record systems	Change records systems to allow better assessment of implementation or clinical outcomes
Change service sites	Change the location of clinical service sites to increase access.

TABLE 6.1 CONTINUED

Strategy	Cluster/Definition
Create or change credentialing and/or licensure standards	Create an organization that certifies clinicians in the innovation or encourage an existing organization to do so. Change governmental professional certification or licensure requirements to include delivering the innovation. Work to alter continuing education requirements to shape professional practice toward the innovation.
Mandate change	Have leadership declare the priority of the innovation and their determination to have it implemented.
Start a dissemination organization	Identify or start a separate organization that is responsible for disseminating the clinical innovation. It could be a for-profit or nonprofit organization.

[a]Reprinted with permission from Powell et al.[3] Italics indicate strategies from Perry et al.[11]

the levels of abstract categorization when specifying implementation strategies.

Implementation strategies can be categorized at the superordinate (ERIC clusters), basic, and subordinate levels. Both *create online learning communities* and *create a learning collaborative* would fall under the superordinate domain of *train and educate stakeholders*, the highest level of abstraction in the ERIC compilation. However, *create an online learning community* strategy is a subordinate category that illustrates a more specific exemplar of the *create a learning collaborative* strategy. A particular project could use multiple subordinate strategies (e.g., both online and in-person learning community activities and supports). When operationalizing implementation strategies for a specific project, attention to the level of abstraction will enhance strategy reporting in ways that will facilitate implementation science meta-analyses. Furthermore, as we emphasize in the following section, Documenting Implementation Strategies, each strategy should be named, defined, and specified in detail.[1] In some cases, it may be useful to further operationalize implementation strategies by specifying the specific behavior change methods and techniques that comprise them.[15–18]

The ERIC compilation can promote the consideration of a more comprehensive range of strategies in implementation research and applied implementation efforts. It can also improve the specification and reporting of implementation strategies used prospectively[19,20] and retrospectively[11,21–23] to provide an accounting of strategies used in a particular project. We hope this compilation will continue to facilitate a more thorough accounting of the strategies employed to support implementation, including those that may be endogenous to an organization (e.g., having an existing clinical reminder system). A discussion of the limitations of the ERIC compilation can be found in Powell et al.[3]

ADAPTING STRATEGIES TO A PROJECT

While adapting specific strategy definitions to reflect a given initiative's specifics, noting the theoretical connection between the specific strategy's operationalization to the established strategy name will help connect the work to the broader literature. As examples, Cook and colleagues took a systematic approach to adapt ERIC strategies to implementing evidence-based mental health practices in schools, and Lyon et al.[24] assessed the importance and feasibility of those strategies among school-based personnel. Others are working to systematically consider the extent to which the ERIC strategies and definitions address needs related to different contexts, such as low- and middle-income countries[25] and community settings,[26] as well as specific aspects of implementation such as dissemination, de-implementation,[27] and sustainment.[28] These studies have generally concluded that relatively minor changes in terms and definitions are necessary to tailor the ERIC compilation's terms and definitions for these contexts and purposes. Box 6.1 describes a seven-step process that aims to both ensure that the strategies are useful for a specific project and remain connected to the ERIC strategy compilation (or other established taxonomy) to facilitate cumulative

BOX 6.1
A SYSTEMATIC APPROACH TO ADAPTING STRATEGIES USING THE ERIC TAXONOMY

1. Project knowledgeable stakeholders review ERIC strategies and make revisions to the language, reference terminology, and ancillary materials to improve the fit of a tailored working definition for the project.
2. Provide descriptive examples of the tailored strategy to increase comprehension of how the strategy is applicable to this specific context.
3. Remove implementation strategies determined to be contextually inappropriate or redundant with other strategies as they manifest in the project.
4. Add novel implementation strategies (i.e., not in the ERIC compilation) that are needed to support implementation in the project.
5. Obtain review and feedback from other implementation experts to support conceptual consistency between tailored strategies and ERIC strategies. Reviewers should attend to the level of abstraction employed when new strategies are proposed to determine whether new strategies represent subordinate applications of strategies or new basic strategies.
6. Additional revision is based on the feedback from the outside implementation experts to ensure conceptual consistency with the original strategies and to increase the comprehension, contextual appropriateness, and utility to the project's context
7. Rereview by outside implementation experts is done to support the connection between the adapted strategies and strategies as they may be identified across studies (i.e., meta-analytically). Steps 6 and 7 are repeated if necessary until the adapted definitions are finalized.

knowledge for the implementation science and practice community.

SELECTING, DEVELOPING, AND TAILORING AN IMPLEMENTATION STRATEGY

Strategy Selection Using Frameworks

With over 70 distinct implementation strategies available for consideration (Table 6.1), researchers and implementers often find it overwhelming to contemplate which strategy (or collection of strategies) to deploy in a given effort to put a new innovation into practice.[29] This task can prove much less daunting by drawing on an implementation science framework or theory to help (a) understand factors or determinants that may influence implementation and (b) select an implementation strategy or strategies.[30,31] Although the value of using a theory or framework to guide implementation has been debated, proceeding without a theory base in implementation has produced mixed results.[30,32–35]

Some implementation science frameworks propose a specific strategy as an integrated component to use in an implementation effort. For example, the integrated Promoting Action on Research Implementation in Health Services (i-PARIHS) framework identifies use of "facilitation" strategies as the "active ingredient" for guiding individuals and clinical teams through change processes or contextual challenges to implementation.[36] Similarly, planned action or "process" models such as replicating effective programs (REP) and quality implementation framework (QIF)[37] may be useful as they specify a stepwise approach to be taken within stages of implementing research into practice. Other frameworks, such as the Consolidated Framework for Implementation Research (CFIR) are more agnostic in terms of proposing a *specific* implementation strategy, but include a domain that explicates broad processes of implementation efforts (i.e., the "process" domain), as well as four domains that identify various determinants that can serve as potential targets for implementation strategies.[38] The CFIR-ERIC Implementation Strategy Matching Tool provides ranked ordered considerations of ERIC strategies given the report of CFIR domain-related barriers.[39,40] This tool can complement other organized approaches to implementation strategy selection.

Some frameworks include the implementation's impact on population health. For example, the Health Equity Impact Assessment is an overarching framework that can be used to identify unintended consequences of an intervention on service delivery or health impact for marginalized groups within a care system.[41] The Health Equity Impact Assessment has a toolkit to guide organizations in health equity evaluations and in implementing strategies to mitigate barriers to equitable care.

Careful consideration of an implementation effort's scope and goals should precede the selection of a particular framework. Selection and tailoring of an implementation strategy, whether guided by a framework/theory (as recommended here) or not, should also be informed by an assessment of the determinants of current practice within the targeted setting, including identification of implementation barriers and facilitators that may exist at the patient, provider, team, clinic, organizational, and system level. Formative evaluation, and more specifically *developmental* formative evaluation, is a rigorous assessment process typically involving the collection of both qualitative and quantitative data to identify the determinants of current practice, barriers and facilitators for a practice change or implementation of a given innovation, and stakeholder perspectives on the feasibility of a proposed implementation strategy.[42] This type of assessment is sometimes referred to as a *needs assessment* or *organizational diagnosis* of factors to be considered and addressed in developing, tailoring, and operationalizing an implementation strategy. For example, facilitation strategies often include elements of formative evaluation as part of the facilitator's responsibilities.[42,43] Similar processes are also included as early "steps" to be completed in numerous planned action models, including REP.[44,45] Assessment findings are used to tailor the implementation strategy and complementary improvement tools to the site's context and needs, taking into account other recommendations for strategies to be multifaceted (when appropriate), feasible, acceptable to stakeholders, trialable, readily adaptable, sustainable, and scalable for spread to similar settings if successful.[13,31]

Note that the assessment processes described above are often applied iteratively, where the implementation strategy and tools may be tailored or adapted multiple times during the course of a given project as needed to enhance fit to the local context or to increase chances for achieving implementation or performance improvement goals. Although the specification and operationalization of the implementation strategy/tools may vary by site (with documented rationale for variability), *the processes for tailoring and adapting the strategy to sites are uniform and replicable.*

User-Centered Designs

Strategies can be selected by considering what the implementers want. Are some strategies preferred over others? Are some strategies considered impractical or unfeasible given the context and resources? Similarly, what is the "fit" of the strategy to implementation approaches used previously? Steffen and team[46] reported that choosing implementation strategies that fit with existing workflow design, in-tact training protocols, and existing time and resources enhances success.[46] Principles of design thinking are increasingly used to select, create, or adapt implementation strategies. Design thinking centers people with the problem, whereby final recipients or consumers of an innovation are sampled about their needs or preferences, asked to create solutions, or engaged in rapid and iterative development of an innovation or implementation strategy.[47] Dopp and colleagues[47] developed a high-level glossary of 30 discrete user-centered design strategies that address problems such as an innovation's ease of use and fit with the delivery context. Many of the 30 user-centered design strategies are specified tasks that can complement strategies within the ERIC clusters "use evaluative and iterative strategies," "adapt and tailor to context," "develop stakeholder interrelationships," "engage consumers," and can provide guidance on methods and processes for engaging stakeholders prior to and during implementation.[48]

Implementation strategies are unlikely to be effective for people who are marginalized without explicit inclusion and attention to their needs. Thus, informing implementation strategies via user-centered design requires clarifying which users are being centered and which users might not be sampled, considered, or invited—specifically people who experience marginalization due to racism, transphobia, or disability discrimination.[49] Design justice, an approach where people who are marginalized are leading and centered in designing solutions, might be highly relevant when selecting, designing, or adapting implementation strategies to reduce disparities or improve equity.[49]

User-centered or human-centered design strategies have been used in a variety of implementation efforts. A design thinking approach was used to develop and organize quality monitoring systems with and for community-based organizations in Ohio to detect infant mortality outcomes.[50] A human-centered design method was used to identify problematic aspects of a multifaceted implementation strategy to increase uptake of measurement-based care among mental health clinicians in US schools that made it ineffective for clinicians.[51] Scholars also used human-centered design strategies to design a care coordination program for young adults with cancer to be more usable and effective with young adults and generated potential implementation strategies with healthcare professionals for its later spread and adoption.[52,53] To summarize, user-centered and human-centered design strategies have been and can be used to complement or adapt implementation strategies (or the innovation).

Strategy Selection Using Structured Methods

Among the highly structured methods for selecting strategies,[54] concept mapping and intervention mapping comprise two of the more accessible approaches. As illustrated in the ERIC project, concept mapping employs a mixed-methods and stakeholder-engaged process that can be used to identify strategies relevant for an implementation initiative, organize them into conceptual themes, and rate them on dimensions like their perceived importance and feasibility.[55] Intervention mapping also employs a mixed-methods and stakeholder-engaged process that involves identifying the behaviors (and their determinants) that need to be targeted for change, specifying related change objectives, and selecting implementation strategies and behavior change techniques to develop practical applications to achieve those objectives. These foundational steps drive the program planning, implementation, and evaluation process.[56]

Strategy Selection Based on Evidence: What Has Worked Where?

The implementation science literature provides, infrequently but importantly, data on what strategies have been used in the adoption of evidence-based strategies. Surveys and key informant interviews can use established compilations such as ERIC to structure implementers' reports of which strategies were used.[57] Rarely does the literature report discrete implementation strategies utilized in broad or system-level initiatives. Rogal et al.[58,59] and Yakovchenko et al.[21,60] provided information from their assessment of site-level implementation strategies used by the US Department of Veterans Affairs sites involved in a national collaborative over a 5-year implementation period. The group identified which individual ERIC strategies changed in frequency of use over time and which were associated with improved process outcomes, including hepatitis C treatment initiation.

Strategies can also be selected based on their reported effectiveness in innovation adoption. To date, most tests of strategies focus on individual or small groups of discrete strategies or the evaluation of a small number of strategies or multifaceted implementation packages, often branded intervention packages. For example, Rogal's team used configurational comparative methods to identify five strategy configurations that perfectly distinguished higher treatment initiation sites from lower sites. Their data also revealed how different, tailored implementation strategy combinations can promote the same outcome. Similarly, configurational analysis[60] identified multiple strategy pathways directly linked to more guideline-concordant cirrhosis care; a subset of eight strategies was determined to comprise "core implementation strategies" to improve care. These articles provided data on the effectiveness of implementation strategies employed system-wide and described important methodologies to consolidate data to a smaller set of the most effective.

Selecting Strategies: How Much Do They Cost?

Implementation strategies require resources, contributing substantially to overall implementation cost, identified as a key outcome in implementation research.[61] The total costs of an implementation strategy include those associated with its development, selection, or adaptation. Moreover, implementation strategies may carry efficiency gains or losses, as when clinicians and other front-line providers take time "off line" from providing direct services to participate in educational activities or training.[62] At the organizational or system level, the costs associated with implementation strategies, especially multicomponent strategies, may be substantial.

Decisions about "how to implement" or choose implementation strategies require assessment of available resources and the comparative costs and benefits of alternative implementation strategies. Cost has been identified as a key implementation outcome,[61] but a factor given insufficient attention. When cost has been addressed, most attention has focused on intervention costs and *not* the costs of implementation strategies required to deploy and sustain them. Nor has cost been adequately addressed at the organizational or system perspective. Cost is a key factor in deciding whether to implement and how to implement; moreover, it can be a rate-limiting factor in the scale-up and sustainment of innovations once implemented.

Stimulated by an economics and implementation science workgroup, resources for cost decisions are increasing. Commonly used in the assessment of health services, economic evaluation is a key tool for making decisions on implementation strategies.[63] Eisman et al. provided guidance for assessing costs in a manner that addresses concerns of various stakeholder groups and identifies agreement and conflict in priorities.[64] Cidav et al. offered a pragmatic approach to systematically estimating detailed, specific resource use and costs of implementation strategies that combine time-driven activity-based costing (TDABC), a business accounting method based on process mapping and known for its practicality, with Proctor's framework for specification and reporting of implementation strategies.[65] Eisman's team[66] estimated the costs and comparative effectiveness comparing different implementation strategies in a sequential, multiple assignment, randomized trial (SMART) to identify the most cost-effective approach. The economic outcome was the incremental cost-effectiveness ratio (ICER) of various combinations and configurations of strategies. As more economic evaluations are performed and decision makers leverage analytic techniques such as modeling and value of implementation analysis, the contribution of economic evaluation to selecting implementation strategies will increase.

DOCUMENTING IMPLEMENTATION STRATEGIES

Implementation strategies often are poorly described, are rarely justified theoretically, lack operational definitions or manuals to guide their use, and are part of "packaged" approaches whose specific elements are poorly understood. Knowledge synthesis through systematic review is difficult when strategies are labeled inconsistently and defined idiosyncratically. Moreover, implementation strategies cannot be used in practice or tested in research without a full description of their components and how they should be used. To date, limitations in strategy specification have thwarted the development of an evidence base for their mechanisms of action, their efficiency, cost, and effectiveness. Conceptual and operational descriptions of implementation strategies must be precise enough to enable measurement and "reproducibility."

The complexity of implementation strategies makes challenging their clear description, operational definition, and measurement. Because they address multifaceted and complicated processes within interpersonal, organizational, and community contexts, implementation strategies inherently are complex social interventions. Several published recommendations can improve the precision with which implementation strategies are reported in research studies. Table 6.2 outlines recommendations for specifying and reporting implementation strategies drawn from Proctor et al.[61,67]

Practical examples of reporting implementation strategies using the Proctor et al.[70] guidelines are beginning to emerge. For example, Bunger et al.[75] used these guidelines to report the key components of a learning collaborative

TABLE 6.2 PROCTOR RECOMMENDATIONS FOR NAMING, DEFINING, AND OPERATIONALIZING STRATEGIES[a]

Recommendation	Description
1. Name it	An implementation strategy must first be named or labeled. We highly recommend implementation strategies be named using the same terms as other researchers in the field, unless the strategy is new and distinct from strategies previously identified in the literature. While the working label used within a project may involve highly localized language (e.g., a specific name for the quality monitoring system used), communication beyond the project for methods and outcome dissemination should reflect strategy labels from existing implementation strategy compilations.
2. Define it	Each strategy needs to be defined conceptually to provide a general sense of what the strategy may involve, which enables readers to discern the strategy's consistency with other uses of the term represented in the literature. Using definitions from established taxonomies such as ERIC provides the basis for a common language.
3. Operationalize it	Operational definitions ensure that strategies are described at a common level of granularity and are readily comparable to other definitions. We propose seven dimensions that, when detailed adequately, constitute adequate operationalization of implementation strategies:
(a) The actors	The "actors" are stakeholders who actually deliver the implementation strategy. A wide range of stakeholders can fill this function, as implementation strategies may be employed or enacted by payers, administrators, intervention developers, outside consultants, personnel within an organization charged with being "implementers," providers/clinicians/support staff, clients/patients/consumers, or community stakeholders.
(b) The actions	Implementation strategies require dynamic verb statements that indicate actions, steps or processes, and sequences of behaviors comprising the strategy. Actions should be behaviorally defined a priori to enable comparison with what was actually done during the implementation process (i.e., measuring fidelity).[68]
(c) Action targets	Implementation strategies are directed or are used to affect various conceptual "targets." For example, strategies such as "realigning payment incentives" target the policy context, while "training" targets front-line providers by increasing knowledge and skill, and "fidelity checklists" target the clarity of the intervention as well as the providers' understanding and ability to break down the intervention into more "doable" steps. Specifying these targets is consistent with calls to identify the mechanisms through which implementation strategies operate.[69–72]
(d) Temporality	The order or sequence of strategy use or strategy components may be critical. For instance, Lyon et al.[73] suggested that strategies to boost providers' motivation to learn new treatments may need to precede other common implementation strategies, such as training and supervision. Authors should report information about the stage or phase of the implementation process at which the strategy was or should be used.
(e) Dose	As with interventions or treatment programs, implementation strategies can vary tremendously in dosage or intensity. Details about the dose or intensity of implementation strategies can include the amount of time spent with an external facilitator, the time and intensity of training, or the frequency of audit and feedback should be designated a priori, tracked, and reported.

TABLE 6.2 CONTINUED

Recommendation	Description
(f) The implementation outcome affected	Strategies impact intermediate outcomes (i.e., acceptability, reach, adoption, appropriateness, feasibility, fidelity, cost, penetration, sustainability) and contribute to more distal outcomes related to consumer health and service system functioning.[61] Certain strategies may target one or more these implementation outcomes (or other outcomes not identified in the taxonomy).
(g) The justification	Advancing or testing theories requires that researchers report and explain the rationale for strategies used to implement a given innovation. Indications of their appropriateness and effectiveness, citing relevant theory,[35,74] empirical evidence,[3] and/or some pragmatic rationale (e.g., using a low-cost, low-intensity intervention when theory and evidence for more intensive strategies are not compelling) comprise ideal justifications.

[a]Reprinted with permission from: Proctor EK, Powell BJ, McMillen JC. Implementation strategies: recommendations for specifying and reporting. *Implement Sci.* 2013;8(1):139. doi:10.1186/1748-5908-8-139

intended to increase the use of Trauma-Focused Cognitive Behavioral Therapy. Similarly, Gold et al.[76] used the guidelines to report a strategy to implement a diabetes quality improvement (QI) intervention within community health centers. Other examples are cited below within the context of efforts to prospectively or retrospectively track and document implementation strategy use. These examples demonstrate the utility of the reporting guidelines for enhancing the clarity of implementation strategies so that they can be replicated in research and practice.

Contemporaneous tracking of implementation strategies is essential given the iterative nature of implementation. Even if implementation strategies are detailed in a study protocol or formal implementation plan using the recommendations above, potential need for alteration should be anticipated as new determinants emerge across implementation phases.[77–80] For example, during the COVID-19 pandemic, implementation strategies such as educational workshops, learning collaboratives, and facilitation that were intended to be delivered using an in-person, live format required adaptation for online or blended synchronous and asynchronous delivery. Other strategy changes arise after substantial turnover in organizational or clinical leadership, necessitating renewed attention to building buy-in and tangible support for an implementation effort, training new staff members, or redefining roles and responsibilities related to the implementation of a program. Departures from planned implementation strategies are likely within and between implementing sites.[81–83] Without rigorous methods for tracking implementation strategy use, efforts to understand which strategies were used and whether or not they were effective are stymied. Miller and colleagues[84] recently extended similar guidance for documenting implementation strategies.[85] Developing approaches for tracking implementation strategies and assessing the extent to which they are pragmatic (e.g., acceptable, compatible, easy, and useful) for both research and applied efforts is a high priority.[29,86] Ideally, evaluators would develop and apply methods to track implementation strategies prospectively using structured forms or surveys[57,87–90]; however, in some cases, evaluators may need to rely on surveys, interviews, or other data sources to assess the use of implementation strategies retrospectively. For example, Bustos and colleagues[91] used survey and interview data to assess implementation strategies used and community partners' satisfaction with those strategies.

IMPLEMENTING AND DOCUMENTING IMPLEMENTATION STRATEGIES: AN EXAMPLE

For the WHAT-IF? study, Edelman and colleagues[4] presented a list of strategies (components) that they named, defined, and operationalized. The study team provided a

TABLE 6.3 COMPONENTS OF WHAT-IF? ADAPTED TO INCLUDE DISCRETE ERIC STRATEGY[a]

Component	General Description	ERIC Strategy	Specifics for WHAT-IF?
External facilitator	Outside content and implementation experts(s) who assist site	Facilitation	Facilitators included members of the investigative team with expertise in internal medicine, addiction medicine and psychiatry, HIV, and implementation science, who led all aspects of IF activities in collaboration with sites.
Formative evaluation	Quantitative and qualitative determination of potential and actual influences on progress and effectiveness of implementation efforts	Access for readiness and identify barriers and facilitators	Guided by the PARIHS framework, web-based survey of clinicians and staff, followed by site visits that included focus groups with stakeholders (including patients), face-to-face meeting with medical directors, HIV clinic tour, review of patient flow and electronic health record documentation, discussion of existing quality improvement (QI) practices, meeting with potential local champions at IF onset. There were two follow-up site visits and additional communication by email, telephone, and video conference.
Local champion	Local site stakeholder(s) who promotes change	Identify and prepare champions	Self-identified individual with expertise and/or interest in promoting practice change to address tobacco, alcohol, and/or opioid use; may have experience in QI and/or be the medical director. Becomes point person(s) for external facilitators.
Education with academic detailing (AD)	Provision of unbiased peer education	Develop educational materials, conduct educational outreach visits, distribute educational materials	After a subset of investigators participated in AD training, AD pamphlets were created, and AD was performed with front-line clinicians and staff during site visits conducted during IF. Information regarding X-waiver training opportunities, professional conferences, relevant journal articles, and clinical guidelines were additionally distributed by external facilitators. Efforts made to facilitate grand rounds and preclinic conferences focused on addressing addiction in HIV with local experts and to facilitate intrainstitutional collaborations for clinical consultation and shadowing opportunities (e.g., observing buprenorphine treatment initiation).
Stakeholder engagement	Aligning goals of implementation and those impacted	Conduct local consensus discussions, develop a formal implementation blueprint	Initial site visits serve to assess interest and perceived relevance in promoting addiction treatment in HIV clinics; based on the initial formative evaluation, the external facilitators share feedback with HIV medical director organized by the PARIHS framework to propose a comprehensive approach for stimulating practice change.

TABLE 6.3 CONTINUED

Component	General Description	ERIC Strategy	Specifics for WHAT-IF?
Tailoring program to site	Addressing site-specific needs based on formative evaluation, problem identification and resolution, assistance with technical issues	Promote adaptability, tailor strategies	Based on local resources and expertise, external facilitators work with local champion to implement most feasible model for enhancing delivery of tobacco, alcohol, and opioid use treatment.
Performance monitoring and feedback	Assess implementation of screening and treatment efforts and inform sites of results	Audit and provide feedback	Provision of electronic health record–based data demonstrating prevalence of diagnoses of tobacco, alcohol, and opioid use disorder and proportion receiving treatment shared with medical director; in addition, half-day site visit is performed to assess performance on care integration as measured by the opioid use disorder and HIV integration (OHI) index.
Establishing a learning collaborative	Shared learning opportunities tailored to stakeholders	Create a learning collaborative	Monthly videoconference hosted by WHAT-IF? team to facilitate mutual learning and clinic updates and included a mixed of didactics and case-based discussion. Monthly newsletter was used to disseminate upcoming learning opportunities (e.g., trainings and conferences) and newly published peer-reviewed articles and guidelines.
Program marketing	Efforts designed to increase attention to availability of on-site and addiction treatment services	Remind clinicians: program marketing	Pins, pads, pens, buttons, and posters with WHAT-IF? logo created and shared with clinic teams to help increase awareness of the project and facilitate patient clinician discussions ("WHAT-IF? what . . ."?)

[a]Reprinted with permission from: Edelman EJ, Dziura J, Esserman D, et al. Working with HIV clinics to adopt addiction treatment using implementation facilitation (WHAT-IF?): rationale and design for a hybrid type 3 effectiveness-implementation study. *Contemp Clin Trials*. 2020;98:106156. doi:10.1016/j.cct.2020.106156

rationale for selecting their multifaceted strategy external facilitation, including flexibility and conduct of a formative evaluation, and embedded the strategy within an implementation framework, PARIHS. We have adapted the WHAT-IF? component table to include a link to discrete ERIC strategies, a widely used strategy typology. In many cases, this is identical to the component in the original publication. We provide the link to ERIC as an example of the value of using an established typology that can allow evaluation of discrete strategies across studies (see Table 6.3). Edelman and colleagues also used an ongoing tracking log to document the strategy action by providing further definition, including the actors (e.g., stakeholders involved), temporality, and dose of discrete implementation strategies.

ASSESSING IMPLEMENTATION STRATEGY FIDELITY

Ensuring appropriate application and spread of successful implementation strategies requires tools and processes to measure fidelity to a given strategy's core components or elements.[68] See Chapter 7 for more detailed discussion of fidelity. When implementing evidence-based practices or other innovations, fidelity must be ensured to both the *innovation* (i.e., ensuring that core components or processes involved with delivering the innovation are included or followed) and to core components of the *implementation strategy*.[39] Despite calls to do so, and recognition of the importance for application and spread, this aspect of implementation science and practice is relatively underdeveloped and infrequently applied.[68]

A recent scoping literature review assessed the extent and quality of documentation of fidelity to implementation strategies in 72 studies. Although 71% of the studies reported at least some details on the extent and/or quality of fidelity to the implementation strategy(ies) used, details were scarce or very limited for many of these studies.[92] Indeed, the authors did not find a single study that included a conceptual framework for fidelity, or even a fidelity definition. Clearly, this is an area that is ripe for research attention.

Stockdale et al. assessed fidelity to an evidence-based quality improvement (EBQI) strategy used to support implementation of patient-centered medical homes (the innovation) in the US Veterans Health Administration (VHA).[93] The authors assessed three core elements of the EBQI strategy—leadership-front-lines priority setting for QI; ongoing access to technical expertise, coaching, and mentoring in QI methods; and data/evidence use to inform QI—finding that higher fidelity to priority setting and ongoing technical expertise correlated with successful QI project completion and spread.[93] Another recent study created and pilot tested a tool for assessing fidelity in use of implementation facilitation (IF) strategies to support use of evidence-based practices or other clinical innovations.[60] IF is a dynamic process of interactive problem-solving and support to help clinical personnel implement and sustain a new program, process, or practice that occurs in the context of a recognized need for improvement and a supportive interpersonal relationship.[8,39,61] Several studies have contributed to a growing evidence base in the literature for the impact of IF strategies to promote use of a new program or practice in healthcare settings.[62,63] A scoping literature review[64] of these studies documented and identified core activities of facilitation through a rigorous, multistage expert panel consensus development process.[94] Results yielded 16 core activities for IF that may be used for assessing fidelity to the strategy. The 16 core activities have been integrated into an implementation facilitation time-tracking log used in previous studies[95] for systematic monitoring of facilitator activities, and two prototype IF fidelity-monitoring tools are currently being piloted[96] for initial testing and refinement.

TESTING STRATEGIES IN RELATION TO IMPLEMENTATION OUTCOMES

As discussed throughout this book, various designs are useful in testing the outcomes of implementation strategies. Tests of strategy outcomes need to specify up front which outcomes are sought. Strategies are typically employed to attain various implementation outcomes, such as an innovation's acceptability, adoption, cost, sustainment, and scale up.[97,98] Equity is another important outcome that strategies may address. Implementation science literature increasingly prioritizes equity through a variety of equity frameworks and lenses. However, equity is rarely measured as an outcome of different implementation strategies. Key implementation outcomes can be defined in ways that emphasize equity, as proposed by Eslava-Schmalbach and colleagues,[99] such as acceptability (equity focused: perception among patients, community, marginalized populations); adoption (equity focused: utilization of a sensitive equity recommendation in the new innovation); or fidelity (equity focused: adherence of marginalized population to the equity-focused implementation strategy). Similarly, strategies can be evaluated employing Reach, Effectiveness, Adoption, Implementation, and Maintenance (RE-AIM) outcomes with an equity lens, which is highlighted in Shelton and colleagues' work.[100] Finally, simulation and modeling approaches can help test the effectiveness of implementation strategies for improving equity-focused outcomes, especially for large-scale implementation initiatives; see McNulty and colleagues for a description and case example.[101]

In the previous version of this book chapter,[102] we presented the Adaptive Implementation of Effective Programs Trial (ADEPT)[103] as a particularly novel SMART design that allowed Kilbourne et al. to assess the efficacy of three implementation strategies. Several outcomes from this study are now published. Below we summarize key factors associated with this innovative work and describe how the design allowed for interpretation of strategy outcomes.

The ADEPT study compared three implementation strategies with increasing intensity of services based on whether or not sites met a preestablished implementation benchmark (see Figure 6.1). The implementation strategies included Replicating Effective Practices (REP),[44,104] a relatively low-intensity multifaceted implementation strategy that focuses on toolkit development and marketing, provider training and limited program assistance, IF[105] using a facilitator who is external to the clinical setting and assists sites in implementing a clinical innovation, and finally adding an implementation facilitator internal to the clinical organization to the existing external facilitator/internal facilitation.[62,67] This design allowed Kilbourne and colleagues to address the questions of (1) who needs more intense levels of assistance and (2) whether internal facilitation increased the uptake of a clinical innovation.[103]

Findings to date indicate that stepping up to the most intensive implementation strategy (REP plus external and internal facilitation) did outperform having external facilitation alone, but that this only occurred in sites that failed to deliver any of the innovation services at a lower level of strategy intensity.[106] Smith et al.[106] noted that these findings suggest that adding strategies to an implementation effort may be most effective when the resources do not duplicate existing efforts or are overly burdensome to the setting within which the implementation effort occurs. These findings were supported with findings from the cost analysis associated with this project. This revealed that to maximize cost-effectiveness, implementation efforts should begin with less intensive, less costly strategies and increase as needed to address contextual and recipient needs.[66] Eisman et al.[66] noted that this approach would allow the most intensive implementation strategies to be allocated to sites with the highest need and thus, potentially, the highest benefit.

Additional innovative designs include the Learn As You Go (LAGO) Designs.[107] These adaptive study designs have been long used in clinical trials and public health but can also be applied to evaluating implementation strategy designs. In an analysis of LAGO studies Nevo et al.[107] compared this type of design to SMART designs, described above. While SMART designs use randomization based on implementation outcomes to optimize implementation strategies, specific implementation strategies or multifaceted bundles of strategies are largely unknown at the beginning of a LAGO design and undergo adaptation and modification based on information gained during the conduct of the study.[107] The first stage of a LAGO study identifies the optimal strategy or strategy bundle, which is refined over time as information emerges from the implementation effort. Thus, the strategy or multifaceted strategy bundle can be considered a random variable that is informed by previous outcomes. While only emerging as a design in implementation science, LAGO studies hold the promise for real-time adaptations that can ultimately increase the rate at which implementation science knowledge is identified and spread.

DISSEMINATING SUCCESSFUL IMPLEMENTATION STRATEGIES

Just as implementation researchers have emphasized the need for studying the implementation of evidence-based *practices and innovations*, we must also turn our attention to the dissemination of evidence-based *implementation strategies.* To initiate lasting changes to care on a broad scale, policymakers and clinical managers must be capable of integrating implementation science knowledge and strategies into initiatives intended to foster adoption and spread of evidence-based practices or other innovations. As one might anticipate, just as there is a gap between evidence-based practices and their routine use in clinical settings, there is likely a similar gap between evidence-based implementation strategies and *their* use in clinical or other organizational change processes.[69]

Kirchner et al. have described the concept of implementation *practitioners* as those that increase the uptake of an EBP into practice by (a) applying strategies and tools developed in implementation research and/or (b) working with those with implementation expertise to contextualize evidence-based implementation strategies and improve clinical processes.[70] Central to increasing the use of evidence-based implementation strategies by implementation practitioners is educating this group about implementation science as well as processes

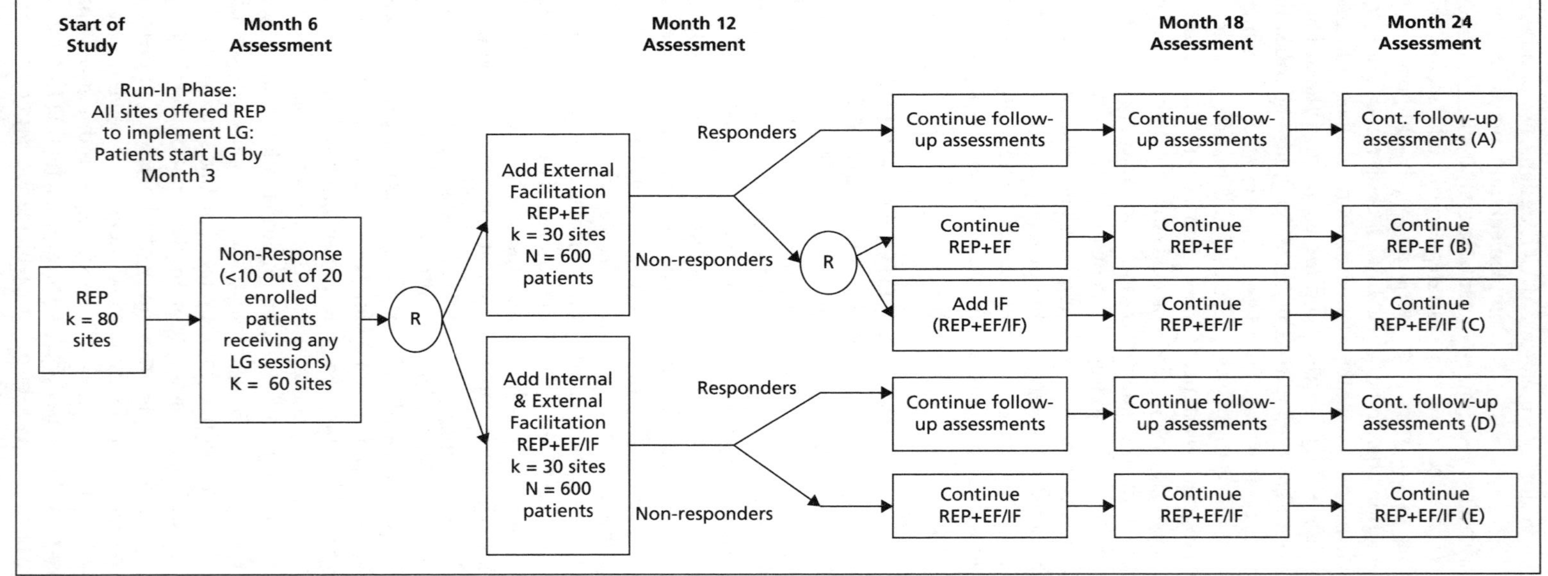

FIGURE 6.1 SMART trial design of REP combined with external (EF, REP+EF) and external and internal facilitation (IF, REP+EF/IF).

Reprinted with permission from: Kilbourne AM, Abraham KM, Goodrich DE, et al. Cluster randomized adaptive implementation trial comparing a standard versus enhanced implementation intervention to improve uptake of an effective re-engagement program for patients with serious mental illness. *Implement Sci.* 2013;8(1):136. doi:10.1186/1748-5908-8-136 through which strategies with a documented evidence base can be transferred.

Several recent publications have focused on describing the foundations of implementation science, its methodology, and ways through which the knowledge gained by this field can be applied by policymakers and clinical managers (i.e., implementation practitioners).[108–110] These articles described how both clinical QI and educational objectives can be achieved by incorporating implementation strategies and products into practice. For example, the Accreditation Council for Graduate Medical Education (ACGME), in conjunction with the American Boards of Medical Specialties, identified six ACGME core competencies, including practice-based learning and improvement and systems-based practice,[111] both central components of implementation.[108,111] In addition, the National Cancer Institute has developed an online resource, Implementation Science at a Glance, that presents a summary of key theories, methods, and considerations intended to help practitioners and policymakers gain familiarity with the building blocks of implementation science.[112]

Yet, as implementation scientists know quite well, education alone is rarely sufficient to effect meaningful or lasting change in clinical behavior. Therefore, an interactive approach to knowledge transfer is needed, with a dedicated focus on skill building. The Society for Implementation Research Collaboration (SIRC) encourages involvement of a wide range of stakeholders, who participate in implementation or QI activities. To support and incentivize such involvement, SIRC has established Practitioner Networks of Expertise, including a Provider Network (leaders and clinicians in clinics and agencies providing direct clinical or prevention services); Intermediaries Network (trainers, consultants, facilitators, or purveyors who provide training and expertise in implementation to provider agencies); and Policy/Funder Network (leaders of governmental, grant, insurance agencies, foundations, and systems of care that fund implementation). In addition, a recent review identified 41 implementation science training opportunities, including formal training institutes focusing on development of implementation science skills, online seminars, and graduate certificate programs courses.[113]

While the availability of training programs and resources noted above is certainly encouraging, an even more integrated approach for the transfer of implementation strategies to implementation practitioners may be warranted. One integrated approach for transferring knowledge and skills for a given implementation strategy would be through interactive training coupled with time-limited consultation with an expert or experienced practitioner of the strategy. Through the Quality Improvement Research Initiative (QUERI), the VHA has developed a network of "learning hubs" that focus on implementation practice to accelerate clinical care improvements.[114] Kirchner et al. recently described the development of one of the QUERI learning hubs focused on IF, with preliminary evaluation of the program showing increased knowledge of and confidence in applying IF strategies among trainees.[115] Finally, the implementation scientist may actually become part of the organization that is applying the evidence-based strategy.

FUTURE RESEARCH

While the evidence base for implementation strategies continues[116–121] to build, there is a need to better understand which strategies may work best for different interventions, stakeholders, settings, and contexts. In addition, emerging literature provides some indication that the need for specific strategies may differ depending on the phase of the implementation process (preimplementation, active implementation, sustainment, or dissemination).[21,77,122,123]

The utility of implementation research would be bolstered through a greater focus on mechanisms, or the processes and events through which an implementation strategy operates to effect desired outcomes, including implementation outcomes.[69] This shifts the focus from simply asking whether or not a strategy was effective, but how, when, where, why, and for what end a strategy was effective.[31] Unfortunately, we know relatively little about the mechanisms of various implementation strategies, as demonstrated by two recent systematic reviews.[71,124] This limits efforts to (1) systematically design and tailor implementation strategies to meet the needs of different interventions, stakeholders, and contexts; (2) replicate positive findings and learn from negative studies; and (3) understand how the effects of an implementation strategy might generalize to another setting and how it might need to be adapted to suit contextual needs.[72] At minimum, we recommend that researchers suggest plausible mechanisms of implementation strategies and document them using causal pathway diagrams,[69] logic models,[125] or another form of mechanism mapping.[126] This makes explicit the researchers' thinking and enables qualitative, quantitative or mixed-methods evaluations of the proposed effects. A conference series funded by the Agency for Healthcare Research and Quality has convened an international group of implementation scientists via a Mechanisms Network of Expertise to develop a research agenda focused on implementation mechanisms. A concept mapping study associated with that effort identified 105 unique challenges to studying implementation mechanisms, including issues related to conceptualization, measurement, methods, designs, the accumulation of knowledge within and across disciplines, and the inherent complexity of implementation problems. The members of the Mechanisms Network of Expertise are currently curating a set of actionable steps that can be taken to enhance knowledge in this area and are developing manuscripts for a special collection that will provide conceptual and methodological guidance.

Implementation research often does not include adequate assessment to determine whether implementation strategies supporting practice innovations are reaching everyone, including the marginalized. Although existing implementation strategies have improved care for the general population,[121] they may not be sufficient to improve care for marginalized populations.[127] One potential solution to reduce healthcare disparities is to engage marginalized consumers (e.g., end users, patients, community members, their families) as a discrete strategy, including their engagement in selecting and tailoring strategies to better meet their needs.[128] These engagement strategies are components of participatory approaches to study design (see chapter 10). Consumer engagement as an implementation strategy has nascent evidence for improving healthcare among marginalized populations,[129] and evidence for involving consumers in selecting and tailoring implementation strategies has not adequately been documented.[130] Woodward and colleagues are developing guidance for implementers to engage marginalized consumers in implementation processes.[131]

SUMMARY

Since the last publication of this book, we have seen significant growth in our understanding of implementation strategies. First, as a field of study, we have better identified the need to incorporate documentation of existing processes that support health equity as a core component of implementation. Inequity in the delivery and receipt of new innovations exists. It is only by documenting the presence or absence of equity and addressing it throughout the implementation process that we will be able to support systematic change. In addition, Perry and colleagues[11] built on the ERIC strategy taxonomy, identifying additional strategies and elaborating on strategy definitions to fit to specific actors, contexts, and outcomes of their project. In this chapter, we provided a systematic approach to adapting strategies using the ERIC taxonomy. We also provided several methods that can be used to select and tailor an implementation strategy for application. This includes the traditional use of conceptual models and frameworks, emerging methods (e.g., the application of user-centered design), highly structured methods (e.g., intervention mapping), post hoc analysis of successful strategies, and incorporating cost as a component of strategy selection.

We continue to call for robust standardized documentation and specification of strategies as a necessary component of implementation science. This advances our understanding of strategy mechanisms of action and supports replicability in future studies. We also challenge those who conduct research in implementation to incorporate an assessment of strategy fidelity in their study design and conduct. Through the incorporation of strategy fidelity assessment, we will better understand the drivers of implementation success or failure. Finally, we continue to call for more work to support the "handoff" of successful, evidence-based strategies to our clinical and operational partners. By supporting transfer of the knowledge we gain, we ensure that arch to become part of the way healthcare and other settings approach change.

ACKNOWLEDGMENTS

We would like to express our gratitude to Nyssa Curtis for her support on this chapter.

SUGGESTED READINGS AND WEBSITES

Readings

Kirchner JE, Smith JL, Powell BJ, Waltz TJ, Proctor EK. Getting a clinical innovation into practice: an introduction to implementation strategies. Psychiatry Res. 2020 Jan;283:112467. doi: 10.1016/j.psychres.2019.06.042. Epub 2019 Jul 2. PMID: 31488332; PMCID: PMC7239693

This manuscript provides an overview of the topic of implementation strategies and is a helpful primer for those who are new to implementation science.

Lewis CC, Klasnja P, Powell BJ, et al. From classification to causality: advancing understanding of mechanisms of change in implementation science. *Front Public Health.* 2017;6:136. doi:10.3389/fpubh.2018.00136

Lewis and colleagues provided a call to identify how different implementation strategies work, noting that the field needs precise, testable theories that describe the causal pathways through which implementation strategies function. This manuscript presents a four-step approach to developing causal pathway models for implementation strategies.

Powell BJ, Beidas RS, Lewis CC, et al. Methods to improve the selection and tailoring of implementation strategies. *J Behav Health Serv Res.* 2017 Apr;44(2):177–194.

Powell and colleagues described four methods to thoughtfully select implementation strategies: concept mapping, group model building, conjoint analysis, and intervention mapping (updated at present as "implementation mapping" in more recent texts). Each method has been shown to be effective in other fields (e.g., marketing, system redesign). Although there are more ways to purposefully align strategies to barriers and facilitators (e.g., evidence-based quality improvement processes), this article provides a helpful overview of some choices and describes their advantages and disadvantages.

Powell BJ, Fernandez ME, Williams NJ, et al. Enhancing the impact of implementation strategies in healthcare: a research agenda. *Front Public Health.* 2019 Jan 22;7:3. doi:10.3389/fpubh.2019.00003. PMID: 30723713; PMCID: PMC6350272

This article provides an overview of implementation strategies and presents priorities for strategies research.

Proctor E, Silmere H, Raghavan R, et al. Outcomes for implementation research: conceptual distinctions, measurement challenges, and research agenda. *Adm Policy Ment Health.* 2011;38(2):65–76. doi:10.1007/s10488-010-0319-7

In this article, the authors proposed a working taxonomy of eight conceptually distinct implementation outcomes—acceptability, adoption, appropriateness, feasibility, fidelity, implementation cost, penetration, and sustainability—along with their nominal definitions that may help guide consideration and selection of measures to assess success of an implementation strategy.

Waltz TJ, Powell BJ, Fernández ME, Abadie B, Damschroder LJ. Choosing implementation strategies to address contextual barriers: diversity in recommendations and future directions. *Implement Sci.* 2019;14(1):42. doi:10.1186/s13012-019-0892-4

This article describes the development of a tool that allows users to specify high-priority CFIR-based barriers and receive a prioritized list of strategies based on endorsements provided by participants. The tool is housed on the CFIR website provided in the Selected Websites and Tools section, below.

Selected Websites and Tools

Consolidated Framework for Implementation Research (CFIR). http://cfirguide.org/

The CFIR provides a menu of constructs that can be used in a range of applications—as a practical guide for systematically assessing potential barriers and facilitators (determinants) and a tool to match these determinants to ERIC strategies.

VA QUERI Learning Hubs. Implementation Strategy Training Opportunities. (va.gov)

The VA QUERI Learning Hubs provide training in specific evidence-based strategies and provide a unique opportunity for leaders, providers, and researchers to gain the practical experience and skills needed to lead care improvements at their sites.

REFERENCES

1. Proctor EK, Powell BJ, McMillen JC. Implementation strategies: recommendations for specifying and reporting. *Implement Sci.* 2013;8(1):139. doi:10.1186/1748-5908-8-139
2. Powell BJ, McMillen JC, Proctor EK, et al. A compilation of strategies for implementing clinical innovations in health and mental health. *Med Care Res Rev.* 2012;69(2):123–157. doi:10.1177/1077558711430690
3. Powell BJ, Waltz TJ, Chinman MJ, et al. A refined compilation of implementation strategies: results from the Expert Recommendations for Implementing Change (ERIC) project. *Implement Sci.* 2015;10(1):21. doi:10.1186/s13012-015-0209-1

4. Edelman EJ, Dziura J, Esserman D, et al. Working with HIV clinics to adopt addiction treatment using implementation facilitation (WHAT-IF?): rationale and design for a hybrid type 3 effectiveness-implementation study. *Contemp Clin Trials.* 2020;98:106156. doi:10.1016/j.cct.2020.106156
5. Weiner BJ, Lewis MA, Clauser SB, Stitzenberg KB. In search of synergy: strategies for combining interventions at multiple levels. *JNCI Monogr.* 2012;2012(44):34–41. doi:10.1093/jncimonographs/lgs001
6. Schilling S, Bigal L, Powell, B. Developing and applying synergistic multilevel implementation strategies: a practical implementation report of an approach to increasing adoption of an evidence based parenting intervention in primary care. *Implement Res Pract.* 2022;3.
7. Effective Practice and Organisation of Care (EPOC). EPOC taxonomy. 2015. Accessed February 10, 2022. https://epoc.cochrane.org/epoc-taxonomy
8. Mazza D, Bairstow P, Buchan H, et al. Refining a taxonomy for guideline implementation: results of an exercise in abstract classification. *Implement Sci.* 2013;8(1):32. doi:10.1186/1748-5908-8-32
9. Mays N, Roberts E, Popay J. Synthesising research evidence. In: Fulop N, Allen P, Clarke A, Black N, eds. *Studying the Organisation and Delivery of Health Services: Research Methods.* Routledge; 2001:188–220. https://researchonline.lshtm.ac.uk/id/eprint/15408
10. Waltz TJ, Powell BJ, Chinman MJ, et al. Expert recommendations for implementing change (ERIC): protocol for a mixed methods study. *Implement Sci.* 2014;9(1):39. doi:10.1186/1748-5908-9-39
11. Perry CK, Damschroder LJ, Hemler JR, Woodson TT, Ono SS, Cohen DJ. Specifying and comparing implementation strategies across seven large implementation interventions: a practical application of theory. *Implement Sci.* 2019;14(32):1–13. doi:10.1186/s13012-019-0876-4
12. Strongwater SL, Pelote VP. *Clinical Process Redesign: A Facilitator's Guide.* Aspen Publishers; 1996.
13. Waltz TJ, Powell BJ, Matthieu MM, et al. Use of concept mapping to characterize relationships among implementation strategies and assess their feasibility and importance: results from the Expert Recommendations for Implementing Change (ERIC) study. *Implement Sci.* 2015;10(1):109. doi:10.1186/s13012-015-0295-0
14. Jones LK, Tilberry S, Gregor C, et al. Implementation strategies to improve statin utilization in individuals with hypercholesterolemia: a systematic review and meta-analysis. *Implement Sci.* 2021;16(1):40. doi:10.1186/s13012-021-01108-0
15. Kok G, Gottlieb NH, Peters GJY, et al. A taxonomy of behaviour change methods: an intervention mapping approach. *Health Psychol Rev.* 2016;10(3):297–312. doi:10.1080/17437199.2015.1077155
16. Michie S, Richardson M, Johnston M, et al. The behavior change technique taxonomy (v1) of 93 hierarchically clustered techniques: building an international consensus for the reporting of behavior change interventions. *Ann Behav Med.* 2013;46(1):81–95. doi:10.1007/s12160-013-9486-6
17. McHugh S, Presseau J, Luecking C, et al. P73 Identifying the active ingredients in implementation: qualitative content analysis of the overlap between behaviour change techniques and implementation strategies. *J Epidemiol Community Health.* 2019;73:A104–A105.
18. McHugh S, Presseau J, Luecking CT, et al. Examining the complementarity between the ERIC compilation of implementation strategies and the behaviour change technique taxonomy: a qualitative analysis. *Implementation Sci.* 2022;17:56. https://doi.org/10.1186/s13012-022-01227-2
19. Finley EP, Huynh AK, Farmer MM, et al. Periodic reflections: a method of guided discussions for documenting implementation phenomena. *BMC Med Res Methodol.* 2018;18(153):1–15. doi:10.1186/s12874-018-0610-y
20. Lyon AR, Connors E, Jensen-Doss A, et al. Intentional research design in implementation science: implications for the use of nomothetic and idiographic assessment. *Transl Behav Med.* 2017;7(3):567–580. doi:10.1007/s13142-017-0464-6
21. Yakovchenko V, Morgan TR, Chinman MJ, et al. Mapping the road to elimination: a 5-year evaluation of implementation strategies associated with hepatitis C treatment in the Veterans Health Administration. *BMC Health Serv Res.* 2021;21(1):1348. doi:10.1186/s12913-021-07312-4
22. Bustos TE, Sridhar A, Drahota A. Community-based implementation strategy use and satisfaction: a mixed-methods approach to using the ERIC compilation for organizations serving children on the autism spectrum. *Implement Res Pract.* 2021;2:263348952110580. doi:10.1177/26334895211058086
23. Rogal SS, Yakovchenko V, Waltz TJ, et al. The association between implementation strategy use and the uptake of hepatitis C treatment in a

national sample. *Implement Sci.* 2017;12(60):1–13. doi:10.1186/s13012-017-0588-6

24. Lyon AR, Cook CR, Locke J, Davis C, Powell BJ, Waltz TJ. Importance and feasibility of an adapted set of implementation strategies in schools. *J Sch Psychol.* 2019;76:66–77. doi:10.1016/j.jsp.2019.07.014
25. Kemp C, Lovero K, Giusto A, Green C, Wagenaar B. Use of the Expert Recommendations for Implementing Change (ERIC) compilation of implementation strategies in low- and middle-income countries; 2021. https://www.crd.york.ac.uk/prospero/display_record.php?ID=CRD42021268374
26. Balis LE, Houghtaling B, Harden SM. Using implementation strategies in community settings: an introduction to the Expert Recommendations for Implementing Change (ERIC) compilation and future directions. *Transl Behav Med.* 2022;16;12(10):965–978. doi:10.1093/tbm/ibac061
27. Ingvarsson S, Hasson H, Von Thiele Schwarz U, et al. Strategies for de-implementation of low-value care—a scoping review. *Implementation Sci.* 2022;17(73).
28. Nathan N, Powell BJ, Shelton RC, et al. Do the Expert Recommendations for Implementing Change (ERIC) strategies adequately address sustainment? *Front Health Serv.* 2022;2:905909. doi:10.3389/frhs.2022.905909
29. Powell BJ, Fernandez ME, Williams NJ, et al. Enhancing the impact of implementation strategies in healthcare: a research agenda. *Front Public Health.* 2019;7(3):1–9. doi:10.3389/fpubh.2019.00003
30. Sales A, Smith J, Curran G, Kochevar L. Models, strategies, and tools: theory in implementing evidence-based findings into health care practice. *J Gen Intern Med.* 2006;21(S2):S43–S49. doi:10.1111/j.1525-1497.2006.00362.x
31. Mittman B. Implementation science in health care. In: Brownson RC, Colditz GA, Proctor EK, eds. *Dissemination and Implementation Research in Health: Translating Science to Practice.* Oxford University Press; 2012:400–418.
32. Bhattacharyya O, Reeves S, Garfinkel S, Zwarenstein M. Designing theoretically-informed implementation interventions: fine in theory, but evidence of effectiveness in practice is needed. *Implement Sci.* 2006;1(1):5. doi:10.1186/1748-5908-1-5
33. Eccles M, Grimshaw J, Walker A, Johnston M, Pitts N. Changing the behavior of healthcare professionals: the use of theory in promoting the uptake of research findings. *J Clin Epidemiol.* 2005;58(2):107–112. doi:10.1016/j.jclinepi.2004.09.002
34. Oxman AD, Fretheim A, Flottorp S. The OFF theory of research utilization. *J Clin Epidemiol.* 2005;58(2):113–116. doi:10.1016/j.jclinepi.2004.10.002
35. The Improved Clinical Effectiveness through Behavioural Research Group (ICEBeRG). Designing theoretically-informed implementation interventions. *Implement Sci.* 2006;1(1):4. doi:10.1186/1748-5908-1-4
36. Harvey G, Kitson A. Translating evidence into healthcare policy and practice: single versus multi-faceted implementation strategies—is there a simple answer to a complex question? *Int J Health Policy Manag.* 2015;4(3):123–126. doi:10.15171/ijhpm.2015.54
37. Meyers DC, Durlak JA, Wandersman A. The quality implementation framework: a synthesis of critical steps in the implementation process. *Am J Community Psychol.* 2012;50(3–4):462–480. doi:10.1007/s10464-012-9522-x
38. Damschroder LJ, Aron DC, Keith RE, Kirsh SR, Alexander JA, Lowery JC. Fostering implementation of health services research findings into practice: a consolidated framework for advancing implementation science. *Implement Sci.* 2009;4(1):50. doi:10.1186/1748-5908-4-50
39. Consolidated Framework for Implementation Research (CFIR). Strategy design. 2022. https://cfirguide.org/choosing-strategies/
40. Waltz TJ, Powell BJ, Fernández ME, Abadie B, Damschroder LJ. Choosing implementation strategies to address contextual barriers: diversity in recommendations and future directions. *Implement Sci.* 2019;14(1):42. doi:10.1186/s13012-019-0892-4
41. *Health Equity Impact Assessment (HEIA) Workbook.* Ministry of Health and Long Term Care; 2012. Accessed March 6, 2017. http://www.health.gov.on.ca/en/pro/programs/heia/docs/workbook.pdf
42. Stetler CB, Legro MW, Wallace CM, et al. The role of formative evaluation in implementation research and the QUERI experience. *J Gen Intern Med.* 2006;21(S2):S1–S8. doi:10.1007/s11606-006-0267-9
43. Owen RR, Drummond KL, Viverito KM, et al. Monitoring and managing metabolic effects of antipsychotics: a cluster randomized trial of an intervention combining evidence-based quality improvement and external facilitation. *Implement Sci.* 2013;8(1):120. doi:10.1186/1748-5908-8-120
44. Kilbourne AM, Neumann MS, Pincus HA, Bauer MS, Stall R. Implementing evidence-based interventions in health care:

application of the replicating effective programs framework. *Implement Sci.* 2007;2(1):42. doi:10.1186/1748-5908-2-42
45. Going Lean in Health Care. *IHI Innovation Series White Paper.* Institute for Healthcare Improvement; 2005. Available at https://www.IHI.org
46. Steffen KM, Spinella PC, Holdsworth LM, et al. Factors influencing implementation of blood transfusion recommendations in pediatric critical care units. *Front Pediatr.* 2021;9:800461. doi:10.3389/fped.2021.800461
47. Dopp AR, Parisi KE, Munson SA, Lyon AR. A glossary of user-centered design strategies for implementation experts. *Transl Behav Med.* 2019;9(6):1057–1064. doi:10.1093/tbm/iby119
48. Chen E, Neta G, Roberts MC. Complementary approaches to problem solving in healthcare and public health: implementation science and human-centered design. *Transl Behav Med.* 2021;11(5):1115–1121. doi:10.1093/tbm/ibaa079
49. Costanza-Chock S. *Design Justice: Community-Led Practices to Build the World We Need.* MIT Press Perspect; 2020.
50. Fareed N, Swoboda CM, Lawrence J, Griesenbrock T, Huerta T. Co-establishing an infrastructure for routine data collection to address disparities in infant mortality: planning and implementation. *BMC Health Serv Res.* 2022;22(1):4. doi:10.1186/s12913-021-07393-1
51. Lyon AR, Bruns EJ. User-centered redesign of evidence-based psychosocial interventions to enhance implementation—hospitable soil or better seeds? *JAMA Psychiatry.* 2019;76(1):3. doi:10.1001/jamapsychiatry.2018.3060
52. Haines ER, Dopp A, Lyon AR, et al. Harmonizing evidence-based practice, implementation context, and implementation strategies with user-centered design: a case example in young adult cancer care. *Implement Sci Commun.* 2021;2(1):45. doi:10.1186/s43058-021-00147-4
53. Haines ER, Kirk MA, Lux L, et al. Ethnography and user-centered design to inform context-driven implementation. *Transl Behav Med.* 2022;12(1):ibab077. doi:10.1093/tbm/ibab077
54. Powell BJ, Beidas RS, Lewis CC, et al. Methods to improve the selection and tailoring of implementation strategies. *J Behav Health Serv Res.* 2017;44(2):177–194. doi:10.1007/s11414-015-9475-6
55. Waltz T. Group concept mapping. In: Nilsen, Birken S, ed. *Handbook on Implementation Science.* Edward Elgar Publishing; 2020:519–526. doi:10.4337/9781788975995
56. Bartholomew Eldredge LK. *Planning health promotion programs: an intervention mapping approach*, 4th ed. San Francisco, CA: Jossey-Bass & Pfeiffer Imprints Wiley; 2016.
57. Proctor E, Hooley C, Morse A, McCrary S, Kim H, Kohl PL. Intermediary/purveyor organizations for evidence-based interventions in the US child mental health: characteristics and implementation strategies. *Implement Sci.* 2019;14(1):3. doi:10.1186/s13012-018-0845-3
58. Rogal SS, Yakovchenko V, Waltz TJ, et al. Longitudinal assessment of the association between implementation strategy use and the uptake of hepatitis C treatment: year 2. *Implement Sci.* 2019;14(1):36. doi:10.1186/s13012-019-0881-7
59. Rogal SS, Yakovchenko V, Waltz TJ, et al. The association between implementation strategy use and the uptake of hepatitis C treatment in a national sample. *Implement Sci.* 2017;12(60) doi:10.1186/s13012-017-0588-6
60. Yakovchenko V, Morgan TR, Miech EJ, et al. Core implementation strategies for improving cirrhosis care in the Veterans Health Administration. *Hepatology.* 2022;76:404–417. doi:10.1002/hep.32395
61. Proctor E, Silmere H, Raghavan R, et al. Outcomes for implementation research: conceptual distinctions, measurement challenges, and research agenda. *Adm Policy Ment Health Ment Health Serv Res.* 2011;38(2):65–76. doi:10.1007/s10488-010-0319-7
62. Gold HT, McDermott C, Hoomans T, Wagner TH. Cost data in implementation science: categories and approaches to costing. *Implement Sci.* 2022;17(1):11. doi:10.1186/s13012-021-01172-6
63. Hoomans T, Severens JL. Economic evaluation of implementation strategies in health care. *Implement Sci.* 2014;9(1):168, s13012-014-0168-y. doi:10.1186/s13012-014-0168-y
64. Eisman AB, Quanbeck A, Bounthavong M, Panattoni L, Glasgow RE. Implementation science issues in understanding, collecting, and using cost estimates: a multi-stakeholder perspective. *Implement Sci.* 2021;16(1):75. doi:10.1186/s13012-021-01143-x
65. Cidav Z, Mandell D, Pyne J, Beidas R, Curran G, Marcus S. A pragmatic method for costing implementation strategies using time-driven activity-based costing. *Implement Sci.* 2020;15(1):28. doi:10.1186/s13012-020-00993-1
66. Eisman AB, Hutton DW, Prosser LA, Smith SN, Kilbourne AM. Cost-effectiveness of the adaptive implementation of effective programs trial (ADEPT): approaches to adopting implementation strategies. *Implement Sci.* 2020;15(1):109. doi:10.1186/s13012-020-01069-w

67. Roberts SLE, Healey A, Sevdalis N. Use of health economic evaluation in the implementation and improvement science fields—a systematic literature review. *Implement Sci.* 2019;14(1):72. doi:10.1186/s13012-019-0901-7
68. Akiba CF, Powell BJ, Pence BW, Nguyen MXB, Golin C, Go V. The case for prioritizing implementation strategy fidelity measurement: benefits and challenges. *Transl Behav Med.* 2022;12(2):335–342. doi:10.1093/tbm/ibab138
69. Lewis CC, Klasnja P, Powell BJ, et al. From classification to causality: advancing understanding of mechanisms of change in implementation science. *Front Public Health.* 2018;6:136. doi:10.3389/fpubh.2018.00136
70. Proctor EK, Powell BJ, McMillen JC. Implementation strategies: recommendations for specifying and reporting. *Implement Sci.* 2013;8(1):139. doi:10.1186/1748-5908-8-139
71. Lewis CC, Boyd MR, Walsh-Bailey C, et al. A systematic review of empirical studies examining mechanisms of implementation in health. *Implement Sci.* 2020;15(1):21. doi:10.1186/s13012-020-00983-3
72. Lewis CC, Powell BJ, Brewer SK, et al. Advancing mechanisms of implementation to accelerate sustainable evidence-based practice integration: protocol for generating a research agenda. *BMJ Open.* 2021;11(10):e053474. doi:10.1136/bmjopen-2021-053474
73. Lyon AR, Cook CR, Duong MT, et al. The influence of a blended, theoretically-informed pre-implementation strategy on school-based clinician implementation of an evidence-based trauma intervention. *Implement Sci.* 2019;14(1):54. doi:10.1186/s13012-019-0905-3
74. Grol RPTM, Bosch MC, Hulscher MEJL, Eccles MP, Wensing M. Planning and studying improvement in patient care: the use of theoretical perspectives. *Milbank Q.* 2007;85(1):93–138. doi:10.1111/j.1468-0009.2007.00478.x
75. Bunger AC, Hanson RF, Doogan NJ, Powell BJ, Cao Y, Dunn J. Can learning collaboratives support implementation by rewiring professional networks? *Adm Policy Ment Health Ment Health Serv Res.* 2016;43(1):79–92. doi:10.1007/s10488-014-0621-x
76. Gold R, Bunce AE, Cohen DJ, et al. Reporting on the strategies needed to implement proven interventions: an example from a "real world" cross-setting implementation study. *Mayo Clin Proc.* 2016;91(8):1074–1083. doi:10.1016/j.mayocp.2016.03.014
77. Aarons GA, Hurlburt M, Horwitz SM. Advancing a conceptual model of evidence-based practice implementation in public service sectors. *Adm Policy Ment Health.* 2011;38:4–23. doi:10.1007/s10488-010-0327-7
78. Dunbar J, Hernan A, Janus E, et al. Implementation salvage experiences from the Melbourne diabetes prevention study. *BMC Public Health.* 2012;12(806):1–9. doi:10.1186/1471-2458-12-806
79. Hoagwood KE, Chaffin M, Chamberlain P, Bickman L, Mittman B. Implementation salvage strategies: maximizing methodological flexibility in children's mental health research. Panel presentation presented at: 4th Annual NIH Conference on the Science of Dissemination and Implementation; March 2011; Washington, DC.
80. Powell BJ, Patel SV, Haley AD, et al. Determinants of implementing evidence-based trauma-focused interventions for children and youth: a systematic review. *Adm Policy Ment Health Ment Health Serv Res.* 2020;47:705–719. doi:10.1007/s10488-019-01003-3
81. Boyd MR, Powell BJ, Endicott D, Lewis CC. A method for tracking implementation strategies: an exemplar implementing measurement-based care in community behavioral health clinics. *Behav Ther.* 2018;49:525–537. doi:10.1016/j.beth.2017.11.012
82. Bunger AC, Powell BJ, Robertson HA, MacDowell H, Birken SA, Shea C. Tracking implementation strategies: a description of a practical approach and early findings. *Health Res Policy Syst.* 2017;15(15):1–12. doi:10.1186/s12961-017-0175-y
83. Haley AD, Powell BJ, Walsh-Bailey C, et al. Strengthening methods for tracking adaptations and modifications to implementation strategies. *BMC Med Res Methodol.* 2021;21(133):1–12. doi:10.1186/s12874-021-01326-6
84. Miller CJ, Barnett ML, Baumann AA, Gutner CA, Wiltsey Stirman S. The FRAME-IS: a framework for documenting modifications to implementation strategies in healthcare. *Implement Sci.* 2021;16(36):1–12. doi:10.1186/s13012-021-01105-3
85. Wiltsey Stirman S, Baumann AA, Miller CJ. The FRAME: an expanded framework for reporting adaptations and modifications to evidence-based interventions. *Implement Sci.* 2019;14(58):1–10. doi:10.1186/s13012-019-0898-y
86. Walsh-Bailey C, Palazzo LG, Jones SMW, et al. A pilot study comparing tools for tracking implementation strategies and treatment adaptations. *Implement Res Pract.* 2021;2:1–14. doi:10.1177/26334895211016028
87. Boyd MR, Powell BJ, Endicott D, Lewis CC. A method for tracking implementation strategies: an exemplar implementing measurement-based care in community behavioral health clinics. *Behav Ther.* 2018;49(4):525–537. doi:10.1016/j.beth.2017.11.012

88. Bunger AC, Powell BJ, Robertson HA, MacDowell H, Birken SA, Shea C. Tracking implementation strategies: a description of a practical approach and early findings. *Health Res Policy Syst.* 2017;15(1):15. doi:10.1186/s12961-017-0175-y
89. Finley EP, Huynh AK, Farmer MM, et al. Periodic reflections: a method of guided discussions for documenting implementation phenomena. *BMC Med Res Methodol.* 2018;18(1):153. doi:10.1186/s12874-018-0610-y
90. Haley AD, Powell BJ, Walsh-Bailey C, et al. Strengthening methods for tracking adaptations and modifications to implementation strategies. *BMC Med Res Methodol.* 2021;21(1):133. doi:10.1186/s12874-021-01326-6
91. Bustos TE, Sridhar A, Drahota A. Community-based implementation strategy use and satisfaction: a mixed-methods approach to using the ERIC compilation for organizations serving children on the autism spectrum. *Implement Res Pract.* 2021;2:1–19. doi:10.1177/26334895211058086
92. Slaughter SE, Hill JN, Snelgrove-Clarke E. What is the extent and quality of documentation and reporting of fidelity to implementation strategies: a scoping review. *Implement Sci.* 2015;10(1):129. doi:10.1186/s13012-015-0320-3
93. Stockdale SE, Hamilton AB, Bergman AA, et al. Assessing fidelity to evidence-based quality improvement as an implementation strategy for patient-centered medical home transformation in the Veterans Health Administration. *Implement Sci.* 2020;15(1):18. doi:10.1186/s13012-020-0979-y
94. Smith J, Ritchie M, Miller C, Chinman M, Kelly P, Kirchner J. Getting to fidelity: scoping review and expert panel process to identify core activities of implementation facilitation strategies. Poster presentation presented at: 2019 HSR&D/QUERI National Conference; October 30, 2019; Washington, DC. https://www.hsrd.research.va.gov/meetings/2019/mobile/abstract-display.cfm?AbsNum=1144
95. Ritchie MJ, Kirchner JE, Townsend JC, Pitcock JA, Dollar KM, Liu CF. Time and organizational cost for facilitating implementation of primary care mental health integration. *J Gen Intern Med.* 2020;35(4):1001–1010. doi:https://doi.org/10.1007/s11606-019-05537-y
96. Landes SJ, Jegley SM, Kirchner JE, et al. Adapting caring contacts for veterans in a Department of Veterans Affairs emergency department: results from a type 2 hybrid effectiveness-implementation pilot study. *Front Psychiatry.* 2021;12:746805. doi:10.3389/fpsyt.2021.746805
97. Proctor EK, Landsverk J, Aarons G, Chambers D, Glisson C, Mittman B. Implementation research in mental health services: an emerging science with conceptual, methodological, and training challenges. *Adm Policy Ment Health Ment Health Serv Res.* 2009;36(1):24–34.
98. Lengnick-Hall R, Proctor EK, Bunger AC, Gerke DR. Ten years of implementation outcome research: a scoping review protocol. *BMJ Open.* 2021;11(6):e049339. doi:10.1136/bmjopen-2021-049339
99. Eslava-Schmalbach J, Garzón-Orjuela N, Elias V, Reveiz L, Tran N, Langlois EV. Conceptual framework of equity-focused implementation research for health programs (EquIR). *Int J Equity Health.* 2019;18(1):80. doi:10.1186/s12939-019-0984-4
100. Shelton RC, Chambers DA, Glasgow RE. An extension of RE-AIM to enhance sustainability: addressing dynamic context and promoting health equity over time. *Front Public Health.* 2020;8:134. doi:10.3389/fpubh.2020.00134
101. McNulty M, Smith JD, Villamar J, et al. Implementation research methodologies for achieving scientific equity and health equity. *Ethn Dis.* 2019;29(suppl 1):83–92. doi:10.18865/ed.29.S1.83
102. Kirchner J, Waltz T, Powell B, Smith J, Proctor E. Implementation strategies. In: Brownson RC, Colditz GA, Proctor EK, eds. *Dissemination and Implementation Research in Health: Translating Science to Practice.* 2nd ed. Oxford University Press; 2018:245–266. doi:10.1093/oso/9780190683214.001.0001
103. Kilbourne AM, Almirall D, Eisenberg D, et al. Protocol: Adaptive Implementation of Effective Programs Trial (ADEPT): cluster randomized SMART trial comparing a standard versus enhanced implementation strategy to improve outcomes of a mood disorders program. *Implement Sci.* 2014;9:132. doi:10.1186/s13012-014-0132-x
104. Kilbourne AM, Abraham KM, Goodrich DE, et al. Cluster randomized adaptive implementation trial comparing a standard versus enhanced implementation intervention to improve uptake of an effective re-engagement program for patients with serious mental illness. *Implement Sci.* 2013;8(1):136. doi:10.1186/1748-5908-8-136
105. Kirchner JE, Ritchie MJ, Pitcock JA, Parker LE, Curran GM, Fortney JC. Outcomes of a partnered facilitation strategy to implement primary care-mental health. *J Gen Intern Med.* 2014;29(suppl 4):904–912. doi:10.1007/s11606-014-3027-2

106. Smith SN, Liebrecht CM, Bauer MS, Kilbourne AM. Comparative effectiveness of external vs. blended facilitation on collaborative care model implementation in slow-implementer community practices. *Health Serv Res.* 2020;55(6):954–965. doi:10.1111/1475-6773.13583
107. Nevo D, Lok JJ, Spiegelman D. Analysis of "learn-as-you-go" (LAGO) studies. *Ann Stat.* 2021;49(2):793–819. doi:10.1214/20-AOS1978
108. Kirchner JE, Woodward EN, Smith JL, et al. Implementation science supports core clinical competencies: an overview and clinical example. *Prim Care Companion CNS Disord.* 2016;18(6). doi:10.4088/PCC.16m02004
109. Bauer MS, Miller C, Kim B, et al. Partnering with health system operations leadership to develop a controlled implementation trial. *Implement Sci.* 2015;11(1):22. doi:10.1186/s13012-016-0385-7
110. Bauer MS, Kirchner J. Implementation science: what is it and why should I care? *Psychiatry Res.* 2020;283:112376. doi:10.1016/j.psychres.2019.04.025
111. Kavic MS. Competency and the six core competencies. *JSLS.* 2002;6(2):95–97.
112. US Department of Health & Human Services. Implementation science at a glance: a guide for cancer control practitioners. United States Government Printing Office; 2019. Accessed February 13, 2022. https://public.ebookcentral.proquest.com/choice/publicfullrecord.aspx?p=5772941
113. Davis R, D'Lima D. Building capacity in dissemination and implementation science: a systematic review of the academic literature on teaching and training initiatives. *Implement Sci.* 2020;15(1):97. doi:10.1186/s13012-020-01051-6
114. QUERI—Quality Enhancement Research Initiative. Implementation strategy training opportunities. December 14, 2021. Accessed February 13, 2022. https://www.queri.research.va.gov/training_hubs/default.cfm
115. Kirchner J, Dollar K, Smith J, et al. Development and preliminary evaluation of an implementation facilitation training program. *Implement Res Pract.* 2022;3. doi.org/10.1177/26334895221087475.
116. Grimshaw JM, Eccles MP, Lavis JN, Hill SJ, Squires JE. Knowledge translation of research findings. *Implement Sci.* 2012;7(1):50. doi:10.1186/1748-5908-7-50
117. Forsetlund L, Bjørndal A, Rashidian A, et al. Continuing education meetings and workshops: effects on professional practice and health care outcomes. Cochrane Effective Practice and Organisation of Care Group, ed. *Cochrane Database Syst Rev.* 2009;2:1–89. doi:10.1002/14651858.CD003030.pub2
118. Ivers N, Jamtvedt G, Flottorp S, et al. Audit and feedback: effects on professional practice and healthcare outcomes. *Cochrane Database Syst Rev.* 2012;(6):CD000259. doi:10.1002/14651858.CD000259.pub3
119. Farmer AP, Légaré F, Turcot L, et al. Printed educational materials: effects on professional practice and health care outcomes. In: Cochrane Collaboration, ed. *Cochrane Database of Systematic Reviews.* John Wiley & Sons, Ltd; 2008:CD004398.pub2. doi:10.1002/14651858.CD004398.pub2
120. Flodgren G, Parmelli E, Doumit G, et al. Local opinion leaders: effects on professional practice and health care outcomes. Cochrane Effective Practice and Organisation of Care Group, ed. *Cochrane Database Syst Rev.* 2011;8:1–66. doi:10.1002/14651858.CD000125.pub4
121. Baker R, Camosso-Stefinovic J, Gillies C, et al. Tailored interventions to address determinants of practice. Cochrane Effective Practice and Organisation of Care Group, ed. *Cochrane Database Syst Rev.* 2015;2015(4):1–114. doi:10.1002/14651858.CD005470.pub3
122. Rogal SS, Yakovchenko V, Waltz TJ, et al. Longitudinal assessment of the association between implementation strategy use and the uptake of hepatitis C treatment: year two. *Implement Sci.* 2019;14(36):1–12. doi:10.1186/s13012-019-0881-7
123. Turner K, Weinberger M, Renfro C, et al. Stages of change: moving community pharmacies from a drug dispensing to population health management model. *Med Care Res Rev.* 2021;78(1):57–67. doi:10.1177/1077558719841159
124. Williams NJ. Multilevel mechanisms of implementation strategies in mental health: integrating theory, research, and practice. *Adm Policy Ment Health Ment Health Serv Res.* 2016;43(5):783–798. doi:10.1007/s10488-015-0693-2
125. Smith JD, Li DH, Rafferty MR. The implementation research logic model: a method for planning, executing, reporting, and synthesizing implementation projects. *Implement Sci.* 2020;15(1):84. doi:10.1186/s13012-020-01041-8
126. Geng EH, Baumann AA, Powell BJ. Mechanism mapping to advance research on implementation strategies. *PLoS Med.* 2022;19(2):e1003918. doi:10.1371/journal.pmed.1003918
127. Lion KC, Raphael JL. Partnering health disparities research with quality improvement science in pediatrics. *Pediatrics.* 2015;135(2):354–361. doi:10.1542/peds.2014-2982

128. Holt CL, Chambers DA. Opportunities and challenges in conducting community-engaged dissemination/implementation research. *Transl Behav Med.* 2017;7(3):389–392. doi:10.1007/s13142-017-0520-2
129. Wells KB, Jones L, Chung B, et al. Community-partnered cluster-randomized comparative effectiveness trial of community engagement and planning or resources for services to address depression disparities. *J Gen Intern Med.* 2013;28(10):1268–1278. doi:10.1007/s11606-013-2484-3
130. Melgar C, Woodward E, True G, Willging C, Kirchner J. Examples and challenges of engaging consumers in implementation science activities: an environmental scan. Presented at: 13th Annual Conference on the Science of Dissemination and Implementation; 2020; Washington, DC.
131. Woodward E, Willging C, Landes S, et al. Determining feasibility of incorporating consumer engagement into implementation activities: study protocol of a hybrid implementation-effectiveness type II pilot. *BMJ Open.* 2022;12(1):e050107. doi:10.1136/bmjopen-2021-050107

7

Fidelity and Its Relationship to Effectiveness, Adaptation, and Implementation

RACHEL C. SHELTON, PRAJAKTA ADSUL, KAREN M. EMMONS, LAURA A. LINNAN, AND JENNIFER D. ALLEN

INTRODUCTION

Effective dissemination and implementation (D&I) of evidence-based interventions (EBIs) necessitates that the intervention will be delivered and replicated with *fidelity*. Fidelity has been defined as the extent to which the intervention was delivered as planned. It represents the quality and integrity of the intervention as intended by the developers.[1–3] In the context of D&I science, there has been growing consideration of fidelity as it relates to the delivery of implementation strategies to support the delivery of EBIs.[4–6]

A focus on fidelity is critical to understanding whether planned interventions and implementation strategies are delivered or implemented as intended, are effective and why, and for whom are they effective.[1,7] Implementing and tracking dose and the extent to which the core elements of the intervention are delivered as planned is central to fidelity[8,9] and can help lay the foundation for future replication, dissemination, and scale-up efforts.[10] Additionally, attention to fidelity can provide insights into feasibility and can help identify potential challenges and considerations when implementing interventions across new settings and populations.[11]

Assessment of fidelity requires researchers and program implementers to evaluate whether the prespecified outcomes of an intervention are related to variability in the quality or extent of implementation, or whether other factors—unrelated to the intervention or its implementation—may account for the observed outcomes.[1,12] In case of interventions that do not achieve expected outcomes, fidelity is critical to understanding whether the failure of an intervention is attributable to poor or inadequate implementation (termed *type III error*) or to intervention program theory failure, or some combination thereof.[13] Additionally, when expected outcomes are observed, it is important to understand if the intervention was delivered with fidelity since there is evidence that the fidelity with which an intervention is implemented is associated with success in achieving change in targeted outcomes.[1,14–16]

Despite the benefits of assessing fidelity to enhance public health impact[17] and growing attention to reproducibility and fidelity in the context of clinical and behavioral interventions,[4,8,9,18–20] there are challenges in implementing interventions with high fidelity when they move from controlled research settings to more complex and dynamic practice settings.[8] There is growing consideration of the value of eliciting stakeholder input and perspectives to enhance program fidelity.[21] Additionally, there is recognition of the importance of balancing fidelity and planned adaptations to interventions and implementation strategies that address health inequities and meet the needs of diverse settings, resources, and populations.[22] Empirical evidence suggests that while assessing fidelity is commonly perceived as an important research goal, most researchers report having limited conceptual and methodological understanding of fidelity.[23]

This chapter seeks to introduce and enhance conceptual and methodological

Rachel C. Shelton, Prajakta Adsul, Karen M. Emmons, Laura A. Linnan, and Jennifer D. Allen, *Fidelity and Its Relationship to Effectiveness, Adaptation, and Implementation* In: *Dissemination and Implementation Research in Health.* Edited by: Ross C. Brownson, Graham A. Colditz, and Enola K. Proctor, Oxford University Press. © Oxford University Press 2023. DOI: 10.1093/oso/9780197660690.003.0007 clarity regarding fidelity in the context of D&I research, propose a framework for factors that influence fidelity, and discuss the relationship between fidelity and adaptation. We describe a case example related to both intervention fidelity and adaptation to share lessons learned from our prior work and conclude with recommendations for practitioners, researchers, and policymakers to advance work in this area.

Defining and Conceptualizing Fidelity

Foundational work on fidelity emerged originally from the fields of community psychology and education[16,24–26] and was typically addressed as part of process evaluation.[2] Over time, several terms have been used interchangeably for this concept (e.g., "implementation fidelity,"[1(p1),27(p531),28(p197),29(p83),30(p77)] "treatment fidelity,"[31(pS381),32(p343)] "treatment integrity"[33(p220)]), leading to a lack of clarity in conceptualization and measurement of fidelity.[34] Here, in the context of D&I research, we focus on fidelity defined as the extent to which the core intervention elements (or implementation strategies) are successfully delivered as intended.[35,36] "Core" [37(p1),38(p1)] intervention elements are components that were tested through rigorous research designs and linked with desired outcomes (e.g., directly responsible for intervention effects).[37,38] While important to recognize that not all intervention developers have identified or tested which components are *core*, these components are typically perceived as the *essential or active ingredients* that represent the internal logic and underlying theory of the intervention.[16] As such, fidelity relates to the extent to which core elements are implemented as originally intended by program developers.[2,39]

Modifications that are "fidelity inconsistent"[40(p398),41(p1)] are often *not planned* (e.g., removing or skipping intervention components) and can potentially reduce intervention impact on prespecified outcomes.[42,43] In contrast, *adaptive* elements of an intervention do not change the internal logic or theoretical foundation of the intervention; changes made to these elements are deemed *fidelity consistent* and are not believed to reduce the intervention's impact.[16] Planned adaptations typically reflect cultural or contextual *translations* (e.g., tailoring, refining, language adaptations) that are critical to successful D&I efforts in nonresearch settings, particularly for addressing health inequities and their root causes. An excellent example of a planned adaptation of an EBI was demonstrated by Handley and colleagues.[44] They presented a fidelity assessment of a bilingual intervention for reducing diabetes risk among English- and Spanish-speaking postpartum women; the researchers used a modified fidelity framework to examine predetermined *core* intervention elements (e.g., systems information technology [IT] integration) as well as *modifiable* intervention components related to equity (e.g., variation by language). We discuss recent developments in relation to fidelity and adaptation[31,43,45,46] further in this chapter.

In our multidimensional conceptualization of fidelity, we build on prior work (e.g., NIH Behavioral Change Consortium, Conceptual Framework of Implementation Fidelity)[1,2,8,16,26] that has commonly described the primary elements: adherence, dose, quality of delivery, participant responsiveness and enactment, and program differentiation. *Adherence* involves consideration of the intervention *dose* or *exposure*—the amount, frequency, and/or duration of intervention delivered. *Quality of delivery* reflects how well an intervention is implemented, in terms of both content and process. Quality is often assessed by comparing actual delivery with a standard or theoretical ideal.[1] *Participant responsiveness* is the extent to which the target audience engages with, understands, or is satisfied with the intervention (e.g., dose of *intervention received*[2]), while *enactment* is whether they use these skills.[12,47] *Program differentiation* reflects the underlying theoretical mechanisms by which the intervention and its unique features and/or core elements exert their influence on outcomes.[1]

There are varying opinions regarding whether comprehensive assessments of fidelity are needed after the initial efficacy of an intervention is demonstrated through empirical research.[1,26,29] Which specific aspects of fidelity are measured may also be influenced by pragmatic considerations (e.g., personnel, resources), as well as the input and priorities of stakeholders within specific settings (e.g., which indicators they value and perceive as being feasible to assess). In D&I research, given that implementation often happens in new settings and populations involving adaptations, we argue that it is ideal to conduct ongoing assessments of fidelity, as well as to document and track adaptations that are made, and examine their potential impact on intervention outcomes. Further, given that fidelity assessments can require intensive time and personnel, we advocate for increased attention to methods by which fidelity can be assessed across a diverse range of clinical and community settings that have varying levels of resources and capacity to do so.[48–51]

Aligned with recent work in D&I science,[4,18,20] we recognize that both implementation and fidelity are strongly influenced by contextual factors, and that fidelity must be understood within the broader socioecological context in which an intervention is situated, including social, economic, structural, and political influences on health.[14,52] To date, contextual factors have not been well accounted for in fidelity frameworks and assessments, but should be considered as potentially important moderators and/or mediators of the impact of fidelity on health outcomes.[44,53–55]

There may be value in approaching fidelity with more specificity depending on the nature, type, or complexity of the EBI being delivered. In particular, there has been increased consideration of the importance of broadening how fidelity is approached for more complex interventions.[56,57] Complex interventions are defined as multi-component interventions in which components interact in synergistic ways, which often require complex behavioral changes across contextual levels and systems. Recent guidance from the Medical Research Council[58] and D&I scientists[59,60] asserted that complex interventions should be delivered and evaluated not only in light of their theoretical basis, but also with regard to the broader contexts in which they will be delivered. In such cases, flexibility in intervention delivery and fidelity may be suitable to allow for the variation in how, where, by whom, and to whom interventions are to be delivered. Thus, it may be appropriate and important to make (and track) adaptations/refinements to the specific "form"[59(p21),60(p1032)] of intervention components based on local context (e.g., providing video vs. manualized protocols), as long as there is fidelity and integrity to the underlying theory[61] or core functions (e.g., core purposes the intervention seeks to change).[59,60] There is value in D&I researchers prespecifying form and function a priori as a way to proactively understand, assess, and ultimately enhance fidelity.

Fidelity is a common implementation indicator in many D&I studies and a common target outcome in the evaluation of implementation strategies.[36,62,63] Implementation strategies (see chapter 6), are active methods or techniques used to enhance the adoption, implementation, and sustainment of new practices, programs, or policies.[64] Specific implementation strategies, such as audit & feedback, training, and facilitation, are commonly used in D&I trials to enhance fidelity in the delivery of EBIs. Recently, researchers have called for greater specification in the measurement and reporting of implementation strategies[64–66] and greater attention to fidelity in the delivery of implementation strategies.[5,6,67] Recent reviews and studies reported that there has been insufficient detail and limited reporting of the fidelity of implementation strategies.[5,6,47,68] For example, Slaughter and colleagues[5] recommended using the Implementation Strategy Fidelity Checklist to enhance the reporting of fidelity; this checklist assesses the quality of the documentation of adherence, dose, and participant responsiveness on a 3-point scale. As with EBIs, it is also important to track adaptations made to implementation strategies to fit the context, setting, or population as part of specification/measurement,[65,69] including ones needed to address health inequities and social determinants of health in lower resource settings and populations (e.g., populations facing stigma, low literacy, transportation challenges, medical mistrust).[53,70–72]

FIDELITY AS A RESEARCH DESIGN ELEMENT

Fidelity is an important consideration for the design of research studies for several reasons. Perhaps most obvious is the impact of fidelity on study validity.[8] *Internal validity* is adversely affected if an intervention is not administered as intended, as it becomes impossible to know if observed effects (or lack thereof) are due to the intervention or to external factors. In essence, if fidelity is not maintained, then internal validity is compromised, and a true test of the intervention cannot be conducted. Described in detail in chapter 16, *external validity* is also impacted by fidelity, in that standardized implementation procedures are needed to ensure that an intervention can be replicated in other (non-research) settings. If the intervention is effective, but the strategies for implementing and/or adapting the intervention occur without attention to fidelity, there may be limits on its generalizability to other settings, populations, and/or health outcomes. Importantly, efforts to enhance one type of validity may result in a diminution of the other[73,74] as more emphasis is placed on controlling core intervention elements to enhance internal validity, such restrictions could make the intervention more difficult to translate or adapt to diverse settings and populations, and thus have lower external validity.

Intervention elements in efficacy studies are typically designed to maximize effects on primary outcomes, and thus may require considerable effort from individual participants, organizations, and staff to replicate. When translating EBIs to *real world* contexts, particularly those designed to reduce health equities, maintaining fidelity to such resource-intensive, complex interventions can be extremely challenging. For example, in a low-resourced community-based setting, such as low-income/subsidized housing or community health centers, implementing complex interventions with high fidelity for one health issue may decrease attention to other health issues that are equally or more important to the population. Further, efforts to maintain high fidelity to a protocol that may be impractical could yield frustration or resentment, or worse, result in unplanned efforts to adapt the intervention to fit the local setting. Any of these situations may ultimately contribute to implementation failure and resistance to using EBIs. Thus, it is critical to identify and monitor the practicality and feasibility of core intervention components from the earliest phases of research and intervention design.[75] Consistent with principles of community-based participatory research (see chapter 10) and "designing for dissemination,"[76(p331)] it is important to meaningfully engage stakeholders and community partners who are the planned beneficiaries of EBIs at the start of the research, in order to maximize effectiveness, reach, implementation,[76] and sustainability once the intervention is applied in a non-research context.[77]

Fidelity is also an important design element by virtue of its impact on *effect size* and *statistical power.* The power to detect a meaningful difference between intervention and control/comparison groups in most study designs, is a function of minimizing random variability and increasing intended variability between study arms.[8] If an intervention is not delivered as intended, particularly if there is more variability, less intervention dose delivered, or intended recipients do not engage with the intervention (e.g., low *participant responsiveness*), all of these factors will likely reduce the potential effect size and diminish statistical power to detect differences between the groups. For D&I research, there are additional considerations to sample size issues, as researchers must consider both the EBI and the implementation strategy-- and the size of its effect-- both of which affect statistical power. Given that the unit for implementation and analysis in D&I research is often the organizational or community level, this may require large numbers of clusters (e.g., clinics, schools, worksites) for studies to be fully-powered to examine outcomes related to both EBIs and implementation strategies.

A key consideration for D&I efforts is to identify the minimal *dose* of the intervention or the implementation strategies (i.e., the "active ingredients"[78(p186)] required to produce desired change), since this has important implications for feasibility, efficiency, and cost-effectiveness.[78] Monitoring fidelity enables estimation of the impact of specific intervention doses.[9] For example, it may be useful to determine whether outcomes were achieved (and done so equitably across different populations and settings) when three of five core elements of an EBI were delivered vs. when all five core elements were delivered. The same considerations apply for researchers selecting and evaluating implementation strategies, as the complexity of strategies selected also has implications for ease of facilitating and monitoring fidelity. As one example, Kilbourne and colleagues[79] use a Sequential Multiple Assignment Randomized Trial (SMART) design to build an adaptive implementation strategy (i.e., providing external and internal facilitation in addition to the original replication strategy) to improve the uptake, fidelity, and effectiveness of an EBI for patients with mood disorders across 80 community-based outpatient clinics. Comparative effectiveness and adaptive research designs[80] may allow investigators to evaluate these empirical questions about dose and advance the evidence-base in this important but understudied area.[81,82]

When fidelity is actively monitored from the onset of implementation in a research context, it is possible to detect problems with intervention quality and/or deviations from protocols, and to subsequently make mid-course corrections, such as by providing encouragement, reward, or recognition for efforts produced. This type of corrective feedback, when incorporated in the study design as a routine part of intervention delivery, is important for maximizing engagement and enhancing intervention impact. As one example, Wang and colleagues[83] conducted an optimization trial evaluating the effects of biweekly monitoring/feedback and site-based assistance/mentorship among 81 low- and moderate-performing teachers on implementation of an evidence-based HIV-risk reduction curriculum for middle-school students. They found that both approaches (monitoring/feedback and mentorship) were significantly associated with higher levels of implementation fidelity (defined as number of core activities taught), and may operate by increasing teacher self-efficacy.[83]

Finally, *assessment of fidelity* plays a key role in the interpretation of study results. If significant intervention results are not found, knowing whether the intervention was delivered as intended makes it possible to eliminate variation in intervention delivery as a contributor to the findings. Null outcomes from research on an EBI that was delivered with high fidelity to the underlying theory and to core implementation strategies would suggest that the intervention itself may not be addressing the key mediators or most salient contextual factors facing the delivery settings and/or intervention participants. Such findings may suggest the need for a fundamental re-evaluation of the intervention theory and/or implementation efforts.

FACTORS THAT INFLUENCE FIDELITY

Understanding factors that influence the fidelity with which interventions or implementation strategies are implemented is vital to efforts to measure and maximize its occurrence. A growing body of literature documents factors that influence implementation processes.[84] Figure 7.1 categorizes potential influences on fidelity over the course of the planning, implementation, evaluation, and dissemination of interventions. Considering these factors during the selection of research designs, methods, and measures may help anticipate potential unintended consequences by considering this broad range of influences upfront, before the expending resources, time, or expertise.

Four categories of influence and their interrelationships are depicted. First, *implementer characteristics* can impact the ability to implement with fidelity. Fidelity may be compromised when an implementer has limited skill, experience, training, or self-efficacy regarding maintaining fidelity, resulting in diminished amount, type or quality of intervention delivered. For example, a novice practitioner may have limited awareness about existing EBIs and therefore be less able to anticipate or solve implementation challenges. Alternatively, highly experienced implementers may be more confident in their abilities to modify intervention elements and therefore, less likely to implement them in a manner consistent with the original EBI. For example, implementation studies of school-based health programs revealed great variability in implementation of *required* curricular components across schools, teachers, and by student characteristics.[85] Implementers may be experienced but may have limits on their cultural or contextual awareness if they differ by socioeconomic status, race or ethnicity of the population for whom an intervention is intended.

Second, *characteristics of the intervention* will influence fidelity. As discussed in chapter 3, factors such as intervention complexity, trialability, flexibility, and the extent to which one intervention provides a relative advantage over others, are all important influences on fidelity (see Rogers's[86] seminal work on Diffusion of Innovations). For example, highly complex interventions or strategies that have a large number of core elements are more difficult to implement with fidelity than those with fewer, less complex elements. Interventions that allow greater flexibility and are amenable to adaptation may be easier for practitioners to implement without omitting or changing core elements. Interventions that are adequately described for the purposes of replication are also more likely to be implemented (*program differentiation*). Similarly, those that are easily accessible to implementers, for example, through online repositories such as interventions posted on the Evidence-Based Cancer Control Programs (EBCCP; a web site with evidence-based cancer prevention and

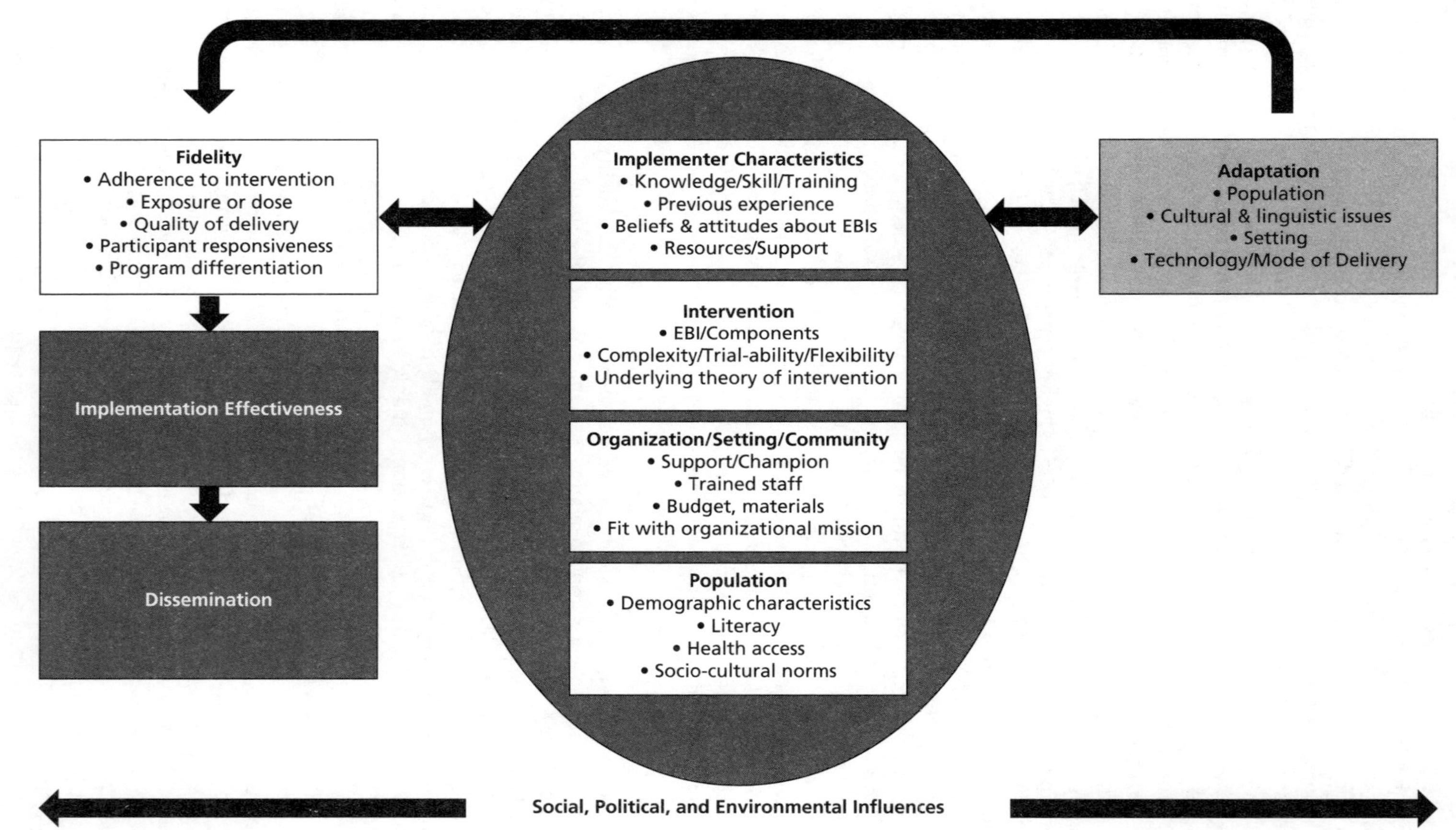

FIGURE 7.1 Factors that influence fidelity.

control interventions),[87] may be more likely to be implemented with fidelity because of the clarity of the underlying theory of change, detailed description of core elements, and/or access to materials provided. Further, the extent to which intervention components fit with the workflow in the implementation setting is critical.[88]

Third, characteristics of the *organization, setting, or community* context in which the intervention is to be implemented or disseminated can have a substantial impact on fidelity. Organizational resources, including the availability of trained staff, financial resources, and presence of a program *champion*, exert a strong impact on implementation. A study by Fagan and colleagues[89] examined adoption and implementation fidelity of science-based prevention programs in 24 communities. Across conditions, results revealed lower rates of implementation fidelity in school-based programs compared to community-based programs. This is consistent with findings from Dariotis and colleagues,[90] who found that schools had more challenges developing program champions and prioritizing prevention strategies than community agencies. Organizational structure, communication channels, and decision-making processes can also affect implementation,[84] including the "readiness"[91(p1)] of an organization to adopt and implement a new intervention.[91]

Fourth, the *population* for whom the intervention was originally developed will impact fidelity. Differences across populations influence the relevance, impact, and appropriateness of EBIs or implementation strategies. Sociodemographic characteristics (e.g., age, gender, socio-economic status, education), socio-cultural norms and values, and literacy levels can all influence *participant responsiveness* to the intervention and are linked to the appropriateness and feasibility of implementing core elements. Such factors will require serious attention when adaptation and more widespread dissemination are considered. Several investigators[18,92] have eloquently discussed the tensions between fidelity and adaptations needed to address sociocultural and ethical/moral issues that influence health equity and justice[51] (see chapter 25). As previously mentioned, engagement with intended beneficiaries or stakeholders across all stages of the implementation and adaptation process will help overcome potential barriers to the equitable delivery and impact of the intervention.

Strategies for Maximizing the Fidelity-Adaptation Balance

Given that it can have a significant moderating effect on intervention impact, concerted efforts to maximize fidelity should be undertaken. While methods to measure and maximize fidelity to core intervention elements have been discussed at length,[93] they are often inconsistently applied.[34,74] We advocate efforts to maximize fidelity by attending to the four categories of influence described in Figure 7.1 (*implementer characteristics, characteristics of the intervention, organizational setting, and population*).

Efforts toward maintaining fidelity should begin with the initial process of intervention development, and consideration of whether such an approach could be scalable for widespread dissemination. *Designing for fidelity* refers both to the consideration of the extent to which tested intervention approaches could be applied in *real world* settings, as well as providing adequate documentation of the theoretical basis, mediating and moderating factors, and description of activities (core components) so that they can be replicated. Not surprisingly, interventions described with a high degree of specificity are more easily and effectively implemented with fidelity than complex interventions that are insufficiently described.[1,16] Checklists like the Template for Intervention Description and Replication (TIDier) and web repositories such as the EBCCP, can play an important role by providing additional specificity to the interventions and implementation strategies.[94–97]

Implementing with fidelity entails putting mechanisms in place to ensure that implementers have the requisite knowledge, skills, and resources required to deliver the intervention as planned (and thus, the *quality of intervention delivery*). This can be accomplished by providing standardized training for implementers, ensuring that implementers have required knowledge/skills following their training (e.g., pre/post assessments, return demonstration), and developing detailed implementation protocols or program manuals that clearly specify core intervention components and strategies, and how they should be implemented.[1,8] Moreover, providing implementers with intervention scripts (e.g., for one-to-one or group interactions), standardized materials that help to ensure consistency of message delivery (e.g., flip charts, tip sheets), or checklists can also be useful. It is also important to anticipate the potential for *intervention drift* (i.e., diminished adherence to or implementer skills in the delivery of interventions over time)[8] by planning booster training sessions, instituting quality control protocols that provide regular feedback to implementers, providing problem-solving support targeted at potential reasons for drift, and engaging stakeholders in the process.

Fidelity measures may be categorized as direct or indirect with varying levels of effort and cost[19] (see Table 7.1). *Direct methods* are generally implemented by trained observers or auditors. This method has traditionally been described as the gold standard for measuring fidelity, because independent observers are less prone to biased reporting.[16,19,98,99] Examples of direct assessment include in-person observation (e.g., completed with a checklist outlining core components), *shadowing* implementers (e.g., as in the case of one-to-one interventions), and audio or video-taping intervention events for subsequent quality assurance. Advantages of direct observation include that they can yield highly accurate and valid data. However, disadvantages include cost and feasibility, particularly for large-scale dissemination initiatives.[19]

Indirect measures may include self-reports by implementers, who may complete intervention logs, diaries or checklists designed to document delivery of core elements, or may involve self-report by program participants. For example, participants may be asked about receipt of core intervention components and/or their level of satisfaction with the intervention (which also reflects *quality of delivery, participant responsiveness*). In-person data collection (e.g., interviews, focus groups) may also be utilized, or participants may be asked to complete self-administered data collection forms (e.g., rating forms or surveys).[19] New technologies and social networking programs offer interesting options for quick feedback from participants via web-based, Facebook, texting, or Twitter.[100]

The main advantages of indirect methods are that they are generally less costly, time-consuming, and labor-intensive. Moreover, the collection of data from implementers or participants can provide helpful insights regarding factors that would not otherwise be available (e.g., factors that influence fidelity, participant responsiveness). Disadvantages relate to the accuracy of data (i.e., potential for over-reporting, social desirability bias) and the possibility of missing data (e.g., either reports not completed or failure to document contextual or situational factors that impact fidelity).

When selecting data collection methods, considerations should include cost, feasibility, efficiency, validity/reliability of data, potential for reactivity (i.e., changed behavior due to observations), and the ability to collect sufficient "samples" [19(p168)] to accurately assess fidelity.[19] Additional considerations include the type of intervention delivery (e.g., in-person, telephone), characteristics and skill levels of implementers, as well as population characteristics (e.g., willingness to be observed). Triangulation across multiple data sources (e.g., interviews, surveys, record review) is ideal to address these challenges,[101] though associated with costs. Additionally, mixed-methods approaches are highly desirable for fidelity assessments.[8,102–106]

A challenge to measuring fidelity and creating fidelity assessments is the limited specificity with which core intervention elements are described and reported in the literature.[107] Measurement instruments for assessing intervention-specific aspects of fidelity have been suggested.[28,30,108–110] However, Breitenstein and colleagues[19] point out that intervention-specific instruments do not allow for standardization or comparison of findings across studies and may hinder the ability to compare similar interventions that share theoretical underpinnings. General fidelity assessments that can be utilized across interventions and settings may be more valuable in D&I science, since they would enable cross-comparison of findings.[19]

There continue to be calls for improvements in the development and use of higher quality fidelity measures.[34,111,112] Reviews indicate that psychometric properties (both reliability and validity) of fidelity measures are not commonly reported[47,113–115] and few studies have assessed implementation quality (e.g., cost, acceptability, feasibility) of such assessments. A recent systematic review by Mettert et al., 2020, identified 18 measures of fidelity used in mental or behavioral health research (excluding ones

TABLE 7.1 DIRECT AND INDIRECT STRATEGIES FOR MEASURING FIDELITY[a]

Direct	Advantages	Disadvantages
Trained observers or independent auditors using checklists, rating scales	-Generally considered most accurate	-Observer variability possible; intensive training may be required -More costly and labor intensive than indirect methods -In vivo observation may alter implementer behaviors -Observer may *miss* seeing subtle events -Difficult to capture rare events -Not feasible for large-scale dissemination -May not be appropriate for some forms of intervention (e.g., counseling)
Audio or videotape	-May be as accurate as in vivo observation -Possible to establish interrater reliability; raters view same video or listen to same audio -Possible to review intervention delivery more than once -Can be used as tool for providing implementers with feedback about their performance -Less likely to impact implementer behaviors than direct observation	-Less costly than having an auditor present at intervention delivery -Potential to miss important nonverbal or contextual cues -Observer variability possible; intensive training may be required -Video recording equipment is costly; audio equipment is less costly -May be logistically difficult to bring equipment to setting of intervention delivery -Equipment malfunction may occur
Indirect		
Data from implementers (e.g., intervention logs, diaries)	-Relatively inexpensive -Less time consuming -Can include implementer insights about factors that influenced fidelity, participant responsiveness	-Prone to bias, overreporting -Completion rates may be low -Recall may be inaccurate, particularly if documentation doesn't occur immediately after intervention delivery
Data collected from intervention participants (e.g., exit interviews, paper-and-pencil surveys, e-based communication (e.g., Twitter, Facebook)	-Enables assessment of participant responsiveness, perceived quality of delivery -Less costly and time consuming than direct methods	-Participants may want to reflect well on implementer; social desirability -Participants may not be able to recognize or distinguish between intervention components -Potential for low completion rates, depending on participant motivation

[a]Adapted with permission from Breitenstein and colleagues.[19]

specific to a single intervention), and found that information about psychometric properties of these measures were infrequently reported. There have also been recent efforts to advance measurement in this area.[47,116–118] For example, Hermes and colleagues[119] have proposed specific considerations and recommendations for measuring fidelity for technology-delivered behavioral interventions (e.g. number of log-ins, clicks, task completions and viewing times as measures of dose; engagement with videos and completion of modules as measures of adherence).[119] Additionally, setting-specific fidelity measures and sample data collection instruments for interventions that take place in a range of community-based settings have been summarized by Linnan and Steckler.[2] To advance work in this area, we recommend engaging community partners and intended beneficiaries in the implementation evaluation process to facilitate the development of valid and pragmatic measures for fidelity.[120]

Monitoring fidelity during initial intervention implementation, after adaptation, and over time prior to dissemination is essential; such fidelity checks can serve as safeguards to help ensure that the EBI or strategy is ready for more widespread dissemination. Monitoring should involve an ongoing review of fidelity data (ideally collected from both direct or indirect measurement) with a feedback loop to ensure that information is provided to those responsible for intervention delivery in a timely manner (see Lyons et al 2020; Duffy et al. 2015).[121,122] Williams and colleagues[105] provide a comprehensive example of fidelity assessment and monitoring in the context of a physical activity intervention to contextualize study findings and inform and improve provider delivery in practice.

Analyzing fidelity, whereby data collected in the process of implementation provides essential information about the extent to which the intervention was implemented as planned, can be valuable in understanding program impact. Berkel and colleagues[123] clarify dimensions of implementation (facilitator and participant dimensions) and offer a thoughtful conceptual and measurement model for understanding interactions between fidelity and implementation, outcomes, and adaptation in the analysis. Several studies have detailed and provided guidance in computing fidelity or implementation scores,[45,50,124] that can be included in analyses to help explain unexpected findings or variability of intervention effects.[19] Future research is needed to advance the development of pragmatic methods and valid/reliable measures for assessing fidelity, and reporting on them in ways that are accessible and sufficiently detailed to enhance implementation research and practice.[5,34]

Researchers are increasingly paying attention to the extent to which availability and implementation of EBIs have been unevenly distributed across diverse settings and populations, since inequitable access and uptake to proven interventions can exacerbate existing health inequities.[22,125–127] To facilitate these efforts, there are several papers that provide initial guidance for collecting data on inequities in implementation indicators (e.g. reach, adoption, fidelity).[22,128] Tracking and examining potential differences in fidelity across settings and groups that experience social and health inequities (e.g., by race, ethnicity; in low resource settings) will help identify barriers to implementation that are not being addressed. Groups or settings experiencing inequities related to fidelity may indicate the need for additional resources/support to build implementer or organizational/community capacity, or adaptations/refinements of the intervention or implementations strategies to meet the needs of diverse cultures or contexts (see ASPIRE Process: Adapting Strategies to Promote Implementation Reach & Equity[126]).

BALANCING THE IMPORTANCE OF FIDELITY WITH NEED FOR ADAPTATION

There are varying perspectives in the field of D&I about the extent to which EBIs can and should be adapted. One view is that complete fidelity, with strict adherence to an intervention protocol, is necessary under all circumstances.[31,115] While some see this as essential to enhancing transparency and validity of intervention evaluation,[129] this approach may reduce the opportunity to learn from the variability that is inherent in implementation across settings and populations.[130] Another view is that 'adaptation happens.' Proponents of this view discourage making major changes in core components or functions (e.g., fidelity-inconsistent modifications), and encourage documenting adaptations that occur so that their impact can be better understood (see chapter 8). Here, we provide an overview of adaptation as it specifically relates to fidelity.

Balancing the need for *fidelity* while maintaining sufficient flexibility to accommodate differences across implementation settings, populations, and situational contexts, is a challenge and a topic of recent increased discussion and study.[20,43,45,46,59,131–133] While high fidelity has been associated with positive program outcomes, it is common for changes to be made when EBIs are implemented outside of controlled, well-resourced settings, and are often necessary to ensure fit and participant responsiveness.[42,90,107] Reviews of EBI implementation across a range of settings demonstrate that 40-80% of programs reported making adaptations to the original program.[43,107,134] There is growing recognition that adaptations are inevitable, particularly for interventions that are complex or for settings/populations that face numerous structural barriers to health and healthcare.[135,136]

Reasons for adaptations may include limited time and resources, competing demands, difficulty engaging or retaining participants, desire to reach specific audiences, and efforts to enhance program fit or health equity.[42,43,137] Adaptation of EBIs may also occur in response to the complexity of characteristics of outer contexts (e.g., service systems) or inner contexts (e.g., organizations). With respect to the long-term sustainability of EBIs, it has also been proposed that some changes to interventions may be important in order to respond to real-world contexts that are dynamic.[138,139] In some cases, there may have to be adaptations to contextual factors in order to facilitate program implementation (e.g., changes in organizational structure, culture, technology).[140]

Many EBIs were not necessarily developed for or tested among populations experiencing health inequities or those facing numerous and intersecting structural barriers to health (e.g., by age, disability, geography, income, race/ethnicity).[22] In this context, adaptations may be necessary to incorporate and reflect the lived experiences, values and beliefs, cultural/linguistic needs, and unique barriers experienced by diverse population sub-groups.[22] Such adaptations may be critical to participant engagement/responsiveness and retention, intervention effectiveness, and to enhance ownership or local buy-in of interventions.[45,141,142] Chambers and colleagues[138] propose that ongoing adaptation and refinement is needed in multi-level interventions to enhance fit with changing context, population needs, and scientific evidence, and question the idea that interventions must be fully optimized prior to implementation.

We recognize that fidelity and adaptation may co-exist, and that it is possible for a program's core components to be implemented with high fidelity, while still making adaptations in response to or to enhance fit with local community needs or context (e.g., fidelity-consistent adaptations where the core elements or functions are preserved). Additionally, we recognize that adaptations should not compromise the essence of the intervention; thus, major changes in the fundamental core components or functions are not desirable. The evidence base is still growing in this area,[143] and empirical work is needed to guide researchers and practitioners. It will be important to make sure that adaptation is measured and examined distinctly from fidelity.[144] Several coding schemas have been proposed to study the full range of adaptations that can be made to interventions and implementation strategies across settings (see chapter 8).[43,143,145]

We believe that fidelity and adaptation should be monitored so that when adaptation occurs, all changes and the effects they have on intervention impact over time are documented. There is growing attention to the relationship between and impacts of both fidelity and adaptation in relation to efficacy/effectiveness, as well as other implementation outcomes that are of value to a range of stakeholders (e.g., acceptability, cost, sustainability, equity).[146] If adaptation occurs and no effort to assess fidelity of the adapted intervention is made, then intervention effectiveness may be compromised. In addition, the positive impact of adaptations may not be documented and therefore, be non-replicable. At a minimum, adaptations should be proactively observed, documented, and understood in order to enhance translation of EBIs into practice.[130,147] The use of frameworks that address both fidelity and adaptation has been limited in the implementation literature and deserves further attention.[5] There has also been growing recognition and discussion of some of the limitations in D&I science of starting with existing EBIs that may not reflect the lived experience of many historically underserved communities and may not be well-equipped to adequately address health inequities or structural barriers to health. In such cases, there may be a need to develop and co-create new EBIs with this focus in collaboration with community partners.[22,127]

CASE EXAMPLE

Fidelity and Adaptation of Cancer Screening Program for African American Women

Here, we introduce a case study which illustrates some of the challenges and considerations associated with fidelity, adaptation, and health equity in the context of nationally implemented, community-led cancer screening program for African American women.

Background: Cancer-related disparities exist and African Americans suffer a disproportionately high incident and mortality burden for nearly all types of cancer nationally. Programs and policies that support the use of community-based lay health advisors (LHAs; trained peers or community members) hold strong promise for reducing cancer disparities. LHA programs have been found to be effective in improving cancer screening and diagnostic follow-up in a range of settings, particularly among racial/ethnic minority women who experience numerous structural barriers to health and healthcare.[148]

Context: The National Witness Project (NWP) is one example of an evidence-based LHA program developed to address cancer disparities and underlying structural barriers to screening with attention to sociocultural context (e.g. stigma, discrimination, mistrust, lack of healthcare access) and adult learning principles. A national trial found that NWP was highly effective in increasing breast and cervical cancer screening among African American women, increasing mammogram rates by 43.3%.[149] NWP uses a robust theory-informed, strengths-based, culturally appropriate and community-led model. During 60–90 minute group-based sessions, trained African American LHAs serve as credible messengers who provide resources, support, navigation, and education. Additionally, African American cancer survivors deliver empowering testimonials and narratives and serve as *Witness Role Models*; faith-based elements (e.g., hymns, prayers, partnerships with churches) are also a foundational part of the program. NWP is identified as one of the National Cancer Institute's Evidence-based Cancer Control Programs. Core components of the program include: 1) group educational sessions conducted by LHAs based on NWP curriculum reflecting screening guidelines; 2) fact sheet on breast/cervical cancer screening guidelines; 3) opening hymn and prayer; 4) NWP video; 5) resources/navigation to access local screening and navigation services; 6) cancer survivor narratives and testimonials.

National Implementation With Attention to Fidelity: Since its original development in 1990, NWP has been replicated and implemented in 40 sites nationally, reaching more than 15,000 women annually; sites often include community non-profits, faith-based organizations, and academic/medical centers, with a site Project Director providing leadership and overseeing recruitment and training. Between 1998 and 2002, the CDC funded a study to assess strategies for replicating and delivering NWP nationally; 25 replication sites were added, over 400 LHAs were trained, and 522 educational sessions were held.[149] To facilitate fidelity in program delivery, researchers created a *Replication Package* that: 1) established implementation protocol standards and identified core components; 2) defined and delivered technical assistance (TA) strategies; and 3) provided sites with written guidance, materials, and implementation manual (e.g. training slides, forms, video, facilitator guide, curricula). Box 7.1 describes the goals of this replication package aimed at supporting fidelity across a range of contexts. To facilitate replication with fidelity across the first 9 months, each site received an in-person site visit, which included a *Train the Trainers* program, as well as coaching and administrative support for new Project Director and staff.

Lessons Learned: Evaluation of fidelity was facilitated through written reports from sites, site visits, and surveys. While it was originally planned to have a *turnkey* system (e.g., toolkit mailed to site), early pilot results indicated that self-guided approach to implementation was insufficient and decreased fidelity. Three key strategies were identified as essential for assuring fidelity to the program and improved outcomes,[149] including: 1) *Establishing Clear Objectives* (sites needed to know exactly what was expected in terms of trained personnel, number of programs conducted, expected outcomes, and development of advisory boards and MOUs; 2) *Technical Assistance and Training* (administrative coaching of staff prior, guidance for staff training, followed by site visits and TA to help problem solve); and 3) *Dual Champions* (crucial importance of having organizational partnerships in place to facilitate both *Administrative* and *Community Champions*; Administrative Champions served as a key resource for securing support and managing grants/resources, while the Community Champion had credibility and recruited and nurtured LHAs and promoted the project in the community).

BOX 7.1

GOALS OF THE REPLICATION PACKAGE TO SUPPORT FIDELITY OF NATIONAL WITNESS PROJECT (NWP) ACROSS A RANGE OF CONTEXTS

1. Explain the NWP model, goals, and evidence
2. Enhance understanding of barriers to screening among African American women
3. Guide staffing needs and the development of steering and advisory committees to support implementation
4. Provide guidance on recruitment, selection, training of LHAs and role models
5. Provide access to guidelines, slides, resources for training team members
6. Help establish MOUs with clinical services/networks providing access to screening
7. Link to resources and forms to monitor, evaluate, measure program delivery and impact
8. Provide videotapes to enhance fidelity to the program
9. Provide platforms to link to the network of NWP programs to enhance TA and shared learning/communication
10. Provide TA as needed from experienced NWP leadership

Fidelity & Adaption Over Time: NWP is one of the longest running and largest community-based LHA programs in the country, and has been sustained for nearly 30 years nationally. Despite its longevity, NWP has also faced challenges to continued delivery and sustainment of the program.[150] Additionally, new challenges have arisen with respect to delivering the program with fidelity while adapting to new scientific evidence over time, given the multiple changes and updates in screening guidelines that inform several of the core components of the program (e.g., curricula, educational sessions); these recommendations differ from the guidelines in place when NWP was developed (e.g. with respect to age of initiation and frequency/interval of mammography screening; and with respect to use of breast self-exam or BSE). For example, BSE is no longer commonly recommended as a screening tool, though American Cancer Society and US Preventive Services Task Force support breast self-awareness.

Between 2017 and 2019, to facilitate adaptation to the new screening guidelines and evolution of the scientific literature (e.g. information about HPV vaccination and cervical cancer), an updated curriculum for NWP reflecting updated scientific evidence was developed and disseminated through an in-person 3-day conference across 18 NWP sites[151]; to support delivery with fidelity to this new curricula, each site received updated Power Point presentations with embedded videos and talking points for LHAs, updated training material and implementation guides, as well as site visits to facilitate TA and *Train the Trainers* program.

Recent research among the sites highlights some of the challenges in maintaining fidelity over time, and the complex relationships between fidelity and adaptation that have implications for health equity. A mixed-methods evaluation at 14 NWP sites nationally among over 200 participants (LHAs and Project Directors) found that while the overwhelming majority have strong attitudes and beliefs about using evidence-based practices and guidelines within NWP and high levels of awareness of the new guidelines and adaptations made to NWP, there were issues raised in implementing these changes in practice.[72] While more than half of participants reported that their site updated messaging about the age of initiation of frequency of mammography screening, fewer sites reported making adaptations related to BSE, and BSE was commonly reported as a core educational component in NWP programming. Survey data and qualitative interviews helped contextualize why changes in screening guidelines may not be embraced at the sites or in the African American communities being served, with concerns related to: 1) high mistrust of medical organizations, providers, and the guidelines themselves; 2) perceptions that African American women in the community were not supportive of the new guidelines; 3) concerns that the guidelines and data informing them do not reflect the lived experiences of Black women (who have higher incidence of aggressive breast cancer at younger ages); 4) misalignment between guidelines and LHA and Project Director personal beliefs and values about screening; 5) wariness to keep adapting the program based on changing guidelines that were inconsistent and confusing across national organizations, and 6) concerns that women in the community will stop listening and trusting them if they keep adapting the messages. Additionally, many LHAs in the program and Role Models found their own cancers through BSE and its importance is ingrained in them; so many participants highlighted the importance of keeping BSE and framing as an empowerment and awareness tool (not screening tool) for women to be familiar with breast changes and facilitate informed decision-making.[72] This case study highlights some of the challenges in maintaining fidelity and promoting adaptation over time based on evolving scientific evidence and community needs, and the importance of documenting both fidelity and adaptation over time. Additionally, it highlights some of the equity considerations of doing so, particularly if the guidelines or scientific evidence are not trusted or not perceived as reflecting the social realities of populations that experience numerous structural barriers (i.e., structural racism, financial hardship) to health.

SUMMARY

There is substantial variability in the implementation of EBIs across the US, which leads to inconsistent access to evidence-based prevention and treatment strategies at a population level.[152] Increased attention to the implementation of interventions should result in significant public health gains and the potential to address persistent health inequities.[152] To achieve the promise and strengthen the impact of implementation research, increased measurement and tracking of fidelity is critically important. Consideration of fidelity is necessary to balance the need for internal and external validity across the research continuum. There is also a need for a more robust empirical work to advance knowledge in a number of areas, including: 1) factors that influence fidelity; 2) strategies for maximizing fidelity and achieving an appropriate balance between fidelity and adaptation; 3) rigorous methods for measuring and analyzing fidelity; and 4) better understanding of the impact of variation identified in implementation fidelity.[130]

We echo the recommendations of others[8,31] who advocate for designing interventions with dissemination in mind,[76] having a comprehensive plan for maximizing fidelity throughout intervention delivery, as well as a system for documenting what, how, and why adaptations are made. As discussed above, there are a growing number of models designed to facilitate adaptation of EBIs while maintaining fidelity. It will be important to study the utility and feasibility of these models across different settings, populations and health issues, and the impact adaptations have on a wider range of program outcomes, including effectiveness and sustainability. We also highlight the critical importance of community and stakeholder partnerships in the implementation, as their ongoing input in these processes could further strengthen fidelity to the interventions and enhance health outcomes (see chapter 10).

Ultimately, efforts to advance the science of D&I with a particular focus on fidelity will require the involvement of researchers, practitioners, intended beneficiaries of an intervention, as well as funders and policy-makers (see Table 7.2). Researchers must lead the charge by: designing interventions that can be implemented with fidelity in practice settings; developing standardized methods and measures for assessing fidelity; evaluating strategies for maximizing fidelity; analyzing the impact of fidelity on program outcomes; making explicit the core elements in interventions; ensuring availability of appropriately *packaged* intervention materials; examining the efficacy of strategies for maximizing fidelity; engaging early and often with intended community partners and intervention beneficiaries; and analyzing emerging models for EBI adaptation. In addition, improvement of methods in tracking and reporting implementation strategies,[70] can contribute towards a comprehensive understanding of intervention effects.[6]

Practitioners, community leaders, and other intended intervention beneficiaries can also be actively involved in identifying available EBIs that are suitable for their populations and settings. They can make significant contributions to D&I research by communicating the challenges they encounter when delivering

TABLE 7.2 ROLES FOR PRACTITIONERS, RESEARCHERS, POLICYMAKERS, AND FUNDERS

Practitioners	Researchers	PolicyMakers/Funders/Journal Editors and Reviewers
• Be proactive in learning about available EBIs; know where to search for information about EBIs (e.g., resources provided here and articles[41,66–69]). • Choose EBIs that are appropriate to specific audience, setting, implementer skills/ knowledge, health issues, available resources. • Engage communities and recipients of the intervention in selection and adapting EBIs. • Contact researchers to gain access to information about core elements and what might be required for effective implementation, adaptation, and/or dissemination. • If adaptations are made, avoid modifying core elements. Consider one of the adaptation models and/or do what is necessary to understand your audience and setting so that adaptation is appropriate and done with fidelity prior to dissemination. • Partner with researchers and/or evaluators to provide input into how EBIs can be implemented in practice and how barriers to implementation may be overcome.	• Design interventions with implementation and dissemination in mind—increased attention to external validity to enhance the ability of practitioners to implement interventions in *real-world* settings. • Depict interventions and implementation strategies with explicit logic models to enhance understanding of the intended process and outcomes. Be sure to clarify core versus adaptive elements. Be explicit about theory that guides the intervention and show key constructs/ elements on the logic model. • Carefully measure and analyze fidelity. Consider undertaking post hoc analyses to examine impact of specific intervention elements. • Consider a conceptual framework for examination of factors that influence fidelity (see Figure 7.1) and integrate specific initiatives to maximize fidelity. • Collect and summarize information and *lessons learned* from *first generation* implementers; provide to *second generation* implementers and integrate their feedback on what is feasible and acceptable for implementation in the settings and for the populations with whom they work. • Package EBIs for implementation and dissemination. Provide access to intervention and implementation protocols; include sufficient detail so that activities can be replicated with fidelity. Develop and make available measures for intervention and implementation strategy fidelity. • Build a more robust literature on fidelity. Specifically address in key publications: Which factors in the logic model are most important in terms of ensuring and maintaining fidelity? What are the best methods for maximizing fidelity?	• Funders: Require assessment of and provide adequate funding for evaluation of fidelity and, if required, adaptations, in all phases of the research continuum. • Policymakers: Advocate for implementation of EBIs with emphasis on initial fidelity as well as allow for measuring/ monitoring fidelity when EBIs are adapted for new health outcomes, settings, or populations. • Journal editors/reviewers: Assess and report fidelity as well as adaptations in guidelines for reporting of interventions (e.g., CONSORT) and implementation strategies.

or receiving EBIs, the reasons for adaptation when this occurs, and for utilizing newly emerging models for adaptation that retain a focus on fidelity to core intervention elements. Such communication, including perceptions of EBI acceptability, appropriateness, and feasibility, will help to build "practice-based evidence" [153(pi20)] that can advance science, practice, and policy.[153]

Policy-makers can play a role in helping to create the infrastructure required for increased communication and exchange between researchers, practitioners and intervention developers. Funders can require attention to fidelity in research applications across the research continuum, and provide targeted funds for examination of the research questions that are needed to build a more robust literature in this field. Journal editors could require increased reporting of issues related to fidelity in publications (along the lines of CONSORT guidelines)[154,155] and reviewers could be asked to pay increased attention to fidelity in the manuscript review process. Such a multi-level approach to advance work on fidelity is critical to both advancing the field and its equitable impact.

ACKNOWLEDGMENTS

This work was supported in part by funding from the National Cancer Institute (NCI) (Emmons, 1 R03 CA256233, 5P30CA006516 supplement, P50CA244433, 1UL1TR002541; Adsul, 3P30CA118100-15S4[NCE] &15S6), and the American Cancer Society (Shelton, 124793-MRSG-13-152-01-CPPB; Adsul, 131567-IRG-17-178-22-IRG). We'd like to thank and acknowledge Savannah Alexander for her support in helping prepare this chapter.

SUGGESTED READINGS AND WEBSITES

Readings

Akiba CF, Powell BJ, Pence BW, Nguyen MXB, Golin C, Go V. The case for prioritizing implementation strategy fidelity measurement: benefits and challenges. *Transl Behav Med.* 2021;12(2):335–342. doi:10.1093/tbm/ibab138

This article focuses on the importance of assessing fidelity for implementation strategies, in addition to intervention fidelity. The authors provide the challenges of measuring fidelity of strategies and present the methodological benefits of doing so, while offering practical recommendations for addressing the challenges.

Bellg AJ, Borrelli B, Resnick B, et al. Enhancing treatment fidelity in health behavior change studies: best practices and recommendations from the NIH Behavior Change Consortium. *Health Psychol.* 2004;23(5):443–451. doi:10.1037/0278-6133.23.5.443

This article describes a multisite initiative by the Treatment Fidelity Workgroup of the National Institutes of Health Behavior Change Consortium to conceptualize and address fidelity and its measurement. They offer recommendations for improving treatment fidelity, including strategies for monitoring and improving provider training, delivery and receipt of treatment, and enactment of treatment skills. The authors emphasized the need for funding agencies, reviewers, and journal editors to make treatment fidelity a standard component in reporting of health intervention research.

Bopp M, Saunders RP, Lattimore D. The tug-of-war: fidelity versus adaptation throughout the health promotion program life cycle. *J Prim Prev.* 2013;34(3):193–207. doi:10.1007/s10935-013-0299-y

This article describes the life cycle (phases) for research-based health promotion programs, the key factors that influence each phase, and issues related to the tension between fidelity and adaptation throughout the process. The authors discuss the importance of reconceptualizing intervention designs, engaging stakeholders, and monitoring fidelity and adaptation across all phases to facilitate implementation fidelity. Consideration is also given to the role of contextual factors in influencing implementation at each phase and the importance of developing a rigorous and flexible definition of implementation fidelity and completeness.

Breitenstein SM, Gross D, Garvey CA, Hill C, Fogg L, Resnick B. Implementation fidelity in community-based interventions. *Res Nurs Health.* 2010;33(2):164–173. doi:10.1002/nur.20373

This article defines implementation fidelity, offers rationale for its importance in implementation science, describes data collection strategies and tools, and provides recommendations for advancing the study of implementation fidelity. The authors provide a comprehensive description of methods for measuring fidelity, including the advantages and limitations of each.

Carroll C, Patterson M, Wood S, Booth A, Rick J, Balain S. A conceptual framework for implementation fidelity. *Implement Sci.* 2007;2:40. doi:10.1186/1748-5908-2-40

This article critically reviews literature on implementation fidelity and presents a new framework for

conceptualizing and evaluating fidelity. They define five elements of fidelity (adherence to intervention; exposure or dose; quality of delivery; participant responsiveness; and program differentiation) and suggest that two additional elements be included in the conceptualization of fidelity: intervention complexity and facilitation strategies.

Chambers DA, Norton WE. The adaptome: advancing the science of intervention adaptation. *Am J Prev Med.* 2016;51(4):S124–S131. doi:10.1016/j.amepre.2016.05.011

This article discusses how the field has been limited by the notion that evidence generation must be complete prior to implementation, which sets up a dichotomy between fidelity and adaptation and limits the science of adaptation to findings from randomized controlled trials of adapted interventions. The authors emphasize the need for advancement of strategies to study the science of adaptation in the context of implementation that would encourage opportunities for ongoing learning over time and propose building an adaptome to serve as a common data platform to capture information about variations in EBI delivery across multiple populations and contexts.

Haynes A, Brennan S, Redman S, et al. Figuring out fidelity: a worked example of the methods used to identify, critique and revise the essential elements of a contextualised intervention in health policy agencies. *Implement Sci.* 2016;11:article 23. doi:10.1186/s13012-016-0378-6

This article highlights challenges in conducting fidelity assessment of novel contextualized interventions, using a worked example to demonstrate how essential elements can be refined without compromising fidelity assessment. The authors discuss how they devised a method for critiquing the construct validity of their intervention's essential elements and modifying how they were articulated and measured, while using them as fidelity indicators. They also highlight how this theoretically and contextually informed process could be used or adapted for other contextualized interventions.

Linnan L, Steckler A. *Process Evaluation for Public Health Interventions and Research.* Jossey-Bass; 2002.

This book provides a rationale and detailed description of how to plan and implement a comprehensive process evaluation effort for a public health intervention that takes place in a wide range of settings. A detailed overview chapter defines key terms of a process evaluation and a process for undertaking the development of process evaluation. Chapters follow that provide detailed examples of process evaluation for worksite, school, and other community settings where sample data collection tools, key results, and lessons learned are offered. Additional chapters on process tracking data management systems and process evaluation for media campaigns are included, which should benefit practitioners and researchers alike.

Perez D, Van der Stuyft P, Zabala MC, Castro M, Lefevre P. A modified theoretical framework to assess implementation fidelity of adaptive public health interventions. *Implement Sci.* 2016;11:91. doi:10.1186/s13012-016-0457-8

This article suggests that classical fidelity dimensions and frameworks do not address the issue of how to adapt an intervention while maintaining its effectiveness. The authors suggest that fidelity and adaptation can coexist, and that adaptations can have positive or negative impacts on program outcomes. The authors discuss adaptive interventions and how an adequate fidelity-adaptation balance can be reached, and modify the Carroll et al. (2007)[1] framework to facilitate a more comprehensive assessment of the implementation fidelity-adaptation balance.

Slaughter SE, Hill JN, Snelgrove-Clarke E. What is the extent and quality of documentation and reporting of fidelity to implementation strategies: a scoping review. *Implement Sci.* 2015;10:129. doi:10.1186/s13012-015-0320-3

In this article, the authors conduct a scoping review and discuss the extent and quality of documentation and reporting of fidelity of implementation strategies that are used to implement evidence-informed interventions. The authors also identify the underreporting of fidelity of implementation strategies and develop and test a simple checklist to assess the reporting of fidelity of implementation strategies.

Toomey E, Hardeman W, Hankonen N, et al. Focusing on fidelity: narrative review and recommendations for improving intervention fidelity within trials of health behaviour change interventions. *Health Psychol Behav Med.* 2020;8(1):132–151. doi:10.1080/21642850.2020.1738935

This article critically reviews the literature around health behavior change interventions to identify the issues concerning fidelity. The authors consider these specific issues (i.e., lack of a standard conceptualization of fidelity, limited focus beyond assessing fidelity, lack of focus on quality and comprehensiveness for fidelity assessments, lack of focus between fidelity and adaptations, and poor reporting of how intervention fidelity is assessed) and provide practical considerations and specific recommendations for researchers proposing behavioral change intervention trials.

Walton H, Spector A, Williamson M, Tombor I, Michie S. Developing quality fidelity and engagement measures for complex health interventions. *Br J Health Psychol.* 2020;25(1):39–60. doi:10.1111/bjhp.12394

This article focuses on complex interventions in which measuring fidelity may not be as straightforward.

They use the definitions of the National Institutes of Health Behaviour Change Consortium framework for fidelity (Bellg et al. 2004)[8] and propose five steps that a researcher could use to develop fidelity measures for complex interventions. These steps are elucidated in the article using an example complex intervention.

Selected Websites and Tools

The Cochrane Collaboration. Cochrane Reviews. http://www2.cochrane.org/reviews/

This site houses systematic reviews of research in human healthcare and health policy conducted by the Cochrane Collaboration, an international network established to assist healthcare providers, policymakers, patients, and their advocates make well-informed decisions about human healthcare by preparing, updating, and promoting the accessibility of evidence.

The Community Guide. https://www.thecommunityguide.org/

The Guide to Community Preventive Services (commonly referred to as The Community Guide) website houses over 25 years' worth of EBIs recommended by the Community Preventive Services Task Force (CPSTF). It complements program planner tools, such as the Healthy People 2030 and the Guide to Clinical Preventive Services.

Compendium of Evidence-Based Interventions and Best Practice for HIV Prevention. https://www.cdc.gov/hiv/research/interventionresearch/compendium/index.html

Curated by the Centers for Disease Control and Prevention, this website provides access to evidence-based or evidence-informed interventions in the form of Info sheets.

Evidence-Based Cancer Control Programs (EBCCP). https://ebccp.cancercontrol.cancer.gov/index.do

The EBCCP is a searchable database of cancer control interventions and program materials and is designed to provide program planners and public health practitioners easy and immediate access to research-tested materials.

Substance Abuse and Mental Health Services Administration Evidence-Based Practices Resource Center. https://www.samhsa.gov/resource-search/ebp

This website provides access to scientifically based resources for communities, clinicians, and policymakers with the toolkits, resource guides, practice guidelines, and protocols that may be needed to incorporate evidence-based practices into the clinical and community settings.

The United States Preventive Services Taskforce. https://www.uspreventiveservicestaskforce.org/uspstf/

This taskforce is an independent panel of national experts in disease prevention and evidence-based medicine that make recommendations about clinical preventive services.

US Department of Health & Human Services: Agency for Healthcare Research and Quality (AHRQ) Evidence-Based Practice. https://www.ahrq.gov/research/findings/evidence-based-reports/index.html

The AHRQ aims to improve the delivery of clinical preventive healthcare by developing tools, resources, and materials to support healthcare organizations and engage the entire healthcare delivery system.

REFERENCES

1. Carroll C, Patterson M, Wood S, Booth A, Rick J, Balain S. A conceptual framework for implementation fidelity. *Implement Sci.* 2007;2:40. doi:10.1186/1748-5908-2-40
2. Linnan L, Steckler A. *Process Evaluation for Public Health Interventions and Research.* Jossey-Bass; 2002.
3. Rabin BA, Brownson RC, Haire-Joshu D, Kreuter MW, Weaver NL. A glossary for dissemination and implementation research in health. *J Public Health Manag Pract.* 2008;14(2):117–123. doi:10.1097/01.PHH.0000311888.06252.bb
4. Haynes A, Brennan S, Redman S, et al. Figuring out fidelity: a worked example of the methods used to identify, critique and revise the essential elements of a contextualised intervention in health policy agencies. *Implement Sci.* 2016;11:23. doi:10.1186/s13012-016-0378-6
5. Slaughter SE, Hill JN, Snelgrove-Clarke E. What is the extent and quality of documentation and reporting of fidelity to implementation strategies: a scoping review. *Implement Sci.* 2015;10:129. doi:10.1186/s13012-015-0320-3
6. Akiba CF, Powell BJ, Pence BW, Nguyen MXB, Golin C, Go V. The case for prioritizing implementation strategy fidelity measurement: benefits and challenges. *Transl Behav Med.* 2021;12(2):335–342. doi:10.1093/tbm/ibab138
7. Abry T, Hulleman CS, Rimm-Kaufman SE. Using indices of fidelity to intervention core components to identify program active ingredients. *Am J Eval.* 2014;36(3):320–338. doi:10.1177/1098214014557009
8. Bellg AJ, Borrelli B, Resnick B, et al. Enhancing treatment fidelity in health behavior change studies: best practices and recommendations from the NIH Behavior Change Consortium. *Health Psychol.* 2004;23(5):443–451. doi:10.1037/0278-6133.23.5.443
9. Resnick B, Bellg AJ, Borrelli B, et al. Examples of implementation and evaluation of treatment fidelity in the BCC studies: where we are and where

we need to go. *Ann Behav Med.* 2005;29(Suppl 2):46–54. doi:10.1207/s15324796abm2902s_8

10. Robb SL, Burns DS, Docherty SL, Haase JE. Ensuring treatment fidelity in a multi-site behavioral intervention study: implementing NIH Behavior Change Consortium recommendations in the SMART trial. *Psychooncology.* 2011;20(11):1193–1201. doi:10.1002/pon.1845
11. Mowbray CT, Holter MC, Teague GB, Bybee D. Fidelity criteria: development, measurement, and validation. *Am J Eval.* 2003;24(3):315–340. doi:10.1016/S1098-2140(03)00057-2
12. Borrelli B. The assessment, monitoring, and enhancement of treatment fidelity in public health clinical trials. *J Public Health Dent.* 2011;71(S1):S52–S63. doi:10.1111/j.1752-7325.2011.00233.x
13. Gearing RE, El-Bassel N, Ghesquiere A, Baldwin S, Gillies J, Ngeow E. Major ingredients of fidelity: a review and scientific guide to improving quality of intervention research implementation. *Clin Psychol Rev.* 2011;31(1):79–88. doi:10.1016/j.cpr.2010.09.007
14. Durlak JA, DuPre EP. Implementation matters: a review of research on the influence of implementation on program outcomes and the factors affecting implementation. *Am J Community Psychol.* 2008;41(3–4):327–350. doi:10.1007/s10464-008-9165-0
15. Johnson-Kozlow M, Hovell MF, Rovniak LS, Sirikulvadhana L, Wahlgren DR, Zakarian JM. Fidelity issues in secondhand smoking interventions for children. *Nicotine Tob Res.* 2008;10(12):1677–1690. doi:10.1080/14622200802443429
16. Dusenbury L, Brannigan R, Falco M, Hansen WB. A review of research on fidelity of implementation: implications for drug abuse prevention in school settings. *Health Educ Res.* 2003;18(2):237–256. doi:10.1093/her/18.2.237
17. Collins FS, Tabak LA. Policy: NIH plans to enhance reproducibility. *Nature.* 2014;505(7485):612–613. doi:10.1038/505612a
18. Bopp M, Saunders RP, Lattimore D. The tug-of-war: fidelity versus adaptation throughout the health promotion program life cycle. *J Prim Prev.* 2013;34(3):193–207. doi:10.1007/s10935-013-0299-y
19. Breitenstein SM, Gross D, Garvey CA, Hill C, Fogg L, Resnick B. Implementation fidelity in community-based interventions. *Res Nurs Health.* 2010;33(2):164–173. doi:10.1002/nur.20373
20. Perez D, Van der Stuyft P, Zabala MC, Castro M, Lefevre P. A modified theoretical framework to assess implementation fidelity of adaptive public health interventions. *Implement Sci.* 2016;11:91. doi:10.1186/s13012-016-0457-8
21. Ramanadhan S, Davis MM, Armstrong R, et al. Participatory implementation science to increase the impact of evidence-based cancer prevention and control. *Cancer Causes Control.* 2018;29(3):363–369. doi:10.1007/s10552-018-1008-1
22. Baumann AA, Cabassa LJ. Reframing implementation science to address inequities in healthcare delivery. *BMC Health Serv Res.* 2020;20:190. doi:10.1186/s12913-020-4975-3
23. McGee D, Lorencatto F, Matvienko-Sikar K, Toomey E. Surveying knowledge, practice and attitudes towards intervention fidelity within trials of complex healthcare interventions. *Trials.* 2018;19:504. doi:10.1186/s13063-018-2838-6
24. Bauman LJ, Stein RE, Ireys HT. Reinventing fidelity: the transfer of social technology among settings. *Am J Community Psychol.* 1991;19(4):619–639. doi:10.1007/BF00937995
25. Blakely CH, Mayer JP, Gottschalk RG, et al. The fidelity adaptation debate—implications for the implementation of public-sector social programs. *Am J Community Psychol.* 1987;15(3):253–268. doi:10.1007/Bf00922697
26. Dane AV, Schneider BH. Program integrity in primary and early secondary prevention: are implementation effects out of control? *Clin Psychol Rev.* 1998;18(1):23–45. doi:10.1016/s0272-7358(97)00043-3
27. Byrnes HF, Miller BA, Aalborg AE, Plasencia AV, Keagy CD. Implementation fidelity in adolescent family-based prevention programs: relationship to family engagement. *Health Educ Res.* 2010;25(4):531–541. doi:10.1093/her/cyq006
28. Gingiss PM, Roberts-Gray C, Boerm M. Bridge-It: a system for predicting implementation fidelity for school-based tobacco prevention programs. *Prev Sci.* 2006;7(2):197–207. doi:10.1007/s11121-006-0038-1
29. Mihalic S. The importance of implementation fidelity. *J Emot Behav Disord.* 2004;4(4):83–105.
30. Rohrbach LA, Gunning M, Sun P, Sussman S. The Project Towards No Drug Abuse (TND) dissemination trial: implementation fidelity and immediate outcomes. *Prev Sci.* 2010;11(1):77–88. doi:10.1007/s11121-009-0151-z
31. Cohen DJ, Crabtree BF, Etz RS, et al. Fidelity versus flexibility: translating evidence-based research into practice. *Am J Prev Med.* 2008;35(5)(suppl):S381–S389. doi:10.1016/j.amepre.2008.08.005
32. Spillane V, Byrne MC, Byrne M, Leathem CS, O'Malley M, Cupples ME. Monitoring treatment fidelity in a randomized controlled trial of a

complex intervention. *J Adv Nurs.* 2007;60(3):343–352. doi:10.1111/j.1365-2648.2007.04386.x
33. DiGennaro FD, Martens BK, McIntyre LL. Increasing treatment integrity through negative reinforcement: effects on teacher and student behavior. *School Psych Rev.* 2005;34(2):220–231.
34. Toomey E, Hardeman W, Hankonen N, et al. Focusing on fidelity: narrative review and recommendations for improving intervention fidelity within trials of health behaviour change interventions. *Health Psychol Behav Med.* 2020;8(1):132–151. doi:10.1080/21642850.2020.1738935
35. Proctor EK, Landsverk J, Aarons G, Chambers D, Glisson C, Mittman B. Implementation research in mental health services: an emerging science with conceptual, methodological, and training challenges. *Adm Policy Ment Health.* 2009;36(1):24–34. doi:10.1007/s10488-008-0197-4
36. Proctor E, Silmere H, Raghavan R, et al. Outcomes for implementation research: conceptual distinctions, measurement challenges, and research agenda. *Adm Policy Ment Health.* 2011;38(2):65–76. doi:10.1007/s10488-010-0319-7
37. Blase K, Fixsen D. *Core Intervention Components: Identifying and Operationalizing What Makes Programs Work.* U.S. Department of Health and Human Services: Office of the Assistant Secretary for Planning and Evaluation; 2021. Accessed April 12, 2022.https://aspe.hhs.gov/reports/core-intervention-components-identifying-operationalizing-what-makes-programs-work-0
38. Kalver EH, McInnes DK, Yakovchenko V, Hyde J, Petrakis BA, Kim B. The CORE (Consensus on Relevant Elements) approach to determining initial core components of an innovation. *Front Health Serv.* 2021;1:752177. doi:10.3389/frhs.2021.752177
39. Prowse PT. A meta-evaluation: the role of treatment fidelity within psychosocial interventions during the last decade. *J Psychiatry.* 2015;18(2):1000251. doi:10.4172/Psychiatry.1000251
40. Stirman SW, Gamarra J, Bartlett B, Calloway A, Gutner C. Empirical examinations of modifications and adaptations to evidence-based psychotherapies: methodologies, impact, and future directions. *Clin Psychol (New York).* 2017;24(4):396–420. doi:10.1111/cpsp.12218
41. Wiltsey Stirman S, Gutner CA, Crits-Christoph P, Edmunds J, Evans AC, Beidas RS. Relationships between clinician-level attributes and fidelity-consistent and fidelity-inconsistent modifications to an evidence-based psychotherapy. *Implement Sci.* 2015;10:115. doi:10.1186/s13012-015-0308-z
42. Carvalho ML, Honeycutt S, Escoffery C, Glanz K, Sabbs D, Kegler MC. Balancing fidelity and adaptation: implementing evidence-based chronic disease prevention programs. *J Public Health Manag Pract.* 2013;19(4):348–356. doi:10.1097/PHH.0b013e31826d80eb
43. Moore JE, Bumbarger BK, Cooper BR. Examining adaptations of evidence-based programs in natural contexts. *J Prim Prev.* 2013;34(3):147–161. doi:10.1007/s10935-013-0303-6
44. Handley MA, Landeros J, Wu C, Najmabadi A, Vargas D, Athavale P. What matters when exploring fidelity when using health IT to reduce disparities? *BMC Med Inform Decis Mak.* 2021;21:119. doi:10.1186/s12911-021-01476-z
45. Castro FG, Barrera M, Martinez CR. The cultural adaptation of prevention interventions: resolving tensions between fidelity and fit. *Prev Sci.* 2004;5(1):41 45. doi:10.1023/B:PREV.0000013980.12412.cd
46. Morrison DM, Hoppe MJ, Gillmore MR, Kluver C, Higa D, Wells EA. Replicating an intervention: the tension between fidelity and adaptation. *AIDS Educ Prev.* 2009;21(2):128–140. doi:10.1521/aeap.2009.21.2.128
47. Walton H, Spector A, Tombor I, Michie S. Measures of fidelity of delivery of, and engagement with, complex, face-to-face health behaviour change interventions: a systematic review of measure quality. *Br J Health Psychol.* 2017;22(4):872–903. doi:10.1111/bjhp.12260
48. Narh-Bana SA, Kawonga M, Chirwa ED, Ibisomi L, Bonsu F, Chirwa TF. Fidelity of implementation of TB screening guidelines by health providers at selected HIV clinics in Ghana. *PLoS One.* 2021;16(9):e0257486. doi:10.1371/journal.pone.0257486
49. Hill JL, Zoellner JM, You W, et al. Participatory development and pilot testing of iChoose: an adaptation of an evidence-based paediatric weight management program for community implementation. *BMC Public Health.* 2019;19:122. doi:10.1186/s12889-019-6450-9
50. Bragstad LK, Bronken BA, Sveen U, et al. Implementation fidelity in a complex intervention promoting psychosocial well-being following stroke: an explanatory sequential mixed methods study. *BMC Med Res Methodol.* 2019;19:59. doi:10.1186/s12874-019-0694-z
51. Alvidrez J, Nápoles AM, Bernal G, et al. Building the evidence base to inform planned intervention adaptations by practitioners serving health disparity populations. *Am J Public*

Health. 2019;109(S1):S94–S101. doi:10.2105/ajph.2018.304915

52. Chaudoir SR, Dugan AG, Barr CH. Measuring factors affecting implementation of health innovations: a systematic review of structural, organizational, provider, patient, and innovation level measures. *Implement Sci.* 2013;8:22. doi:10.1186/1748-5908-8-22
53. Aschbrenner KA, Mueller NM, Banerjee S, Bartels SJ. Applying an equity lens to characterizing the process and reasons for an adaptation to an evidenced-based practice. *Implement Res Pract.* 2021;2(Jan–Dec):1–8. doi:10.1177/26334895211017252
54. Hasson H, Blomberg S, Dunér A. Fidelity and moderating factors in complex interventions: a case study of a continuum of care program for frail elderly people in health and social care. *Implement Sci.* 2012;7:23. doi:10.1186/1748-5908-7-23
55. Hasson H. Systematic evaluation of implementation fidelity of complex interventions in health and social care. *Implement Sci.* 2010;5:67. doi:10.1186/1748-5908-5-67
56. Hawe P, Shiell A, Riley T. Complex interventions: how "out of control" can a randomised controlled trial be? *BMJ.* 2004;328(7455):1561–1563. doi:10.1136/bmj.328.7455.1561
57. Ginsburg LR, Hoben M, Easterbrook A, Anderson RA, Estabrooks CA, Norton PG. Fidelity is not easy! Challenges and guidelines for assessing fidelity in complex interventions. *Trials.* 2021;22:372. doi:10.1186/s13063-021-05322-5
58. Skivington K, Matthews L, Simpson SA, et al. A new framework for developing and evaluating complex interventions: update of Medical Research Council guidance. *BMJ.* 2021;374:n2061. doi:10.1136/bmj.n2061
59. Kirk MA, Haines ER, Rokoske FS, et al. A case study of a theory-based method for identifying and reporting core functions and forms of evidence-based interventions. *Transl Behav Med.* 2021;11(1):21–33. doi:10.1093/tbm/ibz178
60. Perez Jolles M, Lengnick-Hall R, Mittman BS. Core functions and forms of complex health interventions: a patient-centered medical home illustration. *J Gen Intern Med.* 2019;34(6):1032–1038. doi:10.1007/s11606-018-4818-7
61. Keogh A, Matthews J, Hurley DA. An assessment of physiotherapist's delivery of behaviour change techniques within the SOLAS feasibility trial. *Br J Health Psychol.* 2018;23(4):908–932. doi:10.1111/bjhp.12323
62. Wagenaar BH, Hammett WH, Jackson C, Atkins DL, Belus JM, Kemp CG. Implementation outcomes and strategies for depression interventions in low- and middle-income countries: a systematic review. *Glob Ment Health (Camb).* 2020;7:e7. doi:10.1017/gmh.2020.1
63. Lewis CC, Fischer S, Weiner BJ, Stanick C, Kim M, Martinez RG. Outcomes for implementation science: an enhanced systematic review of instruments using evidence-based rating criteria. *Implement Sci.* 2015;10:155. doi:10.1186/s13012-015-0342-x
64. Proctor EK, Powell BJ, McMillen JC. Implementation strategies: recommendations for specifying and reporting. *Implement Sci.* 2013;8:139. doi:10.1186/1748-5908-8-139
65. Powell BJ, Beidas RS, Lewis CC, et al. Methods to improve the selection and tailoring of implementation strategies. *J Behav Health Serv Res.* 2017;44(2):177–194. doi:10.1007/s11414-015-9475-6
66. Lewis CC, Klasnja P, Powell BJ, et al. From classification to causality: advancing understanding of mechanisms of change in implementation science. *Front Public Health.* 2018;6:136. doi:10.3389/fpubh.2018.00136
67. Wolfenden L, Foy R, Presseau J, et al. Designing and undertaking randomised implementation trials: guide for researchers. *BMJ.* 2021;372:m3721. doi:10.1136/bmj.m3721
68. Stockdale SE, Hamilton AB, Bergman AA, et al. Assessing fidelity to evidence-based quality improvement as an implementation strategy for patient-centered medical home transformation in the Veterans Health Administration. *Implement Sci.* 2020;15:18. doi:10.1186/s13012-020-0979-y
69. Walsh-Bailey C, Palazzo LG, Jones SMW, et al. A pilot study comparing tools for tracking implementation strategies and treatment adaptations. *Implement Res Pract.* 2021;2(Jan–Dec):1–14. doi:10.1177/26334895211016028
70. Haley AD, Powell BJ, Walsh-Bailey C, et al. Strengthening methods for tracking adaptations and modifications to implementation strategies. *BMC Med Res Methodol.* 2021;21:133. doi:10.1186/s12874-021-01326-6
71. Mensah GA, Riley WT. Social determinants of health and implementation research: three decades of progress and a need for convergence. *Ethn Dis.* 2021;31(1):1–4. doi:10.18865/ed.31.1.1
72. Shelton RC, Brotzman LE, Johnson D, Erwin D. Trust and mistrust in shaping adaptation and de-implementation in the context of changing screening guidelines. *Ethn Dis.* 2021;31(1):119–132. doi:10.18865/ed.31.1.119
73. Glasgow RE. What types of evidence are most needed to advance behavioral medicine? *Ann*

Behav Med. 2008;35(1):19–25. doi:10.1007/s12160-007-9008-5

74. Glasgow RE, Klesges LM, Dzewaltowski DA, Bull SS, Estabrooks P. The future of health behavior change research: what is needed to improve translation of research into health promotion practice? *Ann Behav Med.* 2004;27(1):3–12. doi:10.1207/s15324796abm2701_2
75. Kerner J, Rimer B, Emmons K. Introduction to the special section on dissemination: dissemination research and research dissemination: how can we close the gap? *Health Psychol.* 2005;24(5):443–446. doi:10.1037/0278-6133.24.5.443
76. Kwan BM, Brownson RC, Glasgow RE, Morrato EH, Luke DA. Designing for dissemination and sustainability to promote equitable impacts on health. *Annu Rev Public Health.* 2022;43:331–353. doi:10.1146/annurev-publhealth-052220-112457
77. Cabassa LJ, Gomes AP, Meyreles Q, et al. Using the collaborative intervention planning framework to adapt a health-care manager intervention to a new population and provider group to improve the health of people with serious mental illness. *Implement Sci.* 2014;9:178. doi:10.1186/s13012-014-0178-9
78. Brownson RC, Fielding JE, Maylahn CM. Evidence-based public health: a fundamental concept for public health practice. *Annu Rev Public Health.* 2009;30:175–201. doi:10.1146/annurev.publhealth.031308.100134
79. Kilbourne AM, Almirall D, Eisenberg D, et al. Protocol: Adaptive Implementation of Effective Programs Trial (ADEPT): cluster randomized SMART trial comparing a standard versus enhanced implementation strategy to improve outcomes of a mood disorders program. *Implement Sci.* 2014;9:132. doi:10.1186/s13012-014-0132-x
80. Almirall D, Nahum-Shani I, Sherwood NE, Murphy SA. Introduction to SMART designs for the development of adaptive interventions: with application to weight loss research. *Transl Behav Med.* 2014;4(3):260–274. doi:10.1007/s13142-014-0265-0
81. Horn SD, Gassaway J. Practice-based evidence study design for comparative effectiveness research. *Med Care.* 2007;45(10)(suppl 2):S50–S57. doi:10.1097/MLR.0b013e318070c07b
82. Brown CH, Curran G, Palinkas LA, et al. An overview of research and evaluation designs for dissemination and implementation. *Annu Rev Public Health.* 2017;38:1–22. doi:10.1146/annurev-publhealth-031816-044215
83. Wang B, Deveaux L, Cottrell L, et al. The effectiveness of two implementation strategies for improving teachers' delivery of an evidenced-based HIV prevention program. *Prev Sci.* 2022;23(6):889–899. doi:10.1007/s11121-022-01335-x
84. Greenhalgh T, Robert G, Macfarlane F, Bate P, Kyriakidou O. Diffusion of innovations in service organizations: systematic review and recommendations. *Milbank Q.* 2004;82(4):581–629. doi:10.1111/j.0887-378X.2004.00325.x
85. Davis M, Baranowski T, Hughes M, Warnecke C, De Moor C, Mullis R. Using children as change agents to increase fruit and vegetable consumption among lower-income African American parents. In: Linnan A, Steckler L, eds. *Process Evaluation for Public Health Interventions and Research.* Jossey-Bass; 2002:249–267.
86. Rogers EM. *Diffusion of Innovations.* 5th ed. Free Press; 2003.
87. National Cancer Institute. Evidence-Based Cancer Control Programs (EBCCP): transforming research into community and clinical practice. Updated October 2, 2020. Accessed February 2, 2022. https://ebccp.cancercontrol.cancer.gov/index.do
88. Grover V. Commentary: implementing interventions: building a shared understanding of why. *New Dir Child Adolesc Dev.* 2016;2016(154):109–112. doi:10.1002/cad.20174
89. Fagan AA, Arthur MW, Hanson K, Briney JS, Hawkins JD. Effects of Communities That Care on the adoption and implementation fidelity of evidence-based prevention programs in communities: results from a randomized controlled trial. *Prev Sci.* 2011;12(3):223–234. doi:10.1007/s11121-011-0226-5
90. Dariotis JK, Bumbarger BK, Duncan LG, Greenberg MT. How do implementation efforts relate to program adherence? Examining the role of organizational, implementer, and program factors. *J Community Psychol.* 2008;36(6):744–760. doi:10.1002/jcop.20255
91. Weiner BJ. A theory of organizational readiness for change. *Implement Sci.* 2009;4:67. doi:10.1186/1748-5908-4-67
92. Kumanyika SK, Yancey AK. Physical activity and health equity: evolving the science. *Am J Health Promot.* 2009;23(6):S4–S7. doi:10.4278/ajhp.23.6.S4
93. Backer TE. Finding the balance: program fidelity and adaptation in substance abuse prevention: a state-of-the-art review. U.S Department of Health and Human Services: Substance Abuse and Mental Health Services Administration: Center for Substance Abuse Prevention. 2001. Accessed April 12, 2022. https://www.csun.edu/sites/default/files/FindingBalance1.pdf

94. Cotterill S, Knowles S, Martindale AM, et al. Getting messier with TIDieR: embracing context and complexity in intervention reporting. *BMC Med Res Methodol.* 2018;18:12. doi:10.1186/s12874-017-0461-y
95. Percy-Laurry A, Adsul P, Uy A, Vinson C. Improving evidence-based program repositories: introducing the Evidence-Based Cancer Control Programs (EBCCP) web repository. *Am J Health Promot.* 2021;35(7):897–899. doi:10.1177/08901171211006589
96. Harden SM, Steketee A, Glasgow T, Glasgow RE, Estabrooks PA. Suggestions for advancing pragmatic solutions for dissemination: potential updates to evidence-based repositories. *Am J Health Promot.* 2021;35(2):289–294. doi:10.1177/0890117120934619
97. Hoffmann TC, Glasziou PP, Boutron I, et al. Better reporting of interventions: Template for Intervention Description and Replication (TIDieR) checklist and guide. *BMJ.* 2014;348:g1687. doi:10.1136/bmj.g1687
98. Schoenwald SK, Garland AF, Chapman JE, Frazier SL, Sheidow AJ, Southam-Gerow MA. Toward the effective and efficient measurement of implementation fidelity. *Adm Policy Ment Health.* 2011;38(1):32–43. doi:10.1007/s10488-010-0321-0
99. Schoenwald SK. It's a bird, it's a plane, it's . . . fidelity measurement in the real world. *Clin Psychol (New York).* 2011;18(2):142–147. doi:10.1111/j.1468-2850.2011.01245.x
100. Lee CY, August GJ, Realmuto GM, Horowitz JL, Bloomquist ML, Klimes-Dougan B. Fidelity at a distance: assessing implementation fidelity of the Early Risers prevention program in a going-to-scale intervention trial. *Prev Sci.* 2008;9(3):215–229. doi:10.1007/s11121-008-0097-6
101. Ledford JR, Gast DL. Measuring procedural fidelity in behavioural research. *Neuropsychol Rehabil.* 2014;24(3–4):332–348. doi:10.1080/09602011.2013.861352
102. Toomey E, Matthews J, Hurley DA. Using mixed methods to assess fidelity of delivery and its influencing factors in a complex self-management intervention for people with osteoarthritis and low back pain. *BMJ Open.* 2017;7(8):e015452. doi:10.1136/bmjopen-2016-015452
103. Smith-Morris C, Lopez G, Ottomanelli L, Goetz L, Dixon-Lawson K. Ethnography, fidelity, and the evidence that anthropology adds: supplementing the fidelity process in a clinical trial of supported employment. *Med Anthropol Q.* 2014;28(2):141–161. doi:10.1111/maq.12093
104. Berry CA, Nguyen AM, Cuthel AM, et al. Measuring implementation strategy fidelity in HealthyHearts NYC: a complex intervention using practice facilitation in primary care. *Am J Med Qual.* 2021;36(4):270–276. doi:10.1177/1062860620959450
105. Williams SL, McSharry J, Taylor C, Dale J, Michie S, French DP. Translating a walking intervention for health professional delivery within primary care: a mixed-methods treatment fidelity assessment. *Br J Health Psychol.* 2020;25(1):17–38. doi:10.1111/bjhp.12392
106. Lorencatto F, West R, Christopherson C, Michie S. Assessing fidelity of delivery of smoking cessation behavioural support in practice. *Implement Sci.* 2013;8:40. doi:10.1186/1748-5908-8-40
107. Fixsen DL, Naoom SF, Blase KA, Friedman M, Wallace F. Implementation research: a synthesis of the literature. University of South Florida, Louis de la Parte Florida Mental Health Institute, National Implementation Research Network; 2010. Accessed April 12, 2022. http://nirn.fpg.unc.edu/sites/nirn.fpg.unc.edu/files/resources/NIRN-MonographFull-01-2005.pdf
108. Keith RE, Hopp FP, Subramanian U, Wiitala W, Lowery JC. Fidelity of implementation: development and testing of a measure. *Implement Sci.* 2010;5:99. doi:10.1186/1748-5908-5-99
109. Nelson MC, Cordray DS, Hulleman CS, Darrow CL, Sommer EC. A procedure for assessing intervention fidelity in experiments testing educational and behavioral interventions. *J Behav Health Serv Res.* 2012;39(4):374–396. doi:10.1007/s11414-012-9295-x
110. Teague GB, Mueser KT, Rapp CA. Advances in fidelity measurement for mental health services research: four measures. *Psychiatr Serv.* 2012;63(8):765–771. doi:10.1176/appi.ps.201100430
111. Lambert JD, Greaves CJ, Farrand P, Cross R, Haase AM, Taylor AH. Assessment of fidelity in individual level behaviour change interventions promoting physical activity among adults: a systematic review. *BMC Public Health.* 2017;17:765. doi:10.1186/s12889-017-4778-6
112. Begum S, Yada A, Lorencatto F. How has intervention fidelity been assessed in smoking cessation interventions? A systematic review. *J Smok Cessat.* 2021;2021:6641208. doi:10.1155/2021/6641208
113. Walton H, Spector A, Williamson M, Tombor I, Michie S. Developing quality fidelity and engagement measures for complex health interventions. *Br J Health Psychol.* 2020;25(1):39–60. doi:10.1111/bjhp.12394
114. Rixon L, Baron J, McGale N, Lorencatto F, Francis J, Davies A. Methods used to address fidelity of receipt in health intervention

research: a citation analysis and systematic review. *BMC Health Serv Res.* 2016;16:663. doi:10.1186/s12913-016-1904-6
115. Elliott DS, Mihalic S. Issues in disseminating and replicating effective prevention programs. *Prev Sci.* 2004;5(1):47–53. doi:10.1023/b:prev.0000013981.28071.52
116. Hankonen N. Participants' enactment of behavior change techniques: a call for increased focus on what people do to manage their motivation and behavior. *Health Psychol Rev.* 2021;15(2):185–194. doi:10.1080/17437199.2020.1814836
117. Bond GR, Drake RE. Assessing the fidelity of evidence-based practices: history and current status of a standardized measurement methodology. *Adm Policy Ment Health.* 2020;47(6):874–884. doi:10.1007/s10488-019-00991-6
118. O'Shea O, McCormick R, Bradley JM, O'Neill B. Fidelity review: a scoping review of the methods used to evaluate treatment fidelity in behavioural change interventions. *Phys Ther Rev.* 2016;21(3–6):207–214. doi:10.1080/10833196.2016.1261237
119. Hermes ED, Lyon AR, Schueller SM, Glass JE. Measuring the implementation of behavioral intervention technologies: recharacterization of established outcomes. *J Med Internet Res.* 2019;21(1):e11752. doi:10.2196/11752
120. Becker-Haimes EM, Klein MR, McLeod BD, et al. The TPOCS-Self-Reported Therapist Intervention Fidelity for Youth (TPOCS-SeRTIFY): a case study of pragmatic measure development. *Implement Res Pract.* 2021;2(Jan–Dec):1–9. doi:10.1177/2633489521992553
121. Lyons VH, Benson LR, Griffin E, et al. Fidelity assessment of a social work-led intervention among patients with firearm injuries. *Res Soc Work Pract.* 2020;30(6):678–687. doi:10.1177/1049731520912002
122. Duffy SA, Cummins SE, Fellows JL, et al. Fidelity monitoring across the seven studies in the Consortium of Hospitals Advancing Research on Tobacco (CHART). *Tob Induc Dis.* 2015;13:29. doi:10.1186/s12971-015-0056-5
123. Berkel C, Mauricio AM, Schoenfelder E, Sandler IN. Putting the pieces together: an integrated model of program implementation. *Prev Sci.* 2011;12(1):23–33. doi:10.1007/s11121-010-0186-1
124. Lobb R, Gonzalez Suarez E, Fay ME, et al. Implementation of a cancer prevention program for working class, multiethnic populations. *Prev Med.* 2004;38(6):766–776. doi:10.1016/j.ypmed.2003.12.025
125. Brownson RC, Kumanyika SK, Kreuter MW, Haire-Joshu D. Implementation science should give higher priority to health equity. *Implement Sci.* 2021;16:28. doi:10.1186/s13012-021-01097-0
126. Gaias LM, Arnold KT, Liu FF, Pullmann MD, Duong MT, Lyon AR. Adapting Strategies to Promote Implementation Reach and Equity (ASPIRE) in school mental health services. *Psychol Sch.* 2021;59(12):2471–2485. doi:10.1002/pits.22515
127. Shelton RC, Adsul P, Oh A, Moise N, Griffith DM. Application of an antiracism lens in the field of implementation science (IS): recommendations for reframing implementation research with a focus on justice and racial equity. *Implement Res Pract.* 2021;2(Jan–Dec):1–19. doi:10.1177/26334895211049482
128. Shelton RC, Chambers DA, Glasgow RE. An extension of RE-AIM to enhance sustainability: addressing dynamic context and promoting health equity over time. *Front Public Health.* 2020;8:134. doi:10.3389/fpubh.2020.00134
129. Holliday J, Audrey S, Moore L, Parry-Langdon N, Campbell R. High fidelity? How should we consider variations in the delivery of school-based health promotion interventions? *Health Educ J.* 2009;68(1):44–62. doi:10.1177/0017896908100448
130. Balu R, Doolittle F. Commentary: learning from variations in fidelity of implementation. *New Dir Child Adolesc Dev.* 2016;2016(154):105–108. doi:10.1002/cad.20173
131. Wiltsey Stirman S, Kimberly J, Cook N, Calloway A, Castro F, Charns M. The sustainability of new programs and innovations: a review of the empirical literature and recommendations for future research. *Implement Sci.* 2012;7:17. doi:10.1186/1748-5908-7-17
132. Greenhalgh T, Papoutsi C. Studying complexity in health services research: desperately seeking an overdue paradigm shift. *BMC Med.* 2018;16:95. doi:10.1186/s12916-018-1089-4
133. Anyon Y, Roscoe J, Bender K, et al. Reconciling adaptation and fidelity: implications for scaling up high quality youth programs. *J Prim Prev.* 2019;40(1):35–49. doi:10.1007/s10935-019-00535-6
134. Durlak JA. Why program implementation is important. *J Prev Interv Community.* 1998;17(2):5–18. doi:10.1300/J005v17n02_02
135. Botvin GJ. Advancing prevention science and practice: challenges, critical issues, and future directions. *Prev Sci.* 2004;5(1):69–72. doi:10.1023/b:prev.0000013984.83251.8b
136. Ennett ST, Haws S, Ringwalt CL, et al. Evidence-based practice in school substance use prevention: fidelity of implementation

under real-world conditions. *Health Educ Res.* 2011;26(2):361–371. doi:10.1093/her/cyr013

137. Hill LG, Maucione K, Hood BK. A focused approach to assessing program fidelity. *Prev Sci.* 2007;8(1):25–34. doi:10.1007/s11121-006-0051-4
138. Chambers DA, Glasgow RE, Stange KC. The Dynamic Sustainability Framework: addressing the paradox of sustainment amid ongoing change. *Implement Sci.* 2013;8:117. doi:10.1186/1748-5908-8-117
139. Lara M, Bryant-Stephens T, Damitz M, et al. Balancing "fidelity" and community context in the adaptation of asthma evidence-based interventions in the "real world." *Health Promot Pract.* 2011;12(6)(suppl 1):63S–72S. doi:10.1177/1524839911414888
140. Green AE, Aarons GA. A comparison of policy and direct practice stakeholder perceptions of factors affecting evidence-based practice implementation using concept mapping. *Implement Sci.* 2011;6:104. doi:10.1186/1748-5908-6-104
141. Bernal G, Saez-Santiago E. Culturally centered psychosocial interventions. *J Community Psychol.* 2006;34(2):121–132. doi:10.1002/jcop.20096
142. Cabassa LJ, Baumann AA. A two-way street: bridging implementation science and cultural adaptations of mental health treatments. *Implement Sci.* 2013;8:90. doi:10.1186/1748-5908-8-90
143. Stirman SW, Miller CJ, Toder K, Calloway A. Development of a framework and coding system for modifications and adaptations of evidence-based interventions. *Implement Sci.* 2013;8:65. doi:10.1186/1748-5908-8-65
144. Marques L, Valentine SE, Kaysen D, et al. Provider fidelity and modifications to cognitive processing therapy in a diverse community health clinic: associations with clinical change. *J Consult Clin Psychol.* 2019;87(4):357–369. doi:10.1037/ccp0000384
145. Chambers DA, Norton WE. The adaptome: advancing the science of intervention adaptation. *Am J Prev Med.* 2016;51(4):S124–S131. doi:10.1016/j.amepre.2016.05.011
146. von Thiele Schwarz U, Aarons GA, Hasson H. The Value Equation: three complementary propositions for reconciling fidelity and adaptation in evidence-based practice implementation. *BMC Health Serv Res.* 2019;19:868. doi:10.1186/s12913-019-4668-y
147. Wingood GM, DiClemente RJ. The ADAPT-ITT model: a novel method of adapting evidence-based HIV interventions. *J Acquir Immune Defic Syndr.* 2008;47(suppl 1):S40–S46. doi:10.1097/QAI.0b013e3181605df1
148. Wells KJ, Luque JS, Miladinovic B, et al. Do community health worker interventions improve rates of screening mammography in the United States? A systematic review. *Cancer Epidemiol Biomarkers Prev.* 2011;20(8):1580–1598. doi:10.1158/1055-9965.Epi-11-0276
149. Erwin DO, Ivory J, Stayton C, et al. Replication and dissemination of a cancer education model for African American women. *Cancer Control.* 2003;10(5)(suppl):13–21. doi:10.1177/107327480301005s03
150. Shelton RC, Charles TA, Dunston SK, Jandorf L, Erwin DO. Advancing understanding of the sustainability of lay health advisor (LHA) programs for African-American women in community settings. *Transl Behav Med.* 2017;7(3):415–426. doi:10.1007/s13142-017-0491-3
151. Rodriguez EM, Jandorf L, Devonish JA, et al. Translating new science into the community to promote opportunities for breast and cervical cancer prevention among African American women. *Health Expect.* 2020;23(2):337–347. doi:10.1111/hex.12985
152. Emmons K, Colditz, GA. Realizing the potential of cancer prevention—the role of implementation science. *N Engl J Med.* 2017;376(10):986–990. doi:10.1056/NEJMsb1609101
153. Green LW. Making research relevant: if it is an evidence-based practice, where's the practice-based evidence? *Fam Pract.* 2008;25(suppl 1):i20–i24. doi:10.1093/fampra/cmn055
154. Zwarenstein M, Treweek S, Gagnier JJ, et al. Improving the reporting of pragmatic trials: an extension of the CONSORT statement. *BMJ.* 2008;337:a2390. doi:10.1136/bmj.a2390
155. Glasgow RE, Huebschmann AG, Brownson RC. Expanding the CONSORT figure: increasing transparency in reporting on external validity. *Am J Prev Med.* 2018;55(3):422–430. doi:10.1016/j.amepre.2018.04.044

8

Adaptation in Dissemination and Implementation Science

ANA A. BAUMANN, SHANNON WILTSEY STIRMAN, AND LEOPOLDO J. CABASSA

INTRODUCTION

The field of dissemination and implementation (D&I) science continues to mature, as more sophisticated evaluations of implementation strategies, their mechanisms, and theory-driven research on factors that predict successful implementation has become more widespread. Recently, researchers have recognized that implementing programs and interventions into systems where health inequities remain is insufficient to achieve health equity.[1–4] We define equity as "providing resources according to the need to help diverse populations achieve their highest state of health and other functioning. Equity is an ongoing process of assessing needs, correcting historical inequities, and creating conditions for optimal outcomes by members of all social identity groups."[5] Despite major advances in research methods, and the increase attention in equity in the field of D&I, we have yet to provide what people, organizations and communities—especially those historically and systematically underserved and marginalized—need to thrive and be successful.[6] Investigators are still calling for increased action in promoting evidence-based interventions in usual care and for testing interventions and designs to optimize outcomes and help achieve health equity.[3,7]

In light of the diversity of communities, patient populations, providers, and service settings into which interventions are delivered, it is unlikely that the same program, techniques, and strategies can be implemented successfully in the exact same way across multiple contexts. In fact, scholars from the fields of implementation science, health disparities research, and cultural adaptation warn of the dangers of implementing evidence-based interventions without attending to the fit of the interventions to the context, in particular to the populations that are being served, the different providers who deliver these interventions, and the diversity of service and public health settings who could benefit from these interventions.[1,7–9] Numerous studies indicate the importance of matching the intervention with the population and context of interest, including attention to race, ethnicity, gender, sexual orientation, religion, disability, location, community norms, service settings and organizational characteristics.[1,7,10] Adaptation needs to be a central aspect of the implementation process to ensure a good fit and promote health equity. In this chapter, we draw from the cultural adaptation, health disparities, and implementation science fields to propose that scholars should carefully consider evaluating, documenting, and rigorously studying the adaptation process, methods, and outcomes at the intervention and at the implementation strategies levels. To begin coverage of key issues, it is important to have a common set of definitions (Table 8.1 and chapter 2).

The term adaptation has been used in different ways in the implementation literature. It has been used to refer as a process or mechanism, as an implementation strategy, or as an outcome (akin to fidelity), or as a characteristic of the intervention (adaptability).[15] Several studies have shown that providers adapt either

Ana A. Baumann, Shannon Wiltsey Stirman, and Leopoldo J. Cabassa, *Adaptation in Dissemination and Implementation Science* In: *Dissemination and Implementation Research in Health*. Edited by: Ross C. Brownson, Graham A. Colditz, and Enola K. Proctor, Oxford University Press.
 DOI: 10.1093/oso/9780197660690.003.0008

TABLE 8.1 KEY DEFINITIONS RELATED TO ADAPTATION AND D&I RESEARCH

Construct	Definition
Adaptation	Thoughtful or deliberate modifications made to the intervention or implementation strategies, with the goal of improving their fit with a given context[11]
Modification	A blanket term that includes changes to the intervention or implementation strategies that can occur through adaptation or in an ad hoc manner[12]
Adaptive interventions or strategies	Those interventions or strategies for which stakeholders are allowed, or even encouraged, to change from the original design. These changes are pre-defined by intervention developers[13] or through the monitoring of outcomes and processes that inform these adaptations (e.g., treat-to-target interventions or strategies)
Systematic adaptation	Adaptations made using a formal process and methods (e.g., with literature review, input of stakeholders)[14]
Unsystematic adaptation	Adaptations made without a formal process [14]
Proactive adaptation	Adaptations made to address an anticipated obstacle/challenge or misfit between the intervention and the context[14,15]
Reactive adaptation	Adaptations made due to an unanticipated challenge/obstacle [14,15]
Adaptability	The degree to which an intervention or strategy can be adapted, tailored, refined, or reinvented to meet local needs[16]
Cultural adaptation	Systematic modification of an intervention or strategy to consider language, culture, and context in such a way that it is compatible with the client's cultural patterns meanings and values[17,18]
Core component of an intervention/strategy	An element of an intervention that is specified and identified to be critical to implementation and intervention success
Intervention Fidelity	Fidelity to core components is the continuation of the elements found to be necessary for intervention effectiveness[19]
Fidelity-consistent modifications	Fidelity-consistent modifications are defined as those that preserve core elements of a treatment that are needed for the intervention to be effective[20]
Fidelity-inconsistent modifications	Fidelity-inconsistent modifications are those that alter the intervention in a manner that fails to preserve its core elements[20]
Core function of an intervention/strategy	Core purposes of the change process that the intervention/strategy seeks to facilitate[21]
Form of an intervention/ strategy	Specific strategies or activities that may be customized to local contexts and that are needed to carry out the core functions[21]
Context	A set of characteristics and circumstances that consist of active and unique factors within which the implementation of an intervention is embedded[13,22]
Adaptive design	A clinical trial design that allows for prospectively planned modification to one or more aspects of the design based on accumulating data from subjects in the trial[23]

the intervention and/or the delivery process from the original during the implementation process, and thus adaptations commonly happen in the implementation process.[24] In fact, adaptation spans all implementation stages (exploration, preparation, implementation, and sustainment).[25,26] The goals of adaptation are usually to increase the fit of the intervention with the context.[1] Thus, adaptation is not inherently good or bad—the value of adaptation lies in whether the intended outcome is achieved when interventions are adapted. Consequently, we could conceptualize adaptation as a strategy that can address the interplay between the fit of the intervention (the what), the process of implementation (the how), and the context in which the intervention is being implemented (the where).[1,15]

This chapter explores the rationale for why we need to adapt interventions and/or implementation strategies and examines our recommendations of best practices of an adaptation study.

WHY SHOULD WE EXPLICITLY ATTEND TO ADAPTATION

As Chambers and Norton[27] mention, the traditional path in science is to develop an intervention, test it, identify the discordance between the intervention and the context or the population, adapt the intervention, and then implement the intervention on a broader scale. However, evidence suggests that interventions that were previously adapted and tested are not being implemented in usual care, and interventions that are being implemented are not necessarily explicitly attending to the adaptation process.[1,27] The field of D&I has recognized the importance of context and scholars have advocated for the fact that the selection of an intervention and its strategies should not be a neutral process but done with care and engagement with the community as partners, and with attention to the historical, political, and systemic forces at play during the implementation process.[1,8,28,29] With the assumption that the implementation process is dynamic, and with the argument that culturally-adapting interventions increases effectiveness and fit,[7,30–33] we outline below the importance for attending to the process of adaptation and its impact on implementation, service, and consumer-level outcomes.

One of the main assumptions of the D&I field is that if an intervention has been proven to be efficacious, the spread of such intervention would decrease the quality gap, reduce cost and/or improve patient, provider and/or service outcomes regardless of the setting where it is being implemented.[27,34–36] However, an intervention is not implemented in a vacuum, and contextual factors at multiple levels (e.g., clients, providers, organizations, communities) influence the implementation process and its success.

There are at least three consequences to not examining contextual factors when planning for implementation. First, assuming that EBIs are the gold-standard of interventions that will improve quality, cost, or outcomes once they are broadly disseminated and implemented overlooks the importance of contextual factors.[34] That is, it is crucial that researchers and practitioners first examine the historical and current context, and the strengths of the community to examine whether the intervention is indeed a good fit for the context.[8] Devoting time and resources in this pre-implementation process is important, especially if we are to not replicate historical discrimination, racism, and trust issues with the communities with whom we collaborate which directly contributes to the sustainment of health inequities.[37]

Consider, for example, parent interventions to improve child externalizing behaviors (e.g., aggressive behaviors, non-compliance). We know that while parenting practices have some universal components, they are heavily culturally-based and dependent on beliefs and orientations (e.g., the role of respect, of gender practices[16,17]). If an intervention developed for a group of parents (e.g., white Americans in urban settings in the U.S.) is delivered for a different group (e.g., Latino parents in rural settings in the U.S.) and engagement or outcomes are not promising, one needs to carefully examine whether the problem was with the implementation process, or rather with the mismatch between the intervention and the population and context into which it was implemented, including experiences with discrimination and adversity with immigration system.[38,39] As another example, consider medical guidelines, which often change depending on new evidence, causing confusion among community members.[40] In the context of medical settings, we need to account for the experiences of medical distrust due to the historical abuse, racism, stigmatization, and discrimination, and how these affect the health and healthcare access of historically underserved populations, especially Black, Native American, Alaskan Native, Asian/Pacific Islanders and Latino communities.[41] Not examining the historical and current contextual aspect of our implementation process and failing to adapt our guidelines and procedures accordingly is dangerous and directly contributes to healthcare inequities.

Not examining context and assuming that any EBI is good for anyone in any context will hinder efforts to effectively address healthcare inequities. While we have made some progress in the last 30 years in detecting healthcare inequities and developing interventions to address them, inequities in health and in the access, use, quality and outcomes of health care have yet to be eliminated.[42] The recent SARS COVID-19 pandemic has made these health and healthcare inequities more explicit.[43–46] Considering such clear historical data, one could argue that, only by developing a science grounded on social-justice approaches and ensuring that interventions are designed and tailored to ensure that they truly fit and meet the needs, context, and culture of the individuals who need them, we will be able to decrease these health and healthcare inequities.[28,29] Health inequity is the result of economic maldistribution, structural violence, colonization, historical trauma, structural racism, and political misrepresentation and therefore health equity entails economic redistribution, structural changes, cultural recognition, and political representation.[47,48] Grounding our argument and implementation science in social justice principles and goal, we state that every person has the right to physical and mental health, and that by promoting health care to all, we will promote the well-being of the community at large.[47,49–52]

Often, however, interventions that have not been evaluated for a given population or context may need to be implemented because there is a pressing need to improve access to quality care. While implementing an intervention that has not been tested in a particular population, culture or setting may not yield the desired outcomes,[53] in such cases of urgency, interventions that are evidence-based may represent the best option available. Especially in these contexts, the engagement with community partners is important to examine how to adapt and implement these interventions with attention to flexibility, cost, feasibility, and community context. More research and investments in services are needed to develop and test interventions across diverse populations, services settings, and communities and to evaluate which implementation strategies for which interventions can reduce health and mental health inequities.[54] The use of strategies to rapidly determine whether and how adaptations are necessary to promote optimal levels of engagement and outcomes are central to the implementation effort. Otherwise, a considerable amount of time could pass before a pattern of disappointing results becomes evident and more effective solutions are identified.[55]

To foster the science of adaptation, we argue that D&I scientists should engage in a careful evaluation of *when, why, and how* adaptation should occur by documenting and studying adaptation during the implementation process. As Rogers[56] explained, an "innovation almost never fits perfectly in the organization in which it is being embedded" (p395). Implementation requires a process of mutual adaptation, in which both the practice innovation being implemented, and the organizations and stakeholders involved in the implementation process must adjust to optimize fit and maximize effectiveness.[57–59] When interventions are adapted with care, there is the potential for optimization of that intervention in context in which it is delivered. However, adapted interventions also have the potential to produce undesired outcomes if not undertaken in the absence of guidance from theory, community input and engagement, rigorous methods and research evidence.[60]

Similar arguments can be made to implementation strategies. As the knowledge around the efficacy components of implementation strategies is still evolving,[61] it is crucial to capture the modifications of the strategies, especially because of their inherent dynamism and complexity.[12] Regardless of the type and level of adaptation (at the health intervention and/or implementation strategy levels), our assumption is that by clearly specifying and evaluating adaptations, we can increase the external validity of the intervention, optimize its expected outcomes across populations, settings, and context, and improve and hopefully accelerate the implementation process. It is by supporting the accumulation of such knowledge and building "the Adaptome"[27] that we will be able to understand what works for whom, under different circumstances and foster the field of adaptation.

Adaptation and Fidelity

When referring to adaptation of intervention and its strategies, it is important to consider the relationship between adaptation and fidelity. Much has been written about the tension between fidelity and adaptation of interventions.[62] We advocate here that attending to adaptation is important as a *complement* to the assessment of fidelity, and not necessarily in conflict with fidelity.[60] While we recognize that fidelity of an intervention is important because it intends to predicts the interventions' desired outcomes,[16,56] it is also important to understand the assumptions underlying the process of conceptualizing and measuring fidelity. That is, fidelity can be a top-down approach, with measures usually developed by treatment developer often based on theoretical assumptions and should be, perhaps, also balanced with a bottom-up approach of examining the fit of the theoretical constructs and core elements or functions of the intervention and centering the intervention with the community.[63] As such, understanding which types of adaptations can occur without eroding the dose and fidelity to key intervention components (e.g., fidelity-consistent adaptations[20,64]) can provide guidance on how to optimize an intervention in a particular setting and population, and center it in the context of the community.[60] By monitoring the adaptation process, researchers can potentially improve the reach, engagement, effectiveness and hopefully the sustainment of the interventions in usual care.[7,65]

Fortunately, there is a developing literature that can provide guidance regarding how to conceptualize the balance of adaptation and fidelity. For example, it is helpful to distinguish between core elements or functions of an intervention,[21] which should be preserved or adapted in such a way that the essence or key function of that component remains evident, and the "adaptable periphery", or forms and aspects of the intervention that can likely be adapted to improve fit without negatively impacting outcomes. Additionally, better outcomes may result by ensuring they reflect stakeholders' needs and preferences that potential unintended consequences are identified and discussed,[14] and that the process of adaptation is iterative, data-driven and preserve the core functions of the intervention.[15] Tools and frameworks have also been developed to track the different forms, goals, and reasons for adaptations to facilitate better understanding of the relationship between adaptation and fidelity,[11,66] and to document the process of adapting implementation strategies with or without fidelity to core elements and functions during the implementation process.[15]

Based on several empirical studies showing that providers adapt interventions when implementing them,[67,68] the field has moved away from dichotomizing adaptation from fidelity and instead recognizing that these two can co-exist and inform each other.[26] It is possible to adapt interventions while preserving fidelity to the aspects of the intervention that are central to the intervention's effectiveness. There is, however, limited empirical evidence on the impact of the different levels and types of adaptations that occur in routine care across the implementation continuum, and their relation with fidelity and efficacy of the interventions and their implementation strategies.[60] While there is evidence that some forms of adaptation can negatively impact health outcomes, even if they improve acceptability or feasibility,[69] several studies have identified adaptations that are associated with similar or better outcomes than the original interventions.[64,70–72]

BEST PRACTICES AND CONSIDERATIONS

As the science of adaptation advances, we advocate for careful conceptualization in the design and methods of adaptation studies or studies that include tracking adaptation as a project aim. Table 8.2 outlines our recommendations for best practices for an adaptation study. These recommendations are based on our collective experience and are therefore subjective; we look forward to the scientific community to test these and develop further recommendations.

WHEN TO ADAPT

A recent review of the adaptation literature indicated that most of the scholars in the adaptation and D&I fields advocate for adaptation to happen after an assessment of the fit of the intervention with the context, but often it occurs throughout the whole endeavor to implement and sustain interventions. If we conceptualize the implementation process in Exploration, Preparation, Implementation and Sustainment phases,[25] the adaptation process starts in the Exploration phase, where the community members, researchers and treatment developers examine the intervention adaptability, fit and appropriateness with the new context.[13,74] In the preparation, implementation and sustainment phases, then, collaborators identify the adaptations that need to be made, develop an adaptation plan, and pilot test the adaptations while also tracking modifications.[75] The Reach, Effectiveness, Adoption, Implementation and Maintenance (RE-AIM)[76] and Replicating Effective Programs (REP)[77,78]

TABLE 8.2 BEST PRACTICES FOR AN ADAPTATION STUDY

Aspects of the Project	Considerations
Frameworks	Use frameworks to guide the process of adaptation as well as to help track important details about adaptations being made during the study.
When to adapt	Plan adaptations before implementation; plan and track adaptations/ modifications during implementation and sustainment
How to adapt	Adapt *with*, not *for*, the community. Involve the community in all levels of adaptation (planning, adaptation, evaluation)[73]
Knowledge and Training Required	Ensure the project team has the necessary knowledge (empirical and/ or theoretical) of the core components of the intervention, and/or strategies to adapt, and/or the setting and community and document appropriately.
Methods	If possible, use mixed methods to inform and track the process and outcomes of the adaptation (minimum of 3) of: - Self-report - Observation - Record Review - Checklist - Real-time tracking/reporting - Interviews - Focus groups - Surveys - Policy documents
Suggestions for Accuracy in Tracking	Create decision rules in codebook that are specific to the intervention and/ or strategies; Meetings to calibrate and ensure rater agreement; Observation. Track what is adapted, what is not adapted, why and who made such decisions
Other data that may need to be collected and adapted	Outcome data, fidelity data, process data
How frequent should tracking happen (e.g., after every session, after the intervention is completed)	As frequent as possible while also considering being pragmatic and cost issues
Who captures the adaptations	If possible, multiple individuals with differing and appropriate levels of visibility (e.g., researcher/observer, administrator, provider) using different methods.
Decision Making about adapting and tracking adaptation	Engage multiple community partners, consider goals and available time, and resources

are other frameworks that similarly suggests an iterative process throughout efforts to pilot, scale, and sustain.

Similarly, frameworks from the cultural adaptation field stipulate for adaptations to occur as early as possible in the implementation process, when deciding which intervention to implement and when preparing for the new context and population. For example, Lau's[79] selective and directive cultural adaptation framework proposes a data driven model, where adaptations are made when there is quantitative and/or qualitative evidence that: (a) the new population has distinctive and unique sociocultural context of risk and resilience that will require consideration or addition of new treatment elements to address these contextual issues and improve the intervention's fit with the new population, and/or (b) when the social validity of an intervention is compromised, thus limiting treatment engagement and the receipt of an adequate exposure to the treatment to achieve its intended effect. Similarly, Barrera and Castro[65] suggest that adaptations are needed when qualitative and/or quantitative evidence indicates that two or more populations differ on: (a) treatment engagement dimensions (e.g. awareness of treatment, treatment initiation, treatment completion); (b) the ability of the treatment to change mediating variables, and (c) the relationships between mediators and treatment outcomes.[7] It is important to note that the adaptation process is not a linear one, and that the adaptations can happen in a parallel fashion and/or with a feedback loop across the implementation process.

WHAT TO ADAPT

Most interventions, especially behavioral health interventions, are multicomponent, and the contexts into which they are implemented will differ. Thus, many different forms of adaptations can occur. Understanding and documenting what these components are can facilitate better understanding of what types of adaptations yield the desired outcomes (e.g., engagement, adoption, improvements in health or functioning). Some work has been done to characterize adaptations made at the individual, organizational, and population levels. The cultural adaptation field has produced many frameworks aimed to guide the adaptation of content of the intervention to enhance cultural fit of the intervention. For example, Bernal and colleagues' Ecological Validity Model[17] was one of the first frameworks that outlined domains that one should consider to enhance cultural congruence between participants and the intervention, including language, persons, metaphors, content, concepts, goals, methods and contexts. Other scholars have suggested that surface-structure adaptations (e.g., translating from English to Spanish) or deep-structure adaptations (e.g., adding sessions, or re-ordering content) that can serve to maintain fidelity to the intervention model while making them more relevant, appealing and effective to cultural groups.[65] Other types of adaptation can happen in the context in which the intervention is being delivered. For example, there could be changes at the organizational level in which the intervention is being delivered (e.g., hiring a new type of workforces, such as peer specialists, or lay health worker, developing new policies or workflows), or at the outer setting (e.g., changes in policy).[80] Below we share frameworks that can help identify and document the types and levels of adaptations for the intervention and their implementation strategies.

HOW TO ADAPT

If adaptation is to be a planned, proactive, data-driven process, rather than a reactive, idiosyncratic process, it should begin during the planning phase of an implementation effort and continue throughout the entire implementation process.

Proactively specifying the nature of adaptations can facilitate better understanding of the elements of the intervention and/context that can be changed, and the elements that must be retained to achieve desired outcomes. Depending on the identified needs, content-level adaptations can be intended for an entire population, community, or they can be made for specific cohorts or individuals.[49] In some contexts, individual providers may also make decisions to adapt interventions for everyone that they serve, if they believe that their changes will enhance outcomes or increase engagement. In such cases, documentation and evaluation is necessary to determine whether these beliefs are correct. There is no single, correct way to adapt all interventions.[9]

Fortunately, D&I science has embraced the science of adaptation and many frameworks have been developed to guide when and how to adapt, and what to track when adapting the interventions and the strategies that accompany them. Scoping reviews, however, have shown that frameworks are not being used to guide the adaptations and/or adaptations are not being reported in empirical studies.[81–83] To foster the science of adaptation, we encourage scholars to use the frameworks to guide their work and report the adaptations. This can lead to a database to capture and classify the adaptations to facilitate learning about what adaptations are effective under different circumstances.[27]

Frameworks to Guide the Process of Adaptation

To complement the framework that describes what is adapted, and the implementation frameworks described in chapter 5, many cultural adaptation frameworks have been developed to guide the process and steps of adaptation as it relates to modifying an existing intervention for a new cultural, racial, or ethnic group. In general, cultural adaptation scholars suggest that one should carefully examine the following issues: (a) what evidence about the intervention is available (e.g., what information does the literature provide about the EBI?), (b) how different is the target population from the original population in the new setting (e.g., adults vs. teenagers), (c) what is the target domain of the intervention (e.g., changing parenting practices, improving coping skills, increasing self-management), and (d) what was the context of the original intervention (e.g., how does the intervention address the needs of the new population in a new setting). It is very likely that one or more of these variables will carefully demand adaptation to fit the intervention to the new context. Other scholars have provided in depth reviews of the cultural adaptation models,[9,62] which in general recommend that the adaptations should (a) be informed by the expertise of stakeholders (e.g., researchers and community representatives) and with collaboration between treatment developer; (b) follow formative research methods to understand population needs, the context of practice and the fit between the population needs and the intervention; (c) be addressed with carefully pilot testing of fidelity; and (d) be formally evaluated with effectiveness trials.[7,9,62]

Some frameworks integrate both the "what" and the "how" of adaptation. These models include the Cultural Adaptation Process (CAP), which was developed to complement Bernal's EVM,[17,18] Barrera and Castro's framework,[65,84] and the tailoring frameworks.[85,86] For example, CAP is influenced by Roger's[56] diffusion of innovation approach. Phase I involves the creation of collaborative approaches between different stakeholders: program developer, the scientist adapting the intervention, the practitioners, local policy makers and those receiving the intervention. A needs assessment including literature review and focus group also take place in Phase I. Phase II consists of making the first iterations of adaptations and pilot testing the measures to be used on Phase III on a large trial. All Phases include feedback loops, and adaptations to the intervention may occur during the large trial. A later iteration of the CAP framework has incorporated Aarons's Dynamic Adaptation Process (DAP)[87] and Forgatch's implementation[88] frameworks to describe the implementation process of a parent intervention in Mexico.[74]

Aarons' DAP framework[87] proposes similar steps in terms of the importance of involving stakeholders during the adaptation process. Within the DAP, decisions about the adaptation are made by an implementation resource team composed of multiple stakeholders (e.g., clinicians, researchers, administrators, clients, intervention developers). This team uses information from a careful assessment of system, organizational, provider and client level characteristics to negotiate system, organization, and intervention adaptations while maintaining core ingredients of the intervention. DAP considers adaptations beyond the intervention, such as modifications to the service context or the organization itself to facilitate implementation. Similarly, a recent scoping review also delineates eight steps for the adaptation process: (1) asses the community, (2) understand the EBI, (3) select the EBI, (4) consult with experts, (5) consult with stakeholders, (6) decide what needs to be adapted, (7) adapt the EBI, (8) train providers. (9) test the adapted materials, (10) implement, and (11) evaluate.[82]

Other frameworks were developed to inform decision-making about, and evaluation of the impacts of the adaptation process. The Iterative Decision-making for Evaluating Adaptations framework (IDEA[15]) provides a data-driven, iterative process that includes ensuring there is sufficient local or empirical evidence that adaptation is needed, consultation with stakeholders around key decision points and potential adaptations, evaluation, and continued refinement. The Model for Adaptation Design and Impact (MADI[14]) encourages the designing of adaptations in a way that anticipates intended and unintended impacts and leverages best practice from research, including specification of potential mediators and moderators that can help explain why and how adaptations are working to impact outcomes. Another approach, advocated by Lyon and Koerner,[89] is embedded in the Usability and User-Centered Design (UCD) approach. The cornerstone of UCS is that adaptations are made considering what people will ultimately use with the goals of (a) clearly identifying the end users (i.e., therapists delivering the intervention, patients receiving the intervention) and their needs, (b) prototyping the intervention with rapid iterations, (c) simplifying existing intervention parameters and procedures, and (d) exploring natural constraints to the implementation of the intervention.[89,90] Intervention mapping and implementation mapping can also be used to guide the adaptation process of interventions and implementation strategies, respectively.[91]

In addition to choosing a framework to guide the adaptation process, it is important to follow recommended strategies for assessing whether the desired outcomes are achieved after adaptation occurs.[60]

DOCUMENTING AND TRACKING ADAPTATIONS

More recently, the adaptation field has been examining strategies to measure adaptation. Choosing the method to track adaptation requires thoughtful thinking about aspects such as (1) the goal of adaptation in the study, (2) the goal of tracking, (3) study design, (4) the study budget,[76] among other aspects. To foster the science of adaptation, we need to have consistent conceptualization about what is and is not an adaptation, comparability in our measures, a comprehensive approach (i.e., multi-method measurement), and coherency across studies. Multi-method measurement is especially important when no single, feasible method is likely to accurately capture every adaptation that occurs. As scholars track adaptations and modifications to their interventions and strategies, it may also be important to track what is *not* being modified and the rationale for not modifying the components of the interventions and/or strategies.

Methods used to track adaptations have varied: scholars have used real-time tracking forms, real-time database tracking, adaptation interview guide,[76] cross sectional surveys,[26] observations,[92] semi-structured interviews and focus groups,[93] summary of meeting and field notes, case logs, email/telephone correspondence, project records, site visits,[94] examination of the EBI manuals and training protocols,[95] and policy documents.[96] In one study, therapists answered session-specific surveys for a specific number of clients to report the adaptations made with simple prompts of "yes" or "no" to the question "in this session, did you adapt (the intervention) for this client?" and had the opportunity to provide an open-ended description of the adaptations they made.[68]

Frameworks for Documenting Adaptations of Interventions

Stirman and colleagues developed the expanded framework for reporting adaptations and modifications to evidence-based interventions (FRAME).[11] According to this framework, adaptations can occur at multiple levels and can be driven by different stakeholders. Thus, complete documentation involves identifying the "Who, What, When, Where (e.g., level of delivery), Why, and How", along with other important factors such as the nature of the adaptation, and whether the adaptations preserved fidelity to the intervention's core elements and functions. Identifying who initiated the adaptation (e.g., the provider, the organization, a coalition of stakeholders, the treatment developer, the clients, or target population) is important, because it is possible that who decides which adaptations to make, and when and how adaptations are made may have an impact on how effective they are. Content-level adaptations focus on the intervention itself. They can vary from very minor changes to an intervention that leaves all major intervention principles or components intact (tailoring) to more significant adaptations such as removing or adding components or integrating other approaches into the intervention. Rather than specifying cultural adaptation as a separate form of content-level adaptation, the FRAME added a code to indicate the broad goal for the adaptation and the reasons why a particular adaptation was made may be necessary to increase clarity about the types of cultural adaptations that are made.[69]

Some of the forms of adaptation described in the framework can be seen as enhancing or augmenting the intervention, while others may reduce or simplify it.[97] These adaptations can be further classified as fidelity-consistent, and fidelity-inconsistent, depending on the requirements of the intervention itself.[20] Whether an adaptation is fidelity-consistent or inconsistent can be determined based on theory that specifies core components for an intervention. The goal of such exploration would be to inform subsequent implementation efforts by specifying which aspects of the intervention are necessary to preserve desired outcomes, and how to adapt in a fidelity-consistent manner for a given population or setting.

Tracking modifications at the strategies level is also important. Based on the FRAME, the FRAME for Implementation Strategies (FRAME-IS)[12] was developed to more specifically document adaptations that are made to implementation strategies. Just as in the case of interventions, differences in context, available resources, or other key factors may necessitate changes to an implementation strategy. Understanding the impact of these adaptations is crucial to ensuring that the field can understand the degree of flexibility with which implementation strategies can be effective. Some implementation strategies have been identified through processes such as the Experts Recommendations for Implementing Change (ERIC) list of implementation strategies,[98] but have not been well-characterized and may vary in how they are executed. The FRAME-IS is best used with implementation strategies that have been developed and specified such that core functions and elements are identifiable, either through the original manual and fidelity assessment materials, or through the procedures that have been set forth in projects designed to research or implement specific strategies. It includes similar elements as the FRAME (e.g., Who, What, When, Why, How), and can be used in a modular fashion to maximize its practicality across implementation projects with a variety of goals, priorities, and available resources.

There is a robust literature in the context of policy and climate change interventions that can provide some learning to implementation scientists. For example, to track adaptations at the policy level, Olazabal et al.[99] developed the Adaptation Policy Credibility (APC) conceptual and operational assessment framework. The APC framework has three main areas: Policy and Economic Credibility, Scientific and Technical Credibility, and Legitimacy, which is common to the first two. Policy and Economic credibility is divided into three components: resources (funding, consistency, prioritization and timing), reliability (past performance, assigned responsibilities), and institutional, public and private support (public opinion, legislation and regulatory nature, network membership, leadership and support). Scientific and technical credibility encompasses usable knowledge (impacts and vulnerability assessment, adaptation options assessment), monitoring, evaluation and reporting processes, adaptive management (learning mechanisms, uncertainty awareness). Finally, Legitimacy entails transparency and dialogue, engagement of stakeholders and civil society, and equity and justice metrics. Figure 8.1 shows an adapted version of FRAME, including components about equity (outcomes) and policy (what is adapted).

EVALUATING THE ADAPTED INTERVENTIONS AND STRATEGIES

The evaluation of the adapted intervention and strategies should be informed by the context and goals of the adaptation. Below we describe considerations regarding assessment of outcomes, measurement issues, and design approaches.

Considerations About Measurement and Measures

When evaluating the adapted interventions or strategies, care should be taken when selecting the measures to be used. Measurement is still an area that needs much attention in the implementation science field as we are still developing and testing psychometric valid measures for several implementation outcomes.[100–102] When selecting the right approach to identify adaptations, it is important to determine which method (e.g., record review, interview, observation) and data source (e.g., client, provider) will yield the most accurate information. No single method is likely to be optimal. For example, observation may capture adaptations that were not documented and therefore missed in record reviews. But record reviews or interviews can shed light on what occurs when observers aren't present—such as extending the length of time or number of sessions over which an intervention occurs or insight into which personnel make adaptations or provide the intervention as a matter of routine. This is why triangulation of methods and data sources is generally recommended, with careful assessment of which approach is likely to provide accurate information about different aspects of the adaptation process. We call attention to the fact that silence in the discussion of measurements in the implementation field is the cultural context of such measures. When selecting measures, it is important to be thoughtful about how these were developed and with which populations they were validated to prevent errors in measurement equivalence.[103]

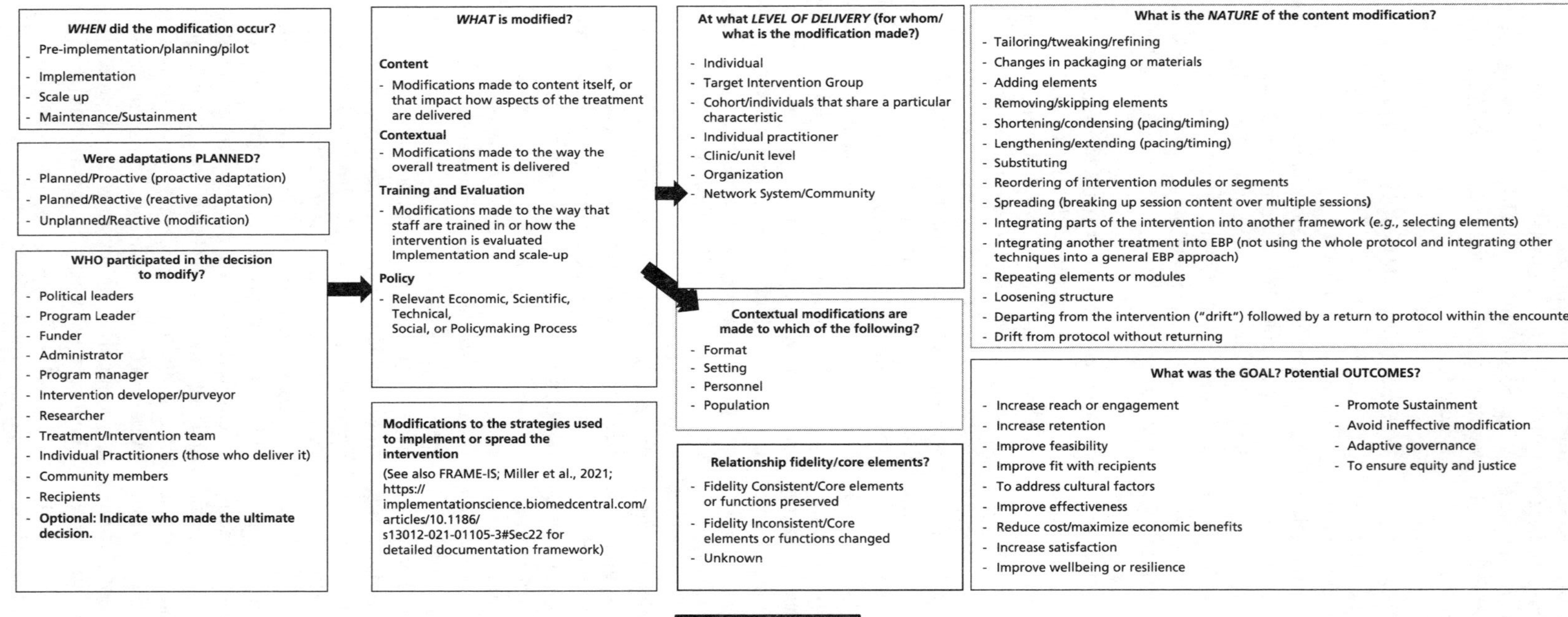

FIGURE 8.1 The Framework for Reporting Adaptations and Modifications-Expanded (FRAME).

Reprinted with permission from: Wiltsey Stirman S, Baumann AA, Miller CJ. The FRAME: an expanded framework for reporting adaptations and modifications to evidence-based interventions. *Implement Sci.* 2019;14(1):58.

Criteria for Evaluation: Outcomes to Consider

To examine the effect of the adapted intervention, an evaluation may occur through a medical record or administrative data review, or through systematically monitoring outcomes. Information on appointment attendance (engagement), satisfaction, and symptoms, functioning, or behaviors that the intervention is intended to target are examples of important recipient-level potential outcomes to consider. By systematically evaluating the effects of the adapted intervention on processes of care and client outcomes, one can ensure that the adaptations are effective, and that the effective core elements or functions of the intervention are maintained. In addition to recipient-level outcomes, several implementation outcomes (e.g., acceptability, equity, adaption, sustainment) can be evaluated to understand the impact of adaptations. Stakeholder input should guide decisions about which health and implementation outcomes to evaluate.

Fidelity, covered in detail in chapter 7, is an implementation outcome that is often assessed, because it helps stakeholders understand the degree to which the essential aspects of the intervention were retained during the implementation process. In light of the tension between fidelity and adaptation that we discussed above, assessing adaptation and fidelity simultaneously allows researchers to better characterize the content of the intervention to be more inclusive and provide a shared language and understanding for how to code intervention elements when changes have occurred. Additionally, it allows for careful consideration of whether adaptations were consistent with the core elements and functions of the intervention, or if they changed the intervention in a more fundamental way. If the health outcomes were not as robust as expected, understanding whether core functions were present even after adaptation is critical to understanding what may need to change in future efforts. It is also important to note that in behavioral interventions, fidelity is evaluated by examining interactions between people, and as such it can be subjective. As such, examining contextual factors when examining fidelity (i.e., the interactions of providers and clients, as well as the contextual factors of fidelity raters) is crucial because, for example, studies that code interactions between parents and children found that coders of different ethnicities and race than the parents viewed the interactions of parents and children differently compared to those with similar ethnicity and race, despite intensive trainings to reach reliability.[104–106] This is an important methodological consideration, since it has implications for how a potential criterion for successful implementation (fidelity) is evaluated.

Other possible outcomes that may matter to key stakeholders include improvement of fit, feasibility, acceptability, or to promote access and equity.[11] Outcomes related to social determinants of health are also important to consider.[107] In a review of climate change interventions that have been adapted, for example, Eriksen and colleagues[73] clearly remind us that, if interventions are adapted in a top-down approach, without engaging the community from the beginning, the adapted interventions may contribute to reinforcing, redistributing or creating yet other sources of inequity. Part of what the field of adaptation needs to grapple with is on how to define the success of adapted interventions.

One perspective in helping examine the effect of the adapted interventions is based on the framework outlined by Singh et al.[108] They propose 11 aspects to help scholars interrogate the effectiveness of climate change adapted interventions, which could be used for other interventions as well, and which we adapt somewhat for implementation of other interventions with our edits in brackets. Their points are: (1) maximizing economic benefits (adaptation should minimize costs and maximize benefits); (2) improved wellbeing (adaptation should support achievement of material, subjective, and relational wellbeing goals); (3) vulnerability reduction or adaptive capacity enhancement (adaptation should reduce vulnerability and/or increase adaptive capacity, especially of the most vulnerable and those most at risk); (4) enhanced resilience (adaptation should increase resilience by building functional persistence over long timescales so that systems have the ability to bounce back from climatic [or political or economic] shocks); (5) sustainable adaptation (adaptation should be economically, ecologically, and socially sustainable, explicitly looking at longer-term, cross-generational viability of adaptation actions); (6) avoiding maladaptation (adaptation should take into account unintended negative consequences and explicitly look at the long-term impacts of adaptation actions); (7) ecosystem-based adaptation (adaptation should invest in ecosystem conservation, management and restoration to enhance ecosystem services, and subsequently reduce impacts of climate change on social and ecological systems [adaptation should reduce the burden of the targeted health problems from the community]); (8) community-based adaptation (adaptation prioritization, implementation, and monitoring should be co-produced with communities to ensure inclusive and sustainable adaptation); (9) adaptive governance (adaptation should be oriented towards achieving transparency, accountability and representation in governance [representation in decision making pre and during the implementation process] through multi-scalar, participatory, and inclusive processes); (10) ensuring equity and justice (adaptation should be oriented toward socially just and equitable processes and outcomes); (11) transformation (adaptation should be a process that generate equity). In summary—it is only by thinking carefully about the goals of adaptation, who is supporting the process and evaluation of adaptation and carefully monitoring the implementation process that we will be able to achieve a social justice approach in the science of adaptations.

Design Considerations

Chapter 14 describes the different designs with details. When considering designs to test the impact of adaptations, it is important to think about the relationships between potential moderators of outcomes and the impact of adaptations designed to address them. Expanding on the selection of the outcomes that may be important to measure, we should not forget about social determinants of health. For example, high levels of psychosocial stressors such as economic instability may require adaptation of a parenting intervention (e.g., adding modules on managing stress) and may in and of themselves impact parenting practices (e.g., harsh discipline). In treatments for depression and other disorders, psychosocial stressors (e.g., unemployment, housing instability, food insecurity) or comorbidities can diminish treatment engagement and participation. Specific adaptations to address such factors may enhance the outcome of these interventions, or it may be the case that moderators of outcomes are not completely addressed by the adaptations. The potential interrelationship between these moderators, adaptations, and outcomes should be considered when designing the methods and analysis. The timing of data collection and identification of adaptations should also be carefully considered when planning for the evaluation of the study to establish temporal precedence of an adaptation and changes in symptoms, functioning, or other outcomes, and to facilitate analyses to explore mediation and moderation.

If examining outcomes in routine care, designs such as the use of plan-do-study-act (PDSA) cycles, which include evaluation of the impact of adaptation[62] may be of interest. This process allows ongoing examination of practice-level data to determine whether the adaptation is having the desired impact and can be used when more formal research is impractical. Ongoing evaluation of this nature allows real-time refinement of interventions through the PDSA process, and when combined with careful documentation of the nature of the adaptations that are made, it can be used optimize outcomes in practice settings. While PDSA cycles can be used in routine care settings, evaluation in the context of implementation research may also be more comprehensive and on a larger scale.

In most of the research on adaptation to date, the efficacy of the adapted intervention has been studied through randomized control trials (RCTs) comparing the adapted intervention to usual care.[109] Because RCTs are designed to control for contextual and patient-level differences, other types of designs have been proposed to test adaptation of interventions in routine care settings. Two of them are the SMART (Sequential Multiple Assignment Randomized Trial; SMART) and the Multiphase Optimization Strategy (MOST). For further details on these designs, we direct the reader to chapter 14 and the review by Collins and al.[110]

Alternatively, methodologies that allow aggregation of evidence from different trials can capitalize on large samples and evaluate what has worked for whom and under which conditions.[111] Coordinated trials of behavioral interventions have been conducted in which the interventions are different, but the targeted outcomes and population groups are similar, allowing the evaluation of different approaches and potential mechanisms of action.[112] By choosing a framework to describe different components of the interventions, one can then link each component with the outcomes, facilitating identification of the active intervention or adaptations that promote behavior change.[111–113] Other scholars have advocated for the use of dashboards to track outcomes metrics and support the evaluation of multiple trials.[87]

Importantly, we advocate for the use of mixed methods should be strongly considered to supplement and enhance quantitative evaluation with qualitative evaluation,[114] both in research and practice contexts. Feedback from stakeholders can inform hypotheses about unexpected results or further adaptation that might be necessary.[115] Qualitative data can also provide information about whether the intent and goals of adaptation were met from the perspective of multiple stakeholders. More details about mixed method designs can be found in chapter 18.

SUMMARY

This chapter focused on adaptations in the context of D&I research and practice. Consistent with the existing literature, we recommend that adaptations be proactively and iteratively determined, informed by a variety of stakeholders, and that efforts be made to carefully describe and document the nature of the adaptations and evaluate their impact on desired service, health, and implementation outcomes.

We expect that in the coming years, more research findings on the impact of adaptations at multiple levels will become available, and that studies of the process of adaptation will elucidate best practices that maximize the likelihood of implementation success. Furthermore, development of methodologies to evaluate the impact of different types of adaptations will eventually provide guidance that can inform efforts to make appropriate adaptations to different forms of interventions and in different practice contexts.[27] Such advances can lead to more rapid and successful implementation of effective interventions in a manner that can fulfill the promise of EBIs for reducing health and health care inequities.

SUGGESTED READINGS AND WEBSITES

Readings

Cabassa, L. J., & Baumann, A. A. (2013). A two-way street: bridging implementation science and cultural adaptations of mental health treatments. *Implementation Science, 8*(1), 90.

This paper discusses how implementation science and the field of cultural adaptation contribute valuable insights and methods on how empirically-supported treatments and/or context can be customized to enhance implementation across routine practice settings and different populations. The development of a two-way street between the fields of implementation science and cultural adaptations of mental health treatments provides a critical avenue for transporting empirically-supported treatments into practice and for reducing racial and ethnic disparities in mental health care.

Chambers, A. & Norton, W. E. (2016). The adaptome: advancing the science of intervention adaptation. *American Journal of Preventive Medicine, 51*(4), S124-S131.

This paper presents a framework and research agenda to advance the science of adaption in the context of implementation. It introduces the idea of developing the adaptome, a data platform used to systematically capture and house information about the variations in the delivery of empirically-supported interventions and programs across multiple settings, populations and communities and provide critical feedback to intervention developers as well as researchers and practitioners involved in implementation efforts.

Baumann, A. A., & Cabassa, L. J. (2020). Reframing implementation science to address inequities in healthcare delivery. *BMC Health Services Research, 20*(1), 1-9.

In this paper the authors show how one implementation science framework (Proctor et al., 2019) could be expanded to have an equity lens through 1) focusing on reach from the very beginning; 2) designing and selecting interventions for vulnerable populations and low-resource communities with implementation in mind; 3) implementing what works and develop implementation strategies that can help reduce inequities in care; 4) developing the science of adaptations; and 5) using an equity lens for implementation outcomes.

Miller, C. J., Barnett, M. L., Baumann, A. A., Gutner, C. A., & Wiltsey-Stirman, S. (2021). The FRAME-IS: a framework for documenting modifications to implementation strategies in healthcare. *Implementation Science, 16*(1), 1-12.

This paper describes the framework for reporting adaptations and modifications to implementation strategies.

Wiltsey Stirman, S., Baumann, A. A., & Miller, C. J. (2019). The FRAME: an expanded framework for reporting adaptations and modifications to evidence-based interventions. *Implementation Science, 14*(1), 1-10.

This paper describes the framework for reporting adaptations and modifications to evidence-based interventions.

Selected Websites and Tools

Webinar about rapid cycle research:

https://pbrn.ahrq.gov/events/using-rapid-cycle-research-reach-goals-awareness-assessment-adaptation-acceleration-resource

This is a webinar supported by the Agency for Healthcare Research and Quality, delivered by Drs. Gustafson and Johnson. The webinar titled "Using rapid-cycle research to reach goals: Awareness, assessment, adaptation, acceleration—a resource document" describes methods for identifying problems and solving issues using a rapid cycle research.

Webinar about the evidence base for implementation: https://cancercontrol.cancer.gov/use_what_works/start.htm

This is a set of materials organized by the National Cancer Institute with four modules: (1) What do we mean by evidence-based?, (2) Needs Assessment, (3) Finding an evidence-based program, (4) Making the evidence-based program fit your needs: adaptation and your program summary, (5) Does it work? Module 4 contains an adaptation guideline and recommendations for pilot testing.

TIDIRC video about adaptation:

Baumann, A. A., & Wiltsey Stirman, S. (April 2021). NCI video training, Module 7: Adaptation & Fidelity of Interventions in Implementation Science. Link: https://cancercontrol.cancer.gov/is/training-education/training-in-cancer/TIDIRC-open-access/module-7

In this video, Drs. Baumann and Wiltsey Stirman talk about context, adaptation and fidelity

Youtube video about FRAME-IS:

Miller, C., Barnett, M. L., Baumann, A., Gutner, C. A., Wiltsey-Stirman, S. (2021). FRAME-IS: Tracking adaptations to implementation strategies. Link: https://www.youtube.com/watch?v=7xTzQukiG6s

In this video, Drs. Miller, Barnett, Baumann, Gutner and Wiltsey Stirman talk about context, adaptation, fidelity and describe how to use FRAME-IS to track implementation strategies

References

1. Baumann AA, Cabassa LJ. Reframing implementation science to address inequities in healthcare delivery. *BMC Health Serv Res.* 2020;20(1):190. doi:10.1186/s12913-020-4975-3
2. Shelton RC, Adsul P, Oh A, Moise A, Griffith D. Application of an anti-racism lens in the field of implementation science: Recommendations for reframing implementation research with a focus on justice and racial equity. *Implement Res Pract.* 2021;2. https://doi.org/10.1177/26334895211049482
3. Brownson RC, Kumanyika SK, Kreuter MW, Haire-Joshu D. Implementation science should give higher priority to health equity. *Implement Sci.* 2021;16(1):28. doi:10.1186/s13012-021-01097-0
4. Kerkhoff AD, Farrand E, Marquez C, Cattamanchi A, Handley MA. Addressing health disparities through implementation science—a need to integrate an equity lens from the outset. *Implement Sci.* 2022;17(1):13. doi:10.1186/s13012-022-01189-5
5. American Psychology Association Task Analysis Force on Psychological Intervention Guidelines. *Inclusive Language Guidelines.* Washington, DC; 2021:27. https://www.apa.org/about/apa/equity-diversity-inclusion/language-guidelines.pdf
6. Paul GL. Strategy of outcome research in psychotherapy. *J Consult Psychol.* 1967;31(2):109.
7. Cabassa L, Baumann A. A two-way street: bridging implementation science and cultural adaptations of mental health treatments *Implement Sci IS.* 2013;8(1):1–14. doi:https://doi.org/10.1186/1748-5908-8-90
8. Shelton RC, Chambers DA, Glasgow RE. An extension of RE-AIM to enhance sustainability: addressing dynamic context and promoting health equity over time. *Front Public Health.* 2020;8:134. https://doi.org/10.3389/fpubh.2020.00134
9. Bernal G, Domenech Rodríguez MM. Cultural adaptations: Tools for evidence-based practice with diverse populations. In: Bernal G, Domenech Rodriguez M, eds. *Cultural Adaptation in Context: Psychotherapy as a Historical Account of Adaptations.* American Psychological Association; 2012:3–22. https://doi.org/10.1037/13752-001
10. Aarons GA, Miller EA, Green AE, Perrott JA, Bradway R. Adaptation happens: a qualitative case study of implementation of The Incredible Years evidence-based parent training programme in a residential substance abuse treatment programme. *J Child Serv.*

Published online 2012;7(4):233–245. https://doi.org/10.1108/17466661211286463
11. Wiltsey Stirman S, Baumann AA, Miller CJ. The FRAME: An expanded framework for reporting adaptations and modifications to evidence-based interventions. *Implement Sci IS.* 2019;14:58. https://doi.org/10.1186/s13012-019-0898-y
12. Miller CJ, Barnett ML, Baumann AA, Gutner CA, Wiltsey-Stirman S. The FRAME-IS: a framework for documenting modifications to implementation strategies in healthcare. *Implement Sci.* 2021;16(1):36. doi:10.1186/s13012-021-01105-3
13. Movsisyan A, Arnold L, Evans R, et al. Adapting evidence-informed complex population health interventions for new contexts: a systematic review of guidance. *Implement Sci.* 2019;14(1):105. doi:10.1186/s13012-019-0956-5
14. Kirk MA, Moore JE, Wiltsey Stirman S, Birken SA. Towards a comprehensive model for understanding adaptations' impact: the model for adaptation design and impact (MADI). *Implement Sci.* 2020;15(1):56. doi:10.1186/s13012-020-01021-y
15. Miller CJ, Wiltsey Stirman S, Baumann AA. Iterative Decision-making for Evaluation of Adaptations (IDEA): A decision tree for balancing adaptation, fidelity, and intervention impact. *J Community Psychol.* 2020;48(4):1163–1177. doi:https://doi.org/10.1002/jcop.22279
16. Damschroder LJ, Aron DC, Keith RE, Kirsh SR, Alexander JA, Lowery JC. Fostering implementation of health services research findings into practice: a consolidated framework for advancing implementation science. *Implement Sci IS.* 2009;4:50. doi:10.1186/1748-5908-4-50
17. Bernal G, Bonilla J, Bellido C. Ecological validity and cultural sensitivity for outcome research: Issues for the cultural adaptation and development of psychosocial treatments with Hispanics. *J Abnorm Child Psychol.* 1995;23(1):67–82.
18. Domenech Rodriguez M, Wieling E. Developing culturally appropriate, evidence-based treatments for interventions with ethnic minority populations. In: Rastogi M, Wieling E, eds. *Voices of Color: First-Person Accounts of Ethnic Minority Therapists.* SAGE; 2005:313–334.
19. Shelton RC, Cooper BR, Stirman SW. The Sustainability of Evidence-Based Interventions and Practices in Public Health and Health Care. *Annu Rev Public Health.* 2018;39(1):55–76. doi:10.1146/annurev-publhealth-040617-014731
20. Wiltsey Stirman S, A Gutner C, Crits-Christoph P, Edmunds J, Evans AC, Beidas RS. Relationships between clinician-level attributes and fidelity-consistent and fidelity-inconsistent modifications to an evidence-based psychotherapy. *Implement Sci.* 2015;10(1):1–10.
21. Perez Jolles M, Lengnick-Hall R, Mittman BS. Core Functions and Forms of Complex Health Interventions: a Patient-Centered Medical Home Illustration. *J Gen Intern Med.* 2019;34(6):1032–1038. doi:10.1007/s11606-018-4818-7
22. Pfadenhauer LM, Gerhardus A, Mozygemba K, et al. Making sense of complexity in context and implementation: the Context and Implementation of Complex Interventions (CICI) framework. *Implement Sci.* 2017;12(1):1–17.
23. U.S. Department of Health and Human ServicesFood and Drug Administration. *Adaptive Designs for Clinical Trials of Drugs and Biologics.* Center for Drug Evaluation and Research (CDER), Center for Biologics Evaluation and Research (CBER); 2019:37. https://www.fda.gov/media/78495/download
24. Kumpfer KL, Alvarado R, Smith P, Bellamy N. Cultural Sensitivity and Adaptation in Family-Based Prevention Interventions. *Prev Sci.* 2002;3:241–246.
25. Aarons GA, Hurlburt M, Horwitz SM. Advancing a Conceptual Model of Evidence-Based Practice Implementation in Public Service Sectors. *Adm Policy Ment Health Ment Health Serv Res.* 2011;38(1):4–23. doi:10.1007/s10488-010-0327-7
26. von Thiele Schwarz U, Giannotta F, Neher M, Zetterlund J, Hasson H. Professionals' management of the fidelity–adaptation dilemma in the use of evidence-based interventions—an intervention study. *Implement Sci Commun.* 2021;2(1):1–9.
27. Chambers DA, Norton WE. The adaptome: advancing the science of intervention adaptation. *Am J Prev Med.* 2016;51(4):S124–S131.
28. Nilsen P, Bernhardsson S. Context matters in implementation science: a scoping review of determinant frameworks that describe contextual determinants for implementation outcomes. *BMC Health Serv Res.* 2019;19(1):189. doi:10.1186/s12913-019-4015-3
29. Woodward EN, Matthieu MM, Uchendu US, Rogal S, Kirchner JE. The health equity implementation framework: proposal and preliminary study of hepatitis C virus treatment. *Implement Sci.* 2019;14(1):26. doi:10.1186/s13012-019-0861-y
30. Perera C, Salamanca-Sanabria A, Caballero-Bernal J, et al. No implementation without cultural adaptation: a process for culturally adapting low-intensity psychological interventions in humanitarian settings. *Confl Health.* 2020;14(1):46. doi:10.1186/s13031-020-00290-0
31. Arundell LL, Barnett P, Buckman JEJ, Saunders R, Pilling S. The effectiveness of adapted psychological interventions for people from

ethnic minority groups: A systematic review and conceptual typology. *Clin Psychol Rev.* 2021;88:102063. doi:10.1016/j.cpr.2021.102063

32. Chowdhary N, Jotheeswaran AT, Nadkarni A, et al. The methods and outcomes of cultural adaptations of psychological treatments for depressive disorders: a systematic review. *Psychol Med.* 2014;44(6):1131–1146. doi:10.1017/S0033291713001785
33. Benish SG, Quintana S, Wampold BE. Culturally adapted psychotherapy and the legitimacy of myth: a direct-comparison meta-analysis. *J Couns Psychol.* 2011;58(3):279–289.
34. Atkins L, Francis J, Islam R, et al. A guide to using the Theoretical Domains Framework of behaviour change to investigate implementation problems. *Implement Sci.* 2017;12(1):77. doi:10.1186/s13012-017-0605-9
35. Tanenbaum SJ. Evidence-based practice as mental health policy: Three controversies and a caveat. *Health Aff (Millwood).* 2005;24(1):163–173.
36. Raghavan R. The role of economic evaluation in dissemination and implementation research. *Dissem Implement Res Health Transl Sci Pract.* 2012;2:89–106.
37. Shelton RC, Adsul P, Oh A. Recommendations for Addressing Structural Racism in Implementation Science: A Call to the Field. *Ethn Dis.* 2021;31(Suppl):357–364. doi:10.18865/ed.31.S1.357
38. Parra-Cardona R, Fuentes-Balderrama J, Vanderziel A, et al. A Culturally Adapted Parenting Intervention for Mexican-Origin Immigrant Families with Adolescents: Integrating Science, Culture, and a Focus on Immigration-Related Adversity. *Prev Sci.* 2022;23(2):271–282. doi:10.1007/s11121-021-01317-5
39. Domenech Rodríguez MM, Baumann AA, Schwartz AL. Cultural adaptation of an evidence based intervention: from theory to practice in a Latino/a community context. *Am J Community Psychol.* 2011;47(1-2):170–186. doi:10.1007/s10464-010-9371-4
40. Shelton RC, Brotzman LE, Johnson D, Erwin D. Trust and Mistrust in Shaping Adaptation and De-Implementation in the Context of Changing Screening Guidelines. *Ethn Dis.* 2021;31(1):119–132. doi:10.18865/ed.31.1.119
41. Smith AC, Woerner J, Perera R, Haeny AM, Cox JM. An investigation of associations between race, ethnicity, and past experiences of discrimination with medical mistrust and COVID-19 protective strategies. *J Racial Ethn Health Disparities.* 2022;9(4):1430–1442.
42. CDC. Data and Statistics on Children's Mental Health | CDC. Centers for Disease Control and Prevention. Published April 19, 2019. Accessed March 15, 2020. https://www.cdc.gov/childrensmentalhealth/data.html
43. Byrd DA, Rivera Mindt MM, Clark US, et al. Creating an antiracist psychology by addressing professional complicity in psychological assessment. *Psychol Assess.* 2021;33(3):279.
44. La Roche MJ. Changing multicultural guidelines: Clinical and research implications for evidence-based psychotherapies. *Prof Psychol Res Pract.* 2021;52(2):111–120. doi:10.1037/pro0000347
45. Denizard-Thompson N, Palakshappa D, Vallevand A, et al. Association of a Health Equity Curriculum With Medical Students' Knowledge of Social Determinants of Health and Confidence in Working With Underserved Populations. *JAMA Netw Open.* 2021;4(3):e210297–e210297. doi:10.1001/jamanetworkopen.2021.0297
46. Galea S. The Price of Health Equity. *JAMA Health Forum.* 2021;2(4):e210720–e210720. doi:10.1001/jamahealthforum.2021.0720
47. Borras AM. Toward an Intersectional Approach to Health Justice. *Int J Health Serv.* 2021;51(2):206–225. doi:10.1177/0020731420981857
48. Fraser N. Chapter one reframing justice in a globalizing world Nancy Fraser. In Julie Connolly, Michael Leach & Lucas Walsh, eds. *Recognition in Politics: Theory, Policy and Practice.* Cambridge Scholars Press; 2007:16.
49. Hodge LM, Turner KM. Sustained implementation of evidence-based programs in disadvantaged communities: A conceptual framework of supporting factors. *Am J Community Psychol.* 2016;58(1-2):192–210.
50. Rawls J. *A Theory of Justice.* Harvard university press; 2020. https://doi.org/10.4159/9780674042605
51. Daniels N. Justice, Health, and Healthcare. *Am J Bioeth.* 2001;1(2):2–16. doi:10.1162/152651601300168834
52. Colditz GA, Emmons KM. The role of universal health coverage in reducing cancer deaths and disparities. *The Lancet.* 2016;388(10045):638–640. doi:10.1016/S0140-6736(16)30376-2
53. Aisenberg E. Evidence-Based Practice in Mental Health Care to Ethnic Minority Communities. *J Child Youth Care Work.* 2012;24:90–106.
54. Cabassa LJ. Implementation science: Why it matters for the future of social work. *J Soc Work Educ.* 2016;52(supl):S38–S50.
55. Weisz JR, Ng MY, Bearman SK. Odd couple? Reenvisioning the relation between science and practice in the dissemination-implementation era. *Clin Psychol Sci.* 2014;2(1):58–74.
56. Rogers EM, Singhal A, Quinlan MM. *Diffusion of Innovations.* Routledge; 2014.

57. Bastida EM, Tseng TS, McKeever C, Jack Jr L. Ethics and community-based participatory research: perspectives from the field. *Health Promot Pract.* 2010;11(1):16–20.
58. Elliott DS, Mihalic S. Issues in disseminating and replicating effective prevention programs. *Prev Sci.* 2004;5(1):47–53.
59. Hogue A, Ozechowski TJ, Robbins MS, Waldron HB. Making fidelity an intramural game: Localizing quality assurance procedures to promote sustainability of evidence-based practices in usual care. *Clin Psychol Sci Pract.* 2013;20(1):60.
60. Stirman SW, Miller CJ, Toder K, Calloway A. Development of a framework and coding system for modifications and adaptations of evidence-based interventions. *Implement Sci.* 2013;8(1):1–12.
61. Waltz TJ, Powell BJ, Fernández ME, Abadie B, Damschroder LJ. Choosing implementation strategies to address contextual barriers: diversity in recommendations and future directions. *Implement Sci.* 2019;14(1):1–15.
62. Chambers DA, Glasgow RE, Stange KC. The dynamic sustainability framework: addressing the paradox of sustainment amid ongoing change. *Implement Sci.* 2013;8(1):1–11.
63. Pérez D, Van der Stuyft P, Zabala M del C, Castro M, Lefèvre P. A modified theoretical framework to assess implementation fidelity of adaptive public health interventions. *Implement Sci.* 2015;11(1):1–11.
64. Marques L, Valentine SE, Kaysen D, et al. Provider fidelity and modifications to cognitive processing therapy in a diverse community health clinic: Associations with clinical change. *J Consult Clin Psychol.* 2019;87(4):357.
65. Barrera M, Berkel C, Castro FG. Directions for the advancement of culturally adapted preventive interventions: Local adaptations, engagement, and sustainability. *Prev Sci.* 2017;18(6):640–648.
66. Edmunds SR, Frost KM, Sheldrick RC, et al. A method for defining the CORE of a psychosocial intervention to guide adaptation in practice: Reciprocal imitation teaching as a case example. *Autism.* 2022;26(3):601–614. https://doi.org/10.1177/13623613211064431
67. Aschbrenner KA, Mueller NM, Banerjee S, Bartels SJ. Applying an equity lens to characterizing the process and reasons for an adaptation to an evidenced-based practice. *Implement Res Pract.* 2021;2:26334895211017252. doi:10.1177/26334895211017252
68. Kim JJ, Brookman-Frazee L, Barnett ML, et al. How community therapists describe adapting evidence-based practices in sessions for youth: Augmenting to improve fit and reach. *J Community Psychol.* 2020;48(4):1238–1257. doi:10.1002/jcop.22333
69. Stanton B, Guo J, Cottrell L, et al. The complex business of adapting effective interventions to new populations: An urban to rural transfer. *J Adolesc Health.* 2005;37(2):163.
70. Wiltsey Stirman S, Gamarra JM, Bartlett BA, Calloway A, Gutner CA. Empirical examinations of modifications and adaptations to evidence-based psychotherapies: Methodologies, impact, and future directions. *Clin Psychol Sci Pract.* 2017;24(4):396.
71. Sundell K, Beelmann A, Hasson H, von Thiele Schwarz U. Novel programs, international adoptions, or contextual adaptations? Meta-analytical results from German and Swedish intervention research. *J Clin Child Adolesc Psychol.* 2016;45(6):784–796.
72. Cabassa LJ, Manrique Y, Meyreles Q, et al. Bridges to Better Health and Wellness: An Adapted Health Care Manager Intervention for Hispanics with Serious Mental Illness. *Adm Policy Ment Health Ment Health Serv Res.* 2018;45(1):163–173. doi:10.1007/s10488-016-0781-y
73. Eriksen S, Schipper ELF, Scoville-Simonds M, et al. Adaptation interventions and their effect on vulnerability in developing countries: Help, hindrance or irrelevance? *World Dev.* 2021;141:105383. doi:10.1016/j.worlddev.2020.105383
74. Baumann AA, Rodríguez MMD, Amador NG, Forgatch MS, Parra-Cardona JR. Parent Management Training-Oregon Model (PMTO™) in Mexico City: Integrating Cultural Adaptation Activities in an Implementation Model. *Clin Psychol Sci Pract.* 2014;21(1):194. doi:10.1111/cpsp.12059
75. Cabassa LJ, Stefancic A, Bochicchio L, Tuda D, Weatherly C, Lengnick-Hall R. Organization leaders' decisions to sustain a peer-led healthy lifestyle intervention for people with serious mental illness in supportive housing. *Transl Behav Med.* 2021;11(5):1151–1159.
76. Rabin BA, McCreight M, Battaglia C, et al. Systematic, Multimethod Assessment of Adaptations Across Four Diverse Health Systems Interventions. *Front Public Health.* 2018;6:102. https://doi.org/10.3389/fpubh.2018.00102
77. Kilbourne AM, Switzer G, Hyman K, Crowley-Matoka M, Fine MJ. Advancing Health Disparities Research Within the Health Care System: A Conceptual Framework. *Am J Public Health.* 2006;96(12):2113–2121. doi:10.2105/AJPH.2005.077628
78. Kraft JM, Mezoff JS, Sogolow ED, Neumann MS, Thomas PA. A technology transfer model for

effective HIV/AIDS interventions: Science and practice. *AIDS Educ Prev.* 2000;12:7–20.
79. Lau AS. Making the case for selective and directed cultural adaptations of evidence-based treatments: Examples from parent training. *Clin Psychol Sci Pract.* 2006;13(4):295–310.
80. Aarons GA, Sklar M, Mustanski B, Benbow N, Brown CH. "Scaling-out" evidence-based interventions to new populations or new health care delivery systems. *Implement Sci.* 2017;12(1):111. doi:10.1186/s13012-017-0640-6
81. Harvey AG, Lammers HS, Dolsen MR, et al. Systematic review to examine the methods used to adapt evidence-based psychological treatments for adults diagnosed with a mental illness. *Evid Based Ment Health.* 2021;24(1):33–40. doi:10.1136/ebmental-2020-300225
82. Escoffery C, Lebow-Skelley E, Haardoerfer R, et al. A systematic review of adaptations of evidence-based public health interventions globally. *Implement Sci.* 2018;13(1):1–21.
83. Stirman SW, Pontoski K, Creed T, et al. A non-randomized comparison of strategies for consultation in a community-academic training program to implement an evidence-based psychotherapy. *Adm Policy Ment Health Ment Health Serv Res.* 2017;44(1):55–66.
84. Barrera Jr M, Castro FG. A heuristic framework for the cultural adaptation of interventions. *Sci Pract.* 2006;13(4):311–316. https://doi.org/10.1111/j.1468-2850.2006.00043.x
85. Kreuter MW, Haughton LT. Integrating culture into health information for African American women. *Am Behav Sci.* 2006; 49(6):794–811.
86. Kreuter MW, Lukwago SN, Bucholtz DC, Clark EM, Sanders-Thompson V. Achieving cultural appropriateness in health promotion programs: targeted and tailored approaches. *Health Educ Behav.* 2003;30(2):133–146.
87. Aarons GA, Green AE, Palinkas LA, et al. Dynamic adaptation process to implement an evidence-based child maltreatment intervention. *Implement Sci.* 2012;7(1):32. doi:10.1186/1748-5908-7-32
88. Forgatch MS, Patterson GR, Gewirtz AH. Looking forward: The promise of widespread implementation of parent training programs. *Perspect Psychol Sci.* 2013;8(6):682–694.
89. Lyon AR, Koerner K. User-Centered Design for Psychosocial Intervention Development and Implementation. *Clin Psychol Publ Div Clin Psychol Am Psychol Assoc.* 2016;23(2):180–200. doi:10.1111/cpsp.12154
90. Courage C, Baxter K. *Understanding Your Users: A Practical Guide to User Requirements Methods, Tools, and Techniques.* Gulf Professional Publishing; 2005.
91. Cabassa LJ, Gomes AP, Meyreles Q, et al. Using the collaborative intervention planning framework to adapt a health-care manager intervention to a new population and provider group to improve the health of people with serious mental illness. *Implement Sci.* 2014;9(1):178. doi:10.1186/s13012-014-0178-9
92. van de Kolk I, Gerards S, Verhees A, Kremers S, Gubbels J. Changing the preschool setting to promote healthy energy balance-related behaviours of preschoolers: a qualitative and quantitative process evaluation of the SuperFIT approach. *Implement Sci.* 2021;16(1):101. doi:10.1186/s13012-021-01161-9
93. Lengnick-Hall R, Willging CE, Hurlburt MS, Aarons GA. Incorporators, Early Investors, and Learners: a longitudinal study of organizational adaptation during EBP implementation and sustainment. *Implement Sci.* 2020;15(1):74. doi:10.1186/s13012-020-01031-w
94. Harrison MB, Graham ID, van den Hoek J, Dogherty EJ, Carley ME, Angus V. Guideline adaptation and implementation planning: a prospective observational study. *Implement Sci.* 2013;8(1):49. doi:10.1186/1748-5908-8-49
95. Smith JD, Berkel C, Rudo-Stern J, et al. The Family Check-Up 4 Health (FCU4Health): Applying Implementation Science Frameworks to the Process of Adapting an Evidence-Based Parenting Program for Prevention of Pediatric Obesity and Excess Weight Gain in Primary Care. *Front Public Health.* 2018;6. doi:10.3389/fpubh.2018.00293
96. Ford JD, Berrang-Ford L. The 4Cs of adaptation tracking: consistency, comparability, comprehensiveness, coherency. *Mitig Adapt Strateg Glob Change.* 2016;21(6):839–859.
97. Lau A, Barnett M, Stadnick N, et al. Therapist report of adaptations to delivery of evidence-based practices within a system-driven reform of publicly funded children's mental health services. *J Consult Clin Psychol.* 2017;85(7):664–675.
98. Powell BJ, Waltz TJ, Chinman MJ, et al. A refined compilation of implementation strategies: results from the Expert Recommendations for Implementing Change (ERIC) project. *Implement Sci.* 2015;10(1):21. doi:10.1186/s13012-015-0209-1
99. Olazabal M, Galarraga I, Ford J, Sainz De Murieta E, Lesnikowski A. Are local climate adaptation policies credible? A conceptual and operational assessment framework. *Int J Urban Sustain Dev.* 2019;11(3):277–296.
100. Rabin BA, Lewis CC, Norton WE, et al. Measurement resources for dissemination and implementation research in health.

Implement Sci. 2016;11(1):42. doi:10.1186/s13012-016-0401-y

101. Mettert K, Lewis C, Dorsey C, Halko H, Weiner B. Measuring implementation outcomes: An updated systematic review of measures' psychometric properties. *Implement Res Pract.* 2020;1:2633489520936644. doi:10.1177/2633489520936644
102. Allen P, Pilar M, Walsh-Bailey C, et al. Quantitative measures of health policy implementation determinants and outcomes: a systematic review. *Implement Sci.* 2020;15(1):47. doi:10.1186/s13012-020-01007-w
103. Davidov E, Meuleman B, Cieciuch J, Schmidt P, Billiet J. Measurement equivalence in cross-national research. *Annu Rev Sociol.* 2014;40:55–75.
104. Costigan CL, Bardina P, Cauce AM, Kim GK, Latendresse SJ. Inter-and intra-group variability in perceptions of behavior among Asian Americans and European Americans. *Cultur Divers Ethnic Minor Psychol.* 2006;12(4):710.
105. Gonzales NA, Cauce AM, Mason CA. Interobserver agreement in the assessment of parental behavior and parent-adolescent conflict: African American mothers, daughters, and independent observers. *Child Dev.* 1996;67(4):1483–1498. doi:https://doi.org/10.1111/j.1467-8624.1996.tb01809.x
106. Yasui M, Dishion TJ. Direct observation of family management: Validity and reliability as a function of coder ethnicity and training. *Behav Ther.* 2008;39(4):336–347.
107. Baumann AA, Long PD. Equity in Implementation Science Is Long Overdue. *Stanf Soc Innov Rev.* 2021;19(3):A15–A17. doi:10.48558/GG1H-A223
108. Singh C, Iyer S, New MG, et al. Interrogating 'effectiveness' in climate change adaptation: 11 guiding principles for adaptation research and practice. *Clim Dev.* 2021;0(0):1–15. doi:10.1080/17565529.2021.1964937
109. Bell EC, Marcus DK, Goodlad JK. Are the parts as good as the whole? A meta-analysis of component treatment studies. *J Consult Clin Psychol.* 2013;81(4):722.
110. Collins LM, Murphy SA, Strecher V. The multiphase optimization strategy (MOST) and the sequential multiple assignment randomized trial (SMART): new methods for more potent eHealth interventions. *Am J Prev Med.* 2007;32(5):S112–S118.
111. Tate DF, Lytle LA, Sherwood NE, et al. Deconstructing interventions: approaches to studying behavior change techniques across obesity interventions. *Transl Behav Med.* 2016;6(2):236–243.
112. Belle SH, Stevens J, Cella D, et al. Overview of the obesity intervention taxonomy and pooled analysis working group. *Transl Behav Med.* 2016;6(2):244–259.
113. Bangdiwala SI, Bhargava A, O'Connor DP, et al. Statistical methodologies to pool across multiple intervention studies. *Transl Behav Med.* 2016;6(2):228–235.
114. Shelton RC, Philbin MM, Ramanadhan S. Qualitative Research Methods in Chronic Disease: Introduction and Opportunities to Promote Health Equity. *Annu Rev Public Health.* 2021;43:1.
115. Palinkas LA, Aarons GA, Horwitz S, Chamberlain P, Hurlburt M, Landsverk J. Mixed method designs in implementation research. *Adm Policy Ment Health Ment Health Serv Res.* 2011;38(1):44–53.

9

The Role of Organizational Processes in Dissemination and Implementation Research

GREGORY A. AARONS, MARK G. EHRHART, REBECCA LENGNICK-HALL, AND JOANNA C. MOULLIN

INTRODUCTION

The science of dissemination and implementation (D&I) is a swiftly growing field that commonly involves change at multiple levels, including both outer (i.e., system) and inner (i.e., organization) contexts.[1–3] The bulk of health, behavioral health, public health, and social services are delivered within or through organizations. This chapter aims to support researchers, implementers, and leaders in attending to and shaping the organizational and interrelated contexts in which implementation takes place to increase the likelihood of implementation success and long-term sustainment. Such attention must be strategic, consistent across organizational levels, goal directed, consider the motivations and needs of individuals and work groups within the participating organizations, and persist over the duration of the implementation process and into sustainment.[1,4,5] Shaping the context should also consider the interplay across contextual levels and the factors that bridge the outer and inner context (bridging factors) as they may be key facilitators of the implementation process.[6]

Although the types of organizations are varied (e.g., for profit, nonprofit, public, private, nongovernmental) and range in size from large (e.g., national health systems, health ministries, health insurance companies, US Veterans Affairs healthcare system, state or county/local health departments) to small (e.g., single-program, community-based, nonprofits), a number of common organizational constructs or processes are likely to be associated with successful D&I of healthcare innovations and evidence-based practices (EBPs).[4,5] Figure 9.1 provides our conceptual model informed by the exploration, preparation, implementation, sustainment (EPIS) framework; it includes outer (system) and inner (organizational) contexts and the bridging factors that connect them.[1,3] For this chapter, we primarily focus on inner context constructs that may operate in ways that are unidirectional or bidirectional or, more likely, have multiple determinants and influences that operate reciprocally or as a function of complex interactions. For example, within a given public or private organization, the organization's culture is influenced by the leadership, structures, and procedures within the organization.[7] While from a "bottom-up" perspective, the nature of the employees and their relationships, motives, and behaviors as well as the upward influence of lower-level leaders also shape the culture of an organization.[7,8]

In a similar way, it is important to consider not only how organizational factors can impact the implementation process, but also how implementation can impact organizational processes and functioning. Such bidirectional effects are key to conceptual models that recognize recipients of new technologies as not passive but as highly likely to react in various ways depending on characteristics of the context, the innovation to be implemented, and individual differences in healthcare providers and patients.[9] For example, it may be that the management style of executives and the climate in the organization can impact the fidelity and integrity with which EBPs are delivered,[10,11] but the process of implementation in combination

Gregory A. Aarons, Mark G. Ehrhart, Rebecca Lengnick-Hall, and Joanna C. Moullin, *The Role of Organizational Processes in Dissemination and Implementation Research* In: *Dissemination and Implementation Research in Health.* Edited by: Ross C. Brownson, Graham A. Colditz, and Enola K. Proctor, Oxford University Press. © Oxford University Press 2023. DOI: 10.1093/oso/9780197660690.003.0009 with the type of EBP may impact the system or organization, its management, and its workforce.[12–14]

Figure 9.1 illustrates the complexity of these interactions and that organizational research is inherently multilevel.[15] In implementation research, relevant levels may reside in both the outer (e.g., system-level) and inner contexts (e.g., teams implementing a particular EBP). Conducting multilevel research involves not only identifying and specifying the levels, but also articulating the top-down and bottom-up factors and processes that explain how those levels are connected to explain a particular outcome. In one study, for example, Becker-Haimes and colleagues specified the cross-level interactions between clinicians' (e.g., knowledge) and organizational characteristics (e.g., climate) that explained EBP use.[16] For conducting rigorous multilevel research, it is critical to consider the level of theory, level of measurement, and level of analysis and the links between them. For example, the referent of items when measuring organizational constructs should indicate the intended level. However, care is needed as "leader," "manager," or "supervisor" could refer to different people or organization levels depending on who is being asked and specific role(s) in an organization. Having accurate and consistent referents (e.g., questions clearly indicate the intended level of theory and analysis) in implementation evaluation is critical when trying to assess shared organizational characteristics and creating a knowledge base that cuts across diverse study settings.

To facilitate our understanding of outer-inner context dynamics, Figure 9.1 also includes the construct of bridging factors. Defined as "relational ties, formal arrangements, and processes that connect outer system and inner organizational contexts" (RLH),[6(p1)] bridging factors are an explicit part of the EPIS framework but apply to any framework where an inner and outer contextual boundary exist.[1,4,6,17] Bridging factors are specific to an implementation effort (e.g., not contracting for a broad suite of services, but contracting for particular EBPs), and they may be critical drivers of sustainment and targets of scale-up strategies.[6] Examples of bridging factors include contracting arrangements, financial reimbursement arrangements, policy-driven fiscal incentives, community-academic partnerships, state-local partnerships, interagency collaborations, data-sharing processes, site-level accreditation processes, and even an individual person.[6,18–20] Although bridging factors are not a major focus of this chapter, they are important to acknowledge as they can play a critical role in many of the organizational factors discussed.

What is not captured in Figure 9.1, but deserving of consideration, is that change in organizational processes or routines (e.g., implementing new interventions) takes time. The proposed phases of the implementation process include exploration (considering what is needed and whether to adopt an innovation); preparation (planning for implementation once the adoption decision is made); implementation (enacting plans and working through emergent issues); and sustainment (creating and supporting the structures and processes that will allow an implemented innovation to be maintained in a system or organization).[1,21,22] Considering D&I as a process with multiple, recursive phases have implications for how the various contextual levels (e.g., country, system, organization, provider, patient) may impact or be impacted by the D&I of EBPs into routine care. Certain organizational factors are likely to be more or less important across the phases of implementation. Some considerations include (1) how much time and effort it takes to create a change, (2) how long it can take to see a change or have an effect when you intervene, and (3) different issues or strategies being more or less important at different times across EPIS phases. For example, effective and committed executive leadership may be particularly important during exploration and preparation phases, whereas team-level leadership may be more critical in the implementation phase once providers have started to actually change their work processes.[1] Changing relatively narrow aspects of organizational support for EBP could involve strategies such as making summaries of peer-reviewed literature available to staff and could be relatively low threshold (i.e., low cost, easily implemented). More complicated goals, such as improving safety in hospital settings, may involve numerous iterative changes or improvement cycles and thus require attention to a broader range of organizational issues across phases. In addition, changes may be slowed or facilitated by the culture of the organization in which practice change is to take

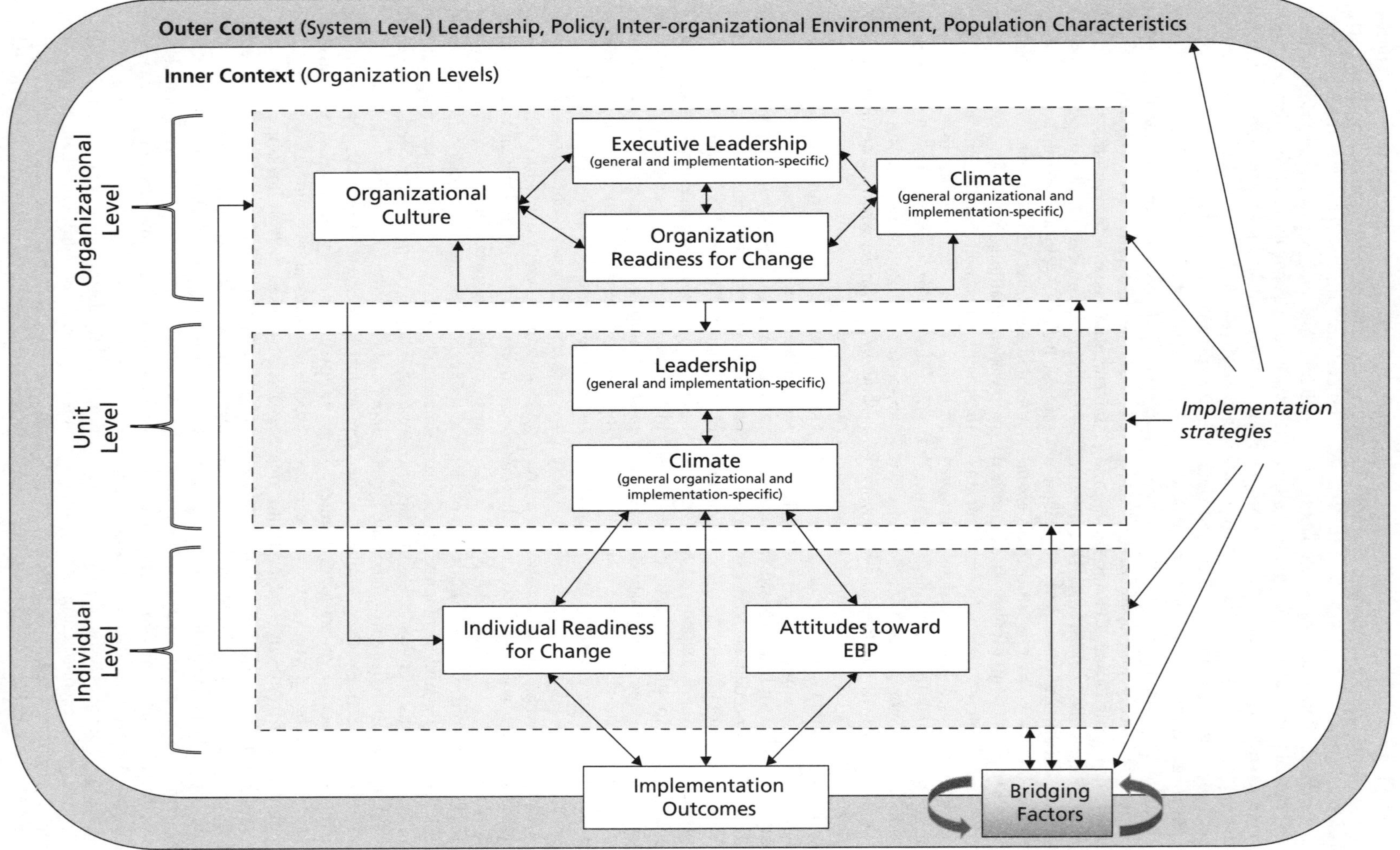

FIGURE 9.1 Multiple levels of organizational factors and processes consistent with exploration, preparation, implementation, sustainment (EPIS) framework.

Adapted with permission from: Aarons GA, Hurlburt M, Horwitz SM. Advancing a conceptual model of evidence-based practice implementation in public service sectors. *Adm Policy Ment Health.* 2011;38(1):4–23.

place.[23] Thus, the type and size of the system or organization and the type and scope of the change target can impact the need for more or less protracted organizational change strategies with the ultimate goal of incorporating evidence and EBP into usual care.

Just as certain organizational factors may be more or less important at certain stages of the implementation process, certain organizational factors may be more relevant or impactful for the implementation of particular EBPs or in particular contexts. Focusing on improving organizational climate for implementation may be more important for a particular team or work group that is implementing an EBP within an organization relative to the rest of the organization that is continuing stable operations. Conversely, if the implementation of an EBP cuts across or impacts the entire organization, then more global organizational culture and climate change strategies may be appropriate to ensure all employees are committed to and focused on the use of the EBP.

Drawing from the implementation science, business, management, and organizational literatures, this chapter focuses on several of the more common and well-researched organizational constructs and processes that may impact uptake and sustainment of EBPs in organizations.

Our discussion begins in the inner context, focusing on two related but distinct organizational-level concepts: organizational culture and organizational climate. After providing a general overview of these two constructs, we distinguish between more general or "molar" organizational climate and the more focused or "strategic" implementation climate, which often functions at the team level. Next, we move to a discussion of leadership, implementation leadership, and readiness for change, which can exist across multiple levels. Finally, we move on to the individual-level construct of attitudes toward EBP. Each factor is considered in relation to the questions and challenges in healthcare, behavioral health, and social service settings, particularly regarding how they can be applied to EBP implementation. To conclude our discussion, we highlight organizational theory and how it may be applied in implementation research. Although most of the focus of this chapter is on the delivery of healthcare, the principles discussed are widely applicable to public health EBP implementation.

ORGANIZATIONAL CULTURE

An organization's culture is essentially what makes that organization unique from all others, including the core values instilled in the organization by its founder(s) and the organization's history of how it has survived through successes and failures. It includes the goals of the organization in terms of the services or products provided, as well as how individuals and groups within the organization treat and interact with one another. Our working definition of organizational culture comes from Schein,[7] who described organizational culture as the "pattern of shared basic assumptions that was learned by a group as it solved its problems of external adaptation and internal integration, and that has worked well enough to be considered valid and, therefore, to be taught to new members as the correct way to perceive, think, and feel in relation to those problems."[7(p6)]

Scholars have often discussed organizational culture in terms of its layers or levels. Two examples are shown in Table 9.1. Frameworks along these lines specify outer layers that are more tangible and easily accessible (e.g., artifacts such as style of dress or the physical arrangement of space) but may have different meanings in different organizations. To truly understand these outer layers, Schein and others have argued that one must gain a deeper understanding of the more deeply held, subjective, and less easily accessed values and assumptions that comprise inner layers.[7,24] Such basic shared assumptions are so deeply ingrained in the organization that its members may not be able to readily articulate them; thus, scholars have argued that both qualitative and quantitative methods must be used to truly understand an organization's culture.[7,25]

Adding to the complexity of defining culture and its levels, scholars vary in their models of the specific components or dimensions of organizational culture. Some scholars have proposed organizational culture categorical types, with the most well known being Cameron and Quinn's four types of clan, adhocracy, hierarchy, and market based on the competing values framework.[26] Culture researchers using survey measures of culture have tended to delineate numerous dimensions of culture.

TABLE 9.1 LAYERS OF ORGANIZATIONAL CULTURE

Source	Number of Layers	Layers
Schein[7]	3	Underlying assumptions Espoused values Artifacts
Rousseau[24]	5	Fundamental assumptions Values Behavioral norms Patterns of behavior Artifacts

Examples include the Denison Organizational Culture Survey,[27] which organizes multiple specific subdimensions into the broad dimensions of involvement, consistency, adaptability, and mission, or the Organizational Culture Profile,[28] which includes a number of specific dimensions, like attention to detail, outcome orientation, and innovation.

Organizational culture has been identified as a key element in EBP adoption, implementation, and sustainment.[1,29–31] It has also been linked to decreased infection rates in a hospital,[32] increased work satisfaction and organizational commitment in long-term care,[33] more positive attitudes toward EBPs,[34] and improved outcomes for youth in child welfare systems.[35] However, a recent systematic review of organizational culture change attempts in healthcare identified only two studies that met criteria for inclusion, suggesting a need for more research in this regard.[36] Interventions that specifically focus on organizational culture change, such as the ARC (Availability, Responsiveness and Continuity) Framework intervention tested in social and mental health services for children and the Advancing Research and Clinical practice through close Collaboration (ARCC) model in nursing,[37] have shown benefits related to EBP attitudes, beliefs, and behaviors, as well as better employee retention, client/patient outcomes, and implementation success.[38,39]

ORGANIZATIONAL CLIMATE

Organizational climate is defined as "the shared meaning organizational members attach to the events, policies, practices, and procedures they experience and the behaviors they see being rewarded, supported, and expected."[40(p69)] Notably, climate is not merely defined by the presence of practices and procedures in the work environment, but rather it is the perceived meaning inferred by employees through management practices and procedures that ultimately define the climate of the organization.[41]

Although organizational culture and climate both address the organizational context, they differ in a number of ways.[40] Organizational culture is a much broader construct, as evidenced by its many layers, whereas climate is more narrowly focused on employees' shared perceptions of the policies, practices, and procedures in the organization. As a result, climate is often considered more malleable or changeable than organizational culture.

Over time, several differences have emerged in how organizational climate has been conceptualized and studied, including in terms of level of analysis (individual vs. organizational unit); content (description vs. evaluation); and type of composition model (climate level vs. climate strength). A key distinction that emerged early in the history of the climate literature is between molar (or generic) climate and focused or "strategic" climate. The molar approach typically involves an attempt to measure climate at a broad level across multiple dimensions, such as role stress, autonomy, leadership support, and warmth.[42] In contrast, the focused climate approach involves employee perceptions of the practices and procedures with regard to a specific criterion, whether it be a strategic outcome (e.g., climate for customer service, climate for safety) or characteristics of organizational processes (e.g., ethics, fairness).[43] While molar climate attempts to capture the general "feel" of the organization (which overlaps more with the construct of organizational culture), the focused or strategic climate approach addresses the extent to which employees perceive that management emphasizes the specific criterion of interest. Most important for this chapter is research and theory related to a focused climate for implementation of innovations in an organization.[44]

IMPLEMENTATION CLIMATE

The strategic climate approach to organizational climate is highly relevant for research on D&I.[45–47] While organizational culture and molar climate are important for successful implementation and for achieving successful clinical outcomes[35,48–50]; their role is important primarily in laying the foundation for the development of an effective implementation climate.[51] An implementation climate is defined as "employees' shared perceptions of the importance of innovation implementation within the organization . . . [that] results from employees' shared experiences and observations of, and their information about and discussions about, their organization's implementation policies and practices".[52(p813)] It is important to note that implementation climate is distinct from a climate for innovation, which involves the extent to which the organization encourages and supports the development of new ideas and technologies[53] but does not capture how those ideas and technologies are actually implemented in the organization. Implementation climate focuses on creating a fertile organizational context for putting a new innovation into practice. When management communicates the importance of the implementation of a new innovation through its policies, procedures, and reward systems, employees can clearly understand that the leaders in the organization care about the implementation and use of the innovation, therefore enabling employees to better focus their energy and motivation for that goal. As a result, overall implementation is more likely to succeed.[52,54,55]

Leaders, managers, and supervisors can communicate the value of successful implementation in many ways. Recent research developing measures of implementation climate provided some insight into potential targets of change. For instance, Jacobs, Weiner, and Bunger (2014) drew from Klein et al.'s definition of implementation climate to measure the three dimensions of implementation climate: expectations, support, and rewards. Alternatively, Ehrhart, Aarons, and Farahnak's (2014) measure captures six dimensions of a climate for EBP implementation: (1) focus on EBP, (2) educational support for EBP, (3) recognition for EBP, (4) rewards for EBP, (5) selection for EBP, and (6) selection for openness. In either case, the idea is that when the organization aligns its policies, practices, and systems in support of implementation, employees have a clear understanding of the organization's priorities and will be more likely to behave accordingly. Research in health and social services has demonstrated a number of positive benefits of a high implementation climate,[56–59] including research showing that improvements in implementation climate over time are linked to increased EBP use,[38] and that the combination of high levels of both implementation climate and molar climate is particularly beneficial with regard to implementation outcomes.[51]

Although implementation climate is the most germane for research on the implementation of EBPs, other focused climates are relevant to research on implementation as well. For instance, research has suggested that workers are more likely to learn about[60] and implement new practices[61] when there is a climate for psychological safety in the work unit. In many cases, providers may be expected to implement prescribed, structured practices, but in other cases, there may be a need for providers to develop new practices or find creative solutions to adapt the practice they are implementing. In that case, a climate for innovation[53] coupled with a climate for implementation may be ideal. Finally, in the context of recent advances in research on health equity and implementation, it may be necessary to have a climate for diversity[62] or inclusion[63] in a given organization to ensure that the new practices that are adopted and implemented are beneficial for all clients or patients. For instance, in organizations with high levels of a climate for diversity or inclusion, staff may be more sensitive during the implementation process if certain groups are reacting negatively to the new practice being implemented, and thus the staff adapt accordingly. This is an area where research is needed to inform the development of strategies to develop and sustain more inclusive policies, practices, and climates in health and allied healthcare organizations.

LEADERSHIP

Leaders are crucial in creating and applying targeted strategies intended to create a positive EBP implementation climate to promote EBP uptake. The history of research on leadership is long and includes leader traits, leader behaviors, contingencies of effective leadership, and leader cognition.[64] Of the many theories of leadership (see Avolio et al.[65] for a review), one particularly useful and well-researched framework is the Full-Range Leadership (FRL) Model.[66,67] According to this model, leadership behaviors fall into three broad categories, with more specific dimensions within each. The first, *transformational* leadership, includes those behaviors by which a leader attends to and develops followers to higher levels of performance and potential (individualized consideration), engages followers in thinking about issues in new ways (intellectual stimulation), communicates an appealing vision for the future (inspirational motivation), and becomes a trusted role model for staff (idealized influence).[68] *Transactional* leadership, the second category in the FRL model, involves exchanges between leaders and followers in which leaders reinforce or reward followers for engaging in certain behaviors and meeting practical and/or aspirational goals (contingent reward) as well as monitoring and correcting performance (passive or active management by exception). The final general category in the FRL model, *passive* or laissez-faire leadership (i.e., non-leadership), refers to withdrawal behaviors on the part of the purported leader in which little exchange between the leader and follower is enacted. It is, however, not merely a nonimpactful or neutral set of behaviors, but is thought to represent an actively destructive abdication of responsibility that is considered to be an ineffective style of leadership.[69] Although the FRL approach is not without its critics,[70] substantial evidence indicated that transformational leadership has numerous positive outcomes for subordinates and organizational effectiveness,[71,72] and that leaders can learn to enact more transformational leadership behaviors.

It is important to note that there are other relevant approaches that we cannot address given space limitations. For instance, leader-member exchange (e.g., relationship between a leader and follower)[73,74] has a large body of research, including in health services, although it also has its critiques.[75] There are also a number of emerging approaches, including ethical leadership,[76] authentic leadership,[77] and servant leadership.[78] In addition, there is increasing attention to leadership for equity and inclusion.[79] For instance, researchers have recently proposed that inclusive leadership involves such behaviors as supporting group members, ensuring justice and equity, promoting shared decision-making, encouraging diverse contributions, and supporting full participation in the group process and activities.[80] Recent meta-analytic evidence suggested that organizational diversity management efforts are positively related to more positive employee attitudes and negatively related to employee withdrawal.[81] One strategy that could be used is for strategic leadership development that equips leaders to support and develop organizational cultures and climates that are more equitable and inclusive.

Across various theories and approaches, leadership has been shown to be a critical factor for organizational effectiveness in healthcare organizations.[82] Positive and effective leadership in healthcare systems can help to create climates that support quality of care and improve other economic, clinical, and humanistic outcomes. For example, leadership has been associated with higher consumer satisfaction and quality of life,[82] more positive work attitudes,[32,33] improved therapeutic alliance and more positive organizational climate,[34] and more positive organizational culture and reduced burnout.[83] Specific to implementation, more effective leadership has been tied to clinicians' receptivity toward the use of EBP,[84] as well as more positive attitudes toward EBP.[85] In addition, promising approaches are being used to integrate FRL—and specifically transformational leadership—in approaches to improve health manager implementation leadership and implementation effectiveness.[86,87]

IMPLEMENTATION LEADERSHIP

Research on leadership and implementation has recently taken a similar approach to the strategic climate literature by focusing on strategic leadership for implementation or "implementation leadership." This research has delineated the specific behaviors leaders perform to support organizational implementation efforts. In developing the concept and measure of implementation leadership, the Implementation Leadership Scale (ILS), Aarons and colleagues (2014) drew from the work of Schein on embedding mechanisms[7] to identify the specific ways that leaders could develop a strategic climate for implementation in their organizations. Using mixed qualitative and quantitative methods, they found that implementation leadership comprised four dimensions: the leader being *knowledgeable* about the practice or innovation to be implemented, being *proactive* in anticipating implementation issues, being *supportive* of direct service providers in their efforts to use a new practice or innovation, and *persevering* through the ups and downs of the implementation process. Although the ILS was originally developed in allied health/mental health service settings, it has now been validated in substance abuse treatment, child welfare, education, and nursing settings.[88–91] Other work has independently formulated a model of implementation leadership for clinical guideline implementation,[92] as well as integration of the Ottawa Model of Implementation Leadership (O-MILe) with the dimensions of the ILS in order to advance theory and ultimately to test these models for effectiveness in supporting implementation.[93] Implementation leadership has been placed within the EPIS framework and linked to implementation in health and in social care.[94,95] More recent research by Williams and colleagues demonstrated that changes in first-level leaders' implementation leadership over a 5-year period were associated with changes in implementation climate, which were then associated with changes in clinicians' EBP use.[96]

One particularly critical issue for understanding how leaders influence implementation efforts is how the role of leadership varies across multiple levels within health and social service organizations.[97] For example, the role of leadership can be considered across multiple levels within the EPIS outer system and inner organizational contexts, including at the level of executives or upper-level management, middle managers, and first-level leaders. There are many commonalities across service sectors in how leadership manifests at different levels that must be considered for effective implementation to occur.[1,21] For example, a recent study across 11 public sector allied health service systems found that outer context or system-level leadership—closely matching dimensions of implementation leadership—was critical in implementation and sustainment, while FRL predicted sustainment at the team level within organizations.[98] At the same time, there may be important differences across levels that should be considered. For instance, strategies and policies often emerge from top management, and thus executive leaders are involved in decision-making processes for the adoption of EBPs, while lower-level supervisors are involved in the day-to-day implementation of EBPs in their teams.[99] In addition, Meza et al. identified "selling the innovation" as a middle manager role that is unique from the first-level leader behaviors in the ILS.[100,101] Thus, leadership at all levels in an organization should be considered so that there is congruence of communication, reinforcement, and direction that is accessible and palpable for staff at the front line of services.[8]

Despite the importance of strong leadership across levels during EBP implementation, first-level leaders are often neglected when it comes to support in how to lead effectively and support organizational change.[8,100,102] Thus, first-level leaders may lack the management and leadership skills and requisite organizational standing and power necessary to develop positive organizational and implementation climates and effectively implement EBPs. This represents a critical gap between workforce readiness for EBP and the need to implement the most effective services for health and mental healthcare. In response to this gap in the literature, the first and second authors have developed the Leadership and Organizational Change for Implementation (LOCI) strategy to simultaneously improve FRL and implementation leadership and provide a positive EBP implementation climate. The LOCI implementation strategy works with multiple levels of leadership using a data-driven approach to leader development, leadership coaching, implementation climate development planning and action at executive and middle management levels, and engagement of leaders at multiple levels in order to align goals and activities. Acceptability and feasibility data for this intervention are promising,[103] and further tailoring and large-scale testing is underway to validate this approach to leadership development and improving organizational readiness and effectiveness in implementing EBPs.[104] Preliminary findings showed more change in implementation leadership and implementation climate and engagement of service providers in the EBP process for LOCI versus control implementation strategies.[105] For instance, an application of the LOCI strategy in Norway found positive effects on first-level implementation leadership and climate in the context of mental health services.[106]

PERCEPTUAL DISTANCE AND ALIGNMENT

In line with the discussion above highlighting the importance of considering multiple levels in the organization, research on leadership in healthcare has specifically begun to address the implications of alignment across levels. Most research in this domain has addressed the perceptual distance between the perceptions of leaders and the perceptions of their subordinates.[107] Alignment of perceptions within organizations occurs when employees, regardless of role, report similar views, values, or beliefs. Recent research suggests that the degree to which employees' perceptions align can have an impact on organizational dynamics and contribute to shaping an organization's culture and climate.[108,109] For example, Hasson and colleagues found that organizational learning improved when a leader and their team agreed on level of organizational learning.[107] Aarons and colleagues found that "humble" leadership, where leaders rated themselves lower than their subordinates, was associated with a more positive climate for performance feedback and organizational involvement compared to groups who agreed or where the leader rated themselves higher on ILS than their followers.[110] In another study, organizational culture was found to suffer more when supervisors rated themselves more positively than providers, in contrast to when supervisors rated themselves lower than the provider ratings of the supervisor.[111] Research along these lines is important because it is apparently not just an average level of leadership that is important, but rather the dynamic relationship between leaders and followers that may impact organizational context. In addition to the perceptual distance between leaders and subordinates, other research has considered the alignment of perceptions across stakeholders in the implementation process. Hasson and colleagues found that staff described their roles and the roles of others in implementation processes differently across various stakeholder groups in the organization.[112] In such cases, implementation strategies should be employed in an attempt to reduce the discrepancy and increase the communication and understanding of the staff's roles and responsibilities.

At a system level, alignment occurs when there is perceptual agreement between stakeholders across organizations. In large system transformations, change may be required across several systems and within several organizations within those systems. A study investigating such a transformation looked at programs to improve the quality of care for the elderly.[113] In such cases, organizational collaboration,[114,115] community-based participatory research[116] or community-academic partnerships,[117] and learning collaboratives[118] are examples of methodologies that may be fruitful to increase perceptual alignment, ensure the perceptions of all stakeholders are accounted for, and select appropriate tailored implementation strategies across all contextual levels.[119]

ORGANIZATIONAL READINESS FOR CHANGE

The concept of organizational readiness for change arose from Lewin's three-stage model of change, which advocates "unfreezing" the workings of an organization and creating the motivation and capacity to change.[120] Organizational readiness is widely regarded as an essential antecedent to successful implementation of change in healthcare and social service organizations.[121,122] However, in implementation research there have been few strategies developed and tested with a specific focus on organizational readiness.

That may be partly due to the fact that organizational readiness for change is the subject of different definitions that focus on various aspects of organizations, including structure, process, equipment and technology, and staff attitudes, intentions, and behaviors.[123,124] Here, we consider organizational readiness for change to involve organization members' psychological and behavioral motivation to implement a new innovation, technology, or EBP; general organizational capacity; and innovation-specific capacity.[9] A number of measures of organizational readiness for change have been developed for services and implementation research and take differing perspectives in regard to comprehensiveness and outer/inner context domains,[121,124–126] some with focus on cultural competency[127] or for specific settings such as surgery.[128]

Organizations are made up of individuals, and their motivation to change is represented by two dimensions, collective commitment and collective efficacy.[124,129] Organizational commitment for change is the shared intention to implement, whereas collective efficacy is the shared belief that the organization members have the capability to implement. Social cognitive theory suggests that when individuals' organizational readiness for change is high, organizational members are more likely to initiate change and exert greater efforts and persistence for change.[130,131] Motivation theory suggests that when individuals' organizational readiness for change is high, members will exhibit prosocial, change-related behaviors that exceed job requirements.[122,132] Several key change beliefs that lead to improved staff commitment and efficacy for change have been identified.[122,126,133] Change valence (e.g., perceived need, benefit, timeliness, and capability) refers to whether employees think the change being implemented is beneficial or worthwhile for them personally.[122,133] Strategies to improve change valence could include discussing with employees the positive results of the change (e.g., improved clinician skills and expertise, better patient/client outcomes) as well as potential negative consequences.[134,135] Change discrepancy refers to employees' belief that implementation or change is needed due to a gap between the organization's current state and a more desired end state. When employees perceive a relevant discrepancy in their workplace, they may be more motivated to lessen the discrepancy.

Change advocates, sometimes referred to as "champions," are types of leaders who can, for example, role model commitment to change and can include employees in activities such as planning meetings in order to increase their buy-in and collective confidence in the ability to implement and manage change.[136] Communicating to employees that training and ongoing support will be available throughout the implementation and sustainment phases can facilitate efficacy.[129] However, system, organizational, and individual capacity must all be considered. For example, funding and service agencies participating in the dynamic adaptation process (DAP) project funded by the Centers for Disease Control and Prevention (CDC) decreased their service providers' caseloads by about 50%, which allowed staff time to prepare for and use the new intervention with clients.[137] In addition, ongoing training and coaching support was part of the implementation strategy and of the innovation being implemented. However, it was also clear that these issues need to be balanced by outer context policies and bridging factors that link outer and inner contexts, including changes to contracts and associated productivity and workflow requirements.[6,138] The DAP is an implementation strategy built on values of stakeholder collaboration, voice, and participation so that relevant outer and inner context adaptations can more effectively support EBP implementation and sustainment.

Structural dimensions of organizational capacity and innovation-specific capacity are also important to consider.[9] General organizational capacity for change refers to the "attributes of a functioning organization . . . and connections with other organizations."[3,9(p486)] Innovation-specific capacity refers to an organization's resources (financial, material, human, and informational); context; and processes that will support the introduction and integration of a specific innovation.[9,139] In order to enhance these two types of capacities, formal leaders and opinion leaders (e.g., clinical supervisors, champions) in the organization can clearly communicate their commitment to the successful implementation of a given change while also adapting workflows, structures, and processes in order to demonstrate commitment and influence and support inner context individual employee motivations and efficacy.

Recent work has identified potential stage-based approaches to address organizational readiness, and while the approach appears useful, it includes the exploration and preparation phases only without considering implementation and sustainment phases.[140] It is important to begin with sustainment as the goal and consider how we enhance readiness across all EPIS phases.[1,3] In change efforts, we recommend considering organizational readiness, individual readiness, and collective motivation and efficacy across EPIS phases while also considering the outer context for change as well as bridging factors linking outer and inner contexts to support readiness.[141–143] Organizational readiness is often considered as a relatively static determinant but is likely to change over the course of implementation.

ATTITUDES TOWARD EVIDENCE-BASED PRACTICE

Staff and leader attitudes toward EBP may be important to consider when implementing in healthcare settings.[144] Early work on attitudes toward EBP identified four primary dimensions (scale names in italics): (1) the intuitive *Appeal* of the EBP; (2) likelihood to adopt if *Requirements* were to do so; (3) the practitioners' *Openness* to new practices; and (4) perceived *Divergence* between EBP and current practice.[145,146] More recent work has identified eight additional dimensions: (1) *Limitations* of EBPs; (2) EBPs' *Fit* with values and needs of client and clinician; (3) perceptions of *Monitoring*; (4) *Balance* between perceptions of clinical skills and science as important in service provision; (5) time and administrative *Burden* with learning EBPs; (6) *Job security* related to expertise in EBP; (7) perceived *Organizational support*; and (8) positive perceptions of receiving *Feedback*.[147,148] Attitudes toward EBP can be predicted by a number of organizational characteristics, including the culture and climate of an organization,[149] leadership,[150,151] and the level of organizational support for EBP that is provided by the organization.[50] It is important to consider the role of attitudes along with other factors, such as behavioral intentions,[152] provider self-efficacy,[134] and intentions to implement.[153] In addition to the effects of attitudes on implementation behaviors, more positive attitudes toward EBP may also be linked to going above and beyond requirements to support implementation. Such "implementation citizenship behaviors" may include offering additional help and assistance to others during the implementation process and keeping up with the latest updates and news on the implementation process and the EBP itself.[154]

APPLYING ORGANIZATIONAL THEORY TO IMPLEMENTATION RESEARCH

Constructs like organizational culture, climate, readiness for change, and attitudes toward EBP help us understand what is going on inside the organization so that we can attend to those inner context factors that have the greatest impact on implementation processes and outcomes. However, organizations are permeable to and shaped and constrained by the broader external environment or outer context; this is referred to as an open systems approach.[155] Examples of how the outer context can shape internal organizational functioning include federal policies that set a reimbursement rate that organizations have to work within when implementing, local legislative agendas that specify a list of EBPs that an organization can implement, or interorganizational relationships that provide infrastructure (e.g., referral and data processes) that ease the burden of a new implementation effort.[4]

Long-standing organizational-level theories in the management literature such as complexity,[156] transaction cost economics,[157] institutional,[158] contingency,[159] and resource dependence theories[160] can help us understand this "open systems" way of approaching organizationally focused D&I work.[161,162] In one example, Leeman and colleagues used institutional theory to reflect on the inner workings of a learning collaborative and identify potential mechanisms that explain how these types of collaboratives can support implementation of evidence-based colorectal cancer screening interventions.[162] The authors specifically applied the constructs of coercive, mimetic, and normative pressures to describe interactions between the American Cancer Society and Federally Qualified Health Centers.[162] In another example, Lengnick-Hall and colleagues invoked resource dependence theory to explain how community-based organizations and county/state systems communicated, interacted, and exchanged resources through contracting arrangements and the way that this impacted SafeCare implementation and sustainment.[138] This theoretical application included articulating specific outer and inner context resources that were exchanged over the course of SafeCare implementation and sustainment.[138] In a third example, Berta and colleagues used organizational learning theory to explain how practice facilitation works.[163] The authors posited that facilitation stimulates learning because it allows organizations to examine, experiment with, and adapt their processes and routines.[163] As is evident in the examples, these types of theories typically position organizations as the unit of analysis and/or focal actor of interest.

SUMMARY

Taken as a whole, both organizational characteristics and specific organizational strategies are important for the effective D&I of EBPs in health and allied healthcare settings. There are many proposed approaches to supporting organizational development and change; this chapter focuses on factors and issues supported by relevant scientific literatures, particularly those relevant to EBP implementation in healthcare and related settings. However, it is important to note that empirical work specifically testing organizational implementation strategies is limited.

With the realization that development of organizational cultures, climates, and contexts supportive of EBP implementation takes time and concerted effort, there is hope that EBP implementation can be effectively pursued in diverse service settings. In order for patients and clients to benefit from care, the best interventions that science has to offer must be implemented effectively. Organizational change can lead to improved implementation outcomes[164,165] and ultimately improved clinical outcomes.[48] These goals can be achieved if we can create the organizational contexts that support EBP implementation.

Although the concepts and constructs discussed in this chapter may appear abstract, it is important to remember that they are created and are maintained by the behaviors, decisions, policies, and procedures developed and supported by people in the organization. In the same vein, they can be changed by individuals, groups, and teams with the vision, determination, and persistence to shepherd the organizational changes needed to implement and sustain EBPs. Any given implementation has the potential to improve the care needed by individuals, groups, and populations. Although there is evidence that EBPs tend to be robust across populations, it is important for organizations to make the changes necessary to deliver those interventions to the right people at the right time. This is done by people in organizations creating organizational contexts open to change and able to implement and sustain that change.

Organizationally focused D&I work continues to evolve. One research stream involves *describing* and *measuring* the organizational context and its connection to outcomes.[47,88,166–168] Another stream focuses on *targeting and modifying* aspects of the organizational context through the use of planned interventions and implementation strategies to introduce and integrate EBPs.[61,102,103,106,140,169] A new frontier is *isolating and activating the mechanisms of implementation strategies* that are most important for creating organizational contexts supportive of EBP implementation and sustainment.[96,170–172] It is imperative that those responsible for the implementation of EBPs take action to first identify the organizational issues to address. Then, effective organizational change strategies must be identified, utilized, and consistently applied to improve the culture and climate of the organization to more effectively implement evidence-based healthcare innovations and practices. The promise of this course of action is improved care, improved health, and improved lives for those we serve.

ACKNOWLEDGMENTS

Preparation of this chapter was supported by National Institute of Mental Health (NIMH) grants R01MH072961 and R01MH092950 (PI: Aarons) and R25MH080916 (PI: Proctor); National Institute on Drug Abuse (NIDA) grants R01DA049891 and R01DA038466 (PI: Aarons); National Center for Advancing Translational Sciences (NCATS) grant UL1TR001442 (PI: Firestein); and Australia Medical Research Future Fund grant MRFF1168155 (PI: Moullin).

SUGGESTED READINGS AND WEBSITES

Readings

Aarons GA, Ehrhart MG, Farahnak LR, Sklar M. Aligning leadership across systems and organizations to develop a strategic climate for evidence-based practice implementation. *Annu Rev Public Health*. 2014 Mar 18;35:255–274.

This article presents a description of how leadership may be considered and used at health and allied health outer context service system and inner context organization levels and how principles of leadership and organizational dynamics can inform shifting systems and organizations in order to be aligned to be more evidence informed.

Ehrhart MG, Schneider B, Macey WH. *Organizational Climate and Culture: An Introduction to Theory, Research, and Practice*. Routledge; 2014.

This book provides a comprehensive review of issues of organizational climate and culture, including definitions, conceptualizations, debates, and research findings.

Klein KJ, Sorra JS. The challenge of innovation implementation. *Acad Manage Rev*. 1996;21:1055–1080.

This seminal article discusses implementation outcomes and presents a model in which implementation effectiveness is a function of organizational climate for implementation and fit of innovations with users' values.

Lee SY, Weiner BJ, Harrison MI, Belden CM. Organizational transformation: a systematic review of empirical research in health care and other industries. *Med Care Res Rev*. 2013 Apr;70(2):115–142.

This article reviews transformational change in health and nonhealthcare settings. The review describes antecedents, processes, and outcomes of change efforts and notes a "multiplicity" of factors that may affect organizational change.

Schein EH, Schein P. *Organizational Culture and Leadership*. 5th ed. John Wiley & Sons, Inc.; 2017.

This book provides a comprehensive review of organizational culture and climate and of leadership. The book describes the "embedding mechanisms" that leaders and organizations can use to demonstrate to employees what is expected, supported, and rewarded in the organization.

Websites and Tools

Exploration, Preparation, Implementation, Sustainment (EPIS) Framework. https://episframework.com/

This site was created to explain and support the EPIS framework and provides resources for using EPIS, including measures and tools (e.g., worksheets, guides). The EPIS framework highlights key phases that guide and describe the implementation process and enumerates common and unique factors, including determinants and mechanisms within and across levels of outer (system) and inner (organizational) context across phases, factors that bridge outer and inner context, and the nature of the innovation or practice being implemented and the role of innovation/practice developers.

Institute for Healthcare Improvement (IHI). http://www.ihi.org/ihi

This site provides resources for process improvement in healthcare, including education, resources, various topics in healthcare improvement, and descriptions of IHI work in the United States and globally.

Leadership and Organizational Change for Implementation (LOCI). http://implementationleadership.com

This site provides description of a leadership and organizational change for implementation intervention and provides related tools, assessments, and other resources. This includes access to the Implementation Leadership Scale (ILS), Implementation Climate Scale (ICS), Implementation Citizenship Behavior Scale (ICBS), and the Evidence-Based Practice Attitude Scale (EBPAS).

Mind Garden. http://www.mindgarden.com/translead.htm#prompt2

This site provides information on the Multifactor Leadership Questionnaire. The authorized measures of the full-range leadership model are available from Mind Garden for research and/or applied purposes.

Veterans Affairs Healthcare System Quality Enhancement Research Initiative (QUERI). http://www.queri.research.va.gov/

This site describes the VA QUERI program, which supports a strategic process for implementing quality improvement initiatives.

REFERENCES

1. Aarons GA, Hurlburt M, Horwitz SM. Advancing a conceptual model of evidence-based practice implementation in public service sectors. *Adm Policy Ment Health*. 2011;38(1):4–23.
2. Rubin RM, Hurford MO, Hadley T, Matlin S, Weaver S, Evans AC. Synchronizing watches: the challenge of aligning implementation science and public systems. *Adm Policy Ment Health*. 2016;43(6):1023–1028.
3. Moullin JC, Dickson KS, Stadnick NA, Rabin B, Aarons GA. Systematic review of the exploration, preparation, implementation, sustainment (EPIS) framework. *Implement Sci*. 2019;14(1):1.
4. Damschroder L, Aron D, Keith R, Kirsh S, Alexander J, Lowery J. Fostering implementation of health services research findings into practice: a consolidated framework for advancing implementation science. *Implement Sci*. 2009;4(1):50–64.
5. Greenhalgh T, Robert G, Macfarlane F, Bate P, Kyriakidou O. Diffusion of innovations in service organizations: systematic review and recommendations. *Milbank Q*. 2004;82(4):581–629.
6. Lengnick-Hall R, Stadnick NA, Dickson KS, Moullin JC, Aarons GA. Forms and functions of bridging factors: specifying the dynamic links between outer and inner contexts during implementation and sustainment. *Implement Sci*. 2021;16(1):1–13.

7. Schein E. *Organizational Culture and Leadership*. 5th ed. John Wiley and Sons; 2017.
8. Priestland A, Hanig R. Developing first-level leaders. *Harv Bus Rev*. 2005;83(6):112–120.
9. Scaccia JP, Cook BS, Lamont A, et al. A practical implementation science heuristic for organizational readiness: R = MC2. *J Community Psychol*. 2015;43(4):484–501.
10. McLeod BD, Southam-Gerow MA, Weisz JR. Conceptual and methodological issues in treatment integrity measurement. *School Psych Rev*. 2009;38(4):541–546.
11. Taxman FS, Friedman PD. Fidelity and adherence at the transition point: theoretically driven experiments. *J Exp Criminol*. 2009;5(3):219–226.
12. Aarons GA, Sommerfeld DH, Hecht DB, Silovsky JF, Chaffin MJ. The impact of evidence-based practice implementation and fidelity monitoring on staff turnover: evidence for a protective effect. *J Consult Clin Psychol*. 2009;77(2):270–280.
13. Aarons GA, Fettes DL, Flores LE, Sommerfeld DH. Evidence-based practice implementation and staff emotional exhaustion in children's services. *Behav Res Ther*. 2009;47(11):954–960.
14. Palinkas LA, Aarons GA. A view from the top: executive and management challenges in a statewide implementation of an evidence-based practice to reduce child neglect. *Int J Child Health Hum Dev*. 2009;2(1):47–55.
15. Klein KJ, Kozlowski SW. *Multilevel Theory, Research, and Methods in Organizations: Foundations, Extensions, and New Directions*. Jossey-Bass; 2000.
16. Becker-Haimes EM, Williams NJ, Okamura KH, Beidas RS. Interactions between clinician and organizational characteristics to predict cognitive-behavioral and psychodynamic therapy use. *Adm Policy Ment Health*. 2019;46(6):701–712.
17. Feldstein A, Glasgow R. A practical, robust implementation and sustainability model (PRISM). *Jt Comm J Qual Patient Saf*. 2008;34(4):228–243.
18. Crable EL, Benintendi A, Jones DK, Walley AY, Hicks JM, Drainoni M-L. Translating Medicaid policy into practice: policy implementation strategies from three US states' experiences enhancing substance use disorder treatment. *Implement Sci*. 2022;17(1):1–14.
19. Aarons GA, Reeder K, Sam-Agudu NA, Vorkoper S, Sturke R. Implementation determinants and mechanisms for the prevention and treatment of adolescent HIV in sub-Saharan Africa: concept mapping of the NIH Fogarty International Center Adolescent HIV Implementation Science Alliance (AHISA) initiative. *Implement Sci Commun*. 2021;2(1):1–11.
20. Lui JH, Brookman-Frazee L, Lind T, et al. Outer-context determinants in the sustainment phase of a reimbursement-driven implementation of evidence-based practices in children's mental health services. *Implement Sci*. 2021;16(1):1–9.
21. Mendel P, Meredith L, Schoenbaum M, Sherbourne C, Wells K. Interventions in organizational and community context: a framework for building evidence on dissemination and implementation in health services research. *Adm Policy Ment Health*. 2008;35(1–2):21–37.
22. Hurlburt M, Aarons GA, Fettes D, Willging C, Gunderson L, Chaffin MJ. Interagency collaborative team model for capacity building to scale-up evidence-based practice. *Child Youth Serv Rev*. 2014;39:160–168.
23. Van Noord I, Bruijne MC, Twisk WR. The relationship between patient safety culture and the implementation of organizational patient safety defences at emergency departments. *Int J Qual Health Care*. 2010;22(3):162–169.
24. Rousseau DM. Normative beliefs in fund-raising organizations: linking culture to organizational performance and individual responses. *Group Organ Stud*. 1990;15(4):448–460.
25. Schein EH. A new era for culture, change, and leadership. *MIT Sloan Manag Rev*. 2019;60(4):52–58.
26. Cameron KS, Quinn RE. *Diagnosing and Changing Organizational Culture: Based on the Competing Values Framework*. 3rd ed. John Wiley & Sons; 2011.
27. Denison D, Nieminen L, Kotrba L. Diagnosing organizational cultures: a conceptual and empirical review of culture effectiveness surveys. *Eur J Work Organ Psy*. 2014;23(1):145–161.
28. Chatman JA, Caldwell DF, O'Reilly CA, Doerr B. Parsing organizational culture: how the norm for adaptability influences the relationship between culture consensus and financial performance in high-technology firms. *J Organ Behav*. 2014;35(6):785–808.
29. Damschroder L, Hall CS, Gillon L, et al. The Consolidated Framework for Implementation Research (CFIR): progress to date, tools and resources, and plans for the future. *Implement Sci*. 2015;10(suppl 1):A12.
30. Gale NK, Shapiro J, McLeod H, Redwood S, Hewison A. Patients-people-place: developing a framework for researching organizational culture during health service redesign and change. *Implement Sci*. 2014;9(106):1–11.
31. Jacobs R, Mannion R, Davies HT, Harrison S, Konteh F, Walshe K. The relationship between organizational culture and performance in acute hospitals. *Soc SciMed*. 2013;76:115–125.

32. Larson EL, Early E, Cloonan P, Sugrue S, Parides M. An organizational climate intervention associated with increased handwashing and decreased nosocomial infections. *Behav Med.* 2000;26(1):14–22.
33. Kinjerski V, Skrypnek BJ. The promise of spirit at work: increasing job satisfaction and organizational commitment and reducing turnover and absenteeism in long-term care. *J Gerontol Nurs.* 2008;34(10):17–25.
34. Aarons GA, Glisson C, Green PD, et al. The organizational social context of mental health services and clinician attitudes toward evidence-based practice: a United States national study. *Implement Sci.* 2012;7(1):56–70.
35. Williams NJ, Glisson C. Testing a theory of organizational culture, climate and youth outcomes in child welfare systems: a United States national study. *Child Abuse Negl.* 2014;38(4):757–767.
36. Parmelli E, Flodgren G, Beyer F, Baillie N, Schaafsma ME, Eccles MP. The effectiveness of strategies to change organisational culture to improve healthcare performance: a systematic review. *Implement Sci.* 2011;6(33):1–8.
37. Melnyk BM, Fineout-Overholt E, Giggleman M, Choy K. A test of the ARCC© model improves implementation of evidence-based practice, healthcare culture, and patient outcomes. *Worldviews Evid Based Nurs.* 2017;14(1):5–9.
38. Williams NJ, Glisson C. Changing organizational social context to support evidence-based practice implementation: a conceptual and empirical review. *Implement Sci.* 2020;30:145–172.
39. Bennett I, Vredevoogd M, Russo J, Grover T, Williams NJ. Organizational culture and climate of community health centers and variation in maternal depression outcomes. Oral presentation at the 48th Annual Meeting of the North American Primary Care Research Group (NAPCRG) Virtual. November, 2020.
40. Ehrhart MG, Schneider B, Macey WH. *Organizational Climate and Culture: An Introduction to Theory, Research, and Practice.* Routledge; 2014.
41. Schneider B, Ehrhart MG, Macey WA. Organizational climate research: achievements and the road ahead. In: Ashkanasy NM, Wilderom CPM, Peterson MF, eds. *Handbook of Organizational Culture and Climate.* 2nd ed. Sage Publications; 2011:29–49.
42. James LA, James LR. Integrating work environment perceptions: explorations into the measurement of meaning. *J Appl Psychol.* 1989;74(5):739–751.
43. Schneider B. *Organizational Climate and Culture.* Jossey-Bass; 1990.
44. Klein KJ, Sorra JS. The challenge of innovation implementation. *Acad Manage Rev.* 1996;21(4):1055–1080.
45. Weiner BJ, Belden CM, Bergmire DM, Johnston M. The meaning and measurement of implementation climate. *Implement Sci.* 2011;6:78.
46. Jacobs SR, Weiner BJ, Bunger AC. Context matters: measuring implementation climate among individuals and groups. *Implement Sci.* 2014;9(1):46.
47. Ehrhart MG, Aarons GA, Farahnak LR. Assessing the organizational context for EBP implementation: the development and validity testing of the Implementation Climate Scale (ICS). *Implement Sci.* 2014;9(157):1–11.
48. Glisson C, Schoenwald SK, Hemmelgarn A, et al. Randomized trial of MST and ARC in a two-level evidence-based treatment implementation strategy. *J Consult Clin Psychol.* 2010;78(4):537–550.
49. Beidas RS, Wolk CL, Walsh LM, Evans AC, Hurford MO, Barg FK. A complementary marriage of perspectives: understanding organizational social context using mixed methods. *Implement Sci.* 2014;9(175):1–15.
50. Aarons GA, Sommerfeld DH, Walrath-Greene CM. Evidence-based practice implementation: the impact of public versus private sector organization type on organizational support, provider attitudes, and adoption of evidence-based practice. *Implement Sci.* 2009;4(1):83–96.
51. Williams NJ, Ehrhart MG, Aarons GA, Marcus SC, Beidas RS. Linking molar organizational climate and strategic implementation climate to clinicians' use of evidence-based psychotherapy techniques: cross-sectional and lagged analyses from a 2-year observational study. *Implement Sci.* 2018;13(1):85.
52. Klein KJ, Conn AB, Sorra JS. Implementing computerized technology: an organizational analysis. *J Appl Psychol.* 2001;86(5):811–824.
53. Newman A, Round H, Wang S, Mount M. Innovation climate: a systematic review of the literature and agenda for future research. *J Occup Organ Psychol.* 2020;93(1):73–109.
54. Drach-Zahavy A, Somech A, Granot M, Spitzer A. Can we win them all? Benefits and costs of structured and flexible innovation–implementations. *J Organ Behav.* 2004;25(2):217–234.
55. Holahan PJ, Aronson ZH, Jurkat MP, Schoorman FD. Implementing computer technology: a multiorganizational test of Klein and Sorra's model. *J Eng Technol Manage.* 2004;21(1):31–50.
56. Pullmann MD, Lucid L, Harrison JP, et al. Implementation climate and time predict intensity of supervision content related to evidence based treatment. *Front Public Health.* 2018;6:280.

57. Jacobs SR, Weiner BJ, Reeve BB, Hofmann DA, Christian M, Weinberger M. Determining the predictors of innovation implementation in healthcare: a quantitative analysis of implementation effectiveness. *BMC Health Serv Res.* 2015;15(1):6.
58. Kratz HE, Stahmer A, Xie M, et al. The effect of implementation climate on program fidelity and student outcomes in autism support classrooms. *J Consult Clin Psychol.* 2019;87(3):270.
59. Woodard GS, Triplett NS, Frank HE, Harrison JP, Robinson S, Dorsey S. The impact of implementation climate on community mental health clinicians' attitudes toward exposure: an evaluation of the effects of training and consultation. *Implement Res Pract.* 2021;2:26334895211057883.
60. Edmondson AC. Psychological safety and learning behavior in work teams. *Admin Sci Q.* 1999;44(2):350–383.
61. Aarons GA, Ehrhart MG, Moullin JC, Torres EM, Green AE. Testing the leadership and organizational change for implementation (LOCI) intervention in substance abuse treatment: a cluster randomized trial study protocol. *Implement Sci.* 2017;12.
62. Holmes IV O, Jiang K, Avery DR, McKay PF, Oh I-S, Tillman CJ. A meta-analysis integrating 25 years of diversity climate research. *J Manage.* 2021;47(6):1357–1382.
63. Nishii LH. The benefits of climate for inclusion for gender-diverse groups. *Acad Manage J.* 2013;56(6):1754–1774.
64. Lord RG, Day DV, Zaccaro SJ, Avolio BJ, Eagly AH. Leadership in applied psychology: three waves of theory and research. *J Appl Psychol.* 2017;102(3):434.
65. Avolio BJ, Walumbwa FO, Weber TJ. Leadership: current theories, research, and future directions. *Annu Rev Psychol.* 2009;60:421–449.
66. Bass BM. Two decades of research and development in transformational leadership. *Eur J Work Organ Psychol.* 1999;8(1):9–32.
67. Avolio BJ, Bass BM, Jung DI. Re-examining the components of transformational and transactional leadership using the Multifactor Leadership Questionnaire. *J Occup Organ Psychol.* 1999;72:441–462.
68. Bass BM, Avolio BJ. *Training Full Range Leadership.* Mind Garden, Inc.; 1999.
69. Skogstad A, Einarsen S, Torsheim T, Aasland MS, Hetland H. The destructiveness of laissez-faire leadership behavior. *J Occup Health Psychol.* 2007;12(1):80–92.
70. Van Knippenberg D, Sitkin S. A critical assessment of charismatic-transformational leadership research: back to the drawing board? *Acad Manag Ann.* 2013;7(1):1–60.
71. Judge TA, Piccolo RF. Transformational and transactional leadership: a meta-analytic test of their relative validity. *J Appl Psychol.* 2004;89(5):755–768.
72. Wang G, Oh I-S, Courtright SH, Colbert AE. Transformational leadership and performance across criteria and levels: a meta-analytic review of 25 years of research. *Group Organ Manag.* 2011;36(2):223–270.
73. Martin R, Guillaume Y, Thomas G, Lee A, Epitropaki O. Leader–member exchange (LMX) and performance: a meta-analytic review. *Pers Psychol.* 2016;69(1):67–121.
74. Aarons GA, Conover KL, Ehrhart MG, Torres EM, Reeder K. Leader–member exchange and organizational climate effects on clinician turnover intentions. *J Health Organ Manag.* 2021;35(1):68–87. https://doi.org/10.1108/JHOM-10-2019-0311
75. Gottfredson RK, Wright SL, Heaphy ED. A critique of the Leader-Member Exchange construct: back to square one. *Leadersh Q.* 2020;31(6):101385.
76. Banks GC, Fischer T, Gooty J, Stock G. Ethical leadership: mapping the terrain for concept cleanup and a future research agenda. *Leadersh Q.* 2021;32(2):101471.
77. Gardner WL, Karam EP, Alvesson M, Einola K. Authentic leadership theory: the case for and against. *Leadersh Q.* 2021;32(6):1–25.
78. Mahon D. Can using a servant-leadership model of supervision mitigate against burnout and secondary trauma in the health and social care sector? *Leadersh Health Serv.* 2021;34(2):198–214.
79. Lee TH, Volpp KG, Cheung VG, Dzau VJ. Diversity and inclusiveness in health care leadership: three key steps. *NEJM Catal Innov Care Del.* 2021;2(3):1–9.
80. Randel AE, Galvin BM, Shore LM, et al. Inclusive leadership: realizing positive outcomes through belongingness and being valued for uniqueness. *Hum Resour Manage Rev.* 2018;28(2):190–203.
81. Mor Barak ME, Lizano EL, Kim A, et al. The promise of diversity management for climate of inclusion: a state-of-the-art review and meta-analysis. *Hum Serv Organ Manag Leadersh Gov.* 2016;40(4):305–333.
82. Corrigan PW, Garman AN. Transformational and transactional leadership skills for mental health teams. *Community Ment Health J.* 1999;35(4):301–312.
83. Corrigan PW, Diwan S, Campion J, Rashid F. Transformational leadership and the

mental health team. *Adm Policy Ment Health.* 2002;30(2):97–108.

84. Aarons GA. Transformational and transactional leadership: association with attitudes toward evidence-based practice. *Psychiatr Serv.* 2006;57(8):1162–1169.
85. Mosson R, Hasson H, Wallin L, Von Thiele Schwarz U. Exploring the role of line managers in implementing evidence-based practice in social services and older people care. *Br J Soc Work.* 2016;47(2):542–560.
86. Richter A, von Thiele Schwarz U, Lornudd C, Lundmark R, Mosson R, Hasson H. iLead—a transformational leadership intervention to train healthcare managers' implementation leadership. *Implement Sci.* 2016;11(1):108.
87. Richter A, Lornudd C, von Thiele Schwarz U, et al. Evaluation of iLead, a generic implementation leadership intervention: mixed-method preintervention–postintervention design. *BMJ Open.* 2020;10(1):e033227.
88. Aarons GA, Ehrhart MG, Torres EM, Finn NK, Roesch SC. Validation of the Implementation Leadership Scale (ILS) in substance use disorder treatment organizations. *J Subst Abuse Treat.* 2016;68:31–35.
89. Finn NK, Torres EM, Ehrhart MG, Roesch SC, Aarons GA. Cross-validation of the Implementation Leadership Scale (ILS) in child welfare service organizations. *Child Maltreat.* 2016;21(3):250–255.
90. Lyon AR, Cook CR, Brown EC, et al. Assessing organizational implementation context in the education sector: confirmatory factor analysis of measures of implementation leadership, climate, and citizenship. *Implement Sci.* 2018;13(1):5.
91. Shuman CJ, Ehrhart MG, Torres EM, et al. EBP implementation leadership of frontline nurse managers: validation of the implementation leadership scale in acute care. *Worldviews Evid Based Nurs.* 2020;17(1):82–91.
92. Tistad M, Palmcrantz S, Wallin L, et al. Developing leadership in managers to facilitate the implementation of national guideline recommendations: a process evaluation of feasibility and usefulness. *Int J Health Policy Manage.* 2016;5(8):477–486.
93. Gifford WA, Graham ID, Ehrhart MG, Davies BL, Aarons GA. Ottawa Model of Implementation Leadership and Implementation Leadership Scale: mapping concepts for developing and evaluating theory-based leadership interventions. *J Healthc Leadersh.* 2017;9:15–23.
94. Mosson R, von Thiele Schwarz U, Richter A, Hasson H. The impact of inner and outer context on line managers' implementation leadership. *Br J Soc Work.* 2018;48(5):1447–1468.
95. Shuman CJ, Liu X, Aebersold ML, Tschannen D, Banaszak-Holl J, Titler MG. Associations among unit leadership and unit climates for implementation in acute care: a cross-sectional study. *Implement Sci.* 2018;13(1):1–10.
96. Williams NJ, Wolk CB, Becker-Haimes EM, Beidas RS. Testing a theory of strategic implementation leadership, implementation climate, and clinicians' use of evidence-based practice: a 5-year panel analysis. *Implement Sci.* 2020;15(1):1–15.
97. Aarons GA, Wells RS, Zagursky K, Fettes DL, Palinkas LA. Implementing evidence-based practice in community mental health agencies: a multiple stakeholder analysis. *Am J Public Health.* 2009;99(11):2087–2095.
98. Aarons GA, Green AE, Trott E, et al. The roles of system and organizational leadership in system-wide evidence-based intervention sustainment: a mixed-method study. *Adm Policy Ment Health.* 2016;43(6):991–1008.
99. Aarons GA, Ehrhart MG, Farahnak LR, Sklar M. Aligning leadership across systems and organizations to develop a strategic climate for evidence-based practice implementation. *Annu Rev Public Health.* 2014;35:255–274.
100. Meza RD, Triplett NS, Woodard GS, et al. The relationship between first-level leadership and inner-context and implementation outcomes in behavioral health: a scoping review. *Implement Sci.* 2021;16(1):1–21.
101. Birken SA, Currie G. Using organization theory to position middle-level managers as agents of evidence-based practice implementation. *Implement Sci.* 2021;16(1):1–6.
102. Proctor E, Ramsey AT, Brown MT, Malone S, Hooley C, McKay V. Training in Implementation Practice Leadership (TRIPLE): evaluation of a novel practice change strategy in behavioral health organizations. *Implement Sci.* 2019;14(1):1–11.
103. Aarons GA, Ehrhart MG, Farahnak LR, Hurlburt MS. Leadership and Organizational Change for Implementation (LOCI): a randomized mixed method pilot study of a leadership and organization development intervention for evidence-based practice implementation. *Implement Sci.* 2015;10(1):11.
104. Aarons GA, Ehrhart MG, Moullin JC, Torres EM, Green AE. Testing the Leadership and Organizational Change for Implementation (LOCI) intervention in substance abuse treatment: a cluster randomized trial study protocol. *Implement Sci.* 2017:12(29):1–11.

105. Sklar M, Ehrhart M, Aarons GA. Change in implementation leadership, climate, and provider reach for motivational interviewing: a cluster randomized trial of the Leadership and Organizational Change for Implementation (LOCI) strategy in substance use disorder treatment. Paper presented at: 14th Annual Conference on the Science of Dissemination and Implementation in Health; December 2021. Virtual.
106. Skar A-MS, Braathu N, Peters N, et al. A stepped-wedge randomized trial investigating the effect of the Leadership and Organizational Change for Implementation (LOCI) intervention on implementation and transformational leadership, and implementation climate. *BMC Health Serv Res.* 2022;22(298):1–15.
107. Hasson H, Von Thiele Schwarz U, Nielsen K, Tafvelin S. Are we all in the same boat? The role of perceptual distance in organizational health interventions. *Stress Health.* 2016;32(4):294–303.
108. Silver Wolf DAP, Dulmus C, Maguin E, Keesler J, Powell BJ. Organizational leaders' and staff members' appraisals of their work environment within a children's social service system. *Hum Serv Organ Manag Leadersh Gov.* 2014;38(3):215–227.
109. Beidas RS, Williams JW Jr., Green AE, et al. Concordance between administrator and clinician ratings of organizational culture and climate. *Adm Policy Ment Health.* 2018;45:142–151.
110. Aarons GA, Ehrhart MG, Torres EM, Finn NK, Beidas RS. The humble leader: association of discrepancies in leader and follower ratings of implementation leadership with organizational climate in mental health organizations. *Psychiatr Serv.* 2017;68(2):115–122.
111. Aarons GA, Ehrhart MG, Farahnak LR, Sklar M, Horowitz J. Discrepancies in leader and follower ratings of transformational leadership: relationships with organizational culture in mental health. *Adm Policy Ment Health.* 2017;.
112. Hasson H, Villaume K, Von Thiele Schwarz U, Palm K. Managing implementation: roles of line managers, senior managers, and human resource professionals in an occupational health intervention. *J Occup Environ Med and Ment Health Serv Res.* 2017;44(4):480–491.
113. Nystrom ME, Strehlenert H, Hansson J, Hasson H. Strategies to facilitate implementation and sustainability of large system transformations: a case study of a national program for improving the quality of care for the elderly people. *BMC Health Serv Res.* 2014;14(1):401.
114. Rycroft-Malone J, Burton CR, Bucknall T, Graham ID, Hutchinson AM, Stacey D. Collaboration and co-production of knowledge in healthcare: opportunities and challenges. *Int J Health Policy Manag.* 2016;5(4):221–223.
115. Kislov R, Harvey G, Walshe K. Collaborations for leadership in applied health research and care: lessons from the theory of communities of practice. *Implement Sci.* 2011;6(64):1–10.
116. Teal R, Bergmire DM, Johnston M, Weiner BJ. Implementing community-based provider participation in research: an empirical study. *Implement Sci.* 2012;7(41):1–15.
117. Kislov R, Waterman H, Harvey G, Boaden R. Rethinking capacity building for knowledge mobilisation: developing multilevel capabilities in healthcare organisations. *Implement Sci.* 2014;9(166):1–12.
118. Bunger A, Hanson RF, Doogan NJ, Powell BJ, Cao Y, Dunn JC. Can learning collaboratives support implementation by rewiring professional networks? *Adm Policy Ment Health.* 2016;43(1):79–92.
119. Powell BJ, Beidas RS, Rubin RM, et al. Applying the policy ecology framework to Philadelphia's behavioral health transformation efforts. *Adm Policy Ment Health.* 2016;43(6):909–926.
120. Lewin K. Frontiers in group dynamics: concept, method and reality in social science; social eqilibria and social change. *Hum Relat.* 1947;1(1):5–41.
121. Lehman WEK, Greener JM, Simpson DD. Assessing organizational readiness for change. *J Subst Abuse Treat.* 2002;22(4):197–209.
122. Weiner BJ. A theory of organizational readiness for change. *Implement Sci.* 2009;4:67.
123. Brooke-Sumner C, Petersen-Williams P, Wagener E, Sorsdahl K, Aarons GA, Myers B. Adaptation of the Texas Christian University Organisational Readiness for Change Short Form (TCU-ORC-SF) for use in primary health facilities in South Africa. *BMJ Open.* 2021;11(12):e047320.
124. Shea CM, Jacobs SR, Esserman DA, Bruce K, Weiner BJ. Organizational readiness for implementing change: a psychometric assessment of a new measure. *Implement Sci.* 2014;9(7):1–15.
125. Helfrich C, Li Y, Sharp N, Sales A. Organizational readiness to change assessment (ORCA): development of an instrument based on the Promoting Action on Research in Health Services (PARIHS) framework *Implement Sci.* 2009;4(38):1–13.
126. Holt DT, Armenakis AA, Feild HS, Harris SG. Readiness for organizational change: the systematic development of a scale. *J Appl Behav Sci.* 2007;43(2):232–255.

127. McAlearney AS, Gregory M, Walker DM, Edwards M. Development and validation of an organizational readiness to change instrument focused on cultural competency. *Health Serv Res.* 2021;56(1):145–153.
128. Hayirli TC, Meara JG, Barash D, et al. Development and content validation of the Safe Surgery Organizational Readiness Tool: a quality improvement study. *Int J Surg.* 2021;89:1–8.
129. Nickel NC, Taylor EC, Labbok MH, Weiner BJ, Williamson NE. Applying organisation theory to understand barriers and facilitators to the implementation of Baby-Friendly: a multisite qualitative study. *Midwifery.* 2013;29(8):956–964.
130. Bandura A. Social cognitive theory: an agentic perspective. *Annu Rev Psychol.* 2001;52:1–26.
131. Gist ME, Mitchell TR. Self-efficacy: a theoretical analysis of its determinants and malleability. *Acad Manage Rev.* 1992;17(2):183–211.
132. Herscovitch L, Meyer JP. Commitment to organizational change: extension of a three-component model. *J Appl Psychol.* 2002;87(3):474–487.
133. Armenakis AA, Harris SG. Reflections: our journey in organizational change research and practice. *J Change Manage.* 2009;9(2):127–142.
134. Bandura A. Self-efficacy mechanism in human agency. *Am Psychol.* 1982;37(2):122–147.
135. Shaw RJ, Kaufman MA, Bosworth HB, et al. Organizational factors associated with readiness to implement and translate a primary care based telemedicine behavioral program to improve blood pressure control: the HTN-IMPROVE study. *Implement Sci.* 2013;8(106):1–13.
136. Armenakis AA, Harris SG, Mossholder KW. Creating readiness for organizational change. *Hum Relat.* 1993;46(6):681–704.
137. Aarons GA, Green AE, Palinkas LA, et al. Dynamic adaptation process to implement an evidence-based child maltreatment intervention. *Implement Sci.* 2012;7(32):1–9.
138. Lengnick-Hall R, Willging C, Hurlburt M, Fenwick K, Aarons GA. Contracting as a bridging factor linking outer and inner contexts during EBP implementation and sustainment: a prospective study across multiple US public sector service systems. *Implement Sci.* 2020;15(1):1–16.
139. Shea CM, Malone R, Weinberger M, et al. Assessing organizational capacity for achieving meaningful use of electronic health records. *Health Care Manage Rev.* 2014;39(2):124–133.
140. Vax S, Farkas M, Russinova Z, Mueser KT, Drainoni M-L. Enhancing organizational readiness for implementation: constructing a typology of readiness-development strategies using a modified Delphi process. *Implement Sci.* 2021;16(1):1–11.
141. Castañeda SF, Holscher J, Mumman MK, et al. Dimensions of community and organizational readiness for change. *Prog Community Health Partnersh.* 2012;6(2):219.
142. Kononowech J, Hagedorn H, Hall C, et al. Mapping the organizational readiness to change assessment to the Consolidated Framework for Implementation Research. *Implement Sci Commun.* 2021;2(1):1–6.
143. Domlyn AM, Wandersman A. Community coalition readiness for implementing something new: using a Delphi methodology. *J Community Psychol.* 2019;47(4):882–897.
144. Aarons GA. Mental health provider attitudes toward adoption of evidence-based practice: the Evidence-Based Practice Attitude Scale (EBPAS). *Ment Health Serv Res.* 2004;6(2):61–74.
145. Aarons GA, Glisson C, Hoagwood K, Kelleher K, Landsverk J, Cafri G. Psychometric properties and United States national norms of the Evidence-Based Practice Attitude Scale (EBPAS). *Psychol Assessment.* 2010;22(2):356–365.
146. Silver Wolf DAP, Dulmus CN, Maguin E, Fava N. Refining the Evidence-Based Practice Attitude Scale: an alternative confirmatory factor analysis. *Soc Work Res.* 2014;38(1):47–58.
147. Aarons GA, Cafri G, Lugo L, Sawitzky A. Expanding the domains of attitudes towards evidence-based practice: the Evidence-Based Practice Attitude Scale-50. *Adm Policy Ment Health.* 2012;39(5):331–340.
148. Rye M, Torres EM, Friborg O, Skre I, Aarons GA. The Evidence-Based Practice Attitude Scale-36 (EPBAS-36): a brief and pragmatic measure of attitudes to evidence-based practice validated in Norwegian and US samples. *Implement Sci.* 2017;12(44):1–11.
149. Aarons GA, Sawitzky AC. Organizational climate partially mediates the effect of culture on work attitudes and staff turnover in mental health services. *Adm Policy Ment Health.* 2006;33(3):289–301.
150. Aarons GA, Sommerfeld DH, Willging CE. The soft underbelly of system change: the role of leadership and organizational climate in turnover during statewide behavioral health reform. *Psychol Serv.* 2011;8(4):269–281.
151. Aarons GA, Palinkas LA. Implementation of evidence-based practice in child welfare: service provider perspectives. *Adm Policy Ment Health.* 2007;34(4):411–419.

152. Ajzen I, Fishbein M. The influence of attitudes on behavior. In: Albarracín D, Johnson BT, Zanna MP, eds. *The Handbook of Attitudes.* Lawrence Erlbaum Associates, Inc.; 2005:173–222.
153. Moullin JC, Ehrhart MG, Aarons GA. Development and testing of the Measure of Innovation-Specific Implementation Intentions (MISII) using Rasch measurement theory. *Implement Sci.* 2018;13(1):89.
154. Ehrhart MG, Aarons GA, Farahnak LR. Going above and beyond for implementation: the development and validity testing of the Implementation Citizenship Behavior Scale (ICBS). *Implement Sci.* 2015;10(65):1–9.
155. Scott WR, Davis GF. *Organizations and Organizing: Rational, Natural and Open Systems Perspectives.* Routledge; 2015.
156. Siegenfeld AF, Bar-Yam Y. An introduction to complex systems science and its applications. *Complexity.* 2020;1–16. Article ID 6105872.
157. Williamson OE. The economics of organization: the transaction cost approach. *Am J Sociol.* 1981;87(3):548–577.
158. DiMaggio PJ, Powell WW. The iron cage revisited: institutional isomorphism and collective rationality in organizational fields. *Am Sociol Rev.* 1983;48(2):147–160.
159. Donaldson L. *The Contingency Theory of Organizations.* Sage; 2001.
160. Salancik GR, Pfeffer J. *The External Control of Organizations: A Resource Dependence Perspective.* Harper & Row; 1978.
161. Birken SA, Bunger AC, Powell BJ, et al. Organizational theory for dissemination and implementation research. *Implement Sci.* 2017;12(1):1–15.
162. Leeman J, Baquero B, Bender M, et al. Advancing the use of organization theory in implementation science. *Prev Med.* 2019;129:105832.
163. Berta W, Cranley L, Dearing JW, Dogherty EJ, Squires JE, Estabrooks CA. Why (we think) facilitation works: insights from organizational learning theory. *Implement Sci.* 2015;10(1): 1–13.
164. Dadich A. From bench to bedside: Methods that help clinicians use evidence-based practice. *Aust Psychol.* 2010;45(3):197–211.
165. Saldana L, Chamberlain P, Wang W, Brown CH. Predicting program start-up using the stages of implementation measure. *Adm Policy Ment Health.* 2011;39(6):419–425.
166. Allen JD, Shelton RC, Kephart L, Jandorf L, Folta SC, Knott CL. Organizational characteristics conducive to the implementation of health programs among Latino churches. *Implement Sci Commun.* 2020;1(1):1–9.
167. Andrew NE, Middleton S, Grimley R, et al. Hospital organizational context and delivery of evidence-based stroke care: a cross-sectional study. *Implement Sci.* 2019;14(1):1–12.
168. Williams NJ, Frank HE, Frederick L, et al. Organizational culture and climate profiles: relationships with fidelity to three evidence-based practices for autism in elementary schools. *Implement Sci.* 2019;14(1):1–14.
169. Powell BJ, Haley AD, Patel SV, et al. Improving the implementation and sustainment of evidence-based practices in community mental health organizations: a study protocol for a matched-pair cluster randomized pilot study of the Collaborative Organizational Approach to Selecting and Tailoring Implementation Strategies (COAST-IS). *Implement Sci Commun.* 2020;1(1):1–13.
170. Johnson JE, Viglione J, Ramezani N, et al. Protocol for a quasi-experimental, 950 county study examining implementation outcomes and mechanisms of Stepping Up, a national policy effort to improve mental health and substance use services for justice-involved individuals. *Implement Sci.* 2021;16(1):1–14.
171. Lewis CC, Boyd MR, Walsh-Bailey C, et al. A systematic review of empirical studies examining mechanisms of implementation in health. *Implement Sci.* 2020;15:1–25.
172. Bunger AC, Birken SA, Hoffman JA, MacDowell H, Choy-Brown M, Magier E. Elucidating the influence of supervisors' roles on implementation climate. *Implement Sci.* 2019;14(1):1–12.

10

Participatory Approaches in Dissemination and Implementation Science

SHOBA RAMANADHAN, MELINDA DAVIS, S. TIFFANY DONALDSON, ELECIA MILLER, AND MEREDITH MINKLER

INTRODUCTION

In contrast to traditional approaches to dissemination and implementation (D&I) science, which consider institutions, communities, and individuals as entities under study, engaged approaches enable academic researchers and community/practice partners to work collaboratively to leverage diverse resources and expertise to close the gap between research and practice. With one such approach, termed *participatory implementation science*, academic researchers and partners engage in an iterative and ongoing manner to coproduce knowledge and create system-level change as they integrate research evidence into practice/community settings to improve health and reduce health inequities.[1] A wide range of terms is used to describe participatory approaches to research, including community-based participatory research (CBPR), community-engaged research, participatory action research, and participatory engagement with learning health systems.[2,3] Embedded in many of these approaches is the notion of community, which has Latin roots denoting the qualities of that which is shared or common.[4] This often refers to a group of individuals who have social relationships, have a shared identity, and are colocated in physical or virtual spaces.[5] In the context of D&I science, several communities may be of interest (e.g., service recipients, implementers, funders, and policymakers). In this chapter, we speak broadly about participatory and engaged approaches to D&I, a group that shares a commitment to combining research, engagement, capacity building, and action to improve health and address health inequities.[6,7] Although attention also is paid, in part, to dissemination, we have intentionally narrowed our main focus to provide more in-depth coverage of our primary concern, namely what participatory approaches add to the implementation components of D&I science.

For many D&I efforts, the goal is to address the challenge that evidence-based interventions (EBIs)—whether programs, practices, policies, or therapeutics—are slow to be integrated as part of routine practice and care and are often inequitably or inappropriately deployed.[8] Challenges with the uptake of the COVID-19 vaccination, diagnostic tools, and other mitigation strategies (e.g., social distancing and masks) in the United States drove home the need to involve practice/community partners in translating novel, life-saving discoveries for diverse community and practice settings. Indeed, the evidence base for COVID-19 vaccines, diagnostics, and therapeutics was generated at a remarkable pace. Yet, greater strategic attention and resource deployment were needed to support the integration of these discoveries into service delivery systems, particularly for communities ineffectively served by typical healthcare and public health systems.[9,10] While this is a common concern raised by implementation scientists, the challenges related to the pandemic response emphasized the inefficiencies and inequities that resulted from the exclusion of the expertise and assets of community and other stakeholders in practice and community settings. Strategic engagement of

Shoba Ramanadhan, Melinda Davis, S. Tiffany Donaldson, Elecia Miller, and Meredith Minkler, *Participatory Approaches in Dissemination and Implementation Science* In: *Dissemination and Implementation Research in Health.* Edited by: Ross C. Brownson, Graham A. Colditz, and Enola K. Proctor, Oxford University Press. © Oxford University Press 2023. DOI: 10.1093/oso/9780197660690.003.0010 diverse experts is critical to deliver appropriate services through the right channels to those that need them—a core tenet of equity-focused D&I.

Engaged approaches to D&I offer the opportunity to center equity, support the development of a relevant and usable evidence base, and improve health impact while producing generalizable knowledge and advancing the field.[11] While there has been a growing emphasis on participatory approaches to bridge the research-practice gap in the last two decades, they are not yet the norm.[12] For example, 2009 data showed that in a pool of 103,250 active National Institutes of Health (NIH) projects, only 294 (0.29%) used participatory approaches (conceptualized broadly to include variations mentioned previously in this chapter and other forms of engaged research).[13] Thus, this chapter seeks to demonstrate the value partners add to the process of designing, conducting, analyzing, disseminating, and translating D&I efforts. We introduce participatory approaches to D&I by describing a range of engagement levels academic researchers and community/practice partners might utilize, from a fully engaged approach to a less-engaged consultative model. We also describe the core benefits and challenges of these approaches and key considerations for projects. We offer a case example illustrating the development and evolution of a rural academic-community research partnership and a series of collaborative studies aligned with regional health system transformation. Finally, we present future directions for the field and additional resources.

DIVERSE PARTNERS AND ENGAGEMENT APPROACHES

To support broad engagement, the team should identify actors who might be impacted by or make decisions about the work and individuals and institutions that can support improved evidence generation and EBI sustainability. The 7 *P*'s Framework for stakeholder identification in outcomes and effectiveness research offers a helpful starting point for considering patients/public, providers, purchasers, payers, policymakers, product makers, and principal investigators.[14] The D&I theory, model, or framework that guides the study may also provide additional prompts. Decisions about which partners to include should ensure that they do not create, reinforce, or maintain existing inequities.[15]

Thought must also be given to the level of engagement needed for a given D&I effort based on the partners involved, timeline, budget, the purpose of the partnership, and other considerations. As seen in Figure 10.1, one way to conceptualize the continuum of engagement from most to least participatory is collegial, collaborative, consultative, and contractual.[16]

We encourage implementation scientists to move away from contractual research models,

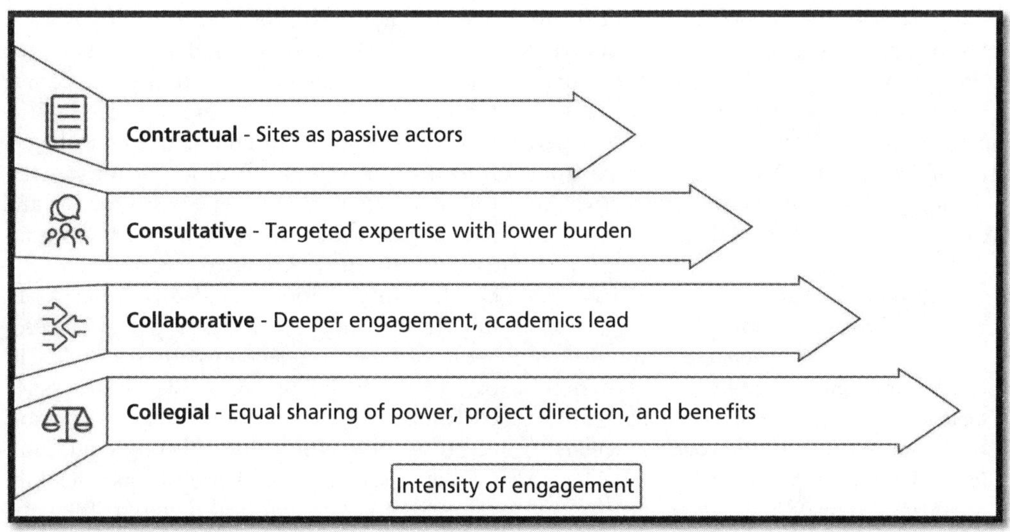

FIGURE 10.1 A range of engagement levels for D&I projects.

Adapted with permission from Minkler and Salvatore.[16]

in which institutions and individuals passively provide a site or data for research. Deloria (a Native American author, theologian, and activist) coined the phrase "helicopter research," which offers an apt metaphor. In the most problematic version of this, academic researchers swoop in, collect data, and leave, privileging scientific inquiry over all else.[17] While not all contractual models produce harm, they do little to improve either the science or the openness to research evidence in a given setting or to build the capacity and skills of community partners. Below, we offer a detailed examination of these levels of partnership in D&I using definitions and examples; we start with collegial, followed by collaborative and consultative approaches.

Collegial/CBPR Approaches to D&I

At the highest level of engagement and action orientation, collegial approaches emphasize power-sharing between academic and community/practice partners. Indeed, explicit attention to power in the development, dissemination, and implementation of research innovations is critical to avoid reproducing broader patterns of inequities. The key is for partners to access and deploy the necessary resources to advance their interests related to the project/issue. That is not always an easy feat given that public health and medical research systems are typically hierarchical in nature, and power and privilege are often concentrated among a narrow set of institutions and individuals.[18] As discussed in the section regarding challenges in engaged approaches to D&I, concrete actions can be taken to move toward meaningful power-sharing. Collegial approaches that emphasize power-sharing are often equated with CBPR traditions. A classic definition from the Kellogg Scholars Program summarizes the core concepts of this approach:

> A collaborative process that equitably involves all partners in the research process and recognizes the unique strengths that each brings. CBPR begins with a research topic of importance to the community with the aim of combining knowledge and action for social change to improve community health and eliminate health disparities.[19]

CBPR approaches aim to involve partners in all phases of research so that a diverse group of actors is involved in both the inquiry and sense-making that underlie the research effort. For D&I science, involvement is particularly important for the dissemination and use of findings to promote more equitable policies and practices.[20,21] CBPR approaches emphasize capacity building, long-term relationships, and local utility of the solutions generated.[22] By minimizing the distance between research and practice, CBPR efforts can develop relevant and impactful solutions for sustained change—a core value of D&I.

Box 10.1 outlines 11 core principles of CBPR—nine from the foundational work by Israel and colleagues and two from Minkler and Wallerstein.[23–26] These principles may provide initial guidance to implementation scientists seeking to utilize participatory approaches in their work.

Example

PLANET MassCONECT is a study aimed at building capacity among the staff of ommunity-based organizations (CBOs) to use EBIs for cancer prevention and control. The name connects resources held in the Cancer Control PLANET (an EBI resource offered by the National Cancer Institute) and the name of a community network launched through a previous grant. The idea for the study originated from leaders of health-focused community coalitions. These leaders noted that organizations in their coalitions were increasingly being asked by funders to use EBIs but did not have the necessary knowledge or skills to find, adapt, and implement such programs. To increase the impact of cancer prevention efforts and improve the ability of CBOs to secure funding, the team began work in this area in 2008, led by Viswanath, Koh and others.[28] The work is still active and has taken various shapes to support continuity, with funding through 2026. The capacity-building intervention included training, tools, minigrants, and a web-based portal (https://www.planetmassconect.org) for trainees. The original PLANET MassCONECT partners led coalitions of CBOs serving three low-income, racially and ethnically diverse communities with strong multisectoral partnerships addressing health and health equity. The partnership has grown and broadened its focus over time but has kept the core CBPR principles as a guide, as detailed below.

BOX 10.1

CBPR PRINCIPLES TO PROMPT DESIGN OF A PARTICIPATORY APPROACH FOR DISSEMINATION AND IMPLEMENTATION

1. Recognizes community as a unit of identity and can be defined based on geographic, sociodemographics, organizational, or other terms.
2. Builds on strengths and resources within the community; operates from an assets focus.
3. Facilitates a collaborative, equitable partnership in all phases of research, involving an empowering and power-sharing process that attends to inequities.
4. Fosters co-learning and capacity building among all partners.
5. Integrates and achieves a balance between knowledge generation and action for the mutual benefit of all partners.
6. Focuses on the local relevance of public health problems and on ecological perspectives that attend to the multiple determinants of health.
7. Involves systems development using a cyclical and iterative process.
8. Disseminates results to all partners and involves them in the broader dissemination of results.
9. Involves a long-term process and commitment to sustainability.
10. Openly addresses issues of race, ethnicity, racism and other social divides, and embodies "cultural humility",[27] recognizing that while one cannot be truly "competent" in another's culture, one can commit to ongoing self-reflection and critique, as well as working to redress power imbalances and to develop authentic partnerships.
11. Works to assure research rigor and validity of the research question (coming from, or being of importance to the community) and that different "ways of knowing," including community- and practice-based knowledge, are valued alongside traditional academic sources of knowledge.

Community definition: The original coalition partners suggested defining communities based on Community Health Network Areas, regions defined by the Massachusetts Department of Health. We note that these regions were meaningful to practitioners but would not resonate with broader community members. A significant benefit was that these were existing networks into which program activity could be integrated. Over time, the participation of communities has changed and so have the ways in which communities have been defined (e.g., the recent addition of a partner serving the Brazilian population in Greater Boston).

Building on strengths and resources: Academic and practice partners co-created the intervention design and content, centering advisory board expertise related to adult learning and the realities of public health practice in low-resource organizations.

Collaborative, equitable partnership: Practice partners identified the issue, and the full team codeveloped potential solutions. The group strived to share power and ownership but sees this as an aspirational and motivating goal rather than something already achieved. Another important aspect of equity was that the project includes stipends for community partners' organizations, funds to cover meeting attendance, and sharing of in-kind resources (e.g., staff time).

Capacity building: In addition to building capacity among CBO practitioners for EBI utilization, the project supported advisory board members in building research capacity and learning about EBIs. The project also supported academic researchers to build capacity related to CBPR and the practical constraints of EBI utilization in historically marginalized and underresourced communities.

Knowledge and action: The intervention under evaluation was a starting point for local action around EBI utilization, ranging from grant-writing supports to efforts to increase public attention to health inequities.

Local relevance: Advisory board coleadership of the project ensured that all activities were conducted with due consideration of the multilevel forces supporting and constraining both CBO practitioners (e.g., the mismatch between needs and EBIs) and potential recipients of services (e.g., inability to capitalize based on competing demands).[29]

Systems development: The project sought to develop broad capacity in the community to leverage research evidence to address priority health equity goals. The intention was to build general capacity to use EBIs rather than innovation-specific capacity, so that CBOs could draw on these resources in the future. The system's focus was also included in the focus on building networks of practitioners to serve as resources for each other.[30]

Dissemination: Dissemination activities have included interactive community discussions, library posters, practice briefs, presentations to policymakers, infographics shared on social media, community events called science cafés, and other formats. Academic and practice partners have also coauthored several journal articles, and one practice partner is a coauthor of this chapter.

Long-term process/sustainability: In CBPR and other forms of participatory research, "staying for the long haul" is critical to building and maintaining authentic partnerships, while also enabling outside partners to be present when some of the action outcomes of the work come to fruition.[31] The work of PLANET MassCONECT has been ongoing for 15 years in two communities and 5 years in another community and has recently expanded to include new partners.

Cultural humility: Consistent with the core principle of cultural humility,[27] the researchers and other outside partners entered the project with an understanding of how much they *did not know* about the communities with which they would be working and reflected on their assumptions while trying to better understand the cultures and realities of the community partners. As relationships strengthened, the group has engaged in open discussions of racism and other social divides. The refinement of a biobanking outreach curriculum offers an example of how this impacted the work. Deep discussions about the historical and current medical mistreatment of African Americans, Native Americans, and other groups resulted in changes to the curriculum to start the outreach sessions with an interactive discussion of mistrust and only then move to a discussion of biobanking.

Rigorous science/diverse ways of knowing: Welcoming myriad ways of knowing requires that outside partners recognize how the lived experience and historical understanding that community/practice partners bring to the table can help improve not only the relevance of the research, but also its rigor (e.g., in fine-tuning research instruments for use in particular cultural contexts) and successful community dissemination or reach.[21] In this project, community-led issue identification and centering practice-based knowledge have been guiding principles for this partnership. That said, the ability to leverage different ways of knowing is an area for continued growth.

Collaborative Approaches to D&I

With this approach, academic and community/practice partners work together, with the former controlling decisions and resources. This approach often includes deep engagement of partners over multiple phases of the research process but does not assume the same level of project co-creation or power-sharing as a collegial approach. In this way, both the investments required by partners and expected benefits are likely to be similar in nature, but not in scale, to collegial levels of engagement. This may better allow for constraints on participation from funders, academic institutions, or competing priorities. For example, a collaborative approach to D&I might include a community advisory board that provides academic researchers with details about implementation context and ensures local benefit and relevance, but the project is fundamentally driven by the research team. Given the similarities to collegial approaches, the example of PLANET MassCONECT is relevant for this type of engagement.

Consultative Approaches to D&I

In consultative approaches to D&I, practice/community partners are consulted once or infrequently with minimal burden for a specific purpose (e.g., facilitate recruitment or advise on dissemination audiences/modalities). The benefits of this type of approach include the ability to access high-level expertise and robust networks, with a decreased investment of time and resources for all partners. However, consultative partnerships can be challenging to develop and maintain, given less frequent and intense interactions. Thus, project teams may not capture the full range of insights offered by a more deeply involved partner. Further, given the history of outside researchers engaging community members of particular communities in exploitative ways, this approach may be equated with tokenism and create further distrust in the community.

A positive and well-known example of the consultative model convenes a panel of experts (using the most inclusive definition) to offer feedback on proposed research activities, ideally early enough to shape the work. An example comes from the Meharry–Vanderbilt Community Engaged Research Core at the Vanderbilt Institute for Clinical and Translational Research, which offered community engagement studios as a service to affiliated academic researchers.[32] This approach relies on a standing pool of community experts to review and offer advice on research presentations. Additional details and a toolkit to support the utilization of this approach are available elsewhere.[33]

As noted previously, the range of potential partners for D&I research is broad. It might include intended recipients of the EBI, implementers, practice leaders and decision makers, and others who can provide insight into the broader implementation context. As with any approach that relies on a subset of experts to represent a larger community, it is critical to utilize a thoughtful process for selection to ensure that certain groups are not excluded from the conversation.

Example

Project Resist is a study addressing tobacco control among young adult sexual minority women in the United States; it used a consultative approach to address two complementary goals: (1) assessing the efficacy of novel health communication strategies to improve tobacco-related outcomes and (2) exploring opportunities to design the resulting intervention for uptake by CBOs and community health centers. For this work, four national leaders in lesbian, gay, bisexual, transgender, and queer (LGBTQ+) health were engaged in the project as members of an advisory committee, meeting every 3 to 6 months. The formative work to understand the needs and preferences of potential adopting organizations offers a helpful illustration. The advisory committee provided rich insight into the practice context, resources, and constraints of LGBTQ+-serving organizations and codeveloped the interview guide for organizational leaders. For example, the advisory committee's insight into the context of LGBTQ+-serving organizations (e.g., funding patterns, emphasis on tobacco control vs. other health issues, and competing demands faced by clients) led to a reframing of the guide and the addition of new topics. The committee also leveraged their rich networks to support maximal diversity in sampling. Committee members offered insight to support the interpretation of findings and coauthored/co-created dissemination products for academic, practice, and community audiences. Connections between advisory committee members and project leadership through other cancer prevention and control activities among LGBTQ+ populations reinforced the relationships and alignment of overarching goals.[34]

As highlighted above and demonstrated in the examples, a range of engagement strategies, whether collegial, collaborative, or consultative, may be appropriate. As partnerships evolve, multiple methods for engagement may be used based on partner interest, capacity, resources, and time. Additionally, partnerships may engage core and ancillary members at different levels and for varied purposes within a given effort. In this vein, several starting points for partnership development are summarized in Figure 10.2. These concepts come from the authors' work and the literature.[35–40]

BENEFITS OF ENGAGED APPROACHES TO D&I SCIENCE

Broadly, the ability to draw from diverse and complementary expertise and skills to create new knowledge and insights should improve the successful execution of research projects while increasing the utility and impact of the

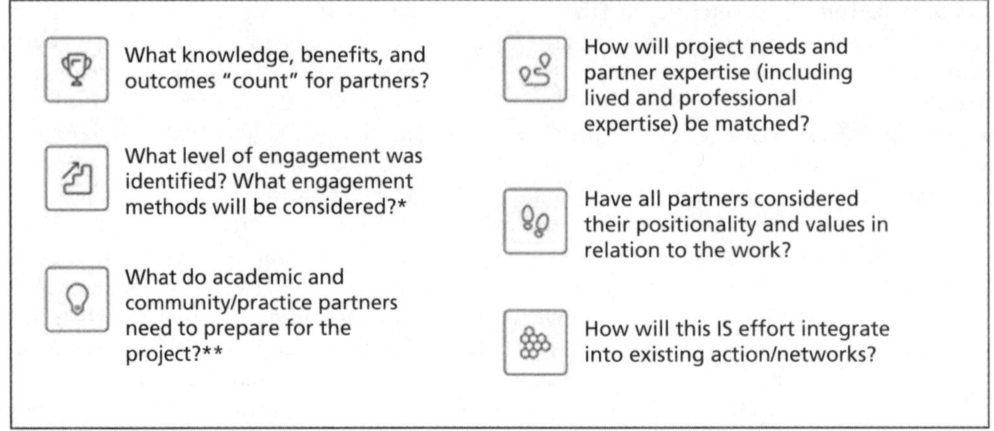

FIGURE 10.2 Starting points for participatory dissemination and implementation projects.
* The DICE Methods tool (https://dicemethods.org/) offers a range of potential methods (e.g., human-centered design approaches) and tools (e.g., network mapping) for examination.[41]
** Resources for examining academic researcher and practice/community partner readiness can support these assessments.[37,42]

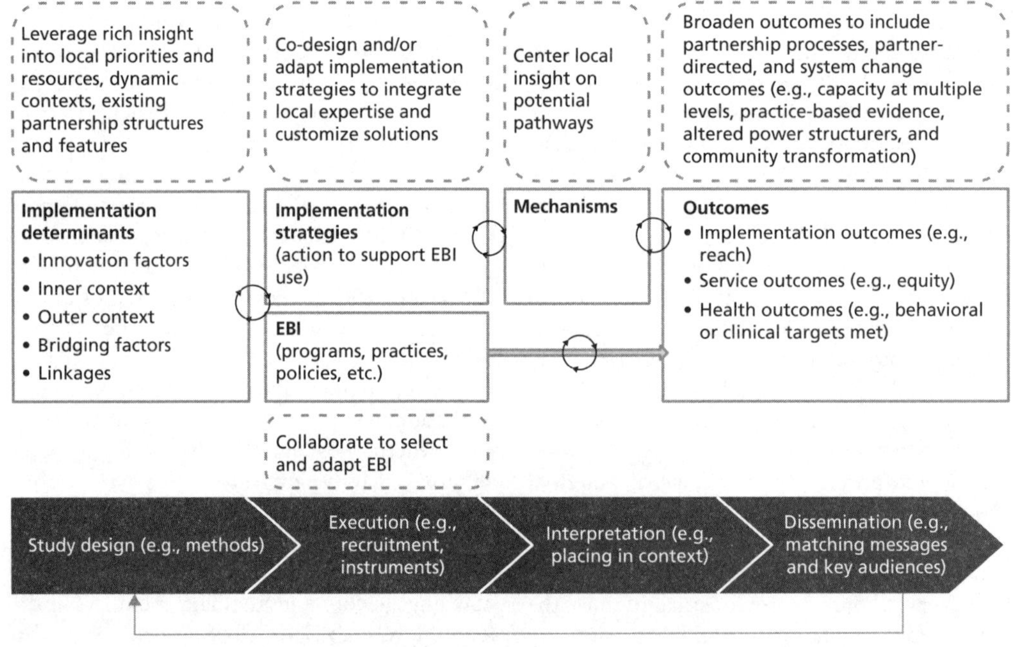

FIGURE 10.3 Opportunities to integrate participatory approaches into D&I studies,[30,48] illustrated with the implementation research logic model[45] and typical study flows.

findings both locally and in the field broadly.[43] Of particular importance for projects focused on advancing health equity, involvement of a range of partners surfaces voices and knowledge that would otherwise remain untapped by the broader scientific and practice fields. Below, we describe the applications and benefits of participatory approaches to D&I, drawing on the Exploration, Preparation, Implementation, and Sustainment Framework[44] and organized by the Implementation Research Logic Model[45] and typical study flows (Figure 10.3). As noted in frameworks and models of adaptation and sustainment,[46,47] logic model components will evolve as the investigation progresses. The expectation of iteration, a hallmark of participatory approaches to D&I, is highlighted in the figure with circular arrows.

Areas of focus for D&I efforts include the following:

1. **Implementation determinants.** The influences that impact implementation outcomes are numerous, interacting, and dynamic,[49] and the deep insight of a range of partners offers the opportunity to track relevant attributes of context. To give a sense of the scale of the effort to examine determinants, a recent review of 17 D&I determinants frameworks found 12 common context domains, each of which includes multiple constructs. For example, the patient/client domain might consist of preferences, expectations, knowledge, attitudes, and resources.[50] A research team could capture these data with formative research but would likely miss key elements and changes in a dynamic system. For example, partners were engaged in a participatory process to co-create a theory of change to introduce mental health services into systems in Ethiopia, India, Nepal, South Africa, and Uganda. This work identified priority characteristics in each site related to the political environment, required resources and capacity, and other drivers of implementation outcomes and health impact.[51] Given the common deficits focus of public health and clinical approaches, engagement offers the opportunity to identify community and practice assets often ignored by academic researchers. At the same time, a participatory approach shifts attention from a narrow consideration of determinants for a given EBI or D&I study to a broader examination of capacity, culture, structures, history, and policy to address the needs of the implementation context as well.[52]
2. **Implementation strategies and mechanisms.** The methods and techniques for increasing the adoption, implementation, and sustainment of EBIs[53] should reflect the needs and preferences of ultimate adopters and implementers. An excellent example comes from the implementation mapping approach, an extension of intervention mapping. This five-step process emphasizes partnership between academic researchers, EBI adopters, and implementers as they (a) assess needs and resources, (b) identify critical determinants of change and core objectives, (c) select or design implementation strategies/theoretical approaches, (d) design implementation protocols and products, and (e) evaluate implementation outcomes.[54] Understanding how implementation strategies affect implementation outcomes is also necessary to advance the field.[55] Partners may have insight into potential mechanisms, such as how particular strategies impact readiness or culture to increase implementation support. These mechanisms of action are likely to be complex and nonlinear and may benefit from mapping using systems science methods.[53,56]
3. **EBI selection and adaptation.** Partnered approaches offer the opportunity to bridge the divide between EBIs and the needs and capacity of implementation settings. In the same way that tailoring D&I interventions through Plan-Do-Study-Act cycles helps integrate research into practice,[57] a parallel argument can be made for participatory approaches. The process by which evidence becomes relevant for local settings may be a core part of moving research into practice across diverse environments. These process steps may be an important aspect of what is generalizable for participatory D&I efforts. The engagement of partners for EBI selection also pushes academic researchers to attend to Hawe's push to focus on the function, rather than the form, of the innovation.[58]
4. **Implementation and other outcomes.** As a complement to typical

implementation outcomes, such as those specified in the Proctor model,[59] there is also an opportunity to engage practice and community partners in outcome definition and prioritization. For example, the Integrative Systems Praxis for Implementation Research (INSPIRE) project used participatory approaches to create systems-focused implementation strategies to reduce global cervical cancer inequities. The process engaged multilevel partners to define and execute monitoring and evaluation strategies that will feed forward into the resulting stages of change.[60] Using a broader set of outcomes supports the opportunity to take a systems perspective and account for the effects of multiple, interacting forces on implementation efforts and individual behavior (see chapter 13). A view of the EBI, implementation strategies, and the implementation effort as events in a system allows for a more nuanced picture.[56,58] This addresses the commonly voiced concern among implementers that D&I efforts focus too narrowly on one issue or one setting, missing the multiple competing demands and influences on potential service recipients and implementation systems.[29] Last, the benefits of engaged approaches to D&I extend to long-term outcomes. Capacity building—a core feature of participatory approaches—is expected to leave partners better able to handle current and future health challenges while building leadership and cohesion and researchers better equipped to produce actionable, relevant knowledge.[61] As described by Wallerstein and colleagues, system and capacity outcomes may include changes in practice/policies, changes in power relations and dynamics, increased ability of community members and leaders to effect change, and community renewal.[42]

5. **Study design, execution, and interpretation of data.** Advantages of participatory approaches for general study activities include more appropriate study design and instruments, improved recruitment and retention, contextualized data analysis, and enhanced interpretation and dissemination.[62] Unique contributions for D&I relate to considering the dynamic implementation context in the design and interpretation phases, leveraging knowledge from a diverse set of experts, and broadening the definition of what "counts" as evidence.[63,64]
6. **Dissemination.** A core obligation of action-oriented, participatory research is sharing study-related information in an accessible, relevant, and action-focused manner to a range of audiences that may benefit. Using a "designing for dissemination" process increases the likelihood that research products match the needs, resources, and requirements of the individuals and systems that will utilize them. As examples, practitioners and policymakers may benefit from toolkits, briefs, knowledge translation platforms and synthesis tools, and training opportunities. For the public, a range of options, including local media, arts-based performances, science cafés, and social media, may be of interest. A collaborative process will increase the likelihood of fit with and utility for target audiences, whatever the set of products. Dissemination impact can be examined by evaluating outcomes (e.g., acceptability appropriateness, utility, sustainability, and satisfaction).[65,66] A planning tool from the Robert Wood Johnson Foundation emphasizes the importance of identifying core dissemination audiences at the outset of a project; developing relationships with them; and understanding what to share with them, how, and when.[67] As Green has emphasized, if we want more evidence-based practice, we need to improve the quality and quantity of practice-based evidence.[68] Participatory approaches offer this opportunity and increase the influence of practice-based expertise in the formal scientific literature.

CHALLENGES OF PARTICIPATORY APPROACHES TO D&I

A subset of relevant challenges applies to participatory research broadly, including the potential for mismatch between policies and structures in academic versus practice settings, insufficient trust or communication among partners, and tensions between the requirements of a rigorous study design, with goals of advancing the field, and the practice-oriented needs of partners.[63,69] Below, we highlight a set of particular interests for D&I science.

1. **Concerns about external validity.** The products of engaged D&I research, such as collaboratively designed implementation strategies, are expected to have greater relevance to users in the settings under study than products developed using standard approaches. At the same time, there is often a concern that these highly customized products will not be relevant to other settings and contexts.[63,70] However, we note that the results of participatory research are useful and relevant elsewhere, given that the studies reflect realities of practice more than those with settings that are artificially constructed and controlled to support internal validity (see also chapters 16–18). Additionally, we draw on concepts of transferability from qualitative research to emphasize the importance of providing enough information about the study, context, and participatory processes to allow others to determine the extent to which findings are relevant for their goals.[71]
2. **Disconnects between worldviews.** Different understandings of research, evidence, and expertise can challenge engaged D&I projects. After all, the critical and action-oriented lenses of participatory research efforts may conflict with the value placed in many public health and medical research environments on technical expertise, objectivity, and uncovering of universal truths.[72] Seward and colleagues described these challenges, drawing on D&I work in low- and middle-income countries and using task shifting as an example.[73] A team member operating from a positivist paradigm might apply a view of reality as a series of observable events to focus on questions about the effectiveness of task shifting to increase uptake of an EBI. By contrast, team members relying on constructivist or critical paradigms might view reality as a function of social, political, and other influences over time that cannot be separated from those participating in the research.[74,75] This may prompt questions of when task shifting is appropriate, for whom, and under what circumstances. Israel noted that participatory research draws on critical and constructivist perspectives but emphasizes the opportunity to find common ground by being transparent about these perspectives and thoughtfully matching methods to study goals, the expected use of the results, the context, local theory, the relevance of measurement tools, and the input of partners and stakeholders.[23]
3. **Diverse conceptualizations of evidence.** There may be disagreement between members of participatory D&I partnerships regarding what "counts" as evidence. As noted in Box 10.1, community- and practice-based knowledge must be integrated with commonly used academic sources of knowledge. As highlighted by Blue Bird Jernigan and colleagues regarding work with a range of Indigenous communities, there can be a tension between knowledge derived from faith plus real-world experience versus learnings derived from a randomized trial.[76] Rather than conceptualizing this as a gap in the research-to-practice pipeline, one can understand the disconnect as a gap in merging academic and practice/community knowledge.
4. **Concerns about power imbalances.** As noted previously, paying particular attention to power and how it may play out in each stage of the research process from study design to implementation,

dissemination, and evidence-based action, is critical in ensuring that we do not unwittingly reproduce and exacerbate health and social inequities. As Stanton and Ali highlighted, it can be helpful to consider three forms of power in the D&I research process: *discursive power* (how implementation issues are defined), *epistemic power* (whose knowledge is valued), and *material power* (how resources are distributed and accessed).[77] Building collaborative relationships is not enough; teams must be transparent and thoughtful about negotiating differential access to resources, knowledge, time for and experience with research, and differing agendas or needs.[72] Coming into a partnership, power imbalances between the academic researchers and community/practice partners may pose a challenge, as can hierarchies within the team. Muhammad and colleagues prompt partners to consider their positionality in relation to other actors in the implementation effort, how power impacts study decision-making, the question of whose voices are privileged as results are shared, and how power impacts the construction of knowledge.[36] With attention to this often-overlooked aspect of implementation systems, teams can explore and reshape the implementation context to be more health and equity promoting.

5. **Tensions balancing action and research.** Typical D&I projects do not have the necessary scope or scale to achieve transformation of practice and community settings, even if the team desires to engage in this way. For example, a D&I effort may improve receipt of a given service in the short term, but staffing challenges or changes to reimbursement in the setting could compromise the service after the funding ends. This can be addressed by focusing on short-term action while planning for sustainability and promoting long-term capacity-building and system development to address future health challenges.[61] Helping practice and community partners bring in their own funding from foundations and other sources to further support capacity building and the continuation and/or broadening of the action component of the work is another way in which researchers can both show their commitment to the community and enhance sustainability.

MEASURING PARTICIPATORY PROCESSES AND OUTCOMES

The literature is still nascent in demonstrating the value and utility of engaged approaches to D&I science (and engaged approaches to research overall). However, recent advances in the field offer the opportunity to build the literature in this area. For example, a recent review by Luger and colleagues identified relevant measures in three main areas. The first set addressed context (e.g., community capacity for research and researcher readiness for participatory research). The second set examined the process of community engagement (e.g., measures of group dynamics, partnership activities and synergy, and satisfaction with the practical aspects of the projects). The third set focused on outcomes (e.g., assessment of system or capacity change, sustainability of the work, or long-term outcomes like policy change).[78] A meta-analytic review covering reviews of participatory research in health is another valuable resource to understand how context, partnership and research processes, and outcomes are examined in the public health literature.[52]

A challenge in identifying outcomes is that academic and community-based partners may define success in research partnerships differently. For example, community/practice partners may be motivated to solve current pressing health challenges in their community—such as improving access to resources to address unmet social needs for low-income patients. At the same time, academic researchers may have a goal of better understanding variation in unmet social needs across racially and ethnically diverse low-income patients in the community. Robust partnerships should discuss partners' needs and prioritize strategies to measure processes and outcomes in ways that honor these perspectives.

Participatory D&I projects must look beyond typical implementation outcomes to examine systems change and long-term impact. The rich literature regarding multilevel, context-appropriate community interventions offers the opportunity to reorient toward an ecological, partnered approach. An essential extension of this perspective is the commitment to identify and examine unintended ripple effects of the implementation efforts in the broader system. These might include broader capacity building, community cohesion, improved relationships between academics and the local practice community, or changes in the priority placed on evidence-based action.[30,79,80] Thus, given that context, relationships, and trust between partners are likely to change and evolve,[23–26] a long-term view is needed.

Recent efforts in this area focus on empirically examining influences on outcomes of participatory research and on matching engagement strategies to goals, resources, and constraints. For example, Wallerstein and colleagues are testing a model that links CBPR contexts, group dynamics/partnerships, interventions, and a series of outcomes (focused on systems/capacity and health/equity).[42] Deeper understanding of the mechanisms by which participatory processes work (e.g., improved tailoring of research evidence or championing findings for a range of practice audiences) will advance this work.[78] Thus, there are both challenges and opportunities for participatory approaches to D&I to (1) balance project- and partner-specific measures with standard measures for evaluating context, process, and outcomes for engagement; (2) examine the mechanisms by which participatory approaches impact D&I studies; and (3) monitor multilevel impacts over time.

CASE STUDY

Partnership Foundation and Emergence

The Community Health Advocacy and Research Alliance (CHARA) is an academic-community partnership initiated in 2014 by a local primary care clinician (Kristen Dillon, MD) and an academic researcher (Melinda Davis, PhD) with roots in the region (see https://www.communityresearchalliance.org/about.html). CHARA is a collaboration of patient, community, health system, and academic partners who are aligned in their mission to "identify, develop, and conduct health research to answer questions that matter [in the Columbia Gorge]." This rural region of 85,000 residents includes seven counties in Oregon and Washington. Drs. Dillon and Davis were interested in creating a research structure to complement health system transformation activities in response to the formation of regional coordinated care organizations (CCOs). CCOs are similar to Medicare accountable care organizations but focus on Medicaid populations.[81] They secured seed funding to develop CHARA, which has enabled the team to secure funding for multiple research collaborations across the spectrum of engagement levels.

Partnership Development and Structure

CHARA development was informed by prior CBPR work with rural community-based health coalitions.[82,83] Activities were designed to align with community priorities by providing research training and information on effective EBIs and implementation/evaluation designs, rather than imposing external agendas.[84] Activities in the first year focused on crafting the organization's mission and vision statements and building an organizational structure that included the core team, a nine-member advisory board, research ambassadors, and academic and organizational partners. Over the next 5 years, activities focused on building capacity and engaging in action through service and research. In 2018, CHARA affiliated with an academic medical center as a regional community hub for clinical and translational science to ensure network sustainability was not dependent on any single actor. We highlight key aspects of these activities and provide examples of the resulting research.[84,85]

Understanding Local Priorities

A first goal in many research collaborations is to show up and listen—ideally becoming part of the complex web that exists, rather than attempting to be the focal point. While Drs. Davis and Dillon were "from the community," early efforts focused on understanding existing regional priorities and networks. Activities included hiring local staff to help manage the network, attending meetings of regional health and social service organizations, engaging key CBO leaders (e.g., Head Start, Rotary), reviewing community health improvement plans and community health needs assessments, conducting appreciative inquiry interviews[86] to understand local health-promoting factors, and engaging the CHARA board.[87]

Building Capacity and Identifying Areas for Research

After discovering that community partners were interested in learning about research, CHARA offered regional research trainings and held a half-day retreat in 2015 for academic and community partners. The retreat was designed to foster partnerships, refine research ideas, and identify next steps. Based on a key community concern that emerged in the retreat, colorectal cancer (CRC), and the fact that effective interventions were available but not routinely practiced, CHARA made studying and addressing CRC the initial focus of its grant applications. The decision was reinforced by community interest, academic partner expertise, and the fact that CRC served as a model system for both implementation science and comparative effectiveness research, which were priorities from target funding agencies.

Action Through Service and Research: Colorectal Cancer Screening Example

Between 2014 and 2019, CHARA advanced numerous health initiatives that leveraged the robust academic-community partnered infrastructure to put research into practice. This included securing 11 grants worth $8.6 million, ranging in size from $14,000 to $5 million, with funding from regional (e.g., Columbia Gorge Health Council, Knight Cancer Institute) and national (e.g., Agency for Healthcare Research and Quality, Patient-Centered Outcomes Institute, Robert Wood Johnson Foundation, National Cancer Institute) agencies. Awards spanned the partnership spectrum: Five used collegial/CBPR approaches, five used collaborative approaches, and one used a consultative approach.

As an example, one award included a community-led investigation of patient preferences for fecal immunochemical tests (FIT) to increase CRC screening. This mixed-methods study called "Finding the Right FIT" was designed to address gaps in the literature and local community needs by (a) evaluating patient preferences for FIT and (b) identifying one FIT to promote across the region.[88] The study found that patients preferred FITs that were single sample, used a probe or brush that allowed a more sanitary-seeming specimen collection process, and had clear instructions. This study, moreover, embodied CBPR practices, including the partners' shared ownership of participation in the design, data collection, analysis, and dissemination of findings. A notable impact of this collaboration was the uptake and impact from regional dissemination, which led to changes in contracting by (a) the local CCO, so clinics were required to use a clinically effective FIT and displayed preferred patient characteristics, and (b) two large health systems in Oregon who reworked their contracts with vendors to use patient preferred FITs.[85]

The Finding the Right FIT study informed subsequent work that engaged CHARA, including (1) a systematic review of effective interventions to improve FIT testing in rural and low-income populations,[89] (2) mapping regional variation in CRC screening across Oregon,[90] (3) a microsimulation study to identify cost-effective interventions for increasing CRC screening in rural Medicaid patients, and (4) implementing a collaborative mailed FIT program in the CHARA region. This work enabled CHARA and partners to secure funding for an Accelerating Colorectal Cancer Screening and Follow-Up Through Implementation Science (ACCSIS) Moonshot award to support the implementation of mailed FIT and patient navigation to colonoscopy following abnormal FIT. The ongoing study involves 29 rural clinics in Oregon. It will ultimately reach 120 rural clinics nationally in a subsequent scale-up trial.[91] CHARA board members and CBO partners have continued to play critical roles in these large-scale studies by helping to design data collection, to support clinic outreach and recruitment, and to help implement program activities via roles on the study advisory board or as implementation partners.

Partnership Sustainability, Impact, and Future Directions

Members of the CHARA core team and advisory board have transitioned over time in alignment with new opportunities or shifts in professional roles. As with any implementation partnership, this creates new opportunities and losses in momentum. In 2019, CHARA aligned with the regional clinical and translational science award program to provide longitudinal support for the collaboration through funding a community research liaison. The liaison supports network maintenance activities and serves as a point of contact for academic researchers and community groups looking for assistance with research or evaluation activities.[85] In the years ahead, CHARA seeks to expand the focus of partnered research in light of emerging regional priorities and serve as a collaborative hub for research and evaluation activities.

RESEARCH OPPORTUNITIES

Several research gaps must be addressed to advance this work. First, the field needs more research to examine the impacts of participatory approaches on the quality and relevance of the science produced and the "cascading" benefits applied to other improvement projects that may occur after the original research funding period ends. This area of inquiry might also examine how engagement impacts EBI implementation and sustainment. As one example, researchers may identify high-impact implementation strategies that explicitly incorporate community/practice engagement as part of the strategy. Only by demonstrating the value of these approaches in ways that speak to a range of audiences, from researchers new to this type of work to funders and academic institutions, can we routinize stakeholder engagement in D&I science. These data will also support models to sustain partnerships outside individual grants and allow for long-term collaboration, sustained capacity for implementation, and system-level change. Second, it will be critical to identify the core factors that should influence the level of engagement for a given partnership and the expected benefits of that type of engagement. Guidance on strategic selection may increase the range of academic researchers and community/practice partners interested in participatory approaches for D&I science. Third, while many academic researchers agree that practice-based evidence is critical for public health impact, it is not always clear how to work with partners to capture that evidence in a manner that supports integration into the academic research literature as well as the practice knowledge base. Fourth, although participatory approaches emphasize the importance of disseminating findings, the question of what, when, and how to share in a manner most beneficial to community/practice audiences deserves more attention.

SUMMARY

Engaging a wide range of partners in D&I efforts supports the broad goal of integrating the best available research evidence with practice and community needs and expertise. Several opportunities are worth considering. First, strategic selection of engagement levels can offer academic, practice, and/or community partners the opportunity to improve the process and utility of D&I efforts. Although there are rich benefits from fully engaged approaches to research, academic researchers will miss opportunities to gain the many benefits described in this chapter if they have a "CBPR-or-bust" mindset. At the same time, examining how best to select an engagement level and what impacts to expect deserve further study. As the field grows, so will the ability to measure the effects of participatory processes on D&I efforts and match engagement levels to resources and desired outcomes. Second, participatory approaches to D&I may require a shift in mindset for academic researchers new to this work as they learn to see practice and community partners not as sources of information or access to communities, but as collaborators who can offer vital, complementary expertise and should benefit directly from the work. Community and practice partners may also need support to engage with research teams and examine the utility of participating in research. By "making the tent bigger," a wider range of available resources can be tapped and a greater range of needs can be met with a given study or project. Third, another shift involves the obligation to identify ways to align the D&I effort with action, networks, and priorities of the implementing system. This systems-focused approach also prompts consideration of a broader set of outcomes, recognition of diverse ways of knowing, and opportunities to reshape the implementation context for equity. The more expansive view of outcomes responds to the long-term iterative nature of participatory D&I collaborations, which can support broader ripple effects and sustained impact on systems.

Engaged approaches to D&I offer the field an opportunity to honor its commitment to connecting the best available evidence with the rich expertise in practice, policy, community, and other settings to advance health equity. For those considering engaging in this way, we offer this wonderful summary of the motivation for participatory approaches from Brydon-Miller and colleagues.[92]

> Messes are complex, multi-dimensional, intractable, dynamic problems that can only be partially addressed and partially resolved. Yet most action researchers have disciplined themselves to believe that messes can be attractive and even exciting. We try not to avoid messy situations despite knowing that we do not have the "magic bullet" because we believe that, together with legitimate community stakeholders, we can do something to improve the situation. (p21)

ACKNOWLEDGMENTS

We are grateful to our partners as we work together to address health equity, including partners linked to CHARA, the Community Advisory Board of the U54 Partnership between the Dana-Farber/Harvard Cancer Center and the University of Massachusetts Boston, and the Project RESIST External Advisory Committee. We also are grateful to Alicia Salvatore and Charlotte Chang, who were coauthors of a related chapter in the previous edition of this volume. We also acknowledge support from the National Cancer Institute (P50 NCA244433, U54CA156732, 2U54CA156734; P50CA244289; and UG3CA244298).

SUGGESTED READINGS AND WEBSITES

Readings on Participatory Approaches

- *Foundations*: Wallerstein N, Duran B, Oetzel J, Minkler M, eds. Community-Based Participatory Research for Health: Advancing Social and Health Equity. 3rd ed. Wiley and Sons; 2017.

The first major volume on CBPR in health in the United States, the third edition of this co-edited text covers a wide range of theoretical, methodological, ethical, and practical issues and tools. Key topics include the theoretical and practice roots of CBPR; a conceptual pathways model of CBPR contexts, dynamics, and outcome; issues of power, race, racism, and trust; ethical and methodological challenges; participatory evaluation; and CBPR as a strategy for policy change. Numerous case studies and practical tools are included.

- *Foundations*: Israel BA, Eng E, Schulz AJ, eds. Methods for Community Based Participatory Research in Health. 2nd ed. Jossey Bass; 2013.

This co-edited book offers an overview of participatory approaches and detailed descriptions of how researchers can apply fundamental principles of participatory research. The book covers methods for CBPR research (qualitative, quantitative, and mixed method) and practical guidance on structuring and supporting partnerships. Each chapter includes a case study with an applied example.

- *Review of measures of engaged research*: Luger TM, Hamilton AB, True G. Measuring community-engaged research contexts, processes, and outcomes: a mapping review. Milbank Q. 2020;98(2):493–553. doi:10.1111/1468-0009.12458.

While not specific to D&I science, this detailed review of participatory research measures offers a useful conceptual frame for identifying measures and an interactive platform to find relevant measures for a given project. The piece covers 28 measures of context that support participatory research (e.g., readiness of the community to engage in research), 43 measures of process (e.g., trust or group dynamics), and 43 measures of outcomes (e.g., system changes or capacity-building impacts).

Readings Connecting Engaged Research and D&I

- *Review of community engagement in D&I frameworks*: Pinto RM, Park S, Miles R, Ong PN. Community engagement in dissemination and implementation models: a narrative review. Implement Res Pract. 2021;2:2633489520985305.

This review examines community engagement constructs in 74 D&I models. The five broad constructs identified are communication, partnership exchange, community capacity building, leadership, and collaboration. The review describes the presence (or lack thereof) of community engagement concepts in D&I frameworks and offers implications for D&I research and practice going forward.

- *Overview of applications of community engagement to D&I research focused on health equity*: Shelton R, Adsul P, Baumann A, Ramanadhan S. Community engagement to promote health equity through implementation science. In: Principles of Community Engagement. US Department of Health and Human Services; Centers for Disease Control and Prevention; in press.

This chapter connects core principles of community engagement and inclusion to implementation science in the context of advancing health equity. The chapter offers an introduction to important considerations, as well as detailed examples. Written for practice and research audiences, it can be a useful prompt for discussion within teams.

Websites and tools

- Stakeholder Engagement Navigator. DICEmethods.org | Dissemination, Implementation, Communication, and Engagement: A Guide for Health Researchers. University of Colorado. https://dicemethods.org/

A web-based tool developed as part of the Data Science to Patient Value Initiative provides education around various types of engagement activities and offers support in identifying methods for partner engagement based on the completion of a brief tool. The tool asks users to clarify purpose, project phase, budget, length and time of interaction, and the types of expertise available. It then produces recommended methods (e.g., human-centered design approaches) and tools (e.g., network mapping) based on responses.

- Putting Public Health Evidence in Action. Cancer Prevention and Control Research Network (CPCRN). https://cpcrn.org/training

An interactive training curriculum that supports public health planners, educators, and practitioners in developing capacity to use EBIs. The six modules can be viewed online or delivered as part of a training workshop to communities. Modules are based on the steps of engagement, assessment/goals, find EBIs, adapt EBIs, implement EBIs, and evaluate impact.

- Community Tool Box. https://ctb.ku.edu/en

The Community Tool Box is a public service developed and managed by the University of Kansas Center for Community and Health Development. It is a free, online resource that provides tools to "learn a skill" or get "help taking action." Materials are designed for those working to build healthier communities and bring about social change. Materials range from conducting community assessments to leadership and developing strategic plans.

- Resources for Stakeholder & Community Engagement. Consortium for Cancer Implementation Science—Community Participation Capacity Building Task Group. July 2021. https://cancercontrol.cancer.gov/sites/default/files/2021-08/CCIS_Engagement-Bibliography_080931_508.pdf

A compilation of resources for academic researchers and community/practice partners interested in participatory approaches to D&I, including key readings, trainings and guidance, tools, and resources.

REFERENCES

1. Ramanadhan S, Davis MM, Armstrong RA, et al. Participatory implementation science to increase the impact of evidence-based cancer prevention and control. *Cancer Causes Control.* 2018;29(3):363–369.
2. Schmittdiel JA, Grant RW. Crossing the research to quality chasm: a checklist for researchers and clinical leadership partners. *J Gen Intern Med.* 2018;33(1):9–10. doi:10.1007/s11606-017-4189-5
3. Schmittdiel JA, Grumbach K, Selby JV. System-based participatory research in health care: an approach for sustainable translational research and quality improvement. *Ann Fam Med.* 2010;8(3):256–259. doi:10.1370/afm.1117
4. Labonte R. Community, community organizing, and the forming of authentic partnerships: looking back, looking ahead. In: Minkler M, Wakimoto P, eds. *Community Organizing and Community Building for Health and Social Equity.* 4th ed. Rutgers University Press; 2022:91–109.
5. Minkler M, Wallerstein N, Wilson N. Improving health through community organization and community building. In: Glanz K, Rimer B, Viswanath K, eds. *Health Behavior and Health Education: Theory, Research and Practice.* 4th ed. Jossey-Bass Inc. Publishers; 2008:287–312.
6. Ramanadhan S, Kohler RK, Viswanath K. Partnerships to support implementation science. In: Chambers D, Vinson C, Norton WE, eds. *Advancing the Science of Implementation Across the Cancer Continuum.* Oxford University Press; 2018:351–367.
7. Minkler M. Community-based research partnerships: challenges and opportunities. *J Urban Health.* 2005;82(2)(Suppl 2):ii3–ii12. doi:10.1093/jurban/jti034
8. Colditz GA, Emmons KM. Accelerating the pace of cancer prevention—right now. *Cancer Prev Res.* 2018;11(4):171–184. doi:10.1158/1940-6207.CAPR-17-0282
9. Wensing M, Sales A, Armstrong R, Wilson P. Implementation science in times of COVID-19. *Implementation Sci.* 2020;15(1):42, s13012-020-01006-x. doi:10.1186/s13012-020-01006-x
10. Dr. Collins reflects on career at NIH, COVID response effort, work on genome sequencing, *PBS NewsHour.* December 20, 2021. Accessed January 26, 2022. https://www.pbs.org/newshour/show/dr-collins-reflects-on-career-at-nih-covid-response-effort-work-on-genome-sequencing
11. Nicolaidis C, Raymaker D. Community-based participatory research with communities defined by race, ethnicity, and disability: translating theory to practice. In: Bradbury H, ed. *The SAGE Handbook of Action Research.* SAGE Publications Ltd.; 2015:167–178. doi:10.4135/9781473921290.n17
12. Westfall JM, Mold J, Fagnan L. Practice-based research—"blue highways" on the NIH roadmap.

JAMA. 2007;297(4):403–406. doi:10.1001/jama.297.4.403

13. Pearson CR, Duran B, Oetzel J, et al. Research for improved health: variability and impact of structural characteristics in federally funded community engaged research. *Prog Community Health Partnersh*. 2015;9(1):17–29. doi:10.1353/cpr.2015.0010
14. Concannon TW, Meissner P, Grunbaum JA, et al. A new taxonomy for stakeholder engagement in patient-centered outcomes research. *J Gen Intern Med*. 2012;27(8):985–991. doi:10.1007/s11606-012-2037-1
15. Travers R, Pyne J, Bauer G, et al. "Community control" in CBPR: challenges experienced and questions raised from the Trans PULSE project. *Action Res*. 2013;11(4):403–422. doi:10.1177/1476750313507093
16. Minkler M, Salvatore AL. Participatory approaches for study design and analysis in dissemination and implementation research. In: Brownson RC, Colditz GA, Proctor EK, eds. *Dissemination and Implementation Research in Health*. Oxford; 2012:192–212.
17. Deloria V. Research, redskins, and reality. *Am Indian Q*. 1991;15(4):457–468. doi:10.2307/1185364
18. Minkler M, Wallerstein N, eds. *Community Based Participatory Research in Health*. 2nd ed. Jossey-Bass; 2008.
19. WK Kellogg Foundation. Kellogg Health Scholars: About Us—Community Health Track. 2001. Accessed April 12, 2010. http://www.kelloghealthscholars.org/about/community.cfm
20. Reason P, Bradbury H. *Handbook of Action Research: Participative Inquiry and Practice*. Sage; 2001.
21. Balazs CL, Morello-Frosch R. The three Rs: how community-based participatory research strengthens the rigor, relevance, and reach of science. *Environ Justice*. 2013;6(1):9–16. doi:10.1089/env.2012.0017
22. Israel BA, Schulz AJ, Parker EA, Becker AB, Allen AJ III, Guzman R. Critical issues in developing and following CBPR principles. In: Minkler M, Wallerstein N, eds. *Community-Based Participatory Research for Health: From Process to Outcomes*. 2nd ed. Jossey-Bass; 2008:47–66.
23. Israel BA, Schulz AJ, Parker EA, Becker AB. Review of community-based research: assessing partnership approaches to improve public health. *Annu Rev Public Health*. 1998;19:173–201.
24. Israel BA, Eng E, Schulz AJ, Parker EA, eds. *Methods for Community-Based Participatory Research for Health*. 2nd ed. John Wiley & Sons; 2012.
25. Minkler M. Enhancing data quality, relevance and use through community-based participatory research. In: Cytron N, Petit K, Kingsley G, eds. *What Counts: Harnessing Data for America's Communities*. Federal Reserve Bank of San Francicso and the Urban Institute; 2014:245–259.
26. Wallerstein N, Duran B, Oetzel J, Minkler M. Introduction to CBPR. In: Wallerstein N, Duran B, Oetzel J, Minkler M, eds. *Community-Based Participatory Research for Health: Advancing Social and Health Equity*. 3rd ed. Wiley and Sons; 2017:3–16.
27. Tervalon M, Murray-Garcia J. Cultural humility versus cultural competence: a critical distinction in defining physician training outcomes in multicultural education. *J Health Care Poor Underserved*. 1998;9(2):117–125.
28. Koh HK, Oppenheimer SC, Massin-Short SB, Emmons KM, Geller AC, Viswanath K. Translating research evidence into practice to reduce health disparities: a social determinants approach. *Am J Public Health*. 2010;100(S1):S72–S80.
29. Ramanadhan S, Galbraith-Gyan K, Revette A, et al. Key considerations for designing capacity-building interventions to support evidence-based programming in underserved communities: a qualitative exploration. *Transl Behav Med*. 2021;11(2):452–461. doi:10.1093/tbm/ibz177
30. Ramanadhan S, Viswanath K. Engaging communities to improve health: models, evidence, and the participatory knowledge translation (PaKT) framework. In: Fisher EB, Cameron L, Christensen AJ, et al., eds. *Principles and Concepts of Behavioral Medicine: A Global Handbook*. Springer Science & Business Media; 2018:679–712.
31. Chang C, Salvatore A, Lee PT, Liu SS, Minkler M. Popular education, participatory research, and community organizing with immigrant restaurant workers in San Francisco's Chinatown: a case study. In: Minkler M, ed. *Community Organizing and Community Building for Health and Welfare*. Vol. 3. Rutgers University Press; 2012.
32. Joosten YA, Israel TL, Williams NA, et al. Community engagement studios: a structured approach to obtaining meaningful input from stakeholders to inform research. *Acad Med*. 2015;90(12):1646.
33. Meharry Vanderbilt Community-Engaged Research Core. Community Engagement Studio Toolkit. 2015. Accessed September 29, 2021. https://www.meharry-vanderbilt.org/community-engagement-studio-toolkit-20

34. Muhammad M, Wallerstein N, Sussman AL, Avila M, Belone L, Duran B. Reflections on Researcher Identity and Power: The Impact of Positionality on Community Based Participatory Research (CBPR) Processes and Outcomes. *Crit Sociol.* 2015;41(7–8):1045–1063. https://doi.org/10.1177/0896920513516025
35. Concannon TW, Stem K, Chaplin J, Girman CJ. Chapter 4: stakeholder engagement in the design and conduct of pragmatic randomized trials. In: Girman CJ, Ritchey ME, eds. *Pragmatic Randomized Clinical Trials.* Academic Press; 2021:33–45. doi:10.1016/B978-0-12-817663-4.00014-3
36. Muhammad M, Wallerstein N, Sussman AL, Avila M, Belone L, Duran B. Reflections on researcher identity and power: the impact of positionality on community based participatory research (CBPR) processes and outcomes. *Crit Sociol (Eugene).* 2015;41(7–8):1045–1063. doi:10.1177/0896920513516025
37. Shea CM, Young TL, Powell BJ, et al. Researcher readiness for participating in community-engaged dissemination and implementation research: a conceptual framework of core competencies. *Transl Behav Med.* 2017;7(3):393–404.
38. Pinto RM, Park S, Miles R, Ong PN. Community engagement in dissemination and implementation models: a narrative review. *Implement Res Pract.* 2021;2:2633489520985305.
39. Brush BL, Mentz G, Jensen M, et al. Success in long-standing community-based participatory research (CBPR) partnerships: a scoping literature review. *Health Educ Behav.* 2020;47(4):556–568. doi:10.1177/1090198119882989
40. Goodman MS, Sanders Thompson VL. The science of stakeholder engagement in research: classification, implementation, and evaluation. *Transl Behav Med.* 2017;7(3):486–491. doi:10.1007/s13142-017-0495-z
41. Kwan BM, Ytell K, Coors M, et al. A stakeholder engagement method navigator webtool for clinical and translational science. *J Clin Trans Sci.* 2021;5(1):e180. doi:10.1017/cts.2021.850
42. Wallerstein N, Oetzel J, Duran B, Tafoya G, Belone L, Rae R. What predicts outcomes in CBPR? In: Minkler M, Wallerstein N, eds. *Community-Based Participatory Research for Health: From Process to Outcomes.* 2nd ed. Jossey-Bass; 2008:371–392.
43. National Research Council; Division of Behavioral and Social Sciences and Education; Board on Behavioral, Cognitive, and Sensory Sciences; Committee on the Science of Team Science. *Enhancing the Effectiveness of Team Science.* National Academies Press; 2015.
44. Aarons GA, Hurlburt M, Horwitz SM. Advancing a conceptual model of evidence-based practice implementation in public service sectors. *Admin Policy Ment Health Ment Health Serv Res.* 2011;38(1):4–23.
45. Smith JD, Li DH, Rafferty MR. The implementation research logic model: a method for planning, executing, reporting, and synthesizing implementation projects. *Implement Sci.* 2020;15(1):84. doi:10.1186/s13012-020-01041-8
46. Stirman SW, Baumann AA, Miller CJ. The FRAME: an expanded framework for reporting adaptations and modifications to evidence-based interventions. *Implement Sci.* 2019;14(1):1–10.
47. Chambers DA, Glasgow RE, Stange KC. The dynamic sustainability framework: addressing the paradox of sustainment amid ongoing change. *Implement Sci.* 2013;8:117. doi:10.1186/1748-5908-8-117
48. Wallerstein N, Duran B, Oetzel J, Minkler M, eds. *Community-Based Participatory Research for Health: Advancing Social and Health Equity.* 3rd ed. Wiley and Sons; 2017.
49. Nilsen P. Making sense of implementation theories, models and frameworks. *Implement Sci.* 2015;10(1):53.
50. Nilsen P, Bernhardsson S. Context matters in implementation science: a scoping review of determinant frameworks that describe contextual determinants for implementation outcomes. *BMC Health Serv Res.* 2019;19(1):189. doi:10.1186/s12913-019-4015-3
51. Breuer E, De Silva MJ, Fekadu A, et al. Using workshops to develop theories of change in five low and middle income countries: lessons from the programme for improving mental health care (PRIME). *Int J Ment Health Syst.* 2014;8(1):15. doi:10.1186/1752-4458-8-15
52. Ortiz K, Nash J, Shea L, et al. Partnerships, processes, and outcomes: a health equity–focused scoping meta-review of community-engaged scholarship. *Annu Rev Public Health.* 2020;41:177–199.
53. Powell BJ, Beidas RS, Lewis CC, et al. Methods to improve the selection and tailoring of implementation strategies. *J Behav Health Serv Res.* 2017;44(2):177–194.
54. Fernandez ME, Ten Hoor GA, van Lieshout S, et al. Implementation mapping: using intervention mapping to develop implementation strategies. *Front Public Health.* 2019;7:158.
55. Lewis CC, Klasnja P, Powell BJ, et al. From classification to causality: advancing understanding of mechanisms of change in implementation science. *Front Public Health.* 2018;6. Accessed

February 4, 2022. https://doi.org/10.3389/fpubh.2018.00136

56. Kenzie ES. *Get Your Model Out There: Advancing Methods for Developing and Using Causal-Loop Diagrams*. PhD thesis. Portland State University; 2021.
57. Davis MM, Gunn R, Kenzie E, et al. Integration of improvement and implementation science in practice-based research networks: a longitudinal, comparative case study. *J Gen Intern Med*. 2021;36(6):1503–1513. doi:10.1007/s11606-021-06610-1
58. Hawe P, Shiell A, Riley T. Theorising interventions as events in systems. *Am J Community Psychol*. 2009;43(3–4):267–276. doi:10.1007/s10464-009-9229-9
59. Proctor E, Silmere H, Raghavan R, et al. Outcomes for implementation research: conceptual distinctions, measurement challenges, and research agenda. *Admin Policy Ment Health Ment Health Serv Res*. 2011;38(2):65–76.
60. Gravitt PE, Rositch AF, Jurczuk M, et al. Integrative Systems Praxis for Implementation Research (INSPIRE): an implementation methodology to facilitate the global elimination of cervical cancer. *Cancer Epidemiol Prev Biomarkers*. 2020;29(9):1710–1719.
61. Hawe P, Noort M, King L, Jordens C. Multiplying health gains: the critical role of capacity-building within health promotion programs. *Health Policy*. 1997;39(1):29–42.
62. Cargo M, Mercer SL. The value and challenges of participatory research: strengthening its practice. *Annu Rev Public Health*. 2008;29:325–350.
63. Wallerstein N, Duran B. Community-based participatory research contributions to intervention research: the intersection of science and practice to improve health equity. *Am J Public Health*. 2010;100(Suppl 1):S40–S46.
64. Glasgow RE, Emmons K. How can we increase translation of research into practice? Types of evidence needed. *Annu Rev Public Health*. 2007;28:413–433.
65. Brownson RC, Jacobs JA, Tabak RG, Hoehner CM, Stamatakis KA. Designing for dissemination among public health researchers: findings from a national survey in the United States. *Am J Public Health*. 2013;103(9):1693–1699.
66. Kwan BM, Brownson RC, Glasgow RE, Morrato EH, Luke DA. Designing for dissemination and sustainability to promote equitable impacts on health. *Annu Rev Public Health*. 2022;43(1):331–353. doi:10.1146/annurev-publhealth-052220-112457
67. Robert Wood Johnson Foundation. *Navigating the Translation and Dissemination of PHSSR Findings*. 2013. Accessed January 31, 2022. https://www.rwjf.org/en/library/research/2013/07/navigating-the-translation-and-dissemination-of-phssr-findings.html
68. Green LW. Making research relevant: if it is an evidence-based practice, where's the practice-based evidence? *Family Pract*. 2008;25(Suppl 1):i20–i24.
69. Carter-Edwards L, Grewe ME, Fair AM, et al. Recognizing cross-institutional fiscal and administrative barriers and facilitators to conducting community-engaged clinical and translational research. *Acad Med*. 2021;96(4):558–567. doi:10.1097/ACM.0000000000003893
70. Green LW, Glasgow RE. Evaluating the relevance, generalization, and applicability of research: issues in translation methodology. *Eval Health Prof*. 2006;29:126–153.
71. Maxwell JA. Why qualitative methods are necessary for generalization. *Qual Psychol*. 2021;8(1):111–118. doi:10.1037/qup0000173
72. Minkler M, Baden AC. Impacts of CBPR on academic researchers, research quality and methodology, and power relations. In Minkler M, Wallerstein N, ed. Community-Based Participatory Research for Health: From Process to Outcomes. Jossey-Bass: 2008:243–262.
73. Seward N, Hanlon C, Hinrichs-Kraples S, et al. A guide to systems-level, participatory, theory-informed implementation research in global health. *BMJ Glob Health*. 2021;6(12):e005365. doi:10.1136/bmjgh-2021-005365
74. Guba EG, Lincoln YS. Competing paradigms in qualitative research. *Handb Qual Res*. 1994;2(163–194):105.
75. Guba EG, Lincoln YS. *Fourth Generation Evaluation*. Sage; 1989.
76. Blue Bird Jernigan V, D'Amico EJ, Keawe'aimoku Kaholokula J. Prevention research with Indigenous communities to expedite dissemination and implementation efforts. *Prev Sci*. 2020;21(1):74–82. doi:10.1007/s11121-018-0951-0
77. Stanton MC, Ali SB, Team the SC. A typology of power in implementation: building on the exploration, preparation, implementation, sustainment (EPIS) framework to advance mental health and HIV health equity. *Implement Res Pract*. 2022;3:26334895211064250. doi:10.1177/26334895211064250
78. Luger TM, Hamilton AB, True G. Measuring community-engaged research contexts, processes, and outcomes: a

mapping review. *Milbank Q*. 2020;98(2):493–553. doi:10.1111/1468-0009.12458
79. Zimmerman EB; H. Assessing the impacts and ripple effects of a community–university partnership: *Mich J Community Serv Learn*. 2019;25(1):62–76. doi:10.3998/mjcsloa.3239521.0025.106
80. Trickett EJ. Multilevel community-based culturally situated interventions and community impact: an ecological perspective. *Am J Community Psychol*. 2009;43(3–4):257–266.
81. McConnell J, Change A, Cohen D, et al. Oregon's Medicaid transformation: an innovative approach to holding a health system accountable for spending growth. *Healthcare*. 2014;2(3):163–167. doi:10.1016/j.hjdsi.2013.11.002
82. Davis MM, Aromaa S, McGinnis PB, et al. Engaging the underserved: a process model to mobilize rural community health coalitions as partners in translational research. *Clin Transl Sci*. 2014;7(4):300–306.
83. McGinnis PB, Hunsberger M, Davis M, Smith J, Beamer BA, Hastings DD. Transitioning from CHIP to CHIRP: blending community health development with community-based participatory research. *Fam Community Health*. 2010;33(3):228–237. doi:10.1097/FCH.0b013e3181e4bc8e
84. Dillon K, Lindberg P, Davis M. Aligning research with action for health and well-being in the Columbia Gorge. In Page-Reeves J, ed. Well-Being as a *Multidimensional Concept:* Understanding *Connections* Among *Culture, Community*, and *Health*. Rowman and Littlefield Publishing Company; 2019:363–385.
85. Davis MM, Lindberg P, Cross S, Lowe S, Gunn R, Dillon K. Aligning systems science and community-based participatory research: a case example of the Community Health Advocacy and Research Alliance (CHARA). *J Clin Transl Sci*. 2019;2(5):280–288. doi:10.1017/cts.2018.334
86. Trajkovski S, Schmied V, Vickers M, Jackson D. Implementing the 4D cycle of appreciative inquiry in health care: a methodological review. *J Adv Nurs*. 2013;69(6):1224–1234. doi:10.1111/jan.12086
87. Spurlock M, Stanley K, Castro Y, Dillon K, Davis M. *Connecting Research to Real Life (CR2L): Findings from Reflective Conversations in the Columbia River Gorge*. Community Health Advocacy and Research Alliance; 2014:20.
88. Pham R, Cross S, Fernandez B, et al. "Finding the Right FIT": rural patient preferences for fecal immunochemical test (FIT) characteristics. *J Am Board Fam Med*. 2017;30(5):632–644. doi:10.3122/jabfm.2017.05.170151
89. Davis MM, Freeman M, Shannon J, et al. A systematic review of clinic and community intervention to increase fecal testing for colorectal cancer in rural and low-income populations in the United States–how, what and when? *BMC Cancer*. 2018;18(1):40.
90. Davis MM, Renfro S, Pham R, et al. Geographic and population-level disparities in colorectal cancer testing: a multilevel analysis of Medicaid and commercial claims data. *Prev Med*. 2017;101:44–52. doi:10.1016/j.ypmed.2017.05.001
91. Coronado G, Leo M, Ramsey K, et al. Mailed fecal testing and patient navigation versus usual care to improve rates of colorectal cancer screening and follow-up colonoscopy in rural Medicaid enrollees: a cluster-randomized controlled trial. *Implement Sci Commun*. 2022;3.
92. Brydon-Miller M, Greenwood D, Maguire P. Why action research? *Action Res*. 2003;1(1):9–28.

11

The Role of Economic Evaluation in Dissemination and Implementation Research

ALEX R. DOPP, SIMON WALKER, AND RAMESH RAGHAVAN

INTRODUCTION

Over the past several decades, considerable research investments have developed and identified many evidence-based practices (EBPs) that can prevent, assess, treat, and support a variety of health problems. Unfortunately, these advances in EBPs have not been accompanied by concomitant improvements in the quality of health-related services and outcomes in practice settings such as medicine, behavioral health, and public health. Bridging this gap between science and practice is a principal goal of dissemination and implementation (D&I) research, the former being concerned with increasing the use of EBPs widely by a target population, and the latter being concerned with the integration of EBPs within service settings such as clinics, schools, or worksites (please see chapter 2 for more formal definitions of these terms). Much of D&I work focuses on processes or activities (i.e., *strategies*) by and through which practices can be spread to, or adopted by, target audiences. For this reason, D&I researchers and/or practitioners have specified distinct dissemination or implementation strategies, which are designed to systematize the process of spreading or integrating target EBPs into community practice settings (also see chapter 6).

This chapter presents an overview of how economic evaluation can be used to study D&I. We argue that the overarching goal of economic evaluation in the field should be to ensure that investments in D&I result in an appropriate, consistent, equitable spread of EBPs that is commensurate with individuals' and communities' needs. Such an orientation requires expanding the focus of economic evaluations beyond elucidating costs of implementation activities that accrue to organizations or provider entities. It also requires that evaluators consider broader societal goals that are not merely aggregates of individual preferences, such as equity or fairness of outcomes between individuals belonging to different demographic groups. This approach has been termed an "extra-welfarist" approach.[1,2] We suggest that such a broadening of perspective is a necessary corrective to a "rich get richer" dynamic, in which only well-resourced provider systems and communities can access the resources needed to consistently implement and sustain a relatively small cohort of EBPs, which may not be the best fit for the community's needs. By asking and answering such questions and by focusing on who asks and answers these questions, economic evaluations can help decision makers understand the *value* (in terms of improved health or other societal outcomes as well as the equity of those outcomes) produced by investing resources in D&I, as well as the conditions and mechanisms through which that value is produced. These methods can also better help mitigate two deleterious developments in D&I research: (1) emphasis on developing and testing intensive, high-resource D&I strategies that produce large effects but are not pragmatic for use in practice—creating an ironic research-to-practice gap *within* D&I; and (2) reliance on research evidence that has marginalized high-need communities and populations, thus underestimating the adaptation and support resources needed for successful, impactful EBP use. In this chapter, we propose

Alex R. Dopp, Simon Walker, and Ramesh Raghavan, *The Role of Economic Evaluation in Dissemination and Implementation Research* In: *Dissemination and Implementation Research in Health.* Edited by: Ross C. Brownson, Graham A. Colditz, and Enola K. Proctor, Oxford University Press.
 DOI: 10.1093/oso/9780197660690.003.0011

a science of D&I economic evaluation that grounds understanding of the resource needs for, and value produced by, EBP D&I within a decision-making framework that (a) places achieving health equity as a central goal alongside health improvement behind D&I activities (rather than minimizing costs) and (b) recognizes the challenges of the distribution of available resources across different settings and populations, both locally and globally.

We begin by recognizing that one major challenge for the target audience of D&I research, whether a population of practitioners, provider organizations, or policymakers, is that many of these activities are highly complex endeavors and, consequently, are likely to be very expensive to deploy within practice settings. Authors of a study costing the implementation of a chronic care model reported that the dominant human resources costs identified in the study were due to the 15 individuals charged with implementing the model,[3] suggesting that ignoring D&I costs can have serious consequences to an organization's bottom line. The service delivery environments for most healthcare and promotion activities in the community do not have access to significant funds or the personnel required to execute these activities within their settings. Furthermore, current reimbursement mechanisms rarely cover the entirety of the costs of disseminating and implementing EBPs. Hence, organizational decision makers that want to deliver new practices should think carefully about the affordability of implementing EBPs in light of the value or benefits produced.

To help support such decisions, economic evaluations of D&I processes and strategies are required, in which one systematically examines what outcomes a strategy—or a set of competing strategies—achieves and the costs of achieving those outcomes. This type of evaluation is best accomplished via a partnership between academic researchers and those disseminating or implementing the EBP. Economic evaluations of competing strategies are one way in which D&I researchers can justify scaling up the use of their dissemination or implementation strategy, by comparing the benefits against the costs to allow for the consideration of the value for money of said strategies. The assessment of value is challenging and could be informed by comparing the benefits of the strategies with the benefits which would be produced by other potential uses of those resources (i.e., the opportunity costs). D&I researchers are interested in both proximal outcomes—such as implementation outcomes (e.g., fidelity to the intended EBP protocol[4,5]) or service outcomes (e.g., timeliness of care)—as well as distal outcomes, like client health and well-being.[6] Outcomes and their measurement are covered in detail in chapter 15. Each of these types of outcomes can be captured in an economic evaluation. As a first step, for example, researchers might quantify the relative costs of different EBP implementation strategies and compare changes in an intermediate outcome, such as fidelity, resulting from the use of those strategies. This type of an analysis provides a researcher with the incremental costs of improving the fidelity to an EBP. The next step might be to examine if these improvements in fidelity have resulted in improvements in a distal outcome, such as improved client health. This type of a sequenced analysis provides information on the costs and benefits of D&I for a provider organization implementing a given EBP and facilitates assessment of value for money.

In this chapter, we use the term *practice* to refer to interventions, treatments, programs, and service delivery approaches. We do not discuss or evaluate specific EBPs that may be disseminated and implemented; we assume the effectiveness and value of those practices for the selected health problems, populations, and contexts. This does not mean that a particular EBP can be deployed, as is, in all populations and within all contexts; some amount of adaptation may be necessary, even imperative. To the extent that adaptation improves outcomes, the value of investing in EBP adaptations is also an object of study for economic evaluation. We recognize that not all adaptations are conducted for implementation purposes; some are conducted for purposes of intervention refinement and, consequently, fall outside the purview of this chapter (though the distinction is not always obvious in practice).

As there are more well-specified implementation strategies whose costs can be assessed, we focus more on implementation strategies in this chapter; the same approach, however, can be also extended to quantifying the costs of dissemination strategies. The chapter begins by providing a brief overview of economic evaluation in D&I science, not only acknowledging its roots in cost and outcome estimation from other disciplines (e.g., health economics, accounting) but also recognizing that all economic evaluations are activities that require collaboration across disciplines. Finally, observations are provided regarding the implications of economic evaluations for the field of D&I research and for policy in general.

FOUNDATIONS OF ECONOMIC EVALUATION

Traditional economic evaluations use a formal methodology to establish whether or not resources used for health-related goods and services (e.g., healthcare and promotion activities) represent the best use of those resources.[7] This kind of information is one among many other factors that inform decision-making, such as availability of a good or service, practitioner familiarity with an intervention, or the goal of reducing an identified health disparity. This information is important for not only payers and other policymakers but also administrators, executive directors, and budget managers within health service organizations or systems, who each day face decisions regarding whether their organizational expenditures are producing the biggest "bang for the buck."

More formally, economic evaluations have been defined as the "comparative analysis of alternative courses of action in terms of both their costs and consequences."[7(p4)] Why is such an analysis necessary? In health, as in all areas of human activity, decisions have to be made under conditions of scarcity. Consider an executive director of a healthcare agency deciding between two EBPs to implement within their setting. Economic evaluation aims to inform whether Practice A or B represents the best use of available resources. (One of these practices could certainly represent what the agency is currently doing, or "usual care"; economic evaluations do not require two entirely novel practices, but rather that the practices being compared are mutually exclusive.) The answer to this question is arrived at by quantifying the costs and consequences of each practice (A and B) within a research design that allows comparison of the incremental differences in costs and consequences (A vs. B).[8] If one practice costs more than another and is also beneficial, then an estimate of the incremental outcome per dollar spent can be produced. The quantification of this dollar amount is the beginning, not the end, of the evaluation. The director now needs to decide whether this represents *value* for money, based on factors such as the outcomes produced from using each practice and the consumers who most benefit from its implementation. If a new practice proves to be more expensive than usual care, activities may need to be forgone elsewhere due to resources being reallocated for this new practice (the *opportunity cost*). Are there any current, but ineffective, practices that could be terminated to free up resources and reduce forgone revenues (this is called de-implementation)? And can these savings then be used to implement the new practice? Clearly, answering such questions requires a consideration of many factors, and economic evaluations represent one input among many for the executive director to consider.

The above discussion suggests that economic evaluations are characterized by two features. First, they are *comparative*, requiring a choice between proposed alternatives. Second, this comparison between the proposed alternatives is based on the analysis of the *costs* and *consequences* (or outcomes) of each alternative.

There are several common types of economic evaluation used in the health literature, which can be distinguished, among other differences, by the method used to calculate each practice's consequences (costs are always measured in monetary terms). We provide a brief overview here since other resources are available for understanding and choosing between economic evaluation types; for example, Table 1.1 of Drummond et al.'s (2015) economic evaluation textbook[7(p11)] summarizes how costs and consequences are measured and valued for each type. *Cost-effectiveness analysis* examines the relative costs of different practices as compared to their effects on outcomes (including health), measured in units such as recipient-reported symptoms, provider-assigned diagnoses, or general health status metrics. Where the unit of outcome in a cost-effectiveness analysis captures practice recipients' health-related quality of life (which can incorporate preferences regarding health outcomes) using standardized measures like quality- or disability-adjusted life years (QALYs and DALYs, respectively), these evaluations are also sometimes termed *cost-utility analyses*.[9] An alternative approach to economic evaluation, *cost-benefit analysis* (or *benefit-cost analysis*), examines outcomes (benefits) that have been quantified in monetary terms, which allows for direct comparison of the monetary benefits and costs of different practices.[10] Cost-benefit analysis may not only be considered simpler to interpret because all costs and consequences are measured with the same metric (money), but also requires assumptions about appropriate monetization of outcomes that cost-effectiveness and cost-utility analyses do not. Further, this approach assumes that a dollar is worth the same in every context.[11] In some settings where constrained budgets are the norm, such as in human services agencies in local government, a dollar may be valued more than in other better resourced agencies. Finally, not all analyses consider costs as well as consequences, but instead may quantify and/or compare costs only (often a useful precursor to full economic evaluation).[12,13] Others examine *cost offsets*, for example, examining if costs of treating depression can be partially recouped by reductions in utilization of general medical services by people with depression.[14]

Regardless of the economic evaluation method chosen, the decision for our executive director is easiest to make in situations like where Practice A is cheaper *and* produces better outcomes than Practice B; in this case, Practice A is the obvious choice (it is said to dominate B). If Practice B is costlier than Practice A but produces better outcomes, then the executive director must choose whether those increased outcomes are worth the added cost. This should be considered in light of other potential uses of those additional resources (i.e., the opportunity cost).[8] For example, this can be done by invoking established cost-effectiveness or cost-per-QALY thresholds or using a decision rule that monetary benefits should exceed costs. Other factors can also be considered, such as the impacts on particular populations and equity.

There is considerable diversity in methods for economic and cost evaluations, not only within health economics but also in other fields, such as accounting and education. To bridge disciplinary perspectives and assumptions, this chapter models transparency in approach. All approaches share an emphasis on identifying the "best" way to achieve an individual-level outcome, such as health status, which can be then aggregated across individuals to capture population-level outcomes. More recently, extensions such as distributional cost-effectiveness analysis[15] have been developed to model the impacts on both overall outcomes and how the distribution of outcomes varies within a population (i.e., modeling health inequities). Furthermore, distributional analyses attempt to quantify trade-offs, such as the extent to which investments in maximizing health outcomes for an entire population can worsen health inequities within that population. These approaches are highly relevant to implementation science, especially in underserved settings with vulnerable populations where a "one-size-fits-all" approach may create real harms.

Economic evaluations are conducted under conditions of uncertainty and often require numerous assumptions. As a result, it is essential to also conduct sensitivity analyses that examine the effects of key sources of uncertainty on analytic conclusions.[16] Sensitivity analyses vary cost and consequence parameters across a plausible range of values, such as best/worst case or most likely scenarios; this checks the robustness of the primary analysis and helps characterize the level of confidence for using results to inform decisions.

This has necessarily been a cursory overview of the area; further details on how to perform economic evaluations in health are available elsewhere.[7,17–19] Of more immediate relevance, the logic behind the theory and practice of economic evaluations of health practices can be extended and applied to D&I strategies for EBPs. Once a provider organization knows how much it will cost them to implement an EBP, for example, and what the returns are likely to be of spending those dollars, it can then make an informed decision regarding whether to participate in such an implementation. A very expensive implementation strategy that produces small improvements in outcomes is likely to be less attractive than another implementation strategy that produces the same improvement but at a fraction of the cost. As we describe next, there are numerous reasons that this extension of traditional economic evaluation methods into D&I science is imperfect, so we are not suggesting that D&I researchers treat the methods as "canon" that should never be changed. We simply recommend that a D&I research team wishing to perform an economic evaluation should be familiar enough with foundational sources to decide when and how established methods should be applied versus modified. D&I teams in this situation often benefit from enlisting the assistance of a health services researcher with expertise in economic evaluations—often someone with training in health economics, public policy, public health, and/or accounting—although we recognize there are numerous challenges to such transdisciplinary work.[20,21]

ECONOMIC EVALUATIONS IN D&I RESEARCH

In the D&I field, economic evaluations are used to answer a different type of question: How can organizations and systems invest in the D&I of EBPs to maximize the value produced? As we alluded to previously in this chapter, such questions are more complex because they acknowledge that (a) costs and consequences result from a combination of the EBP and the D&I strategy (or, more often, multiple strategies) that support it; (b) context matters, with the costs involved and value produced depending on each context's unique needs, assets, and dynamic changes over time; and (c) analyses need to attend to the effects of the findings on subgroups of individuals. Head-to-head comparisons of implementation strategies in terms of implementation outcomes (e.g., EBP uptake) and ultimate EBP recipient outcomes (e.g., improved health) still have a useful logic behind them, but the weight that such analyses have in D&I decision-making is appropriately decreased given how comparative research designs greatly oversimplify the phenomena under study.[22–25] It is rare to find a definitive answer to whether the resources used to deploy a single implementation strategy represents the best use of organizational resources across contexts and across recipients. More expansive methods and data sources are needed to understand the economic impacts of EBP implementation, and at its best D&I science excels at such integrative, transdisciplinary work.

The basic adaptation of the economic evaluation approach described in the previous section to implementation research is as follows:

Now, the analysis quantifies the gains in some outcome (implementation, service, clinical) as compared to the implementation and practice costs required to achieve those gains. The cost of the EBP in the equation excludes its development costs, which are fixed and accrue to different parties than do recurring implementation costs. Implementation Strategy A and B represent two different implementation conditions; in some cases, the condition might represent a bundle of multiple strategies, a single discrete strategy, or even "usual" implementation in that system. There are several named or "branded" implementation strategies, including the Breakthrough Series Collaborative[26]; the Network for the Improvement of Addiction Treatment model[27]; Replicating Effective Programs[28]; Leadership and Organizational Change for Implementation (LOCI)[29]; and Collaborative Organizational Approach to Selecting and Tailoring Implementation Strategies (COAST-IS)[30], among others. The (usually) highly structured nature of these strategies allows them to be subject to an economic evaluation.

There are several scenarios, relatively common in D&I research, where the above equation can become difficult to apply. First, D&I studies cannot always randomly assign receipt of strategies, so Conditions A and B may represent quasi-experimental or pre-post comparisons, which complicates interpretation. Second, dissemination strategies[31] can present greater challenges to economic evaluators because they tend to be more diffuse; each of their elements needs to be operationalized before costs can be attached to them. Third, D&I strategies that are flexible and can be tailored to different contexts[32] are also difficult to evaluate because their costs are so variable. SMART (sequential multiple assignment randomized trial) or quasi-experimental research designs (alongside appropriate causal inference methods[33]) can help to quantify costs for different scenarios with respect to the types and dosage(s) of strategies received, and D&I researchers have started extending economic evaluation methods to effectively analyze outcomes from SMARTs.[34] These scenarios begin to illustrate how D&I science "breaks the mold" and must move beyond wholesale adoption of standard economic evaluation methods.

$$\text{Economic Impact of Implementation} = \frac{(\text{Cost}_{\text{Implementation Strategy A}} + \text{Cost}_{\text{EBP}}\,|A) - (\text{Cost}_{\text{Implementation Strategy B}} + \text{Cost}_{\text{EBP}}\,|B)}{\text{Outcome}_{\text{Implementation Strategy A}} - \text{Outcome}_{\text{Implementation Strategy B}}}$$

In recent years, several key publications have laid out the foundations, methodologies, and values of economic evaluations in D&I.[35,36] Indeed, since the last publication of this chapter, D&I science has sufficiently matured that we now have our own approach to economic evaluations. The different needs of D&I research questions and decisions—more expansive cost and consequence definitions, the need to account for complex systems and contexts, use of pragmatic "minimum acceptable" approaches, shifting perspective to inform decisions of system-level payers who invest in infrastructure—have required radical reshaping of how we understand economic evaluations.[36] This reshaping brings with it not only complexity and challenges, but also new opportunities for economic evaluation researchers. Those who are trained in established methods may benefit from the opportunity to increase the impact of their work, while others with relevant training and expertise are increasingly able to contribute to economic evaluations without extensive formal training. D&I economic evaluations can greatly benefit from transdisciplinary contributions, such as integration of public finance theories or systems science methods. These new perspectives and approaches help to enrich the decision analytic approach, which is an oversimplification for D&I processes.

The remainder of this section provides a detailed orientation to key terminology, methods, and issues in D&I economic evaluations and to the current state of the science. For those new to this area of research, Eisman et al. (2020)[36] offered a useful open-access primer that readers may find beneficial to review first.

Centering Health Equity in the Evaluation

As in economic evaluations of practices, the choice for D&I decision makers depends on their valuation of the different implementation or dissemination strategy options. This valuation is not a wholly objective process, but rather a form of *bounded rationality* in which numerous values, constraints, and sources of information are used to create boundaries within which the logic of economic evaluation can be enacted (e.g., "choose the option that provides the most benefits per dollar spent"). Dominant groups of people and societal systems—including root cause systems of oppression such as racism, sexism, classism, and ableism—structure which peoples' and communities' health is prioritized as worth investing in, which is a major driver of health disparities both globally and locally. People consider *to whom* costs and consequences accrue when determining how they value them, with a recent study on this topic concluding that "self-interest is a prevailing finding" in willingness to pay for public health policies.[37(p74)] Scholars in fields such as health economics and public health economics are beginning to address this tendency, as we briefly described previously in this chapter. Within bounded rationality, it is possible to choose a primary goal of "decision-making under resource scarcity to achieve global health equity," for which economic evaluations are one of several useful inputs for values-based decision-making.

Unless economic evaluations of D&I activities pay explicit attention to health equity implications from the very outset, the resulting analysis has a major risk of reinforcing structural inequalities under the guise of rational cost-reducing or cost-efficiency measures. Consider an economic evaluation scenario in which implementing an EBP with Implementation Strategy B produces worse fidelity and QALY outcomes than Implementation Strategy A, which costs $50,000 more per QALY. Health system administrators will have to decide if they and their service recipients can afford to live with the poorer outcomes given the lowered costs of Strategy B. Is $50,000 in decreased costs enough to justify worse outcomes? Who gets to decide whether an additional QALY is worth $50,000? Can the health system afford to spend $50,000 on purchasing an additional QALY given the other things that they could do with that money (i.e., the opportunity costs)? These can be considered as ethical as well as economic questions,[38] and decision makers consider noneconomic elements that inform their choices regarding adopting a given EBP or strategy. The person or team conducting the economic evaluation needs to decide which costs and consequences are relevant (i.e., from whose perspective the analysis is done) as well as the intended goal (e.g., saving money vs. maximizing health vs. improving the distribution of population health); it is perhaps clear that these analytic choices are unlikely to reduce health disparities unless the team keeps that goal as a consistent focus throughout the evaluation.[39]

Equity concerns are not merely technical or hypothetical, but are fundamental to the ethical practice of economic evaluation. In the United States, for example, cost-benefit analysis became the preferred economic evaluation method for federal policymakers due to its usefulness as an austerity measure; through broad specification of costs and narrow specification of benefits, the analyst can create a compelling and "objective" justification for dis-investment from public programs.[40] At the other extreme, cost-effectiveness analysis based on health outcomes is disallowed in research funded by the Patient-Centered Outcomes Research Institute, though collection of data on costs and economic impacts of care are permitted.[41] Other countries make more judicious use of cost-effectiveness data in policy decisions, with QALYs and DALYs widely used given their generic nature, which facilitates comparisons across diseases. For example, the National Institute for Health and Care Excellence provides evidence on the cost-effectiveness of practices across healthcare and public health in the United Kingdom.[42] However, these metrics have also been criticized because they prioritize disability-free days and thus potentially devalue the provision of healthcare to individuals living with disabilities unless appropriate adjustments are made (e.g., using distributional cost-effectiveness methods to characterize population health across groups by disability status).[43,44] Finally, D&I scholars must contend with the reality that EBPs are more likely to be developed and tested with dominant groups (within a given community or society and globally), and EBPs developed for marginalized groups may still be deprioritized in favor of EBPs that apply to more people.[45] Similarly, D&I strategies are often developed and tested in high-resource organizations and systems and may not promote EBP implementation as effectively in settings with historical disadvantages—especially settings focused on serving marginalized groups.[45] Thus, equity concerns are relevant not only to cost and consequence valuation, but also to decisions about what qualifies as an EBP, which EBPs are selected for dissemination or implementation, and which D&I strategies support those efforts—all of which may already have been made before economic evaluation planning begins.

All that said, economic evaluations also represent a key tool for improving population health and health equity when used appropriately. Examples include use of economic evaluation to study the costs and consequences of (a) strategies for overcoming differential access to health-promoting services; (b) investments in communities and regions that have historically been disinvested in or economically exploited; (c) strategies to achieve sustainment in settings at greatest risk of nonsustainment; and (d) strategies to de-implement ineffective or harmful practices from communities. Of course, examples (c) and (d) are often a subset of (b) for a variety of reasons (e.g., lack of political power or monetary resources, stigma). In all these examples, we can choose to treat benefits from EBPs that accrue to individuals, communities, and regions marginalized by systems of oppression as more desirable than other scenarios—such as through use of distributional cost-effectiveness analysis—depending on what values we let guide our work as researchers.

Perspective

The first analytic choice in an economic evaluation is its perspective, defined as a frame of the evaluation. Perspective should be chosen in line with the decision that is aimed to be informed, reflecting the costs and outcomes of consequence to the decision maker(s). Only costs and consequences relevant to the chosen perspective are included in analyses. The cost of a single day of hospital care, for example, could be the amount of money paid to the hospital by the health plan (payer perspective); the total expenditure undertaken by the hospital on that patient that day, including labor costs, medicines, and overhead (organizational perspective); out-of-pocket payments made to the hospital (patient perspective); or *all* costs associated with the hospital stay, irrespective of who incurs them, including the opportunity costs of all resources donated to the hospital (societal perspective).[19] Similarly, the consequences of a strategy could be limited to implementation outcomes (e.g., fidelity of EBP), distal outcomes (e.g., health of patients), or wider outcomes (e.g., impact on productivity or population health).

Economic evaluations of practices can take a variety of perspectives, from reflecting the entity making the implementation decision (organizational or payer perspective) to those of the social planner (societal perspective).[9] The perspective chosen is important because each considers a different set of outcomes and costs; the societal perspective is considered the most inclusive, but it is difficult to enact fully,[46] offers limited utility for local decisions made by organizations, and is nation bound rather than global in perspective. Implementation studies typically adopt the organizational (or program) perspective instead,[36] which may be appropriate given that organizations bear the costs of implementing EBPs, and third-party payers rarely cover implementation costs in their payment rates.[47] Dissemination studies, by corollary, may take the perspective of the organization disseminating the information—a not-for-profit entity, a professional society, or some other knowledge purveyor (e.g., in the United Kingdom, the National Institute for Health and Care Excellence acts as a disseminator of guidelines). Once the perspective has been chosen for an economic evaluation, selection of measures begins, with the goal of comprehensively tracking all D&I and EBP-relevant costs and consequences contained within the perspective.[48]

Outcomes

As in economic evaluations of practices, economic evaluations of D&I may be concerned with the achievement of EBP recipients' health- and well-being-related outcomes. However, these are but one type of outcome of interest to D&I scientists.[49] Proctor and colleagues defined implementation outcomes as "the effects of deliberate and purposive actions to implement new treatments, practices, and services."[6(p65)] This definition encompasses not only recipient outcomes, but also more proximal implementation and service outcomes (Figure 11.1). Hence, economic evaluations in D&I can examine the costs of achieving gains on a measure of practitioner adoption of an EBP (an implementation outcome), a measure of patient-centeredness (a service outcome), or both. The choice of which should be defined by the perspective and consideration of the decision the evaluation is aiming to inform.

Some D&I scientists may want to compare implementation strategies on gains in QALYs or DALYs, which may be particularly important when the resources used to implement strategies will be taken away from other potential health-generating activities. Scientists interested in capturing changes in practitioner preferences across competing implementation strategies can use an instrument like the Evidence-Based Practice Attitudes Scale[50]; such studies may be useful to D&I scholars seeking ways to examine implementation outcomes such as practitioner acceptability of an EBP. Practitioner-level outcomes can also be measured directly. In mental health,

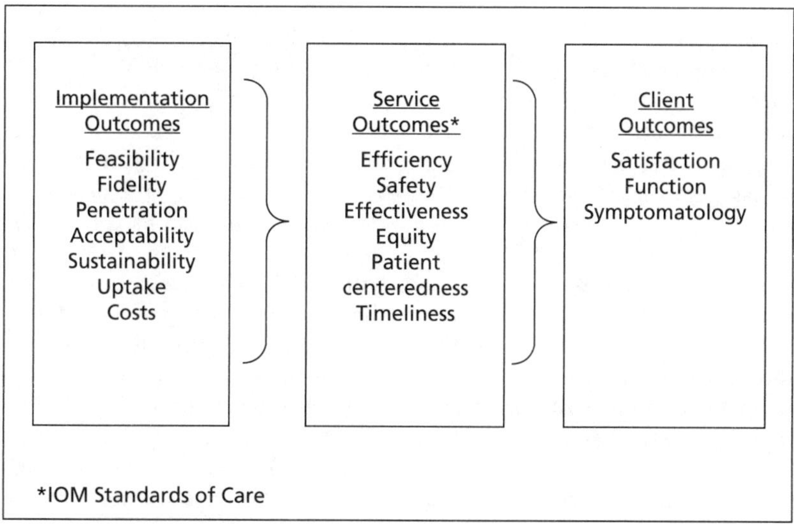

FIGURE 11.1 Implementation outcomes. IOM, Institute of Medicine.

Reprinted with permission from Proctor and colleagues.[6]

for example, practitioner fidelity to an EBP is an important metric. Using fidelity as a practitioner-level outcome, implementation strategies can be compared with respect to the congruence between the deployed EBP and original protocol and the costs that are necessary to achieve such congruence. The choice of outcomes measured should be primarily driven by the research questions and the decision it is aiming to inform, but should also be consistent with the chosen economic evaluation method and perspective. Economic evaluation always relies on a quantitative comparison between the outcome metric and costs, but use of qualitative data within a mixed-method design can greatly strengthen the selection and interpretation of outcomes for a D&I economic evaluation.[35]

Operationalization of D&I outcomes is still relatively new, and more development needs to occur regarding their use in economic evaluations. Conceptually, however, implementation outcomes perhaps may be of more relevance and interest to D&I scholars than are recipient outcomes, and future work that conducts economic evaluations using these consequences may be necessary. However, where D&I activities use resources from other health-generating activities (e.g., displacing service delivery), failure to consider wider outcomes may limit the impact of such research on decisions and limit the ability to inform investment cases for D&I activities. D&I scholars with expertise in economic evaluations have pointed out the lack of credible value-for-money assessments of implementation and service outcomes[36]; such estimates are currently unavailable in health economics literature and will be necessary to monetize implementation outcomes in cost-benefit analysis or determine thresholds for cost-effectiveness ratios based on implementation outcomes.

Cost Estimations

In this chapter, D&I costs are classified into labor and nonlabor costs,[51] which we further subdivide into fixed and variable costs; again, we focus on implementation costs, which are somewhat more concrete than dissemination costs.[52] Activity-based costing methods[53] from the field of accounting are useful for measuring labor costs because it is primarily the *activities* performed by various individuals that consume resources and produce outcomes in terms of D&I strategies (e.g., meeting, learning, planning) and EBP delivery; note that the best way to assign monetary costs to activities will depend on the evaluation perspective. Readers may be interested in practical tools for measuring implementation costs; helpful examples and guidance for developing such tools are now available (see References 52 and 53), although we urge researchers to carefully tailor their cost measurement approach to the particulars of the EBP(s), D&I strategies, and settings under consideration. We return to the need for further costing toolkit development in the last section of this chapter.

Labor costs are the costs associated with discrete EBP implementation and delivery activities, measured by the time cost that each individual spends on the activity. Labor is often the primary cost of EBP implementation efforts, so it is important that time costs are captured comprehensively. This includes time spent in specific, scheduled activities as well as ancillary preparation or follow-up actions. Examples of labor for implementation strategy activities include participation in training or supervision meetings, serving on an implementation planning team, or reading an EBP manual. EBP delivery also involves labor, such as time spent in EBP sessions, scoring a rating instrument, or coordinating care with other providers. When practitioners who typically bill third-party funders for their services engage in nonbillable activities, the lost revenue from billing is another labor cost. *Nonlabor costs* include costs of EBP-specific materials and equipment (e.g., the cost to obtain a rating instrument or EBP manual, travel expenses to attend a training) as well as overhead costs that cannot be assigned to a particular practice (e.g., utilities, administrative support, and building space that are necessary to deliver the EBP but are also used for other purposes). Many nonlabor costs are best measured not with activity-based methods, but by examining the total costs incurred within a relevant time period and assigning some appropriate proportion of those costs to the EBP implementation and delivery activities.

The costs of EBP delivery (i.e., service costs), therefore, are the sum of labor and nonlabor costs associated with delivering that practice, whereas the costs of D&I strategies are the sum of labor and nonlabor costs associated with all dissemination or implementation activities. The key challenges in cost evaluation of implementation are ensuring inclusion of all relevant cost categories (as determined by the perspective) and distinguishing intervention-focused versus implementation-focused activities. D&I researchers have published guidance on incorporating multilevel stakeholder perspectives[54] and using qualitative and mixed (quantitative + qualitative) methods[35] to improve the comprehensiveness and interpretability of cost estimates. The bearers of the costs of D&I efforts are likely to emerge as its key stakeholders; provider organizations currently bear much of the costs of implementation, and information purveyors and health communicators bear much of the costs of dissemination. These organizations will need to be cognizant of the added costs imposed by the use of D&I strategies and clearly distinguish them from EBP delivery costs. The incremental costs of D&I activities are partly a function of an organizations' financial and other resources—that is, the costs will depend on the stakeholders' contexts and perspectives. Qualitative and mixed methods will be invaluable for more accurately and completely understanding the relevant contexts and perspectives.

Another challenge is determining whether to consider a given cost measure as fixed or variable. Certain costs are incurred each time an activity occurs, whereas others last for a certain time regardless of how much (or little) activity occurs. For example, an EBP training produces variable costs if costs are calculated on a per attendee basis, but if the trainer charges the organization a set fee regardless of attendance, that is a fixed cost—at least for the period the training is meant to last. Factors like provider drift or turnover might necessitate repeated trainings, thus making the training fee fixed in a short time span but variable across longer time spans; the time for which a given cost can be considered fixed is not always clear at the outset of a D&I study. This is important because calculations of per provider, per recipient costs, or sometimes per site costs (rather than total costs) require an understanding of how to spread fixed costs across the denominator.

Opportunity Costs

As has been noted previously, a key consideration in using economic evaluation to inform decision-making is to consider the opportunity costs of any additional resources required for D&I strategies. If the benefits exceed the opportunity costs, then a strategy would be considered value for money, although a decision maker could still choose to reject it based on other considerations. Establishing what the opportunity costs are can be challenging and will depend on the context within which a strategy is being implemented. If the costs are to fall onto a fixed budget, for example, within a community provider, then the opportunity costs will be the outcomes of those activities that can no longer be funded. These activities will not necessarily impact the same patients who benefit from the D&I strategy. Alternatively, if the costs can be passed on to the payer, they could result in increased premiums or could displace other care funded by the payer. Consideration should be given to where these opportunity costs are likely to lie to help inform the decision maker about appropriate estimates for them.

In cost-effectiveness analysis, opportunity costs are normally reflected in the choice of cost-effectiveness threshold to which to compare, for example, the incremental cost per QALY. Recent work in the United States has looked at appropriate approaches to considering opportunity costs in US healthcare and potential sources of cost-effectiveness thresholds.[55,56] Within Europe and elsewhere in the world, there has been a great deal of research looking at estimating opportunity cost-based cost-effectiveness thresholds, the first notable example of which being Claxton et al., 2015.[57]

Further Analytic Considerations

Once the costs and consequences for a D&I economic evaluation have been identified, additional steps must be taken before measurement and analysis is complete. First, the evaluation team must select a *time horizon* (or analytic horizon), which is the period within which all costs and consequences will be measured. Intervention researchers commonly use long time horizons because recipient outcomes following the intervention may take decades (e.g., survival after chemotherapy for a malignancy). Many outcomes of interest to D&I researchers take place in a relatively short time horizon (1 or a few years), but research incorporating EBP sustainment outcomes or recipient outcomes can still necessitate much longer time horizons. Second, all monetary values must be adjusted to a common *present value*; this may include adjustment of values for differences in cost of living, year accrued (i.e., adjusting for inflation), or country (i.e., currency conversion). This also requires the application of *discounting*, which adjusts costs and consequences that accrue in the future to their present value. Values are discounted because receiving $1 today is worth more than receiving $1 ten years from now, even if we assume zero inflation; an individual can derive immediate gain from that $1 today or invest it to gain interest that results in a sum greater than $1. Similarly, health outcomes are also discounted because most people would rather enjoy better health now than better health 10 years from now.[58] Discounting is of lesser relevance if D&I researchers focus on D&I costs and on implementation and service outcomes, all occurring within a short time horizon. D&I researchers studying sustainment or long-term recipient outcomes will need to identify and incorporate appropriate cost and health outcome discounting approaches.

Finally, as noted previously, it is essential to use *sensitivity analysis*[16] to examine how sources of uncertainty in the economic evaluation model might be influencing its results. The evaluation team may lack perfect information on how to comprehensively identify the relevant costs and/or outcomes, measure each appropriately (monetizing where warranted), and apply the various analytic steps noted here. Sensitivity analysis helps characterize the extent to which analytic choices made by the team and measurement error in the data contributed to the conclusions and how robust the findings are to uncertainty. Qualitative data can help identify which aspects of the evaluation model are contributing the greatest uncertainty and/or interpret the results of sensitivity analyses.

State of the Literature

The available literature on economic evaluations of D&I remains a small body, but it has begun to grow much more rapidly in recent years. Herein, we provide a brief overview of systematic reviews summarizing many of the published implementation studies available, along with key conclusions drawn from those reviews. We recommend that interested readers refer to the cited systematic reviews for more details, including references for many additional example studies. Unfortunately, no systematic reviews of economic evaluations for EBP dissemination strategies have yet been published.

A systematic review of clinical guideline implementation studies[59] from 1966 to 1998 revealed that 63 of 235 studies provided information on costs of various implementation strategies (e.g., dissemination of educational materials, educational meetings, audit and feedback, use of clinical reminders). Over half of these 63 studies were cost-outcome studies that did not compare alternative implementation strategies, some were cost descriptions, and 11 were cost-effectiveness studies. Many guideline implementation studies published since that review have continued to focus on cost analyses,[60,61] although cost-effectiveness and cost-benefit studies offer support for patient-focused educational strategies in the implementation of practice guidelines in diabetic care[62] and in asthma care.[63] A 2008 systematic review of studies examining implementation of clinical pathways (which are structured intervention protocols also called care protocols or care pathways) for a variety of illnesses also reported modest, though highly heterogeneous and variable, reductions in hospital costs.[64]

Since the last edition of this book, two additional systematic reviews have documented economic evaluations across the D&I landscape. Roberts et al. (2019)[65] reviewed the use of economic evaluation in 30 implementation and improvement science studies published during 2004–2016, almost all of which were cost-effectiveness or cost-utility analyses. The authors rated the quality of the economic evaluations as generally good, though usefulness is limited by the modest amount of literature—most of which was conducted in Europe or North America (75%) and was hospital based (70%). Reeves et al.'s (2019)[66] review focused on implementation of public health interventions and policies from developed countries published during 2000–2017, for which they found 14 economic evaluations (again, almost entirely cost-effectiveness analysis). Evaluation of methodological quality was much more variable in this review; no study met every reporting criterion, and compliance with best practices for measuring costs and resource use were especially poor. Both Roberts et al. and Reeves et al. noted lacking or poor-quality sensitivity analyses as a common methodological weakness. Notably, there was almost no overlap between studies included in the two systematic reviews, suggesting poor consensus around what qualifies as a D&I economic evaluation. Finally, Dopp et al. (2019)[35] attempted to conduct a systematic review of economic evaluations in D&I research that used mixed methods, but were only able to locate one such study, a benefit-cost analysis of the Australian acute care accreditation program.[67] Several mixed-method economic evaluations have since been published,[68–70] and this topic may soon be ripe for its own systematic review.

IMPROVING THE STATE OF THE ART IN ECONOMIC EVALUATIONS OF DISSEMINATION AND IMPLEMENTATION

The relative paucity of studies reporting on economic evaluations of D&I suggests that researchers remain principally focused on developing and refining D&I strategies rather than on evaluating them from an economic perspective. This section outlines some overarching themes we drew from the existing literature. Unfortunately, many of the themes from the previous edition of this chapter still apply today, so the future directions remain largely unchanged despite major conceptual advances in D&I economic evaluations over the past 5 years.[35,36,52,54] The biggest difference in this chapter's approach is the theme of centering health equity in economic evaluation, which has been highlighted throughout.

First, because the consideration of the costs of D&I approaches is already prominent, this cost information can be used to develop a future research agenda on the comparative costs and consequences of D&I strategies. Currently, there are few studies directly comparing one D&I strategy against another on their relative ability to achieve implementation, service, or clinical outcomes. Incorporating costs into the mix will permit researchers not only to ask if a particular strategy works, but also to consider whether the changes in outcomes represent value for money. Those strategies that produce significant change in outcomes at minimal cost are likely to be the ones that are most practicable in everyday use, for example, by reducing the complexity of the D&I process, the various resources necessary for the strategy, and the total duration of D&I while still producing desirable outcomes.[49] Unfortunately, many decision makers and researchers almost exclusively focus on reducing service and D&I costs (assuming "low cost" means "cost-effective"), despite the fact that lower cost alternatives may be less effective and may undermine the health of a marginalized group through austerity measures. Human-centered design approaches can help create EBPs and D&I strategies that better fit within the capacities and resource constraints of targeted settings, while maintaining a focus on health improvement and equity[71]—but the presumed economic benefits must still be confirmed through economic evaluation. Furthermore, the complex interactions between D&I strategies in the multilevel service contexts in which EBPs are implemented will require moving beyond simple randomized trials into methods that are better suited to representing complexity, such as SMART trials,[34] other quasi-experimental approaches and systems science methods (e.g., system dynamics, agent-based modeling) (also see chapters 13 and 14). D&I economic evaluation methods must evolve in parallel to allow use of these methods; for instance, simulation modeling would be well suited for economic evaluation within a systems science approach, but remains rare in D&I studies.[65,66]

Second, the field of D&I needs widespread use of costing toolkits, something that is simple enough to be used by community stakeholders and researchers alike; unifies a common set of costing methodologies suited for D&I; standardizes procedures for capturing costs; is flexible enough to be applicable across varied D&I strategies; is robust across the varied organizations and service settings within which D&I work is being conducted; and serves as a common platform for training and development of economic evaluations in the field. In the area of intervention science, for example, the World Health Organization (WHO), as part of its **Cho**osing **I**nterventions that are **C**ost-**E**ffective (CHOICE) program, has spent the past two decades developing a costing toolkit,[72,73] and the US Institute of Education Sciences funded creation of a similar toolkit called CostOut® for school-based interventions.[74] The European Union recently funded the ProgrammE in Costing resource use measurement and outcome valuation for Use in multisectoral National and International health economic evaluAtions (PECUNIA) to provide standardized, harmonized, and validated methods and tools for assessments of costs.[75] Similar efforts have been underway within D&I science; examples include an approach developed for implementation of sex offender treatment,[76] or the Cost of Implementing New Strategies (COINS) approach,[77] and an adaptation of a cost calculator based on child protection practices in Britain.[78] A common framework for economic evaluations within D&I that builds on these efforts is now necessary because the growth of the field requires that D&I scientists evaluate the same things in much the same ways.

Third, one rate-limiting step in D&I economic evaluations is the cottage industry of D&I strategies, many of which are developed in highly resourced research settings with seemingly little attention being paid to their deployment in lower resource environments, are highly particularistic, appear to be unnecessarily complex and overconceptualized, appear to be indistinguishable from other strategies in terms of focus or intent, and are too poorly described to promote understanding of what actually implementers are supposed to do and what they are supposed to achieve. Activity-based costing—as described elsewhere in this chapter, a key foundation for D&I cost measurement—requires that the activities are clear so that costs can be attached to them; also, the outcomes need to be well operationalized so that the incremental effects of these strategies can be captured. At the present time, reviews of D&I strategies implore the field to name and define these strategies,[79] and the overly complex terminology of the field is referred to as a "Tower of Babel."[80] If it is unclear what a D&I strategy actually is, it is challenging to conduct any rigorous economic evaluation of it. Economic evaluators, therefore, may need to confine themselves to the best operationalized and measured D&I strategies. They might also consider advocating for the culling of several marginal strategies, so that those that remain can be subject to appropriate analysis. Of course, this should not be taken to mean that D&I strategies should be proscriptive or inflexible; in many ways, D&I are fundamentally relational activities, in which partners (e.g., D&I experts and local stakeholders) collaborate to identify emergent needs and tailor their strategies, time, and effort to achieve desired outcomes. These activities cannot be fully specified in advance, but researchers can operationalize the process behind strategy selection and track how the approach unfolds over time to capture all relevant costs.

Fourth, an important contribution of economic evaluations of D&I strategies will be in the ascertainment of the value created by spreading and scaling-up EBPs (see chapter 29). Conceptual frameworks exist to help decision makers decide how best to allocate resources between practices, their implementation, and research—all to maximize a desired goal.[81] As noted at the beginning of this chapter, promotion of health improvement and equity can (and should) be considered a valued goal, even if achieving it requires increased expenses. In an elaboration of a value framework for implementation, Walker and colleagues derived constructs from a payer perspective based on improving overall health outcomes in a population.[82] The *expected value of perfect implementation* represents the highest possible outcome that can be achieved when implementation is "perfect." The *expected value of actual implementation* represents the outcome that would occur under more naturalistic circumstances. The more cost-effective an EBP is, and the more widely applicable it is, the higher is its expected value of actual implementation from a D&I strategy.[83] This is what a payer would be willing to pay in order to secure some desirable health outcome (so, for example, payers should be willing to make considerable investments in implementation strategies that increase the percentage of children vaccinated, based on this model). The *value of the implementation activity* then is the difference between the expected value of actual implementation and its actual implementation cost. If the cost of implementing a practice is small, and the effects of the implementation strategy result in highly desirable outcomes, then this is a high-value implementation strategy that needs to be supported. Empirical investigations using these frameworks have yielded intriguing findings, such as the declining returns to implementation as natural diffusion occurs,[83] suggesting that investments in implementation should be early, intensive, and time limited. More refinement is needed, however, to ensure that the model's assumptions do not de-prioritize health equity—such as by privileging EBPs that can be used with many people over those that can be used with the highest need people.

From a policy perspective, the principal challenge is how to pay for D&I of EBPs, and this is another area where a focus on value can help decision makers.[47] In healthcare, there are efforts focused on twin approaches of *value-based purchasing*[84] (assisting healthcare purchasers to contract with plans that offer greater value rather than merely lower cost) and *pay-for-performance*[85], which involve tying fiscal and nonfiscal rewards and punishments to a variety of performance outcomes, such as health outcomes, patient satisfaction, scores on quality scorecards, screening rates, prescribing practices, adherence to clinical guidelines, and investments in information strategy, among others. Pay-for-performance approaches have also been proposed for population-level health outcomes such as health inequities.[86] Scholars have proposed methods for providing guidance to policymakers on the relative costs and outcomes of implementation strategies and is expressed as a function of the cost-effectiveness of treatment and cost-effectiveness of the practice (organization).[87] But in many disciplines, such as behavioral health, the data necessary to determine these cost-effectiveness ratios are not extant—and provider organizations have limited capacity (e.g., outcomes tracking, billing) to take on new value- or performance-based payment mechanisms, even if available. Paying for implementation of economically viable EBPs, then, is an alternative that policymakers should consider in cases where paying for outcomes is not feasible.[88] In the past few years, researchers have identified and defined 23 financing strategies that can be used to pay for implementation[89] and published guidance on how findings from economic evaluations can be translated into feasible, effective financing strategies in community organizations and systems.[47,90]

SUMMARY

Dissemination and implementation impose costs on EBP purveyors, healthcare and promotion organizations, and payers (including governments). Whether these added costs will result in improved service delivery and, ultimately, improvements in recipient outcomes and population health remains an open question. To be of value in informing a D&I decision, an economic evaluation must provide evidence of the impacts of the alternative strategies under consideration on the relevant outcomes, costs, and opportunity costs for the decision maker(s) involved. This requires careful consideration of the decision maker (who are we informing, what do they care about), the perspective of the analysis (frame of evaluation), the outcomes, the costs, and the opportunity costs. Further, of utmost importance is the approach to capturing the impact on inequities. If emerging studies reveal that defined D&I strategies are more cost-effective than "usual" approaches, then policymakers and service providers will need to resource these added D&I costs to ensure the success and long-term sustainability of high-quality healthcare and public health activities.

SUGGESTED READINGS AND WEBSITES

Readings

Bauer MS, Kirchner JA. Implementation science: what is it and why should I care? *Psychiat Res.* 2020;283:112376. doi:10.1016/j.psychres.2019.04.025

Eisman AB, Kilbourne AM, Dopp AR, et al. Economic evaluation in implementation science: making the business case for implementation strategies. *Psychiat Res.* 2020;283:112433. doi:10.1016/j.psychres.2019.06.008

These articles from a special issue offer overviews of the field of D&I research in general and economic evaluations in D&I science in particular.

Drummond MF, Sculpher MJ, Claxton K, et al. *Methods for the Economic Evaluation of Health Care Programmes.* 4th ed. Oxford University Press; 2015.

Neumann PJ, Sanders GD, Russell LB, et al. *Cost-Effectiveness in Health and Medicine.* 2nd ed. Oxford University Press; 2017.

These are two of the standard texts on conducting economic evaluations in the health sciences.

Sanders GD, Neumann PJ, Basu A, et al. Recommendations for conduct, methodological practices, and reporting of cost-effectiveness analyses: second panel on cost-effectiveness in health and medicine. *JAMA.* 2016;316(10):1093–1103. doi:10.1001/jama.2016.12195

This is a consensus statement that outlines appropriate methodology for the use of cost-effectiveness analyses in health.

Economic evaluation in implementation science. https://www.biomedcentral.com/collections/EconomicEvaluation

This special collection of articles, published in Implementation Science *and* Implementation Science Communications *considers key issues in economic evaluation in implementation science and highlights approaches and examples to inform the field. This collection of papers has been funded in part by the US National Cancer Institute and the US Department of Veterans Affairs. A national Economics and Implementation Science Workgroup provides formative input and an internal review process for all papers in the collection.*

Selected Websites and Tools

The following Internet resources are focused on economic evaluations of interventions, either curative or preventive. The general approach described in these resources, however, can be applied to evaluations of D&I activities.

Chronic Disease Cost Calculator Version 2, Centers for Disease Control and Prevention. https://www.cdc.gov/pcd/issues/2015/15_0131.htm

This tool provides state-level estimates of the cost of several chronic diseases in the United States. Cost is measured as medical expenditures and absenteeism costs. Diseases covered are arthritis, asthma, cancer, cardiovascular diseases, depression, and diabetes.

Cost-Effectiveness Analysis Registry, Center for the Evaluation of Value and Risk in Health, Institute for Clinical Research and Health Policy Studies, Tufts Medical Center. http://healtheconomics.tuftsmedicalcenter.org/cear4/Home.aspx

Originally based on the articles by Tengs et al.,[91,92] *this website includes a detailed database of cost-effectiveness analyses, cost-effectiveness ratios, and QALY weights.*

CostOut.® https://www.cbcsecosttoolkit.org

CostOut is a web-based tool designed to facilitate the estimation of cost- and cost-effectiveness for education programs, funded by the Institute of Education Sciences, US Department of Education. Following the "ingredients" approach that is common in education, the tool allows users to identify all program activities that consume resources, assign prices (national and user-input local values) to each, and calculate costs based on the units per ingredient used with necessary adjustments (e.g., cost of living, inflation, discounting). Cost estimates can be used then to calculate cost-effectiveness ratios within the tool.

Task Force on Community Preventive Services. Economic Reviews. http://www.thecommunityguide.org/about/economics.html#where

The Community Guide provides a repository of the 200+ systematic reviews conducted by the Task Force, an independent, interdisciplinary group with staff support by the Centers for Disease Control and Prevention. This link is for their economic reviews section, which reviews the applications of cost-effectiveness analyses to interventions analyzed by the Community Guide.

REFERENCES

1. Brouwer WBF, Culyer AJ, van Exel NJA, Rutten FFH. Welfarism vs. extra-welfarism. *J Health Econ.* 2008;27(2):325–338. doi:10.1016/j.jhealeco.2007.07.003
2. Coast J, Smith RD, Lorgelly P. Welfarism, extra-welfarism and capability: the spread of ideas in health economics. *Soc Sci Med.* 2008;67(7):1190–1198. doi:10.1016/j.socscimed.2008.06.027
3. Panattoni L, Dillon EC, Hurlimann L, et al. Human resource costs of implementing a tiered team care model for chronically ill patients according to lean management principles. *J Patient Centered Res Reviews.* 2016;3(3):186. https://institutionalrepository.aah.org/jpcrr/vol3/iss3/49/
4. Rabin BA, Brownson RC, Haire-Joshu D, et al. A glossary for dissemination and implementation research in health. *J Public Health Man.* 2008;14(2):117–23. doi:10.1097/01.PHH.0000311888.06252.bb
5. Fixsen AAM, Aijaz M, Fixsen DL, et al. *Implementation Frameworks: An Analysis.* Active Implementation Research Network; 2021.
6. Proctor E, Silmere H, Raghavan R, et al. Outcomes for implementation research: conceptual distinctions, measurement challenges, and research agenda. *Adm Policy Ment Health.* 2011;38(2):65–76. doi:10.1007/s10488-010-0319-7
7. Drummond MF, Sculpher MJ, Claxton K, et al. *Methods for the Economic Evaluation of Health Care Programmes.* 4th ed. Oxford University Press; 2015.
8. Thokala P, Ochalek J, Leech AA, et al. Cost-effectiveness thresholds: the past, the present and the future. *PharmacoEconomics.* 2018;36:509–522. doi:10.1007/s40273-017-0606-1
9. Neumann PJ, Sanders GD, Russell LB, et al. *Cost-Effectiveness in Health and Medicine.* 2nd ed. Oxford University Press; 2017.
10. Clemmer B, Haddix AC. Cost-benefit analysis. In: Haddix AC, Teutsch SM, Shaffer PA, Dunet DO, eds. *Prevention Effectiveness: A Guide to Decision Analysis and Economic Evaluation.* Oxford University Press; 1996:85–102.
11. Finkelstein A, Hendren N. Welfare analysis meets causal inference. *J Econ Perspect.* 2020;34:146–167. doi:10.1257/jep.34.4.146
12. Keel G, Savage C, Rafiq M, Mazzocato P. Time-driven activity-based costing in health care: a systematic review of the literature.

Health Policy. 2017;121:755–763. doi:10.1016/j.healthpol.2017.04.013
13. Levin HM, McEwan PJ, Belfield C, et al. *Economic Evaluation in Education: Cost-Effectiveness and Benefit-Cost Analysis*. SAGE Publications; 2017.
14. Simon GE, Katzelnick DJ. Depression, use of medical services and cost-offset effects. *J Psychosom Res*. 1997;42(4):333–344. doi:10.1016/s0022-3999(96)00367-4
15. Asaria M, Griffin S, Cookson R. Distributional cost-effectiveness analysis: a tutorial. *Med Decis Making*. 2016;36(1):8–19. doi:10.1177/0272989x15583266
16. Briggs AH, Gray AM. Handling uncertainty in economic evaluations of healthcare interventions. *BMJ*. 1999;319:635–638. http://doi.org/10.1136/bmj.319.7210.635
17. Drummond MF, McGuire A. *Economic Evaluation in Health Care: Merging Theory with Practice*. Oxford University Press; 2001.
18. Petitti DB. *Meta-Analysis, Decision Analysis, and Cost-Effectiveness Analysis: Methods for Quantitative Synthesis in Medicine*. 2nd ed. Oxford University Press; 2000.
19. Sanders GD, Neumann PJ, Basu A, et al. Recommendations for conduct, methodological practices, and reporting of cost-effectiveness analyses: Second Panel on Cost-Effectiveness in Health and Medicine. *JAMA*. 2016;316(10):1093–1103. http://doi.org/10.1001/jama.2016.12195
20. Barnett ML, Dopp AR, Klein C, et al. Collaborating with health economists to advance implementation science: a qualitative study. *Implement Sci Commun*. 2020;1:82. doi:10.1186/s43058-020-00074-w
21. Barnett M, Stadnick NA, Proctor EK, et al. Moving beyond Aim Three: a need for a transdisciplinary approach to build capacity for economic evaluations in implementation science. *Implement Sci Commun*. 2021;2:133. doi:10.1186/s43058-021-00239-1
22. Frieden TR. Evidence for health decision making: beyond randomized, controlled trials. *N Engl J Med*. 2017;377(5):465–475. doi:10.1056/NEJMra1614394
23. Jones DS, Podolsky SH. The history and fate of the gold standard. *Lancet*. 2015;385(9977):1502–1503. doi:10.1016/S0140-6736(15)60742-5
24. Rothwell PM. External validity of randomized controlled trials: "To whom do the results of this trial apply?" *Lancet*. 2005;365:82–93. doi:10.1016/S0140-6736(04)17670-8
25. Walker SM, Fox A, Altunkaya J, et al. Programme evaluation of population and system level policies: evidence for decision-making. *Med Decis Making*. 2022;42(1):17–27. doi:10.1177/0272989X211016427
26. Kilo CM. A framework for collaborative improvement: lessons from the Institute for Healthcare Improvement's Breakthrough Series. *Qual Manag Health Care*. 1998;6(4):1–13. doi:10.1097/00019514-199806040-00001
27. McCarty D, Gustafson DH, Wisdom JP, et al. The Network for the Improvement of Addiction Treatment (NIATx): enhancing access and retention. *Drug Alcohol Depen*. 2007;88(2–3):138–145.
28. Kilbourne AM, Neumann MS, Pincus HA, Bauer MS, Stall R. Implementing evidence-based interventions in health care: application of the replicating effective programs framework. Implement Sci. 2007;2:42. doi:10.1016%2Fj.drugalcdep.2006.10.009
29. Aarons GA, Ehrhart MG, Farahnak LR, Hurlburt MS. Leadership and organizational change for implementation (LOCI): a randomized mixed method pilot study of a leadership and organization development intervention for evidence-based practice implementation. *Implement Sci*. 2015;10:11. doi:10.1186/s13012-014-0192-y
30. Powell BJ, Haley AD, Patel SV, et al. Improving the implementation and sustainment of evidence-based practices in community mental health organizations: a study protocol for a matched-pair cluster randomized pilot study of the Collaborative Organizational Approach to Selecting and Tailoring Implementation Strategies (COAST-IS). *Implement Sci Commun*. 2020;1:9. doi:10.1186/s43058-020-00009-5
31. Chapman E, Haby MM, Toma TS, et al. Knowledge translation strategies for dissemination with a focus on healthcare recipients: an overview of systematic reviews. *Implement Sci*. 2020;15:1–14. doi:10.1186/s13012-020-0974-3
32. Baker R, Camosso-Stefinovic J, Gillies C, et al. Tailored interventions to overcome identified barriers to change: effects on professional practice and health care outcomes. *Cochrane Database Syst Rev*. 2010;17:Article CD005470. doi:10.1002/14651858.CD005470.pub2
33. Hernán MA, Robins JM. *Causal Inference: What If?* CRC Press; 2020.
34. Eisman AB, Hutton DW, Prosser LA, et al. Cost-effectiveness of the Adaptive Implementation of Effective Programs Trial (ADEPT): approaches to adopting implementation strategies. *Implement Sci*. 2020;15:109. doi:10.1186/s13012-020-01069-w
35. Dopp AR, Mundey P, Beasley LO, et al. Mixed-method approaches to strengthen economic evaluations in implementation research. *Implement Sci*. 2019;14:2. doi:10.1186/s13012-018-0850-6

36. Eisman AB, Kilbourne AM, Dopp AR, et al. Economic evaluation in implementation science: making the business case for implementation strategies. *Psychiat Res.* 2020;283:112433. doi:10.1016/j.psychres.2019.06.008
37. Bosworth R, Cameron TA, DeShazo JR. Willingness to pay for public health policies to treat illnesses. *J Health Econ.* 2015;39:74–88. doi:10.1016/j.jhealeco.2014.10.004
38. Brock D. Ethical issues in the use of cost effectiveness analysis for the prioritization of health resources. In Khushf G, ed. *Handbook of Bioethics: Taking Stock of the Field From a Philosophical Perspective.* Springer Netherlands; 2004:353–380.
39. Liscow Z. Equity in regulatory cost-benefit analysis. LPE Project. 2021. Accessed January 23, 2023. https://lpeproject.org/blog/equity-in-regulatory-cost-benefit-analysis/
40. Pasquale F. Cost-benefit analysis at a crossroads: a symposium on the future of quantitative policy evaluation. 2021. LPE Project. Accessed January 23, 2023. https://lpeproject.org/blog/cost-benefit-analysis-at-a-crossroads-the-future-of-quantitative-policy-evaluation/
41. PCORI Help Center. What is PCORI's official policy on cost and cost-effectiveness analysis? 2019. Accessed January 23, 2023. https://help.pcori.org/hc/en-us/articles/213716587-What-is-PCORI-s-official-policy-on-cost-and-cost-effectiveness-analysis-
42. National Institute for Health and Care Excellence. Technology appraisal guidance. 2022. Accessed January 23, 2023. https://www.nice.org.uk/about/what-we-do/our-programmes/nice-guidance/nice-technology-appraisal-guidance
43. Mehlman MJ, Durchslag MR, Neuhauser D. When do health care decisions discriminate against persons with disabilities? *J Health Polit Polic.* 1997;22:1385–1411. http://doi.org/10.1215/03616878-22-6-1385
44. Persad G. Priority setting, cost-effectiveness, and the Affordable Care Act. *Am J Law Med.* 2015;41:119–166. http://doi.org/10.1177/0098858815591511
45. Baumann AA, Cabassa LJ. Reframing implementation science to address inequities in healthcare delivery. *BMC Health Serv Res.* 2020;20:190. doi:10.1186/s12913-020-4975-3
46. Kim DD, Silver MC, Kunst N. Perspective and costing in cost-effectiveness analysis, 1974–2018. *PharmacoEconomics.* 2020;38:1135–1145. doi:10.1007/s40273-020-00942-2
47. Dopp AR, Kerns SEU, Panattoni L, et al. Translating economic evaluations into financing strategies for implementing evidence-based practices. *Implement Sci.* 2021;16:66. doi:10.1186/s13012-021-01137-9
48. Walker S, Griffin S, Asaria M, et al. Striving for a societal perspective: a framework for economic evaluations when costs and effects fall on multiple sectors and decision makers. *Appl Health Econ Health Policy.* 2019;17:577–590. doi:10.1007/s40258-019-00481-8
49. Proctor EK, Landsverk J, Aarons G, et al. Implementation research in mental health services: an emerging science with conceptual, methodological, and training challenges. *Admin Policy Ment Health.* 2009;36(1):24–34. doi:10.1007/s10488-008-0197-4
50. Aarons GA. Mental health provider attitudes toward adoption of evidence-based practice: the Evidence-Based Practice Attitude Scale (EBPAS). *Ment Health Serv Res.* 2004;6(2):61–74. doi:10.1023/b:mhsr.0000024351.12294.65
51. Zarkin GA, Dunlap LJ, Homsi G. The substance abuse services cost analysis program (SASCAP): a new method for estimating drug treatment services costs. *Eval Program Plann.* 2004;27(1):35–43. doi:10.1016/j.evalprogplan.2003.09.002
52. Gold HT, McDermott C, Hoomans T, Wagner TH. Cost data in implementation science: categories and approaches to costing. *Implement Sci.* 2022;17:11. doi:10.1186/s13012-021-01172-6
53. Cidav Z, Mandell D, Pyne J, et al. A pragmatic method for costing implementation strategies using time-driven activity-based costing. *Implement Sci.* 2020;15:28. doi:10.1186/s13012-020-00993-1
54. Eisman AB, Quanbeck A, Bounthavong M, et al. Implementation science issues in understanding, collecting, and using cost estimates: a multi-stakeholder perspective. *Implement Sci.* 2021;16:75. doi:10.1186/s13012-021-01143-x
55. Padula WV, Sculpher MJ. Ideas about resourcing health care in the United States: can economic evaluation achieve meaningful use? *Ann Intern Med.* 2021;174:80–85. doi:10.7326/M20-1234
56. Vanness D, Lomas J, Ahn H. A health opportunity cost threshold for cost-effectiveness analysis in the United States. *Ann Intern Med.* 2021;174:25–32. doi:10.7326/M20-1392
57. Claxton K, Martin S, Soares M, et al. Methods for the estimation of the National Institute for Health and Care Excellence cost-effectiveness threshold. *Health Technol Assess.* 2015;19(14):1–503. doi:10.3310/hta19140
58. Brouwer WB, Niessen LW, Postma MJ, Rutten FF. Need for differential discounting of costs and health effects in cost effectiveness analyses. *BMJ.* 2005;331:446–448. doi:10.1136/bmj.331.7514.446

59. Vale L, Thomas R, MacLennan G, et al. Systematic review of economic evaluations and cost analyses of guideline implementation strategies. *Eur J Health Econ.* 2007;8:111–121. doi:10.1007/s10198-007-0043-8
60. Koskinen H, Rautakorpi UM, Sintonen H, et al. Cost-effectiveness of implementing national guidelines in the treatment of acute otitis media in children. *Intl J Technol Assess Health Care.* 2006;22(4):454–459. doi:10.1017/s0266462306051373
61. Hoeijenbos M, Bekkering T, Lamers L, et al. Cost-effectiveness of an active implementation strategy for the Dutch physiotherapy guideline for low back pain. *Health Policy.* 2005;75(1):85–98. doi:10.1016/j.healthpol.2005.02.008
62. Dijkstra RF, Niessen LW, Braspenning JCC, et al. Patient-centred and professional-directed implementation strategies for diabetes guidelines: a cluster-randomized trial-based cost-effectiveness analysis. *Diabetic Med.* 2006;23(2):164–170. doi:10.1111/j.1464-5491.2005.01751.x
63. Tschopp JM, Frey JG, Janssens JP, et al. Asthma outpatient education by multiple implementation strategy. Outcome of a programme using a personal notebook. *Resp Med.* 2005;99(3):355–362. doi:10.1016/j.rmed.2004.07.006
64. Rotter T, Kugler J, Koch R, et al. A systematic review and meta-analysis of the effects of clinical pathways on length of stay, hospital costs and patient outcomes. *BMC Health Serv Res.* 2008;8:265. doi:10.1002/14651858.cd006632.pub2
65. Roberts SLE, Healey A, Sevdalis N. Use of health economic evaluation in the implementation and improvement science fields—a systematic literature review. *Implement Sci.* 2019;14:72. doi:10.1186/s13012-019-0901-7
66. Reeves P, Edmunds K, Searles A, Wiggers J. Economic evaluations of public health implementation-interventions: a systematic review and guideline for practice. *Public Health.* 2019;169:101–113. doi:10.1016/j.puhe.2019.01.012
67. Mumford V, Greenfield D, Hinchcliff R, et al. Economic evaluation of Australian acute care accreditation (ACCREDIT-CBA (acute)): study protocol for a mixed method research project. *BMJ Open.* 2013;3:e002381 doi:10.1136/bmjopen-2012-002381
68. Dopp AR, Mundey P, Silovsky JF, et al. Economic value of community-based services for problematic sexual behaviors in youth: a mixed-method cost-effectiveness analysis. *Child Abuse Negl.* 2020;105:104043. doi:10.1016/j.chiabu.2019.104043
69. Ling VB, Levi EE, Harrington AR, et al. The cost of improving care: a multisite economic analysis of hospital resource use for implementing recommended postpartum contraception programmes. *BMJ Qual Saf.* 2021;30:658–667. doi:10.1136/bmjqs-2020-011111
70. Salloum RG, D'Angelo H, Theis RP, et al. Mixed-methods economic evaluation of the implementation of tobacco treatment programs in National Cancer Institute-designated cancer centers. *Implement Sci Commun.* 2021;2:41. doi:10.1186/s43058-021-00144-7
71. Lyon AR, Munson SA, Renn BN, et al. Use of human-centered design to improve implementation of evidence-based psychotherapies in low-resource communities: protocol for studies applying a framework to assess usability. *JMIR Res Protoc.* 2019;8(10):e14990. doi:10.2196/14990
72. Bertram MY, Lauer JA, Stenberg K, Edejer TTT. Methods for the economic evaluation of health care interventions for priority setting in the health system: an update from WHO CHOICE. *Int J Health Policy Manag.* 2021;10:673–677. doi:10.34172/ijhpm.2020.244
73. Edejer T-T, Baltussen R, Adam T, et al. *WHO Guide to Cost-Effectiveness Analysis.* World Health Organization. 2003.
74. Hollands FM, Hanisch-Cerda B, Levin HM, et al. *CostOut—The CBCSE Cost Tool Kit.* Teachers College, Columbia University, Center for Benefit-Cost Studies of Education; 2015. https://www.cbcsecosttoolkit.org
75. PECUNIA. ProgrammE in Costing, resource use measurement and outcome valuation for Use in multi-sectoral National and International health economic evaluAtions: PECUNIA project. n.d. Accessed January 23, 2023. https://www.pecunia-project.eu/
76. Jennings WG, Zgoba KM. An application of an innovative cost-benefit analysis tool for determining the implementation costs and public safety benefits of SORNA with educational implications for criminology and criminal justice. *J Crim Just Educ.* 2015;26(2):147–162. doi:10.1080/10511253.2014.940057
77. Saldana L, Chamberlain P, Bradford WD, et al. The Cost of Implementing New Strategies (COINS): a method for mapping implementation resources using the stages of implementation completion. *Child Youth Serv Rev.* 2014;39:177–182. doi:10.1016/j.childyouth.2013.10.006
78. Holmes L, Landsverk J, Ward H, et al. Cost calculator methods for estimating casework time in child welfare services: a promising approach for use in implementation of evidence-based practices and other service innovations. *Child*

Youth Serv Rev. 2014;39:169–176. doi:10.1016/j.childyouth.2013.10.003

79. Proctor EK, Powell BJ, McMillen JC. Implementation strategies: recommendations for specifying and reporting. *Implement Sci.* 2013;8:1. doi:10.1186/1748-5908-8-139
80. McKibbon KA, Lokker C, Wilczynski NL, et al. A cross-sectional study of the number and frequency of terms used to refer to knowledge translation in a body of health literature in 2006: a Tower of Babel? *Implement Sci.* 2010;5:16. doi:10.1186/1748-5908-5-16
81. Fenwick E, Claxton K, Sculpher M. The value of implementation and the value of information: combined and uneven development. *Med Decis Making.* 2008;28:21–32. doi:10.1177/0272989x07308751
82. Walker S, Faria R, Whyte S, et al. *Getting Cost-Effective Technologies Into Practice: The Value of Implementation. Report on Framework for Valuing Implementation Initiatives.* Policy Research Unit in Economic Methods in Health & Social Care Interventions; 2014. https://eepru.sites.sheffield.ac.uk/reports-publications/reports
83. Whyte S, Dixon S, Faria R, et al. Estimating the cost-effectiveness of implementation: is sufficient evidence available? *Value Health.* 2016;19(2):138–144. doi:10.1016/j.jval.2015.12.009
84. Chee TT, Ryan AM, Wasfy JH, Borden WB. Current state of value-based purchasing programs. *Circulation.* 2016;133(22):2197–2205. doi:10.1161/circulationaha.115.010268
85. Mendelson A, Kondo K, Damberg C, et al. The effects of pay-for-performance programs on health, health care use, and processes of care: a systematic review. *Ann Intern Med.* 2017;166:341–353. doi:10.7326/m16-1881
86. Asada Y. A summary measure of health inequalities for a pay-for-population health performance system. *Prev Chronic Dis.* 2010;7(4):A72. http://www.cdc.gov/pcd/issues/2010/jul/09_0250.htm
87. Mason J, Freemantle N, Nazareth I, et al. When is it cost-effective to change the behavior of health professionals? *JAMA.* 2001;286(23):2988–2992. doi:10.1001/jama.286.23.2988
88. Raghavan R. Using risk adjustment approaches in child welfare performance measurement: applications and insights from health and mental health settings. *Child Youth Serv Rev.* 2010;32:103–112. doi:10.1016/j.childyouth.2009.07.020
89. Dopp AR, Narcisse MR, Mundey P, et al. A scoping review of strategies for financing the implementation of evidence-based practices in behavioral health systems: state of the literature and future directions. *Implement Res Pract.* 2020. doi:10.1177/2633489520939980
90. Dopp AR, Manuel JK, Breslau J, et al. Value of family involvement in substance use disorder treatment: aligning clinical and financing priorities. *J Subst Abuse Treat.* 2021;132:108652. doi:10.1016/j.jsat.2021.108652
91. Tengs TO, Wallace A. One thousand health-related quality-of-life estimates. *Med Care.* 2000;38:583–637. doi:10.1097/00005650-200006000-00004
92. Tengs TO, Adams ME, Pliskin JS, et al. Five-hundred life-saving interventions and their cost-effectiveness. *Risk Anal.* 1995;15(3):369–390. doi:10.1111/j.1539-6924.1995.tb00330.x

12

Missing the Target—Mis-implementation and De-implementation

VIRGINIA R. MCKAY, CALLIE WALSH-BAILEY, SARA MALONE, COLLIN MCGOVERN, AND DANIEL J. NIVEN

INTRODUCTION

Much of dissemination and implementation (D&I) science is dedicated to examining the uptake and implementation of evidence-based interventions (EBIs), practices, programs, and policies. However, the field increasingly recognizes that interventions are often provided in a suboptimal manner—ineffective interventions are too frequently continued while beneficial EBIs are abandoned. De-implementation and mis-implementation research, which collectively focus on interventions in need of discontinuation or interventions provided suboptimally, is a growing area within D&I science. The presumption that individuals will end or adjust delivery of inappropriate interventions through passive diffusion of scientific knowledge is insufficient for change; active strategies are needed. In this chapter on mis-implementation and de-implementation, we describe the significance of the problem, review relevant concepts and theories, and summarize the current evidence. To help illustrate, we provide two case studies of de-implementation and mis-implementation. The first focuses on mis-implementation and the premature abandonment of a collection of evidence-based mental health interventions disseminated through a major implementation effort, the National Implementing Evidence-Based Practice Project. The second focuses on the de-implementation of public health policies, specifically HIV criminalization laws, which have demonstrated harmful effects for people living with HIV (PLWH), and successful strategies to promote reduction and removal of these laws. We then conclude the chapter by identifying opportunities for further investigations within this emerging area of D&I science.

SIGNIFICANCE OF THE PROBLEM

The significance of this problem for health and well-being is substantial from multiple perspectives within both science and practice. It is not uncommon for the evidence supporting health interventions to change, with initial studies supporting the effectiveness of an intervention and later trials demonstrating no effect.[1] For example, beginning in the 1970s supplemental oxygen for individuals with mild-to-moderate chronic obstructive pulmonary disease (COPD) was a long-standing, common treatment to reduce hospitalization and prolong life. A subsequent randomized control trial decades later did not replicate findings of effectiveness,[2] indicating that thousands of individuals had received unnecessary treatment. Many interventions not only are ineffective but also may cause harm. In a recent examination of a suite of seven low-value procedures conducted in a hospital setting, as many as 15% of individuals experienced hospital-acquired complications, including hospital-associated infection, gastrointestinal bleeding, and falls resulting in fracture or intracranial injury.[3] In addition to poor health outcomes, unnecessary and ineffective treatments, especially expensive or widespread treatments like oxygen for COPD, account for substantial waste of healthcare spending. In the United States alone, costs from overtreatment or low-value care are estimated in the

Virginia R. McKay, Callie Walsh-Bailey, Sara Malone, Collin McGovern, and Daniel J. Niven, *Missing the Target—Mis-implementation and De-implementation* In: *Dissemination and Implementation Research in Health.* Edited by: Ross C. Brownson, Graham A. Colditz, and Enola K. Proctor, Oxford University Press. DOI: 10.1093/oso/9780197660690.003.0012 range of $75–100 billion.[4,5] Furthermore, this burden is shared inequitably, with disadvantaged communities, including low-income and racial/ethnic minorities, experiencing underuse of evidence-based care and overuse of harmful, low-value care depending on the intervention, further exacerbating disparities in addition to providing subquality care.[6,7]

While healthcare has been the primary context of examining suboptimal intervention delivery, particularly in regard to interventions that should be de-implemented, several public health studies highlighted similar problems. Estimates suggest that 30%–50% of health departments end programs that should have continued and 15%–50% continue programs that should end.[8–11] In the instance of premature abandonment of services, initial investments in developing, adopting, and implementing interventions can be substantial in terms of financial and human resources wasted. The benefits of an intervention go unrealized, which can be more diffuse in public health settings, and may not be apparent for weeks, months, or even years of implementation. Further, relationships can be damaged with communities that have received benefits from programs when they are abandoned, especially communities historically abused or neglected by public health and the healthcare system.[12–14]

Finally, an ethical argument can also be made about why reducing low-value care is critical. Healthcare providers have an ethical obligation not to harm patients, to provide beneficial treatment, and to ensure fair use of healthcare resources so that patients have access to care when needed.[15] For public health practitioners, there is an additional responsibility to provide beneficial programs for entire communities while maintaining good stewardship of taxpayer dollars.[16]

CONCEPTUALIZING MIS-IMPLEMENTATION AND DE-IMPLEMENTATION

Mis-implementation refers to both the premature termination of EBIs and ongoing inappropriate continuation of interventions without a solid evidence base capturing all forms of less-than-ideal intervention implementation.[11] De-implementation refers more specifically to one aspect of mis-implementation, namely, the reduction or discontinuation of interventions that are low value.[17] Within clinical settings low-value care was defined by Elshaug and colleagues as "an intervention in which evidence suggests it confers no or very little benefit for patients, or risk of harm exceeds probable benefit, or more broadly, the added costs of the intervention do not provide proportional added benefits."[18(p129)] In other words, interventions should be de-implemented if they are harmful, ineffective, or inefficient to provide. Additionally, within public health circumstances, interventions may no longer be needed, as in the case of recovering from a natural disaster or epidemic, for example.[16]

Many similar and related concepts and terms appear in the broad literature. Within healthcare, the body of literature dedicated to overuse, underuse, and low-value and high-value care has had a heavy contribution to conceptualizing de- and mis-implementation in D&I.[18,19] A scoping review from 2015 identified 43 unique terms, including those mentioned thus far, referring to some aspect of de-adoption—another term within the mis-implementation and de-implementation spectrum.[20] These terms include de-adoption, dis-investment, exnovation, health technology reassessment, and dismantling as the corollary to implementation and similar to de-implementation. Coupled with the fact that many terms may be inappropriately used interchangeably, the terminology used to describe mis-implementation and de-implementation can be confusing. However, there is growing consensus within D&I science of de-implementation as the preferred term to broadly describe the cessation of low-value care.

While the ideal solution for this problem is routinely to encourage total de-implementation or universal sustainment of interventions, other more nuanced outcomes are sometimes warranted. For instance, it may be preferable to restrict an intervention to a narrower, more specific population or reduce the dose of an intervention. Additionally, it is important to consider whether interventions are being provided with fidelity to their core components, whether adaptations have been made, and the impact of fidelity and adaptation on the intended implementation and health outcomes as an indication of sustainability or abandonment. For instance, some adaptations may promote sustainability and safeguard against underuse, while others may render the intervention ineffective and may thus be appropriate to de-implement. A more thorough discussion of these issues can be found in chapter 3.

Paramount to de- and mis-implementation is identifying interventions that are being implemented in a suboptimal manner such that the ultimate effect of the intervention is poor for potential recipients.

Interventions appropriate for de-implementation can occur at all levels of intervention, from individual to policy levels. While singular or collections of EBIs for clinical or public health practice commonly drive implementation initiatives, interventions appropriate for de-implementation or mis-implementation are more often loosely organized within the literature. Some interventions appropriate for de-implementation are sometimes identified within implementation initiatives. More recently, programmatic initiatives such as Choosing Wisely and its derivatives,[21] led by the American Board of Internal Medicine Foundation, systematically identify and prioritize low-value practices. These efforts have successfully contributed to broad awareness of low-value care and de-implementation within medical and mainstream literature.[22]

THEORIES, MODELS, AND FRAMEWORKS

Just as it is valuable and important to use theories, models, and frameworks to guide implementation research, the use of such guidance is essential in conceptualizing, planning, executing, and evaluating de-implementation efforts. We present several examples of how common implementation science models have been applied to de-implementation, as well as examples of models specific to de-implementation.

Perhaps one of the most fundamental theories to D&I science is Roger's diffusion of innovation, which characterizes the spread of a new intervention.[23] The spread of a new intervention is influenced by characteristics of the intervention itself, its adopters, as well as context. Innovators and early adopters, representing about 15%–20% of potential users in a system, are the first to adopt an intervention. After this point, the innovation is rapidly adopted by other users, characterized graphically as an S curve, which ultimately motivates those who are more resistant to change to adopt the intervention, as shown in Figure 12.1 on the left side of the top panel. Dengler and colleagues applied this to de-implementation by posing that, as an intervention wanes in popularity or use, an early small number of users de-implement the intervention, with de-implementation advancing more rapidly after reaching the tipping point among early de-adopters as shown on the right side of the top panel in Figure 12.1.[24] As with strategies targeting adoption and implementation, strategies can expedite this process as represented by the arrows shown in the bottom panel.

To effectively de-implement a low-value intervention, it is important to understand the determinants, or barriers and facilitators, that influence such efforts.[25] Determinants have been well studied in D&I and well-established determinants frameworks, such as the Consolidated Framework for Implementation Research (CFIR),[26] can be applied to de-implementation. A review of medication de-prescribing applied the CFIR and found that studies were limited in their consideration and identification of determinants, potentially hampering the success of de-implementation efforts.[27] This elucidation of determinants can help inform the appropriate selection of strategies to support the successful de-implementation of low-value practices.[28]

As described in chapter 4, process models and frameworks help to describe and/or guide the actions or steps involved in implementation[29] and can also be used to inform the process of de-implementation. One example of a process model empirically applied to de-implementation appeared in Voorn and colleagues' study of the de-implementation of low-value patient blood management practices. They applied a model originally developed by Grol and colleagues,[30] which originally focused on implementation in a process of five activities (see Figure 12.2): development of change targets; analysis of performance, target group, and setting; selection of strategies and measures to change practice; development and execution of (de)implementation plan; and evaluation and adaption of the plan.[31]

Evaluation models can be valuable in identifying and assessing indicators of success in de-implementation efforts (i.e., whether the practice was reduced, removed, restricted, or replaced as intended). In the re-envisioning of RE-AIM (Reach, Effectiveness, Adoption, Implementation, and Maintenance), the authors called for the consideration of

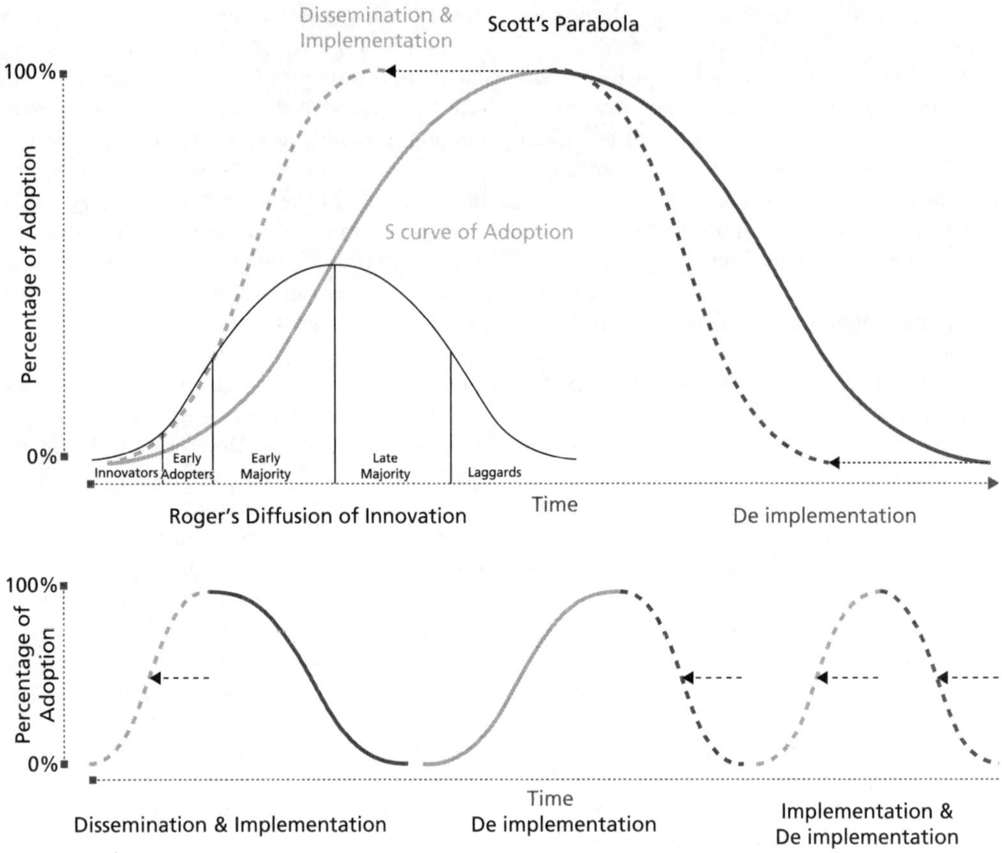

Dissemination & Implementation
Scott's Parabola
100%
Percentage of Adoption
S curve of Adoption
0%
Innovators
Early Adopters
Early Majority
Late Majority
Laggards
Roger's Diffusion of Innovation
Time
De implementation

100%
Percentage of Adoption
0%
Time
Dissemination & Implementation
De implementation
Implementation & De implementation

FIGURE 12.1 Implementation and de-implementation curves.

Reprinted with permission from Dengler et al.[24]

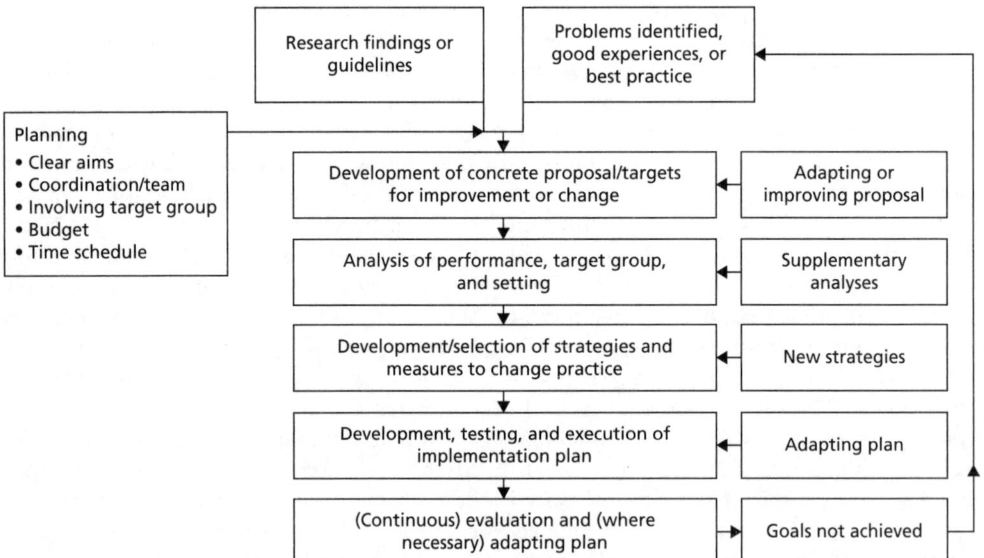

FIGURE 12.2 Conceptualization of the de-implementation process.

Reprinted with permission from Grol et al., 2005, model and Voorn et al.[31]

de-implementation in the EBI life cycle as an extension of maintenance, noting an intervention may no longer be appropriate or effective.[32,33] Prusaczyk and colleagues expanded on Proctor's taxonomy of outcomes and provided guidance on the distinctions and overlap between implementation and de-implementation.[34] These authors suggested that outcomes of both the practice targeted for de-implementation and the de-implementation process itself should be measured and highlighted the importance of considering cultural and historical influences related to the practice that may influence de-implementation. For instance, in an application of Proctor's outcomes to inform the identification and measurement of outcomes for de-implementing detrimental early childhood feeding practices, the authors identified acceptability and feasibility and acknowledged that the process of de-implementation is more than simply undoing implementation and often involves more complex actions.[35]

Models and frameworks like the ones described above and other common examples from D&I can also be used to guide the study of mis-implementation. Determinant frameworks can be used to understand the contextual factors that influence successful implementation and continuation of beneficial practices in real-world settings. Process frameworks that include steps for routine monitoring and reassessment can help guide actions needed after initial implementation to keep a program in place and to ensure it is continuing to have its desired effects. Evaluation frameworks that include maintenance or sustainment can be valuable in identifying outcomes to assess implementation success. Padek and colleagues presented a conceptual framework modeled after the socioecological framework that includes multilevel factors influencing mis-implementation, including determinants, presence or absence of strategies to support successful implementation, evidence for the impact of the intervention, funding, policies, and other external influences.[36]

In addition to the plethora of models and frameworks in D&I,[37–39] there is growing attention toward theories, models, and frameworks developed specifically for de-implementation. In recent reviews,[29,40] authors identified 34 unique theories, models, and frameworks of de-implementation. In another recent scoping review, the most common applications were to guide the identification of determinants and to inform data collection and analysis.[41] The theories found in this review were mainly applicable to cognitive and behavioral processes, indicating a focus in the literature on individual behavior change rather than systemic or policy change. One such example is the synthesis model for the process of de-adoption by Niven and colleagues.[20] This model draws on the knowledge to action framework, a process framework that outlines three stages (research, translation, and institutionalization) and processes needed during each phase to move research-generated knowledge into public health practice.[42,43] This model illustrates a cycle of assessing the low-value practice, assessing determinants to de-implementation, intervening to de-implement the practice, evaluating the process and outcomes of the de-implementation efforts, and sustaining the de-implementation.

Despite decades of policy termination research and efforts analogous to de-implementation in public policy, business, and other fields, few were applied to community and other nonclinical settings.[40] A few frameworks for de-implementation have focused on implementation of another intervention simultaneously, sometimes calling this phenomenon substitution or replacement.[44,45] Table 12.1 presents several examples of de-implementation models and frameworks from these reviews. Discipline/setting indicates the field in which the model was developed and setting in which it was applied per the source reference. Model type appears as reported in two scoping reviews.

Highlighting one of few models focusing on system-level strategies to promote de-implementation through dis-investment, Harris and colleagues developed a framework that combines de-implementation determinants and processes, portraying factors that may influence de-implementation efforts, as well as activities involved in de-implementation efforts.[47] Their framework highlights the complexity of de-implementation by considering influential factors at multiple levels, including necessary predeterminants to de-implementation. The framework also includes eight discrete steps in the de-implementation process (Figure 12.3).

TABLE 12.1 EXAMPLE DE-IMPLEMENTATION AND MIS-IMPLEMENTATION MODELS

Model Name	Discipline/Setting	Model Type
COST (culture, oversight, systems change, training) framework[46]	Healthcare; hospital	Determinant
Conceptual framework for mis-implementation[11]	Public health; state health departments	Determinant
Framework for an organization-wide approach to disinvestment in the local healthcare setting[47]	Healthcare; hospital	Determinant & process
Framework for taking action on overuse[48]	Healthcare; clinical settings	Determinant & process
Process model for termination of public goods[49]	Public policy; US federal government	Process
Synthesis model for the process of de-adoption[20]	Healthcare; clinical settings	Process
Framework for evaluation and explication of disinvestment projects[47]	Healthcare; hospital	Evaluation
PBMA (program budgeting and marginal analysis) evaluation framework[50]	Healthcare; primary care	Evaluation
Potential considerations in prioritizing the testing of unproven medical practice[17]	Healthcare; clinical settings	Evaluation

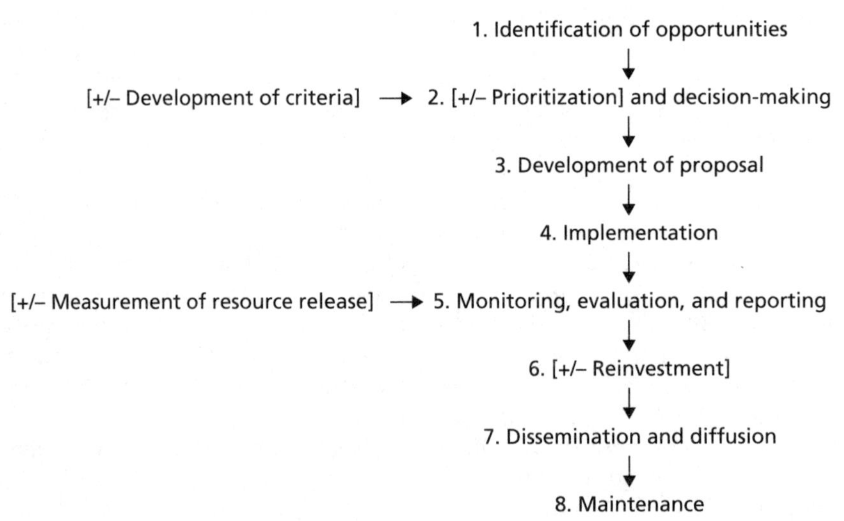

FIGURE 12.3 Steps in the disinvestment process from framework for an organization-wide approach to disinvestment in the local healthcare setting.

Reprinted with permission from Harris et al.[47]

This framework, along with numerous others, has yet to be tested empirically, offering de-implementation researchers many opportunities to contribute to this rapidly budding area of inquiry within D&I.

DETERMINANTS

To fully understand how contextual factors influence de-implementation, it is necessary to address the determinants that influence evidence-based practice and de-implementation. As mentioned, the determinants that influence de-implementation are multilevel, and some examples include the organization, policy, practitioner, patient, and intervention characteristics, indicating a complex web of influences on de-implementation.[51] Reviews of de-implementation determinants suggest that they can either promote and act as a facilitator or hinder and act as a barrier to de-implementation, and they must be assessed to understand the influence that each determinant has on the intervention to be reduced or removed.[52] Furthermore, the determinants impacting overuse and underuse may differ. As an example, the cost awareness of a practitioner has been linked to a reduction in the use of low-value practices, while their fear of malpractice accusations might sustain the use of a low-value practice.[53,54] The same determinant may act as either a barrier or a facilitator, depending on the context within which the intervention exists. For instance, leadership support could act as either a barrier or facilitator depending on the orientation of the leadership team toward the practice. Provider knowledge about a recommendation and belief in the data have been shown to impact their willingness to adopt recommendations regarding reduction of care.[55,56]

Although patient and practitioner determinants have been the focus of de-implementation theory, organization and policy characteristics have also been identified.[24,52,53] The broad categories relevant within the setting include organizational processes, context, and resources. For instance, in a review conducted by van Dulmen and colleagues, clinician time availability was commonly highlighted as a barrier to providing maximally appropriate care.[52] Other organization level determinants identified include the presence of a guideline and the number of handoffs included in the workflow.[24,52,53]

Last, determinants at multiple levels can interact to influence mis-implementation or de-implementation. For example, a study among local health departments found that grant funding ending was the most common reason for mis-implementation; funding impacts budgets for staff salaries and other resources needed for program delivery.[8]

CASE STUDY—ABANDONMENT OF EVIDENCE-BASED MENTAL HEALTH INTERVENTIONS AFTER A NATIONAL IMPLEMENTATION EFFORT

Background

Nearly 1 in 20 adults in the United States suffers from severe mental illnesses, such as major depression, bipolar disorder, and schizophrenia. Access to treatment varies considerably, and 35% of Americans with severe mental illness do not pursue treatment at all.[57] The economic burden is vast as well in terms of both direct and indirect costs. For instance, the unemployment rate for Americans suffering from mental illness is higher than those who do not, and caregivers spend an average of 32 hours a week providing unpaid care to patients with mental disorders.[57] A number of US federal agencies invest in the development and promotion of EBI to address serious mental illness, including the Substance Abuse and Mental Health Services Administration (SAMHSA), the Health Resources and Services Administration (HRSA), and the National Institute of Mental Health (NIMH) to help provide support for people with serious mental illness.

Context

Launched in 1998 in the United States, the National Implementing Evidence-Based Practice Project (NEPP) focused on promoting the implementation of five evidence-based psychosocial practices for adults with schizophrenia and severe mental illness: (1) supported employment, (2) family psychoeducation, (3) illness management and recovery, (4) integrated dual disorders treatment, and (5) assertive community treatment.[58] In an initial phase, packages were created for each of these interventions to support implementation, including training and informational materials, as well as tools to guide implementation and change at local sites. In a second phase, interventions were disseminated among 53 sites across eight states. This effort consisted of several strategies essential for supporting adoption and implementation. There was robust support and collaboration with state health departments to promote adoption and implementation among community mental health agencies, with flexibility among states to tailor their approach to working with agencies and provide consultation.[59] After adoption and initial implementation, several fidelity assessments demonstrated that agencies were able to fully implement interventions and maintain fidelity after 12–24 months.[60] Investigators identified that supportive leadership within agencies contributed to fidelity, and agencies that adequately monitored fidelity were often able to improve.

Unfortunately, follow-up studies showed that many of these interventions had subsequently been abandoned. Eight years post-implementation, approximately 47% of interventions remained in place continuously. An additional 16% restarted the intervention after a period of discontinuation, and 37% of sites abandoned the intervention altogether. There was no association between baseline characteristics and successful sustainment.[61] When implementation leadership was interviewed, major contributing determinants to abandonment included finances, workforce, intervention prioritization, and a lack of reinforcement strategies to help maintain intervention activities. Among reinforcement strategies, fidelity monitoring and supervision approaches that showed success in promoting early fidelity were particularly successful at intervention sustainability. Furthermore, some interventions were more likely to be abandoned than others, suggesting that characteristics of the intervention influenced sustainability. The researchers noted a number of adaptations to the interventions, some required by states and some in response to local contextual factors, but it is unclear whether these adaptations supported sustainability, hindered sustainability, or made no difference.

Lessons for D&I

This case study illustrates the fundamental concept of mis-implementation in public health. Schizophrenia and other serious mental illness will likely persist. As such, providing support for individuals who experience serious mental illness will continue to be beneficial and help avoid more extreme, last-resort intervention, such as institutionalization. While there was a tremendous effort and investment to promote a collection of EBIs to address this significant health issue, wide D&I as well as good initial fidelity to the interventions; there was relatively little attention to the long-term sustainment of these interventions. Subsequently, interventions were steadily abandoned over time, such that after only 8 years, approximately 40% of the interventions had been abandoned. Researchers were able to identify many contributing determinants to abandonment now routinely discussed within de-implementation. This example also represents early thinking within D&I, which emphasized more strict fidelity to interventions and paid relatively less attention to adaptations. Some of the adaptations made to interventions could have plausibly encouraged sustainment and prevented abandonment. Yet, the overall intervention abandonment observed presumably translated into substantial waste of resources used to initially implement interventions and missed opportunities to support individuals who would have benefited from these interventions.

STRATEGIES

The identification of determinants across the individual, organization, policy, and other levels suggests that potential areas for intervention also exist across multiple levels. These intervention points, conceptualized as strategies, aid in the change process to promote intervention optimization. In situations where strategies are used to reduce or eliminate low-value care, we consider them *de-implementation strategies.* Within the domain of mis-implementation, we expect strategies designed to ensure sustainability to appropriately address the additional dimensions of insufficient application or premature abandonment of an intervention. As with implementation strategies, the selection and use of strategies might be different depending on the intervention target, the determinants impacting the intervention and the type of de-implementation that is being planned (e.g., reduction or complete elimination.

To date, comprehensive evaluation of evidence-based de-implementation strategies is limited, and strategies have focused primary on changing provider behavior. Clinician decision support, for example, which leverages the electronic medical record to help provide clinical decision-making at the point of care, has the largest evidence base for the reduction of inappropriate care.[62] This can occur through prompts within the system, which remind the clinician of the appropriate guidelines, or through standard order sets and workflow modifications within the charting system, which help limit the potential for inadvertently delivering inappropriate care. Other strategies that have been successfully used within healthcare include education targeted at the clinician as well as audit and feedback.[44,63,64] Interestingly, many strategies tested have yielded mixed results or no effect.[62] For instance, patient cost sharing, which relies heavily on the patient to be able to distinguish between high- and low-value care and to be able to advocate for high-value care, does not always demonstrate the intended effects.[64]

While many of these strategies have corollaries as implementation strategies, there is indication new strategies are emerging specific to de-implementation. One specific promising strategy highlighted in healthcare is increasing provider comfort with "watchful waiting" and allowing more time to pass without intervention.[65] While many other strategies, like education, decision support tools, or audit and feedback, demonstrate effectiveness as implementation strategies, this particular strategy differs by reframing lack of action as an intervention, increasing the likelihood of other forms of management and observation. Often in clinical settings, this may be the most appropriate intervention given that some diseases and illnesses resolve without intervention. For example, overuse of antibiotics is a growing public health concern, and many efforts have been developed to reduce antibiotic use.[66] Children experiencing pediatric ear infection, or otitis media, have historically been treated excessively with antibiotics, but often improve on their own without treatment. Ongoing efforts to encourage watchful waiting in this circumstance reduced the prescription of antibiotics,[66] while not increasing patient anxiety where there is strong physician-patient communication. This strategy holds promise for reducing intervention that would be designated low value and indicates there may be other strategies more appropriate for de-implementation than other areas of D&I.

Given that determinants at multiple levels may impact the persistence of low-value interventions, de-implementation efforts also leverage multiple strategies in many areas of health.[62,67] Work with state public health officials led to interviews about their perceptions of effective strategies for ending inappropriate programs.[67] Practitioners emphasized the importance of assessment of evidence coupled with communication in the process of ending programs. However, they also discussed the importance of considering what, if any, aspects of the program should be saved before total removal.[67] When multiple strategies are used, they may be targeted at the same actor or different individuals/systems, depending on the intervention. For instance, a multistrategy approach may target the physician and the patient or the medical team and the organization. One review in healthcare identified a handful of effective de-implementation strategies that targeted both the patient and provider.[62,65] A review of strategies used in nursing highlighted that nearly every study with demonstrated effects used more than one strategy.[63] While the use of a single strategy might be sufficient, the use of multiple strategies may be desirable and even necessary.

As mentioned above, de-implementation can co-occur with implementation in some circumstances, which has led to strategies that promote both efforts simultaneously through substitution or replacement. Strategies used for substitution or replacement demonstrate two general approaches. First, strategies can focus on the implementation of the new practice that does not allow for the undesirable intervention to occur. Ho and colleagues described this type of de-implementation as a "reversal with unrelated replacement."[68] For example, antipsychotics in long-term care settings are often prescribed before attempting other interventions but are considered an intense intervention. However, an example of substitution was described as using a new protocol that does not include an option for antipsychotics prescription, but allows for other, milder medication.[68] This implementation of a new, competing protocol reduced inappropriate use of medication through early intervention of a different practice.[69]

A second approach is considering de-implementation and implementation together in a sequential process that has been effective, first focusing on de-implementation, followed by implementation of a new practice.[45,70] This might lead to the use of an initial strategy, such as audit and feedback, to focus on de-implementation followed by education around a new implementation effort. Doing this sequentially can assist with work burden as well as the cognitive load associated with learning and unlearning interventions and related workflows.

CASE STUDY—DE-IMPLEMENTING HIV CRIMINALIZATION LAW

Background

At the end of 2020, nearly 38 million people were living with HIV across the globe, with an estimated 1.5 million acquiring the virus in 2020 alone. The vast majority of new HIV infections occur in sub-Saharan Africa, accounting for slightly more than half of all new infections worldwide. Specifically in the United States, more than 1.2 million Americans are living with HIV, with more than 35,000 new infections each year.[71] Worldwide, only 66% of those living with HIV are virally suppressed due to routine antiretroviral therapies (ARTs) use, and nearly 16% of PLWH were completely unaware of their viral status.[72] To stem the HIV epidemic globally, investments in HIV care are estimated to be between $18 and $20 billion each year,[73] and a robust set of interventions is available to prevent HIV among individuals who may be at risk and treat HIV among those living with HIV.

Context

HIV criminalization laws are intended to reduce transmission through the prosecution of PLWH, who place other individuals at risk for HIV transmission.[74] These statutes were first legislated in the 1980s at a time when the HIV epidemic was still emerging, HIV was highly stigmatized (at the time called gay-related immune deficiency or GRID by the Centers for Disease Control and Prevention), and researchers held a poor scientific understanding of the virus and its transmission or treatment. Under these statutes, individuals can be found guilty of criminal charges for failing to disclose their HIV-positive status or engaging in behaviors that risk transmission. Individuals can face fines and/or imprisonment for several years and, in some jurisdictions, for life.[75]

As of December 2021, there were 35 US states that criminalized the behavior of PLWH through specific laws that target HIV or sexually transmitted infection (STI).[76] HIV criminalization has spread internationally as well; 92 countries have reported to the Joint United Nations Program on HIV/AIDS (UNAIDS) that they criminalize HIV through specific or general statutes.[77] While it is unclear how many individuals have been prosecuted, in the United States alone at least 400 cases were documented from 2008 to 2019.[78] Furthermore, these laws disproportionately affect people of color, lesbian, gay, bisexual, transgender, and queer/questioning (LGBTQ) individuals, and immigrants. For instance, in Canada, researchers observed that there are more than twice the amount of newspaper pictures featuring Black than White defendants in HIV criminalization trials, and that just four immigrant men have dominated nearly half of HIV criminalization coverage since 1989.[79]

Although the intention is to prevent HIV spread, HIV laws do not align with current HIV science, do not have the intended outcome, and cause harm for PLWH. From a biological perspective, HIV-related statutes, which can be vague on what constitutes risky behavior, do not accurately reflect current understanding of HIV transmission. For instance, for people who routinely take ARTs and suppress their viral load of HIV to undetectable levels, transmitting the disease to another person is highly unlikely.[76] Yet, several HIV criminalization laws do not distinguish between behaviors with low and high risk of transmission (e.g., spitting vs. anal sexual intercourse). Generalizations regarding risky behaviors subsequently miscommunicate information surrounding the realities of HIV transmission and undermine existing public health efforts.[80] The Undetectable = Untransmittable (U=U) campaign is one such campaign that promotes ART adherence by highlighting the extremely low likelihood of transmitting HIV after viral suppression through routine usage of ARTs.[81] A number of studies demonstrated that policies do not influence disclosure, curb important behaviors like HIV testing, prevent PLWH from disclosing their behaviors to clinicians and public health practitioners, and have no impact on HIV transmission.[82–84] Thus, by targeting individuals with a specific disease and misrepresenting the modern reality that PLWH can lead a healthy lifestyle, research also demonstrates that HIV criminalization laws exacerbate social stigmas and create barriers to testing, care, and treatment services by associating HIV disclosure with legal risk.[85,86]

Due to demonstratable public health detriments having arisen from HIV criminalization laws, public health, advocacy, legal, and scientific groups currently advocate for the removal or refinement of these laws.[87] Legal efforts to completely de-implement HIV criminalization laws include limiting statutes to focus on serious sex crimes and only prosecuting behaviors with a high chance of transmission and/or clear intent to harm.[80] Other efforts work to modernize HIV criminal laws, for instance rolling HIV into the status of general communicable diseases, requiring prosecutors to demonstrate an intent to transmit, or considering methods used to reduce the risk of HIV transmission (e.g., ART therapy, condom usage) when applying the law and whether transmission actually took place.[76] Since 2014, eight states have modernized their statutes to reflect a proper understanding of the virus, with one state (Illinois) having repealed its HIV nondisclosure law altogether.[76] Globally, UNAIDS, as part of a campaign against "societal enabling," has established a target to reduce the worldwide proportion of countries with HIV criminalization laws to 10% by 2025.[77] These campaigns reflect a growing movement with increasing successes that seeks to dismantle policy that undermines critical public health efforts as well as infringes on human rights to equality and nondiscrimination.

Lessons for D&I

This example demonstrates a problematic policy intervention ripe for de-implementation. HIV criminal laws demonstrate no effect on the intended outcome—that is, they do not reduce behaviors that make HIV transmission more likely—and actually harm the individuals that they target. The scientific community, advocacy groups, and other health organizations at multiple levels have rightly applied a variety of strategies to promote the de-implementation of these laws with a measure of success among early de-implementers. However, many of these laws remain in place in the United States and globally, suggesting that additional strategies will be needed to completely de-implement HIV criminal laws.

FUTURE DIRECTIONS

Opportunities abound for D&I scientists within this line of scientific inquiry, and we expect that a deeper investigation will potentially have significant impact on the D&I field. Along with growing interest, we also expect the literature to change rapidly in the next several years. We propose future directions that will serve the dual purpose of providing a deeper understanding of de-implementation and mis-implementation as well as inform the D&I field as a whole.

Currently, there is growing consensus that implementation and de-implementation are different phenomena. Conceptually, implementation and de-implementation share similar fundamentals in terms of identifying interventions, contextual determinants, and strategies to stimulate change. However, debate in the D&I field remains about why and how de-implementing interventions are different from implementation and to what extent implementation models can be applied to de-implementation.[88] Further study is needed to elucidate key differences between implementation, de-implementation, and mis-implementation, and many proposed de-implementation-specific models and frameworks should be tested to determine their relevance and utility.

Arguably, de-implementation strategies should be based on models of change that consider determinants, are tailored to a specific context, and are evaluated experimentally. As such, the natural initial step is identifying interventions that are being mis-implemented or should be de-implemented.[19] While there are several efforts underway toward this end, particularly in healthcare settings, how to prioritize interventions among the many identified is currently unclear. Cost, extent of delivery, and inequities among intervention recipients may potentially serve as criteria for prioritization.

While research conceptualizing and framing de-implementation has escalated in recent years, there is a pittance of research focusing on determinants and strategies. De-implementation determinant studies have consistently emphasized the role of the patient and patient characteristics in continued practices.[52] A better understanding of the range of determinants across all levels, including the structural and systemic determinants, as well as ways in which they function to influence the continuance of inappropriate practices or removal of effective ones will provide a more comprehensive picture of how and why interventions are implemented in a suboptimal manner. Evidence-based de-implementation strategies have similarly mostly targeted individual clinician behavior change, representing a small fraction of what has been included within implementation strategy taxonomy. In contrast, efforts within D&I to review, categorize, and define implementation strategies that can be generalized across healthcare and public health settings are well established.[89,90] Implementation strategies can be sorted by different implementation factors that they address, their mechanisms of change, and the levels of system targeted.[90] We expect continued exploration of other strategies, such as those focused on policy changes and system-level interventions, theoretically should also function to shift practitioner behavior, but evidence supporting these types of strategies will be beneficial. For instance, Choosing Wisely has championed efforts to reduce overuse in many different healthcare tests and treatments.[91] While the effort has brought attention to the areas that could be considered low-value care, some clinical areas of Choosing Wisely have not demonstrated reduced inappropriate interventions, illustrating mixed success of this strategy.[92] This research agenda will ultimately aid in promotion of appropriate strategies to help with its replacement, reduction, or removal of the incongruous practice.

The unique aspects of de-implementation hold value for D&I science by highlighting different factors that motivate and support behavior change, which result in different types of strategies, such as watchful waiting. It also makes clear opportunities for D&I to learn from other fields, such as the robust literature on policy dismantling, termination, and dis-investment.[19,93,94] For instance, there is a substantial literature outlining models for dis-investment and demonstrating the effectiveness of selective dis-investment targeting low-value procedures and treatments in the context of universal healthcare.

Last, public health research significantly lags behind healthcare research in this area, although it is clear that similar issues occur. Furthermore, equivalent efforts in public health are virtually nonexistent. While it is clear there is substantial cost and undue harm from interventions that are mis-implemented, disparities in this burden are not yet well elucidated either within public health.

Our case study of the NEPP, a single effort to disseminate and implement a collection of EBIs, demonstrated that we likely do not yet know the impact of mis-implementation on public health. However, there will continue to be similar efforts to promote EBI in all areas of public health. We would expect that de-implementation and mis-implementation research in public health would perhaps yield a set of determinants and strategies that are relevant in this setting.

SUMMARY

De-implementation and mis-implementation of interventions are significant problems in both healthcare and public health settings. In recognition of this, D&I science has begun conceptualizing, framing, and empirically examining the extent of the problem. The next major steps in the field will be to test and refine existing de-implementation models, understand major determinants of suboptimal implementation, and identify strategies that promote de-implementation or appropriate sustainment of interventions. The prospect of improving outcomes for patients by removing unnecessary treatment burdens, more judicious use of limited resources in public health practice, and improving equitable health outcomes for communities shows significant promise.

SUGGESTED READINGS AND WEBSITES

Readings

Augustsson H, Ingvarsson S, Nilsen P, et al. Determinants for the use and de-implementation of low-value care in health care: a scoping review. *Implement Sci Commun.* 2021;2(1):1–17. doi:10.1186/S43058-021-00110-3

This is a scoping review of determinants impacting low-value care. Determinants are discussed in relation to the CFIR. It identifies a set of factors unique to de-implementation.

Brownson RC, Allen P, Jacob RR, et al. Understanding mis-implementation in public health practice. *Am J Prev Med.* 2015;48(5):543–551.

This article conceptualizes mis-implementation in public health and distinguishes between overuse and underuse of interventions.

Colla CH, Mainor AJ, Hargreaves C, Sequist T, Morden N. Interventions aimed at reducing use of low-value health services: a systematic review. *Med Care Res Rev.* 2017;74(5):507–550. doi:10.1177/1077558716656970

A systematic review of interventions designed to reduce low-value care is presented. It identifies a number of effective interventions, primarily at the patient and provider levels.

Helfrich CD, Hartmann CW, Parikh TJ, Au DH. Promoting health equity through de-implementation research. *Ethn Dis.* 2019;29(suppl 1):93. doi:10.18865/ED.29.S1.93

The article explores inequity in low-value care for disadvantaged communities and demonstrates how disadvantaged communities receive low-value care in some circumstances. In other circumstances, disadvantaged communities bear an inequitable cost burden when advantaged communities receive more low-value care.

McKay VR, Morshed AB, Brownson RC, Proctor EK, Prusaczyk B. Letting go: Conceptualizing intervention de-implementation in public health and social service settings. *Am J Community Psychol.* 2018;62(1–2):189–202. Doi:10.1002/ajcp.12258

The article conceptualizes de-implementation for D&I science in public health settings and reviews criteria for intervention de-implementation, discusses the application of theoretical models, and provides exemplar cases of de-implementation.

Niven DJ, Mrklas KJ, Holodinsky JK, et al. Towards understanding the de-adoption of low-value clinical practices: a scoping review. BMC Med. 2015;13(1):1–21. doi:10.1186/S12916-015-0488-Z

The article systematically reviews the literature on de-implementation in healthcare. It reviews existing terminology and explores conceptual overlap and differences in terminology. A de-implementation process model based on literature synthesis is presented.

Norton WE, Chambers DA. Unpacking the complexities of de-implementing inappropriate health interventions. *Implement Sci.* 2020;15:2. doi:10.1186/s13012-019-0960-9

Commentary that reviews determinants for de-implementation at multiple levels and types of actions for de-implementation, including removal, replacement, reduction, and restriction, is provided. The article discusses tailoring strategies to promote de-implementation to encourage desired outcomes.

Shrank WH, Rogstad TL, Parekh N. Waste in the US health care system: estimated costs and potential for savings. JAMA. 2019;322(15):1501–1509. doi:10.1001/JAMA.2019.13978

Reviewed in this article is wasteful spending in the US health system, with low-value care as one of six domains. The authors also identify potential cost-saving interventions and their estimated benefit in cost savings.

Walsh-Bailey C, Tsai E, Tabak RG, et al. A scoping review of de-implementation frameworks and models. *Implement Sci.* 2021;16:100. doi:10.1186/s13012-021-01173-5

This review article identifies di-implementation-specific frameworks. It discusses conceptual differences among models and maps models to a socioecological framework.

Websites and Tools

Choosing Wisely. https://www.Choosingwisely.org

An initiative by the American Board of Internal Medicine, this site provides lists of clinical interventions identified as low value by clinical professionfsal organizations. Lists are searchable by disease or by content area.

De-Implementation. The Complexities of Overuse, Overdiagnosis, and De-adoption. https://www.youtube.com/watch?v=Jtad417gCHc&t=2556s

This webinar by the National Cancer Institute provides an overview of de-implementation with cancer-specific examples.

De-implementation Guide. https://evidenceforlearning.org.au/assets/NT/De-implementation-Guide.pdf

This tool developed by the Evidence for Learning Organization is for educators to guide the de-implementation of educational programs.

Dissemination and Implementation Models in Health Research and Practice. https://dissemination-implementation.org

This site describes D&I models, including de-implementation models, and provides a set of tools for model selection based on user need.

The Less Is More Collection. https://jamanetwork.com/collections/44045/less-is-more

This is a collection of over 150 articles describing research in low-value care curated by the Journal of the American Medical Association Internal Medicine (JAMA Internal Medicine).

National Collaborating Centre for Methods and Tools. https://www.nccmt.ca/

Supports evidence-informed decision making for public health practitioners. Provides two tools for guiding de-implementation: Do We Need to De-implement an Existing Program? A Checklist to Inform Decision Making *and* Tool for Assessing Applicability and Transferability of Evidence (A&T Tool), Version B: When Considering Stopping an Existing Program. *Both can be found at the link above.*

REFERENCES

1. Prasad V, Cifu A. Medical reversal: why we must raise the bar before adopting new technologies. *Yale J Biol Med.* 2011;84(4):471–478.
2. Long-Term Oxygen Treatment Trial Research Group. A randomized trial of long-term oxygen for COPD with moderate desaturation. *N Engl J Med.* 2016;375(17):1617–1627. doi:10.1056/NEJMoa1604344
3. Badgery-Parker T, Pearson SA, Dunn S, Elshaug AG. Measuring hospital-acquired complications associated with low-value care. *JAMA*

Intern Med. 2019;179(4):499–505. doi:10.1001/JAMAINTERNMED.2018.7464
4. Berwick DM, Hackbarth AD. Eliminating waste in US health care. *JAMA*. 2012;307(14):1513–1516. doi:10.1001/JAMA.2012.362
5. Shrank WH, Rogstad TL, Parekh N. Waste in the US health care system: estimated costs and potential for savings. *JAMA*. 2019;322(15):1501–1509. doi:10.1001/JAMA.2019.13978
6. Xu WY, Jung JK. Socioeconomic differences in use of low-value cancer screenings and distributional effects in Medicare. *Health Serv Res*. 2017;52(5):1772–1793. doi:10.1111/1475-6773.12559
7. Helfrich CD, Hartmann CW, Parikh TJ, Au DH. Promoting health equity through de-implementation research. *EthnDis*. 2019;29(suppl 1):93. doi:10.18865/ED.29.S1.93
8. Allen P, Jacob RR, Parks RG, et al. Perspectives on program mis-implementation among US local public health departments. *BMC Health Serv Res*. 2020;20(1):1–11. doi:10.1186/S12913-020-05141-5
9. Padek MM, Mazzucca S, Allen P, et al. Patterns and correlates of mis-implementation in state chronic disease public health practice in the United States. *BMC Public Health*. 2021;21(1):1–11. Doi:10.1186/S12889-020-10101-Z/TABLES/4
10. McKay VR, Combs TB, Dolcini MM, Brownson RC. The de-implementation and persistence of low-value HIV prevention interventions in the United States: a cross-sectional study. *Implement Sci Commun*. 2020;1(1):1–10. Doi:10.1186/S43058-020-00040-6
11. Brownson RC, Allen P, Jacob RR, et al. Understanding mis-implementation in public health practice. *Am J Prev Med*. 2015;48(5):543–551.
12. McKay VR, Margaret Dolcini M, Hoffer LD. The dynamics of de-adoption: a case study of policy change, de-adoption, and replacement of an evidence-based HIV intervention. *Transl Behav Med*. 2017;7(4):821–831. doi:10.1007/s13142-017-0493-1
13. Iwelunmor J, Blackstone S, Veira D, et al. Toward the sustainability of health interventions implemented in sub-Saharan Africa: a systematic review and conceptual framework. *Implement Sci*. 2016;11(1):1–27. doi:10.1186/S13012-016-0392-8/FIGURES/3
14. Walugembe DR, Sibbald S, le Ber MJ, Kothari A. Sustainability of public health interventions: where are the gaps? *Health Res Policy Syst*. 2019;17(1):1–7. doi:10.1186/S12961-018-0405-Y/TABLES/2
15. Niven DJ, Leigh JP, Stelfox HT. Ethical considerations in the de-adoption of ineffective or harmful aspects of healthcare. *Health Manage Forum*. 2016;29(5):214–222. doi:10.1177/0840470416666576
16. McKay VR, Morshed AB, Brownson RC, Proctor EK, Prusaczyk B. Letting go: conceptualizing intervention de-implementation in public health and social service settings. *Am J Community Psychol*. 2018;62(1–2):189–202. doi:10.1002/ajcp.12258
17. Prasad V, Ioannidis JPA. Evidence-based de-implementation for contradicted, unproven, and aspiring healthcare practices. *Implement Sci*. 2014;9(1):1–5. doi:10.1186/1748-5908-9-1/TABLES/1
18. Elshaug AG, Rosenthal MB, Lavis JN, et al. Levers for addressing medical underuse and overuse: achieving high-value health care. *Lancet*. 2017;390(10090):191–202. doi:10.1016/S0140-6736(16)32586-7
19. Morgan DJ, Brownlee S, Leppin AL, et al. Setting a research agenda for medical overuse. *BMJ*. 2015;351. https://www.bmj.com/content/351/bmj.h4534.abstract?casa_token=FB7aMf6t6CkAAAAA:qPC48uKsI4iCYi7MKB-41HvptK9OTM8FSE22N3rMofnKCypGAsijoRmLm4v4uoEWTcBWCFVCxhp_
20. Niven DJ, Mrklas KJ, Holodinsky JK, et al. Towards understanding the de-adoption of low-value clinical practices: a scoping review. *BMC Med*. 2015;13(1):1–21. Doi:10.1186/S12916-015-0488-Z
21. ABIM Foundation. Choosing Wisely: home page. 2017. Accessed January 2, 2023. http://www.choosingwisely.org/.
22. Carroll A. It's hard for doctors to unlearn things. That's costly for all of us. *New York Times*. September 10, 2018. Accessed February 27, 2022. https://www.nytimes.com/2018/09/10/upshot/its-hard-for-doctors-to-unlearn-things-thats-costly-for-all-of-us.html
23. Rogers EM. *Diffusion of Innovations*. Free Press; 2003.
24. Dengler J, Padovano WM, Davidge K, McKay V, Yee A, MacKinnon SE. Dissemination and implementation science in plastic and reconstructive surgery: perfecting, protecting, and promoting the innovation that defines our specialty. *Plast Reconstr Surg*. 2021;147(2):303E–313E. doi:10.1097/PRS.0000000000007492
25. Ailabouni NJ, Reeve E, Helfrich CD, Hilmer SN, Wagenaar BH. Leveraging implementation science to increase the translation of deprescribing evidence into practice. *Res Soc Adm Pharm*. 2022;18(3):2550–2555. doi:10.1016/J.SAPHARM.2021.05.018

26. Damschroder LJ, Aron DC, Keith RE, Kirsh SR, Alexander JA, Lowery JC. Fostering implementation of health services research findings into practice: a consolidated framework for advancing implementation science. *Implement Sci.* 2009;4. doi:10.1186/1748-5908-4-50
27. Baumgartner AD, Clark CM, LaValley SA, Monte S v., Wahler RG, Singh R. Interventions to deprescribe potentially inappropriate medications in the elderly: Lost in translation? *J Clin Pharm Ther.* 2020;45(3):453–461. doi:10.1111/JCPT.13103
28. Baker R, Camosso-Stefinovic J, Gillies C, et al. Tailored interventions to address determinants of practice. *Cochrane Database Syst Rev.* 2015;2015(4). https://www.cochranelibrary.com/cdsr/doi/10.1002/14651858.CD005470.pub3/full
29. Nilsen P. Making sense of implementation theories, models and frameworks. *Implement Sci.* 2015;10(1):1–13. doi:10.1186/S13012-015-0242-0/TABLES/2
30. Grol R, Wensing M, Eccles M. *Improving Patient Care: The Implementation of Change in Clinical Practice.* Elsevier; 2005.
31. Voorn VMA, van Bodegom-Vos L, So-Osman C. Towards a systematic approach for (de) implementation of patient blood management strategies. *Transfus Medic.* 2018;28(2):158–167. doi:10.1111/TME.12520
32. Harden SM, Smith ML, Ory MG, Smith-Ray RL, Estabrooks PA, Glasgow RE. RE-AIM in clinical, community, and corporate settings: perspectives, strategies, and recommendations to enhance public health impact. *Front Public Health.* 2018;6(Mar):71. doi:10.3389/FPUBH.2018.00071/BIBTEX
33. Shelton RC, Chambers DA, Glasgow RE. An extension of RE-AIM to enhance sustainability: addressing dynamic context and promoting health equity over time. *Front Public Health.* 2020;8:134. doi:10.3389/FPUBH.2020.00134/BIBTEX
34. Prusaczyk B, Swindle T, Curran G. Defining and conceptualizing outcomes for de-implementation: key distinctions from implementation outcomes. *Implement Sci Commun.* 2020;1(1):1–10. doi:10.1186/S43058-020-00035-3
35. Swindle T, Rutledge JM, Johnson SL, Selig JP, Curran GM. De-implementation of detrimental feeding practices: a pilot protocol. *Pilot Feasibility Stud.* 2020;6(1):1–10. doi:10.1186/S40814-020-00720-Z/TABLES/1
36. Padek M, Allen P, Erwin PC, et al. Toward optimal implementation of cancer prevention and control programs in public health: a study protocol on mis-implementation. *Implement Sci.* 2018;13(1). https://implementationscience.biomedcentral.com/articles/10.1186/s13012-018-0742-9#citeas
37. Strifler L, Cardoso R, McGowan J, et al. Scoping review identifies significant number of knowledge translation theories, models, and frameworks with limited use. *J Clin Epidemiol.* 2018;100:92–102. doi:10.1016/j.jclinepi.2018.04.008
38. Tabak RG, Khoong EC, Chambers DA, Brownson RC. Bridging research and practice: models for dissemination and implementation research. *Am J Prev Med.* 2012;43(3):337–350. doi:10.1016/j.amepre.2012.05.024
39. Nilsen P. Making sense of implementation theories, models and frameworks. *Implement Sci.* 2015;10(1). https://link.springer.com/chapter/10.1007/978-3-030-03874-8_3
40. Walsh-Bailey C, Tsai E, Tabak RG, et al. A scoping review of de-implementation frameworks and models. *Implement Sci.* 2021;16(1):1–18. doi:10.1186/S13012-021-01173-5/TABLES/3
41. Parker G, Shahid N, Rappon T, Kastner M, Born K, Berta W. Using theories and frameworks to understand how to reduce low-value healthcare: a scoping review. *Implement Sci.* 2022;17(1):1–13. doi:10.1186/S13012-021-01177-1/FIGURES/3
42. Graham ID, Logan J, Harrison MB, et al. Lost in knowledge translation: time for a map? *J Contin Educ Health Prof.* 2006;26(1):13–24. doi:10.1002/CHP.47
43. Wilson KM, Brady TJ, Lesesne C, et al. Peer reviewed: an organizing framework for translation in public health: the knowledge to action framework. *Prev Chronic Dis.* 2011;8(2):A46. https://www.ncbi.nlm.nih.gov/pmc/articles/PMC3073439/
44. Helfrich CD, Rose AJ, Hartmann CW, et al. How the dual process model of human cognition can inform efforts to de-implement ineffective and harmful clinical practices: a preliminary model of unlearning and substitution. *J Eval Clin Pract.* 2018;24(1):198–205. doi:10.1111/jep.12855
45. Wang V, Maciejewski ML, Helfrich CD, Weiner BJ. Working smarter not harder: coupling implementation to de-implementation. *Healthcare.* 2018;6(2):104–107. doi:10.1016/j.hjdsi.2017.12.004
46. Gupta A, Brown TJ, Singh S, et al. Applying the "COST" (culture, oversight, systems change, and training) framework to de-adopt the neutropenic diet. *Am J Med.* 2019;132(1):42–47. doi:10.1016/J.AMJMED.2018.08.009
47. Harris C, Green S, Elshaug AG. Sustainability in Health care by Allocating Resources Effectively (SHARE) 10: operationalising disinvestment in a conceptual framework for resource allocation. *BMC Health Serv Res.* 2017;17(1):1–31. doi:10.1186/S12913-017-2506-7

48. Parchman ML, Henrikson NB, Blasi PR, et al. Taking action on overuse: creating the culture for change. *Healthcare*. 2017;5(4):199–203. doi:10.1016/J.HJDSI.2016.10.005
49. Kirkpatrick SE, Lester JP, Peterson MR. The policy termination process. *Rev Policy Res*. 1999;16(1):209–238. doi:10.1111/J.1541-1338.1999.TB00847.X
50. Goodwin E, Frew EJ. Using programme budgeting and marginal analysis (PBMA) to set priorities: reflections from a qualitative assessment in an English Primary Care Trust. *Soc SciMed*. 2013;98:162–168. doi:10.1016/J.SOCSCIMED.2013.09.020
51. Norton WE, Chambers DA. Unpacking the complexities of de-implementing inappropriate health interventions. *Implement Sci*. 2020;15(1):2. doi:10.1186/s13012-019-0960-9
52. Augustsson H, Ingvarsson S, Nilsen P, et al. Determinants for the use and de-implementation of low-value care in health care: a scoping review. *Implement Sci Commun*. 2021;2(1):1–17. doi:10.1186/S43058-021-00110-3
53. Verkerk EW, van Dulmen SA, Born K, Gupta R, Westert GP, Kool RB. Key factors that promote low-value care: views of experts from the United States, Canada, and the Netherlands. *Int J Health Policy Manage*. 2022;11(8):1514–1521. doi:10.34172/IJHPM.2021.53
54. Grover M, Abraham N, Chang YH, Tilburt J. Physician cost consciousness and use of low-value clinical services. *J Am Board Fam Med*. 2016;29(6):785–792. doi:10.3122/JABFM.2016.06.160176
55. Smith ME, Vitous CA, Hughes TM, Shubeck SP, Jagsi R, Dossett LA. Barriers and facilitators to de-implementation of the Choosing Wisely® guidelines for low-value breast cancer surgery. *Ann Surg Oncol*. 2020;27(8):2653–2663. doi:10.1245/s10434-020-08285-0
56. van Dulmen S, Naaktgeboren C, Heus P, et al. Barriers and facilitators to reduce low-value care: a qualitative evidence synthesis. *BMJ Open*. 2020;10(10):e040025. doi:10.1136/bmjopen-2020-040025
57. National Alliance on Mental Illness. Mental health by the numbers. February 2022. Accessed March 30, 2022. https://www.nami.org/mhstats
58. Torrey WC, Lynde DW, Gorman P. Promoting the implementation of practices that are supported by research: the National Implementing Evidence-Based Practice Project. *Child Adolesc Psychiatr Clin N Am*. 2005;14(2):297–306. doi:10.1016/J.CHC.2004.05.004
59. Bond GR, Drake RE, Mchugo GJ, Peterson AE, Jones AM, Williams J. Long-term sustainability of evidence-based practices in community mental health agencies. *Adm Policy Ment Health*. 2014;41(2):228–236. doi:10.1007/s10488-012-0461-5
60. McHugo G, Drake R, Whitley R, et al. Fidelity outcomes in the national implementing evidence-based practices project. *Psychiatr Serv*. 2007;58(10):1279–1284.
61. Peterson AE, Bond GR, Drake RE, Mchugo GJ, Jones AM, Williams JR. Predicting the long-term sustainability of evidence-based practices in mental health care: an 8-year longitudinal analysis. *J Behav Health Serv Res*. 2013;41(3):337–346. doi:10.1007/s11414-013-9347-x
62. Colla CH, Mainor AJ, Hargreaves C, Sequist T, Morden N. Interventions aimed at reducing use of low-value health services: a systematic review. *Med Care Res Rev*. 2017;74(5):507–550. doi:10.1177/1077558716656970
63. Rietbergen T, Spoon D, Brunsveld-Reinders AH, et al. Effects of de-implementation strategies aimed at reducing low-value nursing procedures: a systematic review and meta-analysis. *Implement Sci*. 2020;15(1):38. doi:10.1186/s13012-020-00995-z
64. Bourgault AM, Upvall MJ. De-implementation of tradition-based practices in critical care: a qualitative study. *Int J Nurs Pract*. 2019;25(2):e12723. doi:10.1111/ijn.12723
65. Burton CR, Williams L, Bucknall T, et al. Theory and practical guidance for effective de-implementation of practices across health and care services: a realist synthesis. *Health Serv Deliv Res*. 2021;9(2):1–102. doi:10.3310/hsdr09020
66. Mendelson M, Matsoso MP. The World Health Organization global action plan for antimicrobial resistance. *S Afr Med J*. 2015;105(5):325.
67. Rodriguez Weno E, Allen P, Mazzucca S, et al. Approaches for ending ineffective programs: Strategies from state public health practitioners. *Front Public Health*. 2021;9. https://www.frontiersin.org/articles/10.3389/fpubh.2021.727005/full
68. Ho VP, Dicker RA, Haut ER, Coalition for National Trauma Research Scientific Advisory Council. Dissemination, implementation, and de-implementation: the trauma perspective. *Trauma Surg Acute Care Open*. 2020;5(1):e000423–e000423. doi:10.1136/tsaco-2019-000423
69. Kales HC, Gitlin LN, Lyketsos CG. Management of neuropsychiatric symptoms of dementia in clinical settings: recommendations from a multidisciplinary expert panel. *J Am Geriatr Soc*. 2014;62(4):762–769. doi:10.1111/jgs.12730
70. Davidson KW, Ye S, Mensah GA. Commentary: De-implementation Science: a virtuous cycle of ceasing and desisting low-value care before

implementing new high value care. *EthnDis.* 2017;27(4):463. doi:10.18865/ed.27.4.463

71. Health and Human Services. Global statistics. 2022. Accessed March 30, 2022. https://www.hiv.gov/hiv-basics/overview/data-and-trends/global-statistics
72. Health and Human Services. US Statistics. 2022. Accessed March 30, 2022. https://www.hiv.gov/hiv-basics/overview/data-and-trends/statistics
73. UNAIDS. Investing in HIV really does pay off. 2022. Accessed March 30, 2022. https://www.unaids.org/en/resources/presscentre/featurestories/2020/february/20200224_gow_investments
74. Centers for Disease Control and Prevention. HIV and STD criminalization laws. 2021. Accessed February 1, 2022. https://www.cdc.gov/hiv/policies/law/states/exposure.html
75. Mermin J, Valentine SS, McCray E. HIV criminalisation laws and ending the US HIV epidemic. *Lancet HIV.* 2021;8(1):e4–e6. doi:10.1016/S2352-3018(20)30333-7
76. Centers for Disease Control and Prevention. HIV criminalization and ending the epidemic. 2021. Accessed February 1, 2022. https://www.cdc.gov/hiv/pdf/policies/law/cdc-hiv-criminal-ehe.pdf
77. UNAIDS. HIV criminalization human rights fact sheet series 2021. Accessed January 2, 2022. https://www.unaids.org/en/resources/documents/2021/01-hiv-human-rights-factsheet-criminalization
78. The Center for HIV Law & Policy. Arrests and prosecutions for HIV exposure in the United States, 2008–2019. 2019. Accessed February 4, 2022. https://www.hivlawandpolicy.org/resources/arrests-and-prosecutions-hiv-exposure-united-states-2008%E2%80%932019-center-hiv-law-policy-2019
79. Mykhalovskiy E, Hastings C, Sanders C, Hayman M, Bisaillon L. "Callous, cold and deliberately duplicitous": racialization, immigration and the representation of HIV criminalization in Canadian mainstream media. *SSRN Electronic Journal.* November 30, 2016. https://tspace.library.utoronto.ca/bitstream/1807/107928/1/Mykhalovskiy%2C%20Hastings%2C%20Sanders%20et%20al_2016_%20Callous%2C%20Cold%2C%20Duplicitous.pdf
80. Lehman JS, Carr MH, Nichol AJ, et al. Prevalence and public health implications of state laws that criminalize potential HIV exposure in the United States. *AIDS Behav.* 2014;18(6):997–1006. doi:10.1007/S10461-014-0724-0
81. National Institute of Allergy and Infectious Diseases. HIV undetectable=untransmittable (U=U), or treatment as prevention. 2022. Accessed February 1, 2022. https://www.niaid.nih.gov/diseases-conditions/treatment-prevention
82. Adam BD, Corriveau P, Elliott R, Globerman J, English K, Rourke S. HIV disclosure as practice and public policy. *Crit Public Health.* 2014;25(4):386–397. doi:10.1080/09581596.2014.980395
83. O'Byrne P, Bryan A, Woodyatt C. Nondisclosure prosecutions and HIV prevention: results from an Ottawa-based gay men's sex survey. *J Assoc Nurses AIDS Care.* 2013;24(1):81–87. doi:10.1016/J.JANA.2012.01.009
84. Sweeney P, Gray SC, Purcell DW, et al. Association of HIV diagnosis rates and laws criminalizing HIV exposure in the United States. *AIDS.* 2017;31(10):1483–1488. doi:10.1097/QAD.0000000000001501
85. Patterson S, Nicholson V, Milloy MJ, et al. Awareness and understanding of HIV Non-disclosure Case Law and the Role of Healthcare Providers in Discussions About the Criminalization of HIV Non-disclosure Among Women Living with HIV in Canada. *AIDS Behav.* 2020;24(1):95–113. doi:10.1007/S10461-019-02463-2
86. Baugher AR, Whiteman A, Jeffries WL, Finlayson T, Lewis R, Wejnert C. Black men who have sex with men living in states with HIV criminalization laws report high stigma, 23 US cities, 2017. *AIDS.* 2021;35(10):1637–1645. doi:10.1097/QAD.0000000000002917
87. Barré-Sinoussi F, Abdool Karim SS, Albert J, et al. Expert consensus statement on the science of HIV in the context of criminal law. *J Int AIDS Soc.* 2018;21(7):e25161. doi:10.1002/JIA2.25161
88. van Bodegom-Vos L, Davidoff F, Marang-Van De Mheen PJ. Implementation and de-implementation: two sides of the same coin? *BMJ Quality & Safety.* 2017;26(6):495–501. doi:10.1136/BMJQS-2016-005473
89. Leeman J, Birken SA, Powell BJ, Rohweder C, Shea CM. Beyond "implementation strategies": classifying the full range of strategies used in implementation science and practice. *Implement Sci.* 2017;12(1):125. doi:10.1186/s13012-017-0657-x
90. Powell BJ, Waltz TJ, Chinman MJ, et al. A refined compilation of implementation strategies: results from the Expert Recommendations for Implementing Change (ERIC) project. *Implement Sci.* 2015;10(1):21. doi:10.1186/s13012-015-0209-1
91. Grimshaw JM, Patey AM, Kirkham KR, et al. De-implementing wisely: developing the evidence base to reduce low-value care. *BMJ Qual Saf.* 2020;29(5):409–417. doi:10.1136/bmjqs-2019-010060

92. Wang T, Baskin AS, Dossett LA. Deimplementation of the Choosing Wisely recommendations for low-value breast cancer surgery: a systematic review. *JAMA Surg.* 2020;155(8):759–770. doi:10.1001/jamasurg.2020.0322
93. Jordan A, Bauer MW, Green-Pedersen C. Policy dismantling. *J Eur Public Policy.* 2013;20(5):795–805. doi:10.1080/13501763.2013.771092
94. Bauer MW, Knill C. A conceptual framework for the comparative analysis of policy change: measurement, explanation and strategies of policy dismantling. *J Compar Policy Anal Res Pract.* 2014;16(1):28–44. doi:10.1080/13876988.2014.885186

13

Systems Science Methods in Dissemination and Implementation Research

DOUGLAS A. LUKE, ALEXANDRA B. MORSHED, VIRGINIA R. MCKAY, AND TODD B. COMBS

INTRODUCTION

The still relatively new field of dissemination and implementation (D&I) science is addressing new types of research questions focusing on how society can better reap the benefits of its investments in public health and healthcare research by delivering scientific discoveries into the clinic and community. With these research challenges come requirements for alternative types of analytic methods and study designs.

Systems thinking and research methods have been widely applied in public health,[1–3] focusing on a wide variety of health and public health problems, including infectious disease transmission, chronic disease prevention, healthcare access, and global environmental health. The benefits of these systems science methods are many and move beyond simple prediction of future health outcomes.[4] These benefits include revealing causal mechanisms driving policy and behavioral intervention outcomes, enhancing the connection between theory and intervention planning, modeling even in the absence of data, facilitating understanding intervention impacts over time as well as in different contexts, and improving the design of interventions, producing dissemination tools that engage community stakeholders.[5–7] All of these benefits could apply to implementation science research and evaluation. Moving science from discovery into practice requires integration into and disruption of complex organizational systems,[8] such as healthcare systems, policy systems, and governmental regulatory systems. Although there have been several calls for integrating systems thinking and methods into implementation science,[9,10] progress has been slow. There are likely many reasons for this, including lack of systems-imbued theories, overreliance on intervention- and experimental-focused research designs, and lack of training on systems science methods. In this chapter, we continue this systems dialogue with implementation scholars, first by expanding the general argument for integrating systems thinking and methods into implementation science, then by providing in-depth exploration of three important systems science methods that have started to become more utilized in implementation science.

The Argument From Philosophy of Science

Early methodological work in the social sciences derived from positivist epistemology. The desire to establish firm foundations for causal explanations led to experimental methods and our Popperian approach to hypothesis testing that are common in social and health scientific research.[11] Despite philosophical movement away from positivism, the social sciences have held on to scientific methods that emphasize control and randomization and that value internal validity over external validity. Newer epistemological frameworks that include holism, functionalism, and structuralism that emphasize the influence of multiple social-level forces on individual behavior suggest new methodological approaches that balance internal and external validity and can help identify contextual effects, behavioral dynamics, and causal mechanisms.[12,13] All of these concepts

Douglas A. Luke, Alexandra B. Morshed, Virginia R. McKay, and Todd B. Combs, *Systems Science Methods in Dissemination and Implementation Research* In: *Dissemination and Implementation Research in Health.* Edited by: Ross C. Brownson, Graham A. Colditz, and Enola K. Proctor, Oxford University Press. © Oxford University Press 2023. DOI: 10.1093/oso/9780197660690.003.0013 are relevant and useful for studying the complex, dynamic systems that embody D&I processes and outcomes.

The Argument From Theory

Despite the relative youth of D&I as a distinctive discipline, many important conceptual and theoretical advances have been made and used to guide research (see also chapters 3 and 4).[14] However, the most widely used of these are in the form of conceptual frameworks, rather than more fully fleshed out theories or models.[15] These are still quite useful; for example, RE-AIM (Reach, Effectiveness, Adoption, Implementation, and Maintenance),[16] the Consolidated Framework for Implementation Research (CFIR),[17] and the implementation outcomes framework[18] identify important concepts and conceptual domains (e.g., reach, acceptability, inner and outer settings). These frameworks are mostly silent, however, on how these concepts relate to each other. For example, how exactly do outer settings act to constrain inner-setting behavior, and how do the interactions between inner and outer settings enhance or inhibit successful implementation? Future theoretical development in the D&I sphere would be supported by studies utilizing the sorts of methods that can identify and elaborate on these domain interrelationships.

Figure 13.1 presents a socioecological framework for understanding D&I processes, which is adapted from Glass and McAtee (2006).[19] This framework is also a schematic, much like CFIR.[17] However, it highlights two important characteristics of D&I phenomena

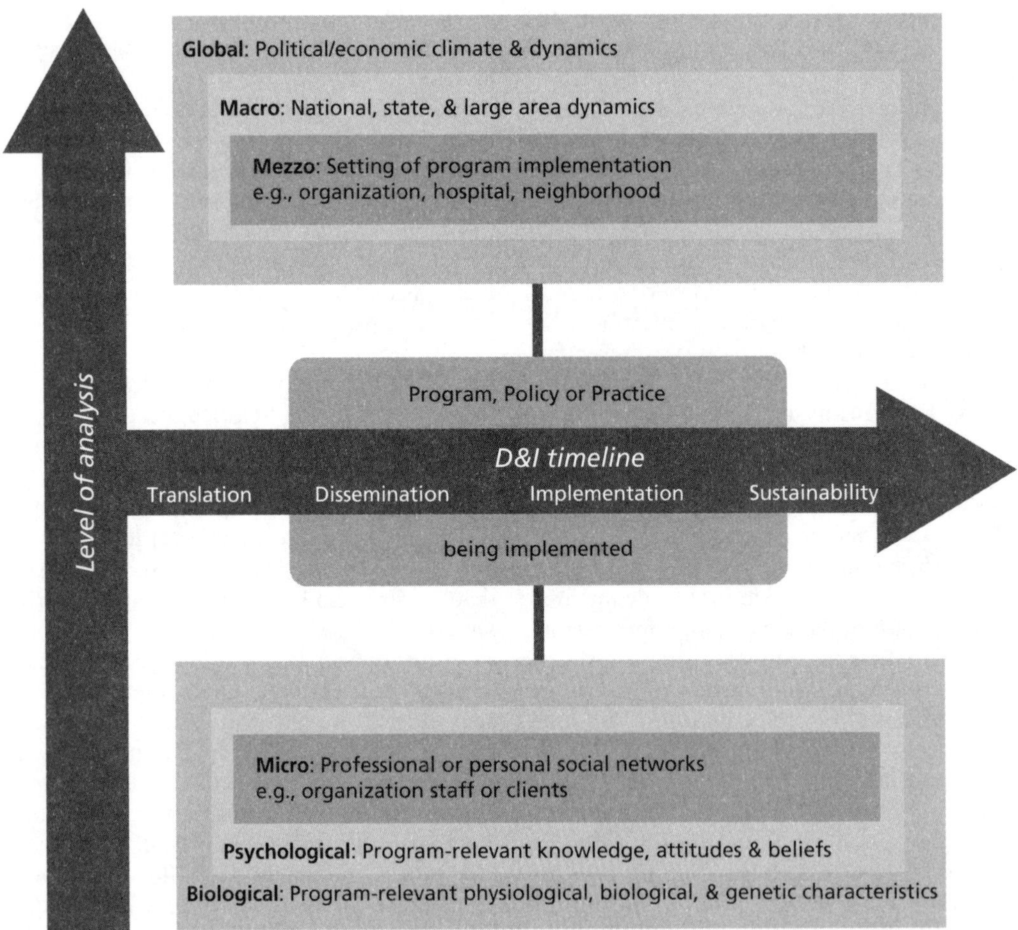

FIGURE 13.1 Socioecologic framework for understanding dissemination and implementation processes.

Adapted with permission Glass TA, McAtee MJ. Behavioral science at the crossroads in public health: extending horizons, envisioning the future. *Soc Sci Med.* 2006;62(7):1650–1671.

that need to be articulated by rich D&I theories and studied using the sorts of methods that are the subject of this chapter. First, D&I processes are embedded in a hierarchical socioecological system (left-hand arrow from lower to higher). Second, these processes play out over time. Traditional analytic methods are fairly limited in their ability to handle these types of multilevel systems, with heterogeneous actors (e.g., persons and organizations) who are interacting and changing dynamically over time. Future theoretical development in implementation science can move even further to incorporate more core concepts and principles from systems science, such as social structure, system dynamics (SD), feedback, information flow, and system evolution.[20]

The Argument From Phenomenology

As suggested above, D&I itself comprises a complex system made up of interacting parts, and those parts are diverse collections of people, settings, and organizations. More so than in many other areas of the social and health sciences, studying these complex systems as phenomena in and of themselves using traditional experimental and quasi-experimental designs is challenging. Even when traditional tools of the experimentalist's art such as randomization can be used, the results are often limited to: "We discovered it worked for this program, at this site, and at this point in time." As Lee Cronbach observed many decades ago: "Generalizations decay," pointing out the strong limitations of being able to generalize from a small set of experiments to broad general principles.[21] Learning about how or why a particular dissemination or implementation approach did in fact work requires a different set of tools, tools that can illuminate dynamic processes; map social and organizational relationships; identify feedback mechanisms; forecast future system behavior; and delineate the interactions between system actors and their social/organizational environments.

Roadmap for the Chapter

Systems science models and methods have been developed in a wide variety of disciplines, including sociology, business, political science, organizational behavior, computer science, and engineering. They have been used increasingly in public health to study and develop new practices and policies in such areas as global pandemics, vaccination system preparation, tobacco control, cancer, and obesity.[22] In public health, three broad types of methods have been used most often: social network analysis, SD modeling, and agent-based modeling (ABM). The rest of this chapter introduces each of these methods, explains how they are appropriate tools for D&I, provides entry points to a broader literature, and illustrates each method with a brief case study.

SOCIAL NETWORK ANALYSIS

Social network analysis focuses on the relationship between objects rather than on the objects themselves—a view of social phenomena fundamentally different from many types of social science investigation.[23] Because of this focus, network analysis is one of the most useful strategies for studying context, social processes, and social structure.[24] Social network analysis has been used widely in public health and health sciences to study infectious disease transmission, information flows, social influences on health behavior, organizational systems, and diffusion of innovations.[1] Suggested by the research translation "pipeline model,"[25] D&I processes can be viewed as a type of information transmission. A new scientific discovery, medical procedure, policy formulation, or other innovation is a piece of information that needs to be transferred to a different part of society and use. A network analytic model of D&I focused on the structural and relational aspects of dissemination or implementation can be used to both *study* and *shape* processes and outcomes.

Social Network Analysis Fundamentals

Social network analysis typically includes three interconnected methodological strategies: description, visualization, and modeling. Network *description* focuses on the nodes (objects) and the ties (relationships) that connect them. Nodes (also called actors, members, or vertexes) can be almost any type of social entity—a person, organization, country, and more. Ties (also called links, arcs, or edges) can be many things—friendship, money exchange, an email, or disease transmission. Networks and their ties can signal directed or nondirected relationships. For example, money is given by one individual (a node) and received by another, typically indicating a directed tie. Many other types of ties are nondirected. For example, two (or more) organizations work together on a common project, and it may not make sense to assign direction to the collaboration. Network structures and characteristics can evolve over time; for example, local departments of health might initially be connected mainly through a centralized department at the state or national level, but over time develop and strengthen ties with other local departments through common programs, goals, or challenges.

Network *visualization* is useful for exploring descriptive properties of nodes and ties and for demonstrating overall analytic network characteristics. Key characteristics of networks include density (proportion of observed ties to total possible ties) and diameter (longest path between any two nodes). Figure 13.2 shows the pattern of dissemination ties that connect the public health agencies making up the tobacco control program in Indiana.[26] Nodes in network graphs can be differentiated by color, and the agencies here are distinguished by agency type. The network has a diameter of two, indicating that information must pass through at most two nodes to travel from any given agency to another. Its density is 0.32, meaning that around one-third of all possible connections are present. This is not to say, however, that perfect density (density = 1) indicates a *better* or more effective network of people or organizations for dissemination or implementation. Network analyses have found the opposite: Relatively less dense networks may be more efficient at disseminating information and implementing prevention programs as denser networks tend to focus inward and are less open to information and community resources provided by weak ties outside the core network.[27]

While both network descriptive statistics and the visualization are important for understanding the structural characteristics of health systems, visualization is especially useful for engaging stakeholders in the analysis. Though social network analysts can provide statistical summaries to accompany network maps, key stakeholders often have stories to tell while viewing the maps that provide important context about how a network is structured, why certain nodes might bridge relationships between others, and more. They can also use information gleaned from the combination of contextual knowledge and network maps to intervene and strengthen the network. In a study on rural cancer networks, Carothers and colleagues shared network maps with stakeholders, who went on to fill gaps identified in the maps, train network members in relationship building, improve health referrals, and plan for the future.[28]

Individual nodes also have analytic characteristics, most of which describe their relative prominence in the network. Key among node

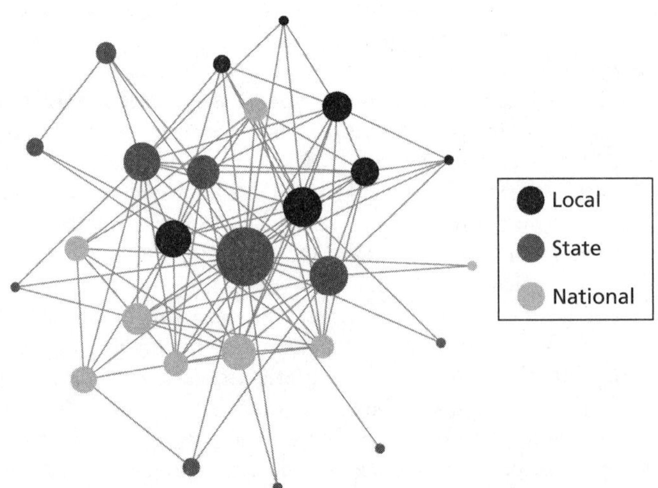

FIGURE 13.2 Indiana Tobacco Control Dissemination Network.

Adapted with permission from Luke DA, Wald LM, Carothers BJ, Bach LE, Harris JK. Network influences on dissemination of evidence-based guidelines in state tobacco control programs. *Health Educ Behav.* 2013;40(1 suppl):33S–42S.

properties are degree (the number of ties) and betweenness centrality (the extent to which a node bridges otherwise-unconnected nodes). In Figure 13.2, the nodes are sized by betweenness centrality, and the lead organization is the largest node, indicating that it bridges more pairs of unconnected nodes than any other, making it a critical element in network sustainability.

Network *modeling* has been made possible through statistical and computational advances over the last few decades that use exponential random graph modeling (ERGM).[29] ERGM predicts the likelihood of ties between nodes using characteristics of individual or pairs of nodes (e.g., people, organizations). Newer modeling strategies incorporate the ability to model changing node and tie characteristics in the longitudinal evolution of networks.[30] For those interested in more in-depth treatment of network analysis, see Wasserman and Faust or Valente.[31,32]

Applications for Dissemination and Implementation Research

Social network analysis has been particularly useful when applied to the theory of diffusion of innovations (see chapter 3),[33] perhaps the most important and influential theoretical framework in D&I research. Pioneering work in diffusion of innovations emphasized different types of members and distinguished them by the time at which they adopted new innovations into clinical or community practice (i.e., early, middle, and late adopters). After some time, observers began to look beyond simple temporal ordering to focus on the structural characteristics that distinguish opinion leaders (individuals who may expedite the diffusion process) from early adopters (those who may adopt an innovation quickly but may not influence others to do so). Network analysis focusing on the structural and relational aspects of diffusion has helped shed light on this issue.[34] As an example, *threshold models* have been developed that suggest that the likelihood of a particular individual (or agency, institution, etc.) adopting an innovation is dependent on the proportion of others in their network who have already done so.[35] One study of healthy cities found that healthcare professionals were more likely to ride bicycles to work if opinion leaders did so *or* if a certain proportion of others in their social networks switched to bicycles for commuting.[36]

More recently, D&I research has turned from examining the adoption of innovations toward long-term implementation and sustainability of innovations.[37] Studies often use Feldstein and Glasgow's practical, robust implementation and sustainability model (PRISM), which incorporates the role of social networks (both organization and patient based) when studying the implementation of interventions as important tools for understanding predictors of adoption, implementation, and maintenance outcomes.[38] In a successful application of the PRISM model, Beck and colleagues further demonstrated the usefulness of network analysis.[39] First, organizational advice-seeking patterns among clinicians and staff at two health maintenance organization sites were identified; next, network maps were used to help drive the subsequent implementation of a new well-child care intervention. More generally, Valente and colleagues illustrated how network analysis might be applied at each of the four stages of program implementation.[40]

Network modeling has also been applied to dissemination in the context of public health. The study from which Figure 13.2 originated found through ERGM that state tobacco control programs and partners were more likely to disseminate Centers for Disease Control and Prevention (CDC) best practices if state organizations, advocacy groups, and advisory agencies had existing contact- or collaboration-based ties.[26] In another study, Harris et al. examined influence within the US Department of Health and Human Services via ERGM and found that certain individual or shared characteristics (e.g., job rank, agency affiliations) were associated with greater organizational influence.[41]

Network Analysis in Dissemination and Implementation Research: A Brief Case Study

During the planning stages for implementing a cancer screening prevention program in the Peel region of Ontario, Canada, Lobb and colleagues[42] observed that reaching South Asian immigrant populations, almost one-third of the region's population, was a challenge for cancer screening programs in the region. Based on this observation, they developed an implementation strategy designed to improve reach. The researchers worked with stakeholders to identify 22 organizations that comprised the cancer screening network for South Asians in the region; these organizations included hospitals, governmental and nongovernmental agencies, clinical service providers, and community service providers who specifically provided social (nonclinical) services to South Asians.

Through surveys of the organizations, three different types of networks were identified and observed: communication, collaboration, and referral networks. Ties in the communications network represented any contact, and ties in the collaboration network were based on organizations that worked together on a common goal. The referral network included directional ties that denoted which organizations referred clients to the others.

Relevance to Dissemination and Implementation Research

Figure 13.3 shows the referral network from the study. The network map shows that the two hospitals in the region were centrally positioned in the referral network, more so than the provincial screening lead. The community service providers as well as the community health centers were on the periphery and not well connected. These were valuable findings to inform intervention planning and increase equity. The provincial lead was intended to lead dissemination of program information, but community health centers are vital in providing services to vulnerable populations who might otherwise not receive any and since community service organizations were explicitly linked to the region's South Asian population. Another specific and important finding was that neither of the two community health centers was linked directly to the provincial cancer screening lead, suggesting that communication of screening program changes from either core agency might take unnecessary time to reach the community health centers.

These system insights would have gone unnoticed in the absence of a focus on the networks and connections among organizations serving South Asians and those providing cancer screening services. Especially important was the knowledge of relationships between community health centers and community service organizations and their place in the greater cancer screening network. Equipped with this information, stakeholders were able to include all relevant types of organizations in intervention planning and focus on strengthening weak ties and utilizing existing ones.

SYSTEM DYNAMICS MODELING

System dynamic models represent complex systems as having underlying generalizable structures that produce specific patterns of system behavior over time. SD experts look for solutions to complex problems from the feedback

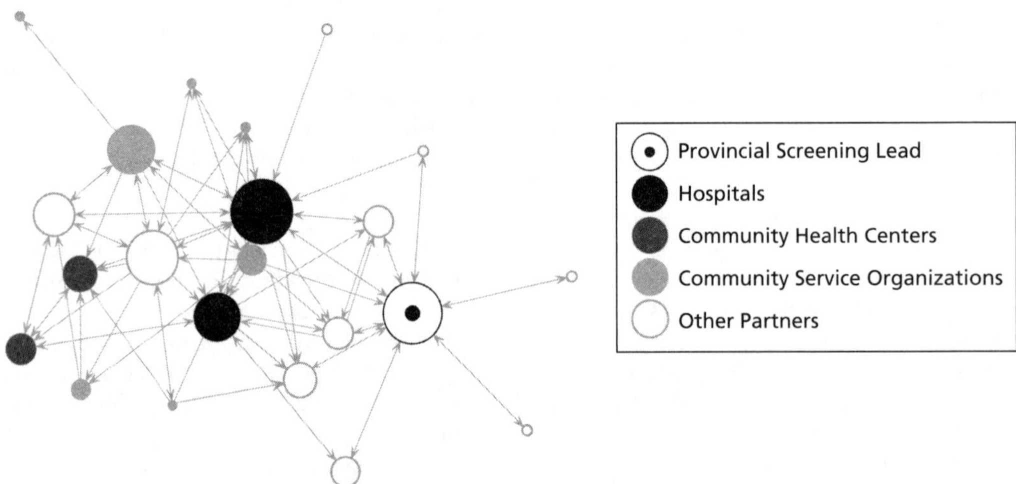

FIGURE 13.3 Referral network in cancer screening intervention planning study.

Adapted with permission from Lobb R, Carothers BJ, Lofters AK. Using organizational network analysis to plan cancer screening programs for vulnerable populations. *Am J Public Health*. 2014;104(2):358–364).

mechanisms within these systems rather than from influences external to the system.[43–45] A D&I research study using traditional analytic approaches may examine whether an implementation strategy results in a greater number of patients receiving evidence-based (EB) treatment. An SD simulation study, on the other hand, may explore the system structure that leads to a sharp increase in patients served followed by a gradual collapse in service reach (an example of a dynamic system behavior) or to identify areas of leverage (i.e., places to intervene in a system) that would most efficiently change the behavior pattern of the system in the desired direction.[44,46] SD is complementary to network analysis and ABM (see further in the chapter), but SD models are typically presented at the aggregate level, tend to have broader boundaries, and can incorporate more variables even in absence the of concrete estimates for parameters.[22,45,47] Developed in the 1950s by Jay W. Forrester,[48] SD has been widely applied to population health; healthcare; and urban, social, ecological, and organizational management problems.[49–52]

System Dynamics Fundamentals

The core elements of SD are the concepts of *endogenous feedback* and *accumulation* of quantities (e.g., information, energy, people, trust) in a system over time.[53,54] Endogenous feedback is present when a change at one point of the system *feeds back* onto itself, creating an endogenous (i.e., within system) feedback loop.[53,55] An example of a feedback loop is the number of infected people in a community increasing the rate of infection, which in turn increases the number of infected people. These feedback loops can be reinforcing (when the original change is amplified by the succeeding changes as in the example, leading to a vicious or virtuous cycle) or balancing (when the succeeding changes balance the initial change). SD models represent accumulation using stocks (levels of accumulation) and flows (rates of change in the stocks). For example, in a mental health treatment system, the number of patients waiting for an intake interview represents a stock, while the rate of intake interviews conducted by the clinic represents a flow of people out of this stock.[56] An important influence on flows within a system are delays (e.g., the average time it takes to conduct an intake interview), which contribute to the dynamic complexity and instability of the system.[53,54] Together feedback, accumulation, and delays are responsible for specific patterns of behaviors of systems, such as exponential growth, overshoot and collapse, oscillation, or S-shaped growth.[53]

System dynamic hypotheses, which posit that given feedback structures result in specific system behaviors over time, can be expressed conceptually using diagrams and mathematically using simulation software. SD simulation models utilize a system of ordinary differential equations to model systems over specific time horizons at an aggregate level. The initial values, relationships between variables, and constants are specified using existing theoretical and empirical literature, surveillance and administrative data, stakeholder estimates, and other sources.[46,54]

The process of problem articulation, dynamic hypothesis formulation, model quantification, confidence building, and policy analysis is iterative and strengthened by the participation of stakeholders.[53,57,58] Group model-building methods have emerged within the broader SD field to provide steps and tools to meaningfully engage stakeholders in creation of system structures and, in some group model-building practices, in development of simulation models.[58,59] Community-based SD, a community participatory practice of group model building, specifically focuses this engagement on community members and the processes of co-creation and empowerment with the goal of building public constituency for addressing root causes of dynamic social problems.[59]

Due to their aggregate and compartmentalized nature, SD models are less able to capture heterogeneity in the system, and adding additional sources of heterogeneity to the model is time intensive as it often changes the system structure. SD models also utilize a top-down perspective that is not well suited to examining how individual-level behaviors generate system-wide behaviors.[60] For those interested in more in-depth treatment of SD methods, see Sterman, Rahmandad, and colleagues, Vennix, or Hovmand.[43,53,58,61]

Applications in Dissemination and Implementation Research

The SD methods are applicable to several areas of D&I research. First, it is useful in developing and testing dynamic D&I theories. Some D&I models and frameworks include recursive influences between processes and concepts (e.g., conceptual model for the diffusion of innovations in service organizations, conceptual model for evidence-based implementation in public service sectors, 4 *E*'s process theory),[62–64] but do not explicitly model them. SD allows for the specification and quantification of the feedback mechanisms, accumulations, and delays that drive the behavior of D&I systems but are normally difficult to conceptualize.[53,65] As stated by Jay Forrester: "A simulation model is a theory describing the structure and interrelationships of a system,"[66(p112)] and through iterative model assessments, modelers can challenge theoretical assumptions, uncover and address flaws, and identify the limitations of the theory.[65] At each step of model specification (e.g., from conceptual models to stock-and-flow diagrams to simulation models), theories are necessarily refined and made more precise. Lich and colleagues illustrated the utility of SD diagramming in understanding complex factors influencing translation efforts of tobacco prevention research at five stages of knowledge translation.[67] The work of Hovmand and Gillespie[68] serves as an example of combining previously quantified theories of organizational change and management to create a new simulated theoretical model of how organizations respond to implementation of evidence-based interventions and what accounts for these responses.

Second, well-developed SD simulation models can serve as virtual laboratories for examining D&I dynamics in a multitude of contexts. Hovmand and Gillespie[68] simulated 2,312 scenarios of organizations with differing initial characteristics to determine what types of organizations were able to improve their performance after implementing evidence-based interventions. In another study, Miller and colleagues[69] examined nine strategies for increasing the reach of an EB HIV prevention program. They found that although some strategies improved reach, they did not stabilize the service delivery system, which was experiencing patterns of overshoot and collapse, placing the service organizations into long-term states of uncertainty. Virtual laboratories capture the feedback and accumulation present in systems and allow for examining how strategies or interventions work under differing conditions that would otherwise be difficult, costly, time consuming, or unethical to manipulate in the real world.[53,65] In addition, contextualizing D&I problems within specific practice contexts using SD produces knowledge that is practice based and thus particularly relevant to D&I science.[10,70,71]

Finally, when modeling is carried out with participation of key stakeholders, SD methods can be useful for building buy-in, developing relationships, and prioritizing implementation actions.[72,73] The strong emphasis in SD on engagement of stakeholders[54,59] lends itself particularly well to meaningful engagement of multidisciplinary actors necessary for producing D&I knowledge,[70,74] and in the case of community-based SD, alignment with existing community-engaged approaches facilitates equitable partnerships necessary for achieving health equity.[75] As a process, group model building is effective in creating individual (e.g., improved insight, commitment to conclusions) and group outcomes (e.g., improved communication, consensus, cohesion, long-term relationships).[62] Models can serve as boundary objects that are tangible representations of structures or processes, partially interpretable across disciplinary, organizational, social, or cultural distinctions, and which all participants can modify.[64] These objects facilitate the negotiation of knowledge, development of shared vocabulary around a problem, and alignment of goals.[60,65] In addition, SD simulation models are useful tools for communication with policymakers, front-line providers, and other decision makers regarding the scope and root causes of health problems, projected magnitude and timing of impact of policy alternatives, and setting of reasonable goals for action.[42,66,67]

System Dynamics in Dissemination and Implementation Research: A Brief Case Study

Zimmerman and colleagues, implementation scientists from the Veterans Health Administration (VA) National Center for Post-Traumatic Stress Disorder (PTSD), carried out a study in partnership with the VA Palo Alto Healthcare System.[68] They used participatory SD modeling to test provider-generated implementation strategies for increasing the number of patients initiating and completing evidence-based treatment for depression and

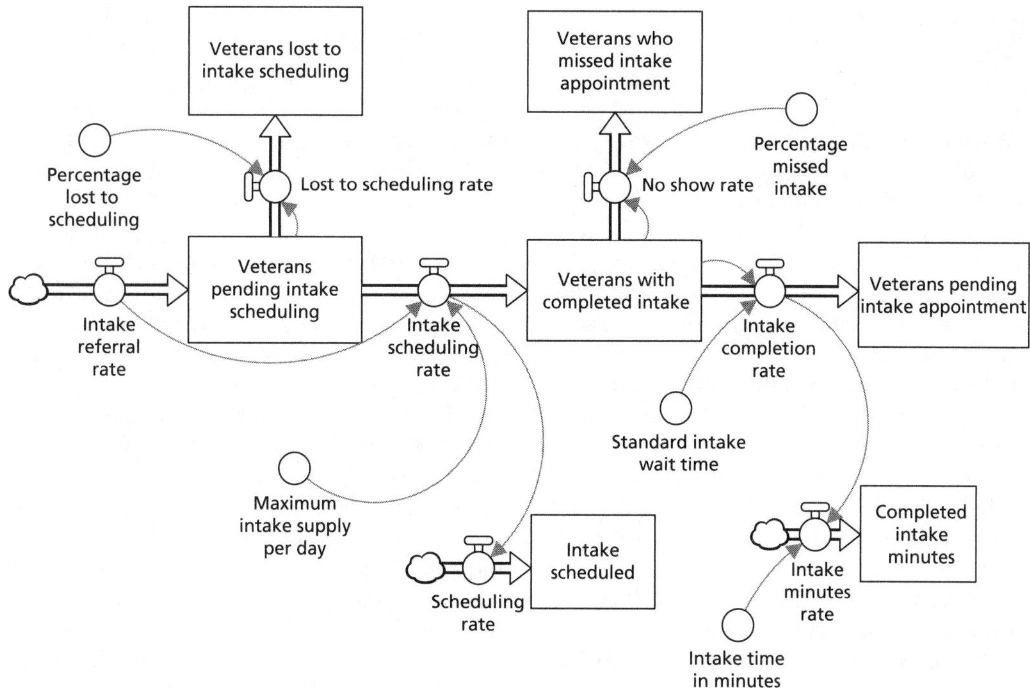

FIGURE 13.4 Stock and flow diagram.

Adapted with permission from Zimmerman L, Lounsbury DW, Rosen CS, Kimerling R, Trafton JA, Lindley SE. Participatory System Dynamics Modeling: Increasing Stakeholder Engagement and Precision to Improve Implementation Planning in Systems. *Adm Policy Ment Health*. 2016;43(6):834–849.

PTSD compared to services as usual. Through repeated engagement with the service delivery teams, the researchers iteratively developed models comprising the accumulation and flow of patients through distinct service provision categories in the clinic over time and included several feedback loops between model elements (Figure 13.4). As part of service delivery, model results allowed provider teams to quickly forecast the level and timing of the impact of potential implementation strategies.[56] Further, the modeling process itself, which the service delivery teams iteratively engaged in, resulted in improvements in overall EB treatment delivery (i.e., dose, course of care) related to mental health when compared to clinics that did not use SD modeling.[76]

Using the above participatory SD modeling approach, Zimmerman and colleagues developed *Modeling to Learn*, a national quality improvement initiative in the VA that provides VA service delivery teams with a suite of SD modeling tools for improving care delivery and trains them in their use.[77] Aligned with values and methods of participatory action and community-based participatory research,[76] Modeling to Learn prioritizes equitable partnerships and building capacity among local service providers in developing, owning, and implementing local solutions in evidence-based practice (EBP) delivery, while leveraging local service delivery data. Two cluster randomized trial studies are underway to assess effectiveness of Modeling to Learn as a multicomponent implementation strategy for improving EBP initiation, dose, completion, and cost through the proposed mechanisms of participatory learning and improved systems thinking among service providers.

Relevance to Dissemination and Implementation Research

This case study illustrates the value of participatory SD modeling for characterizing a service delivery system in its dynamism and complexity and using it to identify and test strategies to improve EBP delivery. Beyond that, it is a rare lesson in how to leverage the power of computational SD modeling by embedding it within service provision systems in a way that empowers local service providers. The process of developing and engaging with mathematically explicit models of a service delivery problem challenges participants to unpack assumptions about the dynamic structure of the implementation context, understand key constraints, and address flaws in how they think about feedback, accumulation, and delays.[65] This leads to what Sterman called double-loop learning,[65] improving participants' mental models, leading to improved decision-making, and ultimately, better implementation. Modeling to Learn demonstrates how to integrate systems science simulation in practice settings in a way that empowers local service delivery teams—building capacity, ensuring equitable access to resources and mutuality, and providing tools for local solutions.[76]

AGENT-BASED MODELING

Agent-based models are computational simulations modeling individual actors that behave according to a set of rules within an environment over time.[22] The models are used to examine how the accumulation of these small individual-level behaviors gives rise to system-level outcomes, often called emergence, that may be qualitatively different from the behavior of any one individual within the system.[78] Early models within the social sciences have illuminated social phenomena, such as emergence of collective social benefit out of cooperation among individuals or neighborhood segregation arising out of slight preferences for others similar to oneself.[79] This generative ability (using simple individual behaviors to generate complex system phenomena) of ABM is a distinguishing feature compared to other simulation approaches. ABMs developed for public health purposes are on the rise, covering a wide range of topics, including infectious disease, chronic disease, health behavior, and health policy.[2,80–84]

Agent-Based Modeling Fundamentals

The basic steps for ABM are (1) model construction, (2) calibration and validation, and (3) analyses.[78,85] ABMs are constructed from three basic components: individuals or agents, their environment, and rules that define how agents interact with one another and with their environment. Agents can represent homogeneous or heterogeneous types of system members, and they exhibit a variety of behaviors defined by a set of decision rules. The environment is the physical or social space where agents engage in the behavior of interest. A key feature of ABMs is explicitly representing the interaction among individuals or between individuals and the environment. Many have modeled interaction between individuals and a physical environment, such as how neighborhood location and household income can influence diet choices and quality.[86] More recently, ABMs representing the interaction between individuals and the social environment, such as how social determinants influence sexual health inequities among sexual and gender minority youth,[87] have been useful for demonstrating the influence of social factors on population health. Aside from these fundamental components, the potential agent characteristics and behaviors, environments, and relationships that can be represented are virtually unlimited. However, researchers must carefully choose the parameters incorporated in a model. The disaggregated nature of ABMs can quickly produce myriad parameters and subsequent growth in complexity that makes interpreting the outcomes of an ABM difficult. Last, time can be represented in ABMs according to any scale (e.g., days, weeks, or years). Although ABMs can be used to model and predict changes in real systems over time, the ability of ABMs to successfully predict real-life outcomes wanes the further out in modeled time due to the dynamic nature of the system represented.[78]

After a baseline ABM is developed, a model is calibrated and validated. These are techniques used to help ensure a model is generating relevant outcomes via plausible mechanisms and that the model is a valid representation of the real system of interest. Empirical data, including qualitative and quantitative data, can be used to inform all aspects of ABM development.[88,89] The amount and specificity of data needed to inform model development reflects the extent to which an ABM is intended to realistically represent a specific system. The realism of ABMs falls along a spectrum that ranges from highly abstract to highly specific (see Figure 13.5).[2] Within public health, ABMs tend toward the specific since public health researchers, including D&I researchers, generally address specific health issues in real contexts. As a rule of thumb, more data are needed to inform ABMs intended to accurately reflect

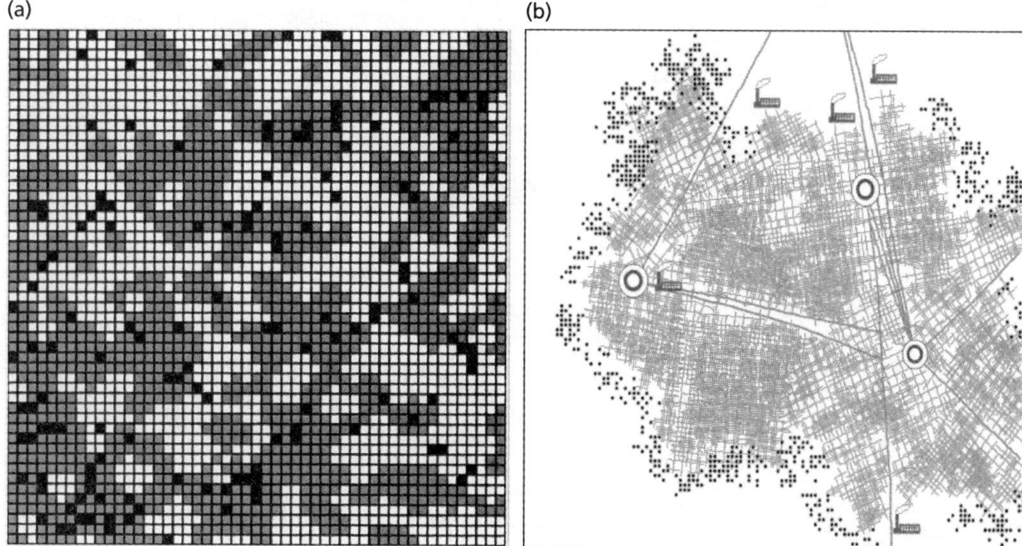

FIGURE 13.5 Illustrations of two ABMs from the Netlogo modeling library demonstrating different levels of abstraction. Model a (left) is a highly abstracted model designed to examine the development of neighborhood segregation where agents are represented by different shades of dots within a grid.[90] Model b (right) is a more realistic model designed to study migrant settlement in a realistic urban landscape based on human geography with centers of commerce (circles), an urban street design (lines), residential settlements (small dark squares) and factory locations (buildings with smoke plumes).[91]

Reprinted with permission from: Wilensky U. NetLogo Segregation model. Published online 1997. http://ccl.northwestern.edu/netlogo/models/Segregation and De Leon FD, Felsen M, Wilensky U. NetLogo Urban Suite—Tijuana Bordertowns model. Published online 2007. http://ccl.northwestern.edu/netlogo/models/UrbanSuite-TijuanaBordertowns.

real contexts, but where data are not available, a researcher may incorporate randomness and error into ABMs to account for uncertainty.

As a final step, the ABM outcomes of interest are analyzed using both descriptive and statistical approaches to identify important aspects of the behavioral dynamics and outcomes of the model. Another analytic approach of ABMs is using the simulation as an experimental laboratory where the researcher can systematically manipulate variables of interest at regular intervals and analyze primary outcomes of repeated iterations.[92] Using this experiment-like approach helps researchers analyze conditions that may be difficult or unethical to conduct in real-life settings. To support these activities, a number of software platforms are available to construct models and conduct analyses, which can also be easily integrated with other software commonly used by scientists.[93] For those interested in more in-depth treatment of ABM, we have provided resources covering these topics in further detail in Table 13.1.

Applications for Dissemination and Implementation Research

Agent-based models relevant to D&I science are increasingly available, and the approach shows promise in its applicability to D&I research questions. D&I of EBPs represents key challenges within D&I where ABM may be particularly relevant and offer several benefits over other experimental or computational designs.

There is a long tradition of using ABMs to examine the diffusion process.[94] ABMs are helpful for investigating how particular actors within a system, such as opinion leaders or innovation champions, improve or hinder the movement of EBPs across a system. ABMs have also been used to understand how different interventions addressing the same issue diffuse differently based on the system structure and intervention characteristics. For example, McKay and colleagues constructed an ABM to examine expanding HIV testing to local pharmacies and impact on linkage to HIV care for diagnosed youth and young adults in Memphis,

TABLE 13.1 USEFUL RESOURCES FOR SYSTEMS SCIENCE METHODS FOR D&I RESEARCH

	Network Analysis	System Dynamics	Agent-Based Modeling
Overview Books	• Scott J & Carrington PJ. 2011. *The SAGE Handbook of Social Network Analysis* • Valente TW. 2010. *Social Networks and Health: Models, Methods & Applications* • Newman MEJ. 2010. *Networks: An introduction.*	• Morecroft JD. 2015. *Strategic Modelling and Business Dynamics: A Feedback Systems Approach* • Rahmandad H & Oliva R. 2015. *Analytical Methods for Dynamic Modelers* • Sterman JD. 2000. *Business Dynamics: Systems Thinking and Modeling in Complex World* • Hovmand PS. 2014. *Community Based System Dynamics*	• Gilbert N. 2008. *Agent-Based Models* • Railsback SF & Grimm V. 2011. *Agent-Based and Individual-Based Modeling: A Practical Introduction* • Wilensky & Rand. 2015 *An Introduction to Agent-Based Modeling*
Professional Associations	• International Network for Social Network Analysis, insna.org	• Systems Dynamics Society, systemdynamics.org	• Network for Computational Modeling in Social & Ecological Sciences, comses.net
Major Conferences	• Sunbelt Conference, insna.org • International Conference on Advances in Social Networks Analysis and Mining, asonam.cpsc.ucalgary.ca	• Conference of the System Dynamics Society, systemdynamics.org/conference	• International Conference on Social Computing, Behavioral-Cultural Modeling & Prediction sbp-brims.org • Social Simulation Conference, openabm.org http://www.essa.eu.org/event-type/conference/
Major Journals	• *Applied Network Science*, appliednetsci.springeropen.com • *Journal of Complex Networks*, comnet.oxfordjournals.org • *Network Science*, cambridge.org/core/journals/network-science	• *System Dynamics Review*, systemdynamics.org/publications/system-dynamics-review • *Systems Research & Behavioral Science*, https://onlinelibrary.wiley.com/journal/10991743a • *Journal of the Operational Research Society*, theorsociety.com/Pages/Publications/JORS.aspx	• *Advances in Complex Systems*, worldscientific.com/page/acs/aims-scope • *Complex Adaptive Systems Modeling*, casmodeling.springeropen.com • *Journal of Artificial Societies and Social Simulation*, jasss.soc.surrey.ac.uk
Software	• R, packages: igraph, RSiena, statnet, visNetwork r-project.org • UCINET, sites.google.com/site/ucinetsoftware/home • Pajek, mrvar.fdv.uni-lj.si/pajek	• Stella/iThink, iseesystems.com/store/products/stella-architect.aspx • Vensim, vensim.com • AnyLogic, http://www.anylogic.com/	• Mason, cs.gmu.edu/~eclab/projects/mason/#Features • NetLogo, ccl.northwestern.edu/netlogo • Repast, repast.github.io/repast_simphony.html

TABLE 13.1 CONTINUED

	Network Analysis	System Dynamics	Agent-Based Modeling
Online Resources	• Social Network Analysis, archived course tutorials, Borgatti sites.google.com/site/mgt780sna • Video Tutorial on Social Network Analysis using R, Goodreau & Hunter rs.resalliance.org/2009/12/16/video-tutorial-on-social-network-analysis-using-r	• System Dynamics Modeling for Health Policy: Collected Videos, Audio, Slides and Examples Models, Osgood, www.cs.usask.ca/faculty/ndo885/Classes/CMPT858LatestSDVersion/index.html • System Dynamics Self Study 15.988, Forrester, ocw.mit.edu/courses/sloan-school-of-management/15-988-system-dynamics-self-study-fall-1998-spring-1999 • Scriptopedia • https://en.wikibooks.org/wiki/Scriptapedia	• Agent-Based Models, various tutorials, http://www.agent-based-models.com/blog/resources/tutorials/ • Modeling Tutorials, OpenABM, openabm.org/page/modeling-tutorials • Online Guide for Newcomers to Agent-Based Modeling in the Social Sciences, Axelrod & Tesfatsion, http://www2.econ.iastate.edu/tesfatsi/abmread.htm#MethodTools • Complexity Explorer, complexityexplorer.org
Trainings	• Systems Science for Social Impact—Washington University in St. Louis, https://systemsscienceforsocialimpact.wustl.edu/ • Participatory Modeling Field School—Michigan State University, https://modeling.engage.msu.edu/	• Systems Science for Social Impact—Washington University in St. Louis, https://systemsscienceforsocialimpact.wustl.edu/ • Participatory Modeling Field School—Michigan State University, https://modeling.engage.msu.edu/ • International System Dynamics Conference Summer School, https://systemdynamics.org/summer-school/	• Systems Science for Social Impact—Washington University in St. Louis, https://systemsscienceforsocialimpact.wustl.edu/ • Participatory Modeling Field School—Michigan State University, https://modeling.engage.msu.edu/

Tennessee.[95] As testing expanded, if the new pharmacies were well integrated with the HIV care system to refer diagnosed individuals to programs supporting linkage to care, individuals expeditiously received care, and fewer were lost to follow up. However, this benefit was not observed in areas where HIV incidence was the highest because these areas of the region had fewer pharmacies relative to other areas. These ABM results illuminate how disparities in the quality of care can arise unintentionally and unexpectedly from a combination of system structure, organization locations, and organizational networks.

Agent-based models are particularly useful because characteristics of physical and social environments influence health outcomes. D&I researchers often work in real contexts where manipulating real settings is difficult and randomization is impossible or unethical. ABMs can aid in understanding differences that might emerge from different implementation choices and the importance of EBP implementation relative to the influence of environmental contexts on individual and community outcomes. ABMs in D&I research in health have focused on the implementation of one policy in multiple contexts,[96–99] the implementation of multiple interventions to address a single problem,[98,100] or the influence of a single intervention on multiple, yet conceptually distinct, outcomes.[101,102]

Agent-Based Modeling in Dissemination and Implementation Research: A Brief Case Study

Yang and colleagues developed an ABM to assess multiple interventions designed to improve active travel to school.[101,102] While they examined multiple approaches and community characteristics relevant to active school travel, the focus here is on their examination of implementation approaches for a walking school bus intervention wherein a group of children walk to school with one or more adults within hypothetical cities of various population densities. The ABM was a simulated city with multiple schools and a grid road system. The primary agents were children who lived within a distance of a designated school. Children decided if they wanted to walk to school based on a personal preference for active travel (i.e., biking or walking), willingness to walk a distance to school, and their parents' perceived safety of the route to school. Children may join the walking school bus, walk on their own, or take some other means to school (e.g., a parent drives the child to school in a car).

The authors used the ABM to assess the influence of a walking school bus route, an education intervention designed to improve attitudes toward active travel to school, or both interventions in combination. The authors tested each approach in a variety of communities with different population densities (and thus varying numbers of students per school). Results suggested that the success of either intervention—alone or in combination—was dependent on community context, and that the magnitude of difference seen across communities varied for interventions (Figure 13.6). While each intervention alone was beneficial for all communities, the walking school bus showed the greatest increase in the least densely populated communities: Student participation in active travel doubled. For the educational intervention alone, results were more equitable, with student participation increasing by about two-thirds across community types. Modeling the potentially synergistic effects of simultaneous interventions in an ABM revealed that all communities enjoyed the most benefits from dual implementation, and this scenario was the only case where at least 20% of students in every type of community engaged in active travel.

Relevance to Dissemination and Implementation Research

This model demonstrates many of the characteristics and strengths of ABM for D&I. The model is made up of multiple heterogeneous actors, in this case children, who make decisions based on personal characteristics, the social environment, and the physical environment. The researchers modeled multiple interventions across multiple community contexts to assess how environment may influence intervention success. The ABM served as an experimental laboratory where researchers could manipulate both the interventions and the community in a systematic way that would otherwise be difficult, costly, or impossible. Although the ABM cannot predict the success of the same or a similar intervention

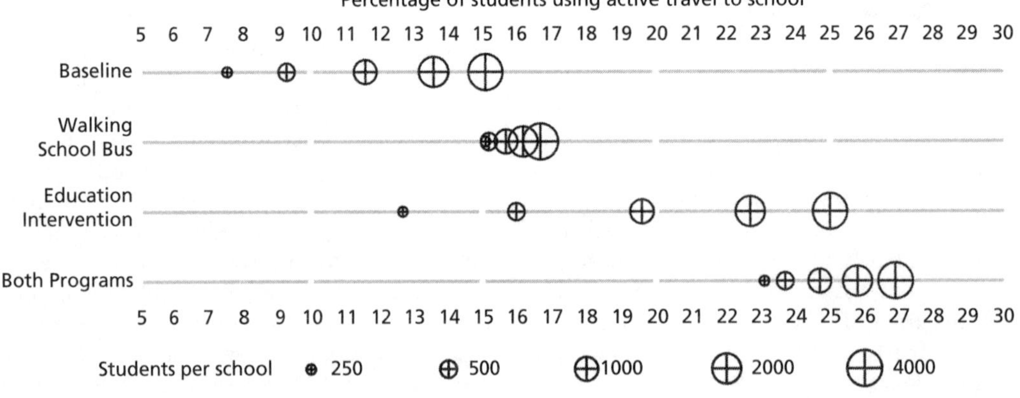

FIGURE 13.6 Results of walking school bus ABM.

Adapted with permission from Yang et al.[102]

in a specific real community, the results could be used to implement interventions that are more likely to be successful, given community characteristics, and eliminate possibilities that show relatively little value. Furthermore, the positive interaction between the intervention, social environment, and individuals to produce a qualitatively different outcome at the community level is a hallmark of ABMs. They demonstrated the potential synergistic benefit of implementing multiple interventions designed to address the same overarching issue but through different approaches.

CONCLUSION

As we have seen, numerous analysis and modeling tools that take into account the natural complexity of systems and D&I processes are available and the use of them is increasing over time.[60] This chapter summarized the characteristics, potential insights, and limitations of each modeling approach and provided a summary in Table 13.2. Computational modeling of any type, like all modeling approaches, requires assumptions about variables to include (or exclude) and hypothesized relationships dictate the quality of the model and the utility of the results. As such, using theory and empirical data to inform model design is paramount.

Systems thinking and methods remain underutilized in D&I despite demonstrations of the utility of incorporating systems thinking and methods into D&I studies (e.g., Miller et al., 2019).[103] How can interested D&I researchers make greater use of these approaches? The following are a number of suggestions based on our own experiences working at the intersection of D&I science and systems science:

- As with any research method, its appropriateness is determined by its fit with the theories and research questions driving the study. Systems methods are more likely to be appropriate when the D&I research is being guided by systems thinking.[44]
- Systems approaches can be integrated into more traditional study designs; however, full-scale integration of systems modeling requires careful attention from the start of the research design process.

TABLE 13.2 SUMMARY OF SYSTEM SCIENCE APPROACHES[a]

	Network Analysis	System Dynamics	Agent-Based Modeling
Characteristics			
Basic building blocks	• Nodes • Ties	• Feedback loops • Stocks and flows	• Agents • Agent behavior
Interactions & dynamics	• Node ↔ node • Tie creation/dissolution • Changing node/tie characteristics	• Feedback structure • Accumulation	• Agent ↔ agent • Agent ↔ environment • Behavioral changes
Insights & outcomes	• Identification and characterization of most efficient information pathways • Social influences on decision-making	• System behavioral patterns • Structural sources of system behavior • Areas of leverage for changing system behavior patterns	• Individual-level adaptations • Emergence of system-level patterns • Unexpected outcomes
Potential challenges & limitations	• Mapping complete networks is dependent on stakeholder participation • Limited ability to model dynamics over time	• Top-down perspective less able to address individual behavior • Difficult to capture large amounts of heterogeneity	• Exponentially growing complexity • Predicting outcomes later in modeled time

[a]Adapted with permission from Luke and Stamatakis[22] and Marshall et al.[60]

- The results of systems modeling are more likely to be valid and useful when they involve a wide variety of stakeholders in all phases of the modeling and incorporate theories, data, and perspectives from multiple disciplines.[59,104]
- Although the systems methods discussed here are presented separately, they are often combined. For example, the Cancer Intervention and Surveillance Monitoring Network combined an ABM that generated individual smoking histories for the entire United States with a higher-level SD model used to forecast effects of cancer control interventions on population health.[105] Modern ABMs often incorporate social network data and knowledge to model the influence of "social spaces" on actor behavior and dynamics.[106,107] In fact, because the three methods reviewed here are complementary modeling approaches, generating solutions to D&I problems using multiple methods is likely to improve the quality of the solutions.[43]
- Finally, there is a wide variety of resources available that can facilitate and accelerate understanding of systems science methods. See Table 13.1 for a concise list of professional associations, major conferences, professional journals, software packages, and important books devoted to the methods covered in this chapter.

SUGGESTED READINGS AND WEBSITES

Readings

Table 13.1.

Selected Websites and Tools

See Table 13.1.

REFERENCES

1. Luke DA, Harris JK. Network analysis in public health: history, methods, and applications. *Annu Rev Public Health.* 2007;28:69–93. doi:10.1146/annurev.publhealth.28.021406.144132
2. Tracy M, Cerdá M, Keyes KM. Agent-based modeling in public health: current applications and future directions. *Annu Rev Public Health.* 2018;39:77–94. doi:10.1146/annurev-publhealth-040617-014317
3. Northridge ME, Metcalf SS. Enhancing implementation science by applying best principles of systems science. *Health Res Policy Syst.* 2016;14(1):74. doi:10.1186/s12961-016-0146-8
4. Epstein JM. Why Model? *J Artif Soc Soc Simul.* 2008;11(4):12.
5. Walker AE, Wattick RA, Olfert MD. The application of systems science in nutrition-related behaviors and outcomes implementation research: a scoping review. *Curr Dev Nutr.* 2021;5(9):nzab105. doi:10.1093/cdn/nzab105
6. Li Y, Kong N, Lawley M, Weiss L, Pagan JA. Advancing the use of evidence-based decision-making in local health departments with systems science methodologies. *Am J Public Health.* 2015;105(suppl 2):S217–S222. doi:10.2105/ajph.2014.302077
7. Luke DA, Ornstein JT, Combs TB, Henriksen L, Mahoney M. Moving from metrics to mechanisms to evaluate tobacco retailer policies: importance of retail policy in tobacco control. *Am J Public Health.* 2020;110(4):431–433. doi:10.2105/AJPH.2020.305578
8. Hawe P, Shiell A, Riley T. Theorising interventions as events in systems. *Am J Community Psychol.* 2009;43(3–4):267–276. doi:10.1007/s10464-009-9229-9
9. Glasgow RE, Chambers D. Developing robust, sustainable, implementation systems using rigorous, rapid and relevant science. *Clin Transl Sci.* 2012;5(1):48–55. doi:10.1111/j.1752-8062.2011.00383.x
10. Northridge ME, Metcalf SS. Enhancing implementation science by applying best principles of systems science. *Health Res Policy Syst.* 2016;14(1):74. doi:10.1186/s12961-016-0146-8
11. Rosenberg A. *Philosophy of Social Science.* 5th edition. Westview Press, a member of the Perseus Books Group; 2016.
12. Hedström P, Ylikoski P. Causal mechanisms in the social sciences. *Annu Rev Sociol.* 2010;36(1):49–67. doi:10.1146/annurev.soc.012809.102632
13. Porpora DV. Four concepts of social structure Douglas v. Porpora. *J Theory Soc Behav.* 1989;19(2):195–211. doi:10.1111/j.1468-5914.1989.tb00144.x
14. Tabak RG, Khoong EC, Chambers DA, Brownson RC. Bridging research and practice. *Am J Prev Med.* 2012;43(3):337–350. doi:10.1016/j.amepre.2012.05.024
15. Ostrom E. Beyond markets and states: polycentric governance of complex economic systems. *Transnatl Corp Rev.* 2010;2(2):12.
16. Glasgow RE, Vogt TM, Boles SM. Evaluating the public health impact of health promotion

interventions: the RE-AIM framework. *Am J Public Health*. 1999;89(9):1322–1327.

17. Damschroder LJ, Hagedorn HJ. A guiding framework and approach for implementation research in substance use disorders treatment. *Psychol Addict Behav*. 2011;25(2):194–205. doi:10.1037/a0022284
18. Proctor E, Silmere H, Raghavan R, et al. Outcomes for implementation research: conceptual distinctions, measurement challenges, and research agenda. *Adm Policy Ment Health*. 2011;38(2):65–76. doi:10.1007/s10488-010-0319-7
19. Glass TA, McAtee MJ. Behavioral science at the crossroads in public health: extending horizons, envisioning the future. *Soc Sci Med*. 2006;62(7):1650–1671. doi:10.1016/j.socscimed.2005.08.044
20. Mobus GE, Kalton MC. *Principles of Systems Science*. Softcover reprint of the original 1st ed. 2015 edition. Springer; 2016.
21. Cronbach LJ. Beyond the two disciplines of scientific psychology. *Am Psychol*. 1975;30(2):116–127. doi:10.1037/h0076829
22. Luke DA, Stamatakis KA. Systems science methods in public health: dynamics, networks, and agents. *Annu Rev Public Health*. 2012;33:357–376. doi:10.1146/annurev-publhealth-031210-101222
23. Monge PR, Contractor NS. *Theories of Communication Networks*. Oxford University Press; 2003.
24. Luke DA. Getting the big picture in community science: methods that capture context. *Am J Community Psychol*. 2005;35(3–4):185–200.
25. Kleinman MS, Mold JW. Defining the components of the research pipeline. *Clin Transl Sci*. 2009;2(4):312–314. doi:10.1111/j.1752-8062.2009.00119.x
26. Luke DA, Wald LM, Carothers BJ, Bach LE, Harris JK. Network influences on dissemination of evidence-based guidelines in state tobacco control programs. *Health Educ Behav*. 2013;40(1)(suppl):33S–42S. doi:10.1177/1090198113492760
27. Brown CH, Kellam SG, Kaupert S, et al. Partnerships for the design, conduct, and analysis of effectiveness, and implementation research: experiences of the prevention science and methodology group. *Adm Policy Ment Health*. 2012;39(4):301–316. doi:10.1007/s10488-011-0387-3
28. Carothers, BJ, Allen P, Walsh-Bailey C, et al. Mapping the lay of the land: using interactive network analytic tools for collaboration in rural cancer prevention and control. *Cance Epidemiol Biomark Prev*. 2022 Jun 1;31(6):1159–1167. doi:10.1158/1055-9965.EPI-21-1446. PMID: 35443033; PMCID: PMC9167755.
29. Harris JK. *An Introduction to Exponential Random Graph Modeling*. Sage; 2014.
30. Snijders TAB, van de Bunt GG, Steglich CEG. Introduction to stochastic actor-based models for network dynamics. *Soc Netw*. 2010;32(1):44–60.
31. Wasserman S, Faust K. *Social Network Analysis: Methods and Applications*. Cambridge University Press; 1994.
32. Valente TW. *Social Networks and Health: Models, Methods, and Applications*. Oxford University Press; 2010.
33. Rogers EM. *Diffusion of Innovations*. 5th ed. Free Press; 2003.
34. Valente TW. *Network Models of the Diffusion of Innovations*. Hampton Press; 1995.
35. Granovetter M. Threshold models of collective behavior. *Am J Sociol*. 1978;83(6):1420–1443. doi:10.1086/226707
36. Benito del Pozo P, Serrano N, Marqués-Sánchez P. Social networks and healthy cities: spreading good practices based on a Spanish case study. *Geogr Rev*. 2017;107:624–639. doi:10.1111/j.1931-0846.2016.12210.x
37. Kwan BM, Brownson RC, Glasgow RE, Morrato EH, Luke DA. Designing for dissemination and sustainability to promote equitable impacts on health. *Annu Rev Public Health*. 2022 Apr 5;43:331–353. doi:10.1146/annurev-publhealth-052220-112457
38. Feldstein AC, Glasgow RE. A practical, robust implementation and sustainability model (PRISM) for integrating research findings into practice. *Jt Comm J Qual Patient Saf*. 2008;34(4):228–243.
39. Beck A, Bergman DA, Rahm AK, Dearing JW, Glasgow RE. Using implementation and dissemination concepts to spread 21st-century well-child care at a health maintenance organization. *Perm J*. 2009;Summer 13(3):8.
40. Valente TW, Palinkas LA, Czaja S, Chu KH, Brown CH. Social network analysis for program implementation. *PLoS One*. 2015;10(6):e0131712. doi:10.1371/journal.pone.0131712
41. Harris JK, Carothers BJ, Wald LM, Shelton SC, Leischow SJ. Interpersonal influence among public health leaders in the United States Department of Health and Human services. *J Public Health Res*. 2012;1(1):67–74. doi:10.4081/jphr.2012.e12
42. Lobb R, Carothers BJ, Lofters AK. Using organizational network analysis to plan cancer screening programs for vulnerable populations. *Am J Public Health*. 2014;104(2):358–364. doi:10.2105/AJPH.2013.301532
43. Hovmand PS, Sato J, Kuhlberg J, Chung S. *Introduction to System Dynamics for Applied Social Sciences*.

44. Meadows DH, Wright D. Thinking in Systems: A Primer. Chelsea Green Publishing; 2008.
45. Hammond RA. Complex systems modeling for obesity research. *Prev Chronic Dis.* 2009;6(3):A97. Accessed February 15, 2020. https://www.ncbi.nlm.nih.gov/pmc/articles/PMC2722404/
46. Meadows DH, Robinson JM. *The Electronic Oracle: Computer Models and Social Decisions.* Wiley; 1985.
47. Homer JB, Hirsch GB. System dynamics modeling for public health: background and opportunities. *Am J Public Health.* 2006;96(3):452–458.
48. Forrester JW. System dynamics—a personal view of the first fifty years. *Syst Dyn Rev.* 2007;23:345–358.
49. Haase D, Schwarz N. Simulation models on human–nature interactions in urban landscapes: a review including spatial economics, system dynamics, cellular automata and agent-based approaches. *Living Rev Landsc Res.* 2009;3. doi:10.12942/lrlr-2009-2
50. Homer J, Milstein B, Wile K, et al. Simulating and evaluating local interventions to improve cardiovascular health. *Prev Chronic Dis.* 2010;7(1):A18.
51. Mingers J, White L. A review of the recent contribution of systems thinking to operational research and management science. *Eur J Oper Res.* 2010;207(3):1147–1161. doi:10.1016/j.ejor.2009.12.019
52. Darabi N, Hosseinichimeh N. System dynamics modeling in health and medicine: a systematic literature review. *Syst Dyn Rev.* 2020;36(1):29–73. doi:10.1002/sdr.1646
53. Sterman J. *Business Dynamics: Systems Thinking and Modeling for a Complex World.* Irwin/McGraw-Hill; 2000.
54. Forrester JW. *Industrial Dynamics.* MIT Press; 1961.
55. Richardson GP. Reflections on the foundations of system dynamics. *Syst Dyn Rev.* 2011;27:219–243. doi:10.1002/sdr.462
56. Zimmerman L, Lounsbury DW, Rosen CS, Kimerling R, Trafton JA, Lindley SE. Participatory system dynamics modeling: increasing stakeholder engagement and precision to improve implementation planning in systems. *Adm Policy Ment Health.* 2016;43(6):834–849.
57. Homer JB. Why we iterate: scientific modeling in theory and practice. *Syst Dyn Rev.* 1996;12(1):1–19.
58. Vennix JAM. Group Model Building: Facilitating Team Learning Using System Dynamics. John Wiley; 1996.
59. Hovmand PS. *Community Based System Dynamics.* Springer; 2014.
60. Marshall DA, Burgos-Liz L, Ijzerman MJ, et al. Selecting a dynamic simulation modeling method for health care delivery research—part 2: report of the ISPOR Dynamic Simulation Modeling Emerging Good Practices Task Force. *Value Health.* 2015;18(2):147–160. doi:10.1016/j.jval.2015.01.006
61. Rahmandad H, Oliva R, Osgood ND, eds. *Analytical Methods for Dynamic Modelers.* MIT Press; 2015.
62. Greenhalgh T, Robert G, Macfarlane F, Bate P, Kyriakidou O. Diffusion of innovations in service organizations: systematic review and recommendations. *Milbank Q.* 2004;82(4):581–629. doi:10.1111/j.0887-378X.2004.00325.x
63. Aarons GA, Hurlburt M, Horwitz SM. Advancing a conceptual model of evidence-based practice implementation in public service sectors. *Adm Policy Ment Health Ment Health Serv Res.* 2011;38(1):4–23. doi:10.1007/s10488-010-0327-7
64. Pronovost P, Berenholtz S, Needham D. Translating evidence into practice: a model for large scale knowledge translation. *Br Med J.* 2008;337(7676):963–965. doi:10.1136/Bmj.A1714
65. Sterman JD. Learning from evidence in a complex world. *Am J Public Health.* 2006;96(3):505–514.
66. Forrester JW. *Urban Dynamics.* MIT Press; 1969.
67. Lich KH, Frerichs L, Fishbein D, Bobashev G, Pentz MA. Translating research into prevention of high-risk behaviors in the presence of complex systems: definitions and systems frameworks. *Transl Behav Med.* 2016;6(1):17–31. doi:10.1007/s13142-016-0390-z
68. Hovmand PS, Gillespie DF. Implementation of evidence-based practice and organizational performance. *J Behav Health Serv Res.* 2010;37(1):79–94.
69. Miller RL, Levine RL, McNall MA, Khamarko K, Valenti MT. A dynamic model of client recruitment and retention in community-based HIV prevention programs. *Health Promot Pract.* 2011;12(1):135–146.
70. Glasgow RE, Emmons KM. How can we increase translation of research into practice? Types of evidence needed. *Annu Rev Public Health.* 2007;28:413–433. doi:10.1146/annurev.publhealth.28.021406.144145
71. Green LW. Public health asks of systems science: to advance our evidence-based practice, can you help us get more practice-based evidence? *Am J Public Health.* 2006;96(3):406–409. doi:10.2105/Ajph.2005.066035
72. Powell BJ, McMillen JC, Proctor EK, et al. A compilation of strategies for implementing clinical innovations in health and mental

health. *Med Care Res Rev*. 2012;69(2):123–157. doi:10.1177/1077558711430690

73. Scott RJ, Cavana RY, Cameron D. Recent evidence on the effectiveness of group model building. *Eur J Oper Res*. 2016;249(3):908–918. doi:10.1016/j.ejor.2015.06.078
74. Brownson RC, Colditz GA, Proctor EK, eds. *Dissemination and Implementation Research in Health: Translating Science to Practice*. 2nd ed. Oxford University Press; 2017.
75. Frerichs L, Lich KH, Dave G, Corbie-Smith G. Integrating systems science and community-based participatory research to achieve health equity. *Am J Public Health*. 2016;106(2):215–222. doi:10.2105/AJPH.2015.302944
76. Zimmerman L. *The How and Why of Modeling to Learn*. Video. PSMG: Implementation and Systems Science Series. Center for Prevention Implementation Methodology for Drug Abuse and HIV. 2021. Accessed February 1, 2022. https://cepim.northwestern.edu/calendar-events/2021-10-12-zimmerman
77. Veterans Health Administration. MTL demo. 2022. Accessed February 1, 2022. https://forio.com/app/va/va-psd-demo/mtl_demo.html
78. Gilbert N. *Agent-Based Models*. Sage; 2008.
79. Retzlaff CO, Ziefle M, Calero Valdez A. The history of agent-based modeling in the social sciences. In: Duffy VG, ed. *Digital Human Modeling and Applications in Health, Safety, Ergonomics and Risk Management. Human Body, Motion and Behavior*. Lecture Notes in Computer Science. Springer International Publishing; 2021:304–319. doi:10.1007/978-3-030-77817-0_22
80. Giabbanelli PJ, Tison B, Keith J. The application of modeling and simulation to public health: assessing the quality of agent-based models for obesity. *Simul Model Pract Theory*. 2021;108:102268. doi:10.1016/j.simpat.2020.102268
81. Cassidy R, Singh NS, Schiratti PR, et al. Mathematical modelling for health systems research: a systematic review of system dynamics and agent-based models. *BMC Health Serv Res*. 2019;19(1):845. doi:10.1186/s12913-019-4627-7
82. Lorig F, Johansson E, Davidsson P. Agent-based social simulation of the COVID-19 pandemic: a systematic review. *J Artif Soc Soc Simul*. 2021;24(3):5.
83. Morshed AB, Kasman M, Heuberger B, Hammond RA, Hovmand PS. A systematic review of system dynamics and agent-based obesity models: evaluating obesity as part of the global syndemic. *Obes Rev*. 2019;20(S2):161–178. doi:10.1111/obr.12877
84. Yang Y. A narrative review of the use of agent-based modeling in health behavior and behavior intervention. *Transl Behav Med*. 2019;9(6):1065–1075. doi:10.1093/tbm/iby132
85. Hammond RA. Considerations and best practices in agent-based modeling to inform policy. In: Wallace R, Geller A, Ogawa VA, eds. *Assessing the Use of Agent-Based Models for Tobacco Regulation*. National Academies Press; 2015:161–193.
86. Auchincloss AH, Garcia LMT. Brief introductory guide to agent-based modeling and an illustration from urban health research. *Cad Saúde Pública*. 2015;31:65–78.
87. Moore TR, Foster EN, Mair C, Burke JG, Coulter RWS. Leveraging complex systems science to advance sexual and gender minority youth health research and equity. *LGBT Health*. 2021;8(6):379–385. doi:10.1089/lgbt.2020.0297
88. Ip EH, Rahmandad H, Shoham DA, et al. Reconciling statistical and systems science approaches to public health. *Health Educ Behav*. 2013;40(1)(suppl):123S–131S. doi:10.1177/1090198113493911
89. Chattoe-Brown E. Using agent based modelling to integrate data on attitude change. *Sociol Res Online*. 2014;19(1):16.
90. Wilensky U. NetLogo segregation model. 1997. Accessed October 21, 2022. http://ccl.northwestern.edu/netlogo/models/Segregation
91. De Leon FD, Felsen M, Wilensky U. NetLogo urban suite—Tijuana bordertowns model. 2007. Accessed October 21, 2022. http://ccl.northwestern.edu/netlogo/models/UrbanSuite-Tijuana Bordertowns
92. Loomis J, Bond C, Harpman D. The potential of agent-based modelling for performing economic analysis of adaptive natural resource management. *J Nat Resour Policy Res*. 2008;1(1):35–48. doi:10.1080/19390450802509773
93. Abar S, Theodoropoulos GK, Lemarinier P, O'Hare GMP. Agent based modelling and simulation tools: a review of the state-of-art software. *Comput Sci Rev*. 2017;24:13–33. doi:10.1016/j.cosrev.2017.03.001
94. Kiesling E, Günther M, Stummer C, Wakolbinger LM. Agent-based simulation of innovation diffusion: a review. *Cent Eur J Oper Res*. 2012;20(2):183–230.
95. Mckay V, Cambey C, Combs T, Stubbs AW, Pichon L, Gaur A. Using a modeling-based approach to assess and optimize HIV linkage to care services. *AIDS Behav*. 2021 Mar;25(3):886–896. doi:10.1007/s10461-020-03051-5
96. Orr MG, Galea S, Riddle M, Kaplan GA. Reducing racial disparities in obesity: simulating the effects of improved education and social network influence on diet behavior. *Ann*

Epidemiol. 2014;24(8):563–569. doi:10.1016/j.annepidem.2014.05.012

97. Auchincloss AH, Riolo RL, Brown DG, Cook J, Diez Roux AV. An agent-based model of income inequalities in diet in the context of residential segregation. *Am J Prev Med.* 2011;40(3):303–311. doi:10.1016/j.amepre.2010.10.033
98. Brookmeyer R, Boren D, Baral SD, et al. Combination HIV prevention among MSM in South Africa: results from agent-based modeling. *PLoS One.* 2014;9(11):e112668. doi:10.1371/journal.pone.0112668
99. Hoffer L, Alam SJ. "Copping" in heroin markets: the hidden information costs of indirect sales and why they matter. In: Greenberg AM, Kennedy WG, Bos ND, eds. *Social Computing, Behavioral-Cultural Modeling and Prediction.* Springer; 2013:83–92.
100. Luke DA, Hammond RA, Combs TB, et al. Tobacco town: computational modeling of policy options to reduce tobacco retailer density. *Am J Public Health.* 2017;107(5):740–746. doi:10.2105/AJPH.2017.303685
101. Yang Y, Diez-Roux A. Using an agent-based model to simulate children's active travel to school. *Int J Behav Nutr Phys Act.* 2013;10(10.1186):1479–5868.
102. Yang Y, Diez-Roux A, Evenson KR, Colabianchi N. Examining the impact of the walking school bus with an agent-based model. *Am J Public Health.* 2014;104(7):1196–1203. doi:10.2105/AJPH.2014.301896
103. Miller WL, Rubinstein EB, Howard J, Crabtree BF. Shifting implementation science theory to empower primary care practices. *Ann Fam Med.* 2019;17(3):250–256. doi:10.1370/afm.2353
104. Institute of Medicine (IOM). *Assessing the Use of Agent-Based Models for Tobacco Regulation.* Washington (DC): National Academies Press (US); 2015.
105. Holford TR, Meza R, Warner KE, et al. Tobacco control and the reduction in smoking-related premature deaths in the United States, 1964–2012. *JAMA.* 2014;311(2):164–171. doi:10.1001/jama.2013.285112
106. Lanham MJ, Morgan GP, Carley KM. Social network modeling and agent-based simulation in support of crisis de-escalation. *IEEE Trans Syst Man Cybern Syst.* 2014;44(1):103–110. doi:10.1109/tsmcc.2012.2230255
107. Alam SJ, Geller A. Networks in agent-based social simulation. In: Heppenstall AJ, Crooks AT, See LM, Batty M, eds. *Agent-Based Models of Geographical Systems.* Springer; 2012:199–216.

SECTION 4

Design and Measurement

14

Design and Analysis in Dissemination and Implementation Research

GEOFFREY M. CURRAN, JUSTIN D. SMITH, JOHN LANDSVERK, WOUTER VERMEER, EDWARD J. MIECH, BO KIM, GRACELYN CRUDEN, MARIA E. FERNANDEZ, AND C. HENDRICKS BROWN

INTRODUCTION

The field of implementation science is growing and changing rapidly. Substantial innovation is occurring in many facets of the field, including the way implementation research is designed and analyzed. The objective of this chapter, and others in this volume covering evaluation approaches (chapters 17 and 18), is to explain why and describe how implementation scientists are incorporating specific design and analytic approaches from the wider scientific method and bringing needed innovation and specificity to their application in dissemination and implementation (D&I) research. In this chapter, we review current design issues in D&I research and present an overview of specific analytic approaches. To encourage continued innovation, in addition to covering more widely used designs and analytic approaches, we also cover emerging D&I-specific research designs and promising D&I applications of analytic approaches from other fields. We also address how implementation designs can be used to address health equity and improve health for all. Finally, the chapter presents a case study demonstrating a novel adaptation of a dynamic wait-listed design for application in D&I research.

Focus of Dissemination and Implementation Research

A useful organizing heuristic is to conceptualize D&I in relation to two other stages of research, efficacy and effectiveness. Nicely captured in the 2009 National Research Council and Institute of Medicine report on *Preventing Mental, Emotional, and Behavioral Disorders Among Young People*[1] (shown in Figure 14.1) and adapted from that report and a recent typology,[2] D&I studies are the last stage of research in the science-to-practice continuum, preceded by efficacy and effectiveness studies that are distinct from and address different questions from D&I studies. The figure also demonstrates that distinct phases (albeit somewhat overlapping) exist within the D&I stage, characterized as exploration, adoption/preparation, implementation, and sustainment, similar to the EPIS (exploration, preparation, implementation, sustainment) model proposed by Aarons and colleagues.[3] In the exploratory phase, we focus on factors including deciding on what evidence-based health intervention would be most appropriate. In the adoption/preparation phase, we are interested in factors related to the formal decision to implement or strategies to increase adoption of a health intervention or program. The next phase is implementation, which often focuses on strategies for improving program delivery/fidelity in the field, and the final phase is sustainment (and moving to scale), involving strategies to maintain delivery of the health intervention or extend its use in communities or organizations. D&I trials are also distinct from efficacy and effectiveness trials with respect to the independent variable that is manipulated, which in this case are the

Geoffrey M. Curran, Justin D. Smith, John Landsverk, Wouter Vermeer, Edward J. Miech, Bo Kim, Gracelyn Cruden, Maria E. Fernandez, and C. Hendricks Brown, *Design and Analysis in Dissemination and Implementation Research* In: *Dissemination and Implementation Research in Health.* Edited by: Ross C. Brownson, Graham A. Colditz, and Enola K. Proctor, Oxford University Press.
DOI: 10.1093/oso/9780197660690.003.0014

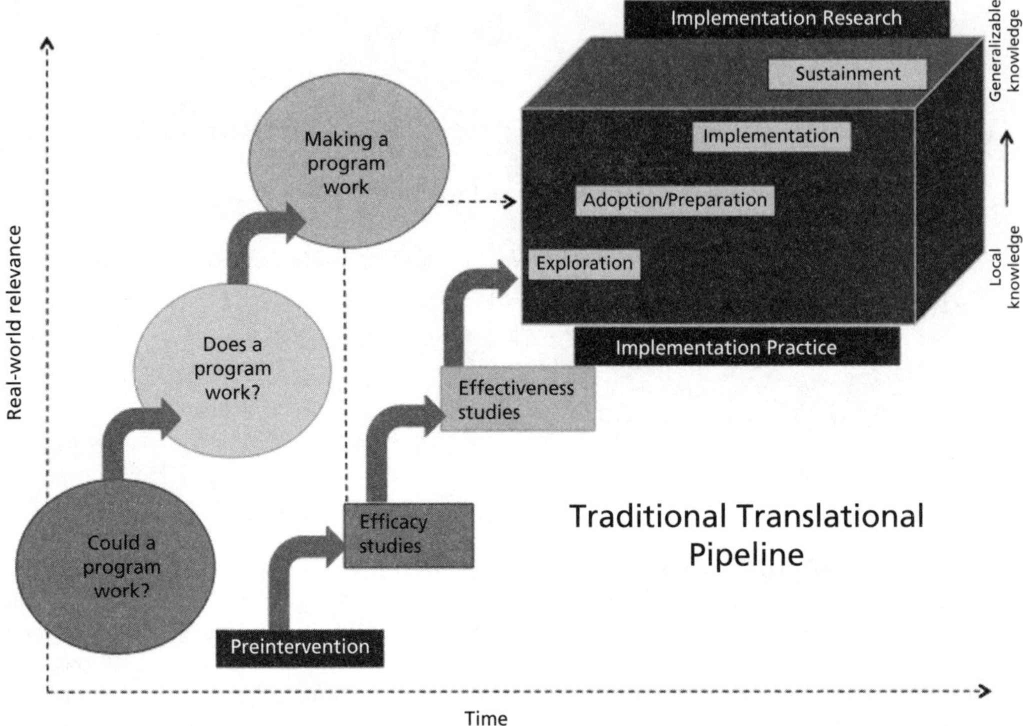

FIGURE 14.1 Stages of research and phases of dissemination and implementation.

Source: Adapted with permission from "Figure 11-1 Stages of research in prevention research cycle" in Chapter 11: Implementation and Dissemination of Prevention Programs (2009) in National Research Council and Institute of Medicine. *Preventing Mental, Emotional, and Behavioral Disorders Among Young People*. Washington, DC: The National Academies Press, p. 326, and Brown CH, et al. (2017). An Overview of Research and Evaluation Designs for Dissemination and Implementation. To appear in *Annual Rev Public Health*.

implementation strategies often addressing providers and/or organizational change.

We note that this research model typology represented in Figure 14.1 is also reflected in the National Institutes of Health (NIH) Roadmap initiative for re-engineering the clinical research enterprise currently driving the translational research initiative at the NIH.[4–6] The Roadmap initiative has identified three types of research leading to improvements in the public health of our nation: basic research that informs the development of clinical interventions (e.g., biochemistry, neurosciences); treatment development that crafts the health interventions and tests them in carefully controlled efficacy trials; and what has come to be known as service system and implementation research, where health interventions are evaluated in usual care and community settings.[7] Based on this tripartite division, the Roadmap further identified two translation steps that would be critical for moving from the findings of basic science to improvements in the quality of healthcare delivered in community, clinical, as well as virtual settings. The first translation step brings together interdisciplinary teams that integrate the work being done in the basic sciences and treatment development science, such as translating neuroscience and basic behavior research findings into new treatments. The focus of the second translation phase is to translate evidence-based health interventions/treatments into service delivery settings, sectors in local communities, or delivered systematically through virtual platforms, and it is this second step that we identify as the D&I research enterprise.[8]

We now briefly define and describe two facets of D&I research—outcomes and research questions—in order to better frame the discussion of evaluation designs and related analytic issues covered in the remainder of this chapter.

In the previous version of this chapter, we also briefly described the concept of implementation strategies, the multicomponent interventions aimed at increasing (or decreasing) implementation of practices/programs that are commonly under investigation in D&I studies. We now direct the reader to chapter 6 in this volume.

Evaluating Implementation Outcomes and Processes

Outcomes of implementation research are covered more fully in other chapters, but an overview is useful here in the context of our discussion of research designs. Inherent in the definition of implementation strategies is the goal of increasing adoption, which can be conceptualized as either a finite event or an ongoing process. However, outcomes in implementation research extend into many areas that affect the adoption and sustained delivery of a new innovation and the efficiency by which adoption and implementation occur. Proctor and colleagues[9] provided a comprehensive taxonomy of implementation outcomes and place them in the greater context of service delivery system outcomes, using the Institute of Medicine's standards of care[10] and the distal clinical outcomes at the level of the individual. Among the implementation outcomes are acceptability, adoption, appropriateness, cost, feasibility, fidelity, reach or penetration, and sustainment. These are viewed as the direct outcomes resulting from the use of implementation strategies, which, in turn, affect service system outcomes and patient-level clinical outcomes, such as symptom severity. Another widely used evaluation framework, RE-AIM,[11] specifies implementation outcomes of reach, adoption, and implementation, effectiveness to cover intervention outcomes, and maintenance to assess sustained changes. A recent update extended the framework to incorporate explicit measurement of health equity and extend its focus on sustainability.[12]

Not explicit in such frameworks is that some implementation outcomes are more germane to particular phases of implementation research.[13] For example, in the early phases of the EPIS model in Figure 14.1, primary outcomes might be acceptability, appropriateness, and feasibility, whereas during implementation, assessments of cost, fidelity, and penetration are possible and considered key outcomes. Likewise, outcomes of acceptability, fidelity, and cost, which are relevant to adoption/preparation and implementation phases, all can have lasting effect on sustainment, the fourth and final phase.

There are additional measures that evaluate the efficiency and success of the implementation process itself. A prime example of this type of measurement system is the Stages of Implementation Completion (SIC).[14] The SIC is intended to be individualized to specific innovations and service contexts as it concerns the stages to be completed and the specific activities within each stage. Some examples of stages include readiness planning, hiring and training of staff, service delivery, and consultation. Each stage contains three or more activities defined by the implementation broker and implementing site, often in consultation with the innovation developer, as being important within a given stage. The SIC measure is focused on critical, observable indicators involving speed, quality, and quantity. These include the completion of key implementation stages, the time spent in each stage, the numbers of the population served, and the proportion of activities completed in each stage. These dimensions can then be used to compare the outcomes between sites. An example of this type of application was provided in the context of the CAL-OH study,[15,16] a cluster randomized trial of two implementation strategies in child county public service systems in California and Ohio.

Research Questions in D&I

The four phases of D&I research in Figure 14.1 correspond to fundamentally different research questions. In particular, the exploration phase focuses on identifying or enlarging the set of organizations or communities that express interest in using or making available a particular innovation (e.g., health intervention or program). One may be interested in the sheer number of settings that express interest through a passive dissemination process or capturing whether some communities, say those serving high proportions of minority or poor populations, are differentially interested in using a certain program.[17] Early D&I research focused extensively on the characterization of barriers and facilitators to implementation. This remains a key consideration today but is often not viewed as a novel research question given the sheer amount of literature in this area. Today, implementation readiness and capacity assessment occurring during the adoption/preparation phase typically identifies barriers and facilitators to inform the choice of implementation strategies.

We can summarize how D&I research is distinct from other research stages. In contrast to the traditional research questions of efficacy research, which routinely examine overall impact in tightly controlled conditions with a relatively homogeneous target population; and of effectiveness research, which routinely asks who benefits and for how long in more realistic settings, D&I research questions focus primarily on whether different strategies for delivery of a health intervention increase the speed of implementation, the quality of program delivery, and/or the quantity or degree of access or penetration of the health intervention. We view these characteristics of speed, quality, and quantity as leading to measurable quantities that can be used to monitor the implementation process. Implementation success would generally be measured by attainment of certain milestones, such as a decision that a community or organization adopts a health program, certification that an agency has been credentialed, or other appropriate milestones that can be measured using standardized measures of implementation. Through these milestone measures, we can assess the speed with which implementation takes place. We also consider the other two dimensions of quality and quantity as critical to evaluating implementation strategies. For example, quality can refer to the fidelity or competence in program delivery, and quantity can refer to how many of the target population are served (similar to concepts of reach covered in chapter 17). Consequently, we recommend that the study designs, assessment instruments, analytical strategies, and analytic tools for D&I research all should relate to speed, quality, or quantity of implementation.

It is useful here to again compare the foci and aims of implementation research with effectiveness research. Figure 14.2, which is an adaptation of a figure that appeared in Smith and Hasan,[18] illustrates the focus of effectiveness research being on the health intervention with lesser attention given to the implementation strategies used and the implementation context. In contrast, implementation research focuses squarely on the implementation strategies and implementation context and, as such, evaluates success by evaluating the impact of implementation strategies on implementation outcomes rather than patient-level behavioral or health metrics that are the primary outcome of effectiveness research. The effectiveness-implementation hybrid approach, described in greater detail further in this chapter, combines elements of both types of research to a greater

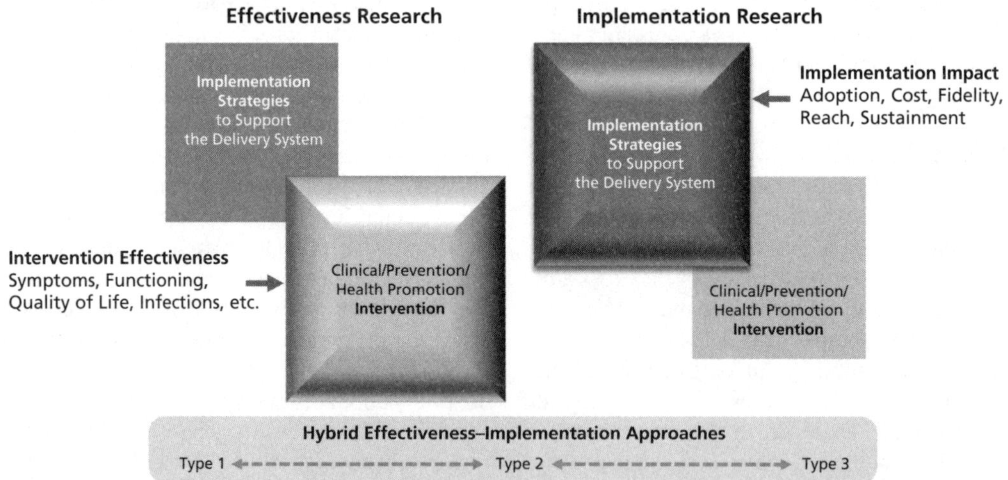

FIGURE 14.2 Emphasis and outcomes evaluated in clinical effectiveness versus implementation research.

Source: Adapted with permission from: "Figure 1: Emphasis and Outcomes Evaluated in Clinical Effectiveness versus Implementation Research" in Justin D Smith, Mohamed Hasan. Quantitative approaches for the evaluation of implementation research studies. *Psychiatry Res.* 2020 Jan;283:112521. doi:10.1016/j.psychres.2019.112521. Epub 2019 Aug 17.

PMID: 31473029 PMCID: PMC7176071 DOI: 10.1016/j.psychres.2019.112521 or lesser degree in a single study. Given the different purposes for D&I research compared to efficacy or effectiveness, it is likely that they may require different research designs or different emphases as they navigate the tension between internal and external validity that exist in all evaluations.

Smith and colleagues[19] developed a useful "continuum" for describing research questions/aims coupled with the broad type of research design that is commonly used. The continuum begins with research questions focused on understanding the contextual barriers and facilitators influencing the implementation of a health intervention. While specific types of trial designs are not usually employed at this point, researchers commonly use qualitative, quantitative, or mixed methods in cross-sectional or longitudinal designs to address these questions. Next are research designs, typically nonexperimental, that aim to develop, select, or adapt implementation strategies for a particular intervention and/or delivery context. Third, an implementation strategy, usually a novel or adapted strategy, is pilot tested to establish feasibility and acceptability and determine either potential impact on the target outcome or, at minimum, that the strategy is affecting the hypothesized mechanism of action. Research designs for piloting a strategy are often single-arm studies, pilot randomized controlled trials (RCTs), or factorial designs (e.g., MOST [multiphase optimization strategy implementation trials]) when the strategy is multicomponent or bundled (see chapter 6). Finally, the last two categories in the continuum involve formal testing and use of experimental (randomized) or quasi-experimental designs. The first, and more common, is testing the impact of a single-strategy condition against implementation as usual. Last, as the field begins to establish the evidence base for certain strategies and moves toward questions of efficiency, cost-effectiveness, and maximizing impact, there is a movement toward comparative implementation trials. Comparative implementation is similar to comparative effectiveness, except the health intervention is the same in all arms of the study and the implementation strategies are being compared. The simplest form of comparative implementation design is the head-to-head trial in which two bona fide strategies are pitted against one another and thought to be more or less likely to be equally effective but perhaps with trade-offs on cost, sustainability, or other outcomes. In such cases, summary metrics like the public health index[20] (effectiveness of the intervention * reach) or cost-effectiveness using a shared-outcome metric can be useful. Many randomized and nonrandomized trial designs can be used to test either a single-strategy or comparative implementation, including cluster randomized, stepped wedge, factorial, and others.

While specific research questions in D&I may most efficiently be addressed by a unique research design, there may remain questions about effectiveness of newly implemented health interventions that are worth answering anew. Indeed, hybrid approaches,[21] which address research questions related to both implementation and effectiveness simultaneously in one study (see Figure 14.2), are frequently used.[22,23] Hybrid approaches are discussed more fully further in this chapter. Finally, we note that the primary focus of this third edition chapter is on implementation without a separate discussion about designs in dissemination research because dissemination research has yet to develop a sufficient body of research designs distinct from or as extensive as that for implementation research.

METHODS IN IMPLEMENTATION PREPARATION

The process of implementing new health interventions in real-world settings is complex and involves numerous decisions on the part of the implementation evaluators and key decision makers in the implementation context. Factors that are commonly considered during implementation preparation, a process that coincides with the exploration and adoption/preparation phases of the EPIS framework in Figure 14.1, include the selection of the health intervention to be implemented, the possible planned adaptation of the intervention, the identification or development of potential implementation strategies, the identification of the target populations, the decision about whether the intervention should be adapted or not, the expected reach of the health intervention within a particular setting given such factors as the characteristics of the population being served and the number of implementers that will deliver it, and other resources being allocated. Each of these factors can affect the overall impact, the effort required, and the speed by which such impact is achieved. Given the plethora of potential decisions facing implementers, including weighting multiple health interventions and implementation strategies and the need to consider costs and efficiency, certain modeling approaches can be useful during implementation preparation. Decision makers face similar questions when crafting legislation, regulations, and other endorsements of specific and general practices. Attention to these factors occurs during exploration when needs and capacities are evaluated for different alternatives.

At times the number of options to be considered in the exploratory phase is small, such as a situation where policymakers have dictated a certain health intervention/program is to be used. One such example is the recent requirement that states must use set-aside funding to implement the coordinated specialty care model, based on the Recovery After an Initial Schizophrenia Episode (RAISE) project[24] to address the mental health needs of adolescents and young adults who are experiencing psychotic symptoms.[25] While this limits the scope in the exploration phase, a wide variety of options on how to actually implement this intervention might be critical to consider in the implementation and sustainment phases.

When exploring a relatively limited number of possible health intervention and implementation strategies, some straightforward tools can help guide decision-making. Often, decision analysis is combined with an economic analysis, supporting not only overall decision analysis, but also cost-effectiveness analyses or benefit analyses that explicitly acknowledge the reality of budget constraints and other limited resources, identifying those health interventions that can feasibly maximize the decision makers' objectives. Economic calculations for different HIV prevention programs, for example, can be compared to provide guidance on efficient use of limited funds[26] or other resources.[27–29] Linear programming tools have been developed to aid health departments in allocating limited resources for HIV prevention, for example.[30]

As the number of health interventions and implementation strategies increases, the exploratory phase becomes more complex. The parameter space of options to consider, whose size is determined by the product of the number of levels considered in each factor, expands due to a factorial explosion in possible health intervention and implementation strategy scenarios. Considering the ways to implement such scenarios requires taking into account interacting processes and agents that often result in nonlinear and highly context-specific behaviors. A full description of such a system with complex behavior requires a scope that is generally infeasible to achieve using traditional experimental methods.[31] There are several complexity-based simulation approaches, under the heading of systems science,[32] that have been used to model such complex behavior in implementation.[33] These include system dynamics,[34] network science, and agent-based modeling[35] (see chapter 13). These methods have informed us about strategies to prevent, for example, the spread of HIV through sexual networks.[36] A wide range of questions can be addressed using these simulation models, yet they mostly consider a variety of scenarios of how an implementation scales from the local to the system level. As these systems science-based simulations are scaled-up, long-term, systemic impacts of a wide range of specified alternative scenarios can be explored, and comparison made among them to provide recommendations about the best actions to take. It is important to note that such analyses provide their greatest value when they are employed in an iterative fashion, allowing policymakers to consider a variety of what-if scenarios and to evaluate multiple decisions holistically.

In this section, we highlight two formal processes through which computer simulations can be leveraged in partnership with policymakers during preimplementation. During each process, decision makers can use simulation modeling to anticipate intervention effects given evidence uncertainty in a low-stakes environment.

Group Model Building

Group model building (GMB) aims to help decision makers specify their assumptions about a problem to create a shared understanding of it and of potential solutions.[37,38] After identifying and characterizing a problem, decision makers collaboratively identify high-impact "leverage points" to be intervened on and explore which policies or health interventions are mostly likely to address those points. GMB employs "scripts," or structured activities to facilitate group learning using both unique and familiar engagement techniques, such as a nominal group technique. Scripts encourage divergence, such as the sharing of heterogeneous mental models about a problem's determinants, followed by convergence, or integration, of these mental models. These processes aim to foster consensus about what needs to be intervened on, by whom, how, and when. Consensus is generated through agreement, not just compromise, thereby increasing commitment to implementation. A compendium of evidence-based and promising scripts exists[39] and is continually expanded. Script adaptations range from surface-level adjustments, such as which examples are used when explaining systems concepts, to deeper adaptations, such as the integration of a particular theoretical framework. For example, Frerichs et al.[40] leveraged critical race theory to refine scripts and to structure their interpretations of community-generated stories about community violence within the context of structural and historical racism. Instead of developing a system dynamics model during GMB, Frerichs et al.[41] adapted GMB scripts to co-develop an agent-based model with youth to learn about how their environment shapes physical activity. In yet another example, Cruden et al.[42] used GMB to support local decision makers to identify which leverage points should be prioritized to prevent child maltreatment in their communities. Using qualitative system dynamics modeling and GMB, decision makers identified three evidence-based interventions that would target their prioritized leverage points or risk and protective factors for child maltreatment: parental peer support, basic needs and health determinants (e.g., transportation, housing, food, hygiene), and positive child behaviors.

Participatory system dynamics[43] (PSD) builds on the rich theoretical and methodological foundation of GMB, but emphasizes embedded, participatory action research principles and processes. PSD aims to facilitate community partner and researcher learning and empower those responsible for implementation decisions—especially those who have previously been left out of key implementation decisions that impact their daily workflow. Modeling to Learn (MTL) is an accredited, nationwide quality improvement initiative that was created with PSD. Because PSD, and thereby MTL, is anchored in participatory action research principles, the intention is to provide valid, useful knowledge through just, inclusive, and equitable processes. Thus, MTL is not a solution or "thing" to be implemented, in and itself. Instead, MTL offers a participatory infrastructure and processes that can be embedded, scaled, and sustained to support implementation decision-making and reduce policy-resistant decisions over time. The infrastructure entails intangible, but critical, resources such as a participatory process for individuals throughout a system to engage with one another, researchers, and the system dynamics model. Tangible resources include a generalizable system dynamics model that can accommodate local data (e.g., historical patient wait times, intake evaluation rates, and delays in treatment initiation). By running simulations that produce output specific to their own context, front-line healthcare workers can be empowered to test their own hypotheses and to select implementation strategies that can be modified through their daily decision-making. Taking a notable step forward in the rigorous evaluation of GMB-inspired efforts,[44] a multisite randomized trial is testing how MTL's deeply interwoven combination of a generalizable method (system dynamics) and generalizable process (participatory engagement) affects implementation outcomes compared to audit and feedback. Although both MTL and audit and feedback strategies leverage local data, MTL's theory of change emphasizes systems thinking and participatory learning. Generalizable qualitative analysis and data visualization methods have been developed to measure change in these proximal outcomes.[45] Prior GMB applications or research studies have not always measured such proximal outcomes or relied on project-specific metrics.

Rapid Cycle Systems Modeling

Rapid cycle systems modeling (RCSM) is a recently developed implementation strategy to increase the use of evidence during decision-making, particularly during preimplementation.[46] RCSM uses three cyclical stages to engage decision makers with simple simulation models to synthesize evidence, make assumptions explicit, reveal contradictions in assumptions, and explore implications of assumptions.

Stage one: identify stakeholders' questions. Questions and outcomes of key importance to decision makers are identified through focus groups and/or semistructured interviews. Through dialogue, the practical knowledge and evidence held by decision makers converges with the scientific knowledge offered by researchers.

Stage two: develop simulation model. Researchers reflect on decision makers' input from step 1 and build a simple simulation model that can be quickly iterated on in order to be responsive to decision timelines. Models are primarily developed by the research team and then presented back to decision makers (in contrast to GMB, for example, during which models might be developed during GMB sessions or asynchronously). The goal is to develop the simplest, most pragmatic model that will foster learning, dialogue, and the critical use of research evidence. Complexity-based simulation models are recommended due to the increased use of systemic, multilevel interventions and initiatives in service systems that address complex needs such as mental health and child welfare. RCSM case studies thus far have relied on Monte Carlo simulation models,[46,47] yet other models are encouraged as appropriate (e.g., system dynamics, discrete event).

Stage three: re-engage stakeholders in dialogue regarding model utility, refinement. The simulation model is then used to facilitate the exchange of ideas between researchers and decision makers about the factors that might be driving system outcomes of interest and to assess model relevance to decision makers' context and implementation decisions.

Community partners can be engaged with systems science modeling processes[48] through less formal processes as well. For example, the HEALing (Helping to End Addiction Long-term[SM]) Communities Initiative is leveraging community-engaged modeling, including GMB-inspired methods, to address the US opioid epidemic.[49] Using a local data-driven approach, coalitions are using modeling to inform action planning, create demand for evidence-based practices, and reduce stigma associated with opioid use. Similarly, use a partnership with the local health department to create an agent-based model to support the local authorities in their decision-making, shedding light on which strategies are and are not likely to achiever there aims to end the HIV epidemic.[50]

During implementation preparation, simulation modeling can serve as a decision support tool well suited to support health and social service policymakers as they confront the challenges of complex, multifaceted, real-world operations,[51] which can help identify policies and health interventions that are most likely to achieve a set of desired objectives given current uncertainties. Indeed, decision analyses have considered the prevention and management of HIV/AIDS, cardiovascular disease, diabetes, and human papilloma virus (HPV) and cervical cancer.[52–57] For example, relying in part on model-based cost-effectiveness analyses, the Institute of Medicine recommended a shift from funding programs based on high AIDS prevalence to targeting prevention efforts to subgroups at high risk of infection.[58]

An excellent illustration of the use of decision analysis was provided by Goldhaber-Fiebert and colleagues.[59] The authors used a simulation model to evaluate the effect of implementing one such evidence-based foster parent training intervention: KEEP (Keeping Foster Parents Trained and Supported).[60] The simulation computed policy-relevant outcomes such as increased rates of adoption and reunification (positive exits) along with improved foster care placement stability (e.g., reduced lateral foster placement changes and reduced negative exits to group care, etc.) resulting from the application of KEEP. The simulation incorporated data on children in foster care from RCTs of KEEP[61,62] as well as large, population-representative longitudinal studies (e.g., National Survey of Child and Adolescent Well-Being [NSCAW-1]), using multivariate Cox proportional hazard models and bootstrapping to provide estimates of the rates of foster care placement change, the main covariates that determine these rates, and their associated uncertainty.

The detailed simulation developed for this analysis simulated large cohorts of individual children whose characteristics matched those of the actual foster care populations within the US child welfare system. The model then followed these "simulated individuals" on their paths through the system, tracking their placement changes and allowing past experiences to influence their future risks of placement change and exit. This approach permitted the consideration of the rich, complex effects of each individual's experience in the system over time, identifying cumulative benefits to KEEP, emphasizing higher-risk groups of children who may differentially benefit from the application of the intervention and gauging the heterogeneous mediating effects that different state child welfare systems could have on KEEP. This research demonstrated decision analytic methods to employ existing data to project policy-relevant child welfare outcomes related to permanence and stability. Decision-analytic simulation modeling is a feasible and useful methodology to inform challenging child welfare policy decisions and can be extended to consider multiple evidence-based interventions and outcomes.

Another recent example highlights how agent-based modeling can be used to study policy impacts.[63] In particular, it focuses on the effects of various Centers for Disease Control and Prevention (CDC) guidelines for PrEP (preexposure prophylaxis) prescription on HIV prevalence. In this study, the authors used existing field data to create a realistic system with interacting agents, men who have sex with men (MSM), and simulate not only how HIV spreads among that population, but also how different implementations of CDC guidelines for PrEP prescription affect this spreading process. The simulation incorporates a heterogeneous population of 10,000 agents with variations in sexual activity, risk behaviors, testing frequencies, and adherence levels. A second agent-based modeling approach highlighted the importance of sexually transmitted infection (STI) testing as a critical factor determining intervention success.[64]

These examples of the use of simulation for implementation preparation highlight this method as a scalable tool for doing virtual experiments, scanning the parameter space, and conducting consequent scenario analysis based on the outcomes, but the potential goes well beyond that. Decision analysis using simulation can also identify the factors critical for successful implementation, inform which populations to target and the differences to be expected for various target populations, and identify tipping points in the system, which can inform the amount of resources needed to achieve the desired impact.

RANDOMIZED AND NONRANDOMIZED IMPLEMENTATION DESIGNS FOR ADOPTION/PREPARATION, IMPLEMENTATION, AND SUSTAINMENT PHASES

Historically, basic science and treatment research have relied heavily on what has come to be known as the "gold standard" of designs, the RCT, which randomizes at the person level. In the efficacy phase, the primary aim is to determine whether a health intervention has impact on its intended target. A great deal of methods development has been devoted to the use of RCTs to evaluate efficacy for medical[65] and behavioral research.[66] While effectiveness research also has played an important role in the science-to-practice continuum, group-based randomized trials are generally needed for these more complex longitudinal designs, which often include multiple levels in the analysis.[67,68] In one of the few comprehensive discussions of the distinction between efficacy and effectiveness trials, Flay in 1986[69] noted that "whereas efficacy trials are concerned with testing whether a treatment or procedure does more good than harm when delivered under optimum conditions, effectiveness trials are concerned with testing whether a treatment does more good than harm when delivered via a real-world program."[69]

It is not accidental that Flay's language on D&I includes a discussion of designs using random assignment to evaluate different approaches for delivery. Flay's perspective then was that randomized trials could be used for such research, but such designs would need to differ from individual participant-level RCTs.[2] There are circumstances where randomization may not be feasible or acceptable,[70] and alternatives may be proposed to the randomized design such as "interrupted time series," "multiple baseline across settings," or "regression-point displacement" designs.[71] But there are options and strengths for implementation designs that incorporate randomization other than at the individual level. Brown and colleagues have argued that incorporating randomization across time and place in rollout trials can be acceptable for both communities and researchers.[22,67,72] Table 14.1, adapted and abridged from Mercer et al. and White and Sabarwal,[73,74] summarizes some trade-offs between randomized, quasi-experimental and related designs for D&I.

This section of the chapter reviews the major issues in designs for D&I research, with a particular focus on randomization and alternatives to randomized designs. The emerging development of hybrid, adaptive, and staging designs is also discussed. This is followed by a discussion of power calculations in multilevel

TABLE 14.1 TRADE-OFFS BETWEEN RANDOMIZED AND QUASI-EXPERIMENTAL DESIGNS FOR DISSEMINATION AND IMPLEMENTATION[a]

Type of Design	Illustrative Use	Common Strengths	Common Weaknesses
Group randomized trial	Randomize clinics to one of two different implementation strategies	High internal validity	If the arms have different strengths (e.g., an "implementation as usual" or encouragement arm), may be unacceptable to communities or organizations Often logistically challenging given large number of sites required for sufficient power
Randomized rollout trial	Randomize when clinics receive a new implementation strategy	Often acceptable to communities as all receive a strategy to enhance delivery of an intervention deemed effective Improved statistical power as it combines within- and between-site measures	Can be expensive to obtain repeated implementation measures across all sites and times
Quasi-experimental designs without controls	Pre-post design of a new dissemination or implementation strategy in one clinic	Cost-effective designs for evaluating a new implementation strategy	Weak causal design since there is no counterfactual comparison
Quasi-experimental designs with controls	Natural experiment comparing those receiving implementation to others without across multiple clinics	Cost-effective comparison design With large numbers of control conditions, group-level propensity score adjustment can reduce biases based on measured covariates[75]	Inferences can be highly biased due to unmeasured selection factors (e.g., readiness), especially with a limited number of controls

[a]Adapted and abridged from Mercer et al. and White and Sabarwal.[73,74]

implementation designs and the use of analytic strategies such as mediation and moderation. Finally, the chapter addresses a rapidly emerging set of tools for D&I research under the labels of "systems science and engineering" and "configurational analysis."

The classification of D&I designs put forth by Brown and colleagues[2] encompasses three overarching categories of designs based on the type of comparison.

Within-site designs involve the evaluation of an implementation project focused on change within a single site or within multiple sites without any cross-site comparisons. This classification includes two types of within-site designs. The weaker design is the postdesign where the system's healthcare processes and utilization are measured and evaluated after the introduction of an evidence-based practice. The more rigorous pre-post design adds an evaluation of preimplementation data, which can then be compared to postimplementation data to infer effects. Interrupted time series designs in the Cochrane Effective Practice and Organization of Care (EPOC) Group framework[76] provide methodological improvements on the within-site design that simply requires additional measurement and analytic techniques that account for trend, serial dependence, and other characteristics of such data.[77] All of these within-site design variants are considered quasi-experimental.

Between-site designs apply for an evaluation that compares outcomes, outputs, and processes between two or more sites where a novel health intervention is being implemented. A basic type of study in this category is a head-to-head comparison of two implementation strategies for a specific health intervention that occurs in two different sites or two groups of sites—randomly assigned when applicable. A variant of this design could be to assign different units or wards within an organization and compare the effectiveness of different implementation strategies. A useful rule of thumb is that randomization should be at the "level of implementation," meaning the level where the full impact of the strategy is designed to occur.[78] Brown and colleagues[2] also discussed special cases of this family of between-site designs: factorial designs; double randomized, two-level nested designs; and site selection of implementation strategies using a decision support strategy, as opposed to an a priori randomization that forces sites to use a certain implementation strategy.

Within- and between-site comparison designs are useful when sites begin as one implementation condition and move to another. The most common example of this design is a rollout randomized implementation trial, which is similar to the stepped-wedge[79] and dynamic wait-listed design[72] that has been used in effectiveness research for decades. In such designs, sites are randomized to a time to crossover from implementation as usual to the use of the implementation strategy. In this way, each site serves as its own control (within site) and can be compared to the performance of other sites while holding chronological time fixed (between site). Statistical power is higher with such a within-between site design than those only involving between site comparisons.

We note that the commonly used term *stepped wedge* implementation design refers to a design where each site in its turn introduces a new implementation strategy. This allows an evaluation of the new implementation strategy with implementation as usual. A number of variants to this design are possible, including those that involve the clustering of sites to start at different time points and pairwise-enrollment rollout designs.[71] Rollout trials, which provide a general term for all these variants where sites are randomized across time to one or a sequence of implementation strategies, is particularly palatable to community organizations as they are assured of receiving the active implementation strategy at some point in the trial as opposed to serving solely as a control site. In situations with few units available for randomization, power can be increased, and the experimental design can be strengthened by using randomized multiple-baseline designs,[80] which come from the single-subject experimental design tradition. Finally, there are circumstances where one or a few sites are chosen for a new implementation strategy, rather than being selected randomly, and then compared to other sites where the novel implementation program is not used. While this nonrandomness places limits on the ability to make rigorous causal inferences, the inclusion of a large number of comparison sites and long implementation measurements in a regression point displacement design can increase the strength of inferential capacity.[71]

The observed dominance of D&I research designs with randomization supports the benefits of such designs for addressing common threats to interpretation of study findings. However, it is important to consider the nature of threats to the integrity of a randomized trial before further reviewing a range of design options for D&I research.

The critical scientific paradigm for assigning observed differences by condition to an implementation's effect is that the only systematic factor that differs by intervention condition is the assigned intervention. For example, an implementation trial can carry out an appropriate randomization of communities to one of two implementation conditions, use valid and reliable measures, and conduct statistical analyses that correctly take into account intraclass clustering within communities. But if community leaders in one arm of the trial are more likely to refuse to be interviewed or drop out more frequently, this effect on the quality of the inferences can never be fully compensated by other good parts of the study. A strong and active partnership between communities, institutions, and researchers is required to reduce the potential for such imbalance and to hold an implementation design in place.[81,82] Below, we list some of the factors that are known to affect the quality of inferences[83] with special attention to D&I research.

Random assignment is the obvious choice for ensuring that an implementation condition is fairly distributed (sometimes with blocking into similar communities followed by random assignment within these blocks). While some have suggested that random assignment is not appropriate for implementation research, our review indicated that there has been a growing number of such randomized implementation trials conducted, and we believe they do have an important place in this research agenda. The usual alternative to randomization is a comparative study design, where one or more select communities apply a specified implementation procedure, while other communities, often selected afterward, are used as comparison. The problem with this design is that it hopelessly confounds two factors: the implementation itself with community readiness since only those communities that are "ready" are prepared to implement. One can never distinguish whether the differences in outcomes in communities are due to one of these factors or both. A good alternative design in this case is a "rollout" design[22] where communities that express their willingness are randomized to the timing of implementation. Such a design[72,84] has been used in the comparison of two implementation strategies for an evidence-based intervention for foster care.[17,85,86] An innovative version of the rollout design is also presented further in this chapter with a case study example.

A second major threat to an implementation trial is a failure to use valid and reliable measures to assess implementation outcomes. Because the implementation process is inherently multilevel, it is critical to assess impact across the appropriate levels. A potential flaw can occur if only distal outcomes on a target population are measured since these may not be comparable across health intervention conditions. For example, suppose an implementation strategy is designed to increase the number of youth who receive an evidence-based program. If we compare findings from those youth in communities randomized to the new implementation strategy to those using implementation as usual, it is quite possible for systematic differences to occur between those target youth who are exposed to different interventions. There is no mechanism to guarantee that those who receive the health intervention are equivalent, and in some cases, it may be that the expansion of service delivery may capture populations that are more challenging (compared to other groups), or less challenging, to serve. When involving a population that may exhibit different characteristics, analytic strategies that use propensity scores to adjust for differences at the nonrandomized level could be considered.[87,88] There is ordinarily no need to adjust for covariates at the higher level where randomization occurs because randomization preserves balance.

While there are important benefits to randomization, the multilevel nature of D&I research creates issues for typical randomization at the individual-level designs. Figure 14.3 shows a classic multilevel structure with four levels that Shortell has suggested for assessing performance improvement in organizations.[89] While randomization in implementation research is most commonly being done at levels higher than the individual, there is an issue in having sufficient power as one moves to higher levels with diminishing numbers of units to be used in a randomized design (see further section on calculation of power in multilevel designs). Since power is so critical to the viable use of randomized designs—and because resource or logistical constraints may eliminate randomization as a valid option—it is reasonable to consider quasi-experimental designs without randomization for D&I research. This clearly was the thrust of Glasgow and colleagues[70] in their 2005 article on practical designs. Another useful source for guidance on alternative designs and the trade-offs between randomized and nonrandomized designs is the *Handbook of Practical Program Evaluation*,[90] edited by Wholey, Hatry, and Newcomer, especially the contrasting chapters on "Quasi-Experimentation"[91] by Reichardt and Mark and the chapter on "Using Randomized Experiments"[92] by St Pierre. We note that Reichardt and Mark described four prototypical quasi-experimental study designs: (1) before-after; (2) interrupted time series; (3) nonequivalent group; and (4) regression-discontinuity. Their rendering of alternative designs is quite comparable to the EPOC classification of designs in implementation research and to the discussion of alternative designs by Glasgow and colleagues.[70]

We would also point to important recent studies that have compared the results between randomized experiments and observational studies. These have included both examples of

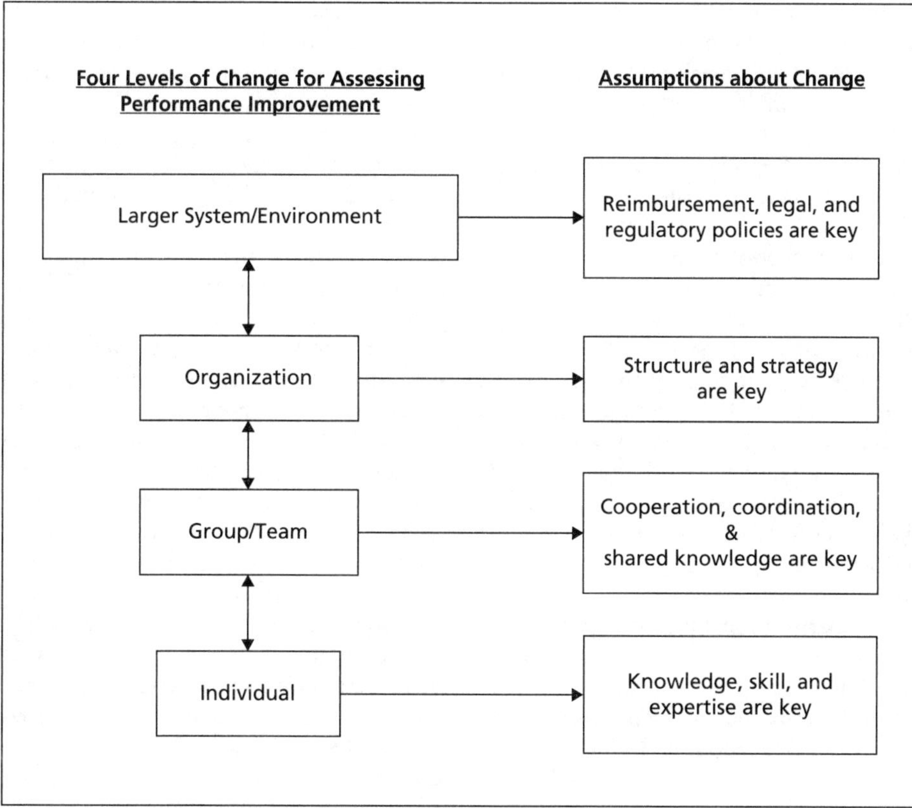

FIGURE 14.3 Four levels of change and assumptions about change.

Source: Adapted with permission from: Shortell SM. Increasing value: a research agenda for addressing the managerial and organizational challenges facing health care delivery in the United States. *Medical Care Research and Review.* 2004;61(3)(suppl):12S–30S.

strong divergence between observational studies and experimental studies, such as found in studies of hormone replacement therapy[93] as well as examples where the results were remarkably consistent. Also notable is the paper published in 2000 by Concato, Shah, and Horwitz[94] that examined meta-analyses of RCTs and meta-analyses of either cohort or case-control studies on the same intervention. Across interventions addressing five very different medical conditions, the authors found remarkable similarity in the results between the two types of designs, which are perceived to be quite different in the hierarchy of evidence. The authors concluded: "The results of well-designed observational studies (with either a cohort or a case-control design) do not systematically overestimate the magnitude of the effects of treatment as compared to those in randomized, controlled trials on the same topic" (p. 1887). A later study published in 2008 by Cook, Shadish, and Wong[95] came to the same conclusion when comparing the results from randomized experiments and regression-discontinuity designs. In both articles, the authors argued that the quality of the observational studies had to be high to be comparable to the results in randomized designs. This line of research informs the emerging field of implementation science by suggesting that observational studies may also be seriously considered.[96]

RETHINKING RANDOMIZED DESIGNS

An alternative approach to problems with use of classic RCT designs, so important in efficacy and effectiveness research stages, is to rethink how randomized designs can be adapted to meet the special needs of research across the four phases of D&I research. Th next section discusses some of this rethinking by considering nontraditional ways of using random assignment in D&I research.

There are three appealing features about rollout designs compared to traditional wait-listed designs. First, the statistical power is substantially greater for the rollout design in answering many relevant research questions.[71,72] Second, it is often not practical to train a large number of communities/organizations in a health intervention all at once, and the rollout feature nicely focuses on a manageable number who can receive the training they need to implement the intervention. Third, the use of multiple times for assignment provides more robustness of the design to influence by exogenous factors, such as economic downturns, that could otherwise destroy any chance to make inferences if its timing occurred at the most critical time in the assignment to training. Some potential drawbacks of the rollout design, compared to parallel group randomized designs, is the ability to withstand unexpected events (e.g., policy change) as they impact both arms equally. Hemming and Taljaard[97] discussed additional considerations for the indication and contraindication for cluster randomized stepped-wedge designs (a particular type of rollout design), which centers on the risk of bias during analysis due to misspecification of the secular trends caused by studies randomizing a small number of heterogeneous clusters. While they conclude, "In situations when a conventional parallel-CRT is feasible, it is likely to be the preferred design" (p. 1043), they provide a number of instances when a stepped-wedge or similar rollout design would be feasible and justified.

We recommend that a rollout design be considered when an implementation program is being introduced into a set of communities as part of a federal, statewide, or local policy change.[22,72,84] As an example of an appropriate use of such a trial, consider examining the following typical strategy for improving the quality and effectiveness of services by improving the training of mental health counselors. There are four levels that we need to pay attention to: the client who receives services, the therapist who delivers the services, the supervisor whose job it is to improve service delivery within a mental health agency, and the agency itself. We first consider an implementation strategy that changes the supervision practices of therapists within agencies. A first question to consider is what level of randomization should be used to provide maximum utility to understanding whether a new supervision strategy is effective relative to that now being used. We can consider randomizing at any and all four levels from the client to the agency, but many of these levels will not be very useful. A key step is to identify the salient "level of intervention" examined; here we are fundamentally interested in how the use of a new supervision program will affect outcomes downstream, and therefore the key level of intervention is at the supervisor level; this is the first level where we would expect behavior to change. An empirically validated rule is the following: Whenever possible, one should randomize at the level of intervention since randomization at lower levels (e.g., therapist) would contort supervisors from using new techniques to train therapists in the standard condition, and randomization at higher levels (e.g., agency) will generally result in major reductions in power.[78] If we do randomize at the level of the supervisor within an agency, then the agency is considered a "blocking factor." Blocking is a well-known way of reducing variability and thereby increasing power. In a rollout design, we would randomly determine the order and timing of training of supervisors and consequently their transmission of new behaviors to their supervisee therapists and in turn their own clients.

To assess impact in this trial design, we would likely want to measure behaviors of the supervising process (supervisor-therapist interactions), as well as of the therapeutic session itself (therapist-client), and perhaps at the level of the client target behavior as well. All three of these measures would normally be assessed over time. Thus, the design in this study would typically involve multiple observation/coding times for supervisors before and after they were trained to deliver a different type of supervision, multiple observation/coding times for their respective therapists, and multiple observation times for different clients across time. Three levels of analysis could be done, with the first examining changes in supervisor behavior across time before and after training; the second involving therapist-client behavior, also coded in terms of how therapist behavior with clients related to the timing of the supervisory training they received; and third the behavior of the clients themselves. To connect these three analyses, we would conduct mediation analyses, which are presented further in this chapter.

The sample size for such a trial may be nested at several levels. For example, sample size determination may include the number of agencies, the number of supervisors in each agency, the distribution of the number of therapists who receive supervision within these agencies, and finally the number of clients served by each therapist. Characteristics of timing include when supervisors in each agency receive training, the number of observation points in each supervision, the number of observation points for each therapist in interacting with a client, and the baseline and follow-up times for assessing client behavior. To ensure that there is sufficient power in this design to answer all three questions of impact on supervisor behavior, on therapist behavior, and on client behavior, as well as on mediational pathways, we would need to carry out a sophisticated study of how statistical power relates to these sample sizes and timing. While there are programs that allow for computation of power in multilevel designs,[98,99] to date the calculations for rollout designs are generally only available to do by simulation[72] (see further section on power calculations).

Rollout Implementation Optimization Design

A novel variation of the rollout design described by Smith and Brown is the rollout implementation optimization (ROIO) design.[100] In most rollout designs, a critical assumption is that the implementation strategy will remain relatively consistent across each cluster such that they can be readily combined to capitalize on the power advantages of a within-and-between site trial design. Analysis of such trials typically involves testing for effect of the cluster sequence (i.e., a learning or sequence effect), in which one might hypothesize that later clusters perform better as a function of the implementation support team having learned from the prior clusters and made adjustments to the implementation for greater impact or efficiency. Even in this situation where a learning effect is found, the strategy itself is functionally similar. Traditional implementation science perspectives would consider wholesale strategy changes as a protocol violation that potentially jeopardizes the internal validity of the trial.

In contrast, the ROIO design prospectively aims for iterative improvement in implementation outcomes and impact via manipulation of the strategy between clusters in the rollout design. Thus, the ROIO shares similar features and goals of quality improvement but with additional design elements to increase rigor and generalizable knowledge. The primary way in which this is accomplished is cluster randomization across time with a sufficient number of units (e.g., clinics, schools) to ensure power to detect effects between clusters. While one could conduct a nonrandomized ROIO, randomization adds to the rigor of the design and aids in the reliability of observed differences between clusters being a result of the optimization of the strategy and not other factors. Similar power considerations for nested data apply, but the power advantage of other rollout designs, such as the stepped wedge, are less pronounced in a ROIO as the clusters are somewhat dependent on one another given that successive clusters use an implementation strategy that is an iteration of the strategy of the prior cluster(s). Thus, the analytic approach and measurement of the primary outcome are of utmost importance for ensuring both power and valid interpretation of observed differences. The case study at the end of the chapter illustrates one potential ROIO design application.

The ROIO design can be used in many of the same circumstances as other rollout designs and shares similar advantages (e.g., all participating sites will eventually implement) and drawbacks (e.g., longer duration and more logistically challenging compared to a concurrent RCT design), but is particularly applicable for testing implementation strategies that are multilevel, multicomponent, or otherwise a complex bundle of discrete strategies that can be both modified, which we define as changes to the specification (e.g., actor, action, temporality, dose), and potentially discontinued if found to be ineffective or infeasible to determine the optimal strategy. For this reason, a highly prescriptive and protocolized implementation strategy might not be suitable as certain modifications and discontinuations might be considered fidelity inconsistent with the overall bundle. As a concrete example of two components in an intervention strategy, consider continued refinement of a monitoring system for clinics that consists of multiple indices of a prevention or care cascade (e.g., proportion of screened positive not linked to care, proportion failing to be retained). With each interim improvement in these monitoring elements, there is a corresponding change called for in the feedback system. Some feedback strategies are known to be counterproductive, so there may need to be continued changes in this system component.

Concerning measurement, four key considerations are part of the ROIO design. First is the primary outcome. While not necessarily required, a primary outcome that is assembled from "lower" levels of clustering, such as the proportion of successfully delivered patient or clinical encounters, improve power due to increasing the number of observations. Second, the strategy modifications with each successive cluster of the ROIO rely on both quantitative and qualitative data from the early periods of each cluster. This design is efficient as improvements are made rapidly between clusters rather than in a sequential manner requiring one cluster to implement for a lengthy period (as is typically the case to obtain sufficient data on the ultimate outcome metric). In the ROIO, selection of a primary outcome that occurs and accumulates rather quickly is preferred, but additional proximal outcomes that can indicate likely later success are also recommended given the importance of data-driven decisions concerning strategy modifications. This is illustrated in the case example. Third, central to the ROIO is interpretation of the effect of the implementation strategy. Whereas a typical implementation trial will typically have few strategy conditions, and for reasons of reliably determining differences in impact, the strategies inevitably have clear differences and are likely to stay relatively constant for the duration of the trial (i.e., most modifications are likely to be minor and in keeping with the a priori strategy). With the ROIO design's intentional modifications, the changes made between conditions are critical to document as they are the main factor in interpreting why a difference is observed between clusters. While there are a number of methods that have been used to track strategy modifications, we recommend a prospective, systematic, and comprehensive method such as the Longitudinal Implementation Strategies Tracking System (LISTS).[101] Last, while there is some inherent scientific value in determining which of the strategy iterations achieves the greatest impact on implementation and clinical outcomes, there is an equal or perhaps greater need to determine the strategy that balances the greatest effect for the resources needed. For this reason, economic analyses such as incremental cost-effectiveness ratios (ICERs), a summary measure representing the economic value of an implementation strategy compared with an alternative, are particularly germane. Computing ICERs requires both careful tracking and specification of the strategies (a la LISTS or some other method) and time-based, activity-driven costing measures at the discrete strategy level (described in chapter 11).

Unsurprisingly, success of a ROIO design is also facilitated by selection and inclusion of delivery systems that possess or can implement data systems capable of rapid and efficient capture of the primary and proximal implementation and clinical outcomes. As will be evident from the case study furtheer in this chapter, the electronic medical record (EMR) can be very useful when the study is conducted in a healthcare setting. Somewhat relatedly, given the underlying quality improvement goal, conducting a ROIO within a learning health system can facilitate success given that data systems and improvement processes are part of the implementation context.

HYBRID EFFECTIVENESS-IMPLEMENTATION APPROACHES

The hybrid effectiveness-implementation approach was introduced in 2012 by Curran et al.[21] The approach, which blends the stages of effectiveness and implementation research, was originally proposed as a way to potentially increase the speed of moving research findings into routine adoption. The authors argued that one did not need to wait for the "perfect" intervention effectiveness data before moving to incorporating aspects of implementation research and that it was possible to "backfill" effectiveness data while evaluating and testing implementation strategies. Further, the hybrid concept sheds light on the critical question of how health intervention outcomes might relate to level of adoption and rate of fidelity, which can only be known when we have data from "both sides," or simultaneously from effectiveness and implementation types of data. The notion to blend effectiveness and implementation research also includes consideration of "designing for dissemination,"[102] which encourages considering the "implementability"[103] of a health intervention as early as you can in its development (e.g., considering service delivery issues such as geographic context, staffing, technology, and "dose"); seeking end user and other stakeholder input and partnership before initiating effectiveness trials; and using determinant implementation frameworks in the design of components (e.g., the Consolidated Framework for Implementation Research [CFIR] framework).[104]

The language of hybrid designs requires some consistency in terminology. We use the term *health intervention* to refer to the various programs, practices, principles, procedures, products, pills, and policies (the "seven *P*'s")[2] designed to effect positive health outcomes. We use the term *implementation strategy* to refer to the support activities/tools to deliver the intervention, as either a single discrete strategy or a package of strategies delivered collectively). We use the term *effectiveness* here when referring to health intervention outcomes (e.g., symptoms/functioning or patient/community member behaviors) and the term *impact* when we describe implementation outcomes (e.g., adoption of or fidelity to an intervention at an implementer or site level).

In 2012, Curran and colleagues[21] proposed three types of hybrid approaches (called "designs" at the time) as a heuristic for what is in reality more of a continuum (see Figure 14.4). On one end of the continuum, hybrid type 1 tests health intervention effectiveness while gathering information on implementation. On the other end, hybrid type 3 tests the impact of implementation strategies while gathering information on effectiveness associated with a health intervention. Hybrid type 2 tests health intervention effectiveness while also studying the impact of strategies. This typology suggests that the emphasis on effectiveness outcomes is greatest in the first type, and the emphasis on implementation outcomes is greatest in the third type, while there is more or less equal emphasis in the middle and varying degrees represented elsewhere on the continuum.

In 2019, Landes, McBain, and Curran[105] published a manuscript with updated guidance concerning the use of hybrids and summaries of published example studies of each type. One key update surrounded the issue of randomization. The initial manuscript focused on gold

Study Characteristic	Hybrid Type I	Hybrid Type II	Hybrid Type III
Research Aims	***Primary Aim:*** Determine effectiveness of a health intervention ***Secondary Aim:*** Assess context for implementation	***Primary Aim:*** Determine effectiveness of a health intervention ***Co-Primary* Aim:*** Determine feasibility and/or (potential) impact of an implementation strategy (or strategies) *or "secondary"...	***Primary Aim:*** Determine impact of an implementation strategy (or strategies) ***Secondary Aim:*** Assess effectiveness outcomes associated with implementation of health intervention

FIGURE 14.4 Research aims by hybrid types.

Source: Adapted with permission from: Curran GM. "Research Questions and Design Considerations: Effectiveness to Implementation." Presented at the University of Wisconsin, Dissemination and Implementation Short Course Program, Madison, WI, October 2016.

standard experimental research designs where randomization was happening somewhere in each hybrid type. As it became clear that the field has embraced the hybrid design concept, many were applying it to nonrandomized evaluation approaches as well. Additionally, since hybrid approaches could include a number of different types of *research* designs (RCTs, group randomized designs, quasi-experimental designs, stepped-wedge designs, and small-scale feasibility studies), perhaps it is best to consider hybrids an "approach" to combining research efforts on interventions and implementation strategies (as we have done in this chapter).

In other updated guidance, Landes et al. offered greater distinction between hybrid types 1 and 2—namely, that hybrid type 2 designs should always have a specifically named implementation strategy (or set of strategies) being evaluated, with a hypothesis, on implementation outcomes.[9] Landes et al. also noted a key potential drawback of a type 2 design—that difficulties can arise if the implementation strategy leads to poor adoption and poor fidelity, as it could compromise the health intervention effectiveness evaluation.[106] However, utilizing implementation strategies with a relevant evidence base, identifying adoption/fidelity benchmarks, building in appropriate measurement and plans to address poor adoption and/or fidelity, and preemptively allotting time to deal with this possibility can reduce the risks of a compromised effectiveness trial. The Landes et al. paper is included in suggested readings for this chapter.

Also in 2019, Kemp et al.[107] expanded the hybrid design concept to include an additional focus on implementation context. They noted that the original hybrid types did not allow for a primary research aim of estimating and understanding the effects of context on implementation process and outcomes. Kemp et al.'s expansion includes a revised hybrid typology to accommodate *three* types of independent variables: [health] intervention, implementation strategy, and context. Their revised typology includes subtypes where any two of the three potential independent variables are simultaneously assessed and subtypes in which all three are assessed, dependent on which of the assessments are specified as primary/secondary.

In light of these updates and extensions, future studies using hybrid approaches would also do well to (1) use implementation theories/frameworks explicitly to guide key aspects of the research (e.g., implementation process, strategy development, and measurements of outcomes[108]); (2) clearly differentiate between health intervention components and implementation strategy components; and (3) fully describe the package of activities making up the implementation strategy (or strategies) under study using published terminology (e.g., Waltz et al., 2015[109]).

SPECIAL ISSUES IN DESIGN AND ANALYSIS OF D&I RESEARCH

Power and sample size calculations. The simpler tables that exist for calculating statistical power and sample size are typically not appropriate for implementation studies because of the multilevel or clustering and longitudinal nature of the data. Two online tools are often useful for these calculations, the Optimal Design (OD) system available through the W. T. Grant Foundation and the RMASS program developed by the Center for Health Statistics at the University of Chicago. Websites for both are listed at the end of this chapter.

Randomization at single versus multiple levels in D&I research. Designs that involve multiple levels of random assignment or allocation are often useful in increasing the precision of inferences. For example, to examine sustainability of a classroom-based intervention, we randomized first-grade teachers and classrooms within schools to the timing of training.[23,110] This was the primary unit of intervention for this study. To compare early versus later training in this classroom-based intervention design, we would essentially rely on the average differences within schools for classrooms that had early versus late training. However, we knew that because schools ordinarily assign students with like ability in the same classrooms, called ability tracking, classrooms within schools would typically not be well matched. Therefore, a design that tried to compare outcomes for the one or two early trained teachers in each school to those who were trained later would require introducing a large heterogeneity in classrooms unless children were matched into similar classrooms within schools. We in fact did this by random assignment of all children to a classroom as they were enrolled in the school,[111] and this design greatly increased the statistical power over a design that did not have balanced classrooms.[78,112] Such designs that use random assignment of groups at one level and random allocation of individuals into these groups can provide substantial improvement in power.

An alternative way to use randomization is to randomize units at two levels. For example, health agencies could be randomized to different implementation strategies, say to business as usual versus a new system for monitoring fidelity and providing correctives. Within each agency, clients could be randomized to a novel client-based intervention versus against standard practice. Such a two-level intervention design is known as a "split plot" and is commonly used in industrial experiments[113] but is suitable for implementation trials as well. It can be used to compare overall impact of the implementation strategy, overall effects of the client-based intervention, and their interaction. An example of such a design for implementation studies was given by Chambers.[114]

Pilot studies and estimating effect size. In developing a new implementation strategy, it is often very sensible to conduct a small-scale study to examine feasibility and assess sources of variation to determine the size one would need to have a fully powered study. While this is a useful approach, we want to convey some caution, especially with the estimation of effect sizes from a pilot study. As pointed out by Kraemer,[115] the precision of an effect size estimate from a pilot study is always lower than that in a fully powered study; consequently, considerable uncertainty in power is introduced when an estimated effect size from the pilot study is entered into power calculation programs. It is possible to use these pilot studies to get some useful information about the magnitude of different sources of variance,[22] but the intended magnitude of the effect that one is aiming to achieve should best be determined by clinical relevance, rather than the estimated value obtained from the pilot study.

There are innovative ways that can be used to fit health intervention effectiveness and implementation design components into the same study. For example, in an eHealth hybrid study delivered through primary care,[116] Prado and colleagues used an initial period prior to delivery of this program to begin enrolling families into the control condition. As this rollout design progresses with more clinics crossing into the implementation condition, families would be differentially enrolled in the new condition. Such a design would have some imbalance in condition across time, but there are sufficient numbers in both conditions at each interval of time, and analytic adjustment for time is appropriate. In particular, random effects for both time and clinic should be included in the analysis, and these random effects effectively diminish statistical power. For complex designs such as this, we recommend computing accurate power analyses using simulation methods.

Analyzing for mechanisms through mediation. A major task for D&I method development is to determine new mediation analysis methods for implementation modeling. There will be many challenging causality questions, particularly around how to best handle protocol deviations in implementation trials. One of these challenges will be to deal with the possibility of differential attrition in intervention agents (i.e., "implementers") in the study arms. For example, teachers who are successfully trained in a practice such as the Good Behavior Game (GBG), which promotes improved classroom behavior, may be less frustrated with teaching and less likely to leave the profession.[117] Such attrition differences can become manifest in a longitudinal comparison of teachers who have been trained in this intervention versus those not trained[23] and may be one explanation of persistent intervention effects.

This work also needs to incorporate innovative developments in causal inference for mediation models, that is, principal stratification (PS).[118–129] Traditional PS causal modeling characterizes subgroups that are responders to an intervention as well as nonresponders[118,121,122] and can assess the magnitude and extent of different impact that these subgroups experience. PS techniques are also closely connected to latent variable modeling and mediation analysis,[130–135] and these latent variable approaches can be used for evaluating intervention impact and examining rates of differential response across intervention conditions.[136] There is, however, a need to extend these methods to take into account repeated measures over time and multilevel modeling. As one example, Brown and colleagues have proposed developing two-level PS to account for different strata of intervention agents' (e.g., teachers') response to training. Like traditional PS, teachers could be classified into always successful managers of their classroom whether or not they received intervention training, always unsuccessful even if given training, and responders to the training. Also like PS, in implementation trials we cannot know any teacher's classification exactly since we can only observe their response to the training or no training condition. However, causal inferences for outcomes of *youth*, who are exposed to these teachers, are indeed possible in randomized trials. We have identified a class of such two-level PS models using the Georgia Gatekeeper Trial[137] and are developing and testing several approaches in implementation research.

"Scaling out" and addressing health equity. One major challenge in designing tests or evaluations of implementation strategies is that they often take a long time to conduct, analyze, and report findings. We note that virtually all implementation frameworks and models identify determinants across large, multiple dimensions, and implementation success depends on their interactions in complex ways. For example, CFIR2.0[138] emphasizes characteristics of innovations, inner context, outer context, individuals, and process. All of these domains have determinants that can affect whether or not a particular intervention (innovation) is successful or not in that context. While we have yet to develop a deep understanding of how constructs in all these domains interact to affect outcomes, there are some helpful design approaches that can help us understand conditions under which an implementation of a tested intervention (health or otherwise) is likely to work when applied to a different population or a different delivery system. We call these adaptations "scaling-out" as opposed to "scaling-up," which is focused on delivery to a population and through a system similar to that which was used to conclude the intervention as evidence based.[139] This chapter outlines a design approach to scaling out an evidence-based intervention to different populations or delivery systems that is based on a hypothesized, sequential, mediational model. It relies on Cook's five pragmatic principles for causal inference, which allows the needed design to "borrow strength" from existing studies. Cook's five principles are (1) surface or proximal similarity, (2) ruling out irrelevancies, (3) making discriminations, (4) interpolation and extrapolation, and (5) causal explanation.[140] Applying this formal method of tracking what needs to be demonstrated anew and what does not in the sequential mediational model allows us to develop an efficient design for a specific scaling out situation.

One area of scaling out that is critical for implementation science is to take the body of knowledge we do have and use it effectively to remove or at least reduce health disparities, particularly among populations that have long histories of experiencing inequities.[141] Comparatively few of the health interventions that have reached the stage of being evidence based have been tested on minoritized populations,[142] relatively few have had even surface, let alone deep, adaptation to address the needs of these communities, and even fewer have to date been tested with implementation strategies designed specifically to remedy inequities in minorities and minoritized communities.[19] There are a number of calls for implementation science to be directed toward equity as a major goal of the field.[142–144] There are also a number of research paradigms that have been identified,[145] as well as new conceptualizations of implementation frameworks,[146] that consider health equity in all its measures and strategies. We envision that the field of D&I science will fully embrace this new equity perspective and will conduct designs with measures that address systemic racism and disparities in social determinants that continue to have powerful effects on the health of vulnerable and disadvantaged populations.[145]

TAKING A SYSTEMS SCIENCE AND ENGINEERING APPROACH IN D&I RESEARCH

The term *systems science* refers to a transdisciplinary approach to understanding how interactions between elementary units produce complex patterns and to take into account the "complexity, dynamic nature, and emergent phenomena."[147] Systems science methods typically include social network analysis, agent-based modeling, and system dynamics (see chapter 13), as well as other tools such as decision analysis and systems engineering. We view these systems science methods as critical to moving implementation research forward as a science for the following reasons. First, implementation is inherently interactional, across multiple levels within systems and between systems, and only when different systems function together can we expect implementation to succeed. The systems science methods we discuss directly deal with interactions, in contrast to, say, traditional statistical modeling involving standard regression modeling, which assumes complete independence or multilevel growth modeling; his allows correlation across persons and time but does not explicitly model these processes. Second, implementation process data, which are essential in research to monitor progress, are heavily dependent on interactions between actors, as exemplified in the development of community-researcher partnerships.[81,82] Third, implementation process data also are essential for communities, organizations, and service systems themselves to provide monitoring and feedback for quality improvement. Most of today's research-level implementation process data are very expensive for these systems to collect. Consequently, we need to develop cost-effective ways to assemble quality implementation process data, conduct analyses on these data, and integrate this into a monitoring and feedback system. We fully anticipate that such systems can be built by automating these steps as much as possible. Systems science methods will need to be used for all these purposes. Below, we describe system science methods not included in chapter 13 and brief illustrations of how they can be used in implementation.

Systems engineering[148] refers to the processes of identifying and manipulating the properties of a system as a whole rather than by its component parts. Systems engineering is both a discipline and a process to guide the development, implementation, and evaluation of complex systems.[149] A system is an aggregation of components structurally organized to accomplish a set of goals or objectives. All systems have the following characteristics: a structure, interacting components, inputs and outputs, goals and objectives. Systems are dynamic in that each system component has an effect on the other components.[150]

System optimization requires design consideration of all components of a system, in contrast to a more traditional reductionist approach focusing on individual components. Attempts to design a system without considering the dynamic physical and social environments where the system operates will degrade system performance. For example, if a school-based prevention program competes for time against instruction, output would be low. *Task analysis* (TA) is one systems engineering tool used to characterize the implementation process and necessary resource and skill requirements. It was successfully applied to describe 15 complex intervention programs in the Resources for Alzheimer's Caregiver Health (REACH) program conducted by Czaja and colleagues.[151] Another system engineering tool is the *analytic hierarchy process* (AHP).[152] This can be used to capture decision-making within systems. By focusing on the decision process and establishing priorities, the AHP can identify critical attributes of an intervention and areas where an intervention might be modified or adapted.[153]

A recent contribution to this general topic is the framework for social systems informatics.[154] By examining feedback loops involving inputs, processes, outputs, and outcomes for delivering an intervention, we can identify where the system is likely to break down (e.g., if a parent is absent from certain parent-training sessions, a large part of the curriculum is missed) and what technologies can be used to aid the delivery, monitoring for fidelity and quality, and provide timely feedback.

Strategies for implementation are numerous and varied, especially when combined into complex combinations.[155–157] We have been struck by the vastly different approaches that have been used. To compare these alternatives, a full characterization of different strategies and their mechanisms of action[158] is required, and that requires the use of a standard procedure for eliciting intended implementation strategies as well as identifying where inefficiencies and other problems exist. The use of TA and the AHP and related techniques provides the ability to develop an ordering of priorities in decision-making to distinguish different implementation models in theory and practice.

Intelligent data analysis refers to advanced computational methods to automate the generation of meaning from text, video, or audio signals. These techniques can be used to reduce large amounts of process data on implementation that come in digitized form. Some implementation process data that are typically collected in agencies, such as number of people attending meetings or self-ratings of fidelity, are relatively weak indicators of the implementation process. However, other sources of information on the implementation process can be converted to analyzable data. Notably, these include audio and videotaped training as well as program delivery sessions. An example is the use of computationally generated evaluation of the fidelity of motivational interviewing in psychotherapy based on natural language processing.[159] Such information can be useful for supervision and can rapidly identify where improvements can be made. Automated signal processing and feature extraction of videotapes are also possible using intelligent data analysis, and the outcomes of such methods would help to identify specific ways to improve facilitator fidelity.

Such computational methods can be used to track implementation process via contact logs, process notes, emails, and other written communications that monitor implementation.[16,144,160] Automated generation of meaning from text is one important tool to convert information that generally requires time-consuming human judgment. By automating the processing of such information into meaningful data on the implementation process, it could lessen the monitoring burden on agencies and service providers.

The transfer of text to meaningful terms involves intelligent data analysis. Similar to psychometrics, computer science research has used latent variables via the hidden Markov model (HMM) to derive meaning from text information. In HMM, there is a time-dependent process governed by state changes and its associated state-dependent distribution, which produces observations at each step (e.g., in speech, a syllable is a state and the sound is the observation). In HMM the goal is to estimate the number of states, the state transition matrix, and the state-dependent distributions of observations.[161] A more advanced latent semantic indexing method models implicit meanings behind texts[162,163] and has been used to classify and categorize documents[164,165] (i.e., automatic groupings). A general assumption is that the documents come from a set of unknown categories and the words and phrases appearing in the documents are produced by category-dependent distributions. Given a set of observed data, these methods explain document generation and word/phrase generation using iterative optimization. We note that completely automated systems for converting text to meaning are not likely to succeed by themselves but require some human coding (i.e., supervised learning). Also, intelligent data analysis provides a probability assessment of this correct classification. Thus we can differentiate texts that are clearly classified and texts that may be incorrectly classified. By human examination of these texts, we can concentrate the high-cost human interaction on those messages that have uncertain classification, greatly limiting the cost involved in producing valid implementation process data.

TWO CONFIGURATIONAL APPROACHES IN D&I: COINCIDENCE ANALYSIS AND THE MATRIXED MULTIPLE CASE STUDY METHOD

Implementation science typically involves complex phenomena, where outcomes arise from several conditions working together rather than due to a single variable operating alone. Implementation outcomes likewise tend to be context dependent: What works for large urban hospitals, for example, may systematically differ from what works for small rural hospitals.

Configurational analysis[166] is a relatively new approach within implementation science that explicitly embraces this complexity, allowing implementation scientists to identify deep patterns within their data-linking conditions with outcomes that might otherwise go undetected. Configurational approaches apply formal logic, Boolean algebra, set theory and systematic observation to explain complex implementation-related phenomena, including what works for whom under what conditions. Using configurational analysis, researchers and evaluators can identify bundles of conditions that *together* yield an outcome of interest, as well as identify when *multiple* paths lead to the same outcome.

The analytic objective of configurational analysis is to identify necessary and sufficient conditions, a fundamentally different search target than that of correlation-based methods. Because it employs Boolean rather than linear algebra, configurational analysis does not require large sample sizes, and an often-cited strength of configurational analysis is its versatility with small *n* studies. As a case-based approach, configurational analysis retains persistent links to individual cases, making it possible to return to original cases at any time throughout the analysis in order to contextualize findings with greater depth and nuance; cases can take on a wide range of values, including individuals, groups, departments, facilities, or organizations. As part of the larger repertoire of mixed-methods approaches, configurational analysis offers implementation science a dynamic and systematic way to account for both complexity and context.

Coincidence Analysis

Coincidence analysis is a mathematical, cross-case approach that algorithmically searches for a "minimal theory," a crucial set of difference-making combinations that is redundancy free and uniquely distinguishes one group of cases from another.[167] Implemented in the R package "cna,"[168] coincidence analysis operates within a regularity framework and applies Boolean algebra and formal logic to identify specific bundles of conditions that distinguish cases that have an outcome of interest from those that do not. Coincidence analysis has the additional capacity to identify causal chains, where a set of initial conditions leads to an intermediary outcome, which in turn combines with additional conditions to yield a final outcome. Data used in coincidence analyses can be dichotomous, multivalue, or fuzzy.

Coincidence analysis has appeared across a wide variety of health-related implementation contexts in the published literature. In a 2020 study, for example, implementation researchers applied coincidence analysis to determine the key subset of implementation strategies directly linked to implementation success across a national sample of 80 Veterans Affairs (VA) medical centers.[169] Instead of analyzing each of the 70 implementation strategies separately, Yakovchenko et al. applied coincidence analysis to consider all possible one-, two-, three-, and four-strategy combinations instantiated in the data set and found that just five strategy configurations distinguished higher-performing VA medical centers from lower-performing sites with 100% consistency.[169]

In another 2020 study, Whitaker et al. applied coincidence analysis to a publicly available data set from Sweden with county-level data on catch-up vaccination uptake in Sweden among fifth- and sixth-grade girls and then compared results to the published regression findings and discovered an entirely new solution pathway not previously identified.[166] In a third example, Miech et al. examined facility-level conditions across a national sample of 102 VA medical centers and found five distinct pathways leading to higher reach in weight-management outcomes, with three of the pathways dependent on the size and complexity of the medical center.[170]

The Matrixed Multiple Case Study Method

The matrixed multiple case study (MMCS) method is a mixed quantitative-qualitative configurational analytical approach that focuses on understanding how and why an implementation strategy works, beyond determining whether it works. MMCS can be used to systematically investigate how sites respond similarly and/or differently to one or more implementation strategies to help identify generalizable principles regarding factors associated with success of those strategies in implementing a health intervention.

The MMCS method was originally conceptualized, developed, and applied in the context of a multisite trial[172] that tested the implementation of interdisciplinary team-based care at nine US Department of Veterans Affairs general mental health clinics, aligning teams to the evidence-based collaborative chronic care model (CCM). CCMs have been extensively tested and found to be effective for medical conditions and depression treated in the primary care setting[173,174] and also for chronic mental health conditions treated in mental health clinics.[175,176] MMCS sought to answer the following research questions: (1) How were the nine sites similar or different in their CCM implementation? (2) What contextual factors were associated with CCM implementation success, in what ways, and under what circumstances? In this work that involved nine sites and an interdisciplinary team of approximately seven staff members per site, conducting MMCS identified the types of sites at which influencing factors (i.e., factors influencing successful implementation) were more or less applicable.[171] For instance, the CCM's difference from current practice contributed to successful CCM implementation at sites where the clinic staff were desiring an improvement to their non-team-based practice, yet hindered implementation success at sites where the clinic staff were not desiring a move away from their established practice.

Then MMCS method arranges data into an array of matrices (Figure 14.5) that can be easily sorted and filtered to test hypothesized patterns (e.g., sites with stronger organizational leadership support implement the health intervention more successfully) and/or identify less expected patterns (e.g., clinic size affects implementation success only when there are no established communication mechanisms between different clinic workgroups). MMCS comprises nine distinct steps, from establishing the research goal to conducting cross-site analysis of matrixed data. Completion of the MMCS steps results in identifying associations between specific influencing factors (and/or their combinations) and the extent of implementation success. Kim et al.[171] provided further detail on the steps and their application to the multisite CCM implementation study mentioned above.

Configurational analytical methods allow identification of combinations of conditions that align to successful implementation. As the number of cases being studied grows, cross-case analysis to identify meaningful combinations becomes difficult without computational algorithms (e.g., Boolean-based algorithms for coincidence analysis). As described above, MMCS provides a formalized sequence of steps leading up to cross-case analysis, such as for specifying the research question, defining "success," identifying potential influences (conditions), and determining the procedure(s) to use for assigning values to conditions and extents of success (e.g., high vs. low). MMCS also proposes a concrete sortable data structure (matrix) that organizes the information/knowledge to be used for cross-case analysis. Hence, the systematized steps of MMCS (often team based and interpretive, e.g., reaching consensus on the strength of a condition's influence based on qualitative analysis of stakeholder interview data) and proposed data structure are applicable for both computational algorithmic methods (e.g., coincidence analysis) and other approaches to cross-case analysis that identify combinations of implementation strategies and contextual factors associated with varying extents of implementation success. The MMCS methodical steps can encourage enhanced rigor and consistency across how different studies approach cross-case analysis, improving comparability across the studies and their findings to build generalizable knowledge for the field of implementation science.

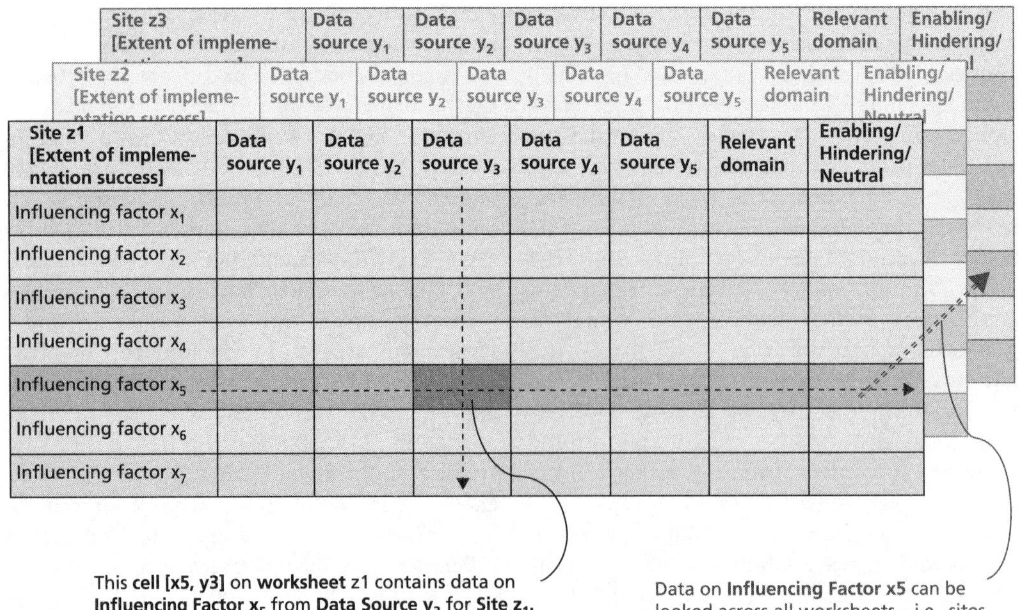

FIGURE 14.5 Matrixed organization of multisite data.

Source: Adapted with permission from: Kim B, Sullivan JL, Ritchie MJ, et al. Comparing variations in implementation processes and influences across multiple sites: what works, for whom, and how? *Psychiatry Res.* 2020;283:112520. doi:10.1016/j.psychres.2019.112520

CASE STUDY: IMPLEMENTATION OF THE CLINICAL PRACTICE GUIDELINES FOR PEDIATRIC HYPERTENSION IN COMMUNITY-BASED PRIMARY CARE USING A RANDOMIZED ROIO DESIGN

Background. Target organ damage, especially left ventricular hypertrophy, which is associated with heightened risk for cardiovascular events in adults, is detectable in children and adolescents with hypertension[177,178] and has been shown to begin in childhood.[177,179] Treating pediatric hypertension (pHTN) would result in lower risk for target organ damage and hypertension-related cardiovascular disease later in life,[180] but the diagnosis is often missed and may not follow the current guidelines released in 2017[180] due to the complexity of measuring blood pressure (BP), interpreting pediatric BP standards, and variable clinician familiarity with treatment.[181,182] Adhering to the pHTN guidelines has been shown to improve identification of youth that will go on to have hypertension as adults.[179,183] A study by Smith's research team using data from eight community health centers in Chicago found that, among 6,233 children aged 3 to 18 years with one or more abnormal BP measurements in a 12-month period, only 14.8% who met diagnostic criteria for either elevated BP (N = 6,178) or primary pHTN (N = 55) were diagnosed, and of those with pHTN, only 13% had guideline-adherent follow-up care.[184] Thus, there is a pressing need to identify effective strategies to ensure implementation of the pHTN guidelines, particularly in primary healthcare systems that serve youth at greatest risk due to social and economic disadvantage and health disparities that underlie pHTN.[185–187]

Context. This study (currently still proposed) would enroll pediatric and family medicine clinic sites within a national health center–controlled network of community health centers that share a common infrastructure for health information technology (HIT), research, and practice transformation. Over the past 2 years, our team[188] has leveraged the Expert Recommendations for Implementing Change (ERIC) protocol[157,189] to deeply engage pediatricians, nurses, medical assistants, and patients/caregivers from our partner community health centers to develop a multilevel implementation intervention to support pHTN guideline adherence. Stakeholders drove the identification of barriers and facilitators to pHTN guideline adherence and the selection of strategies to overcome them, and they then went through a process to prioritize strategies across three tiers characterized by likely impact on the implementation and feasibility considerations.[190] The implementation strategy leverages shared HIT capabilities and infrastructure and incorporates multiple discrete evidence-based strategies[191,192] used to implement HIT tools into clinical workflows: stakeholder involvement, readiness planning, training, and ongoing audit and feedback.[25] The team used the implementation research logic model (IRLM)[193] to ensure conceptual alignment between determinants and strategies for achieving specific primary and secondary implementation outcomes.

Design. The trial proposes using the ROIO design[100] to test whether the components of the implementation strategy improve adherence to clinical practice guidelines for pHTN diagnosis and treatment. Twenty-four pediatric and family medicine clinics that provide care for youth ages 3 to 17 years (the target age range of the pHTN guidelines) would be recruited and randomized using covariate-adjusted randomization to one of four clusters of six clinics each. Training and educational strategies would precede activating HIT tools in the EMR, audit and feedback strategies, and others in the package. Data for optimization of the strategy (described in next section) would be collected for approximately 5 months, which is followed by a period of intensive mixed-methods analysis and engagement of stakeholders to interpret the findings and modify strategies through a process of pruning ineffective or infeasible strategies; modifying strategies (changes to the dose, actor, actions, etc.); and offering suggestions for strategy additions to address unexpected barriers. Implementation continues in the first cluster of clinics with few modifications, and the revised implementation strategy is introduced to the second cluster of clinics. This process is repeated for the third and then fourth clusters.

Measurement and analytic framework. Central to the ROIO design is stakeholder-driven mixed-methods analysis. EMR measures include guideline-adherent pHTN diagnosis and proximal indicators to obtain data to inform optimization early in each cluster (e.g., when BP equals the 95th percentile or greater, a follow-up visit occurs within 2–4 weeks). Interviews or focus groups with implementing pediatric clinicians and operational and clinical leadership focus on the impact of each discrete strategy on the hypothesized outcomes as specified in the IRLM. Triangulation of data, interpreted by stakeholders and the study team, determines the strategy modifications for the next cluster.

The analysis strategy to determine the optimal strategy package involves four complementary methods: (1) nonparametric Kruskal-Wallis tests comparing time to criterion of a single cluster to another cluster or to all other clusters combined; (2) nonlinear growth curves with mixed-effects modeling based on binomial proportions that use random effects to account for heterogeneity in the initial starting rate and growth trajectory in the sites over time; (3) growth mixture models (GMMs)[67,194,195] to examine heterogeneity in the response of sites over time that is not accounted for by routine mixed-effects modeling (key to inferring that change in outcomes occurred as a result of strategy optimization); and (4) incremental cost-effectiveness analyses to assess the incremental economic benefit associated with each subsequent cluster (2 vs. 1, 3 vs. 2, 4 vs. 3), as each cluster may entail additional discrete strategies or modifications to strategies used in the prior cluster to increase intensity or improve efficiency. In this type of cost-effectiveness analysis, the difference in mean costs between two or more strategies is compared with the difference in mean effectiveness of the same strategies. If one strategy is both less costly and more effective, then that strategy will be "dominant." If neither strategy is dominant, the trade-off between cost and effectiveness must be calculated via an ICER, where ICER = $(\text{cost}_{\text{Strategy J}} - \text{cost}_{\text{Strategy J-1}})/(\text{effectiveness}_{\text{Strategy J}} - \text{effectiveness}_{\text{Strategy J-1}})$, *cost* is the implementation cost per 100 children (because clinics are of different sizes), and *effectiveness* is the percentage improvement in guideline-adherent pHTN diagnosis rate. We will estimate the precision of the analysis using the bootstrapping approach.[196]

Finally, accurate measurement of the implementation strategies in each cluster is critical for valid costing of each strategy and for interpreting the strategy differences between clusters. This still will use the LISTS.[101] As LISTS collects data on the personnel who enact each discrete strategy and the amount of time required, the data can be easily transformed into a time-driven, activity-based costing approach.[197] To facilitate processing of qualitative data sources in a timely manner, we will employ framework-guided rapid qualitative analysis using a structured template based on the IRLM already developed by the study team.[198]

SUMMARY

A wide variety of D&I research designs are now being used to evaluate and improve health systems and outcomes. This chapter discusses research questions in D&I, methods for implementation preparation, and randomized and nonrandomized designs for the traditional translational research continuum or pipeline, which builds on existing efficacy and effectiveness trials to examine how one or more health interventions are adopted, scaled up, and sustained in community or service delivery systems. The chapter also considers other designs, including hybrid approaches that combine effectiveness and implementation research and designs that use simulation modeling and configurational analysis. A case example of a novel large scale ROIO implementation study is also presented. The chapter also provides suggested readings and websites useful for design decisions.

SUGGESTED READINGS AND WEBSITES

Readings

Anderson DE, Vennix JAM, Richardson GP, Rouwette EAJA. Group model building: problem structuring, policy simulation and decision support. *J Oper Res Soc.* 2007;58(5):691–694.

This article was written by some of the key founders of GMB. It provides an overview of the intentions and methods behind GMB; the interrelationship between simulation models and the modeling process; similarities and distinctions with five other problem-structuring methods; and a brief history of GMB. The authors share their thoughts on how GMB aims to avoid participatory problem-solving processes being just an"add-on" to system dynamics modeling. They call for more effectiveness studies and dialogue between other problem-solving methods.

Brown CH, Curran G, Palinkas LA, et al. An overview of research and evaluation designs for dissemination and implementation. *Annu Rev Public Health.* 2017;38(1):1–22.

This article provides an overview of state-of-the-science experimental and quasi-experimental research designs for D&I. Three broad categories are discussed: (1) within-site designs; (2) between-site designs; and (3) within- and between-site comparison designs.

Hwang S, Birken SA, Melvin CL, Rohweder CL, Smith JD. Designs and methods for implementation research: advancing the mission of the CTSA program. *J Clin Transl Sci.* 2020;4(3):159–167. Epub March 4, 2020. doi:10.1017/cts.2020.16

This article provides an overview of research designs and methods for implementation science situated within the aims of the NIH's Clinical and Translational Science Awards (CTSAs) for rapid translation of new discovery from bench to bedside to community impact and population health.

Kim B, Sullivan JL, Ritchie MJ, et al. Comparing variations in implementation processes and influences across multiple sites: what works, for whom, and how? Psychiatry Res. 2020;283:112520. doi:10.1016/j.psychres.2019.112520

This article outlines the MMCS method, which allows for understanding how implementation processes and contextual influences similarly or differently interact with outcomes across multiple sites at which an evidence-based practice is implemented. An example of applying MMCS is provided using data from a multisite trial that tested the implementation of the evidence-based CCM at nine US Department of Veterans Affairs medical centers.

Landes SJ, McBain SA, Curran GM. An introduction to effectiveness-implementation hybrid designs. Psychiatry Res. 2019 Oct;280:112513. Epub 2019 Aug 9. PMID: 31434011; PMCID: PMC6779135. doi:10.1016/ j.psychres.2019.112513

This article presents the concept of hybrid designs that are especially appropriate for implementation research and discusses the three basic types of such designs. Included as well are updates and new recommendations associated with the types since the original publication in 2012.

Reichardt C, Mark M. Quasi-experimentation. In: Wholey J, Hatry H, Newcomer K, eds. *Handbook of Practical Program Evaluation.* Jossey-Bass Inc.; 2004:126–149.

In this chapter, Reichardt and Mark consider four quasi-experimental designs: before-after, interrupted time series, nonequivalent group, and regression-discontinuity. They describe the strengths and weaknesses of each design, as well as threats to validity.

Smith JD, Li DH, Rafferty MR. The implementation research logic model: a method for planning, executing, reporting, and synthesizing implementation projects. *Implement Sci.* 2020;15(1):84. doi: 10.1186/s13012-020-01041-8

This article provides an implementation research-specific logic model that can be used to plan, execute, report, and synthesize implementation projects. A number of variations are provided for specific research designs and the principles-driven approach to its use encourages users to adapt the model to fit their research design and implementation project.

Vennix, Jac AM. *Group Model Building.* John Wiley & Sons: Chichester; 1996.

This book offers a comprehensive guide to the theory, practical motivations, and early methods behind GMB. Case studies and practical guidance for facilitation sessions and using scripts are presented. It is authored by one of the founders of this methodology.

West SG, Duan N, Pequegnat W, et al. Alternatives to the randomized controlled trial. *Am J Public Health.* 2008;98(8):1359–1366.

The authors consider alternatives to the randomized controlled trial that also allow for drawing causal inferences. They describe the strengths and weaknesses of each design, including threats to validity and the strategies that can be used to diminish those threats.

Wolfenden L, Foy R, Presseau J, et al. Designing and undertaking randomised implementation trials: guide for researchers. BMJ. 2021;372:m3721. doi:10.1136/bmj.m3721

This article provides guidance to researchers on developing, conducting, and reporting randomized trials that test implementation strategies. Authored by an international group of researchers, current limitations of randomized implementation trials are thoroughly outlined. In an effort to address these limitations, topics discussed include aims articulation, recruitment/retention strategies, design selection, theories/frameworks usage, measures, sample size, ethical considerations, and reporting of findings.

Selected Websites and Tools

https://wtgrantfoundation.org/resource/optimal-design-with-empirical-information-od

https://www.healthstats.org/index.php/our-work/

Center for Prevention Implementation Methodology for Drug Abuse and HIV (CePIM). http://cepim.northwestern.edu

*The Center for Prevention Implementation Methodology for Drug Abuse and HIV (Ce-PIM) website provides a range of publications and presentations on implementation principles, measures, designs, and analyses. A central resource on the Ce-PIM website is the Prevention Science and Methodology Group (PSMG) (*https://cepim.north

western.edu/psmg*), which hosts weekly virtual grand rounds during the academic year and curates an online repository of past presentations on implementation science methodology and other related topics. Resources for the implementation research logic model (IRLM; Smith, Li, & Rafferty, 2020, Implement Sci.) are also available on the Ce-PIM website (*https://cepim.northwestern.edu/implementationresearchlogicmodel*).*

Cochrane Effective Practice and Organization of Care (EPOC) Group. http://epoc.cochrane.org/
The Cochrane Effective Practice and Organization of Care (EPOC) Group is a review group of the Cochrane Collaboration—an international network of people helping healthcare providers, policymakers, patients, and their advocates and carers—make well-informed decisions about human healthcare by preparing and publishing systematic reviews. The research focus of the EPOC Group are interventions designed to improve the delivery, practice, and organization of healthcare services. The EPOC editorial base is located in Ottawa, Canada, with satellite centers in Norway, Australia, and England.

Implementation Science Webinar Series. https://cyberseminar.cancercontrolplanet.org/implementationscience/
The Implementation Science Webinar Series is sponsored by the National Cancer Institute (NCI) Division of Cancer Control and Population Sciences. In 2013, the Implementation Science team started a webinar series focused on advanced dissemination and implementation research topics, including design and analysis issues. *Each session includes approximately 40 minutes for presentation(s) by leaders in the field as well as 20 minutes for engaged discussion and Q&A. The website lists topics and session titles for upcoming sessions or archived sessions.*

Modeling to Learn (MTL). https://github.com/lzim/mtl
Modeling to Learn (MTL) is open-access science. This github-based website makes MTL content readily available, including MTL html code, MTL's manual, content for the 12-session quality improvement initiative, and the full instruments being used in ongoing randomized controlled trials. Numerous resources for learning more about MTL are also available, including a demonstration model, references, and team members' stories.

Optimal Design. http://www.wtgrantfoundation.org/resources/overview/research_tools/
Optimal Design is a software package, developed by Stephen Raudenbush and colleagues, that helps researchers determine sample size, statistical power, and optimal allocation of resources for multilevel and longitudinal studies. This includes group-randomized trials, also called setting-level experiments. Version 2.0 was released in summer 2009. The software, a description of the updates from the previous version, and a manual containing software documentation are available for download.

RMASS. http://www.healthstats.org/rmass/
The RMASS program computes sample size for three-level, mixed-effects, linear regression models for the analysis of clustered longitudinal data. Three-level designs are used in many areas, but in particular multicenter randomized longitudinal clinical trials in medical or health-related research. In this case, level 1 represents measurement occasion, level 2 represents subject, and level 3 represents center. The model allows for random effects of the time trends at both the subject level and the center level. The sample size determinations in this program are based on the requirements for a test of treatment by time interaction(s) for designs based on either subject-level or cluster-level randomization. The approach is general with respect to sampling proportions and number of groups, and it allows for differential attrition rates over time.

Scriptapedia. https://en.wikibooks.org/wiki/Scriptapedia
Scriptapedia is a compendium of GMB scripts or "structured small group exercises." It is maintained through a wikibook in order to be open access and edited by diverse practitioners to refine and develop scripts and to advance practice through "discussion of what works and what doesn't, and internationalization of group model building practice."

REFERENCES

1. National Research Council and Institute of Medicine, Committee on Prevention of Mental Disorders and Substance Abuse Among Children Youth and Young Adults: Research Advances and Promising Interventions; Mary Ellen O'Connell, Thomas Boat, Warner KE, Board on Children Y, and Families, Division of Behavioral and Social Sciences and Education, eds. *Preventing mental, emotional, and behavioral disorders among young people: progress and possibilities.* Washington, DC: National Academy Press; 2009.
2. Brown CH, Curran G, Palinkas LA, et al. An overview of research and evaluation designs for dissemination and implementation. *Annu Rev Public Health.* 2017;38(1):1–22.
3. Aarons GA, Hurlburt M, Horwitz SM. Advancing a conceptual model of evidence-based practice implementation in public service sectors. *Adm Policy Ment Health.* 2011;38(1):4–23.

4. Zerhouni E. The NIH roadmap. *Science(Washington)*. 2003;302(5642):63–72.
5. Zerhouni E. Translational and clinical science—time for a new vision. *N Engl J Med*. 2005;353(15):1621.
6. Culliton B. Extracting knowledge from science: a conversation with Elias Zerhouni. *Health Aff*. 2006;25(3):w94.
7. Westfall J, Mold J, Fagnan L. Practice-based research—"Blue Highways" on the NIH Roadmap. *JAMA*. 2007;297(4):403.
8. Spoth R, Rohrbach LA, Greenberg M, et al. Addressing core challenges for the next generation of type 2 translation research and systems: the translation science to population impact (TSci impact) framework. *Prev Sci*. 2013;14(4):319–351.
9. Proctor E, Silmere H, Raghavan R, et al. Outcomes for implementation research: conceptual distinctions, measurement challenges, and research agenda. *Adm Policy Ment Health*. 2011;38(2):65–76.
10. Institute of Medicine Committee on Crossing the Quality Chasm: Adaptation to Mental Health and Addictive Disorders. *Improving the Quality of Health Care for Mental and Substance-Use Conditions*. National Academy Press; 2006.
11. Gaglio B, Shoup JA, Glasgow RE. The RE-AIM framework: a systematic review of use over time. *Am J Public Health*. 2013;103(6):e38–e46.
12. Shelton RC, Chambers DA, Glasgow RE. An extension of RE-AIM to enhance sustainability: addressing dynamic context and promoting health equity over time. *Front Public Health*. 2020;8:134.
13. Smith J, Polaha J. Using implementation science to guide the integration of evidence-based family interventions into primary care. *Fam Syst Health*. 2017;35(2):125–135.
14. Chamberlain P, Brown CH, Saldana L. Observational measure of implementation progress in community based settings: the stages of implementation completion (SIC). *ImplementSci*. 2011;6(1):116.
15. Brown CH, Chamberlain P, Saldana L, Wang W, Padgett C, Cruden G. Evaluation of two implementation strategies in fifty-one counties in two states: results of a cluster randomized implementation trial. *Implement Sci*. 2015;9:134.
16. Wang D, Ogihara M, Gallo C, et al. Automatic classification of communication logs into implementation stages via text analysis. *Implement Sci*. 2016;11(1):119.
17. Wang W, Saldana L, Brown CH, Chamberlain P. Factors that influenced county system leaders to implement an evidence-based program: a baseline survey within a randomized controlled trial. *Implement Sci*. 2010;5(1):72.
18. Smith JD, Hasan M. Quantitative approaches for the evaluation of implementation research studies. *Psychiatry Res*. 2020;283:112521.
19. Smith JD, Li DH, Hirschhorn LR, et al. Landscape of HIV implementation research funded by the National Institutes of Health: a mapping review of project abstracts. *AIDS Behav*. 2020;24(6):1903–1911.
20. Glasgow RE, Klesges LM, Dzewaltowski DA, Estabrooks PA, Vogt TM. Evaluating the impact of health promotion programs: using the RE-AIM framework to form summary measures for decision making involving complex issues. *Health Educ Res*. 2006;21(5):688–694.
21. Curran GM, Bauer M, Mittman B, Pyne JM, Stetler C. Effectiveness-implementation hybrid designs: combining elements of clinical effectiveness and implementation research to enhance public health impact. *Med Care*. 2012;50(3):217.
22. Brown CH, Ten Have TR, Jo B, et al. Adaptive designs for randomized trials in public health. *Annu Rev Public Health*. 2009;30:1–25.
23. Poduska J, Kellam S, Brown C, et al. Study protocol for a group randomized controlled trial of a classroom-based intervention aimed at preventing early risk factors for drug abuse: integrating effectiveness and implementation research. *Implement Sci*. 2009;4(1):56.
24. Dixon LB, Goldman HH, Bennett ME, et al. Implementing coordinated specialty care for early psychosis: the RAISE Connection Program. *Psych Serv*. 2015;66(7):691–698.
25. Kane JM, Robinson DG, Schooler NR, et al. Comprehensive versus usual community care for first-episode psychosis: 2-year outcomes from the NIMH RAISE early treatment program. *Am J Psychiatry*. 2015;173(4):362–372.
26. Holtgrave DR. *Handbook of Economic Evaluation of HIV Prevention Programs*. Springer Science & Business Media; 1998.
27. Baltussen R, Niessen L. Priority setting of health interventions: the need for multi-criteria decision analysis. *Cost Effect Resour Alloc*. 2006;4(1):14.
28. Alonso-Coello P, Schünemann HJ, Moberg J, et al. GRADE evidence to decision (EtD) frameworks: a systematic and transparent approach to making well informed healthcare choices. 1: Introduction. *BMJ*. 2016;353:i2016.
29. Haddix AC, Teutsch SM, Corso PS. *Prevention Effectiveness: A Guide to Decision Analysis and Economic Evaluation*. Oxford University Press; 2003.
30. Yaylali E, Farnham PG, Schneider KL, et al. From theory to practice: implementation of a resource allocation model in health departments. *J Public Health Manag*. 2016;22(6):567.

31. Sterman J. *Business Dynamics, Systems Thinking and Modeling for a Complex World.* McGraw-Hill, Inc.; 2000.
32. Lich KH, Ginexi EM, Osgood ND, Mabry PL. A call to address complexity in prevention science research. *Prev Sci.* 2013;14(3):279–289.
33. Northridge ME, Metcalf SS. Enhancing implementation science by applying best principles of systems science. *Health Res Policy Syst.* 2016;14(1):74.
34. Lich KH, Frerichs L, Fishbein D, Bobashev G, Pentz MA. Translating research into prevention of high-risk behaviors in the presence of complex systems: definitions and systems frameworks. *Transl Behav Med.* 2016;6(1):17–31.
35. Weiss CH, Poncela-Casasnovas J, Glaser JI, et al. Adoption of a high-impact innovation in a homogeneous population. *Phys Rev X.* 2014;4(4):041008.
36. Liljeros F, Edling CR, Amaral LAN, Stanley HE, Åberg Y. The web of human sexual contacts. *Nature.* 2001;411(6840):907–908.
37. Andersen DF, Vennix JAM, Richardson GP, Rouwette EAJA. Group model building: problem structuring, policy simulation and decision support. *J Oper Res Soc.* 2007;58(5):691–694.
38. Vennix JAM. *Group Model Building: Facilitating Team Learning Using System Dynamics.* John Wiley; 1996.
39. Hovmand P, Rouwette E, Andersen D, et al. Scriptapedia: a handbook of scripts for developing structured group model building sessions. *Soc Sci Med.* 2011.
40. Frerichs L, Lich KH, Funchess M, et al. Applying critical race theory to group model building methods to address community violence. *Prog Community Health Partnersh.* 2016;10(3):443–459.
41. Frerichs L, Smith N, Kuhlberg JA, et al. Novel participatory methods for co-building an agent-based model of physical activity with youth. *PLoS One.* 2020;15(11):e0241108.
42. Cruden G, Frerichs L, Lanier P, Powell BJ, Brown CH, Hassmiller Lich K. Supporting the selection of evidence based interventions to prevent child neglect for community implementation. Paper presented at: International Conference of the System Dynamics Society; July 2019; Albuquerque, NM.
43. Zimmerman L, Lounsbury DW, Rosen CS, Kimerling R, Trafton JA, Lindley SE. Participatory system dynamics modeling: increasing stakeholder engagement and precision to improve implementation planning in systems. *Adm Policy Ment Health.* 2016;43(6):834–849.
44. Rouwette EAJA, Vennix JAM, Mullekom Tv. Group model building effectiveness: a review of assessment studies. *Syst Dynam Rev.* 2002;18(1):5–45.
45. Zimmerman LE. The how and why of Modeling to Learn: participatory system dynamics to improve evidence-based addiction and mental health care. Paper presented at: Prevention Science and Methodology Group PSMG: Implementation and Systems Science Series; October 12, 2021; Northwestern University, Chicago.
46. Sheldrick RC, Cruden G, Schaefer AJ, Mackie TI. Rapid-cycle systems modeling to support evidence-informed decision-making during system-wide implementation. *Implement Sci Commun.* 2021;2(1):116.
47. Barnett ML, Sheldrick RC, Liu SR, Kia-Keating M, Negriff S. Implications of adverse childhood experiences screening on behavioral health services: a scoping review and systems modeling analysis. *Am Psychol.* 2021;76(2):364–378.
48. Vermeer WH, Smith JD, Wilensky U, Brown CH. High-fidelity agent-based modeling to support prevention decision-making: an open science approach. *Prev Sci.* 2022;23:832–843.
49. El-Bassel N, Gilbert L, Hunt T, et al. Using community engagement to implement evidence-based practices for opioid use disorder: a data-driven paradigm & systems science approach. *Drug Alcohol Depend.* 2021;222:108675.
50. Vermeer W, Benbow N. Ending the HIV epidemic in Chicago: evidence from high-fidelity local agent-based model. Prevention Science and Methodology Virtual Grand Rounds Series; September 22, 2020; Northwestern University, Chicago.
51. Gold MR, Siegel JE, Russell LB, Weinstein MC, eds. *Cost-Effectiveness in Health and Medicine.* New York: Oxford University Press; 1996.
52. Frazier AL, Colditz GA, Fuchs CS, Kuntz KM. Cost-effectiveness of screening for colorectal cancer in the general population. *JAMA.* 2000;284(15):1954.
53. Gaspoz JM, Coxson PG, Goldman PA, et al. Cost effectiveness of aspirin, clopidogrel, or both for secondary prevention of coronary heart disease. *N Eng J Med.* 2002;346(23):1800.
54. Goldhaber-Fiebert JD, Stout NK, Salomon JA, Kuntz KM, Goldie SJ. Cost-effectiveness of cervical cancer screening with human papillomavirus DNA testing and HPV-16, 18 vaccination. *J Natl Cancer Inst.* 2008;100(5):308.
55. CDC Diabetes Cost-effectiveness Group. Cost-effectiveness of intensive glycemic control, intensified hypertension control, and serum cholesterol level reduction for type 2 diabetes. *JAMA.* 2002;287(19):2542–2551.

56. Sanders GD, Bayoumi AM, Sundaram V, et al. Cost-effectiveness of screening for HIV in the era of highly active antiretroviral therapy. *N Engl J Med.* 2005;352(6):570.
57. Tosteson ANA, Stout NK, Fryback DG, et al. Cost-effectiveness of digital mammography breast cancer screening. *Ann Intern Med.* 2008;148(1):1.
58. Ruiz MS. *No Time to Lose: Getting More From HIV Prevention.* National Academies Press; 2001.
59. Goldhaber-Fiebert JD, Snowden LR, Wulczyn F, Landsverk J, Horwitz SM. Economic evaluation research in the context of child welfare policy: a structured literature review and recommendations. *Child Abuse Negl.* 2011;35(9):722–740.
60. Price JM, Chamberlain P, Landsverk J, Reid J. KEEP foster parent training intervention: model description and effectiveness. *Child Fam Soc Work.* 2009;14(2):233–242.
61. Price J, Chamberlain P, Landsverk J, Reid J, Leve L, Laurent H. Effects of a foster parent training intervention on placement changes of children in foster care. *Child Maltreat.* 2008;13(1):64.
62. Chamberlain P, Price J, Reid J, Landsverk J. Cascading implementation of a foster and kinship parent intervention. *Child Welfare.* 2008;87(5):27–48.
63. Jenness SM, Goodreau SM, Rosenberg E, et al. Impact of the Centers for Disease Control's HIV preexposure prophylaxis guidelines for men who have sex with men in the United States. *J Infect Dis.* 2016;214(12):1800–1807.
64. Beck EC, Birkett M, Armbruster B, Mustanski B. A data-driven simulation of HIV spread among young men who have sex with men: the role of age and race mixing, and STIs. *J Acq Immun Def Synd.* 2015;70(2):186.
65. Friedman LM, Furberg C, DeMets DL. *Fundamentals of Clinical Trials.* 3rd ed. Springer; 1998.
66. Torgerson D, Torgerson C. Designing randomised trials in health, education, and the social sciences: An introduction. Palgrave Macmillan; 2008.
67. Brown CH, Wang W, Kellam SG, et al. Methods for testing theory and evaluating impact in randomized field trials: intent-to-treat analyses for integrating the perspectives of person, place, and time. *Drug Alcohol Depend.* 2008;95(suppl 1):S74–S104; Supplementary data associated with this article can be found, in the online version, at doi:110.1016/j.drugalcdep.2008.1001.1005
68. Murray DM. *Design and Analysis of Group-Randomized Trials.* Vol. 29: Oxford University Press; 1998.
69. Flay B. Efficacy and effectiveness trials (and other phases of research) in the development of health promotion programs. *Prev Med.* 1986;15(5):451–474.
70. Glasgow R, Magid D, Beck A, Ritzwoller D, Estabrooks P. Practical clinical trials for translating research to practice: design and measurement recommendations. *Med Care.* 2005;43(6):551.
71. Wyman PA, Henry D, Knoblauch S, Brown CH. Designs for testing group-based interventions with limited numbers of social units: the dynamic wait-listed and regression point displacement designs. *Prev Sci.* 2015;16(7):956–966.
72. Brown CH, Wyman PA, Guo J, Peña J. Dynamic wait-listed designs for randomized trials: new designs for prevention of youth suicide. *Clin Trials.* 2006;3(3):259–271.
73. Mercer SL, DeVinney BJ, Fine LJ, Green LW, Dougherty D. Study designs for effectiveness and translation research: identifying trade-offs. *Am J Prev Med.* 2007;33(2):139–154.
74. White H, Sabarwal S. *Quasi-experimental Design and Methods.* UNICEF Office of Research; 2014.
75. Hong G. Marginal mean weighting through stratification: adjustment for selection bias in multilevel data. *J Educ Behav Stat.* 2010;35(5):499–531.
76. Effective Practice and Organisation of Care (EPOC). EPOC resources for review authors. 2015. http://epoc.cochrane.org/epoc-specific-resources-review-authors
77. Smith JD. Single-case experimental designs: a systematic review of published research and current standards. *Psychol Methods.* 2012;17(4):510.
78. Brown CH, Liao J. Principles for designing randomized preventive trials in mental health: an emerging developmental epidemiology paradigm. *Am J Commun Psychol.* 1999;27(5):673–710.
79. Brown CA, Lilford RJ. The stepped wedge trial design: a systematic review. *BMC Med Res Methodol.* 2006;6(1):54.
80. Kratochwill TR, Levin JR. Enhancing the scientific credibility of single-case intervention research: randomization to the rescue. *Psychol Methods.* 2010;15(2):124.
81. Brown CH, Kellam SG, Kaupert S, et al. Partnerships for the design, conduct, and analysis of effectiveness, and implementation research: experiences of the Prevention Science and Methodology Group. *Adm Policy Ment Health.* 2012;39(4):301–316.
82. Chamberlain P, Roberts R, Jones H, Marsenich L, Sosna Tww, Price JM. Three collaborative models for scaling up evidence-based practices. *Adm Policy Ment Health.* 2012;39(4):278–290.
83. Brown CH, Berndt D, Brinales JM, Zong X, Bhagwat D. Evaluating the evidence of

effectiveness for preventive interventions: using a registry system to influence policy through science. *Addict Behav.* 2000;25(6):955–964.
84. Brown CH, Wyman PA, Brinales JM, Gibbons RD. The role of randomized trials in testing interventions for the prevention of youth suicide. *Int Rev Psychiatr.* 2007;19(6):617–631.
85. Chamberlain P, Saldana L, Brown CH, Leve LD. Implementation of multidimensional treatment foster care in California: a randomized trial of an evidence-based practice. In: Roberts-DeGennaro M, Fogel S, eds. *Empirically Supported Interventions for Community and Organizational Change.* Lyceum Books, Inc.; 2010:218–234.
86. Chamberlain P, Brown C, Saldana L, et al. Engaging and recruiting counties in an experiment on implementing evidence-based practice in California. *Admin Policy Ment Health Ment Health Res.* 2008;35:250–260.
87. Marcus SM, Gibbons RD. Estimating the efficacy of receiving treatment in randomized clinical trials with noncompliance. *Health Services & Outcomes Research Methodology.* 2001;2(3–4):247–257.
88. Stuart EA, Green KM. Using full matching to estimate causal effects in nonexperimental studies: examining the relationship between adolescent marijuana use and adult outcomes. *Dev Psychol.* 2008;44(2):395–406.
89. Shortell SM. Increasing value: a research agenda for addressing the managerial and organizational challenges facing health care delivery in the United States. *Med Care Res Rev.* 2004;61(3)(suppl):12S–30S.
90. Wholey J, Hatry H, Newcomer K, eds. *Handbook of Practical Program Evaluation.* Jossey-Bass Inc.; 2004.
91. Reichardt C, Mark M. Quasi-experimentation. In: Wholey J, Hatry H, Newcomer K, eds. Handbook of *Practical Program Evaluation.* Jossey-Bass Inc.; 2004:126.
92. Pierre R. Using randomized experiments. In: Wholey J, Hatry H, Newcomer K, eds. Handbook of *Practical Program Evaluation.* Jossey-Bass Inc.; 2004:150.
93. Barrett-Connor E, Grady D, Stefanick M. The rise and fall of menopausal hormone therapy. *Annu Rev Public Health.* 2005;26:115–140.
94. Concato J, Shah N, Horwitz R. Randomized, controlled trials, observational studies, and the hierarchy of research designs. *N Engl J Med.* 2000;342(25):1887.
95. Cook T, Shadish W, Wong V. Three conditions under which experiments and observational studies produce comparable causal estimates: new findings from within-study comparisons. *J Policy Anal Manage.* 2008;27(4):724–750.
96. Concato J, Lawler EV, Lew RA, Gaziano JM, Aslan M, Huang GD. Observational methods in comparative effectiveness research. *Am J Med.* 2010;123(12):e16–e23.
97. Hemming K, Taljaard M. Reflection on modern methods: when is a stepped-wedge cluster randomized trial a good study design choice? *Int J Epidemiol.* 2020;49(3):1043–1052.
98. Raudenbush SW, Liu X. Statistical power and optimal design for multisite randomized trials. *Psychol Methods.* 2000;5(2):199–213.
99. Bhaumik DK, Roy A, Aryal S, et al. Sample size determination for studies with repeated continuous outcomes. *Psychiatr Ann.* 2008;38(12):765–771.
100. Smith JD, Brown CH. The roll-out implementation optimization (ROIO) design: rigorous testing of a data-driven implementation improvement aim. Presented at: Academy Health/NIH 13th Annual Conference on the Science of Dissemination and Implementation in Health; 2020; Washington, DC.
101. Smith JD, Norton W, DiMartino L, et al. A Longitudinal Implementation Strategies Tracking System (LISTS): development and initial acceptability. Paper presented at: 13th Annual Conference on the Science of Dissemination and Implementation; 2020; Washington, DC.
102. Brownson RC, Jacobs JA, Tabak RG, Hoehner CM, Stamatakis KA. Designing for dissemination among public health researchers: findings from a national survey in the United States. *Am J Public Health.* 2013;103(9):1693–1699.
103. Shekelle P, Woolf S, Grimshaw JM, Schunemann HJ, Eccles MP. Developing clinical practice guidelines: reviewing, reporting, and publishing guidelines; updating guidelines; and the emerging issues of enhancing guideline implementability and accounting for comorbid conditions in guideline development. *Implement Sci.* 2012;7:62.
104. Damschroder LJ, Aron DC, Keith RE, Kirsh SR, Alexander JA, Lowery JC. Fostering implementation of health services research findings into practice: a consolidated framework for advancing implementation science. *Implement Sci.* 2009;4:50.
105. Landes SJ, McBain SA, Curran GM. An introduction to effectiveness-implementation hybrid designs. *Psychiatry Res.* 2019;280:112513.
106. Basch CE, Gold RS. The dubious effects of type V errors in hypothesis testing on health education practice and theory. *Health Educ Res.* 1986;1(4):299–305.
107. Kemp CG, Wagenaar BH, Haroz EE. Expanding hybrid studies for implementation research:

intervention, implementation strategy, and context. *Front Public Health.* 2019;7:325.

108. Nilsen P. Making sense of implementation theories, models and frameworks. *Implement Sci.* 2015;10(1):53.
109. Waltz TJ, Powell BJ, Matthieu MM, et al. Use of concept mapping to characterize relationships among implementation strategies and assess their feasibility and importance: results from the Expert Recommendations for Implementing Change (ERIC) study. *Implement Sci.* 2015;10(1):109.
110. Wilcox HC, Petras H, Brown HC, Kellam SG. Testing the impact of the whole-day good behavior game on aggressive behavior: results of a classroom-based randomized effectiveness trial. *Prev Sci.* 2022 Aug;23(6):907–921.
111. Brown CH, Kellam SG, Ialongo N, Poduska J, Ford C. Prevention of aggressive behavior through middle school using a first grade classroom-based Intervention In: Tsuang MT, Lyons MJ, Stone WS, eds. *Towards Prevention and Early Intervention of Major Mental and Substance Abuse Disorders.* American Psychiatric Publishing, Inc.; 2007:347–370.
112. Kellam SG, Brown CH, Poduska JM, et al. Effects of a universal classroom behavior management program in first and second grades on young adult behavioral, psychiatric, and social outcomes. *Drug Alcohol Depend.* 2008;95(suppl 1):S5–S28. Supplementary data associated with this article can be found in the online version: doi:10.1016/j.drugalcdep.2008.1001.1004
113. Jones B, Nachtsheim CJ. Split-plot design: what, why, and how. *J Qual Technol.* 2009;41(4):340–361.
114. Chambers DA. Advancing the science of implementation: a workshop summary. *Adm Policy Ment Health.* 2008;35(1–2):3–10.
115. Kraemer HC, Mintz J, Noda A, Tinklenberg J, Yesavage JA. Caution regarding the use of pilot studies to guide power calculations for study proposals. *Arch Gen Psychiatry.* 2006;63(5):484–489.
116. Prado G, Estrada Y, Rojas LM, et al. Rationale and design for eHealth Familias Unidas primary care: a drug use, sexual risk behavior, and STI preventive intervention for Hispanic youth in pediatric primary care clinics. *Contemp Clin Trials.* 2019;76:64–71.
117. Kellam SG, Ling X, Merisca R, Brown CH, Ialongo N. The effect of the level of aggression in the first grade classroom on the course and malleability of aggressive behavior into middle school. *Develop Psychopathol.* 1998;10(2):165–185.
118. Frangakis CE, Rubin DB. Principal stratification in causal inference. *Biometrics.* 2002;58:21–29.
119. Greenland S, Lanes S, Jara M. Estimating effects from randomized trials with discontinuations: the need for intent to treat design and G-estimation. *Clin Trials.* 2007;5:5–13.
120. Robins JM, Greenland S. Identifiability and exchangeability for direct and indirect effects. *Epidemiology.* 1992;3:143–155.
121. Barnard J, Frangakis CE, Hill JL, Rubin DB. Principal stratification approach to broken randomized experiments: a case study of school choice vouchers in New York City/comment/rejoinder. *J Am Stat Assoc.* 2003;98(462):299–323.
122. Frangakis CE, Brookmeyer RS, Varadham R, Safaeian M, Vlahov D, Strathdee SA. Methodology for evaluating a partially controlled longitudinal treatment using principal stratification, with application to a needle exchange Program. *J Am Stat Assoc.* 2004;99(465):239–250.
123. Barnard J, Frangakis C, Hill J, Rubin DB. School choice in NY City: a Bayesian analysis of an imperfect randomized experiment. In: Gatsonis C, Kass RE, Carriquiry A, Gelman A, Higdon D, Pauler DK, Verdinelli I, eds. *Case Studies in Bayesian Statistics.* Springer; 2002:3–97.
124. Muthén BO, Jo B, Brown CH. Comment on the Barnard, Frangakis, Hill & Rubin article, principal stratification approach to broken randomized experiments: a case study of school choice vouchers in New York City. *J Am Stat Assoc.* 2003;98(462):311–314.
125. Frangakis CE, Rubin DB, Frangakis CE, Rubin DB. Principal stratification in causal inference. *Biometrics.* 2002;58(1):21–29.
126. Frangakis CE, Varadham R. Systematizing the evaluation of partially controlled studies using principal stratification: from theory to practice. *Stat Sin.* 2004;14:945–947.
127. Jin H, Rubin DB. Principal stratification for causal inference with extended partial compliance. *J Am Stat Assoc.* 2008;103(481):101–111.
128. Rubin DB. Direct and indirect causal effects via potential outcomes. *Scand J Stat.* 2004;31(2):161–170.
129. Angrist JD, Imbens GW, Rubin DB. Identification of causal effects using instrumental variables. *J Am Stat Assoc.* 1996;91(434):444–455.
130. Asparouhov T, Muthén BO. Multilevel mixture models. In: Hancock GR, Samuelsen KM, eds. *Advances in Latent Variable Mixture Models.* Information Age Publishing, Inc.; 2008:27–51.
131. Muthen B. Latent variable mixture modeling. In: Marcoulides GA, Schumacker RE, eds.

Advanced Structural Equational Modeling: New Development and Techniques: Lawrence Earlbaum Associates; 2000:1–33.

132. Muthen B. Second-generation structural equation modeling with a combination of categorical and continuous latent variables. In: Collins LM, Sayer AG, eds. *New Methods for Analysis of Change*. Washington DC, APA; 2001:291–323.
133. Muthen B. Statistical and substantive checking in growth mixture modeling. *Psychol Methods*. 2003;8:369–377.
134. Muthen B. Latent variable modeling of longitudinal and multilevel data. *Sociol Methodol*. 2005;27:453–480.
135. Muthén B. Latent variable modeling of longitudinal and multilevel data. *Sociol Methodol*. 1997;27:453–480.
136. Muthén B, Brown CH. Estimating drug effects in the presence of placebo response: causal inference using growth mixture modeling. *Stat Med*. 2009;28(27):3363–3395.
137. Guo J. *Extending the Principal Stratification Methods to Multi-Level Randomized Trials*. Doctoral dissertation. University of South Florida; 2010.
138. Damschroder LJ, Reardon CM, Opra Widerquist MA, Lowery J. Conceptualizing outcomes for use with the Consolidated Framework for Implementation Research (CFIR): the CFIR Outcomes Addendum. *Implement Sci*. 2022;17(1):7.
139. Aarons GA, Sklar M, Mustanski B, Benbow N, Brown CH. "Scaling-out" evidence-based interventions to new populations or new health care delivery systems. *Implement Sci*. 2017;12(1):111.
140. Cook TD, Campbell DT, Shadish W. *Experimental and Quasi-experimental Designs for Generalized Causal Inference*. Houghton Mifflin; 2002.
141. Smith JD, Davis P, Kho AN. Community-driven health solutions on Chicago's south side. *Stanf Soc Innov Rev*. 2021;19(3):A27–A29.
142. Perrino T, Beardslee W, Bernal G, et al. Toward scientific equity for the prevention of depression and depressive symptoms in vulnerable youth. *Prev Sci*. 2015;16(5):642–651.
143. Mensah GA, Cooper RS, Siega-Riz AM, et al. Reducing cardiovascular disparities through community-engaged implementation research: a National Heart, Lung, and Blood Institute workshop report. *Circ Res*. 2018;122(2):213–230.
144. Brown CH, Mohr DC, Gallo CG, et al. A computational future for preventing HIV in minority communities: how advanced technology can improve implementation of effective programs. *J Acquir Immune Defic Syndr*. 2013;63(suppl 1):S72–S84.
145. McNulty M, Smith JD, Villamar J, et al. Implementation research methodologies for achieving scientific equity and health equity. *Ethn Dis*. 2019;29(suppl 1):83–92.
146. Woodward EN, Matthieu MM, Uchendu US, Rogal S, Kirchner JE. The health equity implementation framework: proposal and preliminary study of hepatitis C virus treatment. *Implement Sci*. 2019;14(1):26.
147. Mabry PL, Marcus SE, Clark PI, Leischow SJ, Mendez D. Systems science: a revolution in public health policy research. *Am J Public Health*. 2010;100(7):1161–1163.
148. Czaja SJ, Valente TW, Nair SN, Villamar JA, Brown CH. Characterizing implementation strategies using a systems engineering survey and interview tool: a comparison across 10 prevention programs for drug abuse and HIV sexual risk behavior. *Implement Sci*. 2016;11(1):70.
149. Kossisakoff A, Sweet WN. *Systems Engineering Principles and Practice*. John Wiley & Sons Inc.; 2003.
150. Czaja SJ, Nair SN. Human factors engineering and systems design. In: Salvendy G, ed. *Handbook of Human Factors and Ergonomics*. 3rd ed. John Wiley & Sons, Inc.; 2006:32–49.
151. Schulz R, Belle SH, Czaja SJ, Gitlin LN, Wisniewski SR, Ory MG. Introduction to the special section on Resources for Enhancing Alzheimer's Caregiver Health (REACH). *Psychol Aging*. 2003;18(3):357–360.
152. Saaty TL. The analytic hierarchy process in conflict management. *Int J Conflict Manage*. 1990;1(1):47–68.
153. Czaja SJ, Schulz R, Lee CC, Belle SH. A methodology for describing and decomposing complex psychosocial and behavioral interventions. *Psychol Aging*. 2003;18(3):385–395.
154. Gallo CG, Berkel C, Mauricio A, et al. Implementation methodology from a social systems informatics and engineering perspective applied to a parenting training program. *Fam Syst Health*. 2021;39(1):7–18.
155. Powell BJ, Fernandez ME, Williams NJ, et al. Enhancing the impact of implementation strategies in healthcare: a research agenda. *Front Public Health*. 2019;7:3.
156. Powell BJ, McMillen JC, Proctor EK, et al. A compilation of strategies for implementing clinical innovations in health and mental health. *Med Care Res Rev*. 2012;69(2):123–157.
157. Powell BJ, Waltz TJ, Chinman MJ, et al. A refined compilation of implementation strategies: results from the Expert Recommendations

for Implementing Change (ERIC) project. *Implement Sci.* 2015;10(1):21.

158. Lewis CC, Klasnja P, Powell BJ, et al. From classification to causality: advancing understanding of mechanisms of change in implementation science. *Front Public Health.* 2018;6:136.
159. Imel ZE, Pace BT, Soma CS, et al. Design feasibility of an automated, machine-learning based feedback system for motivational interviewing. *Psychotherapy.* 2019;56(2):318–328.
160. Brown CH. Three flavorings for a soup to cure what ails mental health services. *Adm Policy Ment Health.* 2020;47(5):844–851.
161. Rabiner LR. A tutorial on hidden Markov models and selected applications in speech recognition. *Proc IEEE.* 1989;77(2):257–286.
162. Deerwester S, Dumais ST, Furnas GW, Landauer TK, Harshman R. Indexing by latent semantic analysis. *J Am Soc Info Sci.* 1990;41(6):391–407.
163. Hofmann T. Probabilistic latent semantic indexing. Presented at: Proceedings of the 22nd Annual International ACM SIGIR Conference on Research and Development in Information Retrieval; 1999; Berkeley, CA.
164. Li T, Zhu S, Ogihara M. Hierarchical document classification using automatically generated hierarchy. *J Intell Inf Syst* 2007;29(2):211–230.
165. Li T, Zhu S, Ogihara M. Text categorization via generalized discriminant analysis. *Inf Process Manag.* 2008;44(5):1684–1697.
166. Whitaker RG, Sperber N, Baumgartner M, et al. Coincidence analysis: a new method for causal inference in implementation science. *Implement Sci.* 2020;15(1):108.
167. Baumgartner M, Falk C. Boolean difference-making: a modern regularity theory of causation. *Br J Philos Sci.*
168. Ambühl M, Baumgartner M, Epple R, Parkkinen VP, Thiem A. *Cna: causal Modeling With Coincidence Analysis.* 2021. https://cran.r-project.org/web/packages/cna/cna.pdf
169. Yakovchenko V, Miech EJ, Chinman MJ, et al. Strategy configurations directly linked to higher hepatitis C. *Med Care.* 2020;58(5):e31–e38.
170. Miech EJ, Freitag MB, Evans RR, et al. Facility-level conditions leading to higher reach: a configurational analysis of national VA weight management programming. *BMC Health Serv Res.* 2021;21(1):797.
171. Kim B, Sullivan JL, Ritchie MJ, et al. Comparing variations in implementation processes and influences across multiple sites: what works, for whom, and how? *Psychiatry Res.* 2020;283:112520.
172. Bauer MS, Miller CJ, Kim B, et al. Effectiveness of implementing a collaborative chronic care model for clinician teams on patient outcomes and health status in mental health: a randomized clinical trial. *JAMA Netw Open.* 2019;2(3):e190230.
173. Coleman K, Austin BT, Brach C, Wagner EH. Evidence on the chronic care model in the new millennium. *Health Aff (Millwood).* 2009;28(1):75–85.
174. Gilbody S, Bower P, Fletcher J, Richards D, Sutton AJ. Collaborative care for depression: a cumulative meta-analysis and review of longer-term outcomes. *Arch Intern Med.* 2006;166(21):2314–2321.
175. Woltmann E, Grogan-Kaylor A, Perron B, Georges H, Kilbourne AM, Bauer MS. Comparative effectiveness of collaborative chronic care models for mental health conditions across primary, specialty, and behavioral health care settings: systematic review and meta-analysis. *Am J Psychiatry.* 2012;169(8):790–804.
176. Miller CJ, Grogan-Kaylor A, Perron BE, Kilbourne AM, Woltmann E, Bauer MS. Collaborative chronic care models for mental health conditions: cumulative meta-analysis and metaregression to guide future research and implementation. *Med Care.* 2013;51(10):922–930.
177. Sun SS, Grave GD, Siervogel RM, Pickoff AA, Arslanian SS, Daniels SR. Systolic blood pressure in childhood predicts hypertension and metabolic syndrome later in life. *Pediatrics.* 2007;119(2):237–246.
178. Kelly RK, Thomson R, Smith KJ, Dwyer T, Venn A, Magnussen CG. Factors affecting tracking of blood pressure from childhood to adulthood: the Childhood Determinants of Adult Health Study. *J Pediatr.* 2015;167(6):1422–1428.e1422.
179. Du T, Fernandez C, Barshop R, Chen W, Urbina EM, Bazzano LA. 2017 Pediatric hypertension guidelines improve prediction of adult cardiovascular outcomes. *Hypertension.* 2019;73(6):1217–1223.
180. Flynn JT, Kaelber DC, Baker-Smith CM, et al. Clinical practice guideline for screening and management of high blood pressure in children and adolescents. *Pediatrics.* 2017;140(3):e20171904. doi:10.1542/peds.2017-1904. Epub 2017 Aug 21. PMID: 28827377.
181. Rao G. Diagnosis, epidemiology, and management of hypertension in children. *Pediatrics.* 2016;138(2):e20153616.
182. Hwang KO, Aigbe A, Ju H-H, Jackson VC, Sedlock EW. Barriers to accurate blood pressure measurement in the medical office. *J Prim Care Community Health.* 2018;9:2150132718816929.

183. Khoury M, Khoury P, Bazzano L, et al. Prevalence implications of the 2017 American Academy of Pediatrics hypertension guideline and associations with adult hypertension. *J Pediatrics.* 2021;241:22–28.e4.
184. Moin A, Mohanty N, Tedla YG, et al. Underrecognition of pediatric hypertension diagnosis: examination of 1 year of visits to community health centers. *J Clin Hypertension.* 2021;23(2):257–264.
185. Ogden CL, Carroll MD, Kit BK, Flegal KM. Prevalence of childhood and adult obesity in the United States, 2011–2012. *JAMA.* 2014;311(8):806–814.
186. Mhanna MJ, Iqbal AM, Kaelber DC. Weight gain and hypertension at three years of age and older in extremely low birth weight infants. *J Neonatal Perinatal Med.* 2015;8(4):363–369.
187. Crump C, Howell EA, Stroustrup A, McLaughlin MA, Sundquist J, Sundquist K. Association of preterm birth with risk of ischemic heart disease in adulthood. *JAMA Pediatrics.* 2019 Aug 1;173(8):736–743.
188. Go VF, Morales GJ, Mai NT, Brownson RC, Ha TV, Miller WC. Finding what works: identification of implementation strategies for the integration of methadone maintenance therapy and HIV services in Vietnam. *Implement Sci.* 2016;11(1):54.
189. Waltz TJ, Powell BJ, Chinman MJ, et al. Expert recommendations for implementing change (ERIC): protocol for a mixed methods study. *Implement Sci.* 2014;9:39.
190. Knapp AA, Carroll AJ, Mohanty N, et al. A stakeholder-driven method for selecting implementation strategies: a case example of pediatric hypertension clinical practice guideline implementation. *Implement Sci Commun.* 2022;3:25.
191. Holtrop JS, Rabin BA, Glasgow RE. Dissemination and implementation science in primary care research and practice: Contributions and opportunities. *J Am Board Fam Med.* 2018;31(3):466–478.
192. Bao Y, Druss BG, Jung H-Y, Chan Y-F, Unützer J. Unpacking collaborative depression care: Examining two essential tasks for implementation. *Implementation Science.* 2015;10(1):A33.
193. Smith JD, Li DH, Rafferty MR. The Implementation Research Logic Model: a method for planning, executing, reporting, and synthesizing implementation projects. *Implement Sci.* 2020;15(1):84.
194. Muthén BO, Muthén LK. Integrating person-centered and variable-centered analyses: Growth mixture modeling with latent trajectory classes. *Alcoholism: Clinical and Experimental Research.* 2000;24(6):882–891.
195. Muthén B, Brown CH, Masyn K, et al. General growth mixture modeling for randomized preventive interventions. *Biostatistics.* 2002;3(4):459–475.
196. Efron B, Tibshirani RJ. *An introduction to the bootstrap.* CRC Press; 1994.
197. Cidav Z, Mandell D, Pyne J, Beidas R, Curran G, Marcus S. A pragmatic method for costing implementation strategies using time-driven activity-based costing. *Implement Sci.* 2020;15(1):28.
198. Knapp AA, Mohanty N, Carroll AJ, et al. Identifying contextual barriers and potential strategies to increase adoption of pediatric hypertension guidelines using framework-guided rapid analysis. Paper presented at: 13th Annual Conference on the Science of Dissemination and Implementation 2020; Washington, DC.

15

Measurement Issues in Dissemination and Implementation Research

CARA C. LEWIS, KAYNE METTERT, ENOLA K. PROCTOR, AND ROSS C. BROWNSON

INTRODUCTION

New fields are often beset with measurement challenges given the dearth of measures and psychometric studies, inconsistent and evolving use of constructs, underdeveloped theories, and isolated research teams.[1] In 2013, the National Institutes of Health acknowledged the issues threatening dissemination and implementation (D&I) research in health and held a 2-day working meeting on measurement and reporting standards.[2] Twenty-three leaders of large-scale initiatives were charged with establishing the current state of the field and articulating a research agenda.[2,3] Now, almost a decade later, this chapter provides an overview of work to date that attempts to advance D&I measurement.

The language of D&I is highly varied, as even these key processes (dissemination and implementation) may be described as diffusion, translation, and numerous other terms; indeed, McKibbon et al.[4] identified 100 different terms with which to refer to D&I. The chapter follows the definitions of D&I offered by Rabin and colleagues[5] in this book. Dissemination is an active approach of spreading evidence-based interventions (EBIs) to target audiences via determined channels using planned strategies. Implementation is the process of putting to use, or integrating, EBIs within a specific setting.

The constructs for D&I measurement derive from conceptual models. The framework of D&I reflected in Figure 15.1 makes a number of key distinctions that carry implications for conceptualizing and measuring implementation processes and outcomes. First, the model distinguishes between the EBI being introduced and the *dissemination strategies* for spreading information about them and *implementation strategies* for putting those programs and policies in place in usual settings of prevention or care. For more information on D&I strategies and how they are measured, please see chapter 6. Grimshaw et al.[6] reported that meta-analyses of the effectiveness of implementation strategies have been thwarted by measurement issues, notably lack of detailed information about outcomes, use of widely varying constructs, reliance on dichotomous rather than continuous measures, and unit of analysis errors.[7] Second, these D&I strategies are different from their *outcomes*, which in turn need to be distinguished according to their several types. D&I outcomes serve as intermediate outcomes, or the proximal effects that are presumed to contribute to more distal outcomes, such as changes in service systems, in consumer health, behavior change, and larger population health. Service system outcomes reflect the six quality improvement aims set out in the Institute of Medicine Crossing the Quality Chasm reports: the extent to which services are safe, effective, patient centered, timely, efficient, and equitable.[8,9] D&I outcomes along with service system outcomes are viewed as contributing to individual and population health outcomes.[10]

Clearly the progress of D&I science *and* practice requires the development of reliable, valid, and pragmatic measures of contexts and outcomes. Psychometrically and pragmatically

Cara C. Lewis, Kayne Mettert, Enola K. Proctor, and Ross C. Brownson, *Measurement Issues in Dissemination and Implementation Research* In: *Dissemination and Implementation Research in Health.* Edited by: Ross C. Brownson, Graham A. Colditz, and Enola K. Proctor, Oxford University Press.
 DOI: 10.1093/oso/9780197660690.003.0015

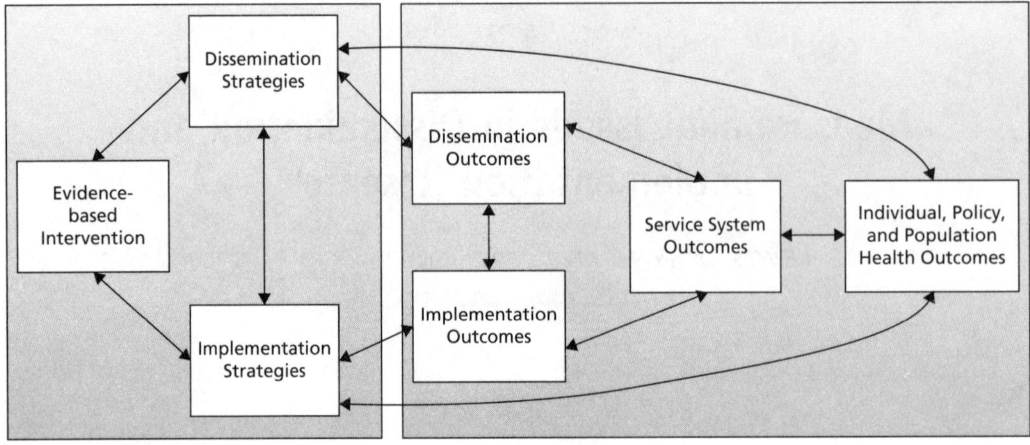

FIGURE 15.1 A framework for dissemination and implementation.

strong D&I context and outcome measures will enable empirical testing of the success of efforts to disseminate and implement new interventions and identification of D&I mechanisms of change (i.e., how strategies exert their effects) and pave the way for comparative effectiveness research on D&I strategies. Moreover, measures have the potential to provide actionable information for adapting and tailoring D&I strategies to the context. Unfortunately, measurement issues undermine this potential. The current literature reflects a wide array of constructs that are used when discussing D&I processes and outcomes, terms that are often used inconsistently, reflecting issues of homonymy (i.e., measures that purportedly assess the same construct but do so with substantively different items); synonymy (i.e., measures that have similar items that purportedly assess different constructs); and instability (i.e., items in a measure that shift or are modified over time in an unpredictable manner). When these constructs have been studied, they are measured in different ways—ranging from qualitative, quantitative survey, and record archival[7,11]—but often without any reporting of their measurement properties or rigor. What follows is an overview of the current state of D&I context and outcome measurement.

CURRENT STATE OF D&I MEASUREMENT: CONTEXTUAL FACTORS

Theories, models, and frameworks derive the D&I constructs and their definitions for process evaluation. Striffler and colleagues[12] identified over 150 such models in their 2018 review, some with overlapping or redundant constructs and others with distinct constructs for evaluation. Content validity measurement issues such as homonymy, synonymy, and instability arise due to diversity in operationalization of D&I constructs across models.[13] Systematic reviews of D&I measures can summarize the psychometric quality of measures, including their content validity. Nineteen systematic reviews of contextual factors have been conducted in the past 15 years[14–32]; see Rabin et al.[2] for a summary of several of these studies and related measurement resources.

Three of these reviews focused on single constructs (i.e., fidelity and clinician behavior,[14,15] organizational readiness to change[16]); one on five key organization-level constructs (i.e., leadership, vision, managerial relations, climate, and absorptive capacity[17]); and eleven on numerous constructs depicted in an established D&I model (i.e., framework for effective implementation[18]; Consolidated Framework for Implementation Research[19] (CFIR); theoretical framework for 27 predictors of adoption[20]). Unfortunately, only two studies evaluated content validity of the measures and found that 56% and 58.14% of the measures, respectively, had established content validity evidence,[15,16] indicating that nearly half of the included measures had not ensured that the items represented all facets of a known construct. However, in a recent special collection of measurement systematic reviews,[21–25,31,32] experts reviewed item content—as a proxy for a formal content validity assessment—as an inclusion criterion, a practice that focuses the product of these reviews on most promising measures. In measurement systematic reviews published prior to 2020, most common was that these studies reported broadly on the psychometric strength of the measures, as in the Chor et al.[20] review, wherein they simply stated "yes" or "no" with respect to whether a measure had demonstrated reliability or validity. More recently, Lewis and colleagues published the Psychometric and Pragmatic Evidence Rating Scale (PAPERS) for measure development and evaluation,[33] which has been applied internationally by research teams[26–28] to offer a quality profile across nuanced properties of included measures that improves interpretability of systematic review findings. Two crosscutting findings emerged from both generations of reviews: (1) The majority of measures are not psychometrically strong or they have never been tested for their psychometric quality, and (2) measures are typically used only in a single study. These findings suggest that the majority of D&I studies are reporting on measures that may not be assessing their intended construct, all facets of the known construct, and may not operate consistently within and across studies. Accordingly, D&I reports on contextual factors should *still* be interpreted with caution, and much more work needs to be done to establish evidence for the psychometric properties of measures.

CURRENT STATE OF D&I MEASUREMENT: OUTCOMES

Dissemination outcomes are defined here as the effects of dissemination strategies, that is, the consequences of targeted distribution of information and intervention materials to a specific public health or clinical practice audience. Similarly, implementation outcomes are defined as the effects of deliberate and purposive actions to implement new interventions, guidelines, preventive strategies, and/or innovations. D&I outcomes are proximal reflections of their respective processes and thus serve as intermediate outcomes in larger efforts to improve the service system, and ultimately individual or population health.[7] Distinguishing D&I effectiveness from program or intervention effectiveness is critical. When efforts to transport new programs, or the information about them, from laboratory settings to community health and mental health venues fail—as they often do (2/3 of efforts fail[34])—we must be able to determine if failure occurred because the intervention was ineffective in the new setting (intervention failure), or if a good intervention was conveyed and deployed incorrectly (dissemination/implementation failure). Important to acknowledge is that attenuated effects are often observed when interventions are implemented in new contexts or outside of a research trial, which does not constitute failure.

Table 15.1 provides an initial taxonomy of D&I outcomes that may appropriately evolve as conceptual distinctiveness emerges for constructs like *equity* and *scale*. For each outcome, the table (a) nominates a level of analysis, (b) identifies the theoretical basis to the construct from literature, (c) offers different terms that are used for the construct in the literature, (d) suggests the point or phase within D&I processes at which the outcome may be most salient, (e) indicates whether the outcome is appropriate for latent variable conceptualization, (f) lists the types of existing measures for the construct, and (g) health equity considerations for each outcome. Level of analysis is an important consideration because it has implications for the measure's target (e.g., provider, middle manager, administrator); language (e.g., intended to capture individual perspective vs. that of the larger group); and analysis (e.g., aggregated to reflect a group or organization). The theoretical basis should delineate the interrelations among constructs and inform its definition to ensure that item development reflects the content of what the construct is and is not (i.e., to establish construct and content validity). Different terms are offered, but it remains an empirical question whether these terms are actually synonyms or reflective of unique constructs worthy of evaluation.

Of the more than 150 theories, frameworks, and models,[12] few indicate when in an implementation process each outcome is most relevant for measurement. That is, D&I outcomes are likely to differ in importance across phases. For example, feasibility may be most important once organizations and providers try new interventions. Later, it may be a "moot point," once the intervention—initially considered novel or unknown—has become part of normal routine. However, feasibility could once again become highly salient if resources or context changed. The literature suggests that studies

TABLE 15.1 TAXONOMY OF DISSEMINATION AND IMPLEMENTATION OUTCOMES

Dissemination and Implementation Outcome	Level of Analysis	Theoretical Basis	Other Terms in the Literature	Salience by D&I Phase Informed by the EPIS Model[39]	Latent Variable Y/N	Example Method of Measurement	Health Equity Considerations
Reach	Individual	RE-AIM	Participation	Exploration	N	Surveys Administrative data	Assess whether all populations are reached by the intervention and remove barriers related to social determinants of health
Acceptability	Individual	Rogers: complexity and relative advantage Greenhalgh: user orientation	Satisfaction with the innovation System readiness	Primarily exploration, secondarily implementation and sustainment	Y	Survey Key informant interviews Administrative data	Ensure representation of subpopulations who are intended to benefit from the EBI
Appropriateness	Individual Organization Policy	Rogers: compatibility	Perceived fit Relevance Compatibility Suitability Usefulness Practicability	Primarily exploration and secondarily preparation	Y	Surveys Key informant interviews Focus groups	Ensure representation of subpopulations who are intended to benefit from the EBI
Feasibility	Individual Organization Policy	Rogers: compatibility, trialability, observability	Actual fit or utility Suitability Practicability Community readiness	Primarily exploration and secondarily preparation	Y	Surveys Administrative data	Assess feasibility in a given context where unique constraints may undermine feasibility
Adoption	Individual Organization Policy	Rogers: trialability, observability RE-AIM	Uptake Utilization Intention to try Use of the innovation Knowledge transfer	Preparation	N	Surveys Observation Key informant interviews Focus groups Administrative data	Assess whether all settings were able to adopt the intervention and whether adaptations need to be made to support lower resource settings

Fidelity	Individual	RE-AIM: part of implementation	Delivered as intended Adherence Integrity Quality of program delivery	Implementation and sustainment	N	Observation Checklists Content analyses Self-report	Examine whether fidelity is appropriate as a central outcome based on representativeness of research sample on which EBI is based
Cost	Individual Organization Policy	RE-AIM Texas Christian University program change model: costs and resources	Marginal cost Cost-effectiveness Cost-benefit Economic evaluation	Primarily exploration and secondarily implementation and sustainment	N	Administrative data	Center cost of EBI implementation to support equitable implementation
Penetration	Organization Policy	RE-AIM necessary for reach	Spread Access to services Level of utilization	Primarily implementation and secondarily sustainment	N	Surveys Case studies Key informant interviews	Assess whether all populations are reached by the intervention and remove barriers related to social determinants of health
Sustainability	Organization Policy	Rogers: confirmation RE-AIM: maintenance	Maintenance Institutionalization Continuation Sustained use Standard of practice or care	Primarily sustainment and secondarily exploration	Y	Surveys Case studies Record & policy reviews Key informant interviews	Assess whether all settings and populations are being reached by the intervention over a long period of time

*Note. Latent variable refers to a variable that itself cannot be directly observed but can be inferred through measurable indicators.

usually capture measures of fidelity prior to, or during, initial implementation, while adoption is often assessed at 6,[35] 12,[36,37] or 18 months[38] after initial implementation. But, most studies fail to specify a time frame or are inconsistent in choice of a time point in the implementation process for measuring each implementation outcome. Clearer specification of the time frame chosen for measurement and the rationale for the choice is needed. The EPIS model (exploration, preparation, implementation, sustainment[39]) is one of the few models that provides some guidance regarding the temporal relations of the D&I outcomes, and their 2019 systematic review of its use offers empirical examples regarding which phase-relevant constructs were measured.[40] Although a review of the EPIS model is beyond the scope of this chapter, we use it to illustrate where each D&I outcome would fall across the four phases to inform strategic assessment (see Table 15.1).

Finally, as can be seen in Table 15.1, many of the D&I outcomes can be inferred or measured in terms of expressed attitudes and opinions, intentions, or perspectives as is often the target of survey measurement methods. However, several of the D&I outcomes are not best conceptualized as latent variables and should instead be measured directly through observation (e.g., adoption), objective rating (e.g., fidelity), concrete information tracking (e.g., cost), or administrative data collection (e.g., penetration). As can be seen in Table 15.1, methods of measurement for each outcome do not always adhere to that which is most appropriate, as surveys tend to be the approach favored by researchers (despite likely issues of shared method variance undermining the accuracy of one's findings).

DISSEMINATION OUTCOMES

The literature on dissemination outcomes is sparse and scattered, reflecting no conceptual typology or list of dissemination outcomes, and there have not been any systematic reviews of dissemination outcome measures. Rabin and colleagues[41] reported that nearly half of all published reports of dissemination research in cancer failed to report any outcomes. However, several constructs reflecting potential outcomes are mentioned in articles that discuss dissemination approaches, the most frequent of which is *change in attitude/behavior.*[41] Other commonly referenced desired effects (outcomes) of dissemination include *awareness, receipt, acceptance, engagement with materials,* and *use of information.*[42,43] Dingfelder and Mandell's[44] definition of dissemination strategies reflect such dissemination outcomes as *awareness of an innovation* and an *inclination to use* the innovation. Similarly, *intentions* emerged as one of the 14 domains delineated in the Theoretical Domains Framework,[45] a social psychology-informed listing of 84 constructs relevant to the kind of behavior change that occurs in implementation. The RE-AIM framework's constructs of *reach, adoption, implementation,* and *maintenance* are sometimes referenced as outcomes, although Rabin et al.[46] presented them as mediators of the extent and speed of dissemination. Clearly, *reach* may reflect the breadth with which health information spreads and offer critical equity-related information about "success," and thus serves as a key dissemination outcome. The diffusion of innovations theory[47] is often used for dissemination planning and practice, which includes a list of four innovation-specific constructs—relative advantage, compatibility, complexity, trialability—that may moderate or mediate dissemination outcomes and for which a recent systematic review of measures exists.[32] Finally, a recent systematic review of quantitative measures featured policy determinants and outcomes that may be conceptualized as dissemination outcomes, such as *communication of policy* and *visibility of policy actors.*[26]

IMPLEMENTATION OUTCOMES

The literature reflects at least eight conceptually distinct implementation outcomes—*acceptability, appropriateness, feasibility, adoption, fidelity, implementation cost, penetration,* and *sustainability.*[7,11] Proctor and colleagues[11] developed a taxonomy of implementation outcomes, offered conceptual definitions, and addressed their measurement challenges (Table 15.1). A recent review of measurement of implementation outcomes published as part of a special collection of systematic reviews identified 150 measures of implementation outcomes in the literature. These measures were unevenly distributed across outcomes and had mostly unknown psychometric quality.[21] A few promising measures were identified, but more work needs to be done to systematically develop and validate measures that can be used by implementation researchers and practitioners.

Acceptability is the perception among implementation stakeholders that a given intervention or innovation is agreeable, palatable, or satisfactory. The referent of the implementation outcome "acceptability" (or *"what" is acceptable*) may be a specific intervention, practice, technology, or service within a particular setting of care. Acceptability should be assessed based on the stakeholder's knowledge of or direct experience with various dimensions of the EBI to be implemented, such as its content, complexity, or comfort. Acceptability may be measured from the perspective of various stakeholders, such as administrators, payers, providers, and consumers, and acceptability is likely to be dynamic, changing with experience. Thus ratings of acceptability may be different when taken, for example, in the exploration phase and again in later phases of implementation.

Appropriateness is the perceived fit, relevance, or compatibility of the innovation or EBI for a given practice setting, provider, or consumer and/or perceived fit of the innovation to address a particular issue or problem. "Appropriateness" is conceptually similar to acceptability, and the literature reflects overlapping and sometimes inconsistent terms when discussing these constructs. Indeed, a series of laboratory and field studies recently revealed that although these terms are conceptually distinct, they are not meaningfully distinct in that rarely would it be the case that an intervention or innovation would be acceptable but not appropriate or vice versa.[48] More empirical work is needed to determine whether measurement of both acceptability and appropriateness is advantageous.

Feasibility is the extent to which a new program or policy can be successfully used or carried out within a given agency, in a particular setting, or in a certain population.[49] Typically, the concept of feasibility is invoked retrospectively as a potential explanation of an implementation's success or failure, as reflected in poor recruitment, retention, or participation rates. While feasibility is related to appropriateness, the two constructs are conceptually and meaningfully distinct. For example, a program may be appropriate for a service setting—in that it is compatible with the setting's mission or service mandate—but may not be feasible due to resource or training requirements.

Acceptability, appropriateness, and feasibility are predictors of adoption.[50] *Adoption* is the intention, initial decision, or action to try or employ an innovation or EBI.[46,51] Adoption also may be referred to as "uptake." Adoption could be measured from the perspective of provider or organization. Shelton et al. provided health equity considerations related to adoption that inspire a more nuanced approach to measurement.[52] Health equity-informed, adoption-specific questions include the following: Did all settings equitably adopt the EBI? Which settings and staff adopted and applied the EBI? Which did not and why? Were low-resourced settings able to adopt the EBI to the same extent as higher-resourced settings? What adaptations might be needed to facilitate adoption?[52]

Incremental implementation cost is the additional expense of implementing an EBI. Chapter 11 on economic aspects of D&I provides a fuller exposition of this outcome and details the ways in which implementation costs vary. Direct measures of implementation cost are essential for studies comparing the costs of implementing alternative interventions and of various implementation strategies. From a health equity perspective, low-resourced settings may face higher costs if they do not have a quality improvement or related infrastructure to serve as a foundation for implementing new EBIs unless policy-related supports can offset implementation costs. Moreover, incremental implementation cost is likely critical information for low-resourced settings in making an adoption decision, demanding much more work in this space.

Fidelity is the most common implementation outcome, defined as the degree to which an intervention was implemented as it was prescribed in the original protocol or as it was intended by the program developers.[46,53] Fidelity is typically measured by comparing the original EBI and the disseminated/implemented intervention in terms of (1) adherence to the program protocol, (2) dose or amount of program delivered, and (3) quality of program delivery. The literature identifies five implementation fidelity dimensions: adherence, quality of delivery, program component differentiation, exposure to the intervention, and participant responsiveness or involvement.[54,55] Provider fidelity is often of most interest, but there is evidence that providers are poor reporters of their intervention delivery, particularly when the intervention is new to them, whereas objectively rated measures of fidelity remain the gold standard.[56] From a health equity perspective, fidelity may be a somewhat questionable construct to measure in isolation given the valid criticisms that many EBIs are established with nonrepresentative samples and the commonly held belief that there is no implementation without adaptation.[57]

Penetration is defined as the integration of a practice within a service setting and its subsystems,[58] and is similar to Rabin et al.'s[46] notion of niche saturation. Stiles et al.[58] applied the concept of service penetration to service recipients (the number of eligible persons who use a service divided by the total number of persons eligible for the service). Penetration also can be calculated in terms of the number of providers who deliver a given intervention divided by the total number of providers trained in or expected to deliver the service. From a service system perspective, the construct is also similar to "reach" in the RE-AIM framework.[59] Shelton et al. posed a set of questions related to reach motivated by health equity considerations[52]: Are all populations equitably reached by the EBI? Who is not reached by the intervention (in terms of a range of social dimensions and social determinants of health) and why? How can we better reach those who are not receiving the intervention and ensure we are reaching those who experience inequities related to social dimensions and social/structural determinants of health?

Sustainability is the extent to which a newly implemented intervention is maintained or institutionalized within a service setting's ongoing, stable operations. The literature reflects quite varied uses of the term *sustainability*.[4,46,60–63] Rabin et al.[46] emphasized the integration of a given program within an organization's culture through policies and practices and distinguishes three stages that determine institutionalization: (1) passage (a single event, e.g., transition from temporary to permanent funding); (2) cycle or routine (i.e., repetitive reinforcement of the importance of the EBI through including it into organizational or community procedures and behaviors such as the annual budget and evaluation criteria); and (3) niche saturation (the extent to which an EBI is integrated into all subsystems of an organization). Thus, the outcomes of "penetration" and "sustainability" may be related conceptually and empirically in that higher penetration may contribute to long-term sustainability. Shelton et al. provided a series of questions related to health equity considerations that should inform measurement of sustainability[52]:

- Is the EBI being equitably sustained?
- What settings and populations continue to be reached long term by the EBI and continue to receive benefits over time—why or why not?
- Do adaptations to EBIs reduce or exacerbate health inequities over time?
- Do all settings have continued capacity and partnerships to maintain delivery of EBIs?
- Are the determinants of sustainability the same across low-resource and high-resource settings?
- How do social determinants of health shape inequitable implementation and sustainability of EBIs over time?

A recent review by Mettert et al. identified more than 160 measures of implementation outcomes used in mental and behavioral health that were unevenly distributed across the eight outcomes: 32 measures of acceptability, 26 measures of adoption, 6 measures of appropriateness, 31 measures of cost, 18 measures of feasibility, 18 measures of fidelity, 23 measures of penetration, and 14 measures of sustainability were identified. Overall, there was limited psychometric information available for all measures identified. Norms was the most commonly reported psychometric criterion (N = 63, 52%), followed by internal consistency (N = 58, 48%). Responsiveness was the least reported psychometric property (3%), despite the fact that, for implementation outcomes, responsiveness (or sensitivity to change) is a critically important property. Finally, limited evidence of measures' reliability and validity was found. Psychometric ratings using PAPERS[33] ranged from −1 to 14, with a possible minimum of score of −9 and a possible maximum score of 36, illustrating a profound need for measurement studies in this field. Compared with a previous review of implementation outcome measures (Lewis et al.[46]), 66 new measures were identified—with a continued uneven distribution of measures across implementation outcomes. This proliferation of measures suggests increasing focus on measurement of implementation outcomes, but validation of psychometric quality remains largely scant.

Modeling Interrelationships Among D&I Outcomes

The literature has only begun to address the ways in which D&I outcomes are interrelated.[7,11] Dingfelder and Mandell's model[44] positions dissemination as a contributor to successful implementation outcome. Yet dissemination outcomes are likely interrelated in dynamic and complex ways, as are implementation outcomes.[64–67] For example, the perceived feasibility and implementation cost associated with an intervention will likely bear on ratings of the intervention's acceptability. Acceptability, in turn, will likely affect adoption, penetration, and sustainability. Similarly, consistent with Rogers's diffusion of innovations theory, the ability to adopt or adapt an innovation for local use may increase its acceptability.[47]

Important work needs to be done to model these interrelationships, and this work will likely inform definitions and thus shape our D&I language. For example, if two outcomes that we now define as distinct concepts are shown through research to always occur together, the empirical evidence would suggest that the concepts are really the same thing and should be combined, as is likely the case for acceptability and appropriateness. Similarly, if two of the outcomes are shown to have different empirical patterns, evidence would confirm their conceptual distinction. Refining the D&I contextual factors and outcomes taxonomy is critical to the advancement of the field.

MEASURING STAKEHOLDER PERSPECTIVES: CONTEXTUAL FACTORS AND OUTCOMES

Advancing methods to capture stakeholder perspectives is essential for D&I research.[68,69] A US federal report, the "Road Ahead Report," calls for assessing the perspectives of multiple stakeholders in order to improve the sustainability of EBIs in real-world care.[70] Successful D&I of EBIs depends largely on the fit of EBIs with the preferences and priorities of those who shape, deliver, and participate in care. For equitable implementation, careful attention must be paid to the methods and messaging used to engage stakeholders that is culturally sensitive and inclusive. Several groups of D&I stakeholders can be distinguished, within which rich diversity exists that demands representation to achieve health equity. *Community members* may include (1) *healthcare consumers*, who comprise the primary beneficiaries in the successful D&I of evidence-based health services, and (2) the *whole population* in a community, which benefits from dissemination of a population-level public health intervention (e.g., water fluoridation). Many dissemination efforts target health consumers directly, as in marketing campaigns designed to increase consumer demand for a particular program, drug, or service. *Families* and *caregivers* comprise another group of D&I stakeholders, often sharing consumer desires for quality care and similarly affected by successful D&I. Service recipients and family members bring different perspectives to the evaluation of health care,[71] underscoring the importance of systematically assessing their perspectives on D&I of evidence-based healthcare.

Intervention developers constitute a third group of stakeholders. Many engage in D&I efforts, fueled by a desire that their interventions be used in real-world care and are then also known as intermediaries or purveyors. For example, many intervention developers (including nurse in-home visitation program developers) have launched their own implementation "shops," many of which are proprietary. Many provide direct training, supervision, and consultation. Those who develop health policies, such as smoking bans, launch advertising campaigns, as do pharmaceutical firms, who also provide academic detailing aimed at changing provider prescribing behavior. Another set of stakeholders, *public health and healthcare advocates*, engage in similar efforts. Intervention developers and/or their marketing enterprises highly value the implementation outcomes of penetration, fidelity, and sustainability.

Many, if not most, D&I efforts target the *front-line practitioners* who deliver healthcare and prevention services or *agency administrators* through organizational implementation strategies. Healthcare providers themselves can serve important dissemination roles. For example, Kerner et al.[72] suggested that primary care physicians, dentists, and community health workers have high potential for exposing the broader public to evidence-based health promotion and disease prevention. Personnel in public health agencies have an obligation to survey the evidence carefully and decide when the science base is sufficient for widespread dissemination. Finally, *policymakers* at the local, regional, state, national, and international levels are an important audience for D&I efforts. These individuals are often faced with macro-level decisions on how to allocate the public resources for which they have been elected stewards. This often raises important dissemination issues related to balancing individual and social good or deciding on costs for implementing evidence-based policies.

A variety of established quantitative approaches for stakeholder preference assessment derive from medical decision-making and health services research[73,74] (standard gamble and time trade-off); psychophysics and psychology[75] (category rating and magnitude estimation); marketing[76] (conjoint analysis); cognitive anthropology[77] (cultural domain analysis [CDA] and cultural consensus analysis); and sorting and ranking approaches common to multiple disciplines. Research is needed to test these methods for assessing the feasibility, acceptability, and validity of stakeholder perspectives using, for example, cognitive interviewing techniques such as "think aloud"[78] and quantitative measures of method performance. The Sawtooth Software Conjoint Value Analysis web system software can be used for conjoint analysis. ANTHROPAC 4.98,[79] a menu-driven DOS program, can be used to conduct metric and nonmetric multidimensional scaling and cluster analyses in exploratory analyses of stakeholder preference domains.

Salience of D&I Outcomes to Stakeholders: Pragmatic Measures

As noted above, any effort to change care involves a range of stakeholders, including the intervention developers, who design and test the intervention effectiveness; policymakers, who design and pay for service; administrators, who shape program direction; providers and supervisors; patients/clients/consumers and their family members; and community members interested in healthcare. The success of efforts to implement EBIs may rest on their congruence with the preferences and priorities of those who shape, deliver, and participate in care. D&I outcomes may be differentially important to various stakeholders, just as the salience of clinical outcomes varies across stakeholders.[80] For example, implementation cost may be most important to policymakers and program directors, feasibility may be most important to direct service providers, and fidelity may be most important to intervention developers. To ensure applicability of implementation outcomes across a range of healthcare settings and to maximize their external validity and health equity, all stakeholder groups and priorities should be represented in this research.

Moreover, measures of D&I context, process, and outcomes should be pragmatic. Glasgow and Riley[81] described pragmatic measures as those that measure constructs that are important to stakeholders, are low burden, have broad applicability, are sensitive to change, and are actionable. Until pragmatic measures are prioritized, stakeholders will remain limited in terms of their ability to conduct implementations independently of researchers. As noted above, Lewis and colleagues[19] developed PAPERS[33] via a synthesis of findings from a systematic literature review and stakeholder interviews, followed by a concept-mapping process to establish stakeholder-driven domains of relevance and a Delphi activity to come to consensus on stakeholder priorities for pragmatic measure qualities. The goal is that PAPERS will inform measure development and evaluation going forward, increasing the likelihood that measures are useful to and used by a broad range of stakeholders.

CONCEPTUAL AND METHODOLOGIC CHALLENGES

Although it was published almost a decade ago, we invite readers to review an article, "Instrumentation Issues in Implementation Science," for an in-depth consideration of conceptual and methodologic challenges of D&I measurement[82]; a concise overview of the outstanding issues follows. Conceptualizing and measuring implementation outcomes will advance understanding of implementation processes, enhance efficiency in implementation research, and pave the way for studies of the comparative effectiveness of D&I strategies. Advancing the nominal and operational measurement of D&I outcomes requires work on several fronts. First, accurate measurement of D&I outcomes requires more consistent nominal definition, including the use of consistent terminology. Studies often use different labels for what appear to be the same construct or use one term for the outcome's label or nominal definition but a different term for operationalizing or measuring the same construct. While language inconsistency is typical in most still-developing fields, implementation research may be particularly susceptible to this problem. No single discipline is "home" to D&I research. Studies are conducted across a broad range of disciplines, published in a scattered set of journals, and consequently are rarely cross-referenced.[7] The field now has the beginnings of a common language to characterize implementation outcomes, with much work to be done with dissemination outcomes. Continued progress is essential to our field's conceptual and empirical advancement. Those developing taxonomies serve to organize the key variables and frame research questions required to advance implementation science. Their measurement and empirical test helps specify the mechanisms and causal relations within D&I processes and advance a base of empirical evidence about successful D&I. Researchers should also clearly report and describe their role in measurement and analysis of implementation outcomes.[83]

Measurement Approaches

The literature reflects a wide array of approaches for measuring implementation outcomes, ranging from qualitative to quantitative survey to record archival to administrative.[7,11] Examples of the often used measurement approaches for each implementation outcome are provided in Table 15.1. The preferred approach is (quantitative) survey, regardless of whether it is most appropriate. Unfortunately, much of the existing quantitative measurement has been "homegrown," often leading to this one-time use phenomenon, with virtually no work on the psychometric properties or measurement rigor. Importantly, as discussed by Martinez et al.,[82] these measurement approaches should be used strategically depending on the research question, design, context in which the study is being conducted, and the state of the measurement literature regarding the specific outcome(s) in question. Careful attention paid to selecting the measurement approach can help with the measure development and evaluation issues noted throughout this chapter.

Level of Analysis for Outcomes

Dissemination of health information and the implementation of new preventive practices involve change at multiple levels, ranging from the individual (health consumer, provider) to the organization, to the community and in policy.[7,84] Some outcomes, such as attitude change and acceptance, may most appropriately be assessed at the individual level, while others, such as spread or penetration, may be more appropriate for aggregate analysis, such as at the level of the organization. Currently, very few studies reporting D&I outcomes specify the level at which measurement was taken. In one of the existing systematic reviews, Emmons et al.[17] found that the level of the measure and analysis did not always match. Specification and appropriate matching of the measure with its intended target is critical to advancing D&I theory.

Construct Validity

Construct validity is the degree to which a measure "behaves" in a way consistent with theoretical hypotheses[85] and is predictive of some external attribute (e.g., rate of smoking). Establishing construct validity for a measure begins in the development process by creating a nomological network that establishes the theoretical relations among constructs (e.g., antecedents, predicted outcomes).[19] Despite the existence of 150+ D&I models, there are few that delineate interrelations between constructs and outcomes, making construct validity difficult to test. Additionally, qualitative data, reflecting language used by various stakeholders as they think and talk about D&I processes, is important for validating outcome constructs. Through in-depth interviews, stakeholders' cognitive representations and mental models of outcomes can be analyzed using such methods as CDA.[86]

Criterion-Related Validity

Criterion-related validity (sometimes considered a subset of construct validity) is the degree to which a measure is predictive of some "gold standard" measure of the same attribute,[79] as is the case for concurrent validity. Assessment of criterion validity is common in many areas of medical and public health research. For example, for concurrent validity, to gauge the accuracy of self-reported smoking behavior one might compare self-reported data with biochemical measures of cotinine (a nicotine breakdown product). However, in most areas of D&I research the gold standard does not exist to assess concurrent validity. Similarly, to assess accuracy of staff self-report of use of a new intervention, records might be audited for evidence of the intervention's delivery, and supervisors might be queried. Currently, neither dissemination research nor implementation research adequately discusses or explores the validity of outcome measurement.

Perhaps of most interest to D&I researchers is the predictive validity component of criterion-related validity. As the term suggests, this is an evaluation to determine whether a D&I construct predicts an outcome that is measured at a later time interval. For example, one might explore whether organizational readiness to change predicts provider fidelity to an EBI postdeployment of an implementation strategy. Surprisingly, the minority of D&I measures have evidence of predictive validity, ranging from 10% of measures, as in the case of structural characteristics of the setting,[24] to 51.61% of Chaudoir et al.'s[18] review of measures across five levels of analysis. It is unclear the reason for so few tests of predictive validity. One likely explanation is that studies are not designed to prospectively test the impact of determinants on implementation outcomes subsequent to an implementation intervention. The majority of the D&I literature to date simply characterizes barriers and facilitators at a single time point.

Using Implementation Outcomes to Model Success

Success in D&I is probably a function of a "portfolio" of factors, including the effectiveness of the intervention itself and the skillful use of D&I strategies.[7,11] For example, implementation strategies could be employed to increase provider acceptance, improve penetration, reduce implementation costs, and achieve sustainability of the intervention being implemented. It is important to conceptually and empirically address how various D&I outcomes contribute to success. For example, an EBI may be highly effective, but it may be largely unknown to potential adopters; this poor dissemination outcome (low awareness) would undermine the likelihood of its implementation. This scenario may be modeled as follows:

Implementation success = function of effectiveness (= high) + awareness (= low)

As another example, a program may be highly effective but only mildly acceptable and costly, making it difficult to sustain. The overall potential success of implementation in this case might be modeled as follows:

Implementation success = function of effectiveness (= high) + acceptability (= moderate) + cost (high) + sustainability (low)

In a third situation, a given intervention might be only moderately effective but highly acceptable to stakeholders because current care is poor, the intervention is inexpensive, and current training protocols ensure high penetration through providers. This intervention's potential might be modeled in the following equation:

Implementation success = function of intervention effectiveness (moderate) + acceptability (high) + potential to improve care (high) + penetration (high).

These examples suggest that successful change in public health and health delivery can be understood and modeled using the concepts of D&I outcomes, thereby making decisions about what to implement more explicit and transparent. It is critical to specify these interrelations a priori to ensure psychometrically strong and pragmatic measures are available and administered at the appropriate time point in the implementation process (e.g., exploration, preparation, implementation, or sustainment[39]).

SUMMARY

The National Institutes of Health, the Agency for Healthcare Research and Quality (AHRQ), the Centers for Disease Control and Prevention (CDC), and a number of private foundations have expressed the need for advancing the science of D&I. Interest in D&I research is present in many countries, including the UK Center for Reviews and Dissemination, the UK Medical Research Council, and the Canadian Institutes of Health Research. Improving healthcare requires not only effective programs and interventions, but also effective strategies to move them into community-based settings of care. But before discrete strategies can be tested for effectiveness, comparative effectiveness, or cost-effectiveness, context and outcome constructs must be identified and defined in such a way that enables their manipulation and measurement. Measurement is underdeveloped, with few psychometrically strong measures and very little attention paid to their pragmatic nature. A variety of tools are needed to capture healthcare access and quality, and no measurement issues are more pressing than those for D&I science.

ACKNOWLEDGMENTS

Preparation of this chapter was supported by R01CA262325, R01MH106510, P30MH068579, and UL1RR024992.

The authors acknowledge the following individuals, who contributed ideas or insights about measurement of dissemination and implementation outcomes: Graham Colditz, Lauren Gulbas, Curtis McMillen, Susan Pfefferle, Martha Shumway, Caitlin Dorsey, and Bryan Weiner.

SUGGESTED READINGS AND WEBSITES

Readings

Glasgow RE, Vogt TM, Boles SM. Evaluating the public health impact of health promotion interventions: the RE-AIM framework. *Am J Public Health*. 1999;89(9):1322–1327.

In this seminal article, Glasgow et al. evaluated public health interventions using the RE-AIM framework. The model's five dimensions (reach, efficacy, adoption, implementation, and maintenance) act together to determine a particular program's public health impact. The article also summarizes the model's strengths and limitations and suggests that failure to evaluate on all five dimensions can result in wasted resources.

Lewis, C. C., Mettert, K. D., Dorsey, C. N., Martinez, R. G., Weiner, B. J., Nolen, E., . . . Powell, B. J. An updated protocol for a systematic review of implementation-related measures. *Syst Rev.* 2018);7(1):1–8.

Lewis and her team have contributed significant advancements to the D&I measurement literature through their enhanced systematic reviews of measures assessment constructs of the Consolidated Framework for Implementation Research and Implementation Outcomes. Consider their special collection of articles in which they present the Psychometric and Pragmatic Rating Scale (PAPERS) and the results of their systematics reviews in which they applied PAPERS. https://journals.sagepub.com/topic/collections-irp/irp-1-systematic_reviews_of_methods_to_measure_implementation_constructs/irp

Proctor E, Landsverk J, Aarons G, Chambers D, Glisson C, Mittman B. Implementation research in mental health services: an emerging science with conceptual, methodological, and training challenges. *Adm Policy Ment Health.* 2009;36(1):24–34.

The conceptual framework proposed in this article by Proctor et al. identifies the key components in implementation science—an EBI or quality improvement to be implemented, an implementation strategy for putting the EBI into place in a new setting or healthcare context, and three types of outcomes that are conceptually related: implementation outcomes, service system outcomes, and health outcomes. Proctor et al. address the training needs for the D&I field and offer a research agenda for advancing the field.

Proctor E, Silmere H, Raghavan R, et al. Outcomes for implementation research: conceptual distinctions, measurement challenges, and research agenda. *Adm Policy Ment Health.* 2011;38(2):65–76.

Proctor et al. offer a groundbreaking summary of issues in the design and evaluation of implementation research, setting out a model that defines steps in the process and discusses a model for quantifying the benefits of program implementation. The ability to measure implementation outcomes leads to better understanding of the implementation process and improves efficiency.

Rabin BA, Lewis CC, Norton WE, et al. Measurement resources for dissemination and implementation research in health. *Implement Sci.* 2016;11:42.

This article presents results from an environmental scan of published systematic reviews of D&I measures and publicly available web resources. This work stemmed from the 2014 invited meeting sponsored by the National Institutes of Health that focused on advancing D&I measurement and reporting standards.

Shelton RC, Chambers DA, & Glasgow RE. An extension of RE-AIM to enhance sustainability: addressing dynamic context and promoting health equity over time. Front Public Health. 2000;8:134.

This article offers a reconsideration of the widely utilized RE-AIM framework to address current conceptualizations of sustainability and dynamic context while promoting health equity. The addendums to this framework serve to guide planning, measurement, and adaptations to promote intervention sustainability.

Selected Websites and Tools

Cancer Control P.L.A.N.E.T. https://toolsofchange.com/en/topic-resources/detail/69

Cancer Control P.L.A.N.E.T. acts as a portal to provide access to data and resources for designing, implementing, and evaluating evidence-based cancer control programs. The site provides five steps (with links) for developing a comprehensive cancer control plan or program.

CDC Behavioral Risk Surveillance System (BRFSS). https://www.cdc.gov/brfss/

The BRFSS, an ongoing data collection program conducted in all states, the District of Columbia, and three US territories, and the world's largest telephone survey, tracks health risks in the United States. Information from the survey is used to improve the health of the American people. The CDC has developed a standard core questionnaire so that data can be compared across various strata.

CDC WONDER. http://wonder.cdc.gov

CDC WONDER is an easy-to-use system that provides a single point of access to a wide variety of CDC reports, guidelines, and numeric public health data. It can be valuable in public health research, decision-making, priority setting, program evaluation, and resource allocation.

Center for Evaluation and Implementation (CEIR). http://www.queri.research.va.gov/ceir/

The Veterans Affairs (VA) Center for Evaluation and Implementation (CEIR) is a Quality Enhancement Research Initiative (QUERI) resource center that provides time-sensitive consultation and support to VA healthcare delivery system leaders to enable scale-up and spread of effective policies, practices, and programs aligned with VA priorities. CIPRS programs include consultation to VA implementation practitioners and researchers, and web-based guides and training opportunities.

Group Evaluated Measures (GEM). https://www.gem-beta.org/Public/Home.aspx

The Group Evaluated Measures (GEM) Database represents a wiki platform dedicated to increasing access and harmonization of measures used in D&I.[88] *GEM enables its users to add constructs and measures, contribute to and update measure metadata (e.g., psychometric quality), rate and comment on measures, access and share harmonized data, and access measures.*

Implementation Science. http://implementationscience.biomedcentral.com/

Implementation Science is an open-access, peer-reviewed online journal that aims to publish research relevant to the scientific study of methods to promote the uptake of research findings into routine healthcare in both clinical and policy contexts. The website provides links to articles, many of which address measurement issues in implementation research, as well as links to questionnaires for measuring key constructs in implementation research.

National Center for Health Statistics. http://www.cdc.gov/nchs/

The National Center for Health Statistics (NCHS) is the principal vital and health statistics agency for the US government. NCHS data systems include information on vital events as well as information on health status, lifestyle and exposure to unhealthy influences, the onset and diagnosis of illness and disability, and the use of healthcare. NCHS has two major types of data systems: systems based on populations, containing data collected through personal interviews or examinations (e.g., National Health Interview Survey and National Health and Nutrition Examination Survey), and systems based on records, containing data collected from vital and medical records. These data are used by policymakers in the US Congress and the administration, by medical researchers, and by others in the health community.

Society for Implementation Research Collaboration (SIRC). https://societyforimplementationresearchcollaboration.org/

The Society for Implementation Research Collaboration (SIRC) is a free-standing society that grew out of a R13 conference series grant funded by the National Institute of Mental Health (NIMH) and led by principal investigator Kate Comtois. SIRC aims to advance rigorous methods and measurement for the evaluation and practice of D&I, primarily with respect to behavioral health. SIRC served as the springboard for the Instrument Review Project, which includes a systematic review of measures pertaining to constructs of the CFIR[87] *and the implementation outcomes framework*[7,11] *via an NIMH-funded R01 to principal investigator Cara Lewis.*

REFERENCES

1. Sallis JF, Owen N, Fotheringham MJ. Behavioral epidemiology: a systematic framework to classify phases of research on health promotion and disease prevention. *Ann Behav Med.* Fall 2000;22(4):294–298.
2. Rabin BA, Lewis CC, Norton WE, et al. Measurement resources for dissemination and implementation research in health. *Implement Sci.* Mar 22 2016;11:42. doi:10.1186/s13012-016-0401-y
3. Neta G, Glasgow RE, Carpenter CR, et al. A framework for enhancing the value of research

for dissemination and implementation. *Am J Public Health*. Jan 2015;105(1):49–57. doi:10.2105/AJPH.2014.302206

4. McKibbon KA, Lokker C, Wilczynski NL, et al. A cross-sectional study of the number and frequency of terms used to refer to knowledge translation in a body of health literature in 2006: a Tower of Babel? *Implement Sci*. Feb 12 2010;5:16. doi:10.1186/1748-5908-5-16
5. Rabin BA, Brownson RC. Developing the terminology for dissemination and implementation research in health. In: Brownson RC, Colditz GA, Proctor EK, eds. *Dissemination and Implementation Research in Health: Translating Science to Practice*. 2nd ed. Oxford University Press; 2017.
6. Grimshaw J, Eccles M, Thomas R, et al. Toward evidence-based quality improvement. Evidence (and its limitations) of the effectiveness of guideline dissemination and implementation strategies 1966–1998. *J Gen Intern Med*. Feb 2006;21(suppl 2):S14–S20. doi:10.1111/j.1525-1497.2006.00357.x
7. Proctor E, Landsverk J, Aarons G, Chambers D, Glisson C, Mittman B. Implementation research in mental health services: an emerging science with conceptual, methodological, and training challenges. *Adm Policy Ment Health*. Jan 2009;36(1):24–34. doi:10.1007/s10488-008-0197-4
8. Institute of Medicine (IOM). *Crossing the Quality Chasm: A New Health System for the 21st Century*. Institute of Medicine, National Academy Press; 2001.
9. Institute of Medicine Committee on Crossing the Quality Chasm. *Adaption to Mental Health and Addictive Disorder: Improving the Quality of Health Care for Mental and Substance-Use Conditions*. Institute of Medicine, National Academies Press; 2006.
10. Brownson RC, Chriqui JF, Stamatakis KA. Understanding evidence-based public health policy. *Am J Public Health*. Sep 2009;99(9):1576–1583. doi:10.2105/AJPH.2008.156224
11. Proctor E, Silmere H, Raghavan R, et al. Outcomes for implementation research: conceptual distinctions, measurement challenges, and research agenda. *Adm Policy Ment Health*. Mar 2011;38(2):65–76. doi:10.1007/s10488-010-0319-7
12. Strifler L, Cardoso R, McGowan J, et al. Scoping review identifies significant number of knowledge translation theories, models, and frameworks with limited use. *J Clin Epidemiol*. Aug 2018;100:92–102. doi:10.1016/j.jclinepi.2018.04.008
13. Gerring J. *Social Science Methodology: A Criterial Framework*. Cambridge University Press; 2001.
14. Hrisos S, Eccles MP, Francis JJ, et al. Are there valid proxy measures of clinical behaviour? A systematic review. *Implement Sci*. Jul 03 2009;4:37. doi:10.1186/1748-5908-4-37
15. Ibrahim S, Sidani S. Fidelity of intervention implementation: a review of instruments. *Health Aff*. 2015;7(12):1687–1695. doi:10.4236/health.2015.712183
16. Weiner BJ, Amick H, Lee SY. Conceptualization and measurement of organizational readiness for change: a review of the literature in health services research and other fields. *Med Care Res Rev*. Aug 2008;65(4):379–436. doi:10.1177/1077558708317802
17. Emmons KM, Weiner B, Fernandez ME, Tu SP. Systems antecedents for dissemination and implementation: a review and analysis of measures. *Health Educ Behav*. Feb 2012;39(1):87–105. doi:10.1177/1090198111409748
18. Chaudoir SR, Dugan AG, Barr CH. Measuring factors affecting implementation of health innovations: a systematic review of structural, organizational, provider, patient, and innovation level measures. *Implement Sci*. Feb 17 2013;8:22. doi:10.1186/1748-5908-8-22
19. Lewis CC, Stanick CF, Martinez RG, et al. The Society for Implementation Research Collaboration Instrument Review Project: a methodology to promote rigorous evaluation. *Implement Sci*. 2016;10(1):1–18. doi:10.1186/s13012-014-0193-x
20. Chor KH, Wisdom JP, Olin SC, Hoagwood KE, Horwitz SM. Measures for predictors of innovation adoption. *Adm Policy Ment Health*. Sep 2015;42(5):545–573. doi:10.1007/s10488-014-0551-7
21. Mettert K, Lewis C, Dorsey C, Halko H, Weiner B. Measuring implementation outcomes: an updated systematic review of measures' psychometric properties. *Implement Res Pract*. 2020;1:2633489520936644. doi:10.1177/2633489520936644
22. Weiner BJ, Mettert KD, Dorsey CN, et al. Measuring readiness for implementation: a systematic review of measures' psychometric and pragmatic properties. *Implementation Res Pract*. 2020;1:2633489520933896. doi:10.1177/2633489520933896
23. Powell BJ, Mettert KD, Dorsey CN, et al. Measures of organizational culture, organizational climate, and implementation climate in behavioral health: a systematic review. *Implement Res Pract*. 2021;2:26334895211018862. doi:10.1177/26334895211018862
24. Dorsey CN, Mettert KD, Puspitasari AJ, Damschroder LJ, Lewis CC. A systematic

review of measures of implementation players and processes: summarizing the dearth of psychometrics evidence. *Implement Res Pract.* 2021;2:26334895211002474.

25. McHugh S, Dorsey CN, Mettert K, Purtle J, Bruns E, Lewis CC. Measures of outer setting constructs for implementation research: a systematic review and analysis of psychometric quality. *Implement Res Pract.* 2020;1:2633489520940022. doi:10.1177/2633489520940022
26. Allen P, Pilar M, Walsh-Bailey C, et al. Quantitative measures of health policy implementation determinants and outcomes: a systematic review. *Implement Sci.* 2020;15(1):47. doi:10.1186/s13012-020-01007-w
27. McLoughlin GM, Allen P, Walsh-Bailey C, Brownson RC. A systematic review of school health policy measurement tools: implementation determinants and outcomes. *Implement Sci Commun.* 2021;2(1):67. doi:10.1186/s43058-021-00169-y
28. Khadjesari Z, Boufkhed S, Vitoratou S, et al. Implementation outcome instruments for use in physical healthcare settings: a systematic review. *Implement Sci.* 2020;15(1):66. doi:10.1186/s13012-020-01027-6
29. Allen JD, Towne SD, Maxwell AE, et al. Measures of organizational characteristics associated with adoption and/or implementation of innovations: a systematic review. *BMC Health Serv Res.* 2017;17(1):591. doi:10.1186/s12913-017-2459-x
30. Moullin JC, Sklar M, Green A, et al. Advancing the pragmatic measurement of sustainment: a narrative review of measures. *Implement Sci Commun.* 2020;1(1):76. doi:10.1186/s43058-020-00068-8
31. Stanick C, Halko H, Mettert K, et al. Measuring characteristics of individuals: an updated systematic review of instruments' psychometric properties. *Implement Res Pract.* 2021;2:26334895211000458. doi:10.1177/26334895211000458
32. Lewis CC, Mettert K, Lyon AR. Determining the influence of intervention characteristics on implementation success requires reliable and valid measures: results from a systematic review. *Implement Res Pract.* 2021;2:2633489521994197. doi:10.1177/2633489521994197
33. Lewis CC, Mettert KD, Stanick CF, et al. The Psychometric and Pragmatic Evidence Rating Scale (PAPERS) for measure development and evaluation. *Implement Res Pract.* 2021;2:26334895211037391. doi:10.1177/26334895211037391
34. Burnes B. Emergent change and planned change—competitors or allies? The case of XYZ construction. *International Journal of Operations & Production Management.* 2004;24(9):886–902. doi:doi:10.1108/01443570410552108
35. Waldorff FB, Steenstrup AP, Nielsen B, Rubak J, Bro F. Diffusion of an e-learning programme among Danish general practitioners: a nationwide prospective survey. *BMC Fam Pract.* Apr 25 2008;9:24. doi:10.1186/1471-2296-9-24
36. Adily A, Westbrook J, Coiera E, Ward J. Use of on-line evidence databases by Australian public health practitioners. *Med Inform Internet Med.* Jun 2004;29(2):127–136. doi:10.1080/14639230410001723437
37. Fischer MA, Vogeli C, Stedman MR, Ferris TG, Weissman JS. Uptake of electronic prescribing in community-based practices. *J Gen Intern Med.* Apr 2008;23(4):358–363. doi:10.1007/s11606-007-0383-1
38. Cooke M, Mattick RP, Walsh RA. Implementation of the "Fresh Start" smoking cessation programme to 23 antenatal clinics: a randomized controlled trial investigating two methods of dissemination. *Drug Alcohol Rev.* 2001;20(1):19–28. doi:10.1080/09595230124432
39. Aarons GA, Hurlburt M, Horwitz SM. Advancing a conceptual model of evidence-based practice implementation in public service sectors. *Adm Policy Ment Health.* Jan 2011;38(1):4–23. doi:10.1007/s10488-010-0327-7
40. Moullin JC, Dickson KS, Stadnick NA, Rabin B, Aarons GA. Systematic review of the Exploration, Preparation, Implementation, Sustainment (EPIS) framework. *Implement Sci.* 2019;14(1):1. doi:10.1186/s13012-018-0842-6
41. Rabin BA, Glasgow RE, Kerner JF, Klump MP, Brownson RC. Dissemination and implementation research on community-based cancer prevention: a systematic review. *Am J Prev Med.* Apr 2010;38(4):443–456. doi:10.1016/j.amepre.2009.12.035
42. Rabin BA, Brownson RC, Kerner JF, Glasgow RE. Methodologic challenges in disseminating evidence-based interventions to promote physical activity. *Am J Prev Med.* Oct 2006;31(4)(suppl):S24–S34. doi:10.1016/j.amepre.2006.06.009
43. Purtle J, Crane ME, Nelson KL, Brownson RC. Disseminating information about evidence-based interventions. In: Weiner BJ, Lewis CC, Sherr K, eds. *Practical Implementation Science: Moving Evidence into Action.* Springer Publishing; 2022:227–252.
44. Dingfelder HE, Mandell DS. Bridging the research-to-practice gap in autism intervention: an application of diffusion of innovation theory. *J Autism Dev Disord.* May 2011;41(5):597–609. doi:10.1007/s10803-010-1081-0

45. Cane J, O'Connor D, Michie S. Validation of the theoretical domains framework for use in behaviour change and implementation research. *Implement Sci.* Apr 24 2012;7:37. doi:10.1186/1748-5908-7-37
46. Rabin BA, Brownson RC, Haire-Joshu D, Kreuter MW, Weaver NL. A glossary for dissemination and implementation research in health. *J Public Health Manag Pract.* Mar-Apr 2008;14(2):117–123. doi:10.1097/01.PHH.0000311888.06252.bb
47. Rogers EM. *Diffusion of Innovations.* 4th ed. Free Press; 1995.
48. Lewis CC, Mettert KD, Stanick CF, et al. The psychometric and pragmatic evidence rating scale (PAPERS) for measure development and evaluation. *Implement Res Pract.* 2021;2:26334895211037391.
49. Karsh BT. Beyond usability: designing effective technology implementation systems to promote patient safety. *Qual Saf Health Care.* Oct 2004;13(5):388–394. doi:10.1136/qhc.13.5.388
50. Lewis CC, Weiner BJ, Stanick C, Fischer SM. Advancing implementation science through measure development and evaluation: a study protocol. *Implement Sci.* Jul 22 2015;10:102. doi:10.1186/s13012-015-0287-0
51. Rye CB, Kimberly JR. The adoption of innovations by provider organizations in health care. *Med Care Res Rev.* Jun 2007;64(3):235–278. doi:10.1177/1077558707299865
52. Shelton RC, Chambers DA, Glasgow RE. An extension of RE-AIM to enhance sustainability: addressing dynamic context and promoting health equity over time. *Front Public Health.* 2020;8:134. doi:10.3389/fpubh.2020.00134
53. Dusenbury L, Brannigan R, Falco M, Hansen WB. A review of research on fidelity of implementation: implications for drug abuse prevention in school settings. *Health Educ Res.* Apr 2003;18(2):237–256.
54. Mihalic S. The importance of implementation fidelity. *J Emot Behav Disord in Youth.* 2004;4(4):83–105.
55. Dane AV, Schneider BH. Program integrity in primary and early secondary prevention: are implementation effects out of control? *Clin Psychol Rev.* Jan 1998;18(1):23–45.
56. Schoenwald SK, Garland AF, Chapman JE, Frazier SL, Sheidow AJ, Southam-Gerow MA. Toward the effective and efficient measurement of implementation fidelity. *Adm Policy Ment Health.* Jan 2011;38(1):32–43. doi:10.1007/s10488-010-0321-0
57. Perera C, Salamanca-Sanabria A, Caballero-Bernal J, et al. No implementation without cultural adaptation: a process for culturally adapting low-intensity psychological interventions in humanitarian settings. *Conflict Health.* 2020/07/14 2020;14(1):46. doi:10.1186/s13031-020-00290-0
58. Stiles PG, Boothroyd RA, Snyder K, Zong X. Service penetration by persons with severe mental illness: how should it be measured? *J Behav Health Serv Res.* May 2002;29(2):198–207.
59. Glasgow RE. The RE-AIM model for planning, evaluation and reporting on implementation and dissemination research. Presented at: NIH Conference on Building the Science of D & I in the Service of Public Health; 2007; Bethesda, MD.
60. Johnson K, Hays C, Center H, Daley C. Building capacity and sustainable prevention innovations: a sustainability planning model. *Eval Prog Plann.* 2004;27(2):135–149. doi:10.1016/j.evalprogplan.2004.01.002
61. Turner KMT, Sanders MR. Dissemination of evidence-based parenting and family support strategies: learning from the Triple P—Positive Parenting Program system approach. *Aggress Violent Behav.* 2006;11(2):176–193. doi:10.1016/j.avb.2005.07.005
62. Glasgow RE, Vogt TM, Boles SM. Evaluating the public health impact of health promotion interventions: the RE-AIM framework. *Am J Public Health.* Sep 1999;89(9):1322–1327.
63. Goodman RM, McLeroy KR, Steckler AB, Hoyle RH. Development of level of institutionalization scales for health promotion programs. *Health Educ Q.* Summer 1993;20(2):161–178.
64. Woolf SH. The meaning of translational research and why it matters. *JAMA.* 2008;299(2):211–213. doi:10.1001/jama.2007.26
65. Repenning NP. A simulation-based approach to understanding the dynamics of innovation implementation. *Org Sci.* 2002;13(2):109–127. doi:10.1287/orsc.13.2.109.535
66. Hovmand PS, Gillespie DF. Implementation of evidence-based practice and organizational performance. *J Behav Health Serv Res.* Jan 2010;37(1):79–94. doi:10.1007/s11414-008-9154-y
67. Klein KJ, Knight AP. Innovation implementation. *Curr Dir Psychol Sci.* 2005;14(5):243–246. doi:doi:10.1111/j.0963-7214.2005.00373.x
68. Chambers DA. Advancing the science of implementation: a workshop summary. *Adm Policy Ment Health.* Mar 2008;35(1–2):3–10. doi:10.1007/s10488-007-0146-7
69. Kimberly J, Cook JM. Organizational measurement and the implementation of innovations in mental health services. *Adm Policy Ment Health.* Mar 2008;35(1–2):11–20. doi:10.1007/s10488-007-0143-x

70. US Department of Health and Human Services. *The road ahead: Research partnerships to transform services A report by the National Advisory Mental Health Council's Workgroup on Services and Clinical Epidemiology Research*. Bethesda, MD: National Institutes of Health, National Institute of Mental Health; 2006.
71. Coyne I, McNamara N, Healy M, Gower C, Sarkar M, McNicholas F. Adolescents' and parents' views of Child and Adolescent Mental Health Services (CAMHS) in Ireland. *J Psychiatr Ment Health Nurs.* Oct 2015;22(8):561–569. doi:10.1111/jpm.12215
72. Kerner J, Rimer B, Emmons K. Introduction to the special section on dissemination: dissemination research and research dissemination: how can we close the gap? *Health Psychol.* Sep 2005;24(5):443–446. doi:10.1037/0278-6133.24.5.443
73. Lambooij MS, Hummel MJ. Differentiating innovation priorities among stakeholder in hospital care. *BMC Med Inform Decis Mak.* Aug 16 2013;13:91. doi:10.1186/1472-6947-13-91
74. Wahlster P, Goetghebeur M, Kriza C, Niederlander C, Kolominsky-Rabas P, National Leading-Edge Cluster Medical Technologies' Medical Valley EMN. Balancing costs and benefits at different stages of medical innovation: a systematic review of multi-criteria decision analysis (MCDA). *BMC Health Serv Res.* Jul 09 2015;15:262. doi:10.1186/s12913-015-0930-0
75. Preston CC, Colman AM. Optimal number of response categories in rating scales: reliability, validity, discriminating power, and respondent preferences. *Acta Psychol (Amst).* Mar 2000;104(1):1–15.
76. Sándor Z, Wedel M. Heterogeneous conjoint choice designs. *J Mark Res.* 2005;42(2):210–218. doi:10.1509/jmkr.42.2.210.62285
77. Wierenga SJ, Kamsteeg FH, Simons RJ, Veenswijk M. Teachers making sense of result-oriented teams: a cognitive anthropological approach to educational change. *J Educ Change.* 2015;16(1):53–78. doi:10.1007/s10833-014-9240-2
78. Shumway M, Sentell T, Chouljian T, Tellier J, Rozewicz F, Okun M. Assessing preferences for schizophrenia outcomes: comprehension and decision strategies in three assessment methods. *Ment Health Serv Res.* Sep 2003;5(3):121–135.
79. Palinkas LA. Nutritional interventions for treatment of seasonal affective disorder. *CNS Neurosci Ther.* Spring 2010;16(1):3–5. doi:10.1111/j.1755-5949.2009.00123.x
80. Shumway M, Saunders T, Shern D, et al. Preferences for schizophrenia treatment outcomes among public policy makers, consumers, families, and providers. *Psychiatr Serv.* Aug 2003;54(8):1124–1128. doi:10.1176/appi.ps.54.8.1124
81. Glasgow RE, Riley WT. Pragmatic measures: what they are and why we need them. *Am J Prev Med.* Aug 2013;45(2):237–243. doi:10.1016/j.amepre.2013.03.010
82. Martinez RG, Lewis CC, Weiner BJ. Instrumentation issues in implementation science. *Implement Sci.* Sep 04 2014;9:118. doi:10.1186/s13012-014-0118-8
83. Lengnick-Hall R, Gerke DR, Proctor EK, et al. Six practical recommendations for improved implementation outcomes reporting. *Implement Sci.* 2022;17(1):16. doi:10.1186/s13012-021-01183-3
84. Raghavan R, Bright CL, Shadoin AL. Toward a policy ecology of implementation of evidence-based practices in public mental health settings. *Implement Sci.* May 16 2008;3:26. doi:10.1186/1748-5908-3-26
85. Frost MH, Reeve BB, Liepa AM, Stauffer JW, Hays RD, Mayo FDA Patient-Reported Outcomes Consensus Meeting Group. What is sufficient evidence for the reliability and validity of patient-reported outcome measures? *Value Health.* Nov–Dec 2007;10(suppl 2):S94–S105. doi:10.1111/j.1524-4733.2007.00272.x
86. Luke DA. *Multilevel Modeling.* Sage University Papers Series on Quantitative Applications in the Social Sciences. Sage; 2004.
87. Damschroder LJ, Aron DC, Keith RE, Kirsh SR, Alexander JA, Lowery JC. Fostering implementation of health services research findings into practice: a consolidated framework for advancing implementation science. *Implement Sci.* Aug 07 2009;4:50. doi:10.1186/1748-5908-4-50
88. Rabin BA, Purcell P, Naveed S, et al. Advancing the application, quality and harmonization of implementation science measures. *Implement Sci.* Dec 11 2012;7:119. doi:10.1186/1748-5908-7-119

16

Furthering Dissemination and Implementation Research

Paying More Attention to External Validity Through an Equity Lens

KATY E. TRINKLEY, DEMETRIA M. MCNEAL, MEREDITH P. FORT, LAWRENCE W. GREEN, AND AMY G. HUEBSCHMANN

INTRODUCTION

Channels and tools of disseminating medical and public health literature have become more efficient, accessible, and omnipresent in their capacity to index, distribute, and search for publications. Clinicians, policymakers, and community practitioners seldom complain anymore that they cannot find something published on their issue at hand. Their complaint now is more often that they are drowning in information but starved for relevance. This disconnect between the growing volume of available medical and public health literature and its limited relevance to practitioners, populations, or settings is a concerning indictment of the research establishment's lack of attention to external validity.[1–3] Indeed, perceived lack of relevance is a frequently stated reason that evidence-based interventions are not adopted[3–6] and a barrier to achieving the visionary goals of a learning health system in which research informs practice and practice informs research.[7–9] Despite recognition of this problem as a driving force for development of the field of dissemination and implementation (D&I) science and calls by ourselves and others to address this issue for over two decades, external validity is still underemphasized relative to internal validity for many researchers, journal editors, reviewers, and funders.[3,10–14]

Achieving greater research relevance requires us to question the assumptions of traditional efficacy trials that prioritize internal validity to generate data on causal associations.[13] The generalizability of "proven" efficacy studies is limited to the narrow range of populations, settings, treatment conditions, and outcomes they sample and observe.[13] For example, the gold standard, a randomized controlled efficacy trial, often occurs in an academic setting, typically with higher levels of resources than are found elsewhere. Yet, the majority of healthcare and public health services happen in nonacademic hospitals, health centers, clinics, schools, worksites, and community settings. This begs the question: How do outcomes realized in a high-resourced academic setting consisting of a mostly homogeneous group of participants and staff translate, or compare, to the outcomes expected in a diverse community-based setting? The usual answer, "Not very well," thus limiting the external validity.[14–17] This challenge has led to the pithy observation that in order to increase the rate of translation of evidence-based practice, we need more practice-based evidence, gathered with attention to external validity by drawing from diverse and representative settings and populations.[13–15,18]

Research that attends to external validity also holds promise for addressing the critical problem of health inequities, including disparities in mortality, chronic disease management, and the delivery of healthcare and public health services among certain populations and communities. We consider

Katy E. Trinkley, Demetria M. McNeal, Meredith P. Fort, Lawrence W. Green, and Amy G. Huebschmann, *Furthering Dissemination and Implementation Research* In: *Dissemination and Implementation Research in Health.* Edited by: Ross C. Brownson, Graham A. Colditz, and Enola K. Proctor, Oxford University Press. © Oxford University Press 2023. DOI: 10.1093/oso/9780197660690.003.0016 populations experiencing inequities broadly as those who have experienced health inequities related to historical, cultural, and social barriers/discrimination and based on race/ethnicity, gender, sexual orientation, disability, income, immigration status, living in geographically remote areas, or other factors.[19–23]

The World Health Organization, National Institutes of Health (NIH), American Heart Association, Centers for Disease Control and Prevention (CDC), and others have recently intensified their push for more attention to the role that social and environmental determinants of health play in propagating health inequities.[24–32] These include the role of the built environment, food deserts, neighborhood segregation, and environmental injustice in fostering differential rates of diabetes, hypertension, asthma, and other chronic diseases in low-income communities as a form of structural racism.[24,25,27,33,34] Spurred by greater societal attention to structural racism, organizations around the globe have acknowledged and declared a commitment to dismantling racial discrimination, including the need to address this issue among scientists, health policymakers, and health practitioners. Specifically, on March 1, 2021, the director of the NIH launched an initiative aimed at helping to bring an end to structural racism in biomedical research.[30,35] Shortly thereafter, the director of the CDC released a statement declaring racism a "serious public health threat that directly affects the well-being of millions of Americans."[36] Taken together, there is a clear call to action for the scientific community to consciously and proactively highlight and address systemic acts of oppression and inequity due to race/ethnicity, class, gender, and many other forms of discrimination across the healthcare and public health continuum—as well as at higher policy levels.

The field of D&I science has responded to this call to action by doubling down on the importance of considering health equity when applying D&I approaches to deliver evidence-based programs across all phases of research—spanning the preimplementation, implementation, and evaluation/sustainment phases.[28,29,31,37–39] With all of these factors in mind, in this chapter we underscore opportunities within the field of D&I science to plan, implement, and evaluate research with attention to external validity through an equity lens. The use of an equity lens emphasizes the inclusion and representation of low-resource and marginalized communities in the research process.

The lack of attention to external validity is a key contributor to another major health research problem: the failure to replicate findings.[10,40–42] This replication problem impedes the goals of learning health systems to support a symbiosis of reciprocal relevance between evidence-based practice and practice-based evidence.[7–9,13,43] Part of the failure to disseminate evidence-based programs is because researchers have not reported enough information to allow for replicability or programs are not applicable when exported into real-world, non-academic settings.[3,13,15,44] Failure to replicate or adapt is especially problematic in applied T3/T4 translational research that is conducted in highly heterogeneous, real-world settings that are inherently more complex; the high degree of contextual variability in these pragmatic studies may influence the intervention response across settings to a greater degree than in highly controlled explanatory studies.[40–42] To understand replicability of findings, adequate reporting of the following is needed: the intervention's form and function,[17,45] the context of settings, participants and communities, and adaptations needed to fit the context.[3,6,46] Without adequate reporting it is difficult to attribute inconsistent results across studies to a failure to replicate faithfully or whether they occur because effects are conditioned on important contextual factors.[6,17,45,47–49]

This discourse does not seek to denigrate or sacrifice efficacy trials—explanatory research that prioritizes internal validity over external validity.[3,13] Rather, we seek to place a greater emphasis on external validity and examine the natural consequences of limited attention to external validity. One overarching consequence of limited attention to external validity is that if clinicians, communities, and policymakers do not see evidence-based programs generated in environments relevant to where they live, work, study, play, and worship, they will remain skeptical of adopting such programs due to the limited applicability, relevance, and fit.[5,10,14,16]

In our third edition update to this chapter, our two key goals are *(1) to highlight the importance of paying attention to threats to external validity through an equity lens and (2) to showcase opportunities to enhance the relevance and reproducibility of studies by engaging diverse invested partners (or stakeholders) to generate equitable practice-based evidence.* The rationale for adding this equity lens is to promote the equitable translation of evidence to low-resource settings and the equitable impact of research on low-resource populations. In particular, we propose specific ways to engage diverse invested partners and settings throughout the research life cycle: from the early planning phases through the evaluation and sustainment phases. Concrete examples that we feature include *community-based participatory research (CBPR) and learning health systems approaches*, among others.

To meet our goals, this chapter first provides a discussion of key conceptual and methodological issues related to external validity with an emphasis on health equity; next, we include an outline of approaches to enhance external validity in each of the three key project phases within D&I process models (the preimplementation phase of study design and planning, implementation phase, and evaluation/sustainment phases, shown in Figure 16.1); finally, we conclude with concrete recommendations for those who influence the conduct of research and its later translation, including grant funders, researchers, journal editors, clinical and public health practitioners, and policymakers.

EXTERNAL VALIDITY: WHAT IT IS

External validity asks: To what populations, settings, treatment variables, and measurement variables can this effect be generalized? External validity is concerned with whether a causal effect generalizes to most, if not all, units of people, treatments, observations, or settings.[10,50] For pragmatic research that is intended to provide relevant, applied data to inform health organization decisions, external validity is particularly important.[36,49–51] One must ask the So what? question if a study is airtight with its internal validity but has nowhere to go with its lack of external validity. External validity is diminished when an experiment is less representative of real-world participants, practitioners, interventions, outcome measures, and settings where it is expected to apply.[3,52] In addition, external validity is also diminished when research does not represent those populations and settings that are historically marginalized or difficult to reach. The places and populations seen as hardest to reach, late adopters, and the underserved are often underrepresented in much of the research that generates the "evidence-based practices" we are seeking to disseminate. The logical conclusion is that in order to increase the *representativeness* of our research findings to future potential adopters, it is key to seek *representation* proactively in research of low-resource settings, as well as the populations experiencing inequities who are disproportionately served within low-resource settings. It may also be necessary, at least to confer again with such populations, when the historical circumstances have changed since the original study was conducted.

Threats to External Validity

Common threats to external validity that can diminish the impact or generalizability of research have been defined in the previous edition of this textbook,[53] based on seminal publications of internal and external validity, as the (1) "interaction of the intervention and any pre-intervention testing" or run-in periods; (2) "interaction of the intervention and participant selection"; (3) "reactive arrangements due to the settings"; (4) "interaction of treatment variations with the causal relationship" (failure to replicate); (5) and "context-dependent mediation". (pp303–304). We further simplify the description of these threats to external validity in the following bulleted list, with consideration of other recent publications on factors known to influence external validity,[10,49] such as priority/relevance to invested partners:

- *Unrealistic resource expectations/selection bias of settings*: Research is too seldom tested with realistic expectations of the staff and organizational resources of future adopters. Specifically, interventions and implementation strategies that require large amounts of research staff training, time, and/or resources are often infeasible for public health or community practice settings—particularly for low-resource settings, such as Federally Qualified Health Centers. Instead, randomized controlled trials (RCTs) are often conducted within urban academic settings—driven partly by ease of resource availability and a culture that more readily embraces research. Overall, we would frame

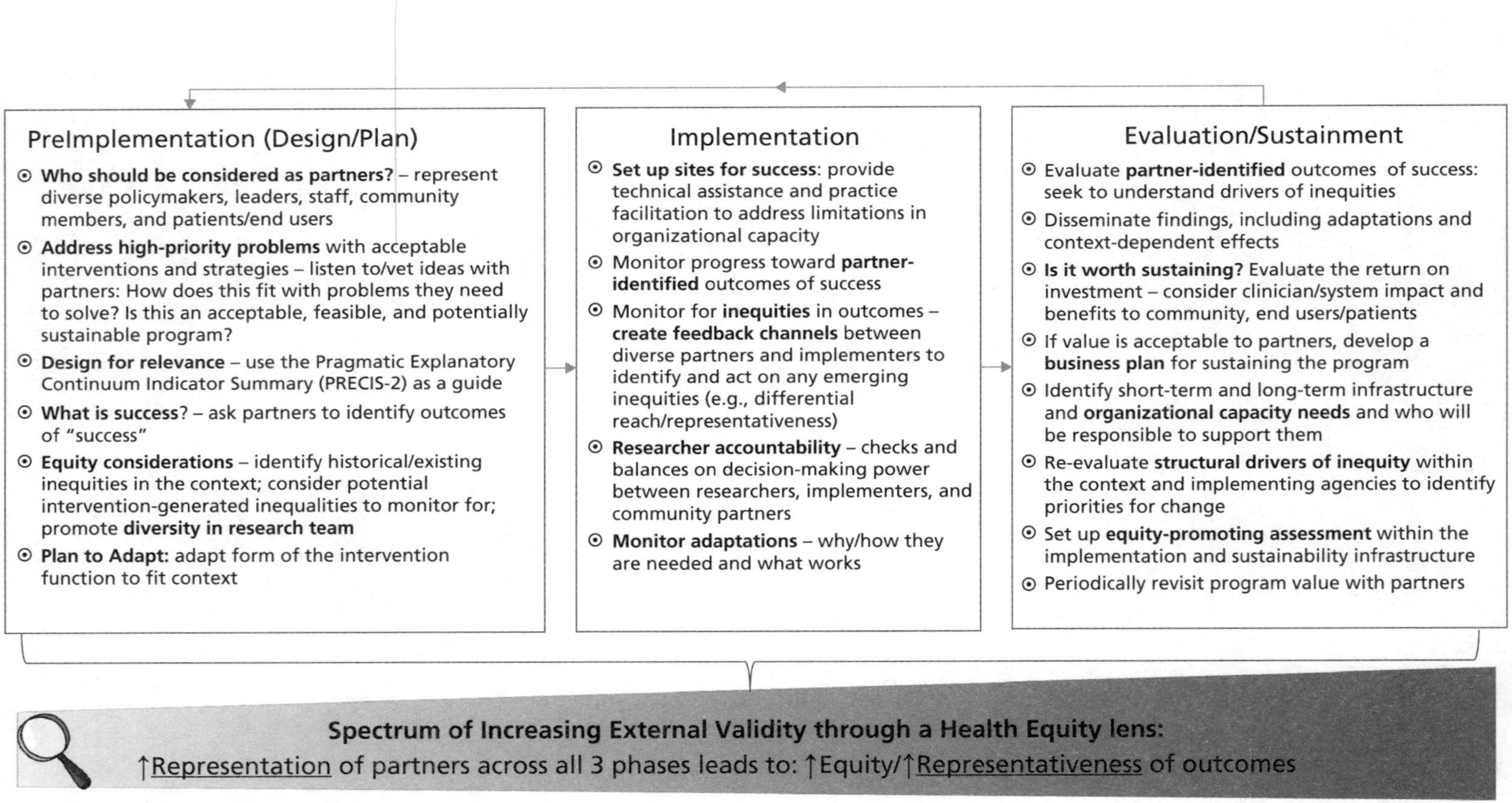

PreImplementation (Design/Plan)

- **Who should be considered as partners?** – represent diverse policymakers, leaders, staff, community members, and patients/end users
- **Address high-priority problems** with acceptable interventions and strategies – listen to/vet ideas with partners: How does this fit with problems they need to solve? Is this an acceptable, feasible, and potentially sustainable program?
- **Design for relevance** – use the Pragmatic Explanatory Continuum Indicator Summary (PRECIS-2) as a guide
- **What is success**? – ask partners to identify outcomes of "success"
- **Equity considerations** – identify historical/existing inequities in the context; consider potential intervention-generated inequalities to monitor for; promote **diversity in research team**
- **Plan to Adapt:** adapt form of the intervention function to fit context

Implementation

- **Set up sites for success**: provide technical assistance and practice facilitation to address limitations in organizational capacity
- Monitor progress toward **partner-identified** outcomes of success
- Monitor for **inequities** in outcomes – **create feedback channels** between diverse partners and implementers to identify and act on any emerging inequities (e.g., differential reach/representativeness)
- **Researcher accountability** – checks and balances on decision-making power between researchers, implementers, and community partners
- **Monitor adaptations** – why/how they are needed and what works

Evaluation/Sustainment

- Evaluate **partner-identified** outcomes of success: seek to understand drivers of inequities
- Disseminate findings, including adaptations and context-dependent effects
- **Is it worth sustaining?** Evaluate the return on investment – consider clinician/system impact and benefits to community, end users/patients
- If value is acceptable to partners, develop a **business plan** for sustaining the program
- Identify short-term and long-term infrastructure and **organizational capacity needs** and who will be responsible to support them
- Re-evaluate **structural drivers of inequity** within the context and implementing agencies to identify priorities for change
- Set up **equity-promoting assessment** within the implementation and sustainability infrastructure
- Periodically revisit program value with partners

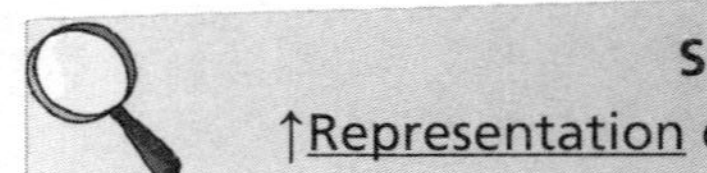

Spectrum of Increasing External Validity through a Health Equity lens:

↑Representation of partners across all 3 phases leads to: ↑Equity/↑Representativeness of outcomes

FIGURE 16.1 Factors to consider across research phases to promote external validity through a health equity lens.

Source: Adapted from the VA Quality Enhancement Research Initiative (QUERI) Roadmap[87] and other process models (Exploration, Preparation, Implementation, Sustainment[39]; Replicating Effective Programs[84]), with attention to health equity and community-based participatory research principles (Wallerstein et al.[92]).

this issue as a failure to test programs with representative staff and delivery conditions (e.g., supervision, feedback, and measurement).

- *Low-priority or externally imposed topics*: Research topics that are selected for studies may not be priorities for communities where they are intended to be implemented in the future. Communities are often not consulted or engaged adequately in defining the research problem; furthermore, study teams often lack diversity and expertise in community context. Limited relevance of the research problem to invested partners can lead to low levels of uptake or support, especially in settings where more basic and high-priority needs have not been met. The problem of limited relevance may become most evident once funding no longer supports an initial testing and implementation phase.
- *Unrepresentative participants/selection bias of participants*: Research is too seldom tested with representative participants. Participants in research studies are often less diverse than in the real world, in terms of the comorbidities allowed, as well as the cultural, demographic, and health literacy differences; these factors often influence program effectiveness. Research that "cherry-picks" participants based on their likelihood of success also suffers from a "cooperativeness" selection bias that lessens external validity. While RCTs are the so-called gold standard on which many therapeutic decisions and clinical practice guidelines are based, these trials have often underrepresented certain subgroups, such as older adults, youth, and people of color, and others less likely to consent to participation.
- *Interventions and strategies too tightly controlled*: Research interventions that are planned as highly controlled studies and inflexible to local site adaptation might require redesign or increased observational resources to monitor processes and adaptations of implementation. Tightly controlled interventions often do not generate results that apply to real-world people and settings that are highly heterogeneous and dynamically changing.
- *Interventions and strategies too tailored for a specific setting*: In an effort to create contextually relevant research at a specific location, interventions and implementation strategies can become less externally relevant. Research that depends on resources or stems from values/priorities that are unique to the local setting will be less generalizable to other settings.
- *Subject engagement in research conduct*: In a traditional RCT design that includes informed consent, subjects are aware they are being observed. The response bias that occurs when subjects act differently because of this awareness, termed the Hawthorne effect, limits the generalizability of study findings to real-world situations where the Hawthorne effect is not present. Similarly, "close distancing," in which the researchers engage with subjects, can also result in subjects acting differently and bias study findings toward greater effectiveness than would be seen in real-world situations.[54]

In Table 16.1, we address potential solutions to each of these threats, with attention to how these solutions map to the domains of the Pragmatic Explanatory Continuum Indicator Summary 2 (PRECIS-2) framework.[50] The PRECIS-2 framework is addressed in further detail in a further section of this chapter; briefly, PRECIS-2 includes several domains, developed through consensus with multiple, diverse partners, that influence the degree to which a research study is *pragmatic* and intended to generate data on effectiveness that are broadly generalizable, as compared to *explanatory* and intended to demonstrate efficacy for highly selected populations.[50]

The overarching threats to external validity included in this section are particularly relevant in the preimplementation phase of research that includes study design and planning (Figure 16.1). Paying attention to external validity in this phase is a critical first step. However, an important next step is to continue to attend to external validity across the implementation and evaluation/sustainment phases of research (see Figure 16.1). In

TABLE 16.1 POTENTIAL SOLUTIONS TO ADDRESS COMMON THREATS TO EXTERNAL VALIDITY[a]

Threat to External Validity	Potential Solutions to Enhance External Validity
Unrealistic resource expectations/ selection bias of settings	*PRECIS-2 domains of settings and organization capacity/resources*: • Seek representation from diverse and low-resource settings in the design of interventions/programs and when planning implementation strategies in order to ensure fit with the setting • Engage invested partners to select a relevant and representative range of settings to use for testing
Low-priority or externally imposed topics	*PRECIS-2 domain of primary outcome*: • Conduct multilevel partner engagement to understand priorities for the topic and outcomes and gauge ability and interest to participate
Unrepresentative participants/selection bias of participants	*PRECIS-2 domains of eligibility and recruitment*: • Align inclusion criteria with who the intended target audience or recipients are, with consideration of their real-world heterogeneity
Interventions and strategies too tightly controlled	*PRECIS-2 domain of flexibility*: • Design with consideration of the needs of a heterogeneous group of participants, staff, and settings • Plan for and allow adaptations that are consistent with the core functions of the program
Interventions and strategies too tailored for a specific setting	*PRECIS-2 domains of flexibility, settings, and organization*: • Design with dissemination in mind from the beginning ("Design for Dissemination") considering (1) the values and resources of heterogeneous participants, staff, and settings and (2) how others could flexibly adapt the intervention and strategies
Subject engagement in research conduct	*PRECIS-2 domain of follow-up*: • Select a pragmatic study design that can be integrated within routine clinical, public health, and community settings in a manner that does not require informed consent • Consider how different types of researcher engagement with subjects could bias findings

Abbreviation: PRECIS-2, Pragmatic Explanatory Continuum Indicator Summary, version 2.[50]
[a]This table is intended to illustrate ways to address common threats to external validity with attention to PRECIS-2 domains and is not an all-inclusive list of threats or potential solutions.

the next section, we go into further detail on approaches that promote external validity across each of these research phases. Before we transition to that section, in order to motivate attention to these elements, we first provide a case example (Box 16.1) that highlights how certain threats to external validity and failure to report on contextual factors affected the generalizability of a body of research related to social skills training for patients with autism spectrum disorder.

Methods and Approaches to Enhance External Validity

There are measures that researchers can take at each phase of research to promote the external validity of studies. In addition, there are also specific recommendations and resources to assist researchers in anticipating, identifying, and mitigating existing structures and systems of oppression that threaten to stifle the translation of evidence-based programs to low-resource health settings and marginalized

BOX 16.1

EXAMPLE OF THE INFLUENCE OF THREATS TO EXTERNAL VALIDITY ON RESEARCH GENERALIZABILITY

A systematic review was conducted to evaluate the external validity of RCTs that studied the effects of social skills group interventions for school-aged children and adolescents with autism spectrum disorder.[55] Among 15 RCTs, the authors found that internal validity was high, but that determinants of external validity were either skewed or inadequately reported: The inclusion criteria restricted the sample to highly functional children, the intervention delivery was tightly controlled, and there were limited data on the characteristics of participants and settings. Accordingly, the reviewers concluded that these RCTs suggested social skills interventions were efficacious for a narrow subgroup of highly functional children and adolescents with autism spectrum disorder and when delivered in a highly controlled manner. However, the relevance and generalizability of these findings for delivery of this intervention in schools is unclear, as schools serve children with autism with a range of functional abilities, and many schools lack resources to deliver the program as it was delivered in the research. Based on the available contextual factors reported in the RCTs, the authors noted the following potential limitations, which we frame within the threats to external validity itemized in Table 16.1:

- *Unrealistic resource expectations/selection bias of settings*: The feasibility of implementing the interventions may not be possible across real-world settings. Further, the studies did not report the cost of delivering the interventions, which limits the ability to understand the feasibility of resource allocation for settings that would be interested in adopting a social skills group intervention. It would have been optimal to assess both costs of intervention delivery and the implementation strategies used,[56,57] as well as consider the evaluation of other factors that contribute to feasibility and sustainability.[58,59]
- *Low-priority or externally imposed topics*: There was no discussion of whether the outcomes addressed were informed by any input from invested partners, other than the expertise available within the research team. Key partner perspectives in this case would include a socioeconomically diverse set of potential program end users (patient/family partners and school staff/other staff who commonly implement these types of therapies) as well as leaders of organizations that implement these types of therapies.[60,61]
- *Unrepresentative participants/selection bias of participants*: The inclusion criteria for study subjects was biased toward selecting high-functioning, school-aged children and adolescents and their parents who were highly educated, which is not at all representative of the full spectrum of youth with autism. The education status of the parents may have introduced selection bias by including guardians of higher socioeconomic status who had greater means to support the intervention delivery to their children and may have resulted in the inequitable exclusion of racial/ethnic minority participants.
- *Interventions and strategies too tightly controlled*: The intervention was not delivered to subjects in their usual care environments, but rather in a controlled clinical setting, which does not account for the effects of dynamic interactions of the real-world context on the intervention.

communities.[62] In this section of the chapter, we dive into ways to enhance external validity at each phase of research: the preimplementation phase of study design and planning, the implementation phase, and the evaluation/sustainment phase, as illustrated in Figure 16.1. We also address other considerations, including secondary data analyses and the role of funders.

Phase 1: Preimplementation During Study Design/Planning

Study Design

Multiple tools exist to support researchers to attend to external validity in the preimplementation phase. One key resource that was addressed in Table 16.1 is the Pragmatic Explanatory Continuum Indicator Summary (PRECIS) tool[63] and the more recently updated and validated PRECIS-2 tool (accessible at http://www.precis-2.org).[50] The rationale for developing PRECIS and PRECIS-2 was to guide researchers to consider domains related to external validity explicitly when designing a study. These domains were developed with representation from diverse partners, including clinical trialists, clinicians, and policymakers.[50] PRECIS-2 visually summarizes the extent to which a trial is more versus less pragmatic for each of the nine domains. More recently, the PRECIS-2-PS was also developed to provide further consideration of cluster-randomized trials in which clinicians (vs. patients) are the subjects.[51] We recommend inclusion of a PRECIS-2 or PRECIS-2-PS graphic when developing a study to allow both reviewers and potential adopters to interpret the degree to which design decisions are prioritizing pragmatic choices that are more generalizable to invested partners, and to what extent design decisions are giving due attention to external validity. Figure 16.2 depicts a PRECIS-2 graphic in which researchers would evaluate each of the nine domains on a scale from 1 to 5, where a score of 5 indicates maximal pragmatism, and a score of 1 indicates minimal pragmatism on the continuum. No one study is typically fully pragmatic or explanatory, and this is an opportunity for researchers and invested partners to consider the trade-offs of design decisions on the study's findings and application. Guidance on rating studies have been developed, and inter-rater reliability is good when using these approaches.[50,64] Many of these approaches, including PRECIS-2, are quantitative assessments, which are important to use in tandem with qualitative assessments to evaluate external validity. Quantitative assessments, such as PRECIS-2 ratings, are useful as an initial means of evaluating and reporting external validity, but might need adaptation to nonclinical public health settings. Qualitative assessments that provide rich descriptions of contextual issues offer a deeper understanding of factors that influence the external relevance of a study. Chapter 18 provides further guidance on different qualitative and mixed-methods approaches that could be used. We have highlighted here some ways to promote external validity for trials that are predominantly explanatory in focus, as well as approaches to promote external validity for trials that are more pragmatic in focus (Table 16.2).

In addition to PRECIS-2, the 5Rs model for pragmatism can inform elements of pragmatic study design and outcome selection.[65] The 5 *R*'s model informs research that is relevant, rapid, recursive (iterative), reports on resources required, and is replicable. As a qualitative assessment approach, the 5 *R*'s model can be used to augment PRECIS-2 quantitative assessments. To give an example, a health system could apply both the PRECIS-2 tool and 5 *R*'s model to vet the vast array of digital health programs they could potentially integrate with their electronic health record to support chronic disease prevention. In the case of digital health programs, the PRECIS-2 domain of organisation and the 5 *R*'s domain of resources each relate to the available infrastructure to implement and sustain a digital health program across a diverse number of settings; this relates to a number of elements: interoperability with the electronic health record, as well as information technology resources and staff time available. The external validity of a given digital health program would be diminished if the resources required for implementation and sustainment are only present in a limited number of high-resource settings. When considered from the perspective of a specific learning health system that has a rather homogeneous set of resources available across its satellite clinics, the PRECIS-2 domain of outcome relevance and the 5 *R*'s model elements of rapid and relevant take on particular significance because of the limited capacity to implement

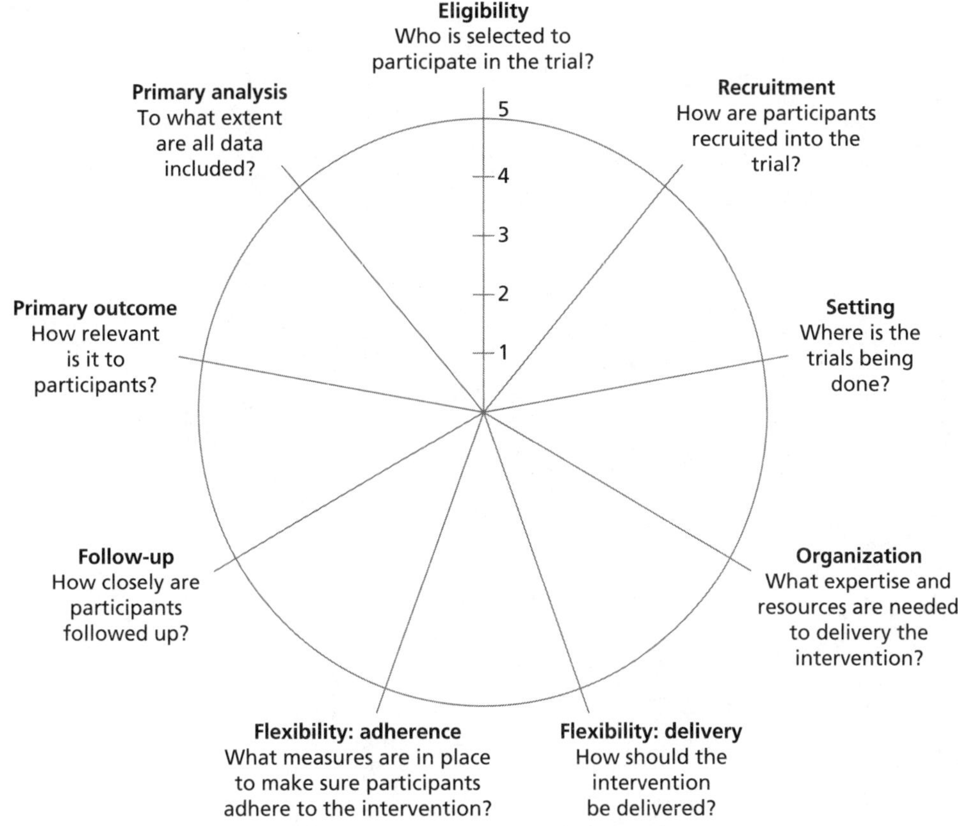

FIGURE 16.2 The Pragmatic Explanatory Continuum Indicator Summary 2 (PRECIS-2) wheel.

Source: Reproduced with permission from: Loudon et al. *BMJ* 2015.[50]

numerous digital health programs across all clinics. Accordingly, the system leaders would strategically select relevant, high-priority digital health programs that address the pressing problems and inequities facing the system. Conducting a formal needs assessment could also assist in identifying the topmost digital health priorities, as well as other priorities, and to ensure the candidate digital health interventions that address these priorities are feasible for the resources of the setting.

Researchers should also consider study designs beyond the gold standard RCT. Pragmatic study designs such as the stepped wedge trial design, adaptive trial designs, and natural experiments/observational designs allow for more seamless integration of research in real-world settings (see chapter 14). Such pragmatic trial designs enhance external validity by allowing for rigorous evaluation in usual care settings without the tightly controlled constraints of traditional RCTs and can mitigate biases seen with the Hawthorne effect.[10] Further, on-site, evaluative studies of the adaptation and implementation of components of efficacy-tested interventions to make them fit local circumstances and enhance their relevance are needed.[10] The notion of a type 1 hybrid-effectiveness implementation trial[66] is another example of including implementation outcomes that reflect the acceptability and feasibility of an evidence-based program for the settings and populations involved, even at a stage when the effectiveness is still being verified.

Representation of Interests of Invested Partners

The perspectives of diverse invested partners—including those who design, deliver, and receive a program—are crucial to consider in the preimplementation phase. In Figure 16.1, we have highlighted the importance of including partner perspectives during the planning,

TABLE 16.2 RECOMMENDATIONS TO ENHANCE EXTERNAL VALIDITY IN EFFICACY-FOCUSED AND PRAGMATIC RESEARCH

Element of research design	Common explanatory (efficacy-focused) research methods that emphasize internal validity	Recommendations for efficacy-focused research to enhance external validity while prioritizing internal validity	Recommendations for pragmatic studies to enhance external validity through a health equity lens
Participating units, settings and populations	Uses exclusion criteria to identify homogeneous participants and settings: minimal noise/complexity and most likely to respond to treatment; often not representative of intended target audience	Use exclusion criteria to identify relatively homogeneous participants from settings that still reflect the target audience Compare the similarity of participants, settings, and delivery staff with the intended target audience Analyze the differences between participants and those who decline	Most relevant for pragmatic trials: • Enroll participants/settings that represent the intended target audience, including populations that have experience inequities • Assess the reach (participation rate) among potential participants/settings, and representativeness to the intended target audience • Analyze differences between participants and those who decline • Investigate how/why differences occur
Development of evidence-based intervention (or program or policy)	Developed from prior evidence published in the literature or basic science research	If seeking future translation to health organizations, also seek to draw on input from invested partners in terms of the feasibility, acceptability, future sustainability, and equity considerations of the program studied	Developed from prior evidence published in the literature or existing guidelines Multilevel input from partners: • Feasibility to deliver program given typical organizational infrastructure, especially in low-resource settings • Acceptability and feasibility of program to all relevant partner types (e.g., participants, staff, system leaders) • Potential sustainability of program-consider ongoing staff needs

Implementation and adaptation of evidence-based intervention	Fidelity is paramount: strict protocol adherence enforced by highly trained and carefully supervised intervention staff	The type of intervention staff utilized should be feasible for downstream target settings	Emphasize fidelity to core components or functions, but allow (and report) adaptations to ensure flexibility to site/participant context • Site context includes: priorities, workflow, organizational capacity, change capability, local site/staff experience and resources • Participant context includes: cultural/social factors, literacy, and individual motives
Outcomes for decision making	Focus on a single primary outcome, usually a biological intermediate outcome to prove efficacy	The efficacy focus is reasonable, but if seeking future translation to health settings, cost and resource demands for settings should be reported, as well as feasibility and acceptability to program end-users	Outcomes assess generalizability and context: • The primary outcome(s) should equitably impact population health and be relevant to low- and high-resource settings • State the relevance of the outcomes to clinical guidelines and public health goals • Outcomes should include long-term effects, such as sustainment, and a description of any attrition
Maintenance and sustainability	Not assessed	Not typically necessary to assess maintenance during an explanatory trial, but intent to maintain (or adapt) should be reported and the potential downstream sustainability should be considered if the program is ultimately intended for clinical use	Utilize designing for dissemination principles to inform the dissemination strategies: • Identify systems and communication channels needed for dissemination • Obtain multilevel partner input throughout the project—from planning through to evaluation/sustainment • Develop a value proposition for the program for future adopters

Adapted with permission from the Annual Review of Public Health, Volume 40 © 2019 by Annual Reviews, http://www.annualreviews.org[10]

conduct, and evaluation of studies as a key way to enhance external validity.[67] In addition, chapters 10 and 27 of this text and others provide further details on the benefits of participatory research processes[68] to produce public health impact.[42,49,69–71] In brief, we also provide some specific recommendations and details about which invested partners to engage and how engaging a diverse set of partners throughout the life cycle of a research study enhances the external validity of the findings.

Engaging a diverse set of partners will vary to some extent based on those "touched" directly or indirectly by a research project; it may include community members, patients, front-line clinicians, public health practitioners, and/or policy-level leaders. Studies should optimally engage each of the relevant types of partners touched by the research, as the project scope and budget permit. For example, patients were historically regarded as "subjects" who had research performed "on" them, but community-engaged research seeks to involve populations experiencing inequities to help design and plan research studies to address those inequities.[72] The International Association for Public Participation (IAP2) standards have been developed to showcase a spectrum across which partners can be engaged, which ranges from low-to-moderate engagement such as serving as advisors or consultants, and ranging up to high levels of engagement where invested partners are major collaborators who are empowered to make decisions, such as in CBPR.[73,74] On the less intensive end of the partner engagement spectrum, consultative approaches to this could include community advisory boards and the development of partnerships with existing aligned community organizations by identifying shared goals. The advantage of specifying a particular level of partner engagement within the IAP2 spectrum is to formalize the goals of community/public participation and to commit to the level that the public will be involved. Another tool to consider using with IAP2, is the Health Equity Impact Assessment tool, which can support planners and implementers in identifying, prior to starting a new program, people who are routinely excluded.[75] Engagement of invested partners can assist in understanding how different approaches may be needed for different groups with attention to addressing inequities. Figure 16.1 illustrates the benefits of enhanced partner engagement at the bottom of the diagram: A greater extent of engagement and representation across the continuum of research phases enhances both external validity and equitable outcomes.

Figure 16.1 also illustrates a range of participatory research processes with invested partners. These include defining high-priority problems with acceptable interventions, guiding the planning and implementation approaches, identifying priority "outcomes of success," providing feedback during implementation, and giving input on the value and sustainability of the research findings.[14,73] By engaging partners, researchers will better understand the context relevant to a specific issue. This will benefit equitable implementation and dissemination in several ways:

- *Promoting representative reach among participants*: Partners representing diverse population segments can identify appropriate communication channels to reach vulnerable populations and those who have been historically excluded/marginalized in their communities. Greater representation also often leads to better acceptability and feasibility of the program among diverse segments of the target audience, which in turn yields more equitable and representative program reach.
- *Understanding organizational capacity/infrastructure across "typical" and low-resource settings*: To accomplish this, an environmental scan or needs assessment of the types of settings that would deliver the intervention is useful. This may identify potential inequities in resources and capacity across the target settings that could contribute to inequitable intervention outcomes. Practice-based research networks (PBRNs), public health research networks, and schools of public health offer opportunities for researchers to conduct these environmental scans as they represent a diverse set of community-based clinics and public health settings.[76] A growing emphasis on practice-based and participatory research among the prevention research centers funded by CDC has suggested ways to build greater reality testing and

representativeness into multisite D&I studies.[77]

- *Identifying interventions and strategies acceptable to settings*: To promote equitable implementation among low-resource settings, invested partners should evaluate the acceptability of the intervention and implementation strategies proposed. Some specific goals for vetting implementation strategies with partners include identifying:
  - o The relative importance and feasibility of the interventions and strategies proposed.
  - o Approaches needed to build sufficient organizational capacity and infrastructure for low-resource settings to adopt and equitably implement/sustain the program.[37,39]

Lest the process of engaging invested partners seems overwhelming, we highlight a number of methods and approaches that may be used to support engagement:

- *Engagement methods tailored to budget and stakeholder availability*: A key tool to support engagement is the Stakeholder Engagement Navigator website (https://dicemethods.org/), which guides researchers to identify engagement strategies to fit the budget, resources, and the availability of partners for a given research project.[38,78]
- *Use of frameworks*: Other ways to engage with partners to understand more about the context of settings, staff, and populations include utilizing D&I frameworks to guide assessments of the local context. D&I frameworks can guide efforts to understand these key elements of context[6,79]; in fact, use of frameworks in the preimplementation planning phase has improved the rates of successful implementation and sustainment.[53] See chapters 27 and 29 and our suggested resources for more details regarding the use of frameworks to design for implementation, sustainability, and dissemination. As described in chapter 4, a website compiling most of the D&I frameworks, their associated constructs, and relevant measures for each may be accessed online (http://www.dissemination-implementation.org), and chapter 4 also reviews several frameworks that address contextual factors related to external validity, including the practical Robust Implementation and Sustainability Model (PRISM)[48]; the Research, Effectiveness, Adoption, Implementation and Maintenance (RE-AIM) model[80]; the Consolidated Framework for Implementation Research (CFIR)[81]; the Exploration, Preparation, Implementation, and Sustainment (EPIS) Model[60]; and others.[82–84]
- *Logic models and implementation manuals*: Pulling together the big picture for invested partners and implementation teams is also a key part of the planning phase. To this end, it is useful to develop both logic models and implementation manuals (see chapter 27). A logic model is a depiction of all parts of a program (i.e., contextual determinants, intervention functions, implementation strategies, and their relationship to outcomes).[85] It is a valuable communication tool to share the program overview and a specific theory of change with a variety of invested partners. For certain partners that require a more detailed understanding, implementation manuals provide further specificity on the forms and functions and the implementation strategy specifics. By including a detailed protocol for all program core functions and checklists for activities for implementers, this simplifies the reporting and evaluation of the program, including identifying adaptations that were necessary. Finally, implementation manuals also represent "knowledge-to-action" products that are critical for future translation and for increasing the replicability of a program.[86(pA46)]

In addition to engagement of diverse invested partners, it is ideal for the research team to include researchers with lived experience from the communities that the research is intended to benefit. Specifically, studies have shown that inclusion of populations who have experienced inequities as team members may improve the equity and sustainability of research.[87–90] In addition, it is common for participatory research to include community principal investigators, community co-investigators, or consultants with community expertise, in line with a CBPR approach.[91,92] This collaborative approach recognizes the limitations of relying primarily on research- or disease-content expertise and the importance of representing those with appropriate lived experience.

In summary, a key lesson from this section is that representation of diverse partners in the preimplementation phase informs the delivery of the study in a way that makes it more likely to be adopted by representative settings and to reach representative populations; this is a prerequisite to the ultimate end goal of achieving equitable outcomes among participants and replicability across diverse settings. In other words, involving invested partners more collaboratively promotes greater attention to external validity through an equity lens. In Box 16.2, we provide two examples that demonstrate the influence of engagement with invested partners on external validity.

Phase 2: Research Implementation

As displayed in Figure 16.1, there are several elements to consider related to external validity

BOX 16.2

CASE EXAMPLES WITH VARYING DEGREES OF PARTNER ENGAGEMENT

EXAMPLE 1: HIGH DEGREE OF ENGAGEMENT: COLLABORATE

Boot Camp translation is an engagement tool that moves beyond invested partners informing the research and involves them as collaborators, partnering with the research team in each aspect of decision-making.[73,74] Such a collaborative approach to engaging partners has demonstrated particular benefits in addressing inequities in improving colon cancer screening rates among overall settings.[93] By partnering with rural clinic and community partners, the root issues deterring colon cancer screening were identified, and strategic solutions that were appropriate for the intended recipients in the rural settings were designed. The end result of this partnership with stakeholders was a rapid 10% increase in colon cancer screening. Because of the success of this community-engaged partnership approach, the Boot Camp translation process has been applied in other rural settings to address disparities in colon cancer screening. One caveat to this approach is that although Boot Camp translation includes a high degree of engagement with invested partners, the engagement is often more intense during the implementation phase of research as compared to the preimplementation or evaluation/sustainment phases.

EXAMPLE 2: MODERATE DEGREE OF ENGAGEMENT: CONSULT

For a variety of reasons, including competing demands for invested partners, a less intensive approach of engaging invested partners as consultants rather than collaborators may also be selected. In these situations, a diverse set of invested partners may still serve an important consultative role. This is often seen in human- or user-centered design of new interventions, such as health-related technologies. For example, implementers seeking to design an inpatient navigation aid for patients with dementia conducted focus groups of patients with dementia or their caregivers who would be the anticipated users of the aid.[94] In this example, the findings from these focus groups informed the design of a technology-enabled navigation aid, but these partners were not fully involved in the actual design decisions. In these types of human-centered design approaches, an approach to optimize external validity is to iteratively retest prototypes of the new intervention with invested partners in order to revise the product until a diverse set of partners finds it to be usable and acceptable.

and health equity during the implementation phase of a study. These include equipping sites and staff for successful implementation, developing feedback channels with invested partners to monitor what is working and what is not, acting to correct any emerging inequities, and tracking adaptations that are needed.[48,60,95–97] Key elements to consider include the following:

- *Setting up sites and staff for success*: As noted in Figure 16.1 and outlined in the Veterans Affairs Quality Enhancement Research Initiative (VA QUERI) roadmap,[95] implementation strategies need to address the contextual needs and resources of each site. If there are meaningful variations in capacity across sites, an implementation strategy of "tailoring to context" may also be warranted.
- *Setting up feedback channels*: Although adaptations are often avoided and suppressed in efficacy-focused research to preserve homogeneity and fidelity of the intervention delivered, in pragmatic research there is a need to set up feedback channels with invested partners to obtain data on any "midcourse corrections" needed.[61,65,98] Such midcourse corrections may be required due to feasibility/acceptability challenges with implementers or due to emerging inequities, such as an inequitable program reach among certain participant subgroups (e.g., lower reach to men, lower reach to racial/ethnic subpopulations).
- *Taking action to correct health inequities*: Revisiting the Health Equity Impact Assessment[75] during implementation can encourage the team to address emerging inequities in either effectiveness or implementation outcomes. Applying the periodic reflections[99] method engages implementers to reflect on how best to ensure equitable delivery of interventions. Taking action to address inequities will require adaptation of the implementation strategies and/or intervention form. When changes to the intervention are necessary, approaches to preserve internal validity include adapting the form of intervention components, such as mode of delivery,[100,101] while maintaining fidelity to the core function of the intervention.[45] There are resources available to help inform adaptations[102–104] (see chapter 8, Adaptation in Dissemination and Implementation Science) and some approaches that encourage iterative implementation and evaluation, such as the iterative RE-AIM[98] and Plan-Do-Study-Act (PDSA) cycles within quality improvement programs.
- *Tracking adaptations*: Adaptations that occur and contextual factors driving these adaptations should be documented, and there are several recommended approaches for this process.[102–104] The overarching goal of tracking adaptations is to support a better mechanistic understanding of how and why certain adaptations may be warranted for different types of settings and populations, what Chambers et al. have described as an aspirational "adaptome" model.[101] The Model for Adaptation Design and Impact (MADI) is particularly useful in this regard as it guides researchers to track the ripple effects of adaptations on outcomes.[104]

Phase 3: Research Evaluation/Sustainment

As summarized in Figure 16.1, it is important in the evaluation/sustainment phase to report on the value of a program to a diverse set of invested partners. This includes reporting context-dependent benefits that inform the "ultimate use question" of what works for which participants in which settings to produce which outcomes, under which circumstances, at what cost, and with what means. Program benefits are an important element of program value, but the costs of implementing and sustaining the program are another key element. To address these issues, we suggest the following approaches:

- *Benefits* reported should include
  - *Partner-identified outcomes of success*: Considering the results of any partner-identified or -preferred outcomes of success, as these are particularly important to program sustainment.[49,50] These often include patient, community, or sponsor outcomes that are

economic- or health-related, such as behavior change, functioning, cost savings, or disease status.

- o *Representativeness of implementation and health outcomes*: As developed by Proctor and colleagues,[105] implementation outcomes, include adoption (uptake by the organization), penetration (reach within the community), acceptability, appropriateness, feasibility of implementation, and costs. It is important to assess for equity and representativeness of implementation outcomes across the participating settings and populations. Were the health outcome benefits observed equally and representatively across different subpopulations by race, ethnicity, and socioeconomic status/neighborhood?[106] The RE-AIM framework and Predisposing, Reinforcing, and Enabling Constructs in Educational Diagnosis and Evaluation-Policy, Regulatory, and Organizational Constructs in Educational and Environmental Development (PRECEDE-PROCEED) model[107,108] specifically consider equity in terms of the representativeness of implementation outcomes and also identify contextual factors that may influence inequities.[80,109]
- o *Understanding context-dependent outcomes*: When disseminating the findings, it is important to report on variability in effects that may be attributed to contextual factors and what types of adaptations were necessary to yield the benefits observed. To measure how and why context influences inequities in outcomes, mixed methods are often necessary, as further described in a review by Leviton et al.[6] and in chapter 18. Attention to this approach will overcome the current dearth of reporting on the representativeness of participants and settings for research interventions,[70,110–112] including information on the race and ethnicity of clinical trial participants.[113]

- *Costs* reported should include the following general domains:
  - o *Staffing costs and other resources* necessary to implement and sustain programs.[112,114–116]
  - o Reporting *contextual factors* that influenced the costs and sustainability of an intervention.
  - o Estimating *replication costs* for a range of future adopters important to the reproducibility of a program or intervention.[58,59]
  - o The time required to complete each phase of program implementation.
  - o For further details on recommended elements of cost assessments, see chapter 11.[56]
- *Was the program sustained?* Although these types of data on decisions to sustain an intervention after research funding ends are critically important to future adopters, they are very scarce; it is estimated that fewer than 10% of studies report on sustainment or factors related to program sustainability.[114,117] We recommend following standard recommendations for external validity reporting of sustainment and sustainability[14,118] in order to guide clinicians, community members, health system leaders, and policymakers who are considering the future adoption of these programs.[70,112,114–117,119]
- *Developing plans for sustainment*: For studies where a health organization's leadership determines that a program is worth sustaining, it is key to plan for ongoing financial sponsorship and infrastructure to sustain the program (e.g., business plan, memorandum of understanding). Any elements of training or technical assistance that were supported by the research team during implementation must be taken on by designated teams to sustain the program. Ongoing review of the costs and benefits (including the equity of outcomes) should be undertaken by implementing organizations to ensure it remains worthy of sustainment. Such ongoing review should also consider whether further adaptations are needed due to changes in context that occur over time.
- *Broad dissemination*: Another critical piece is to disseminate research findings and context in clear language through the communication channels used by policymakers, health system

leaders, and communities.[38,120,121] In particular, it is important to report context transparently to make it easy to interpret. For reporting context in academic publications, a resource that is particularly helpful is the expanded Consolidated Standards of Reporting Trials (CONSORT) diagram, which aims to encourage more transparent reporting of original research.[47] To assist researchers in using the expanded CONSORT diagram, a user's guide and fillable template are available (https://re-aim.org/resources-and-tools/figures-and-tables/). The expanded CONSORT diagram can be used with the CONSORT-equity framework[122] to emphasize equity issues. Figure 16.3 provides an example of how the expanded CONSORT diagram can be used in conjunction with the principles of the CONSORT-equity framework.

Other Considerations

External Validity of Secondary Data Analyses

When designing secondary data analyses, such as systematic and nonsystematic reviews, meta-analyses or subgroup analyses (a priori planned or post hoc), context should be considered just as it is for primary research. Such secondary research can also be a powerful means to understand the external validity of primary research, facilitating an understanding of the effectiveness of the interventions across different populations, contexts, treatment variations, and outcomes. The issues and solutions addressed in prior sections of this chapter also apply to enhancing the external validity of secondary investigations.

The Role of Funders

Another important way that researchers, funders, and policymakers can enhance external validity is by addressing the problem of systemic underrepresentation of racial/ethnic minorities and women in the receipt of research funding; for example, recent funding announcements have prioritized funding research projects that collaborate with community partners to improve health inequities,[123] and to link minority-serving institutions with partner academic organizations.[124] However, these efforts are somewhat dampened by the systemic underrepresentation of racial/ethnic minorities and women in senior academic research positions and policymaking roles.[125–129] The NIH has published its commitment to addressing diversity, equity, and inclusion of populations that have experienced inequities as a funding agency, and other national organizations are considering similar approaches.[30,130]

SUMMARY

Throughout this chapter, we have (a) described what external validity is and why it matters; (b) summarized common threats to external validity and highlighted how inattention to external validity impedes translation and can exacerbate health inequities; and (c) provided some specific recommendations, resources, and tools that can be used to enhance external validity and thereby the relevance, equity, and translation of research. We echo again the often-quoted refrain that more practice-based evidence is critical to generate more evidence-based practice,[12–14,18,130] and we now add an updated verse to that chorus: If we want to see representative and equitable translation of evidence-based interventions, we must have meaningful representation of diverse partners in the research process (Figure 16.1).[38,39] Indeed, bringing this idea to reality would also go a long way toward accomplishing the visionary goals of learning health systems to test and refine solutions with ongoing input and feedback from invested partners.[8,9,95] Achieving relevance in research requires a shift from traditional efficacy studies with exquisite internal validity to a new mindset in which threats to external validity are equally and carefully valued. Making the shift requires involvement from multiple invested partners; researchers, journal editors, funders, and policymakers all need to have a role and responsibility. Here we reprise our previous calls to action for researchers, journal editors, funders, and policymakers to lean into their role-specific responsibility to address the crisis of failure to replicate research by prioritizing external validity[10,12,13] and add further specificity to the need for attention to health equity.[31,37–39,130]

- For researchers, we call for additional consideration of study design elements related to external validity for both efficacy-focused research and pragmatic

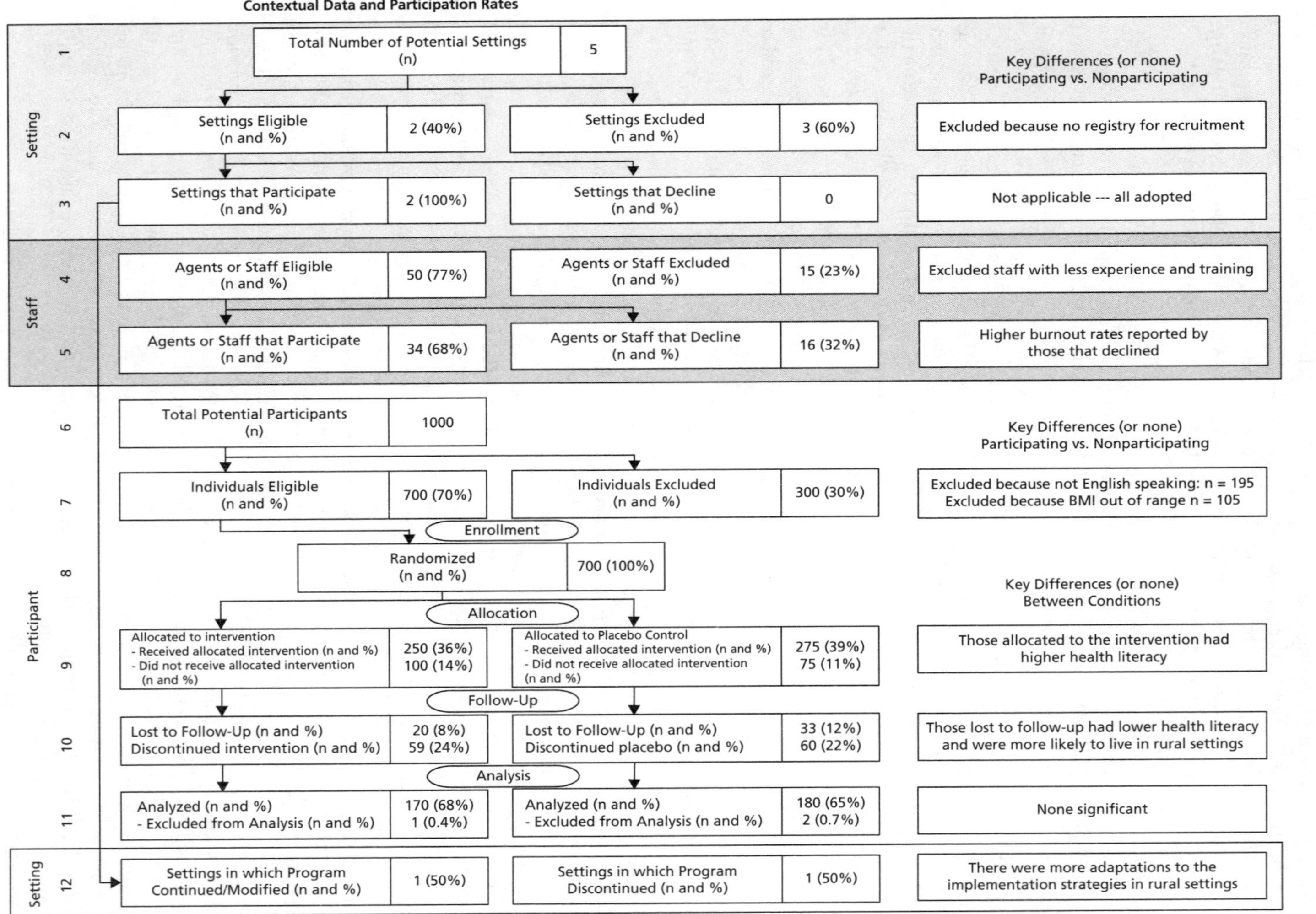

FIGURE 16.3 Example of an expanded CONSORT diagram.

studies, as outlined in Table 16.2. For researchers conducting traditional efficacy-focused studies, the point of considering external validity prior to proving efficacy is to maximize the relevance of the findings. For pragmatic research, we recommend the use of PRECIS-2[50] or PRECIS-2-PS[51], the expanded CONSORT extension,[70] and a D&I science framework to support planning, implementing, and reporting findings in a way that addresses the key external validity issues put forth in the Standards for Reporting Implementation studies.[71] In addition, it is important to design research with the goals of sustainability, broad dissemination, and health equity in mind. As such, it is key to have meaningful engagement and representation of the perspectives of diverse partners across all phases of research (Figure 16.1). Greater representation of invested partners ensures that the research questions asked are of relevance and importance to our invested partners, the implementation strategies utilized are feasible and acceptable, partner-identified outcomes of success are measured and evaluated, and the programs developed are likely to be scalable across diverse settings and populations.

- For journal editors and reviewers, we call for standards that hold researchers accountable to report on the internal and external validity factors that influence researchers' findings. One concrete element of this call to editors is to provide space to publish such findings; a simple approach would be to require an expanded CONSORT diagram that illustrates potential inequities in participation of settings, staff, or participants (or alternative presentation of these types of data) in lieu of the standard CONSORT diagram.[122] The points of such requirements are to provide simple ways to inform future adopters about the potential relevance of this work to their practice and to incentivize researchers to measure these factors that are related to the replication and impact of their findings.
- For funders, we call for requirements for grant applications to provide data or descriptions on the applicability and relevance of the proposed research to a range of diverse potential future adopters, including those in low-resource settings and populations. One simple way to approach this would be to require a PRECIS-2 or PRECIS-2-PS diagram[50,51] or an alternative visual method. We applaud recent steps by funders to prioritize funding research led by a diverse set of researchers,[25,26,30] including research teams led by and inclusive of women and other populations experiencing inequities, researchers from minority-serving institutions, and community partners. Including equity and representation of invested partners as explicit review criteria will encourage researchers to expand the diversity of their proposed teams and the extent to which their research assesses for and reports on inequities.
- For policymakers, we call for further promotion of the need for researchers and publishers to collect and report data on external validity in a way that public health organizations may readily interpret, as these data are necessary to inform decisions for real-world application.

Working together with a greater emphasis on external validity and representation of invested partners in research, the caliber of research produced will be elevated to be more widely generalizable, relevant, and equitable. This approach will help to address the ultimate use question: Which programs/policies work for which participants in which settings in order to produce which outcomes, under which circumstances, at what cost, and with what means? It is not necessary to sacrifice internal validity to anticipate, design for, and report on external validity issues; however, we do need to rectify the well-documented current imbalance. As PRECIS-2 demonstrates visually, there is a continuum of external validity, and we must carefully consider our priorities.[50,51] If we are serious about translating more than the reputed 14% of evidence-based research into practice, and if we would like it to take fewer than 17 years for these findings to be translated,[118] then we need to respond collectively to this call to action. Failure to act will constitute a waste of time, money, effort, human capital, and opportunities to improve public health.

SUGGESTED READINGS AND WEBSITES

Readings

Green LW, Gielen AC, Ottoson JM, Peterson D, Kreuter M., eds. *Health Program Planning, Implementation, and Evaluation: Creating Behavioral, Environmental and Policy Change.* Johns Hopkins University Press; 2022.

This book provides practical guidance to those planning, implementing, and evaluating programs in real-world settings with an emphasis on participation and external validity.

Loudon K, Treweek S, Sullivan F, Donnan P, Thorpe KE, Zwarenstein M. The PRECIS-2 tool: designing trials that are fit for purpose. *BMJ.* 2015 May 8;350:h2147.

This article presents a tool developed to map the extent to which a clinical trial aims to be pragmatic or explanatory. PRECIS-2 was developed by multiple invested partners *to represent their diverse perspectives, including clinical trialists, clinicians, and policymakers.*

Norton WE, Loudon K, Chambers DA, Zwarenstein M. Designing provider focused implementation trials with purpose and intent: introducing the PRECIS-2-PS tool. *Implement Sci.* 2021 Jan 7;16(1):7.

This article describes the PRECIS-2-PS, which is an adaptation of the original PRECIS-2 tool. The PRECIS-2-PS was developed to provide further consideration of clinical trials in which clinicians "versus patients" are the recipients of the intervention.

Selected Websites and Tools

CONSORT-equity. https://www.equator-network.org/reporting-guidelines/consort-equity/

The CONSORT extension aims to improve more transparent reporting of health equity when relevant to clinical trials.[122] *The website includes useful resources, including a checklist and flow diagram that can be downloaded.*

Expanded CONSORT. https://re-aim.org/resources-and-tools/figures-and-tables/

The expanded CONSORT aims to encourage more transparent reporting of original research. To assist researchers in using the expanded CONSORT, a user's guide and fillable expanded CONSORT diagram are available.

PRECEDE-PROCEED. https://www.lgreen.net

The two acronyms PRECEDE-PROCEED refer for health planning and evaluation to Predisposing, Enabling, and Reinforcing Constructs in Educational/Economic Diagnosis and Evaluation and *Policy, Regulatory, and Organizational Constructs in Educational and Environmental Development.*

PRECIS-2 tool. https://re-aim.org/resources-and-tools/figures-and-tables/

Developed to guide researchers to explicitly consider nine factors (originally 10) related to external validity when designing a study, PRECIS-2 visually summarizes the extent to which a trial is more versus less pragmatic for each of the nine factors, recognizing that no study is entirely pragmatic or entirely explanatory. It can be used when proposing or reporting on a study to allow both reviewers and potential adopters to interpret the relative strengths and weaknesses of the study from an external validity perspective.

RE-AIM. http://www.RE-AIM.org

The acronym RE-AIM refers to Reach, Effectiveness, Adoption, Implementation, and Maintenance, all important dimensions in the consideration of D&I research and in the external validity or applicability of research results in original studies for the alternative settings and circumstances in which they might be applied.

Stakeholder Engagement Navigator. https://Dicemethods.org

This is an interactive web tool that can assist researchers in selecting engagement approaches for collaborating with a variety of types of invested partners, and methods aligned with their resources and purpose.

Task Force on Community Preventive Services. http://www.thecommunityguide.org

The Community Guide provides a repository of the more than 200 systematic reviews conducted by the task force, an independent, interdisciplinary group with staff support by the CDC. Each review gives attention to the "applicability" of the conclusions beyond the study populations and settings in which the original studies were conducted.

REFERENCES

1. Alonso-Coello P, Schünemann HJ, Moberg J, et al. GRADE Evidence to Decision (EtD) frameworks: a systematic and transparent approach to making well informed healthcare choices. 1: introduction. *BMJ.* 2016;353:i2016. doi:10.1136/bmj.i2016
2. Burchett H, Umoquit M, Dobrow M. How do we know when research from one setting can be useful in another? A review of external validity, applicability and transferability frameworks.

J Health Serv Res Policy. 2011;16(4):238–244. doi:10.1258/jhsrp.2011.010124

3. Green L, Nasser M. Furthering dissemination and implementation research: the need for more attention to external validity. In: Brownson R, Colditz G, Proctor E, eds. *Dissemination and Implementation Research in Health: Translating Science to Practice.* 2nd ed. Oxford University Press; 2018:301–316.
4. Rothwell PM. External validity of randomised controlled trials: "To whom do the results of this trial apply?" *Lancet.* 2005;365:82–93. doi:10.1016/S0140-6736(04)17670-8
5. Nguyen QD, Moodie EM, Desmarais P, et al. Appraising clinical applicability of studies: mapping and synthesis of current frameworks, and proposal of the FrACAS framework and VICORT checklist. *BMC Med Res Methodol.* 2021;21(1):248. doi:10.1186/s12874-021-01445-0
6. Leviton LC. Generalizing about public health interventions: a mixed-methods approach to external validity. *Annu Rev Public Health.* 2017;38:371–391. doi:10.1146/ANNUREV-PUBLHEALTH-031816-044509
7. Olsen LA, Aisner D, McGinnis JM. The Learning Healthcare System. National Academies Press; 2007. doi:10.17226/11903
8. Lindsell CJ, Gatto CL, Dear ML, et al. Learning from what we do, and doing what we learn. *Acad Med.* 2021;96(9):1291–1299. doi:10.1097/acm.0000000000004021
9. Trinkley K, Ho M, Glasgow R, Huebschmann A. How Dissemination and Implementation Science Can Contribute to the Advancement of Learning Health Systems. *Acad Medicine.* 2022;97(10):1447–1458. doi:10.1097/ACM.0000000000004801
10. Huebschmann AG, Leavitt IM, Glasgow RE. Making health research matter: a call to increase attention to external validity. *Ann Rev Public Health.* 2019;40:45–63. doi:10.1146/annurev-publhealth-040218-043945
11. Green LW. From research to "best practices" in other settings and populations. *Am J Health Behav.* 2001;25(3):165–178. doi:10.5993/AJHB.25.3.2
12. Green L, Glasgow R, Atkins D, Stange K. Making evidence from research more relevant, useful, and actionable in policy, program planning, and practice: slips "twixt cup and lip." *Am J Prev Med.* 2009;37(6):187–191.
13. Green L. Public health asks of systems science: to advance our evidence-based practice, can you help us get more practice-based evidence? *Am J Public Health.* 2006;96(3):406–409. doi:10.2105/AJPH.2005.066035
14. Ammerman A, Smith T, Calancie L. Practice-based evidence in public health: improving reach, relevance, and results. *Annu Rev Public Health.* 2014;35:47–63. doi:10.1146/ANNUREV-PUBLHEALTH-032013-182458
15. Green L, Ottoson J, Garcia C, Hiatt R. Diffusion theory and knowledge dissemination, utilization, and integration in public health. *Annu Rev Public Health.* 2009;30:151–174. doi:10.1146/ANNUREV.PUBLHEALTH.031308.100049
16. Green LW. Public health asks of systems science: to advance our evidence-based practice, can you help us get more practice-based evidence? *Am J Public Health.* 2006;96(3):406–409. doi:10.2105/AJPH.2005.066035
17. Esmail LC, Barasky R, Mittman BS, Hickam DH. Improving comparative effectiveness research of complex health interventions: standards from the Patient-Centered Outcomes Research Institute (PCORI). *J Gen Intern Med.* 2020;35(suppl 2):875–881. doi:10.1007/s11606-020-06093-6
18. Green L. From research to "best practices" in other settings and populations. *Am J Health Behav.* 2001;25(3):165–178. doi:10.5993/AJHB.25.3.2
19. Weinstein JN, Geller A, Negussie Y, Baciu A. Communities in Action: Pathways to Health Equity. National Academies Press; 2017. doi:10.17226/24624
20. Yu Z, Kowalkowski J, Roll AE, Lor M. Engaging underrepresented communities in health research: lessons learned. *West J Nurs Res.* 2021;43(10):915–923. doi:10.1177/0193945920987999
21. McNair T, Bensimon E, Malcom-Piqueux L, Pasquerella L, eds. *From Equity Talk to Equity Walk: Expanding Practitioner Knowledge for Racial Justice in Higher Education.* John Wiley & Sons; 2020.
22. Walden S, Trytten D, Shafab RL, Foor C. ASEE PEER—critiquing the "underrepresented minorities" label. 2018. Accessed March 25, 2022. https://peer.asee.org/critiquing-the-underrepresented-minorities-label
23. Bensimon E. The misbegotten URM as a data point. Center for Urban Education, Rossier School of Education, University of Southern California. 2016. Accessed March 29, 2022. https://www.google.com/url?sa=t&rct=j&q=&esrc=s&source=web&cd=&ved=2ahUKEwjy2sixsO72AhU5JTQIHSayAcEQFnoECBEQAQ&url=https%3A%2F%2Fcue.usc.edu%2Ffiles%2F2016%2F01%2FBensimon_The-Misbegotten-URM-as-a-Data-Point.pdf&usg=AOvVaw2QiyJkvvS14AbbT5p74UOe
24. Byhoff E, Kangovi S, Berkowitz SA, et al. A Society of General Internal Medicine position statement on the internists' role in social determinants of

health. *J Gen Intern Med*. 2020;35(9):2721–2727. doi:10.1007/S11606-020-05934-8

25. Carnethon MR, Pu J, Howard G, et al. Cardiovascular health in African Americans: a scientific statement from the American Heart Association. *Circulation*. 2017;136(21):e393–e423. doi:10.1161/CIR.0000000000000534
26. Dankwa-Mullan I, Rhee KB, Williams K, et al. The science of eliminating health disparities: summary and analysis of the NIH summit recommendations. *Am J Public Health*. 2010;100(suppl 1):S12–S18. doi:10.2105/AJPH.2010.191619
27. Marmot M, Friel S, Bell R, Houweling TA, Taylor S. Closing the gap in a generation: health equity through action on the social determinants of health. *Lancet*. 2008;372(9650):1661–1669. doi:10.1016/S0140-6736(08)61690-6
28. Yousefi Nooraie R, Kwan BM, Cohn E, et al. Advancing health equity through CTSA programs: opportunities for interaction between health equity, dissemination and implementation, and translational science. *J Clin Transl Sci*. 2020;4(3):168–175. doi:10.1017/cts.2020.10
29. Mazzucca S, Arredondo EM, Hoelscher DM, et al. Expanding implementation research to prevent chronic diseases in community settings. *Annu Rev Public Health*. 2021;42:135–158. doi:10.1146/ANNUREV-PUBLHEALTH-090419-102547
30. Collins FS, Adams AB, Aklin C, et al. Affirming NIH's commitment to addressing structural racism in the biomedical research enterprise. *Cell*. 2021;184(12):3075–3079. doi:10.1016/J.CELL.2021.05.014
31. Brownson RC, Kumanyika SK, Kreuter MW, Haire-Joshu D. Implementation science should give higher priority to health equity. *Implement Sci*. 2021;16(1):28. doi:10.1186/S13012-021-01097-0
32. Centers for Disease Control and Prevention. Health Equity. CDC core health equity science and intervention strategy. 2022. Accessed February 1, 2022. https://www.cdc.gov/healthequity/core/index.html
33. National Academy of Medicine. *Integrating Social Care Into the Delivery of Health Care: Moving Upstream to Improve the Nation's Health*. National Academies Press; 2019.
34. National Institute on Minority Health and Health Disparities. NIMHD research framework. 2017. Accessed March 26, 2022. https://www.nimhd.nih.gov/about/overview/research-framework/
35. Kaiser J. NIH apologizes for "structural racism," pledges change. *Science*. 2021;371(6533):977. doi:10.1126/SCIENCE.371.6533.977
36. Centers for Disease Control and Prevention. CDC Newsroom. Media Statement from CDC Director Rochelle P. Walensky, MD, MPH, on Racism and Health. 2021. Accessed January 19, 2022. https://www.cdc.gov/media/releases/2021/s0408-racism-health.html
37. Shelton RC, Adsul P, Oh A. Recommendations for addressing structural racism in implementation science: a call to the field. *Ethn Dis*. 2021;31(suppl 1):357–364. doi:10.18865/ed.31.S1.357
38. Kwan BM, Brownson RC, Glasgow RE, Morrato EH, Luke DA. Designing for dissemination and sustainability to promote equitable impacts on health. *Annu Rev Public Health*. 2022;43(1):331–353. doi:10.1146/ANNUREV-PUBLHEALTH-052220-112457
39. Shelton RC, Chambers DA, Glasgow RE. An extension of RE-AIM to enhance sustainability: addressing dynamic context and promoting health equity over time. *Front Public Health*. 2020;8:134. doi:10.3389/fpubh.2020.00134
40. Ioannidis JPA. How to make more published research true. *PLoS Med*. 2014;11(10):e1001747. doi:10.1371/JOURNAL.PMED.1001747
41. Ioannidis JPA. Why most published research findings are false. *PLoS Med*. 2005;2(8):e124. doi:10.1371/JOURNAL.PMED.0020124
42. Hoffmann TC, Glasziou PP, Boutron I, et al. Better reporting of interventions: template for intervention description and replication (TIDieR) checklist and guide. *BMJ*. 2014;348:g1687. doi:10.1136/BMJ.G1687
43. Etheredge LM. A rapid-learning health system. *Health Aff*. 2007;26(2):w107–w118. doi:10.1377/hlthaff.26.2.w107
44. De Maeseneer JM, Van Driel ML, Green LA, Van Weel C. The need for research in primary care. *Lancet*. 2003;362(9392):1314–1319. doi:10.1016/S0140-6736(03)14576-X
45. Perez Jolles M, Lengnick-Hall R, Mittman BS. Core functions and forms of complex health interventions: a patient-centered medical home illustration. *J Gen Intern Med*. 2019;34(6):1032–1038. doi:10.1007/s11606-018-4818-7
46. Mcleroy KR, Bibeau D, Steckler A, Glanz K. An ecological perspective on health promotion programs. *Health Educ Q*. 1988;15(4):351–377. doi:10.1177/109019818801500401
47. Damschroder LJ, Aron DC, Keith RE, Kirsh SR, Alexander JA, Lowery JC. Fostering implementation of health services research findings into practice: a consolidated framework for advancing implementation science. *Implement Sci*. 2009;4(1):50. doi:10.1186/1748-5908-4-50
48. Feldstein AC, Glasgow RE. A practical, robust implementation and sustainability

model (PRISM) for integrating research findings into practice. *Jt Comm J Qual Patient Saf.* 2008;34(4):228–243. doi:10.1016/S1553-7250(08)34030-6

49. Tomoaia-Cotisel A, Scammon DL, Waitzman NJ, et al. Context matters: the experience of 14 research teams in systematically reporting contextual factors important for practice change. *Ann Fam Med.* 2013;11(suppl 1):S115–S123. doi:10.1370/AFM.1549
50. Loudon K, Treweek S, Sullivan F, Donnan P, Thorpe KE, Zwarenstein M. The PRECIS-2 tool: designing trials that are fit for purpose. *BMJ.* 2015;350:h2147. doi:10.1136/BMJ.H2147
51. Norton WE, Loudon K, Chambers DA, Zwarenstein M. Designing provider-focused implementation trials with purpose and intent: introducing the PRECIS-2-PS tool. *Implement Sci.* 2021;16(1):7. doi:10.1186/s13012-020-01075-y
52. Cook T, Campbell D. *Quasi-Experimentation: Design and Analysis Issues for Field Settings.* Rand McNally & Company; 1979.
53. Brownson R, Colditz G, Proctor E. *Dissemination and Implementation Research in Health: Translating Science to Practice.* 2nd ed. Oxford University Press; 2018.
54. Nzinga K, Rapp DN, Leatherwood C, et al. Should social scientists be distanced from or engaged with the people they study? *Proc Natl Acad Sci U S A.* 2018;115(45):11435–11441. doi:10.1073/PNAS.1721167115
55. Jonsson U, Choque Olsson N, Bölte S. Can findings from randomized controlled trials of social skills training in autism spectrum disorder be generalized? The neglected dimension of external validity. *Autism.* 2016;20(3):295–305. doi:10.1177/1362361315583817
56. Cidav Z, Mandell D, Pyne J, Beidas R, Curran G, Marcus S. A pragmatic method for costing implementation strategies using time-driven activity-based costing. *Implement Sci.* 2020;15(1):28. doi:10.1186/s13012-020-00993-1
57. Wagner TH, Yoon J, Jacobs JC, et al. Estimating costs of an implementation intervention. *Med Decis Making.* 2020;40(8):959–967. doi:10.1177/0272989X20960455
58. Malone S, Prewitt K, Hackett R, et al. The Clinical Sustainability Assessment Tool: measuring organizational capacity to promote sustainability in healthcare. *Implement Sci Commun.* 2021;2(1):77. doi:10.1186/S43058-021-00181-2
59. Luke DA, Calhoun A, Robichaux CB, Moreland-Russell S, Elliott MB. The Program Sustainability Assessment Tool: a new instrument for public health programs. *Prev Chronic Dis.* 2014;11(2014):130184. doi:10.5888/PCD11.130184
60. Moullin JC, Dickson KS, Stadnick NA, Rabin B, Aarons GA. Systematic review of the Exploration, Preparation, Implementation, Sustainment (EPIS) framework. *Implement Sci.* 2019;14(1):1. doi:10.1186/s13012-018-0842-6
61. Glasgow RE, Harden SM, Gaglio B, et al. RE-AIM planning and evaluation framework: adapting to new science and practice with a 20-year review. *Front Public Health.* 2019;7(Mar):64. doi:10.3389/fpubh.2019.00064
62. Burchett HED, Blanchard L, Kneale D, Thomas J. Assessing the applicability of public health intervention evaluations from one setting to another: a methodological study of the usability and usefulness of assessment tools and frameworks. *Health Res Policy Syst.* 2018;16(1):88. doi:10.1186/S12961-018-0364-3
63. Thorpe K, Zwarenstein M, Oxman A, et al. A pragmatic–explanatory continuum indicator summary (PRECIS): a tool to help trial designers. *J Clin Epidemiol.* 2009;62(5):464–475. doi:10.1016/J.JCLINEPI.2008.12.011
64. Loudon K, Zwarenstein M, Sullivan FM, et al. The PRECIS-2 tool has good interrater reliability and modest discriminant validity. *J Clin Epidemiol.* 2017;88:113–121. doi:10.1016/J.JCLINEPI.2017.06.001
65. Peek CJ, Glasgow RE, Stange KC, Klesges LM, Peyton Purcell E, Kessler RS. The 5 R's: an emerging bold standard for conducting relevant research in a changing world. *Ann Fam Med.* 2014;12(5):447–455. doi:10.1370/afm.1688
66. Curran GM, Bauer M, Mittman B, Pyne JM, Stetler C. Effectiveness-implementation hybrid designs: combining elements of clinical effectiveness and implementation research to enhance public health impact. *Med Care.* 2012;50(3):217–226. doi:10.1097/MLR.0b013e3182408812
67. Nápoles AM, Stewart AL. Transcreation: an implementation science framework for community-engaged behavioral interventions to reduce health disparities. *BMC Health Serv Res.* 2018;18(1):710. doi:10.1186/s12913-018-3521-z
68. Wallerstein N, Duran B, Oetzel J, Minkler M, eds. *Community-Based Participatory Research for Health: Advancing Social and Health Equity.* 3rd ed. Jossey-Bass; 2018.
69. Barbour V, Bhui K, Chescheir N, et al. CONSORT statement for randomized trials of nonpharmacologic treatments: A 2017 update and a CONSORT extension for nonpharmacologic trial abstracts. *Ann Intern Med.* 2017;167(1):40–47. doi:10.7326/M17-0046
70. Glasgow RE, Huebschmann AG, Brownson RC. Expanding the CONSORT figure: increasing

transparency in reporting on external validity. *Am J Prev Med.* 2018;55(3):422–430. doi:10.1016/j.amepre.2018.04.044

71. Pinnock H, Barwick M, Carpenter CR, et al. Standards for Reporting Implementation Studies (StaRI): explanation and elaboration document. *BMJ Open.* 2017;7(4):e013318. doi:10.1136/bmjopen-2016-013318
72. Delbanco T, Berwick DM, Boufford JI, et al. Healthcare in a land called peoplepower: nothing about me without me. *Health Expect.* 2001;4(3):144–150. doi:10.1046/j.1369-6513.2001.00145.x
73. International Association for Public Participation. Core values, ethics, spectrum—the 3 pillars of public participation. 2021. Accessed March 26, 2022. https://www.iap2.org/page/pillars
74. Norman N, Bennett C, Cowart S, et al. Boot Camp translation: a method for building a community of solution. *J Am Board Fam Med.* 2013;26(3):254–263. doi:10.3122/JABFM.2013.03.120253
75. Sadare O, Williams M, Simon L. Implementation of the Health Equity Impact Assessment (HEIA) tool in a local public health setting: challenges, facilitators, and impacts. *Can J Public Health.* 2020;111(2):212–219. doi:10.17269/s41997-019-00269-2
76. Green L, Hickner J. A short history of primary care practice-based research networks: from concept to essential research laboratories. *J Am Board Fam Med.* 2006;19(1):1–10. doi:10.3122/JABFM.19.1.1
77. Katz D, Murimi M, Gonzalez A, Njike V, Green L. From controlled trial to community adoption: the multisite translational community trial. *Am J Public Health.* 2011;101(8):e17. doi:10.2105/AJPH.2010.300104
78. DICEMethods.org. Stakeholder engagement navigator: a guide for health researchers. 2022. Accessed January 3, 2022. https://dicemethods.org
79. Fisher EB. The importance of context in understanding behavior and promoting health. *Ann Behav Med.* 2008;35(1):3–18. doi:10.1007/S12160-007-9001-Z
80. Glasgow RE, Vogt TM, Boles SM. Evaluating the public health impact of health promotion interventions: the RE-AIM framework. *Am J Public Health.* 1999;89(9):1322–1327. doi:10.2105/AJPH.89.9.1322
81. Concannon TW, Fuster M, Saunders T, et al. A systematic review of stakeholder engagement in comparative effectiveness and patient-centered outcomes research. *J Gen Intern Med.* 2014;29(12):1692–1701. doi:10.1007/S11606-014-2878-X
82. Graham ID, Logan J, Harrison MB, et al. Lost in knowledge translation: time for a map? *J Contin Educ Health Prof.* 2006;26(1):13–24. doi:10.1002/CHP.47
83. Greenhalgh T, Robert G, Macfarlane F, Bate P, Kyriakidou O. Diffusion of innovations in service organizations: systematic review and recommendations. *Milbank Q.* 2004;82(4):581–629. doi:10.1111/J.0887-378X.2004.00325.X
84. Kilbourne AM, Neumann MS, Pincus HA, Bauer MS, Stall R. Implementing evidence-based interventions in health care: application of the replicating effective programs framework. *Implement Sci.* 2007;2(1):42. doi:10.1186/1748-5908-2-42
85. Smith JD, Li DH, Rafferty MR. The implementation research logic model: a method for planning, executing, reporting, and synthesizing implementation projects. *Implement Sci.* 2020;15(1):84. doi:10.1186/S13012-020-01041-8
86. Wilson K, Brady T, Lesesne C, NCCDPHP Work Group on Translation. An organizing framework for translation in public health: the Knowledge to Action Framework. *Prev Chronic Dis.* 2011;8(2):A46. Accessed December 3, 2021. https://pubmed.ncbi.nlm.nih.gov/21324260/
87. Rasmus SM, Whitesell NR, Mousseau A, Allen J. An intervention science to advance underrepresented perspectives and indigenous self-determination in health. *Prev Sci.* 2020;21(suppl 1):83–92. doi:10.1007/S11121-019-01025-1
88. Kogan JN, Bauer MS, Dennehy EB, et al. Increasing minority research participation through collaboration with community outpatient clinics: the STEP-BD community partners experience. *Clin Trials.* 2009;6(4):344–354. doi:10.1177/1740774509338427
89. Gray JS, Carter PM. Growing our own: building a native research team. *J Psychoactive Drugs.* 2012;44(2):160–165. doi:10.1080/02791072.2012.684632
90. Polanco FR, Dominguez DC, Grady C, et al. Conducting HIV research in racial and ethnic minority communities: building a successful interdisciplinary research team. *J Assoc Nurses AIDS Care.* 2011;22(5):388–396. doi:10.1016/J.JANA.2010.10.008
91. Luger TM, Hamilton AB, True G. Measuring community-engaged research contexts, processes, and outcomes: a mapping review. *Milbank Q.* 2020;98(2):493–553. doi:10.1111/1468-0009.12458
92. Wallerstein N. Engage for equity: advancing the fields of community-based participatory research and community-engaged research in community psychology and the social sciences. *Am J Community Psychol.* 2021;67(3-4):251–255. doi:10.1002/AJCP.12530

93. Westfall JM, Zittleman L, Felzien M, et al. Reinventing the wheel of medical evidence: how the boot camp translation process is making gains. *Health Aff.* 2016;35(4):613–618. doi:10.1377/hlthaff.2015.1648
94. Kowe A, Köhler S, Görß D, Teipel S. The patients' and caregivers' perspective: in-hospital navigation aids for people with dementia—a qualitative study with a value sensitive design approach. *Assist Technol.* 2021:1–10. doi:10.1080/10400435.2021.2020378
95. Kilbourne AM, Goodrich DE, Miake-Lye I, Braganza MZ, Bowersox NW. Quality enhancement research initiative implementation roadmap: toward sustainability of evidence-based practices in a learning health system. *Med Care.* 2019;57(10)(suppl 3):S286–S293. doi:10.1097/MLR.0000000000001144
96. McCreight MS, Rabin BA, Glasgow RE, et al. Using the practical, robust implementation and sustainability model (PRISM) to qualitatively assess multilevel contextual factors to help plan, implement, evaluate, and disseminate health services programs. *Transl Behav Med.* 2019;9(6):1002–1011. doi:10.1093/tbm/ibz085
97. Safaeinili N, Brown-Johnson C, Shaw JG, Mahoney M, Winget M. CFIR simplified: pragmatic application of and adaptations to the Consolidated Framework for Implementation Research (CFIR) for evaluation of a patient-centered care transformation within a learning health system. *Learn Health Syst.* 2020;4(1):e10201. doi:10.1002/lrh2.10201
98. Glasgow RE, Battaglia C, McCreight M, Ayele RA, Rabin BA. Making implementation science more rapid: use of the RE-AIM framework for mid-course adaptations across five health services research projects in the Veterans Health Administration. *Front Public Health.* 2020;8:194. doi:10.3389/fpubh.2020.00194
99. Finley EP, Huynh AK, Farmer MM, et al. Periodic reflections: a method of guided discussions for documenting implementation phenomena. *BMC Med Res Methodol.* 2018;18(1):153. doi:10.1186/S12874-018-0610-Y
100. Stirman SW, Miller CJ, Toder K, Calloway A. Development of a framework and coding system for modifications and adaptations of evidence-based interventions. *Implement Sci.* 2013;8(1):1–12. doi:10.1186/1748-5908-8-65/TABLES/2
101. Chambers DA, Norton WE. The adaptome: advancing the science of intervention adaptation. *Am J Prev Med.* 2016;51(4):S124–S131. doi:10.1016/j.amepre.2016.05.011
102. Miller CJ, Barnett ML, Baumann AA, Gutner CA, Wiltsey-Stirman S. The FRAME-IS: a framework for documenting modifications to implementation strategies in healthcare. *Implement Sci.* 2021;16(1):36. doi:10.1186/s13012-021-01105-3
103. Stirman SW, Baumann AA, Miller CJ. The FRAME: an expanded framework for reporting adaptations and modifications to evidence-based interventions. *Implement Sci.* 2019;14(1):58. doi:10.1186/s13012-019-0898-y
104. Kirk MA, Moore JE, Wiltsey Stirman S, Birken SA. Towards a comprehensive model for understanding adaptations' impact: the model for adaptation design and impact (MADI). *Implement Sci.* 2020;15(1):1–15. doi:10.1186/S13012-020-01021-Y/FIGURES/3
105. Proctor E, Silmere H, Raghavan R, et al. Outcomes for implementation research: conceptual distinctions, measurement challenges, and research agenda. *Admin Policy Ment Health Ment Health Serv Res.* 2011;38(2):65–76. doi:10.1007/s10488-010-0319-7
106. Murray CJL, Kulkarni SC, Michaud C, et al. Eight Americas: investigating mortality disparities across races, counties, and race-counties in the United States. *PLoS Med.* 2006;3(9):e260. doi:10.1371/JOURNAL.PMED.0030260
107. Green LW. Toward cost-benefit evaluations of health education: some concepts, methods, and examples. *Health Educ Monogr.* 2016;2(1)(suppl):34–64. doi:10.1177/10901981740020S106
108. Green LW, Kreuter MW, Green LW. *Health Program Planning: An Educational and Ecological Approach.* McGraw-Hill Higher Education; 2005.
109. Green L, Gielen A, Ottoson J, Peterson D, Kreuter M. *Health Program Planning, Implementation and Evaluation.* Johns Hopkins University Press; 2022.
110. Ahmad N, Boutron I, Dechartres A, Durieux P, Ravaud P. Applicability and generalisability of the results of systematic reviews to public health practice and policy: a systematic review. *Trials.* 2010;11(1):1–9. doi:10.1186/1745-6215-11-20/TABLES/2
111. Gaglio B, Shoup JA, Glasgow RE. The RE-AIM framework: a systematic review of use over time. *Am J Public Health.* 2013;103(6):e38–e46. doi:10.2105/AJPH.2013.301299
112. Harden SM, Gaglio B, Shoup JA, et al. Fidelity to and comparative results across behavioral interventions evaluated through the RE-AIM framework: a systematic review. *Syst Rev.* 2015;4(1):155. doi:10.1186/S13643-015-0141-0
113. Rochon PA, Mashari A, Cohen A, et al. The inclusion of minority groups in clinical trials: problems of under representation and under

reporting of data. *Account Res.* 2004;11(3–4):215–223. doi:10.1080/08989620490891412

114. Luoma KA, Leavitt IM, Marrs JC, et al. How can clinical practices pragmatically increase physical activity for patients with type 2 diabetes? A systematic review. *Transl Behav Med.* 2017;7(4):751–772. doi:10.1007/S13142-017-0502-4
115. Sanchez MA, Rabin BA, Gaglio B, et al. A systematic review of eHealth cancer prevention and control interventions: new technology, same methods and designs? *Transl Behav Med.* 2013;3(4):392–401. doi:10.1007/S13142-013-0224-1
116. Thomson HJ, Thomas S. External validity in healthy public policy: application of the RE-AIM tool to the field of housing improvement. *BMC Public Health.* 2012;12(1):1–6. doi:10.1186/1471-2458-12-633/TABLES/2
117. Klesges L, Dzewaltowski D, Glasgow R. Review of external validity reporting in childhood obesity prevention research. *Am J Prev Med.* 2008;34(3):216–223. doi:10.1016/J.AMEPRE.2007.11.019
118. Balas E, Boren S. Managing clinical knowledge for health care improvement. *Yearb Med.* 2000;1(1):65–70.
119. Compernolle S, De Cocker K, Lakerveld J, et al. A RE-AIM evaluation of evidence-based multi-level interventions to improve obesity-related behaviours in adults: a systematic review (the SPOTLIGHT project). *Int J Behav Nutr Phys Act.* 2014;11(1):1–13. doi:10.1186/S12966-014-0147-3/FIGURES/2
120. Tricco AC, Zarin W, Rios P, et al. Engaging policy-makers, health system managers, and policy analysts in the knowledge synthesis process: a scoping review. *Implement Sci.* 2018;13(1):31. doi:10.1186/S13012-018-0717-X
121. Purtle J, Lê-Scherban F, Wang X, Shattuck PT, Proctor EK, Brownson RC. Audience segmentation to disseminate behavioral health evidence to legislators: an empirical clustering analysis. *Implement Sci.* 2018;13(1):121. doi:10.1186/S13012-018-0816-8
122. Welch VA, Norheim OF, Jull J, Cookson R, Sommerfelt H, Tugwell P. CONSORT-Equity 2017 extension and elaboration for better reporting of health equity in randomised trials. *BMJ.* 2017;359:j5085. doi:10.1136/BMJ.J5085
123. Department of Health and Human Services. Disparities Elimination through Coordinated Interventions to Prevent and Control Heart and Lung Disease Risk (DECIPHeR) (UG3/UH3 clinical trial optional). 2019. Accessed March 22, 2022.https://grants.nih.gov/grants/guide/rfa-files/rfa-hl-20-003.html
124. Thompson B, O'Connell M, Löest H, Anderson J, Westcott R. Understanding and reducing obstacles in a collaboration between a minority institution and a cancer center. *J Health Care Poor Underserved.* 2013;24(4):1648–1656. doi:10.1353/hpu.2013.0167
125. Fox RL, Lawless JL. If only they'd ask: gender, recruitment, and political ambition. *J Polit.* 2010;72(2):310–326. doi:10.1017/S0022381609990752
126. Ashe J, Stewart K. Legislative recruitment: using diagnostic testing to explain underrepresentation. *Party Politics.* 2011;18(5):687–707. doi:10.1177/1354068810389635
127. Ceci SJ, Williams WM. Understanding current causes of women's underrepresentation in science. *Proc Natl Acad Sci U S A.* 2011;108(8):3157–3162. doi:10.1073/PNAS.1014871108/-/DCSUPPLEMENTAL
128. Whittaker JA, Montgomery BL, Martinez Acosta VG. Retention of underrepresented minority faculty: strategic initiatives for institutional value proposition based on perspectives from a range of academic institutions. *J Undergrad Neurosci Educ.* 2015;13(3):A136. Accessed January 25, 2022. https://www.ncbi.nlm.nih.gov/pmc/articles/PMC4521729/
129. NIH Extramural Nexus. Inequalities in the distribution of National Institutes of Health Research Project Grant Funding— January 18, 2022. Accessed February 1, 2022. https://nexus.od.nih.gov/all/2022/01/18/inequalities-in-the-distribution-of-national-institutes-of-health-research-project-grant-funding/
130. Churchwell K, Elkind MSV, Benjamin RM, et al. Call to action: structural racism as a fundamental driver of health disparities: a presidential advisory from the American Heart Association. *Circulation.* 2020;142(24):E454–E468. doi:10.1161/CIR.0000000000000936

17

Evaluation Approaches for Dissemination and Implementation Research

BRIDGET GAGLIO AND RUSSELL E. GLASGOW

INTRODUCTION

This chapter focuses on evaluation approaches for dissemination and implementation (D&I) science research. An important take-home point is that evaluation should be considered an ongoing process, rather than a one-time, post hoc activity. Like planning for dissemination, best results are obtained by an integrated series of evaluation activities stretching from initial needs assessment to formative evaluation, ongoing process evaluation, and finally summative evaluation, all of which are interactive and provide feedback to key stakeholders and decision makers. Overlap exists between this chapter and others on related topics, particularly the ones on models and frameworks for D&I research (chapter 4), adaptation (chapter 8), measurement issues in D&I research (chapter 15), external validity (chapter 16), economic evaluation (chapter 11), and mixed-methods evaluation (chapter 18).

Evaluation is defined in authoritative papers and texts as the systematic collection of information about the activities, characteristics, and results of programs to make judgments about the program, improve or further develop program effectiveness, inform decisions about future programming, and/or increase understanding.[1,2] Evaluation research is a multidisciplinary field; has its own professional organization (American Evaluation Association) and journals (*American Journal of Evaluation and Research Evaluation*); and includes a broad range of conceptual models, frameworks, perspectives, and measurement approaches. Importantly, evaluation research includes multimethod approaches, which can be used to inform program planning, iteratively assess progress and guide adaptations, and comprehensively assess program outcomes. In the remainder of the chapter, we use the umbrella term *program* to refer to interventions, guidelines, policies, and products to be disseminated or implemented unless otherwise specified.

This chapter is limited in scope and focuses on evaluation methods and approaches most relevant to D&I science. We first review how evaluation has been used in D&I research along with key D&I evaluation issues, then discuss the predominant evaluation models and frameworks that have guided D&I research; we end with a case study. Finally, we summarize the status of current research/practice and future directions in D&I-related evaluation. Further, an appendix includes suggested readings and selected websites and tools.

EVALUATION IN DISSEMINATION AND IMPLEMENTATION RESEARCH

In contrast to more standard program evaluation[3] and effectiveness evaluations, D&I research focuses on issues related to the wide-scale adoption, implementation, maintenance, and generalizability of program impacts. Although overlap and lack of a clear boundary between effectiveness outcomes research, quality improvement research,[4] and D&I evaluations exist,[5] the purposes of these types of evaluations are different. Instead of focusing on the results of an intervention in a specific setting when an intervention is evaluated under well-controlled conditions[6] or rapid

Bridget Gaglio and Russell E. Glasgow, *Evaluation Approaches for Dissemination and Implementation Research* In: *Dissemination and Implementation Research in Health.* Edited by: Ross C. Brownson, Graham A. Colditz, and Enola K. Proctor, Oxford University Press. © Oxford University Press 2023.
DOI: 10.1093/oso/9780197660690.003.0017

improvement when developing new innovations,[4] D&I evaluation seeks to understand implementation processes, identify contextual influences, and assess external validity (see chapter 16).[6,7] Implementation outcomes are also different from those in efficacy, effectiveness, and often quality improvement research, which are often focused on a single primary outcome. Implementation research, in contrast, is focused on multiple outcomes, including acceptability, adoption, appropriateness, costs, feasibility, fidelity, penetration, and sustainability,[8] or stated differently, on the RE-AIM dimensions of reach, effectiveness across subgroups (including unintended outcomes), adoption, implementation (including costs and adaptations), and maintenance.[9,10] In summary, the ultimate goal of D&I evaluation (although usually not possible to answer in a given study) is to determine: What programs (interventions, guidelines, products, or policies) and what components, conducted under what conditions and in what settings, using what strategies, conducted by which agents, produce which outcomes, for which populations (and subgroups) via which processes, and how much does it cost?[11,12]

Planning and Program/Policy Design

Evaluation approaches, usually termed formative or evaluability assessments,[7,13] have been productively used to iteratively design and evaluate programs that will be robust across different settings and over time. A frequent mantra in D&I research, although seldom practiced in depth, is that it is never too early to "design for dissemination" (and equity and successful implementation). More recently, such planning has also come to focus on planning for sustainability.[14] Evaluation models and tools such as diffusion of innovations,[15] PRECEDE-PROCEED (defined in a separate section in this chapter),[16] RE-AIM,[17] or system dynamics modeling[18] can be used with stakeholders and implementation staff to do a priori estimates of impacts on different D&I outcomes and help plan interventions to maximize their reach, effectiveness, and sustainability.[19,20] More iterative approaches to evaluate program implementation and initial effects during program delivery have recently been used.[21] However, with the exception of informal, rapid assessments in quality improvement methods such as the Plan-Do-Study-Act (PDSA) cycle efforts,[22] there have been few reports of iterative use of D&I evaluation models. It is hoped that as the field of D&I science continues to grow and evolve, there will be sufficient literature on such iterative approaches to conduct reviews of their use and derive lessons learned from such applications.

Application of D&I models and evaluation methods during a program brings up another important evaluation issue. Such applications can inform program adjustments or modifications to enhance impact and to decrease the likelihood that possible "negative results" are not due to insufficient implementation or fidelity.[23,24] Fidelity issues are discussed in greater detail in chapter 7. Here we briefly describe a rapidly evolving area of evaluation termed *adaptation research*.[25,26] The genesis for this area of evaluation is the universal experience that in real-world applications, programs are never delivered in exactly the same way across different settings or how they were in efficacy or effectiveness studies.[27]

Some adaptations are undoubtedly not advisable, for example, if they result in failure to deliver essential effective components of a program. However, some adaptations are increasingly being found to be useful and maybe even necessary for successful application in different settings.[26,28] In particular, adaptations to make programs culturally appropriate, feasible to conduct in low-resource settings, and to be compatible with existing workflow are likely to be important. Paradoxically and somewhat provocatively, recent conceptual approaches have suggested that adaption to changing context may even be necessary and should be encouraged to produce (or even exceed prior effectiveness study outcomes) sustainable programs in a rapidly changing healthcare environment.[26,29] Adaptations are discussed in greater detail in chapter 8.

Pragmatic and Comparative Effectiveness Evaluations

Pragmatic[11,30] and realist[12] approaches to evaluation have become more common over the last several years. These approaches focus on questions relevant to D&I, such as the conditions under which different results can be obtained, and address generalizability concerns related to reach and breadth of effects, especially among subgroups (e.g., low-income or minority participants).[31] Pragmatic and realist approaches have also been part of comparative effectiveness research (CER) evaluations.[32,33]

D&I evaluation approaches have also been prominently featured in pragmatic trials, especially those supported by the Patient-Centered Outcomes Research Institute (PCORI) and some National Institutes of Health (NIH) programs (e.g., NIH Collaboratory, https://rethinkingclinicaltrials.org/).[34] Pragmatic investigations are concerned with the conduct of studies under more representative conditions rather than ideal or efficacy conditions. Tools and evaluation methods have been developed to help plan, guide, and evaluate pragmatic studies.[30,35,36] In addition to effectiveness and heterogeneity of effects, these approaches are concerned with issues of costs of different, real-world approaches and their feasibility under different conditions and in different settings. Most prominent among these, is the Pragmatic Explanatory Continuum Indicator Summary-2 (PRECIS-2) and its extension, PRECIS-2 Provider Strategies (PRECIS-2-PS).[35,36] These tools focus on nine domains on which a proposed or delivered program can be rated according to its degree of pragmatism as it relates to patient-focused (PRECIS-2) or provider-focused (PRECIS-2-PS) intervention trials.

Related reporting standards for implementation research have been published by Pinnock et al.[37] Called the Standardized Reporting Implementation studies (StaRI) statement, these recommendations resulted from a systematic review and multistage e-Delphi process involving international experts in D&I to identify the most important types of data to report in D&I studies. This international effort builds on both the Consolidated Standards of Reporting Trials (CONSORT)[38] and other reporting criteria for traditional outcomes research as well as earlier recommendations for reporting on contextual and external validity issues.[39] The 27 items in StaRI are intended to promote standard, transparent, and accurate reporting to describe implementation strategies and the effectiveness of the intervention on key implementation outcomes.[37] The annotated bibliography at the end of this chapter provides further description, but in brief the StaRI criteria include reporting on context and contextual changes, process, cost, representativeness, fidelity, and adaptation that apply across a broad range of research designs.

Finally, discussion of pragmatic research should address the issue of the practicality of using the evaluation methods. Many D&I assessments, and especially those often cited as exemplary evaluations, are very comprehensive, detailed, and expensive. This is appropriate and necessary for definitive or large-scale investigations or when detailed knowledge of outcomes will determine public policies or substantial investment of scarce resources. However, there is substantial need for "pragmatic measures"[11,40,41] that are more feasible and widely applicable and can be acted on to produce more rapid results exists.

KEY DISSEMINATION AND IMPLEMENTATION EVALUATION ISSUES

Understanding Context

Context has been defined as any factors (e.g., organization, policies, workflow) that are not part of the evidence-based intervention or program.[42] Others define context as the dynamic and diverse array of forces working for or against implementation efforts.[43] Understanding the context for which a program is delivered is critical for the success of D&I and has major implications for fidelity and adaptions (see chapters 7 and 8). Context is dynamic and iterative; therefore identifying and assessing contextual factors at multiple levels and over time throughout the course of program implementation are important (see Table 17.1).[44] In addition, assessment of how the program interacts with the settings over time is necessary so one can assess how much of the outcomes are attributable to the program and how much to the context. To address this issue, Damschroder et al. have proposed an Outcomes Addendum to the Consolidated Framework for Implementation Research (CFIR) to assist researchers in stating which outcomes their studies are proposing to address, judiciously consider the determinants (i.e., setting level barriers and facilitators) that can affect those outcomes, and thus design studies that can collect the best data for evaluating both outcomes and their determinants.[45]

Sustainment

A literature review highlighted the lack of a working definition for sustainability in many research studies. The authors suggested that

TABLE 17.1 KEY EVALUATION ISSUES IN DISSEMINATION AND IMPLEMENTATION SCIENCE

Key Issue	Recommendations and Comments
Understanding context	• Evaluate the influence of multilevel contextual factors in diverse settings. • Specify, hypothesize, and test models of contextual factors related to outcomes. • Use context and determinants frameworks to assess context and changes over time. • Use mixed methods to understand the complex issues involved.
Sustainment	• Consider evolution across the dynamic life cycle of the evidence-based intervention within a broader context with the goal of sustainable and equitable health impact. • Assess who (both individual and setting level) is and is not being reached by the intervention/program over time. Measure sustainability over time and evaluate changes in use of the intervention, context, and implementation strategies.
Stakeholder engagement	• Identify the appropriate stakeholders to engage and assess at what points in time. • Determine level of stakeholder engagement and key issues on which to assess stakeholder perspectives. • Include stakeholders in all aspects of the research process to ensure that results are relevant and can lead to greater use and uptake. • Evaluate representation of different types of stakeholders (see below).
Health equity	• Routinely assess equity using measures and approaches tailored to the particular issue and program. • Requires attention to reach, adoption, and representativeness of the participants and settings. Are all populations and settings equitably reached by the intervention/program? Who is not reached (in terms of a range of social dimensions and social determinants of health) and why? • How can we better reach those who are not receiving the program and ensure we are reaching those who experience inequities related to social needs and social/structural determinants of health? • Context of studies should reflect settings where vulnerable populations seek healthcare, work, and live.
Use of qualitative methods	• Use to identify and explain which aspects of the program and implementation strategies are working (or not) and for which populations and/or contexts. • Use to evaluate the implementation process and sustainment. • Use to elicit perspectives from stakeholders, implementers, participants, and potential adopters.
Evaluation of costs	• Evaluate costs from the perspective of the adopting organization and individuals such as employers, healthcare providers, patients, or families. • Evaluate costs beyond monetary costs. Consider additional costs, such as resources and staff needed, time involved, and patient burden. • Consider opportunity costs and degree of disruption to usual workflows.
External validity	• Evaluate representation and representativeness of community/organizational settings, decision makers, intervention agents, patients/end users. • Evaluate outcomes compared across different groups of participants (heterogeneity of effects). • Evaluate unintended adverse consequences and nonhealth impacts. • Evaluate implementation, fidelity, and adaptations. • Evaluate long-term effects at least 12–24 months following conclusion of active intervention. • Evaluate sustainment, long-term adaptation or integration (see below).

TABLE 17.1 CONTINUED

Key Issue	Recommendations and Comments
Adaptations	• Track adaptations of evidence-based interventions and implementation strategies to enhance fit within different contexts, populations, and settings. • Note whether the adaptation is fidelity consistent (preserve core elements of intervention) or fidelity inconsistent (change the core elements of the intervention). • Apply form-function concepts and evaluations of adaptations.

researchers consider the following factors when choosing a definition for sustainment: (1) whether and to what extent core elements of the program are maintained; (2) extent to which health outcomes are maintained or improved on after initial support is withdrawn; (3) the extent, nature, and impact of modifications to the core elements; and (4) capacity to continue to maintain desired benefits.[46] Whereas significant advancements have been made in understanding the adoption and implementation of evidence-based interventions across a range of community and healthcare settings, less is known about their sustainability. Sustained practice changes of programs are infrequently investigated, often due to the constrained time frames for research that are set by grant mechanisms and the budgetary and political necessity of many decision makers to take a short-term perspective. Evaluation of sustainment needs to take into consideration changes in the program and implementation strategies over time and contextual characteristics.[29,47] The dynamic sustainability framework (DSF) and the exploration, preparation, implementation, and sustainment (EPIS) framework both conceptualize the need to move away from thinking about sustainability as a linear process toward one that needs to be evaluated in a dynamic and continual manner to understand the factors that influence sustainment.[29,48] See chapter 27 for a more detailed discussion of sustainability.

Stakeholder Engagement

There continues to be a shift from clinical research traditionally driven by investigators, to one more inclusive and driven by patient and stakeholders across the research project continuum—from generation of research questions, to implementation, to evaluation and interpretation of outcomes, and to dissemination of study results.[49,50] Inclusion of stakeholders can help to ensure the relevance of the research topic, focus the evaluation questions asked, and improve the potential for dissemination of findings and sustainment.[51,52] In addition, inclusions of stakeholder perspectives and priorities can enhance relevance to intended end users, identify cultural issues that should be included when designing the study, identify and prioritize outcome measures, and advise on the appropriateness of design and recruitment strategies.[52] However, despite the growing number of stakeholder-engaged research projects, more work is needed to advance evaluation of the quality of engagement and the overall impact.[53] Evaluation of what stakeholders are involved in what ways over time for what purposes and what outcomes are produced is needed to advance D&I research beyond a simplistic mantra that "stakeholder engagement is good." More information on participatory approaches in D&I research can be found in chapter 10.

Health Equity

There has been increasing acknowledgment of the importance of the equitable implementation of evidence-based programs across a range of diverse populations and settings.[54–56] To achieve health equity, implementation and dissemination of effective evidence-based programs that account for the complex and multilayered social determinants of health among marginalized groups and across healthcare settings are needed.[56] Health equity is increasingly being included in D&I science models and includes issues of representation (e.g., stakeholders) and representativeness (of participation and outcomes).[47,57] Health equity considerations include questions such as the following: Are all populations equitably reached by the program? Are the health impacts experienced equitably across all groups on the basis of various social determinants of health? Did all settings equitably adopt the program? Were the program and implementation strategies equitably delivered across staff/settings? What settings and populations continue to be reached long term by the program and continue to receive benefits over time?[47] See chapter 25 for a more focused review of D&I efforts among racial/ethnic minorities and disadvantaged populations.

Use of Qualitative Methods

Qualitative evaluation methods are essential tools that evaluators can draw on (see chapter 18). Certain questions, problems, and purposes are more fitting with qualitative methods than with others, and these approaches can almost always be used to help understand and explain quantitative findings. Qualitative methods can be used in evaluation work to provide detail and context to the interpretation of statistical data.[58] Qualitative approaches to evaluation are themselves diverse. They can range from formative studies to outcome evaluation, to process studies, and to implementation evaluation, program comparisons, documentation of program development over time, investigation of system change, and conduct of "postmortem" exams to explore unanticipated results.[59,60] Qualitative evaluations often rely on a variety of data collection methods. These methods include focus groups, case studies, in-depth interviews, and observational field notes. Integrating qualitative methods with more traditional quantitative evaluation methods in mixed-methods research lends depth and clarity to understanding outcomes.

In D&I research, mixed-method designs have been increasingly used to understand and overcome barriers to implementation. More recently, they have been used in the design and implementation of strategies to facilitate the implementation of evidence-based practices.[61] Mixed-method designs focus on collecting, analyzing, and merging both quantitative and qualitative data. The central premise of these designs is that the use of quantitative and qualitative approaches in combination provides a better understanding of research issues than either approach alone.[62,63] In mixed-method evaluation designs, qualitative methods are used to explore and obtain depth of understanding about the reasons for success or failure to implement an evidence-based practice or to identify strategies for facilitating implementation, while quantitative methods are used to test and confirm hypotheses based on a conceptual model and obtain breadth of understanding of predictors of successful implementation.[62,63]

Evaluation of Costs

Information on cost issues is often a primary consideration in whether a potential program will be adopted or sustained. Information on costs anticipated during planning stages, experienced during implementation, and projected during dissemination phases is an important aspect of evaluation and has been identified as a key outcome in implementation research.[8] Although receiving increasing attention, costs are one of the least often captured components of D&I evaluations, and lack of cost information has been cited as a barrier to implementation.[64,65] Chapter 11 presents an overview of economic evaluation in D&I science.

The perspective and concerns of the adopting organizations and individuals such as employers, healthcare clinics or providers, implementers or delivery staff, or patients and families are often different from that most often reported in economic reports[66] and differ across different stakeholders. As in other areas of D&I, understanding what implementing partners and potential adoptees value and the types of costs they are most concerned about is central to conducting relevant economic evaluations likely to be useful to consumers.[65] For example, rather than formal business or societal definitions of "return on investment," healthcare clinics and patients/families are often primarily concerned about time involved and the burden and degree of disruption in usual workflows or daily patterns (as well as opportunity costs, although often not articulated as such).[65]

External Validity

Dissemination and implementation research emphasizes external validity (see chapter 16), in contrast to the main emphasis on internal validity in traditional randomized efficacy and effectiveness trials.[39] In the last several years, there has been a call for a shift from research under ideal conditions to research conducted in real-world settings with participants who would receive a program if it became usual care: pragmatic or practical trials.[32,35,36,67] Tools such as PRECIS-2 were designed to be used at the design stage of a trial to help researchers make the purpose of their trial explicit and to ensure that their design choices were concordant with their intended purpose.[35] However, this tool can also be used on trial completion to objectively evaluate how close the trial was conducted to the original intent. Moreover, use of the RE-AIM framework was created to help balance the traditional focus on internal over external validity as discussed in greater detail further in this chapter.[17,68] RE-AIM and D&I perspectives focus on key issues for external validity: representativeness at multiple levels (patient, intervention agent, and setting); generalization of effects (Were different results produced for different types of patients or settings? Did findings produce unintended or deleterious outcomes and for whom?); and replication (Can the results of the program be duplicated in settings in addition to those in which they were originally produced?).[69]

Adaptations

Implementation strategies are often used to ensure that an intervention is adopted into, successfully delivered, and sustained within target settings.[70] These strategies, like the program or intervention, are often changed or modified to fit the setting or target population. A critical area of emerging research is to better understand what adaptations are made, assess reasons why and when they are made, and what impact they have on the program being implemented.[71] Two frameworks are widely used: (a) to guide tracking adaptations to interventions (Framework for Reporting Adaptations and Modifications–Expanded [FRAME]), and (b) adaptations to implementation strategies (Framework for Reporting Adaptions and Modifications to Evidence-Based Implementation Strategies [FRAME-IS]).[25,72] In addition, the form-function framework is increasingly used to conceptualize, differentiate, and assess adaptations.[73] See chapter 8 for additional information on adaptations.

KEY EVALUATION MODELS AND FRAMEWORKS

Many programs found to be effective in health services research studies fail to translate into meaningful patient care or public health outcomes or across different contexts.[74] Complex interventions are increasingly used in the health service and public health practice, but they pose a number of evaluation challenges.[75] A key question in evaluating complex interventions is about practical effectiveness, whether the intervention works in everyday practice, in which case it is important to understand the whole range of effects; how they vary among recipients of the program, across sites, over time; and causes of variation.[76] Barriers to implementation arise at multiple levels of healthcare delivery: the patient, the provider team or group, the organizational, and the policy levels.[77,78] While this chapter does not provide an exhaustive list (see chapter 4), the following is a summary of several key and widely used evaluation models and frameworks that have been proven to be practical in guiding and evaluating translation of research findings (see Table 17.2).

PRECEDE-PROCEED Model

PRECEDE is an acronym for *p*redisposing, *r*einforcing, and *e*nabling *c*onstructs in *e*ducational/*e*cological *d*iagnosis and *e*valuation. PROCEED is an acronym for *p*olicy, *r*egulatory, and *o*rganizational *c*onstructs in *e*ducation and *e*nvironmental *d*evelopment. The PRECEDE-PROCEED model is one of the most comprehensive models in that it combines the causal assessment and the intervention planning and evaluation into one overarching framework.[16,79,80] The goals of the model are to explain health-related behaviors and environments and to design and evaluate the programs needed to influence both the behaviors and the social and contextual conditions that influence them. Due to the flexibility and scalability of this classic model, it has been extensively applied and tested in a wide variety of settings, especially for public health programs, and policies.[81–83]

The PRECEDE-PROCEED model has two main components. The first component, PRECEDE, consists of four phases aimed at generating information. The original PRECEDE model was developed in the 1970s and has probably been more widely used than any other model to plan and evaluate public health interventions (https://www.lgreen.net). This part of the model recognizes the need for

TABLE 17.2 SUMMARY OF SELECTED EVALUATION APPROACHES FOR DISSEMINATION AND IMPLEMENTATION RESEARCH

Evaluation Approach	Acronym	Emphasis on Planning, Evaluation, or Both	Summary and Key Features	Key Recommended References
PRECEDE-PROCEED model	PRECEDE-PROCEED	Planning and evaluation	Links intervention planning and evaluation into one integrated framework. Comprehensive model emphasizing a multidisciplinary approach to assessing the multiple factors that impact and influence health. Eight-phase model: 1. Social assessment: identifying the ultimate desired goal or result; 2. Epidemiological assessment: identify the genetics, behavioral, and/or environmental indicators that may contribute to or interact with overall desired goal or result; 3. Educational and ecological assessment: identifying predisposing, reinforcing, and enabling factors that can affect the behaviors, genetic, and environmental indicators identified in prior phase; 4. Identifying the administrative and policy factors that influence what can be implemented. 5. Implementation: conducting the intervention; 6. Process evaluation: determines the extent to which the program components were implemented as planned; 7. Impact evaluation: how well the intended audiences were reached; and 8. Outcome evaluation: determines the effect of the program on the overall goal or result as well as quality-of-life indicators.	Green LW, Kreuter MW. *Health Program Planning: An Education and Ecological Approach.* 4th ed. McGraw-Hill; 2005. https://www.lgreen.net
Realist evaluation	n/a	Evaluation	The premise is that programs work (outcomes) through mechanisms acting in contexts. Realist evaluation emphasizes understanding what program works for whom in what circumstances. Outcomes = Mechanisms + Context *Context* is the characteristics of the conditions in which a program is introduced. The context in which it operates makes a difference to and thus shapes the mechanism(s) through which it works and thus the outcomes it achieves. *Mechanisms* describe what it is about the program that brings about any effects or changes. *Outcomes* include the intended and unintended consequences of the program resulting from the activation (or lack thereof) of different mechanisms in different contexts.	Pawson R, Tilley N. *Realistic Evaluation*. Sage Publications; 1997. Pawson R. *The Science of Evaluation: A Realist Manifesto.* Sage Publications; 2013.

Reach, Effectiveness, Adoption, Implementation, and Maintenance framework *Plus* Practical, robust implementation and sustainability model	RE-AIM + PRISM	Planning and evaluation	Emphasizes five dimensions that together determine public health impact. Places equal emphasis on external and internal validity. Evaluates results at both the setting/contextual and individual levels. *Reach* is the absolute number, proportion, and representativeness of individuals who are willing to participate in a given initiative. *Effectiveness* is the impact of a program on outcomes, including potential negative effects, quality of life, and economic outcomes. *Adoption* is the absolute number, proportion, and representativeness of settings and intervention agents are willing to initiate a program. *Implementation* refers to the intervention agents' fidelity to the various elements of an intervention's protocol. It includes consistency of delivery as intended, adaptations made, and the time and cost of the program. *Maintenance* is the extent to which a program or policy becomes institutionalized or part of the routine organizational practices and policies. At the individual level, it is defined as the long-term effects of a program on outcomes, ideally at 24 or more months after the most recent program contact. PRISM expands RE-AIM by adding increased focus on multilevel contextual factors, specifically how intervention design, external environment, organizational characteristics, and the intended population influence intervention effectiveness when implementing evidence-based practices.	Glasgow RE, Vogt TM, Boles SM. Evaluating the public health impact of health promotion interventions: the RE-AIM Framework. *Am J Public Health.* 1999;89(9):1322–1327. https://www.re-aim.org Feldstein AC, Glasgow RE. A practical, robust, implementation and sustainability model (PRISM) for integrating research findings into practice. *Jt Comm J Qual Patient Saf.* 2008;34(4):228–243.
Implementation outcomes framework	IOF	Evaluation	This framework provides eight distinct implementation outcomes as well as highlights the differences between implementation, service, and client outcomes to provide better understanding of how and why implementation succeeds or fails. *Implementation Outcomes*: 1. Acceptability 2. Adoption 3. Appropriateness 4. Costs 5. Feasibility 6. Fidelity 7. Penetration 8. Sustainability	Proctor E, Silmere H, Raghavan R, et al. Outcomes for implementation research: conceptual distinctions, measurement challenges, and research agenda. *Adm Policy Ment Health.* 2011;38:65–76.

(*continued*)

TABLE 17.2 CONTINUED

Evaluation Approach	Acronym	Emphasis on Planning, Evaluation, or Both	Summary and Key Features	Key Recommended References
Medical Research Council Guidance for Evaluating Complex Interventions	n/a	Planning and evaluation	This framework for developing and evaluating complex interventions emphasizes four phases: development or identification of an intervention, assessment of feasibility of the intervention and evaluation design, evaluation of the intervention, and impactful implementation. At each phase, there are six core elements that should be considered: • Consider context • Develop, refine, and (re)test program theory • Engage stakeholders • Identify key uncertainties • Refine intervention • Economic considerations	Skivington K, Matthews L, Simpson SA, et al. A new framework for developing and evaluating complex interventions: update of Medical Research Council guidance. *BMJ*. 2021;374:n2061.

Abbreviation: n/a, not applicable.

assessment prior to program planning. The following are the phases of PRECEDE:

1. Social assessment: identifying the ultimate desired goal or result;
2. Epidemiological assessment: identify the genetics, behavioral, and/or environmental indicators that may contribute to or interact with overall desired goal or result;
3. Educational and ecological assessment: identifying predisposing, reinforcing, and enabling factors that can affect the behaviors, genetic, and environmental indicators identified in prior phases; and
4. Identifying the administrative and policy factors that influence what can be implemented.

This is followed by the second component, PROCEED, added in the early 1990s, which highlights the importance of environmental, contextual, and genetic factors (added later in 2005) as determinants of health and health inequities. PROCEED consists of four additional phases that focus on the actual implementation of the program and evaluation of it. The phases in this part of the model are the following:

5. Implementation: conducting the intervention;
6. Process evaluation: determining the extent to which the program components were implemented as planned;
7. Impact evaluation: evaluating how well the intended audiences were reached; and
8. Outcome evaluation: determining the effect of the program on the overall goal or result that was proposed in phase 1 as well as quality-of-life indicators.[16]

The PRECEDE-PROCEED model provides a structured framework to apply health behavior theories at all levels. Although developed prior to the establishment of D&I science as a field of inquiry, PRECEDE-PROCEED is still very relevant to most D&I issues, and it stresses a transdisciplinary approach and evaluation of the multitude of factors that impact implementation and health outcomes.

Realist Evaluation

A realist evaluation as espoused by Pawson and Tilley is somewhat of a contrarian perspective.[12,84] In particular, it rejects the notion that the goal of evaluation should be to determine "average effects" across patients, settings, time, staff, and so on. Instead, realist evaluation is based on the assumption that the same intervention will not work everywhere and for everyone. Realist evaluation is highly contextual and uses a complexity theory and systems thinking approach to evaluate complex interventions in complex situations. At the heart of realist evaluation is a focus on context (C), mechanism (M), and outcomes (O) relationships in the form of C + M = O.

Context, in realist evaluation, is the characteristics of the conditions in which a program is introduced. The context in which it operates makes a difference to and thus shapes the mechanism(s) through which it works and the outcomes it achieves. Mechanisms describe what it is about the program that brings about any effects or changes. Outcomes include the intended and unintended consequences of the program, resulting from the activation (or lack thereof) of different mechanisms in different contexts.

This approach recommends developing an adaptable "program theory" (this need not be a formal theory but can be a working logic model identifying mechanisms, contexts, and outcomes) and then forming and testing hypotheses related to what might work for whom (or not) and in what circumstances with what results.[84] Then both quantitative and qualitative data are collected to evaluate the mechanisms, context, and outcomes, which in turn help refine the program theory, and the process continues until the complexities are understood. Thus, the highly contextual question realist evaluation addresses is What (complex) interventions operating through what underlying process mechanisms produce what outcomes for whom and under what conditions?

RE-AIM and PRISM Frameworks

The RE-AIM framework, which is an acronym for reach, effectiveness, adoption, implementation, and maintenance, is over 20 years old.[68] RE-AIM has helped to balance the focus between internal and external validity. It is one of the most frequently used frameworks for planning and evaluation of NIH-funded D&I research grants.[85]

The dimensions of the multilevel framework are defined as follows[11,12,65]: *Reach* is the absolute number, proportion, and representativeness of individuals who are willing to participate in a given initiative. *Effectiveness* is the impact of a program on outcomes, including potential negative effects, heterogeneity of effects, quality of life, and economic outcomes. *Adoption* is the absolute number, proportion, and representativeness of (a) settings and (b) intervention agents who are willing to initiate a program. *Implementation* refers to the intervention agents' fidelity to and adaptation of the various elements of a program protocol. This includes consistency of delivery as intended and the time and costs of the intervention. *Maintenance* at the setting level is the extent to which a program or policy becomes institutionalized or part of routine organizational practices and policies. At the individual level, it is defined as the long-term effects of a program on outcomes 6 or more months after the most recent intervention contact. Resources for using the RE-AIM framework can be found online (https://re-aim.org).

RE-AIM has evolved over the last two decades to include more qualitative and mixed-methods assessments (see chapter 18), assessment of adaptions prior to and during implementation, assessment of costs from the perspective of multiple stakeholders and across the RE-AIM dimensions, and a focus on specific contextual factors with the practical, robust implementation and sustainability model (PRISM) (see Figure 17.1).[68] PRISM is an extension of RE-AIM that was developed to help identify and assess contextual factors and influences needed to successfully implement and sustain a program in a given setting.[86] It looks at how program design, external environment, organizational characteristics, and the intended population influence program effectiveness when implementing evidence-based practices. PRISM posits that the "implementation and sustainability infrastructure" (factors such as resources and systems to monitor and support program success) is an important determinant of program success and sustainment). PRISM was developed using several models: diffusion of innovations, the chronic care model, the model for improvement, and the RE-AIM framework. As can be seen in Figure 17.1, PRISM focuses on multilevel contextual factors related to a program and incorporates RE-AIM dimensions to evaluate program effects.

Implementation Outcomes Framework

Dissemination and implementation research, which has evolved from numerous and diverse fields, has struggled to come to consensus on how to conceptualize and evaluate successful implementation.[45] Proctor et al. proposed a taxonomy for eight distinct implementation outcomes as well as differentiated among implementation, service, and client outcomes to provide better understanding of how and why implementation succeeds or fails.[8] Their eight implementation outcomes and definitions are as follows:

1. *Acceptability*: the perception among implementation stakeholders that a given treatment, service, practice, or innovation is agreeable, palatable, or satisfactory.
2. *Adoption*: the intention, initial decision, or action to try or employ an innovation or evidence-based practice.
3. *Appropriateness*: the perceived fit, relevance, or compatibility of the innovation or evidence-based practice for a given practice setting, provider, or consumer and/or perceived fit of the innovation to address a particular issue or problem.
4. *Cost*: the cost impact of an implementation effort. Of note: implementation costs will vary due to the variability in complexity of treatments, complexity of an implementation strategy selected, and setting variability.
5. *Feasibility*: the extent to which a new treatment or an innovation can be successfully used or carried out within a given agency or setting.
6. *Fidelity*: the degree to which an intervention was implemented as it was prescribed in the original protocol or as it was intended by the program developers. Measuring fidelity in usual care has been plagued with numerous challenges.

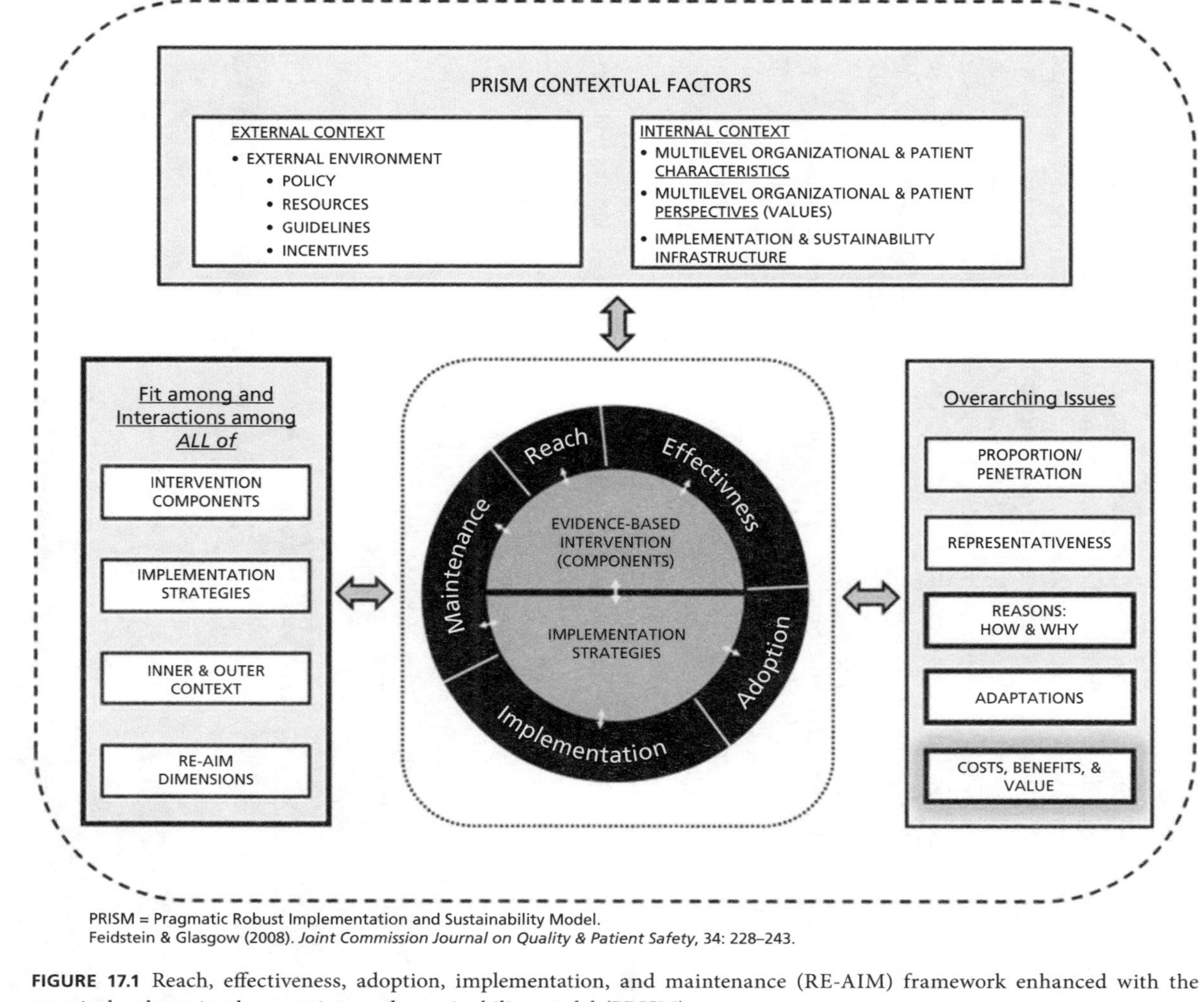

PRISM = Pragmatic Robust Implementation and Sustainability Model.
Feidstein & Glasgow (2008). *Joint Commission Journal on Quality & Patient Safety*, 34: 228–243.

FIGURE 17.1 Reach, effectiveness, adoption, implementation, and maintenance (RE-AIM) framework enhanced with the practical, robust, implementation, and sustainability model (PRISM).

Source: Reprinted with permission from Glasgow RE, Harden SM, Gaglio B, Rabin B, Smith ML, et al. RE-AIM planning and evaluation framework: adapting to new science and practice with a 20-year review. *Front Public Health*. 2019;7:64.

7. *Penetration*: the integration of a practice within a service setting and its subsystems.
8. *Sustainability*: the extent to which a newly implemented treatment is maintained or institutionalized within a service setting's ongoing stable operations.

Lengnick-Hall et al. recently conducted a scoping review to describe how the field has conceptualized, measured, and advanced theory around implementation outcomes since the publication of the implementation outcomes framework.[87] They identified six problems related to rigor and consistency in reporting of implementation outcomes and propose recommendations to prevent them in future work.

Medical Research Council Guidance for Evaluating Complex Interventions

The Medical Research Council (MRC) of the United Kingdom has produced periodic guidance from panels of experts on the design and evaluation of complex interventions.[76,88] Recently, they have updated their previous guidance with a new framework, commissioned jointly by the MRC and the National Institute for Health Research; the update focuses on inclusion of stakeholders to identify key questions about complex interventions and to design and conduct research with a diversity of perspectives and corresponding methods.[89] This is especially relevant to D&I science since the vast majority of interventions evaluated in D&I are complex and should include a variety of stakeholders.

The new MRC guidance considers the complexity that arises from both the intervention's components and from its interaction with the context in which it is being implemented.[89] The framework divides complex intervention research into four phases: (1) development or identification of the intervention; (2) assessment of feasibility of the intervention and evaluation design; (3) evaluation of the intervention; and (4) impactful implementation. The phases are not necessarily linear. At each phase, there are six core elements that should be considered to decide whether the research should proceed to the next phase, return to a previous phase, repeat a phase, or stop (see Figure 17.2).[89]

1. *Consider context*: How does the intervention interact with its context?

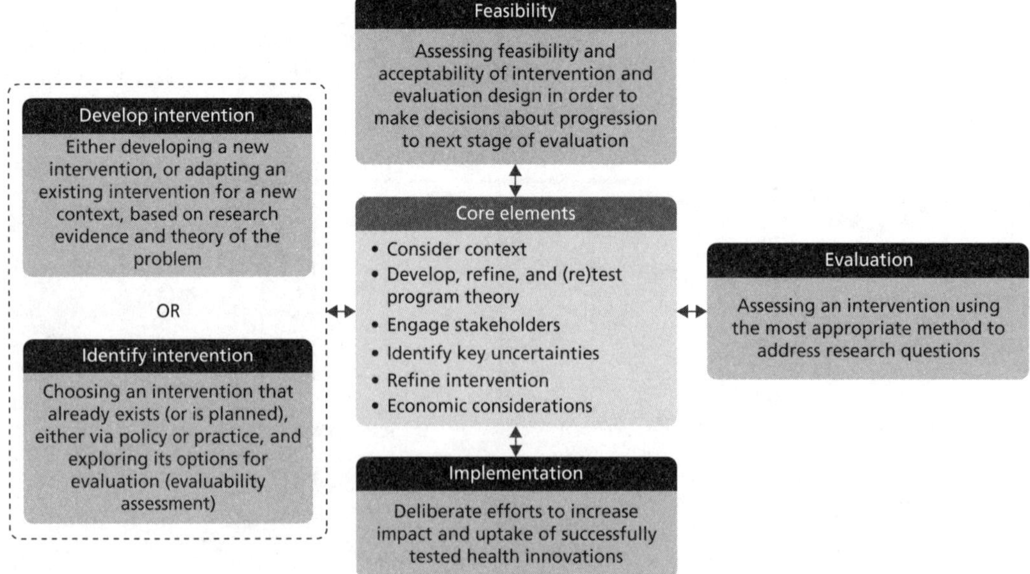

FIGURE 17.2 Phases and core elements of complex intervention research from the United Kingdom's Medical Research Council.

Source: Reprinted with permission from Skivington K, Matthews L, Simpson SA, Craig P, et al. A new framework for developing and evaluating complex interventions: update of Medical Research Council guidance. *BMJ*. 2021;374:n2061.

2. *Develop, refine, and (re)test program theory*: What is the underpinning program theory?
3. *Engage stakeholders*: How can diverse stakeholder perspectives be included in the research?
4. *Identify key uncertainties*: What are the key uncertainties?
5. *Refine intervention*: How can the intervention be refined?
6. *Economic considerations*: What are the comparative resource and outcome consequences of the intervention?

Commonalities Across Evaluation Frameworks

The frameworks above constitute some of the most widely used evaluation approaches in D&I science, but this list is not exhaustive, and frameworks continue to evolve.[90] While evaluation frameworks such as those above may be considered in a category of their own, models and frameworks such as the CFIR,[43,45] Promoting Action on Research Implementation in Health Research (PARIHS),[91] and the Theoretical Domains Framework[92] can also be applied for evaluation purposes. While each evaluation framework and model has its unique strengths and limitations, evaluation approaches for D&I share several common themes.[93,94] First, implementation is heavily dependent on context, and one needs to understand and be sensitive to local conditions, history, and resources. Second, as discussed in more detail in chapter 7 on fidelity-adaptation, quality of implementation is a frequent challenge, and programs are almost never implemented exactly as they were designed or tested in efficacy studies.[95] Third, both implementation and dissemination are complex, multilevel undertakings, not easily explained by simplistic models or appropriately evaluated by reductionistic designs. Finally, traditional evaluation and research methods tend to ignore or underemphasize the importance of key D&I factors such as reach and engagement of the target audience[64]; the need to operationalize and provide practical assessments of setting, delivery staff, and organizational and individual factors and their interactions[93,96]; issues of cost and economic outcomes[97]; and external validity.[39] The important point is not to argue about the minor differences among approaches or to say which one is "best," but rather to have program developers and evaluators select a framework, or combination of frameworks, that fits their question and needs and then *use* the framework(s) consistently to evaluate results—including collecting data on factors hypothesized by the model to produce different outcomes.

CASE STUDY

Table 17.3 illustrates the example of how RE-AIM was used to evaluate the Faith, Activity, and Nutrition (FAN) D&I study.[98–100] FAN was an evidence-based program designed to promote physical activity and healthy eating through church policy, systems, and environmental change. It was a group randomized trial in which churches from a medically underserved and rural county were invited to participate in the study. Committees from 40 churches were trained by community health advisors. The training focused on helping churches create healthier church environments for physical activity and healthy eating. Each church committee participated in a full-day training. Churches received materials to support implementation of the program. After the full-day training, trained churches received 12 monthly technical assistance calls to help them implement their program plan. The church coordinator received 8 calls, and the pastor received 4 calls over 12 months. Primary outcomes were adoption, reach, implementation/fidelity, and maintenance. Secondary outcomes were self-reported physical activity, self-reported fruit and vegetable intake, self-efficacy for physical activity, and self-efficacy for fruit and vegetable intake for members of participating churches.

The estimated weekly worship attendance of the 132 churches in the county was 8,484. The estimated weekly worship attendance of the 55 trained churches was 3,527. Thus, more than 42% of regular church attendees and 15% of county residents were reached.[100] Of the 132 active churches in Fairfield County, South Carolina, 59 were interested, eligible, and randomized. Thirty-six of the 39 intervention churches and 18 of the 20 control churches were trained. One church ineligible because of size was also trained and considered an adopting church. Adoption was 42% of churches (55/132). Of the churches randomized, 92% (54/59) of church FAN coordinators

TABLE 17.3 CASE STUDY: EXAMPLE OF APPLYING THE RE-AIM FRAMEWORK TO EVALUATE THE FAITH, ACTIVITY, AND NUTRITION DISSEMINATION AND IMPLEMENTATION STUDY

	RE-AIM Dimension	Application
Wilcox S, Saunders RP, Kaczynski AT, et al. Faith, activity, and nutrition randomized dissemination and implementation study: countywide adoption, reach, and effectiveness. *Am J Prev Med.* 2018;54:776–785.	REACH: Defined as the pastor-reported number of individuals who typically attended worship services among churches that adopted the program as compared to both the number of attendees at nonadopting churches and the total county population.	The estimated weekly worship attendance of the 132 churches in the county was 8,484. The estimated weekly worship attendance of the 55 trained churches was 3,527. Thus, > 42% of regular church attendees and 15% of county residents were reached.
	EFFECTIVENESS: Assessment of member-perceived changes in opportunities, messages, and pastor support for physical activity and healthy eating.	Questionnaires were completed by 1,423 attendees; 115 were not used because they were missing a covariate, leaving a sample of 1,308. Intervention and control churches did not differ on church-level characteristics. Intervention church attendees were younger, and more self-reported cancer. Intervention church attendees reported more frequent physical activity opportunities, healthy eating and physical activity messages, and pastor support for healthy eating and physical activity than control church attendees.
Saunders RP, Wilcox S, Jake-Schoffman DE, et al. The faith, activity, and nutrition (FAN) dissemination and implementation study, phase 1: implementation monitoring methods and results. *Health Educ Behav.* 2019;46:388–397.	ADOPTION: The percentage of churches (both intervention and control/delayed intervention) in the county that attended a FAN training and the percentage of pastors and church FAN coordinators from enrolled churches who were trained.	Of the 132 active churches in Fairfield County, 59 were interested, eligible, and randomized. Thirty-six of the 39 intervention churches and 18 of the 20 control churches (delayed intervention) were trained. One church ineligible because of size was also trained and considered an adopting church. Thus, adoption was 42% of churches (55/132) in the target county. Churches with predominantly black/African American attendees and those that had participated in an earlier tobacco-free county initiative were significantly more likely to adopt. Church size and denomination were unrelated to adoption.

Wilcox S, Saunders RP, Jake-Schoffman D, Hutto B. The faith, activity, and nutrition, dissemination and implementation study: 24-month organizational maintenance in a countywide initiative. *Front Public Health.* 2020;8:171.	IMPLEMENTATION: The fidelity of delivering the intervention to the church committees and the degree to which church committees implemented the intervention as intended in their churches.	Two community health advisors trained 142 committee members from the 36 intervention churches and 60 church committee members from the 18 control churches. University staff observed the trainings and rated nearly complete coverage of all content areas. Over 90% of calls were delivered, and calls averaged around 7 minutes in duration. In a sample of 1,308 church members (811 from intervention and 497 from control), members from the intervention churches reported significantly greater implementation than members from the control churches for physical activity and healthy eating at 12 months.
	MAINTENANCE: Church coordinator-reported 24-month implementation of the four FAN components (providing opportunities, setting guidelines, sharing messages, and engaging pastor).	Church coordinators reported significantly greater implementation of both physical activity and healthy eating FAN components at 12 and 24 months compared to baseline. Most churches (58% for physical activity and 97% for healthy eating) were maintaining at least one FAN component at 24 months.

and 64% (38/59) of pastors attended training.[100] The intervention was effective, with intervention church members reporting greater postintervention church-level physical activity opportunities, physical activity and healthy eating messages, and physical activity and healthy eating pastor support.[100] Two community health advisors trained 142 committee members from the 36 intervention churches and 60 church committee members from the 18 control churches. University staff observed the trainings and rated nearly complete coverage of all content areas. Over 90% of calls were delivered, and calls averaged around 7 minutes in duration.[98] Church coordinators reported significantly greater implementation of both physical activity and healthy eating FAN components at 12 and 24 months compared to baseline. Most churches were maintaining at least one FAN component at 24 months.[99]

SUMMARY

Considerable progress has been made in evaluation of D&I research; however, we still lack knowledge in several key areas. The complex, inherently multilevel and contextual nature of D&I science and the always and sometimes rapidly changing environment present ongoing challenges. Given these challenges, evaluation of D&I efforts need more adapted, novel, responsive, and sophisticated approaches to evaluation and, especially, more pragmatic measures.

As evaluation of D&I science continues to evolve, several new areas must be considered. Engaging patients, stakeholders, and communities in research continues to gain momentum and popularity in pragmatic, real-world studies; however, evaluation of engagement and its impact on study outcomes as well as impact on D&I efforts need further attention. Future work should consider if understanding context is enough to capture the impact of engagement on D&I efforts or if existing models and frameworks will need to be revised to account for this change to how research is conducted. Genomic methods[101] and precision medicine[102] applications will continue to progress. Evaluation of precision medicine applications will be challenging but needs to be undertaken, especially to assess costs, outcomes, adaptations, and importantly, equity and unintended consequences. Evaluations of multilevel programs will continue to challenge the field because of not only the complexity of the programs and related implementation strategies, but also their interactions and how each changes over time. How this is reported in a transparent manner should continue to be a priority for the field.

As D&I science continues to evolve, we will be able to more conclusively answer the key, ultimate use question mentioned at the beginning of this chapter: What programs (interventions, guidelines, products, or policies) and what components, conducted under what conditions and in what settings, using what strategies, conducted by which agents, produce which outcomes, for which populations (and subgroups) via which processes, and how much does it cost?

SUGGESTED READINGS AND WEBSITES

Readings

Glasgow RE, Harden SM, Gaglio B, et al. RE-AIM planning and evaluation framework: adapting to new science and practice with a 20-year review. *Front Public Health.* 2019;7:64.

The article summarizes key issues in applying and the evolution of the RE-AIM framework over time. It discusses continued focus on representativeness, equity, transparency, population impact, and external validity, as well as more recent inclusion of issues of pragmatic use, adaptations, and costs and use of RE-AIM for planning and iterative evaluation.

Lewis CC, Mettert KD, Stanick CF, et al. The Psychometric and Pragmatic Evidence Rating Scale (PAPERS) for measure development and evaluation. *Implement Res Pract.* 2021;2. doi:10.1177/26334895211037391

This article presents a rating scale for implementation science measures that considers their psychometric and pragmatic properties and the evidence available: the Psychometric and Pragmatic Evidence Rating Scale (PAPERS) that evaluates implementation science measures on both their traditional psychometric criteria and several criteria for widespread pragmatic use.

Loudon K, Treweek S, Sullivan F, Donnan P, Thorpe KE, Zwarenstein M. The PRECIS-2 tool: designing trials that are fit for purpose. *BMJ.* 2015;350:h2147; and

Norton WE, Loudon K, Chambers DA, Zwarenstein M. Designing provider-focused implementation trials with purpose and intent: introducing the PRECIS-2-PS tool. *Implement Sci.* 2021;16:7.

These articles give guidance on how to use an updated version of the Pragmatic-Explanatory Continuum

Indicator Summary (PRECIS) that more directly addresses issues relevant to implementation science. PRECIS-2-PS focuses on provider/implementer level factors rather than predominantly on individual participant level issues. It now has nine domains scored from 1 (very explanatory) to 5 (very pragmatic), and although developed for planning of evaluations, it can also be used to review the literature and report implementation research.

Pinnock H, Barwick M, Carpenter CR, et al. Standards for Reporting Implementation Studies (StaRI) statement. *BMJ*. 2017;356:i6795.

This article presents a 27-item checklist to prompt researchers to describe both the implementation strategy and the effectiveness of the intervention being implemented. The checklist applies to a broad range of research methodologies employed in implementation science.

Proctor EK, Silmere H, Raghavan R, et al. Outcomes for implementation research: conceptual distinctions, measurement challenges, and research agenda. *Adm Policy Ment Health*. 2011;38(2):65–76.

The article proposes a heuristic, working "taxonomy" of eight conceptually distinct implementation outcomes—acceptability, adoption, appropriateness, feasibility, fidelity, implementation cost, penetration, and sustainability—along with their nominal definitions. A two-prong agenda is proposed for research on implementation outcomes. This framework has been widely used for conceptualizing and measuring implementation outcomes to help understand implementation processes, enhance efficiency in implementation research, and evaluate the effectiveness of implementation strategies.

Skivington L, Matthews L, Simpson SA, et al. A new framework for developing and evaluating complex interventions: update of Medical Research Council guidance. *BMJ*. 2021;374:n2061.

The article presents an updated framework for planning and process evaluation of complex interventions focused on three themes: implementation, mechanisms, and context. This guidance from the British Medical Research Counsel argues for a systematic approach to designing and conducting evaluations, drawing on clear descriptions of program theory and identification of key evaluation questions and hypotheses. It includes a nice checklist for guidance.

Websites and Tools

Grid-Enable Measures Database (GEM). https://www.gem-beta.org/Public/MeasureList.aspx?cat=2&viewall=false&scont=35

This site uses a wiki platform to provide a compendium of measures considered for inclusion in a battery of pragmatic measures for use in implementation science and especially primary care settings. A separate section on very brief validated items that can be included in electronic health records is provided. It includes information on length, psychometric characteristics, sensitivity to change and other criteria and the option for users to provide feedback on measure use.

National Cancer Institute, Division of Cancer Control and Population Sciences (DCCPS). Webinars.https://cancercontrol.cancer.gov/is/training-events/webinars

A subsection of the overall NCI implementation science website, this page contains searchable repositories of webinars on implementation science evaluation issues and links to articles, trainings, and current events related to evaluation.

PRECEDE-PROCEED model for health planning and evaluation. http://www.lgreen.net

This is a resource that provides full citation of references that use the PRECEDE-PROCEED model. Many of the references have direct links to Medline or PubMed abstracts.

RE-AIM website. https://www.re-aim.org

The RE-AIM website provides an explanation of and resources for those wanting to apply the RE-AIM framework. It has been recently updated and revised to include more examples, guidance, resources, and recommended slides for use in explaining and applying RE-AIM and its contextual extension of PRISM.

Society for Implementation Research Collaboration (SIRC). https://societyforimplementationresearchcollaboration.org/measures-collection/

The Society for Implementation Research Collaboration (SIRC) has conducted a comprehensive instrument review project using the CFIR constructs and Proctor et al. implementation outcomes, the results of which are presented on this website. This website uses the PAPERS criteria described above to evaluate measures. One must be a SIRC member to access the database.

US Department of Veterans Affairs Quality Enhancement Research Initiative (QUERI). http://www.queri.research.va.gov/

This page summarizes QUERI, whose mission is to improve the health of veterans by supporting the more rapid implementation of effective clinical practices into routine care. It includes their roadmap approach to planning, implementation, and sustainability and a focus on implementation strategies and their evaluation.

REFERENCES

1. Patton MQ. *Utilization-Focused Evaluation*. 5th ed. Sage Publications; 2021.
2. Trochim WM, Rubio DM, Thomas VG, Evaluation Key Function Committee of the CTSA Consortium. Evaluation guidelines for the Clinical and Translational Science Awards (CTSAs). *Clin Transl Sci*. Aug 2013;6(4):303–309.
3. Wholey JS, Hatry HP, Newcomer KE, eds. *Handbook of Practical Program Evaluation*. 4th ed. Jossey-Bass; 2015.
4. Ogrinc G, Davies L, Goodman D, Batalden P, Davidoff F, Stevens D. SQUIRE 2.0 (Standards for QUality Improvement Reporting Excellence): revised publication guidelines from a detailed consensus process. *BMJ Qual Saf*. Dec 2016;25(12):986–992.
5. Curran GM, Bauer M, Mittman B, Pyne JM, Stetler C. Effectiveness-implementation hybrid designs: combining elements of clinical effectiveness and implementation research to enhance public health impact. *Med Care*. Mar 2012;50(3):217–226.
6. Shadish WR, Cook TD, Campbell DT. *Experimental and Quasi-experimental Designs for Generalized Causal Inference*. Houghton Mifflin Company; 2002.
7. Leviton LC, Khan LK, Rog D, Dawkins N, Cotton D. Evaluability assessment to improve public health policies, programs, and practices. *Annu Rev Public Health*. 2010;31:213–233.
8. Proctor E, Silmere H, Raghavan R, et al. Outcomes for implementation research: conceptual distinctions, measurement challenges, and research agenda. *Adm Policy Ment Health*. Mar 2011;38(2):65–76.
9. Gaglio B, Shoup JA, Glasgow RE. The RE-AIM framework: a systematic review of use over time. *Am J Public Health*. Jun 2013;103(6):e38–e46.
10. Kessler RS, Purcell EP, Glasgow RE, Klesges LM, Benkeser RM, Peek CJ. What does it mean to "employ" the RE-AIM model? *Eval Health Prof*. Mar 2013;36(1):44–66.
11. Glasgow RE. What does it mean to be pragmatic? Pragmatic methods, measures, and models to facilitate research translation. *Health Educ Behav*. Jun 2013;40(3):257–265.
12. Pawson R, Tilley N. *Realistic Evaluation*. Sage Publications; 1997.
13. Trevisan MS, Walser TM. *Evaluability Assessment: Improving Evaluation Quality and Use*. Sage Publications; 2015.
14. Calhoun A, Mainor A, Moreland-Russell S, Maier RC, Brossart L, Luke DA. Using the program sustainability assessment tool to assess and plan for sustainability. *Prev Chronic Dis*. Jan 23 2014;11:130185.
15. Rogers EM. *Diffusion of Innovations*. Free Press; 2003.
16. Green LW, Kreuter MW. *Health Program Planning: An Educational and Ecological Approach*. 4th ed. McGraw-Hill; 2005.
17. Glasgow RE, Vogt TM, Boles SM. Evaluating the public health impact of health promotion interventions: the RE-AIM framework. *Am J Public Health*. Sep 1999;89(9):1322–1327.
18. Hovmand PS. *Community-Based System Dynamics*. Springer; 2014.
19. Klesges LM, Estabrooks PA, Dzewaltowski DA, Bull SS, Glasgow RE. Beginning with the application in mind: designing and planning health behavior change interventions to enhance dissemination. *Ann Behav Med*. Apr 2005;29)(suppl):66–75.
20. RE-AIM website. https://www.re-aim.org. January 29, 2022. Accessed March 20, 2022.
21. Shah N, Mathew S, Pereira A, Nakaima A, Sridharan S. The role of evaluation in iterative learning and implementation of quality of care interventions. *Glob Health Action*. Jan 1 2021;14(1):1882182.
22. Institute for Healthcare Improvement. Plan-Do-Study-Act (PDSA) worksheet. December 2012. Accessed January 28, 2022. http://www.ihi.org/resources/Pages/Tools/PlanDoStudyActWorksheet.aspx
23. JaKa MM, Haapala JL, Trapl ES, et al. Reporting of treatment fidelity in behavioural paediatric obesity intervention trials: a systematic review. *Obes Rev*. Dec 2016;17(12):1287–1300.
24. Breitenstein SM, Gross D, Garvey CA, Hill C, Fogg L, Resnick B. Implementation fidelity in community-based interventions. *Res Nurs Health*. Apr 2010;33(2):164–173.
25. Stirman SW, Miller CJ, Toder K, Calloway A. Development of a framework and coding system for modifications and adaptations of evidence-based interventions. *Implement Sci*. Jun 10 2013;8:65.
26. Chambers DA, Norton WE. The adaptome: advancing the science of intervention adaptation. *Am J Prev Med*. Oct 2016;51(4)(suppl 2):S124–S131.
27. Glasgow RE, Emmons KM. How can we increase translation of research into practice? Types of evidence needed. *Annu Rev Public Health*. 2007;28:413–433.
28. Castro FG, Barrera M Jr, Holleran Steiker LK. Issues and challenges in the design of culturally adapted evidence-based interventions. *Annu Rev Clin Psychol*. 2010;6:213–239.

29. Chambers DA, Glasgow RE, Stange KC. The dynamic sustainability framework: addressing the paradox of sustainment amid ongoing change. *Implement Sci.* Oct 2 2013;8:117.
30. Gaglio B, Phillips SM, Heurtin-Roberts S, Sanchez MA, Glasgow RE. How pragmatic is it? Lessons learned using PRECIS and RE-AIM for determining pragmatic characteristics of research. *Implement Sci.* Aug 28 2014;9:96.
31. Bennett GG, Glasgow RE. The delivery of public health interventions via the Internet: actualizing their potential. *Annu Rev Public Health.* 2009;30:273–292.
32. Chalkidou K, Tunis S, Whicher D, Fowler R, Zwarenstein M. The role for pragmatic randomized controlled trials (pRCTs) in comparative effectiveness research. *Clin Trials.* Aug 2012;9(4):436–446.
33. Kairalla JA, Coffey CS, Thomann MA, Shorr RI, Muller KE. Adaptive designs for comparative effectiveness research trials. *Clin Res Regul Aff.* 2015;32(1):36–44.
34. Glasgow RE, Vinson C, Chambers D, Khoury MJ, Kaplan RM, Hunter C. National Institutes of Health approaches to dissemination and implementation science: current and future directions. *Am J Public Health.* Jul 2012;102(7):1274–1281.
35. Loudon K, Treweek S, Sullivan F, Donnan P, Thorpe KE, Zwarenstein M. The PRECIS-2 tool: designing trials that are fit for purpose. *BMJ.* May 8 2015;350:h2147.
36. Thorpe KE, Zwarenstein M, Oxman AD, et al. A pragmatic-explanatory continuum indicator summary (PRECIS): a tool to help trial designers. *J Clin Epidemiol.* May 2009;62(5):464–475.
37. Pinnock H, Sheikh A. Standards for reporting implementation studies (StaRI): enhancing reporting to improve care. *NPJ Prim Care Respir Med.* Jun 26 2017;27(1):42.
38. Moher D, Hopewell S, Schulz KF, et al. CONSORT 2010 explanation and elaboration: updated guidelines for reporting parallel group randomised trials. *Int J Surg.* 2012;10(1):28–55.
39. Green LW, Glasgow RE. Evaluating the relevance, generalization, and applicability of research: issues in external validation and translation methodology. *Eval Health Prof.* Mar 2006;29(1):126–153.
40. Glasgow RE, Riley WT. Pragmatic measures: what they are and why we need them. *Am J Prev Med.* Aug 2013;45(2):237–243.
41. Rabin BA, Purcell EP, Glasgow RE. Harmonizing measures for implementation science using crowd-sourcing. *Clin Med Res.* 2013;11(3):158.
42. Ovretveit J. Understanding the conditions for improvement: research to discover which context influences affect improvement success. *BMJ Qual Saf.* Apr 2011;20)(suppl 1:i18–i23.
43. Damschroder LJ, Aron DC, Keith RE, Kirsh SR, Alexander JA, Lowery JC. Fostering implementation of health services research findings into practice: a consolidated framework for advancing implementation science. *Implement Sci.* Aug 7 2009;4:50.
44. McCreight MS, Rabin BA, Glasgow RE, et al. Using the practical, robust implementation and sustainability model (PRISM) to qualitatively assess multilevel contextual factors to help plan, implement, evaluate, and disseminate health services programs. *Transl Behav Med.* Nov 25 2019;9(6):1002–1011.
45. Damschroder LJ, Reardon CM, Opra Widerquist MA, Lowery J. Conceptualizing outcomes for use with the consolidated framework for implementation research (CFIR): the CFIR outcomes addendum. *Implement Sci.* Jan 22 2022;17(1):7.
46. Wiltsey Stirman S, Kimberly J, Cook N, Calloway A, Castro F, Charns M. The sustainability of new programs and innovations: a review of the empirical literature and recommendations for future research. *Implement Sci.* Mar 14 2012;7:17.
47. Shelton RC, Chambers DA, Glasgow RE. An extension of RE-AIM to enhance sustainability: addressing dynamic context and promoting health equity over time. *Front Public Health.* 2020;8:134.
48. Moullin JC, Dickson KS, Stadnick NA, Rabin B, Aarons GA. Systematic review of the exploration, preparation, implementation, sustainment (EPIS) framework. *Implement Sci.* Jan 5 2019;14(1):1.
49. Goodman MS, Sanders Thompson VL. The science of stakeholder engagement in research: classification, implementation, and evaluation. *Transl Behav Med.* Sep 2017;7(3):486–491.
50. Knoepke CE, Ingle MP, Matlock DD, Brownson RC, Glasgow RE. Dissemination and stakeholder engagement practices among dissemination & implementation scientists: results from an online survey. *PLoS One.* 2019;14(11):e0216971.
51. Domecq JP, Prutsky G, Elraiyah T, et al. Patient engagement in research: a systematic review. *BMC Health Serv Res.* Feb 26 2014;14:89.
52. Brett J, Staniszewska S, Mockford C, et al. Mapping the impact of patient and public involvement on health and social care research: a systematic review. *Health Expect.* Oct 2014;17(5):637–650.
53. Esmail L, Moore E, Rein A. Evaluating patient and stakeholder engagement in research: moving from theory to practice. *J Comp Eff Res.* Mar 2015;4(2):133–145.

54. Brownson RC, Kumanyika SK, Kreuter MW, Haire-Joshu D. Implementation science should give higher priority to health equity. *Implement Sci.* Mar 19 2021;16(1):28.
55. Yousefi Nooraie R, Kwan BM, Cohn E, et al. Advancing health equity through CTSA programs: opportunities for interaction between health equity, dissemination and implementation, and translational science. *J Clin Transl Sci.* Jan 28 2020;4(3):168–175.
56. Sterling MR, Echeverria SE, Commodore-Mensah Y, Breland JY, Nunez-Smith M. Health equity and implementation science in heart, lung, blood, and sleep-related research: emerging themes from the 2018 Saunders-Watkins Leadership Workshop. *Circ Cardiovasc Qual Outcomes.* Oct 2019;12(10):e005586.
57. Woodward EN, Matthieu MM, Uchendu US, Rogal S, Kirchner JE. The health equity implementation framework: proposal and preliminary study of hepatitis C virus treatment. *Implement Sci.* Mar 12 2019;14(1):26.
58. Patton MQ. *Qualitative Research and Evaluation Methods: Integrating Theory and Practice.* 4th ed. Sage Publications; 2015.
59. Webster LA, Ekers D, Chew-Graham CA. Feasibility of training practice nurses to deliver a psychosocial intervention within a collaborative care framework for people with depression and long-term conditions. *BMC Nurs.* 2016;15:71.
60. Huntink E, Wensing M, Timmers IM, van Lieshout J. Process evaluation of a tailored intervention programme of cardiovascular risk management in general practices. *Implement Sci.* Dec 15 2016;11(1):164.
61. Proctor EK, Landsverk J, Aarons G, Chambers D, Glisson C, Mittman B. Implementation research in mental health services: an emerging science with conceptual, methodological, and training challenges. *Adm Policy Ment Health.* Jan 2009;36(1):24–34.
62. Creswell JW, Clark VLP. *Designing and Conducting Mixed Methods Research.* 3rd ed. Sage Publication; 2018.
63. Teddlie C, Tashakkori A. *Foundations of Mixed Methods Research: Integrating Quantitative and Qualitative Approaches in Social and Behavioral Sciences.* 2nd ed. Sage Publications; 2021.
64. Harden SM, Gaglio B, Shoup JA, et al. Fidelity to and comparative results across behavioral interventions evaluated through the RE-AIM framework: a systematic review. *Syst Rev.* Nov 8 2015;4:155.
65. Gold HT, McDermott C, Hoomans T, Wagner TH. Cost data in implementation science: categories and approaches to costing. *Implement Sci.* Jan 28 2022;17(1):11.
66. Neumann PJ, Sanders GD, Russell LB, Siegel JE, Ganiats TG, eds. *Cost-effectiveness in Health and Medicine.* Oxford University Press; 2017.
67. Kessler R, Glasgow RE. A proposal to speed translation of healthcare research into practice: dramatic change is needed. *Am J Prev Med.* Jun 2011;40(6):637–644.
68. Glasgow RE, Harden SM, Gaglio B, et al. RE-AIM planning and evaluation framework: adapting to new science and practice with a 20-year review. *Front Public Health.* 2019;7:64.
69. Glasgow RE. RE-AIMing research for application: ways to improve evidence for family medicine. *J Am Board Fam Med.* Jan–Feb 2006;19(1):11–19.
70. Powell BJ, Beidas RS, Lewis CC, et al. Methods to improve the selection and tailoring of implementation strategies. *J Behav Health Serv Res.* Apr 2017;44(2):177–194.
71. Kirk MA, Moore JE, Wiltsey Stirman S, Birken SA. Towards a comprehensive model for understanding adaptations' impact: the model for adaptation design and impact (MADI). *Implement Sci.* Jul 20 2020;15(1):56.
72. Wiltsey Stirman S, Baumann AA, Miller CJ. The FRAME: an expanded framework for reporting adaptations and modifications to evidence-based interventions. *Implement Sci.* Jun 6 2019;14(1):58.
73. Perez Jolles M, Lengnick-Hall R, Mittman BS. Core functions and forms of complex health interventions: a patient-centered medical home illustration. *J Gen Intern Med.* Jun 2019;34(6):1032–1038.
74. Glasgow RE, Lichtenstein E, Marcus AC. Why don't we see more translation of health promotion research to practice? Rethinking the efficacy-to-effectiveness transition. *Am J Public Health.* Aug 2003;93(8):1261–1267.
75. Moore GF, Audrey S, Barker M, et al. Process evaluation of complex interventions: Medical Research Council guidance. *BMJ.* Mar 19 2015;350:h1258.
76. Craig P, Dieppe P, Macintyre S, et al. Developing and evaluating complex interventions: the new Medical Research Council guidance. *BMJ.* Sep 29 2008;337:a1655.
77. McLeroy KR, Bibeau D, Steckler A, Glanz K. An ecological perspective on health promotion programs. *Health Educ Q.* Winter 1988;15(4):351–377.
78. Purtle J, Brownson RC, Proctor EK. Infusing science into politics and policy: the importance of legislators as an audience in mental health policy dissemination research. *Adm Policy Ment Health.* Mar 2017;44(2):160–163.

79. Bartholomew-Eldredge LK, Markham Cm, Ruiter RAC, Fernandez ME, Kok G, Parcel GS. *Planning Health Promotion Programs: An Intervention Mapping Approach.* Jossey-Bass; 2016.
80. Gielen AC, McDonald EM, Gary TL, Bone LR. Using the PRECEDE-PROCEED model to apply health behavior theories. In: Glanz K, Rimer BK, Viswanath K, eds. *Health Behavior and Health Education: Theory, Research, and Practice.* Jossey-Bass; 2008:407–433.
81. Weir C, McLeskey N, Brunker C, Brooks D, Supiano MA. The role of information technology in translating educational interventions into practice: an analysis using the PRECEDE/PROCEED model. *J Am Med Inform Assoc.* Nov–Dec 2011;18(6):827–834.
82. Tramm R, McCarthy A, Yates P. Using the PRECEDE-PROCEED model of health program planning in breast cancer nursing research. *J Adv Nurs.* Aug 2012;68(8):1870–1880.
83. Pocetta G, Votino A, Biribanti A, Rossi A. Recording non communicable chronic diseases at risk behaviours in general practice. A qualitative study using the PRECEDE-PROCEED model. *Ann Ig.* May–Jun 2015;27(3):554–561.
84. Pawson R. *The Science of Evaluation: A Realist Manifesto.* Sage Publications; 2013.
85. Vinson CA, Stamatakis KA, Kerner JF. Dissemination and implementation research in community and public health settings. In: Brownson RC, Colditz GA, Proctor EK, eds. *Dissemination and Implementation Research in Health: Translating Science to Practice.* Oxford University Press ;2018:chap 21.
86. Feldstein AC, Glasgow RE. A practical, robust implementation and sustainability model (PRISM) for integrating research findings into practice. *Jt Comm J Qual Patient Saf.* Apr 2008;34(4):228–243.
87. Lengnick-Hall R, Gerke DR, Proctor EK, et al. Six practical recommendations for improved implementation outcomes reporting. *Implement Sci.* Feb 8 2022;17(1):16.
88. Campbell M, Fitzpatrick R, Haines A, et al. Framework for design and evaluation of complex interventions to improve health. *BMJ.* Sep 16 2000;321(7262):694–696.
89. Skivington K, Matthews L, Simpson SA, et al. A new framework for developing and evaluating complex interventions: update of Medical Research Council guidance. *BMJ.* Sep 30 2021;374:n2061.
90. Kislov R. Engaging with theory: from theoretically informed to theoretically informative improvement research. *BMJ Qual Saf.* Mar 2019;28(3):177–179.
91. Harvey G, Kitson A. PARIHS revisited: from heuristic to integrated framework for the successful implementation of knowledge into practice. *Implement Sci.* Mar 10 2016;11:33.
92. Atkins L, Francis J, Islam R, et al. A guide to using the theoretical domains framework of behaviour change to investigate implementation problems. *Implement Sci.* Jun 21 2017;12(1):77.
93. Neta G, Glasgow RE, Carpenter CR, et al. A framework for enhancing the value of research for dissemination and implementation. *Am J Public Health.* Jan 2015;105(1):49–57.
94. Rabin BA, Lewis CC, Norton WE, et al. Measurement resources for dissemination and implementation research in health. *Implement Sci.* Mar 22 2016;11:42.
95. Harden SM, McEwan D, Sylvester BD, et al. Understanding for whom, under what conditions, and how group-based physical activity interventions are successful: a realist review. *BMC Public Health.* Sep 24 2015;15:958.
96. Brimhall KC, Fenwick K, Farahnak LR, Hurlburt MS, Roesch SC, Aarons GA. Leadership, organizational climate, and perceived burden of evidence-based practice in mental health services. *Adm Policy Ment Health.* Sep 2016;43(5):629–639.
97. Ritzwoller DP, Sukhanova A, Gaglio B, Glasgow RE. Costing behavioral interventions: a practical guide to enhance translation. *Ann Behav Med.* Apr 2009;37(2):218–227.
98. Saunders RP, Wilcox S, Jake-Schoffman DE, et al. The faith, activity, and nutrition (FAN) dissemination and implementation study, phase 1: implementation monitoring methods and results. *Health Educ Behav.* Jun 2019;46(3):388–397.
99. Wilcox S, Saunders RP, Jake-Schoffman D, Hutto B. The faith, activity, and nutrition (FAN) dissemination and implementation study: 24-month organizational maintenance in a countywide initiative. *Front Public Health.* 2020;8:171.
100. Wilcox S, Saunders RP, Kaczynski AT, et al. Faith, activity, and nutrition randomized dissemination and implementation study: countywide adoption, reach, and effectiveness. *Am J Prev Med.* Jun 2018;54(6):776–785.
101. Khoury MJ, Clauser SB, Freedman AN, et al. Population sciences, translational research, and the opportunities and challenges for genomics to reduce the burden of cancer in the 21st century. *Cancer Epidemiol Biomarkers Prev.* Oct 2011;20(10):2105–2114.
102. Collins FS, Varmus H. A new initiative on precision medicine. *N Engl J Med.* Feb 26 2015;372(9):793–795.

18

Mixed-Methods Evaluation in Dissemination and Implementation Science

LAWRENCE A. PALINKAS, BRITTANY RHOADES COOPER, JESSENIA DE LEON, AND ERIKA SALINAS

INTRODUCTION

Mixed-methods evaluation is a methodology that focuses on collecting, analyzing, and mixing both quantitative and qualitative data in a single study or multiphase study. Its central premise is that the use of quantitative and qualitative approaches in combination provides a better understanding of research problems than either approach alone.[1] The critical feature of mixed methods is the integration of quantitative and qualitative methods; conducting one or more qualitative studies and one or more quantitative studies in the same project without integrating the methods or the results (i.e., engaging in "parallel play") is not mixed methods per se,[2] but is perhaps better described as a multimethod design. In a mixed-method design, each set of methods plays an important role in achieving the overall goals of the project and is enhanced in value and outcome by its ability to offset the weaknesses inherent in the other set and through its "engagement" with the other set of methods. Consequently, mixed methods represent both a model of and a model for transdisciplinary research.[3]

Mixed methods have come to play a critical role in the field of dissemination and implementation (D&I) science. This role has emerged from both necessity and opportunity. Similar to the use of hybrid designs in which evidence-based practice effectiveness and implementation are addressed simultaneously,[4] mixed methods are often used to simultaneously answer confirmatory and exploratory research questions and therefore verify and generate theory in the same study.[2] Some of the theories, frameworks, and models used in implementation science explicitly call for the use of both quantitative and qualitative methods due to the complexity of the subject matter, the importance of understanding both general principles and specific context, and the need to acquire depth as well as breadth of understanding of D&I.[5]

In D&I science, mixed methods are most frequently used to identify barriers and facilitators to successful implementation but may also be used as a tool for developing strategies and conceptual models of implementation and sustainment, monitoring the implementation process, and enhancing the likelihood of successful implementation and sustainment. Qualitative methods are generally used inductively to examine the context and process of implementation with depth of understanding, while quantitative methods are commonly used deductively to examine the content and outcomes of implementation with breadth of understanding.

The aims of this chapter are to (1) provide a brief overview as to the structure, function, and process of mixed methods; (2) describe what quantitative and qualitative methods can and cannot do within the context of D&I science; and (3) provide examples of what mixed methods can accomplish in D&I science.

Lawrence A. Palinkas, Brittany Rhoades Cooper, Jessenia De Leon, and Erika Salinas, *Mixed-Methods Evaluation in Dissemination and Implementation Science* In: *Dissemination and Implementation Research in Health.* Edited by: Ross C. Brownson, Graham A. Colditz, and Enola K. Proctor, Oxford University Press. © Oxford University Press 2023. DOI: 10.1093/oso/9780197660690.003.0018

CHARACTERISTICS OF MIXED-METHODS DESIGNS

Structure

Mixed-method designs in D&I research can be categorized in terms of their structure, function, and process.[6–8] Quantitative and qualitative methods may be used simultaneously or sequentially, with one method viewed as dominant or primary and the other as secondary, although equal weight can be given to both methods.[1] A review of published studies of D&I found that most studies involved the simultaneous use of quantitative and qualitative methods, and most used quantitative methods as the primary or dominant method and qualitative methods as the secondary or subordinate method.[6] However, a little less than half of the studies used balanced designs in which quantitative and qualitative methods were used simultaneously and given equal weight. For instance, Lewis and colleagues[9] conducted mixed-methods analyses following the simultaneous use of quantitative and quantitative (QUAN + QUAL) methods to identify implementation barriers for the purpose of developing a blueprint for tailoring implementation strategies.

Function

In D&I research, mixed methods have been used to achieve one or more of five different functions (Table 18.1). First, qualitative and quantitative methods may be used sequentially or simultaneously to answer the same question; this is known as *convergence*. There are two specific forms of convergence: triangulation and transformation. Triangulation involves the use of one type of data to validate or confirm conclusions reached from analysis of the other type of data. Kerins and colleagues[10] used a triangulation protocol to integrate findings from multiple sources in exploring factors influencing fidelity to a calorie posting policy in Irish acute public hospitals. Data on influencing factors and fidelity were then combined using joint displays for within and cross-case analysis. Hemler and colleagues[11] used a mixed-methods convergent design to explore the

TABLE 18.1 FUNCTIONS OF MIXED-METHOD DESIGNS

Design Type	Purpose
Convergence	• Corroboration of findings (data + interpretation) generated through quantitative methods with findings generated through qualitative designs (triangulation). • Conversion of one type of data into another (quantitizing/qualitizing).
Complementarity	• Findings generated through qualitative methods answer exploratory questions, while findings generated through quantitative methods answer confirmatory questions. • Qualitative methods provide depth of understanding to complement breadth of understanding afforded by quantitative methods. • Qualitative methods used to study process and context and quantitative methods to study outcomes.
Expansion	• Findings from a qualitative study used to expand the depth of understanding of issues addressed in a quantitative study. • Findings from a quantitative study used to expand the breadth of understanding of issues addressed in a qualitative study.
Exploratory/ development	• Findings from a qualitative study used to develop questions or items for a quantitative survey or instrument, develop or modify a conceptual framework used to generate hypotheses for quantitative analyses, or develop an intervention or program that can be evaluated quantitatively.
Sampling	• Use of one set of methods to identify participants who will provide data using the other set of methods (e.g., purposeful sampling of research participants for semistructured interviews based on information collected from a quantitative survey; random sampling of a subpopulation of participants identified from interviews, or participant observation as being of particular interest.

relationship between disruptions in primary care practices and practice participation using data collected from a large-scale, facilitation-based quality improvement initiative in small and medium primary care practices. One team of investigators examined associations between disruptions during interventions and practice participation in facilitation, measured by in-person facilitator hours in 987 practices, which were examined using multivariate regression, while another team analyzed qualitative data on 40 practices that described disruptions. Qualitative and quantitative teams iterated analyses based on the emergent findings discovered by the other team.

Transformation involves the sequential quantification of qualitative data or the use of qualitative techniques to transform quantitative data. For instance, Moniz and colleagues[12] embedded the constructs of the Consolidated Framework for Implementation Research (CFIR)[5] in semistructured interviews in a comparative case study of the implementation of inpatient postpartum contraceptive care at 11 US maternity hospitals. Numerical ratings were then assigned that reflected their valence (positive or negative influence) and their magnitude or strength. Another example of transformation is the technique of concept mapping,[13] where qualitative data elicited from a brainstorming process are "quantitized" using multidimensional scaling and hierarchical cluster analysis. Concept mapping was used by Malone and colleagues[14] to identify stakeholder perceptions of factors that lead to sustained clinical practices. Using concept mapping analyses, items were grouped into meaningful domains to develop a clinical sustainability assessment tool.

Second, quantitative and qualitative methods may be used to answer related questions for the purpose of evaluation or elaboration; this is known as *complementarity.* In evaluative designs, quantitative data are used to evaluate outcomes, while qualitative data are used to evaluate process. In elaborative designs, qualitative methods are used to provide depth of understanding, and quantitative methods are used to provide breadth of understanding. This includes studies that present descriptive quantitative data on subjects and studies that used qualitative data to focus on beliefs and perspectives. Swindle et al.[15] used mixed methods to achieve complementarity in their evaluation of the implementation of an intervention for the early care and education setting to support children's exposure to and intake of fruits and vegetables. Quantitative data were used to assess Reach, Effectiveness, Adoption, Implementation, and Maintenance (RE-AIM) implementation outcomes, while qualitative data from semistructured interviews were used to conduct formative evaluations of implementation process.

Third, one method may be used in sequence to answer questions raised by the other method; this is known as *expansion* or *explanation.* Kaelin and colleagues[16] reported plans to employ a hybrid type 1 effectiveness-implementation study design to evaluate an evidence-based measure and decision support tool as an option for use within routine early intervention care, on service quality and child outcomes (Aim 1). Following trial completion, they will characterize stakeholder perspectives of facilitators and barriers to its implementation across multiple early intervention programs and to explain Aim 1 results (Aim 2).

Fourth, one set of methods may be used to answer questions that will enable use of the other method to answer other questions; this is known as development. In implementation research, there are three distinct forms of development: instrument development, conceptual development, and intervention development or adaptation. Informed by interview themes derived from analysis of semistructured interviews with an anticoagulation nurse or pharmacist staff at five anticoagulation clinics, Barnes and colleagues[17] developed and administered a survey to all anticoagulation clinical staff about their self-reported utilization of less-frequent international normalized ratio (INR) testing and specific barriers to de-implementing the standard (more frequent) INR testing practice. Lengneck-Hall et al.[18] used an iterative qualitative inquiry process to develop and refine a list of dimensions of relational ties, formal arrangements, and processes that connect or "bridge" outer system and inner organizational contexts in implementation frameworks. Mousa and colleagues[19] used a mixed-method approach, which included a qualitative analysis of the barriers and facilitation strategies used by change facilitators during implementation of a health destination pharmacy program and a quantitative analysis of the effectiveness (based on predictive resolution percentage) of the facilitation strategies used, to tailor facilitation strategies to overcome implementation barriers in community pharmacies in Australia.

Finally, there is the sequential use of one method to identify a sample of participants for use of the other method; this is known as *sampling*. In a study designed to achieve mixed-methods functions of both sampling and expansion, Lyon and colleagues will qualitatively explore unexplained residuals (i.e., implementation behavior that is insufficiently accounted for by a mediation model) by conducting semistructured interviews with clinicians with favorable implementation outcomes, but who demonstrate low levels of use of an implementation strategy.[20] Participants will include those whose predicted probability score is greater than 1.0 standard deviation of the mean from their predicted behavior, balanced between implementers and nonimplementers and intervention conditions.

Qualitative comparative analysis (QCA)[21] is another form of mixed method that can be used to examine complex combinations of explanatory factors associated with implementation outcomes when traditional statistical methods are not possible because of the limited number of cases. It can also be used to systematically combine quantitative and qualitative data.[22] As an analytic technique, QCA can be used to achieve several of the functions described above. For example, it can be used to examine convergence of quantitative and qualitative data to answer configural research questions about combinations of conditions that are necessary or sufficient to achieve desired outcomes.[23] Holtrop and colleagues[24] used this approach to determine the combination of program components necessary for successful care management across diverse physician organizations and patient populations. Quantitative survey data collected from staff, patients, and medical records were collected alongside observations of delivery settings and interviews with physician organization leaders, clinicians, and other staff in five physician organizations. Qualitative data on program quality were transformed into quantitative outcomes scores. For the conditions, the research team examined both quantitative survey data and themes discovered through the qualitative analysis to identify program components most likely to influence program success and include in the QCA. The analysis revealed that the combination of having a high-quality care manager on site with provider support was consistently present in successful care management sites.[24]

Qualitative comparative analysis can also be used "as a point of connected integration" in exploratory and explanatory sequential designs.[23] For example, quantitative data can be collected first and analyzed using QCA to provide insights into combinations of implementation conditions leading to program success. These results could then inform the development of interview protocols to collect more in-depth information and answer additional questions that help expand and further contextualize the quantitative results. This approach was used in a mixed-methods study by Cragun et al.[25] that aimed to better understand factors associated with variability in universal tumor screening (UTS) implementation and patient follow-through for Lynch syndrome testing. In explanatory sequential designs, QCA can be used in a similar way—by analyzing quantitative data collected using QCA to uncover profiles or types of cases present in the data. Then, these results can inform the selection of a subsample representing the types of cases uncovered via the QCA to provide more in-depth qualitative data to further understand explanatory factors underlying the types of cases.[23]

Process

The process of integrating quantitative and qualitative data occurs in three forms: merging the data, connecting the data, and embedding the data (Figure 18.1).[1] In D&I research, merging the data occurs when qualitative and quantitative data are brought together in the analysis phase to answer the same question through triangulation or related questions through complementarity.[13] Connecting the data occurs when the analysis of one data set leads to (and thereby connects to) the need for the other data set, such as when quantitative results lead to the subsequent collection and analysis of qualitative data (i.e., expansion) or when qualitative results are used to build to the subsequent collection and analysis of quantitative data (e.g., development). Embedding the data occurs when qualitative or mixed-method studies of treatment or implementation process or context are embedded within larger quantitative studies of treatment or implementation

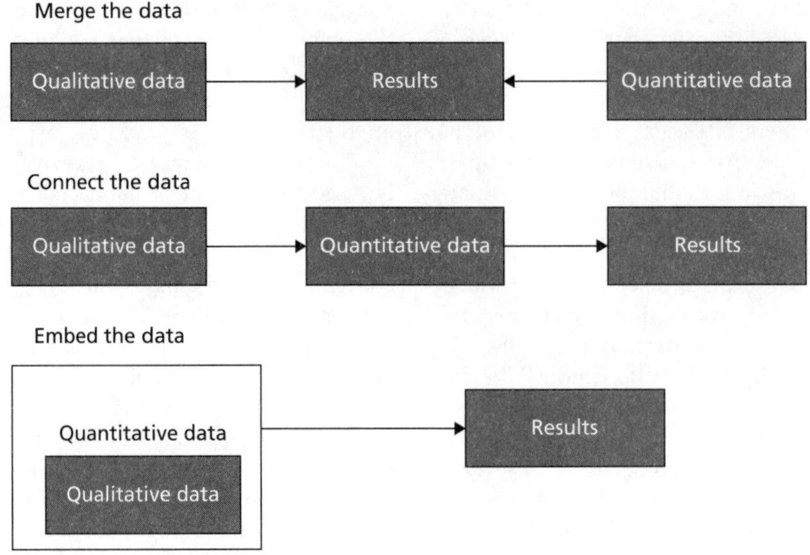

FIGURE 18.1 Three ways of mixing quantitative and qualitative data.

Source: Reprinted with permission from Creswell JW, Klassen AC, Plano Clark VL, Smith KC; for the Office of Behavioral and Social Sciences Research. Best practices for mixed methods research in the health sciences. August 2011. National Institutes of Health.

outcome for the purpose of complementarity, convergence, or expansion. In general, quantitative and qualitative data are merged when the two sets of data are used to provide answers to the same questions, connected when they are used to provide answers to related questions sequentially, and embedded when they are used to provide answers to related questions simultaneously.

Operation

An illustration of how and why quantitative and qualitative methods are mixed can be found in a randomized cluster trial study of routine implementation of shared decision-making in cancer care.[26] In a stepped wedge design, three departments of a comprehensive cancer center sequentially received the implementation program in a randomized order. In this study, quantitative and qualitative data were collected simultaneously, with priority given to the quantitative outcome measures and qualitative data embedded in the randomized controlled trial (RCT) to evaluate implementation process (QUAN + qual) for the purpose of complementarity and explanation. A mixed-methods process evaluation was conducted to evaluate RE-AIM outcomes of reach and implementation fidelity. Data were analyzed using mixed linear models, qualitative content analysis, and descriptive statistics. The process evaluation provided possible explanations for the lack of statistically significant effects in the primary and most of the secondary outcomes.

To understand the implementation-as-usual processes of community-based organizations (CBOs) delivering services to individuals with autism spectrum disorders, Drahota and colleagues[27] utilized a convergent mixed-methods design in which qualitative and quantitative data were collected simultaneously, with priority given to the qualitative methods (quan + QUAL). Twenty agency leaders and 26 direct providers from 21 CBOs completed an implementation survey battery, including demographic and agency process questions relating to implementation as usual. Surveys were analyzed through descriptive and content analyses. A subset of 10 agency leaders provided qualitative interview data that were analyzed using coding, consensus, and comparison methods to allow for a more comprehensive understanding of the implementation process within their organizations. Quantitative analyses and qualitative coding were merged utilizing a joint display and compared to draw convergent and/or divergent conclusions from the quantitative and qualitative results.

WHAT QUANTITATIVE METHODS CAN AND CANNOT DO IN DISSEMINATION AND IMPLEMENTATION SCIENCE

Quantitative methods have specific characteristics that affect the role they play in D&I research. As the name implies, quantitative methods focus on the quantity of the phenomenon being studied, mostly through the analysis of numeric data to determine statistical significance of the associations between constructs or the differences across groups.[28] Given the numerous conceptual models and frameworks proposed to explain the characteristics of and processes by which successful D&I occurs,[5,29] quantitative methods are often used deductively to test assertions and confirm hypotheses based on existing conceptual frameworks and models.

Many of these frameworks and models describe implementation in terms of key stages or processes.[30] One reason to use quantitative methods is to quantify or characterize these stages and processes. For example, McIntosh and colleagues[31] found four distinct patterns of implementation in a large sample of schools implementing a school-wide positive behavioral support framework across 5 years: sustainers (schools likely to meet fidelity criterion all 5 years), slow starters (schools with inconsistent fidelity across the first 3 years, but higher likelihood of meeting fidelity criterion in Years 4 and 5), late abandoners (schools likely to meet fidelity criterion in the first 3 years and unlikely in Years 4 and 5), and rapid abandoners (schools likely to meet fidelity criterion during the first year, followed by rapid decline across the remaining 4 years).

Quantitative methods are also used to test hypotheses related to predictors of successful implementation and to quantify implementation barriers and facilitators.[32–35] Aarons and colleagues[32] used quantitative methods to survey service providers about the factors predictive of continued use of a parenting intervention. The authors used ordinal regression analyses to determine how different types of administration leadership (e.g., transformational, transactional, passive-avoidant) within the inner and outer context of the intervention were associated with the organizations' level of program sustainment (full, partial, or nonsustainment).

The theoretically based assertions about how different aspects of implementation lead to intervention outcomes can also be tested using quantitative methods.[31,36] Berkel et al.[36] used structural equation modeling (SEM) to test a cascade model of implementation in the New Beginnings Program for divorcing families. Program fidelity and quality of program delivery predicted participant responsiveness (i.e., attendance and home practice), and the association between program fidelity and improvements in child and parent outcomes was significantly mediated by parents' home practice of the skills learned in the program.

Another goal of D&I science is to develop and evaluate discrete strategies aimed at effectively moving evidence-based health interventions into routine care settings.[37,38] Quantitative methods, especially within the context of randomized controlled designs, are used to determine the impact implementation strategies have on measurable implementation (e.g., adoption, fidelity, sustainability) and intervention outcomes (e.g., participant health outcomes).[39] For example, Chinman and colleagues[37] conducted a cluster-randomized hybrid type II effectiveness-implementation trial to test the impact of minimal versus facilitated implementation support on the deployment of Veterans Health Administration peer specialists in patient-aligned care teams (PACTs) over 2 years. Twenty-five VA medical centers in three successive cohorts over 6-month blocks were matched and randomized to each study condition. A general linear mixed model was used to compare the two conditions on quantitative measures of peer specialist workload data and veteran measures of activation, satisfaction, and functioning over time (baseline, 6 months, 12 months), with veteran age, race, and gender as covariates and site as a random effect. In a hybrid type III effectiveness-implementation trial using a longitudinal cluster randomized design, Beidas and colleagues[38] will test the comparative effectiveness of two implementation strategies to support clinicians' use of an evidence-based firearm safety practice, *S.A.F.E. Firearm*, in 32 pediatric practices across two health systems. Half of the practices will be randomized to receive a behavioral economic-informed implementation strategy (Nudge); the other half will be randomized to receive the strategy plus 1 year of facilitation to target additional practice and clinician implementation barriers (Nudge+). The primary implementation outcome is parent-reported clinician fidelity to the S.A.F.E. Firearm program.

Another reason quantitative methods are used in D&I science is for summarizing quantitative findings across multiple studies in systematic reviews and meta-analyses.[40,41] These reviews are often used to determine the degree to which specific types of implementation strategies or interventions are effective across studies and settings. For example, Lowther and colleagues[42] conducted a systematic review of 11 studies testing the effectiveness of quality improvement collaboratives (QICs) in improving stroke care. They used vote counting to determine the proportion of studies that found statistically significant positive results of the strategy on implementation or clinical outcomes. Meta-analysis uses more formalized quantitative techniques to summarize quantitative findings across studies. For example, Jones and colleagues[43] identified 86 RCT studies (N = 42,236 participants) assessing implementation strategies to improve utilization of statins in patients with hypercholesterolemia. Standardized mean differences (SMDs) with corresponding 95% confidence intervals (CIs) were estimated for continuous outcomes, and odds ratios (ORs) and 95% CIs were calculated for binary outcomes from included studies. Publication bias was evaluated by Egger's test. Variability between included studies was assessed by heterogeneity tests using the I^2 statistic. Their analysis found the number of implementation strategies used per study positively influenced the efficacy outcomes. Systematic reviews and meta-analyses are also helpful in determining how similar or different results are across studies and synthesizing findings related to specific implementation frameworks and models.[40,44]

As illustrated in the studies described, quantitative methods play an important role in D&I science. However, if used in isolation, they are likely to hinder the field's advancement due to several important limitations. Some of these limitations are driven by the fact that quantitative methods are only as good as the research designs, measures, and statistical analyses available to D&I researchers.[45] Quantitative methods emphasize breadth and generalizability of findings, and therefore they are also limited in their ability to provide depth of understanding for how and why implementation varies across different circumstances and settings. This is especially true when the subgroup of interest is small.[46,47] Few quantitative methods are well suited to examine quantitative phenomena with low variability or in small samples. Fortunately, as discussed in the following section, many of the limitations associated with quantitative methods can be addressed with qualitative methods.

WHAT QUALITATIVE METHODS CAN AND CANNOT DO IN DISSEMINATION AND IMPLEMENTATION SCIENCE

As with quantitative methods, there are certain things that can and cannot be done with qualitative methods in D&I science. One of the most frequently cited reasons for using qualitative methods in implementation research is to understand barriers and facilitators to implementation[48] and sustainment.[49] While the findings of these studies point to several commonly occurring barriers and facilitators, thus increasing the generalizability of these qualitative findings, other studies have highlighted barriers and facilitators that are context or setting specific. For instance, in using data from focus groups and individual semistructured interviews, Fox and colleagues[50] ascertained barriers and facilitators of implementing an evidence-based quality improvement intervention that have been identified in settings with other interventions (e.g., scheduling trainings for busy providers) and barriers and facilitators that were specific to both the setting and the intervention (e.g., audiovisual equipment that sometimes failed, space not being optimal at some sites, and complexities inherent in adapting a training initially developed for individual completion to a group setting).

Another reason for using qualitative methods is to document implementation processes. For instance, in a three-arm hybrid type I RCT evaluating a health coaching intervention and a text messaging intervention, Wong and colleagues[51] used an implementation planning framework, the PRACTical planning for Implementation and Scale-up (PRACTIS), to guide the process evaluation for the trial. Semistructured interviews and focus groups with trial participants, health coaches, and health service stakeholders will explore expectations, factors influencing the delivery of the

Coaching and Exercise for Better Walking (ComeBACK) intervention, and potential scalability within existing health services. In an evaluation of the implementation and effectiveness of the electronic Patient-Reported Outcome (ePRO) mobile app and portal system, Gray and colleagues[52] conducted ethnographic case studies over a 15-month period in six comprehensive primary care practices in Canada to reveal a complex implementation process in which the meaningfulness (or coherence) of the technology to individuals' lives and work acted as a key driver of adoption and tool appraisal.

Related to an understanding of process is the use of qualitative methods to evaluate implementation success by identifying and explaining which aspects of the program are working or not working, for whom, and in what circumstances[53] and to understand how interventions are sustained.[49] As Albright et al. observed: "Qualitative approaches are also useful when seeking to understand why evidence-based practices were successfully or unsuccessfully implemented, or when seeking strategies for facilitating implementation."[8(p202)]

Qualitative methods are used in implementation research to confirm or validate quantitative analyses through the technique of triangulation or convergence. In a pragmatic study comparing a nurse-administered tobacco tactics intervention to usual care, Duffy and colleagues[54] triangulated quantitative data from recruitment logs, chart audits, and surveys administered to study participants, with qualitative data collected from structured interviews to cross-verify the same information from different sources. Use of qualitative methods to confirm or validate quantitative analyses is especially important in implementation research because the unit of analysis is the organization at which implementation occurs, resulting in sample sizes that are often too small to provide adequate statistical power for traditional quantitative analyses.[6–8] In a comparison of barriers and facilitators between pharmacies that implemented a physician-approved protocol for dispensing of naloxone in pharmacies versus pharmacies that did not, Hincapie et al.[55] used a convergent parallel mixed-method design in which qualitative data collected via semistructured interviews were used to confirm findings from quantitative data collected via survey.

Qualitative methods are also well suited for understanding the context in which implementation occurs. For instance, Theis and colleagues[56] conducted qualitative interviews with patients and focus groups with providers in two primary care clinics to inform the implementation of a module that collects and integrates patient-reported social needs information into the electronic health record. Their aim was to understand the contextual factors that impact implementing these interventions in clinical settings.

Qualitative methods can also be used to develop and establish construct validity of quantitative implementation outcome measures. According to Proctor and colleagues: "Qualitative data, reflecting language used by various stakeholders as they think and talk about implementation processes, is important for validating implementation outcome constructs."[39(p71)] Haroz and colleagues[57] used a vignette-based validation process for the validation of implementation measures, free listing, and focus group discussions to better understand local mental health and psychosocial problems and their solutions in adapting an implementation measure for use in Ukraine. Walker and colleagues[58] are conducting a series of qualitative interviews to adapt a measure of implementation readiness for use in Federally Qualified Health Centers and schools.

Qualitative methods have increasingly been used to reduce the duration required to collect and analyze data for implementation research. The length of time and labor-intensive resources required to collect and analyze qualitative data often make their use somewhat problematic in implementation research.[59–60] Palinkas and Zatzick[59] developed the Rapid Assessment Procedure-Informed Clinical Ethnography (RAPICE) to assess the processes of implementation of clinical guidelines for screening and treatment of comorbid conditions of trauma patients in acute care settings. RAPICE used data from multiple sources, including study team intervention documentation, as well as recruitment, regulatory, and other clinical trial logs. The RAPICE approach also embedded participant observation by clinician investigators pragmatic trial implementation coupled with periodic mixed-method consultation.[61] A community ethnography version of RAPICE was used to assess policy and practice implementation of mental health services delivery for children and adolescents during the COVID pandemic.[62]

Rapid methods for analysis of qualitative data have also been developed. One approach summarizes data into a matrix where predefined categories from the data are directly abstracted into an analytic database with supporting quotes.[63] In implementation research, frameworks such as CFIR are commonly used to create such templates.[7,64] Brown-Johnson and colleagues[65] conducted qualitative rapid ethnography at a community-based test clinic to identify implementation themes related to team-based care and specifically the integration of roles purposively designed to enhance coordination for better patient outcomes, including preventive screening and mental health. Rapid analysis involved coding of research memos summarizing observations and semistructured interviews.

The benefits of using such methods were demonstrated in a study conducted by Nevedal and colleagues,[60] which found that a rapid deductive approach to analyzing semistructured interview transcripts guided by the CFIR was less time intensive and eliminated transcription costs compared to the traditional CFIR deductive approach of directed content analysis. In the rapid approach, a primary analyst wrote detailed notes during interviews and immediately "coded" notes into a Microsoft Excel CFIR construct matrix, followed by a secondary analyst who listened to the audio recordings and edited the matrix. Other studies of rapid qualitative analytical techniques have demonstrated similar results as traditional methods but in a shorter time with reduced expense.[64,66]

Qualitative methods have also been used as an implementation strategy to facilitate increased likelihood of implementation success through periodic formative evaluations. Palinkas and Zatzick[59] proposed the use of RAPICE to influence outcomes of hybrid implementation-effectiveness pragmatic clinical trials. Finley and colleagues[67] used a method of guided "periodic reflections" to assess implementation of innovative care models in Veterans Affairs women's health for high-priority health concerns: prediabetes, cardiovascular risk, and mental health. The reflections provided detailed, near-real-time information on projects' dynamic implementation context, including characteristics of implementation settings and changes in the local or national environment, adaptations to the intervention and implementation plan, and implementation team sense-making and learning. Reflections also provide an opportunity for implementation teams to engage in recurring reflection and problem-solving. Glasgow and colleagues[68] conducted qualitative and quantitative assessments of implementation progress using the RE-AIM framework for midcourse adaptations across five health services research projects in the Veterans Health Administration.

In each of these instances, qualitative methods are used to elicit the perspectives of implementation stakeholders, including administrators, providers, and patients/clients[17] as well as researchers. As Proctor and colleagues observed:

> Any effort to implement change in care involves a range of stakeholders, including the treatment developers who design and test the effectiveness of ESTs [empirically supported treatments], policy makers who design and pay for the service, administrators who shape program direction, providers and supervisors, patients/clients/consumers and their family members, and interested community members and advocates. The success of efforts to implement evidence-based treatment may rest on their congruence with the preferences and priorities of those who shape, deliver, and participate in care.[39(p72)]

It is in its ability to elicit the perspectives of the beneficiaries of evidence-based interventions that have been successfully implemented that qualitative methods are especially useful in addressing issues of health equity. For example, Shelton and colleagues[69] concluded that qualitative methods are important tools for enabling the field of implementation science to address health inequities because they can offer a thorough understanding of underlying factors that form health inequities that may be otherwise overlooked when solely relying on quantitative measures by enabling those who have experienced such disparities to exercise their voice in addressing them. Specifically, qualitative data can provide the opportunity to understand how contextual factors, such as structural racism, that perpetuate health inequities can impact a specific population and thus inform researchers how to effectively address inequities.[70] Cabassa and colleagues[71] used qualitative methods (e.g., focus groups) to explore the experiences of Latino patients with serious mental health issues using the Bridges to Better Health and Wellness intervention, a culturally adapted healthcare manager intervention delivered in a public outpatient mental health clinic. Focus groups enabled participants to discuss what they most liked about the intervention; the benefits they perceived to have received; and how they perceived the relationship with their healthcare managers. Oluwoye and colleagues[72] will use intervention mapping (IM),[73] often used in implementation science to iteratively develop interventions and implementation strategies that are rooted in theory and incorporate stakeholder perspectives, to develop, implement, and evaluate a culturally informed FAmily Motivational Engagement Strategy (FAMES) and implementation toolkit for specialty care providers. A mixed-methods approach will be used to comprehensively examine the feasibility, acceptability, and implementation outcomes, as qualitative data themes could be compared to trends found in the quantitative data. Qualitative methods have played and can continue to play an important role in addressing inequities beyond the healthcare field.

While qualitative methods have important roles to play in the scientific endeavor that extends from identification of a phenomenon to active intervention, they are also limited in certain respects. For instance, while qualitative methods are often used to generate hypotheses related to D&I, they are rarely used for hypothesis testing. Some researchers have argued that qualitative data can be used to test hypotheses.[2,74] Deductive approaches to analyzing the content of qualitative data where themes are identified a priori can be viewed as one form of hypothesis testing. Colon-Emeric et al.[49] analyzed interview transcripts using framework analysis[75] of a priori concepts, combined with inductive analyses. Sommerbakk and colleagues[76] used a combination of thematic analysis using an inductive approach and theoretical thematic approach, applying codes to Grol and Wensing's[77] multilevel model of barriers and facilitators. Still other studies have relied on theoretical models to inform use of qualitative methods in mixed-method implementation studies. However, other researchers have noted that qualitative methods are better suited to inductively generating hypotheses than deductively testing them.[78] Still others take a "pragmatic approach," arguing that inductive and deductive techniques can be employed in the same study in an iterative fashion. As Patton observed:

> The extent to which a qualitative study is inductive or deductive varies along a continuum. As evaluation fieldwork begins, an evaluator may be open to whatever emerges from the data, a discovery, or inductive approach. Then, as the inquiry reveals patterns and major dimensions of interest, the evaluator will begin to focus on verifying and elucidating what appears to be emerging—a more deductively oriented approach to data collection and analysis.[79(p253)]

Second, qualitative methods are generally not used to produce generalizable findings due to the lack of samples that are selected at random from a larger population and of insufficient size to provide adequate power for statistical analysis. Occasionally, efforts are made to ensure that the information gained from one sample or study is "transferable" to another sample or setting, which is not the same as claiming that the findings obtained from a sample of a population is "generalizable" to other members of the population not sampled.[78] However, although some forms of purposive sampling are designed to identify a range of variation in participant or organizational characteristics and behavior,[80] such methods are not designed to eliminate known or unknown potential sources of bias that may limit generalizability. Nevertheless, as Padgett asserted, "findings can have generalizability and resonance without being generalizable in a statistical sense based on how the sample was selected."[78(p183)]

As noted at the beginning of this chapter, qualitative methods are intended to provide a depth of understanding to complement the breadth of understanding afforded by quantitative methods. As such, it relies on different standards for determining the sample size necessary for attaining "saturation," the qualitative equivalent of statistical power. Saturation refers to the point at which the data show redundancy and reveal no new information.[78] The number of participants necessary to produce sufficiently valid and reliable results cannot be calculated using standard formulas for statistical analysis. Nevertheless, previous studies relying on this methodology have typically found that saturation may be reached after analyses of data collected from as few as 12 respondents.[81] However, because the criteria for defining saturation are often vague and ill defined,[78] transparency in defending sample size in qualitative studies and situating sample size efficiency within broader and more encompassing assessments of data adequacy is highly recommended.[82]

Third, when quantifying and analyzing qualitative data using statistical methods, caution must be exercised in adhering to the assumption associated with the conduct of such analyses. It must be remembered that despite their numerical form, findings from the analysis of quantitized qualitative data are primarily exploratory and descriptive.

CASE STUDY

Palinkas and colleagues[83] developed a protocol for the development and evaluation of a system measuring sustainment of prevention programs supported by the US Substance Abuse and Mental Health Services Administration (SAMHSA) that target substance abuse or HIV prevention at the state or single-community level, suicide prevention, and prevention of aggressive/disruptive behavior in elementary schools. The mixed-method design was sequential, giving priority to the development of the quantitative measurement system (qual ≥ QUAN) through convergence and development by merging and connecting the data. In the first phase of the study, researchers interviewed 45 representatives of 10 grantees and 9 program offices within four SAMHSA programs (Strategic Prevention Framework—State Initiative Grants, Sober Truth on Preventing Underage Drinking [STOP-Act], Garrett Lee Smith Suicide Prevention Program, and Prevention Practices in Schools) to identify key domains of sustainability indicators (i.e., dependent variables) and requirements or predictors (i.e., independent variables).[84] The conceptualization of "sustainability" was captured using three approaches: semistructured interviews to identify experiences with implementation and sustainability barriers and facilitators; a free list exercise to identify how participants conceptualized sustainability, program elements they wished to sustain, and requirements to sustain such elements; and a checklist of CFIR[5] constructs assessing how important each item was to sustainment. Interviews were analyzed using a grounded theory approach, while free lists and CFIR items were quantitized; the former consisted of rank-ordered weights applied to frequencies of listed items, and the latter used a numeric scale ranging from 0 (not important) to 2 (very important). Four sustainability elements were identified by all three data sets (ongoing coalitions, collaborations, networks, and partnerships; infrastructure and capacity to support sustainability; community need for the program; and ongoing evaluation of performance and outcomes), and 11 elements were identified by two of three data sets (availability of funding, consistency with organizational culture, evidence of positive outcomes, development of a plan for implementation and sustainment, presence of a champion, institutionalization and integration of program, institutional support and commitment, community buy-in and support, program continuity, supportive leadership, and opportunities for staff training).

Based on these findings, a 42-item scale was administered to 186 representatives of 145 programs funded by 7 SAMHSA prevention grant initiatives.[85] Cronbach alphas were used to determine interitem reliability. Convergent validity was assessed by comparisons of a global measure of sustainment with current SAMHSA-funding status and continued operation in the same form. Discriminant validity was assessed by comparisons of sustainability determinants with whether the program had undergone adaptations. Confirmatory factor analysis provided support for a 35-item model fit to the data. Cronbach alpha was .84 for the sustainment outcome construct and ranged from .70 to .93 for the sustainability determinants constructs. All the determinant constructs were significantly associated with sustainment outcome individual and global measures for the entire sample ($p < .01$ to .001) and for community-based programs and programs with a substance abuse focus ($p < .05$ to .001). Convergent validity was supported by significant associations between the global sustainment measure and current SAMHSA-funding status and continued operation in the same form ($p < .001$). Four of the sustainability determinant constructs (responsive to community needs; coalitions, partnerships, and networks; organizational staff capability; and evaluation, feedback, and program outcomes) were also significantly associated with current SAMHSA-funding status ($p < .5$ to .01). Except for organizational staff capability, all sustainability determinants were unrelated to program adaptation as predicted.

The third phase of the study identified configurations of determinants sufficient for producing sustainment of 145 grantees funded by the 7 SAMHSA programs.[86] Sustainment was assessed by the extent to which grantees (1) continued to operate as described in the original application, (2) continued to deliver preventive services to the intended population, (3) continued to deliver evidence-based services, and (4) periodically measured fidelity of services delivered. Fuzzy-set QCA (fsQCA) was conducted to assess configurations of five determinants derived from the CFIR: financial stability; responsiveness to community needs and values; coalitions, partnerships, and networks; organizational capacity and staff capability; and characteristics of the implementation process. Two configurational pathways with high consistency and moderate coverage were identified as sufficient to produce sustainment: (1) community responsiveness and organizational capacity when combined with process and (2) community responsiveness and organizational capacity when combined with coalitions, networks, and partnerships. This study moved beyond identifying individual factors that predict sustainment by using a configurational approach to identify how these factors work in combination. Knowing which pathways are sufficient for sustainment will provide guidance on selection of implementation strategies.

FUTURE DIRECTIONS IN MIXED METHODS

As with any field of inquiry, scientific advancements often dictate or capitalize on advancements in methodology. This principle also applies to the use of mixed methods in D&I science. The Qualitative Research in Implementation Science (QUALRIS) report[7] identified five needs: (1) bring greater transparency to and documentation of team-based analysis; (2) continue to strengthen tools and techniques for conducting rapid qualitative assessment and analysis; (3) explore methods of qualitative data collection and analysis not commonly used in implementation research; (4) contribute to the development of a common language while remaining "true" to a qualitative approach; and (5) develop meaningful approaches for cross-context comparison and synthesis of qualitative data.

One potential focus of innovation in mixed methods lies in the development of a comprehensive understanding of implementation that links process to outcomes and both process and outcomes to context. Understanding the process of D&I is believed to be critical to understanding its outcome,[8] but new causal models linking the two may require broader application of specific mixed methods such as QCA.[87] While qualitative methods are appropriately used to gain an in-depth understanding of the context in which D&I occurs, some generalization of process and outcomes is necessary to achieve a level of understanding that extends beyond merely a collection of unique experiences and circumstances. Further efforts are required to identify the "sweet spot" that exists between the generalizable and the specific characteristics of D&I processes and outcomes.

A second focus of mixed-methods innovation is the identification of new strategies to support implementation of innovative evidence-based programs and practices. For instance, Curtis and colleagues[88] used an exploratory convergent mixed-method approach to examine facilitators and barriers to implementation of a clinical handover tool to increase safety when transferring patients from the emergency department to the inpatient ward. The implementation process model[89] was used to guide data collection and development of implementation strategies. In the first phase, surveys informed by the Theoretical Domains Framework (TDF)[89] were administered to nursing staff to assess the primary factors (i.e., barriers and facilitators) influencing uptake of the handover tool. For each survey item, respondents could also add open-ended comments, and these were analyzed using inductive thematic analysis. The qualitative results showed that most barriers were related to the environment where the tool was being used, the content and usability of the form, and beliefs about the benefits of the tool. Next, the authors mapped the TDF domains identified via the quantitative and qualitative analysis to their corresponding intervention functions and behavior change techniques as suggested by the behavior change wheel.[90] Finally, key stakeholders (nurses, nurse managers, nurse educators) helped evaluate and prioritize the functions and techniques by using the APEASE (affordable, practical, effective, acceptable, had side-effects, and were safe and equitable) criteria.[91] Based on this systematic, stakeholder-informed, and theory-driven process, seven of the nine functions and 18 behavior change techniques were determined to be a good fit for this context. These results were then used as the foundation for developing specific implementation strategy recommendations, which were summarized in an implementation checklist aimed at increasing uptake, quality of implementation, and sustainment of the handover tool.

SUMMARY

In reviewing the rapidly growing literature on the use of mixed methods to address important issues confronting the science of D&I, we conclude with three observations. The first observation is that mixed methods reflect an iterative process of data collection and analysis that involves both inductive and deductive approaches to understanding complex phenomena. As such, researchers may be forced to alter or abandon a priori strategies for data collection and analysis. How these activities actually occur may bear little resemblance to how they were imagined to occur when a grant application was prepared and submitted. This is especially true during the exploratory phases of a multiphase project, where determining the most appropriate means for collecting and analyzing data may lead to some form of methodological trial and error.

Second, this chapter began with the observation that using mixed methods is more than parallel play involving separate quantitative and qualitative studies. One of the implications of the defining characteristic that the methods must somehow be integrated is that the standards for ensuring the rigor and appropriateness of each method when conducted as part of a mixed-method strategy may not be the same as the standards when conducted independently. In a mixed-method design, it is conceivable, if not necessarily desirable, that qualitative data may be analyzed quantitatively despite their failure to adhere to the assumptions of sufficient sample size, normality, and generalizability required for use of statistical tests. Such a practice may run counter to the disciplinary traditions of both quantitative and qualitative methodologists. The point here is that mixed methods represent both naturalistic inquiry and experimentation. The nature of D&I requires innovation in use of both quantitative and qualitative methods, and not every innovation will be successful.

Third, mixed methods can play a significant role in promoting health equity through the application of implementation science. In health, vulnerable groups are more likely to experience health disparities and, in research, may need additional protection from risk.[92] This can be done through research strategies implemented by the researcher. One is to focus on effective recruitment strategies as vulnerable populations may be hard to reach.[93] Additional strategies include the involvement of a diverse research team consisting of members similar to the vulnerable populations, spending time with the vulnerable groups, holding informational sessions to introduce the research, and establishing community partnerships.[94] It is recommended that the researcher engage disadvantaged individuals and communities in the research process from recruitment to data collection, data analysis, and dissemination.[95] Incorporating vulnerable persons in research provides an opportunity for such groups to raise concerns, voice opinions, and ensure they are appropriately represented, thus promoting greater equality between researchers and participants.[96] Overall, researchers must pay careful attention when interpreting data to not lose the voices of vulnerable populations.[97] Therefore, qualitative and mixed methods are important in understanding the nuance, subtlety, and depth of individuals' experiences from an emic perspective.[1,79]

Both the iterative nature of D&I science and the likely debate and compromises involved in selection and application of quantitative and qualitative methods in a mixed-method design demand attention on the part of the investigators to document and detail the rationale for the selection of methods and the process and outcomes of their use. Without such documentation, the strengths and weaknesses of mixed-method designs will be as context specific with limited generalizability and utility as the phenomena of D&I to which these methods are applied.

ACKNOWLEDGMENTS

Support for this chapter was provided by the following grant funded by the National Institute on Mental Health: P50 MH113662-01A1.

SUGGESTED READINGS AND WEBSITES

Readings

Albright K, Gechter K, Kempe A. Importance of mixed methods in pragmatic trials and dissemination and implementation research. *Acad Pediatr.* 2013;13:400–407.

This article discusses a number of dimensions of mixed-methods research, utilizing at least one qualitative method and at least one quantitative method, that may be helpful when designing projects or preparing grant proposals for conducting pragmatic trials and D&I research.

Creswell JW, Klassen AC, Plano Clark VL, Smith KC; for the Office of Behavioral and Social Sciences Research. *Best Practices for Mixed Methods Research in the Health Sciences.* National Institutes of Health; August 2011.

This report provides guidance to National Institutes of Health investigators on how to rigorously develop and evaluate mixed-methods research applications.

Cresswell JW, Plano Clark VL. *Designing and Conducting Mixed Method Research.* 3rd ed. Sage; 2018.

This textbook provides an introduction to mixed-methods research, discusses the steps involved in design and execution, and focuses on three types of core mixed-methods designs.

Palinkas LA, Aarons GA, Horwitz SM, Chamberlain P, Hurlburt M, Landsverk J. Mixed method designs in implementation research. *Adm Policy Ment Health.* 2011;38:44–53.

This article describes seven different structural arrangements of qualitative and quantitative methods, five different functions of mixed methods, and three different ways of linking quantitative and qualitative data in implementation research.

Websites and Tools

Center for Qualitative and Mixed Methods. http://www.rand.org/capabilities/methods-centers/qualitative-and-mixed-methods.html

The RAND Center for Qualitative and Mixed Methods (C-QAMM) develops and promotes tools for generating empirically based insights through iterative, exploratory data collection and analysis.

Journal of Mixed Methods Research. http://journals.sagepub.com/home/mmr

The Journal of Mixed Methods Research *(JMMR) focuses on empirical, methodological, and theoretical articles about mixed-methods research across the social, behavioral, health, and human sciences.*

Mixed Methods Research Training Program for the Health Sciences. http://www.jhsph.edu/academics/training-programs/mixed-methods-training-program-for-the-health-sciences/

This program nationally recruits 14 investigators (called scholars) in each cohort representing diverse interests in the health sciences and including individuals representing underrepresented minorities. Scholars participate in a 3-day training program supplemented with other activities.

Online Certificate Program in Mixed Methods Research. https://ssw.umich.edu/offices/continuing-education/certificate-courses/mixed-methods-research

The Certificate Program in Mixed Methods Research is designed for researchers and practitioners who are interested in ways to integrate qualitative and quantitative research methods and data, commonly used qualitative and quantitative data collection methods and procedures, popular data analysis techniques used in the applied professions, and effective approaches to research conducted in practice settings

REFERENCES

1. Cresswell JW, Plano Clark VL. *Designing and Conducting Mixed Method Research.* 3rd ed. Sage; 2018.
2. Teddlie C, Tashakkori A. Major issues and controversies in the use of mixed methods in the social and behavioral sciences. In: Tashakkori A, Teddlie C, eds. *Handbook of Mixed Methods in the Social and Behavioral Sciences.* Sage; 2003:3–50.
3. Palinkas LA, Soydan H. *Translation and Implementation of Evidence Based Practice.* Oxford University Press; 2012.
4. Curran GM, Bauer M, Mittman B, Pyne JM, Stetler C. Effectiveness-implementation hybrid designs: combining elements of clinical effectiveness and implementation research to enhance public health impact. *Med Care.* 2012;50(3):217–226.
5. Damschroeder LJ, Aron DC, Keith RE, Kirsh SR, Alexander JA, Lowery JC. Fostering implementation of health services research findings into practice: a consolidated framework for advancing implementation science. *Implement Sci.* 2009;4:50.
6. Palinkas LA, Aarons GA, Horwitz SM, Chamberlain P, Hurlburt, M., Landsverk J. Mixed method designs in implementation research. *Adm Policy Ment Health.* 2011;38:44–53.

7. US Department of Health and Human Services National Cancer Institute. *National Cancer Institute. Qualitative Research in Implementation Science (QualRIS)*. 2020. Accessed January 20, 2022. https://cancercontrol.cancer.gov/IS/docs/NCI-DCCPS-ImplementationScience-WhitePaper.pdf
8. Albright K, Gechter K, Kempe A. Importance of mixed methods in pragmatic trials and dissemination and implementation research. *Acad Pediatr.* 2013;13:400–407.
9. Lewis CC, Scott K, Marriott BR. A methodology for generating a tailored implementation blueprint: an exemplar from a youth residential setting. *Implement Sci.* 2018;13:68.
10. Kerins C, Kelly C, Reardon CM, et al. Factors influencing fidelity to a calorie posting policy in public hospitals: a mixed methods study. *Front Public Health.* 2021;9:707668. doi:10.3389/fpubh.2021.707668
11. Hemler JR, Edwards ST, Valenzuela S, et al. The effect of major disruptions on practice participation in facilitation during a primary care quality improvement initiative. *J Am Board Fam Med.* 2022 Jan–Feb;35(1):124–139. doi:10.3122/jabfm.2022.01.210205
12. Moniz MH, Bonawitz K, Wetmore MK, et al. Implementing immediate postpartum contraception: a comparative case study at 11 hospitals. *Implement Sci Commun.* 2021;2:42.
13. Trochim WM. An introduction to concept mapping for planning and evaluation. *Eval Prog Plan.* 1989;12:1–16.
14. Malone S, Prewitt K, Hackett R, et al. The Clinical Sustainability Assessment Tool: measuring organizational capacity to promote sustainability in healthcare. *Implement Sci Commun.* 2021;2(1):77.
15. Swindle T, McBride NM, Selig JP, et al. Stakeholder selected strategies for obesity prevention in childcare: results from a small-scale cluster randomized hybrid type III trial. *Implement Sci.* 2021;16:48.
16. Kaelin V, Villegas V, Chen YF, High Value Early Intervention Research Group. Effectiveness and scalability of an electronic patient-reported outcome measure and decision support tool for family-centred and participation-focused early intervention: PROSPECT hybrid type 1 trial protocol. *BMJ Open.* 2022;12(1):e051582. doi:10.1136/bmjopen-2021-051582
17. Barnes GD, Misirliyan S, Kaatz S, et al. Barriers and facilitators to reducing frequent laboratory testing for patients who are stable on warfarin: a mixed methods study of de-implementation in five anticoagulation clinics. *Implement Sci.* 2017;12:87.
18. Lengnick-Hall R, Stadnick NA, Dickson KS, Moullin JC, Aarons GA. Forms and functions of bridging factors: specifying the dynamic links between the outer and inner contexts during implementation and sustainment. *Implement Sci.* 2021;16:34.
19. Moussa L, Benrimoj S, Musial K, Kocbek S, Garcia-Cardenas V. Data-driven approach for tailoring facilitation strategies to overcome implementation barriers in community pharmacy. *Implement Sci.* 2021;16:73.
20. Lyon AR, Pullmann MD, Dorsey S, et al. Protocol for a hybrid type 2 cluster randomized trial of trauma-focused cognitive behavioral therapy and a pragmatic individual-level implementation strategy. *Implement Sci.* 2021;16:3.
21. Ragin CC. *Redesigning Social Inquiry: Fuzzy Sets and Beyond.* University of Chicago Press; 2009.
22. Kane H, Lewis MA, Williams PA, Kahwati LC. Using qualitative comparative analysis to understand and quantify translation and implementation. *Transl Behav Med.* 2014;4:201–208.
23. Kahwati LC, Kane HL. *Qualitative Comparative Analysis in Mixed Methods Research and Evaluation.* Vol. 6. SAGE Publications; 2020.
24. Holtrop JS, Potworowski G, Green LA, Fetters M. Analysis of novel care management programs in primary care: an example of mixed methods in health services research. *J Mixed Methods Res.* 2019;13(1):85–112. doi:10.1177/1558689816668689
25. Cragun, D, Pal T, Vadaparmpil ST, Baldwin J, Hampel H, DeBate RD. Qualitative comparative analysis: a hybrid method for identifying factors associated with program effectiveness. *J Mixed Methods Res.* 2016;10(3):251–272.
26. Scholl I, Hahlweg P, Lindig A, et al. Evaluation of a program for routine implementation of shared decision-making in cancer care: results of a stepped wedge cluster randomized trial. *Implement Sci.* 2021;16(1):106. doi:10.1186/s13012-021-01174-4
27. Drahota A, Meza RD, Bustos TE, et al. Implementation-as-usual in community-based organizations providing specialized services to individuals with autism spectrum disorder: a mixed methods study. *Adm Policy Ment Health.* 2021;48(3):482–498. doi:10.1007/s10488-020-01084-5
28. Creswell JW, Klassen AC, Plano Clark VL, Smith KC; for the Office of Behavioral and Social Sciences Research. Best practices for mixed methods research in the health sciences. National Institutes of Health; August 2011. https://obssr.od.nih.gov/sites/obssr/files/Best_Practices_for_Mixed_Methods_Research.pdf

29. Tabak RG, Khoong EC, Chambers D, Brownson RC. Bridging research and practice: models for dissemination and implementation research. *Am J Prev Med*. 2012;43(3):337–350.
30. Aarons GA, Hurlburt M, Horwitz SM. Advancing a conceptual model of evidence-based practice implementation in public service sectors. *Adm Policy Ment Health*. 2011;38(1):4–23.
31. Mcintosh K, Mercer SH, Nese RNT, Ghemraoui A. Identifying and predicting distinct patterns of implementation in a school-wide behavior support framework speed and patterns of implementation. *Prev Sci*. 2016;17(8):992–1001.
32. Aarons GA, Green AE, Trott E, et al. The roles of system and organizational leadership in system-wide evidence-based intervention sustainment: a mixed-method study. *Adm Policy Ment Health*. 2016;43(6):991–1008.
33. Welsh JA, Chilenski SM, Johnson L, Greenberg MT, Spoth RL. Pathways to sustainability: 8-Year follow-up from the PROSPER project. *J Prim Prev*. 2016;37(3):263–286.
34. Green AE, Trott E, Willging CE, Finn NK, Ehrhart MG, Aarons GA. The role of collaborations in sustaining an evidence-based intervention to reduce child neglect. *Child Abuse Negl*. 2016;53:4–16.
35. Kostick KM, Trejo M, Bhimaraj A, et al. A principal components analysis of factors associated with successful implementation of a LVAD decision support tool. *BMC Med Inform Decis Mak*. 2021;21(1):106. doi:10.1186/s12911-021-01468-z
36. Berkel C, Mauricio AM, Sandler IN, Wolchik SA, Gallo CG, Brown CH. The cascading effects of multiple dimensions of implementation on program outcomes: a test of a theoretical model. *Prev Sci*. 2018;19(6):782–794.
37. Chinman M, Goldberg R, Daniels K, et al. Implementation of peer specialist services in VA primary care: a cluster randomized trial on the impact of external facilitation. *Implement Sci*. 2021;16:60.
38. Beidas RS, Ahmedani BK, Linn, KA, et al. Study protocol for a type III hybrid effectiveness-implementation trial of strategies to implement firearm safety promotion as a universal suicide prevention strategy in pediatric primary care. *Implement Sci*. 2021;16:89.
39. Proctor E, Silmere H, Raghavan R, et al. Outcomes for implementation research: conceptual distinctions, measurement challenges, and research agenda. *Adm Policy Ment Health*. 2011;38(2):65–76.
40. Kirk MA, Kelley C, Yankey N, Birken SA, Abadie B, Damschroder L. A systematic review of the use of the Consolidated Framework for Implementation Research. *Implement Sci*. 2016;11(1):72.
41. Tang MY, Rhodes S, Powell R, et al. How effective are social norms interventions in changing the clinical behaviours of healthcare workers? A systematic review and meta-analysis. *Implement Sci*. 2021;16:8.
42. Lowther HJ, Harrison J, Hill JE, et al. The effectiveness of quality improvement collaboratives in improving stroke care and the facilitators and barriers to their implementation: a systematic review. *Implement Sci*. 2021;16:95.
43. Jones LK, Tilberry S, Gregor C, et al. Implementation strategies to improve statin utilization in individuals with hypercholesterolemia: a systematic review and meta-analysis. *Implement Sci*. 2021;16:40.
44. Moullin JC, Dickson KC, Stadnick NA, Rabin B, Aarons GA. Systematic review of the exploration, preparation, implementation and sustainment (EPIS) framework. *Implement Sci*. 2019;14:1.
45. Brown CH, Curran G, Palinkas LA, et al. An overview of research and evaluation for dissemination and implementation. *Annu Rev Public Health*. 2017;38(March):1–48.
46. Brownson RC, Allen P, Jacob RR, et al. Understanding mis-implementation in public health practice. *Am J Prev Med*. 2015;48(5):543–551.
47. Shapiro CJ, Prinz RJ, Sanders MR. Sustaining use of an evidence-based parenting intervention: practitioner perspectives. *J Child Fam Stud*. 2015;24:1615–1624.
48. Kozica SL, Lombard CB, Harrison CL, Teede HJ. Evaluation of a large healthy lifestyle program: informing program implementation and scale-up in the prevention of obesity. *Implement Sci*. 2016;11:151.
49. Colon-Emeric C, Toles M, Cary Jr. MP, et al. Sustaining complex interventions in long-term care: a qualitative study of direct care staff and managers. *Implement Sci*. 2016;11:94.
50. Fox AB, Hamilton AB, Frayne SN, et al. Effectiveness of an evidence-based quality improvement approach to cultural competence training: the Veterans Affairs "Caring for Women Veterans" program. *J Contin Educ Health Prof*. 2016;36:96–103.
51. Wong S, Hassett L, Koorts H, et al. Planning implementation and scale-up of physical activity interventions for people with walking difficulties: study protocol for the process evaluation of the ComeBACK trial. *Trials*. 2022;23(1):40. doi:10.1186/s13063-021-059960-3
52. Gray CS, Chau E, Tahsin F, et al. Assessing the implementation and effectiveness of the

Electronic Patient-Reported Outcome Tool for older adults with complex care needs: mixed methods study. *J Med Internet Res.* 2021; 23(12):e29071v.

53. McHugh S, Tracey ML, Riordan F, O'Neill K, Mays N, Kearney PM. Evaluating the implementation of a national clinical programme for diabetes to standardize and improve services: a realist evaluation protocol. *Implement Sci.* 2016;11:7.
54. Duffy SA, Ronis DL, Ewing LA, et al. Implementation of the Tobacco Tactics intervention versus usual care in Trinity Health community hospitals. *Implement Sci.* 2016;11:147.
55. Hincapie AL, Hegener M, Heaton PC, et al. Challenges and facilitators of implementing a physician-approved naloxone protocol: a mixed-methods study. *J Addict Med.* 2021;15(1):40–48. doi:10.1097/ADM.0000000000000672
56. Theis RP, Blackburn K, Lipori G, et al. Implementation context for addressing social needs in a learning health system: a qualitative study. *J Clin Trans Sci.* 2021;5:e201. doi:10.1017/cts2021.842
57. Haroz EE, Bolton P, Nguyen AJ, et al. Measuring implementation in global mental health: validation of a pragmatic implementation science measure in eastern Ukraine using an experimental vignette design. *BMC Health Serv Res.* 2019;19(1):262. doi:10.1186/s12913-019-4097-y
58. Walker TJ, Brandt HM, Wandersman A, et al. Development of a comprehensive measure of organizational readiness (motivation × capacity) for implementation: a study protocol. *Implement Sci Commun.* 2020;1:103. doi:10.1186/s43058-020-00088-4
59. Palinkas LA, Zatzick D. Rapid Assessment Procedure Informed Clinical Ethnography (RAPICE) in pragmatic clinical trials of mental health services implementation: methods and applied case study. *Adm Policy Ment Health.* 2019 Mar;46(2):255–270.
60. Nevedal AL, Reardon CM, Opra Widerquist MA, et al. Rapid versus traditional qualitative analysis using the Consolidated Framework for Implementation Research (CFIR). *Implement Sci.* 2021 Jul 2;16(1):67. doi:10.1186/s13012-021-01111-5
61. Zatzick D, Jurkovich G, Heagerty P, et al. Stepped collaborative care targeting posttraumatic stress disorder symptoms and comorbidity for US trauma care systems: a pragmatic randomized clinical trial. *JAMA Surg.* 2021;156(5):462–470.
62. Palinkas LA, De Leon J, Salinas E, et al. Impact of the COVID-19 pandemic on child and adolescent mental health policy and practice implementation. *Int J Environ Res Public Health.* 2021;21:9622. doi:10.3390/ ijerph18189622
63. McCarthy MS, Ujano-De Motta LL, Nunnery MA, et al. Understanding adaptations in the Veteran Health Administration's Transition Nurse Program: refining methodology and pragmatic implications for scale up. *Implement Sci.* 2021;16:71.
64. Gale RC, Wu J, Erhardt T, et al. Comparison of rapid vs in-depth qualitative analytic methods from a process evaluation of academic detailing in the Veterans Health Administration. *Implement Sci.* 2019;14(1):11. doi:10.1186/13012-019-0853-y
65. Brown-Johnson C, Shaw JG, Safaeinili N, et al. Role definition is key—rapid qualitative ethnography findings from a team-based primary care transformation. *Learn Health Syst.* 2019;3(3):e10188.
66. Holdsworth LM, Safaeinili N, Winget M, et al. Adapting rapid assessment procedures for implementation research using a team-based approach to analysis: a case example of patient quality and safety interventions in the ICU. *Implement Sci.* 2020;15(1):1–12.
67. Finley EP, Huynh AK, Farmer MM, et al. Periodic reflections: a method of guided discussions for documenting intervention phenomena: *BMC Med Res Methodol.* 2018;18(1):153. doi:10.1186/s12874-018-0610-y
68. Glasgow RE, Battaglia C, McCreight M, Ayele RA, Rabin BA. Making implementation science more rapid: use of the RE-AIM framework for mid-course adaptations across five health services research projects in the Veterans Health Administration. *Front Public Health.* 2020 May 27;8:194. doi:10.3389/fpubh.2020.00194
69. Shelton RC, Philbin MM, Ramanadhan S. Qualitative research methods in chronic disease: introduction and opportunities to promote health equity. *Annu Rev Public Health.* 2022;43:37–57. doi:10.1146/annurev-publhealth-012420-105104
70. Shelton RC, Adsul P, Oh A. Recommendations for addressing structural racism in implementation science: a call to the field. *Ethn Dis.* 2021;31(suppl 1):357–364. doi:10.18865/ed.31.S1.357
71. Cabassa LJ, Manrique Y, Meyreles Q, et al. "Treated me . . . like I was family": qualitative evaluation of a culturally-adapted health care manager intervention for Latinos with serious mental illness and at risk for cardiovascular disease. *Transcult Psychiatry.* 2019;56(6):1218–1236. doi:10.1177/1363461518808616
72. Oluwoye O, Dyck D, McPherson SM, et al. Developing and implementing a culturally informed FAmily Motivational Engagement Strategy (FAMES) to increase family engagement in first episode psychosis programs: mixed methods pilot

study protocol. *BMJ Open.* 2020;10(8):e036907. doi:10.1136/bmjopen-2020-036907

73. Bartholomew LK, Parcel GS, Kok G. Intervention mapping: a process for developing theory and evidence-based health education programs. *Health Educ Behav.* 1998;25:545–63. doi:10.1177/109019819802500502
74. Miles MB, Huberman AM. *Qualitative Data Analysis: An Expanded Sourcebook.* 2nd ed. Sage; 1994.
75. Gale NK, Heath G, Cameron E, Rashid S, Redwood S. Using the framework method for the analysis of qualitative data in multi-disciplinary health research. *BMC Med Res Methodol.* 2013;13:117.
76. Sommerbakk R, Haugen DF, Tjora A, Kaasa S, Hjermstad MJ. Barriers to and facilitators for implementing quality improvements in palliative care—results for a qualitative interview study in Norway. *BMC Palliat Care.* 2016;15:61. doi:10.1186/s12904-016-0132-5
77. Grol R, Wensing M. What drives change? Barriers to and incentives for achieving evidence-based practice. *Med J Aust.* 2004;180(6)(suppl):S57–S60.
78. Padgett DK. *Qualitative Methods in Social Work Research.* 3rd ed. Sage; 2017.
79. Patton MQ. *Qualitative Research and Evaluation Methods.* 4th ed. Sage; 2015.
80. Palinkas LA, Horwitz SM, Green CA, Wisdom JP, Duan N, Hoagwood KE. Purposeful sampling for qualitative data collection and analysis in mixed method implementation research. *Adm Policy Ment Health.* 2015;42:533–544.
81. Guest G, Bunce A, Johnson L. How many interviews are enough? An experiment with data saturation and variability. *Field Meth.* 2006;18(1):59–82.
82. Vasileiou K, Barrett J, Thorpe S, Young T. Characterising and justifying sample size sufficiency in interview-based studies: systematic analysis of qualitative health research over a 15-year period. *Implement Sci.* 2018;18:148. doi:10.1186/s12874-018-0594-7
83. Palinkas LA, Spear SE, Mendon SJ, et al. Measuring sustainment of prevention programs and initiatives: a study protocol. *Implement Sci.* 2016;11:95. doi:10.1186/s13012-016-0467-6
84. Palinkas LA, Spear SW, Mendon SJ, et al. Conceptualizing and measuring sustainability of prevention programs, policies and practices. *Translat Behav Med*; 2020;10:136–145. pii:ibz170. doi:10.1093/tbm/ibz170. PMID:31764968
85. Palinkas LA, Chou CP, Spear SE, Mendon SJ, Villamar J, Brown CH. Measurement of sustainment of prevention programs and initiatives: the Sustainment Measurement System Scale. *Implement Sci.* 2020;15:71. doi:10.1186/s13012-020-01030-x
86. Mendon-Plasek S, Palinkas LA, Hurlburt M, Villamar J, Brown CH. Sufficient pathways for maintaining prevention programs long-term: a configurational approach using fuzzy-set qualitative comparative analysis. *Implement Sci.* 2021;16(suppl 1):S86.
87. Hill LG, Cooper BR, Parker LA. Qualitative comparative analysis: a mixed-method tool for complex implementation questions. *J Prim Prev.* 2019 Feb;40(1):69–87.
88. Curtis K, Elphick TL, Eyles M, et al. Identifying facilitators and barriers to develop implementation strategy for an ED to ward handover tool using behaviour change theory (EDWHAT). *Implement Sci Commun.* 2020;1:71. doi:10.1186/s43058-020-00045-1
89. French S, Green S, O'Connor D, et al. Developing theory-informed behaviour change interventions to implement evidence into practice: a systematic approach using the theoretical domains framework. *Implement Sci.* 2012;7(38):16.
90. Michie S, van Stralen M, West R. The behaviour change wheel: a new method for characterising and designing behaviour change interventions. *Implement Sci.* 2011;6:42.
91. Michie S, Atkins L, West R. *The Behaviour Change Wheel—A Guide to Designing Interventions.* Silverback Publishing; 2014.
92. Mollard E, Hatton-Bowers H, Tippens J. Finding strength in vulnerability: ethical approaches when conducting research with vulnerable populations. *J Midwifery Womens Health.* 2020;65(6):802–807. doi:10.1111/jmwh.13151
93. Ellard-Gray A, Jeffrey NK, Choubak M, Crann SE. Finding the hidden participant: solutions for recruiting hidden, hard-to-reach, and vulnerable populations. *Int J Qual Methods.* 2015;14(5):1–10. doi:10.1177/1609406915621420
94. Webber-Ritchey KJ, Simonovich SD, Spurlark RS. COVID-19: qualitative research with vulnerable populations. *Nurs Sci Q.* 2021;34(1):13–19. doi:10.1177/0894318420965225
95. von Benzon N, van Blerk L. Research relationships and responsibilities: "doing" research with "vulnerable" participants: introduction to the special edition. *Soc Cult Geogr.* 2017;18(7):895–905. doi:10.1080/14649365.2017.1346199
96. Cook K. *Marginalized Populations. The SAGE Encyclopedia of Qualitative Research Methods.* SAGE Publications; 2008.
97. Ravindran V. Data analysis in qualitative research. *Ind J Contin Nurs Educ.* 2019;20(1):40–45. doi:10.4103/IJCN.IJCN_1_19

SECTION 5

Setting- and Population-Specific Dissemination and Implementation

19

Dissemination and Implementation Research in Community and Public Health Settings

STEPHANIE MAZZUCCA-RAGAN, ERIC M. WIEDENMAN, AND CYNTHIA A. VINSON

INTRODUCTION

Community and public health settings are uniquely structured and well poised to support the implementation of evidence-based programs and policies (EBPPs) to support population-wide health, including the prevention and treatment of infectious diseases, chronic diseases, mental illness, substance use, and physical injuries. Public health-focused EBPPs may take the form of programs and policies that intervene broadly at national levels or that address specific regional, local, or organizational issues. For example, the implementation of sugar-sweetened beverage taxes and zoning laws to increase access to physical activity opportunities have contributed to the progress against the obesity epidemic.[1–4] Dissemination and implementation (D&I) research conducted in these settings can support the delivery of programs and policies by characterizing the key contextual factors operating in these settings and identifying effective strategies for the adoption, implementation, scale-up, and sustainability of EBPPs. Also, the field of D&I has developed and adapted theoretical models focused on health equity that can ensure that research is focused on relevant contextual factors and strategies that have the greatest potential to impact health equity outcomes. Thereby, D&I research can close the gap between scientific evidence and the use of EBPPs by the organizations and policymakers responsible for promoting health and improving health equity and in the long term contribute to widespread improvements in population health.

As is demonstrated in this book, D&I research is conducted across multiple settings, spanning clinical and nonclinical settings. Nonclinical settings relevant for public health include those described in this chapter as well as in detail in other chapters of this book: social services (chapter 20), schools (chapter 22), workplaces (chapter 23), and policymaking settings (chapter 24). D&I research conducted outside of clinical settings is an important complement to that done in clinical settings, which have a primary mission for the delivery of health services and are discussed in chapter 21. Previous reviews have highlighted that D&I research outside health settings is relatively underdeveloped compared with implementation research in clinical healthcare and public health settings.[5,6] Figure 19.1 depicts the many opportunities to support health outside of clinical settings. In this chapter, we focus on governmental public health agencies; municipal institutions (e.g., city planning, transportation); and other community-based organizations, such as faith-based organizations (FBOs) and recreational organizations. These settings are very diverse in their missions, services delivered, and organizational structures, but they represent settings of daily life for most individuals and can have a strong influence on individuals' and their surrounding community's behaviors.[7] These settings also serve as crucial entrance points for D&I research to address health equity through meaningful engagement and partnership with community stakeholders and emphasizing their needs, culture, and history.[8] Table 19.1 highlights the strengths, opportunities, and challenges for D&I research in community and public health settings.

Stephanie Mazzucca-Ragan, Eric M. Wiedenman, and Cynthia A. Vinson, *Dissemination and Implementation Research in Community and Public Health Settings* In: *Dissemination and Implementation Research in Health.* Edited by: Ross C. Brownson, Graham A. Colditz, and Enola K. Proctor, Oxford University Press. © Oxford University Press 2023. DOI: 10.1093/oso/9780197660690.003.0019

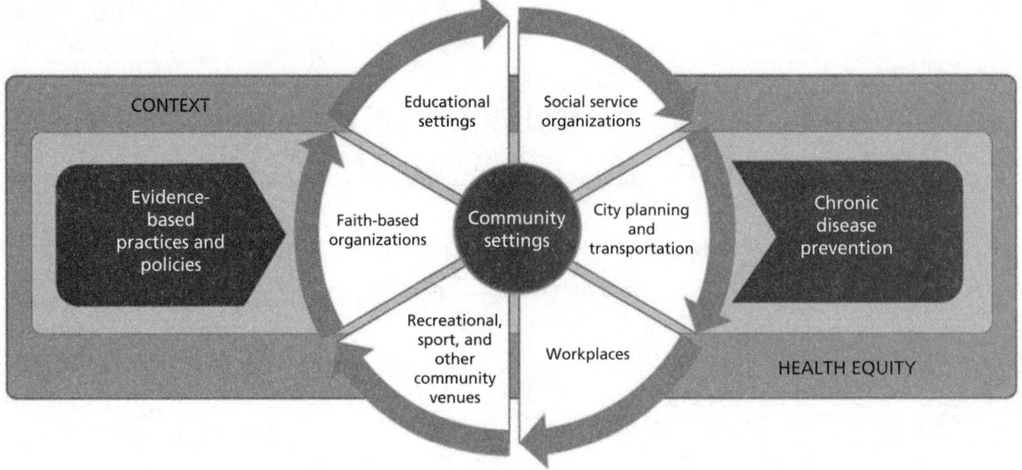

FIGURE 19.1 Dissemination and implementation research in community settings.

Source: Reprinted with permission from: Mazzucca S, Arredondo EM, Hoelscher DM, et al. Expanding Implementation Research to Prevent Chronic Diseases in Community Settings. *Annu Rev Public Health*. Apr 1 2021;42:135–158d.

TABLE 19.1 SUMMARY OF STRENGTHS, OPPORTUNITIES, AND CHALLENGES TO DISSEMINATION AND IMPLEMENTATION RESEARCH IN COMMUNITY SETTINGS

Strengths and Opportunities	Challenges
• Individuals across the life span spend much of their time in community settings[6,7,9] • Potential to reach historically marginalized communities served by these organizations[10,11] • Organizations and staff are viewed as trustworthy,[10,12] which can lend credibility to implementation efforts • Alignment of health promotion with principles or other outcomes of focus (e.g., social cohesion, community development, religious texts)[13] • Availability of existing physical space, infrastructure resources (e.g., rooms, kitchens), and communication outlets to support dissemination and implementation[14–17] • System of volunteers who can implement programs and provide social support[18] • Staff and volunteers in these organizations are knowledgeable of the needs of the populations they serve, which is crucial to understanding the local context for implementation • Social networks can enhance EBPP uptake (e.g., peer influence)	• Willingness of organizations to implement EBPPs may be limited because their primary focus is not on health • Wide variation in capacity, and resources needed to implement EBPPs[12,13] • Many are volunteer-run organizations that may have limited capacity to implement EBPPs • Forming new relationships with stakeholders who are different from the research team may be difficult and time consuming[19] • Knowledge of the social and environmental context is needed to improve fit of implementation strategies and EBPPs but may be difficult to obtain[12,20,21] • Staff issues related to turnover, motivation, and commitment • Typical research funding structures may restrict flexibility in implementation approaches (e.g., mode) • Large-scale strategies with potential for wide impact across a community may be costly and require coordination of multiple governmental departments and policymakers[22]

Public health settings are a natural fit for D&I research, as the delivery of population-level programs and policies is central to the mission of public health agencies. Among public health settings, resources and infrastructure vary considerably. In this chapter, the focus is primarily on governmental public health systems in the United States, although we draw on literature from multiple parts of the world (especially Australia and Canada), and the research and discussion points presented here are mainly applicable to governmental public health agencies outside the United States. For research exclusively taking place in global settings, see chapter 26.

Within the United States, three levels of governmental public health agencies—national, state, and local—operate "to protect and promote the health of all people in all communities."[23] At the national level, the Department of Health and Human Services and the Centers for Disease Control and Prevention set the nation's agenda for public health (e.g., through Healthy People objectives), establish funding priorities, and distribute public funds to state and local health departments for specific disease prevention and treatment activities (e.g., cancer screening, tobacco control, healthy eating, physical activity promotion).[24] The primary authority for public health in the United States resides at the state and territorial level.[25] Often, state health departments serve as pass-through agencies to distribute national-level funds to contracted partner organizations (e.g., local health departments or community-based organizations). Local health departments are front-line organizations responsible for delivering public health programs to their communities, either directly to individuals or in partnership with other local organizations. As such, local health departments often serve as a bridge linking state and federal infrastructure and resources with local communities. This complex system works to promote equity by "actively [promoting] policies, systems, and overall community conditions that enable optimal health for all and [seeking] to remove systemic and structural barriers that have resulted in health inequities."[23]

In addition to D&I research in governmental public health agencies, D&I research in community settings is needed to support the delivery of EBPPs in organizations or institutions that are often not designed specifically for health-related programming but are natural partners for health-related activities. Implementation of health-related programs in these settings is challenging because these organizations typically do not have a primary focus on health or accountability for health outcomes.[26] For example, the financial standing of an FBO is not dependent on the delivery of tobacco cessation programming. Also, D&I research in community settings is challenging because the diversity of these settings necessitates careful adaptation of evidence-based practices to fit the context and the need to obtain evaluation data on implementation and health-related outcomes that are not typically measured during the usual operations of the organization. Despite these challenges, community settings are valuable for health promotion because they influence the everyday life of individuals and are settings in which people spend much more of their time relative to time spent in healthcare organizations. They also represent key entrance points to direct health equity through community organizations. Because community settings contribute so greatly to the basic survival and psychosocial needs of individuals, these settings have a major role in reaching populations who have disproportionate chronic and infectious disease risks because of inequities in social determinants of health, such as employment, access to food, and transportation.

This chapter discusses the evidence base, tools and resources, and other important themes guiding current D&I research in community and public health settings. We provide examples that highlight important considerations for research in this area, as well as research gaps and opportunities for future work in these settings. The chapter provides multiple examples focused on chronic disease prevention and control; however, the principles described in the examples extend to research in other areas of public health.

EVIDENCE-BASED PRACTICES AND POLICIES FOR COMMUNITY AND PUBLIC HEALTH SETTINGS

A number of resources and tools are available to enhance the ease with which public health and clinical practitioners and researchers can find and use evidence-based programs and practices. These resources and tools include systematic reviews of public health intervention and policy approaches and web-based tools to help researchers and practitioners find evidence-based programs and associated resources for planning and implementation. These resources themselves are sometimes the focus of D&I research in studies to understand how and to what extent practitioners use these tools and to identify effective strategies to enhance the dissemination and integration of these tools in public health decision-making.[27] Some of the tools designed for use by practitioners and policymakers are described briefly in the following section and in Table 19.2.

The Community Guide

In 1996, the US Department of Health and Human Services established the Task Force for Community Preventive Services to develop guidelines for evidence-based practice based on the systematic review of community-based health promotion and disease prevention interventions.[28] The Guide to Community Preventive Services (known as the Community Guide)[36] is an online resource based on the task force's findings, which can be used to select from evaluated interventions. The web-based tool lists the intervention effect, the intervention aspects that users can identify as most appropriate for their respective communities, and the intervention cost and return on investment. Interventions are rated as "recommended," "recommended against," or "insufficient evidence," with those that are recommended also rated according to the strength of the evidence as "strong" or "sufficient." Topics include health behaviors and outcomes, as well as a specific section on health equity, which focuses on addressing social determinants of health.

Evidence-Based Practices Resource Center

In 1997, the Substance Abuse and Mental Health Services Administration (SAMHSA) launched the National Registry of Effective Prevention Programs (NREPP)[32] as a resource to help practitioners identify and implement substance abuse prevention programs. The NREPP site expanded to include mental health and substance use prevention and treatment interventions in 2004 and also updated their rating and review criteria. As of 2015, outcome ratings of "effective," "promising," "ineffective," and "inconclusive" are displayed as a stoplight and were assigned based on rigorous peer-review criteria. In 2018, SAMHSA released the Evidence-Based Practices Resource Center, which aims to "provide communities, clinicians, policy-makers and others in the field with the information and tools they need to incorporate evidence-based practices into their communities or clinical settings."[37] The website includes evidence-based strategies as well as toolkits, guidelines, and evidence reviews that can support implementation of programs that address behavioral health issues. The resource center is intended to be used by a variety of audiences, including clinicians, prevention professionals, patients, policymakers, and family and caregivers.

Evidence-Based Cancer Control Programs Website

In 2002, the National Cancer Institute (NCI) began developing the Research-Tested Interventions Programs (RTIPs) website[33] to provide cancer control practitioners access to programs that had been conducted in peer-reviewed, grant-funded studies; had positive outcomes published in peer-reviewed journals; and had materials that could be disseminated and adapted for use in community or clinical settings. The next year, the Cancer Control P.L.A.N.E.T. (Plan, Link, Act, Network With Evidence-Based Tools) web portal was launched by the NCI, which was designed to provide cancer control practitioners with access to data and evidence-based resources to assist in planning and implementation of EBPPs. In 2020, the NCI launched a new resource, the Evidence-Based Cancer Control Programs (EBCCP) website, which combines elements of RTIPs and Cancer Control P.L.A.N.E.T. At the time of this publication, the EBCCP website has more than 200 behavioral, psychosocial, and policy programs across a range of health topics (e.g., breast, cervical, colorectal, and prostate cancer screening; diet/nutrition; and human papilloma virus [HPV] vaccination). For each program, the website includes detailed information about the program (e.g., delivery location) and ratings of RE-AIM (Reach, Effectiveness, Adoption, Implementation, and Maintenance) constructs, research integrity, intervention impact, dissemination capability, and tools and materials that program planners and public health practitioners can use.

TABLE 19.2 RESOURCES FOR IDENTIFYING EVIDENCE-BASED PRACTICES AND POLICIES FOR COMMUNITY SETTINGS

Resource	Host Organization	Description
The Guide to Community Preventive Services (The Community Guide)[28–31]	Task Force for Community Preventive Services, US Department of Health and Human Services	• Web-based tool describing programs to improve health behaviors, health outcomes, and health equity • Tool lists the intervention effect; intervention components; intervention cost and return on investment; whether the intervention is "recommended," is "recommended against," or has "insufficient evidence"; and relevant Healthy People 2030 objectives
Evidence-Based Practices Resource Center (formerly National Registry of Effective Prevention Programs [NREPP])[32]	Substance Abuse and Mental Health Services Administration (SAMHSA)	• Website includes information about evidence-based practices for mental health and substance use prevention and treatment with outcome ratings of "effective," "promising," "ineffective," and "inconclusive" displayed as a stoplight • Site contains a learning center with resources (e.g., toolkits, guidelines, and evidence reviews) to help with program planning, evaluation, and implementation
Evidence-Based Cancer Control Programs (EBCCP) (formerly Research-Tested Interventions Programs [RTIPs])[33]	National Cancer Institute (NCI)	• Website contains behavioral, psychosocial, and policy programs addressing cancer screening; diet/nutrition; human papilloma virus vaccination; obesity; physical activity; public health genomics; sun safety; cancer survivorship; and tobacco control • Programs are from grant-funded studies, have had positive outcomes published in peer-reviewed journals, and have materials that could be disseminated and adapted in real-world settings • The website includes program components and ratings of RE-AIM constructs, research integrity, intervention impact, and dissemination capability • Tools and materials that program planners and public health practitioners can use to select, plan for, implement, and evaluate a program are provided

(*continued*)

TABLE 19.2 CONTINUED

Resource	Host Organization	Description
High-Impact HIV/AIDS Prevention Project (formerly [DEBI])[34]	Centers for Disease Control and Prevention, US Department of Health and Human Services	• Compendium of tested interventions proven effective in research studies, utilized experimental or quasi-experimental study design, and have materials packaged and ready for dissemination • Project staff provides training and technical assistance for the programs posted in the compendium • HIV prevention efforts are guided by five major considerations to improve the efficient translation of research into practice: effectiveness and cost; feasibility of full-scale implementation; coverage in the target populations; interaction and targeting when combining interventions; and prioritization of interventions with the greatest overall potential to reduce HIV infections and improve health equity
Health Evidence[35]	McMaster University, the National Collaborating Center for Methods and Tools, and the McMaster Optimal Aging Portal	• Free, searchable database of reviews for health promotion programs • The website prioritizes programs that practitioners can adapt for their local settings and uses specific criteria for inclusion and to summarize study characteristics, including requirements that the level of evidence used in the review (e.g., randomized trial) be disclosed; and a minimum assessment of four of seven quality components of included primary studies

High Impact HIV/AIDS Prevention Project

HIV prevention researchers and practitioners have been pioneers in D&I of evidence-based interventions (EBIs). Beginning in 1999, the CDC sponsored High Impact HIV/AIDS Prevention Project (HIP) (formerly known as DEBI) and conducted a systematic review of evidence-based HIV prevention interventions. A compendium of tested interventions was published and currently includes over 80 programs proven effective in research studies, that utilized experimental or quasi-experimental study design, and have materials packaged and ready for dissemination.[34] To enhance the dissemination process, the project staff provides training and technical assistance for the programs posted in the compendium, which is seen as essential for building the capacity of individuals, organizations, and communities.[38]

Health Evidence

In 2005, Health Evidence, a free, searchable database of reviews, was released by McMaster University, the National Collaborating Center for Methods and Tools, and the McMaster Optimal Aging Portal to help the public health workforce and policymakers identify high-quality evidence for health promotion programs and use evidence-informed public health decision-making to apply research evidence in their local context. The group of academics who run the website also offer training and consultation services. The website prioritizes programs that practitioners can adapt for their local settings and uses specific criteria for inclusion and to summarize study characteristics, including requirements that the level of evidence used in the review (e.g., randomized trial) be disclosed, and a minimum assessment of four of seven quality components are required of included primary studies. Seven bibliographic databases are searched (e.g., Cumulated Index to Nursing and Allied Health Literature, PsycINFO, and SPORTDiscus), from 1995 to present.

OVERVIEW OF RESEARCH IN COMMUNITY AND PUBLIC HEALTH SETTINGS

Governmental Public Health Agencies

Dissemination and implementation research in governmental public health settings broadly focuses on how EBPPs are disseminated to agencies and how to increase the capacity of agencies and their staff to conduct evidence-based public health (EBPH). EBPH is an approach to public health practice in which public health practitioners identify, implement, and evaluate EBPPs. EBPH is characterized by the use of evidence-based decision-making (EBDM), the process of integrating the best available research evidence, practitioner expertise, and the characteristics, needs, and preferences of the community.[39,40] The use of EBDM is associated with the use of EBPPs, improved public health agency performance, and efficient use of finite resources.[41–45] To use EBDM, agency staff need the relevant skills, and their organizations need to have sufficient resources, infrastructure, and leadership in place.[46]

Descriptive and measurement development research conducted in governmental health agencies has identified several domains of administrative evidence-based practices that can facilitate EBDM, including workforce development, organizational climate and culture, leadership, relationships and partnerships, and financial processes and developed quantitative measures to assess the use of these practices.[47,48] Experimental studies have been conducted by Brownson and colleagues in the United States[41,49] and Dobbins and colleagues in Canada[50] to test the effectiveness of implementation strategies such as staff training, ongoing technical assistance, leadership development, and organizational change on the adoption and implementation of EBPPs focused on chronic disease prevention and management.[51–58] These studies have highlighted several features of governmental public health agencies that are key to the successful implementation of EBPPs:

- Leaders at multiple levels (e.g., deputy directors, division directors, program managers) play a specific role in promoting a culture of EBPH and need to work together to communicate a consistent message to employees and facilitate EBPH use.[59,60] The influence of a leader may differ by level; for example, Birken and colleagues identified specific roles of middle managers (e.g., program managers), including mediating between strategy and day-to-day operations.[61]

- Creating and maintaining partnerships are critical to successful EBDM and EBPP implementation because agencies rely heavily on partner organizations to directly implement programs within a local community. In particular, forming partnerships with private and nonhealth sector organizations holds promise to improve public health.[62]
- For successful implementation to occur, individuals within organizations should have skills to use EBDM, and the organization should be supportive of EBDM. As such, D&I strategies are needed to facilitate individual and organizational-level change. These two types of changes likely require different strategies, and the time frame for observing these changes is likely longer for organizational change.

A strategy to improve capacity for EBPH in governmental public health agencies that has received growing recognition is an academic-health department partnership, which is a type of community-academic partnership between an academic institution and a governmental public health agency that provides mutual benefits in teaching, research, and service.[63–67] These partnerships offer a structure to deliver the training, technical assistance, and other supports needed to implement EBPPs that can be sustained in real-world settings. Cross-sectional work led by Erwin and colleagues demonstrated that local health departments engaged in an academic-health department partnership were 2.3 times more likely to implement EBPPs compared to local health departments not in a partnership.[68] Although academic-health department partnerships are recognized as important for public health practice and education, research about these partnerships is emerging, and additional work is needed to understand how to structure these partnerships best to facilitate EBPP implementation.[69]

Another area of research focus in public health agencies is mis-implementation, defined as the inappropriate continuation of programs or policies that are not evidence based or the inappropriate termination of EBPPs.[70] Mis-implementation is similar to the work done to de-implement low-value programs and practices in clinical and public health settings (chapter 12); however, it is important to study mis-implementation as a unique phenomenon since it may occur as a result of mechanisms beyond the absence of EBH and distinct from the mechanisms by which ineffective programs can be de-implemented. Cross-sectional studies have quantified the extent to which mis-implementation occurs in public health settings[70,71] and identified practitioner- and organizational-level correlates of mis-implementation, with the strongest correlates and predictors of mis-implementation at the organizational level.[71] Examples of correlates include individuals having the skills to modify programs or policies to a new population, number of organizational layers impeding decision-making, loss of funding, lack of support from key stakeholders, and the use of economic evaluation in decision-making about programs.[71–73] Qualitative studies have identified key characteristics of agency leaders (e.g., being transparent and facilitating bidirectional communication) that can prevent mis-implementation[74] and reasons public health staff perceive mis-implementation occurs, including factors related to a program itself; relational factors with partners, champions, and decision-makers; and higher-level factors (e.g., ongoing funding, agency capacity). An ongoing study led by Brownson and colleagues seeks to understand mis-implementation using a systems science lens by developing an agent-based model to describe mis-implementation and identify potentially effective strategies to reduce mis-implementation among state public health programs.[75]

City Planning, Transportation, and Parks and Recreation Departments

In addition to governmental public health agencies, other governmental departments can support the implementation of health-focused EBPPs and programs and policies that can address social determinants of health, such as transportation, access to a health-promoting built environment, and economic opportunities. For example, policies to improve the built environment through zoning and land use, and active travel opportunities can improve eating and physical activity behaviors.[9,76] From an equity standpoint, the presence of accessible, safe, and affordable transportation routes to employment opportunities, healthcare, and other community resources can improve the health of individuals who do not have access to private transportation and address social determinants of health in the community.[77] This type of implementation can be challenging because it often requires the coordination of multiple departments and partnering organizations within communities that all have different organizational dynamics and priorities. Also, funding is typically allocated by policymakers who make decisions based on factors such as cost, which is not always available for research-tested EBPPs to promote health.[22,78–81] These challenges also extend to programs addressing social determinants of health, with lack of political will and the complexity of factors cited as limiting progress in this area.[82]

A well-recognized example of an evidence-based program that has been implemented with coordination from many municipal governmental agencies is a ciclovía (open streets), a community event where streets are closed to motor vehicles and exclusively used for nonmotorized transit and walking. Ciclovías can increase leisure time physical activity and have other benefits, including decreasing unequal access to recreational opportunities, promoting social capital, improving the population's quality of life, reducing particulate pollution and street noise, and increasing business activity.[83] Ciclovías have been implemented across a variety of urban and rural communities worldwide, most notably in urban Latin American communities like Bogotá, where ciclovías originated.[83]

The scale-up of ciclovías has taken place largely outside of research studies, and as such, D&I research has focused on understanding the contextual factors that contribute to the scale-up and sustainability of ciclovías. For example, Sarmiento and colleagues conducted a mixed-methods evaluation of the sustained implementation of ciclovías across Latin America to understand the extent to which they had been implemented and what contributed to their sustained implementation.[83] Commonly cited factors that contributed to sustainability fell into individual (e.g., perceived benefits by users, citizen support, committed champions); organizational (e.g., compatibility with host organization's mission, organizational capacity, flexibility); and external (e.g., alliances, funding stability, government support) levels, even though the ciclovías differed in characteristics such as the funding source.[83] These factors supported the continued implementation of ciclovías even in the midst of political changes that reduced government support, in which cases community partner groups were able to take more of an active role in implementation to ensure long-lasting success of the program.

Beyond the implementation of individual EBPPs, coordination among governmental agencies to promote health has been recognized through efforts such as the World Health Organization's Health in All Policies approach. Health in All Policies calls on all levels of government to commit to chronic disease prevention and health equity by systematically accounting for the health-related implications of policy decisions and avoiding unintended negative health-related consequences of policy decisions.[84,85] This approach is facilitated by the presence of stable funding mechanisms; strong, long-term political support; open communication channels; and legal obligations, whereas the perception of interorganizational collaboration as an extra task and siloed organizational structures can hinder implementation.[86] Identifying common ground between health and the goals of other governmental agencies, such as dual benefits of nonmotorized transit for physical activity and climate change, may facilitate implementation. To date there have been notable successes in the implementation of EBPPs to support health through governmental agencies with a focus on health equity, and future research can demonstrate the long-term benefits of these approaches and identify the best implementation approaches.[78]

Faith-Based Organizations

Faith-based organizations are well recognized as key settings to promote health for a variety of reasons: FBOs are important in the lives of their congregants and local communities; there is an alignment of health and well-being with religious doctrines; and organizational characteristics of FBOs such as physical space and social networks can support EBPP implementation.[13–18,87,88] For example, the strong social ties between leaders and among members in an FBO can support the implementation of programs with an interpersonal focus. Research conducted in FBOs has focused on a range of health topics (e.g., healthy eating and physical activity promotion, cancer screening) and within a variety of religious denominations.[12,13,20,21,89,90]

Much of the research in FBOs has focused on churches with predominantly racial or ethnic minority congregations, which offers an opportunity to address health disparities.[10,20,91–95] The strong social networks within FBOs positions leaders well as trustworthy sources of information, including health-related information, and they can advocate for participation in EBPPs implemented in FBOs. As such, forming relationships with leaders and members of a faith-based setting should be done carefully and with recognition that congregations may be skeptical of outsiders or researchers based on historical abuses of minority groups. Gaining leadership support for health programs, especially by demonstrating that there is a good fit between the program to be implemented and the values of the FBO can improve both implementation effectiveness and reach.[94–96]

Many programs in FBOs are implemented by lay community health workers (CHWs), who typically have existing connections within the FBO community. They often have insider knowledge of the local context of the FBO that can be used to adapt a program to fit better within the setting, and they are viewed as trustworthy sources of information. Frequently, CHWs join research studies as volunteers. However, this may hinder the sustainability of a program, and it may be necessary to identify stable funding streams to pay CHWs as they continue to implement a program.[97] Also, CHWs are not expected to have formal training in health or behavior change, so the quality of trainings and ongoing technical assistance for CHWs to build the skills required to deliver complex health interventions are critical to implementation fidelity and success.[98] In-person trainings for CHWs that have been delivered in efficacy and effectiveness trials may not be designed for scalability. Other approaches, such as asynchronous, self-paced online trainings, have been explored, as in the example described below, which can support widespread use of CHW-delivered programs.[99]

One example of an intervention that has been implemented in FBOs is Faith in Action, which was designed to increase physical activity among churchgoing Latinas through changes at the individual, interpersonal, organizational, and environmental levels.[10] The yearlong intervention was delivered by promotoras, the Spanish term for community health workers, hired from participating churches and trained to lead free physical activity classes and provide social support to participants. The promotoras also advocated for improvements to the social and built environment by conducting walkability audits of the church grounds and mobilizing the congregation to develop projects to address aspects of the built environment that should be improved.[10] In an effectiveness trial, Faith in Action showed significant increases in accelerometer-measured moderate-to-vigorous physical activity (MVPA, 22 minutes per week) and self-report leisure-time MVPA (40 minutes per week) among Latinas versus a cancer screening comparison arm.[100]

Case studies were conducted to understand the determinants of implementation effectiveness at the organization level, which identified the innovation-values fit, leadership support, and resource availability as key participant-identified factors influencing implementation success.[94] Qualitative interviews with FBO leaders, community members, and physical activity advocates were conducted to inform implementation strategies to scale up Faith in Action.[101] Analysis of these interviews identified several promising implementation strategies to scale up Faith in Action: the importance of supporting health behavior change training for pastors and staff; tailored/targeted messaging; and developing local and national community collaborations.[101] These interviews highlighted the importance of focusing on organizational-level change and supporting sustainment throughout implementation. In an ongoing trial (R01HL158538), the research team is testing the standard Faith in Action intervention compared to two enhanced implementation arms: (1) Faith in Action plus organizational strategies and (2) Faith in Action plus organizational and sustainment strategies (https://reporter.nih.gov/).

Other Community Settings

There are a number of other types of organizations, typically nonprofit, community-based organizations that focus on a variety of areas, such as family and youth development (e.g., YMCAs, Boy Scouts of America) or sports and recreation programs. These community organizations are diverse in terms of their focus, size, and capacity to implement EBPPs, but they share strong social networks and a potential for wide reach because they are trusted organizations in their communities where individuals spend much of their recreational time. For example, the Diabetes Prevention Program, a lifestyle modification program to prevent type 2 diabetes, has been disseminated widely in the United States through community settings such as the YMCA.[102,103] Disseminating this program has faced similar challenges as other areas of D&I research; its reach and effectiveness in individuals with low income and racial or ethnic minorities is lower than higher-income and racial or ethnic majority individuals.[104] Additional work is needed to understand how to effectively adapt, disseminate, and implement the Diabetes Prevention Program equitably in different communities.

These organizations, by their structure, often find implementing EBPPs to be more challenging. Economos and colleagues reported the effects of voluntary healthy eating and physical activity standards, which had been challenging for volunteer-led programs like the Boy Scouts of America and 4-H clubs to implement compared to more structured organizations that provide afterschool care.[105] The three standards were (1) Drink Right: choose water over sugar-sweetened beverages; (2) Move More: boost movement and physical activity in all programs; and (3) Snack Smart: fuel up on fruits and vegetables. D&I strategies were designed with stakeholder input so that they could easily integrate into each organization's culture and leverage existing policies and communication channels. A multimodal approach, including volunteer training, technical assistance, and supporting materials such as water bottles, physical activity games, recipes, and educational activities, including an interactive sugar quiz showing amounts of sugar in popular beverages. A quasi-experimental study was conducted to evaluate the D&I of these standards. The program showed success 6 months postimplementation with the beverage and move standards, which is notable as these were cost-neutral or cost-negative changes. Subsequently, program materials were integrated on the Boy Scouts of America and 4-H websites, demonstrating buy-in from top leadership, which can contribute to sustained support for implementation of these standards. Future work is needed to address the barriers to implementation that were identified, including parent pushback, child pushback, cost and time associated with fresh fruit and vegetable snacks, inclement weather, and adequate space available for physical activity.

CHALLENGES AND OPPORTUNITIES FOR DISSEMINATION AND IMPLEMENTATION IN COMMUNITY AND PUBLIC HEALTH SETTINGS

Infrastructure and Workforce Issues

Community and public health settings play an important role in the widespread application of EBPPs, although there are many differences in these organizations based on size, resources, and capacity to implement public health services.[106] Governmental public health agencies are positioned well to serve as a link between producers of research evidence (i.e., federal agencies and academia) and users and beneficiaries of knowledge (e.g., local practitioners, community members)[107] by cultivating community advocacy and partnerships[108] and developing and adapting programs and policies to the unique context of the organizations and communities they serve. Either in partnership with public health agencies or on their own, community settings play a key role in directly delivering programs (e.g., the Diabetes Prevention Program); promoting the utilization of public health services (e.g., screening referrals); advocating for public health policy change (e.g., increased tobacco excise taxes); and promoting health equity. The relationship between government, public health agencies, and community organizations varies greatly by community, and as such, it is critical to understand the structure and capacity of the public health system of the community in which D&I is occurring. Understanding this context will allow researchers and practitioners to select and/or adapt D&I strategies that match the context and have the greatest potential to support the use of EBPPs in communities.

A central issue within the public health systems of communities that can impact implementation relates to the workforce available. Public health and community settings have high turnover of employees over time, which can impact implementation in a number of ways, including changes in leadership support for a program and the loss of individuals who have the necessary skills and training to implement a particular program. Turnover in governmental public health agencies and the impact of funding cuts to public health agencies were concerns prior to the COVID-19 pandemic, and the pandemic has brought even more attention to these issues.[109] For example, prior to the pandemic, only 14% of state health department employees surveyed by Eyler and colleagues agreed that there was a good pool of replacements for employees who retire or move to different job amidst an aging public health workforce.[110] Since 2020, many individuals in public health and community organizations retired or took positions within other sectors, which will have long-term impacts on the capacity of the public health infrastructure to effectively deliver EBPPs. From an equity standpoint, it is important to ensure that those who are tasked with implementing EBPPs are appropriately compensated for their work, either because the work fits into their job or by receiving a stipend or salary for their time. Sustained, impactful change cannot rest on volunteers in lower-resourced agencies.

Stakeholder Engagement and Supporting Strong Community Partnerships

Involving stakeholders in the conceptualization, implementation, and evaluation of D&I research is not unique to public health and community settings, but it is critical to create ownership and facilitate fit of EBPP efforts.[111,112] Within public health and community settings, there are many diverse groups of stakeholders, from policymakers to organizational staff to individuals who are recipients of programs. The specific set of stakeholders for each research initiative will differ depending on the setting, so it is important to first define the group of relevant stakeholders so that D&I strategies can be chosen and tailored to address the priorities and needs of each stakeholder group.[11,12,78,113] Working with stakeholders can help researchers learn about and understand aspects of the local organizational and community context and the perspectives and experiences of stakeholders. The partnerships that form from engaging with stakeholders over time can improve the success of D&I research efforts and support equitable implementation,[114] especially if partnerships are intentionally and carefully formed and maintained. Strong partnerships with community groups should be built on trust, especially in cases when practitioners in community settings and community members are skeptical of working with researchers based on perceptions of research and historical abuses of groups by research and medical institutions.[19,115] Also, particularly in community organizations, researchers may need to make a case for how health-related EBPPs align with the organizational priorities and values.[26,115] While outside the scope of this chapter, it is important to consider how feasible it is for academics to spend the amount of time it takes to form and maintain partnerships given current standards for tenure and promotion. Research institutions should consider how they incentivize or disincentivize researchers to prioritize this important aspect of D&I research, and the impact that can have on communities, depending on how those partnerships are valued by academics and their subsequent institutions.

Building Capacity for Health Equity-Focused D&I Research

The field of implementation science has acknowledged that health equity needs to be centered on research to make meaningful, timely progress toward health equity outcomes.[114,116,117] The research presented in this chapter highlights many examples of research that can reduce disparities and address inequities; however, to achieve health equity at a population level, additional investments to build sufficient capacity to conduct health equity-focused research are needed.

Brownson and colleagues highlighted several limitations within implementation science that can undermine progress toward health equity goals. They discussed limitations of the evidence base itself—that too few EBIs address upstream social and systems-level factors and the lack of diversity in study participants and organizations.[116] There is a need to consider the multiple levels of influence on implementation,[117] especially the upstream social and structural factors that are key contributors to inequities but are rarely addressed with implementation strategies.[114] Research in community and public health settings often acknowledges that there are multiple levels of influence on health behaviors and outcomes, but there should be a more careful examination of the contextual factors that influence equity-related outcomes.

Additionally, research methods to directly address health equity-related research questions need to be improved. It is important to support the use of pragmatic approaches to trial design, that is, conducting research in real-world conditions and not relying only on a highly internally valid randomized control trial to generate evidence that likely does not generalize to diverse populations.[114,116] While there has been notable progress to develop health equity-focused frameworks[118] and measures, more work is needed to integrate health equity into the variety of settings and EBIs on which implementation science focuses. Careful attention should also be paid to assessing any unintended negative consequences of implementing a single EBI, for example, if disparities are widened because the only individuals who can access an EBI are those who do not experience inequities. This is especially of concern in community and public health settings, which involve organizations that have the potential to reach a broad, diverse population (i.e., state public health departments that decide to implement one EBI across an entire state). The improvements in the evidence base and research methods required to conduct high-quality health equity research will be costly and will take dedication from funders and the implementation science community; however, ignoring these needs will perpetuate or even worsen current disparities.

CASE STUDY: PROMOTING CANCER SCREENING THROUGH FAITH-BASED ORGANIZATIONS—PROJECT HEAL

Background

Project HEAL (Health Through Early Awareness and Learning) is a program that was initially designed to deliver an evidence-based set of spiritually based print materials about early detection of breast, prostate, and colorectal cancer that were distributed through a series of in-person workshops in Black congregations in Maryland, United States.[99,119] An efficacy trial demonstrated improved knowledge of cancer screening behaviors.[99] The interventions were developed separately for each cancer type using the health belief model, and a combined intervention was developed and pilot tested using a community-engaged process, including an advisory panel of faith leaders, healthcare system leaders, and cancer survivors.[120] The workshops were designed to be delivered by CHWs with little to no health background, and an initial implementation question was how best to train and certify the CHWs to prepare them for implementing Project HEAL in a manner that could be scaled widely.

Context

Since initial efficacy testing and refinement of the implementation and intervention approaches, research studies have focused on the implementation and sustainability of Project HEAL. In the first implementation study, the research team used a cluster-randomized trial with 15 churches to test two implementation strategies to train CHWs to deliver the workshop series. These implementation strategies were (1) a traditional approach that used in-person, group-based training along with self-study modules and (2) a technology-based training that began with a short introductory meeting in person but then was delivered online and completed in an asynchronous, self-paced manner.[99] CHWs in both groups were certified with the same knowledge exam to ensure the training topics were mastered before leading Project HEAL workshops, although the exams were delivered in different formats (i.e., paper and pencil for the in-person group and online for technology group). The RE-AIM framework was used to understand if the technology-based training and workshops were feasible and effective at the church and individual levels, beyond effectiveness at the individual level.[120] This evaluation used multiple quantitative and qualitative data sources that represented the perspectives and experiences of individual participants, CHWs, and church leaders. The study team operationalized and measured reach, adoption, and implementation as follows:

- **Reach:** number of workshop participants enrolled in Project HEAL divided by the number of eligible participants in the church, which was estimated by the pastor
- **Adoption:** number of churches agreeing to participate and who began the program divided by the number of churches approached for recruitment

- **Implementation:** three dimensions of implementation were evaluated: *adherence* (e.g., the time to complete the workshops), *dosage* (e.g., how much of the educational print materials participants read), and *quality* (e.g., participants' willingness to recommend the program to their peers)

Lessons Learned

This implementation study showed statistically significant increases in participants' cancer knowledge and cancer screening behaviors over time, but few differences by implementation strategy. CHWs in both arms of the study demonstrated similar increases in their knowledge of and ability to lead the intervention, showing that a low-touch, less-resource-intensive training model is a promising approach to guide implementation.[99] The RE-AIM evaluation highlighted many similarities in the adoption and implementation of Project HEAL between the two implementation strategies. Notable differences between the two training modes were a higher reach in the in-person training group compared to the technology-based training group (43% vs. 21%, respectively; $p < .10$).[120] Although not statistically significant, the churches with CHWs in the technology-based training group completed the workshops faster than those in the in-person training group (64 vs. 84 days, respectively).[120]

In addition to the question of how best to train the CHWs to deliver Project HEAL, another important question considered by the research team was how to maximize the fit of the program within the local context of an individual church so that health promotion could be institutionalized into the organization. The research team refined the implementation approach through the NCI-funded SPRINT (SPeeding Research tested INTerventions) program focused on transforming behavioral interventions into successful, market-ready products that can be implemented in real-world settings.[119] An expanded implementation approach was developed using theories of institutionalization to include three additional components: (1) a memorandum of understanding with implementation strategies chosen by church leaders; (2) a training module for CHWs focused on how to integrate health promotion activities into their church organizational practices; and (3) check-in sessions with churches to track and support their progress.[121] Church leaders selected implementation strategies that fit their church's context from a list of 20 strategies, including the formation of a health ministry, allocating dedication of one person to be in charge of health activities, or incorporating health into church newsletters.[121] The tailored implementation approach was tested compared to a standardized approach in a cluster randomized trial of 17 churches.[121]

The trial results showed increases in the institutionalization of health promotion practices in both groups, which was the study's primary outcome assessed by a self-report measure developed and validated by the research team.[122] Few differences in institutionalization were detected between the two implementation approaches, and the study team noted the possibility of a testing effect since churches in the standardized implementation group implemented several of the health promotion activities. The team also assessed seven dimensions of sustainability over time, such as continued benefits for intervention recipients, changes in organizational policies or structures, or unplanned consequences of the intervention. Sustainability estimates varied from 0% sustainability (whether the churches replicated the Project HEAL three-workshop series) to 92% (participants sharing Project HEAL intervention content with peers),[123] which highlights the variation in how sustainability can be operationalized. In a study using coincidence analysis, the research team identified dimensions of organizational capacity that separated churches who were successful in implementation (specifically reach and time to intervention completion from those who were not successful in implementing Project HEAL).[124] For example, organizational capacity metrics that contributed to implementing the intervention in fewer days included having conducted one or two health promotion activities in the past 2 years; having one to five part-time staff and a pastor without additional outside employment; or churches with a highly educated pastor and a weekly attendance of 101–249 congregants.

This example highlights many of the central issues of implementation research in public health and community settings: how to engage with tight-knit organizations to reach historically marginalized populations, how to support lay individuals as program implementers, and how to adapt programs and implementation strategies to meet the real-world conditions in which implementation occurs. The research team took the time to build rapport with church leaders and CHWs in their studies, even adding an additional orientation to the CHW training to allow for time to build relationships with church members and facilitate timely completion of the training modules.[121] The way the research team engaged stakeholders to support the modification of intervention and implementation materials likely contributed to an improved fit of Project HEAL within participating churches.

DIRECTIONS FOR FUTURE RESEARCH

Based on the review for this chapter and prior work,[113,125] we provide these recommendations for future research and practice that apply broadly to D&I research in community and public health settings:

- Evaluate the D&I of effective interventions delivered in diverse populations and various community settings. The use of active, multimodal D&I strategies that account for the complex nature of these settings based on input from stakeholder groups is likely to be more effective than passive, single-modal strategies developed by researchers in isolation. Develop and tailor strategies focused on health equity.
- Continue to expand the notion of what is a health-related program or policy to progress toward equity and justice. Until factors like the social determinants of health and systemic oppression are addressed, a focus exclusively on health behaviors and outcomes will have limited impact on health for those who experience inequities.
- Develop and use reliable and valid measures of D&I constructs that can accurately and pragmatically assess relevant constructs across a variety of community and public health settings.
- Use a combination of quantitative and qualitative methods and data from multiple sources to understand D&I from the perspectives of the many stakeholder groups involved. Use equity-relevant metrics when appropriate.
- Employ methods that use systems thinking approaches (e.g., agent-based modeling, system dynamics, and social network analyses), which can account for the structural, dynamic factors that influence D&I.
- Measure the real-world impact of D&I studies using standardized measures of stages of the D&I process, moderators, mediators, and outcomes, moving beyond adoption as the primary outcome of interest as has been done in previous work.
- Apply relevant study designs that balance rigor, relevance, and pragmatism. Randomized controlled trials are not always the most appropriate or feasible to generate generalizable information or to learn from ongoing practice efforts.

SUMMARY

There are many opportunities to disseminate and implement EBPPs through public health and community settings to support health and work toward health equity and justice. This chapter highlights the breadth of these opportunities. However, making the most of these opportunities will require significant prioritization and investment of time and financial resources on the part of funders, research institutions, public health agencies, community partners, and policymakers. The US National Institutes of Health and Centers for Disease Control and Prevention have supported D&I research, although there is a need for increased funding to address the remaining and future challenges of this line of research. These funding agencies, along with others internationally, have also created and supported infrastructures to increase access to information about evidence-based programs and linkages between researchers and practitioners in public health and community organizations. However, these relatively small steps at their current level of support will be insufficient to accelerate closing the discovery–delivery gap.[126] Closing this gap necessitates an increase in funding for this type of D&I research beyond the typical, disease-specific funding structures and an increase in the support for collaborations between researchers and practitioners, such as the recognition of community-focused research activities and products in tenure and promotion standards and value placed on practice-based research. Absent a significant effort at redesigning and increasing investments in D&I research and knowledge translation on the part of science and service-funding agencies, and a similar change in the academic rewards for research, practice, and policy partnerships, integrating the lessons learned from research with those learned from practice and policy, the ideal of research influencing practice and policy and vice versa will remain a side show to our seemingly unquenchable thirst for discovery.

ACKNOWLEDGMENT

Parts of this chapter were adapted with permission from the *Annual Review of Public Health*, Volume 42 ©2021 by Annual Reviews www.annualreviews.org

SUGGESTED READINGS AND WEBSITES

Readings

Brownson RC, Fielding JE, Green LW. Building capacity for evidence-based public health: reconciling the pulls of practice and the push of research. *Annu Rev Public Health.* Apr 1 2018;39:27–53.

This review describes the principles of EBPH, the importance of capacity building to advance evidence-based approaches, emerging approaches for capacity building, and recommendations for future areas for research and practice.

Carmichael L, Townshend TG, Fischer TB, et al. Urban planning as an enabler of urban health: challenges and good practice in England following the 2012 planning and public health reforms. *Land Use Policy.* 2019;84:154–162.

This article discusses the challenges faced by the English urban/spatial planning system to integrate health-focused programs and practices and highlights the many issues that arise when implementing health-related programming through cross-sectoral initiatives.

Koorts H, Eakin E, Estabrooks P, et al. Implementation and scale up of population physical activity interventions for clinical and community settings: the PRACTIS guide. *Int J Behav Nutr Phys Act.* 2018;15:51.

This article describes the PRACTIS (PRACTical planning for Implementation and Scale-up) guide to support the development of an implementation approach through four iterative steps: (1) characterize the implementation setting; (2) identify and engage key stakeholders across multiple levels within the delivery system(s); (3) identify contextual barriers and facilitators to implementation, and (4) address potential barriers to effective implementation.

McCrabb S, Lane C, Hall A, et al. Scaling-up evidence-based obesity interventions: a systematic review assessing intervention adaptations and effectiveness and quantifying the scale-up penalty. *Obes Rev.* 2019;20(7):964–982.

This systematic review was conducted to understand the effects of scale-up on intervention success for community-wide obesity prevention and treatment interventions, adaptations made for scale up, and differences in individual-level effectiveness between the effectiveness and scale-up trials.

Riley BL, Garcia JM, Edwards NC. 2007. Organizational change for obesity prevention—perspectives, possibilities and potential pitfalls. In: Kumanyika S, Brownson RC, eds. *Handbook of Obesity Prevention.* Springer; 2007:239–261.

This book chapter discusses dimensions of organizational change to implement and institutionalize health-related programs and practices and the processes required for organizational change to occur.

Rosas LG, Espinosa PR, Jimenez FM, King AC. The role of citizen science in promoting health equity. *Annu Rev Public Health.* 2022;43(1):215–234.

This review summarizes efforts using citizen science to address health equity in the conduct of health-related interventions, which can be a powerful, equity-focused strategy for improving the success of D&I efforts.

Selected Websites and Tools

Evidence-Based Cancer Control Programs (EBCCP). https://ebccp.cancercontrol.cancer.gov/index.do

The Evidence-Based Cancer Control Programs (EBCCP) provide a searchable database of cancer control interventions and program materials designed to provide program planners and public health practitioners easy and immediate access to research-tested materials.

Evidence-Based Practices Resource Center. https://www.samhsa.gov/resource-search/ebp

The Evidence-Based Practices Resource Center is an online registry of tested interventions that support mental health promotion, substance abuse prevention, and mental health and substance abuse treatment.

Guide to Community Preventive Services. http://www.thecommunityguide.org/index.html

The Guide to Community Preventive Services is a federally sponsored website that provides guidance on selecting community-based programs and policies to improve health and prevent disease based on systematic reviews.

Health Evidence. https://www.healthevidence.org/

Health Evidence provides a searchable database of quality-rated systematic reviews evaluating the effectiveness and cost-effectiveness of public health interventions.

High-Impact HIV/AIDS Prevention Project (HIP) website. http://www.effectiveinterventions.org/en/home.aspx

This website is designed to bring science-based, community, group, and individual-level HIV prevention interventions to community-based service providers and state and local health departments.

REFERENCES

1. de Leeuw E. Engagement of sectors other than health in integrated health governance, policy, and action. *Annu Rev Public Health.* Mar 20 2017;38:329–349. doi:10.1146/annurev-publhealth-031816-044309
2. Kumanyika SK, Parker L, Sim LJ. *Institute of Medicine (US) Committee on an Evidence Framework for Obesity Prevention Decision Making. Bridging the Evidence Gap in Obesity Prevention: A Framework to Inform Decision Making.* Washington (DC): National Academies Press (US); 2010. PMID: 25032376.
3. Wisham SL, Kraak VI, Liverman CT, Koplan JP. *Progress in Preventing Childhood Obesity: How Do We Measure Up?* National Academies Press; 2007.
4. Lee BY, Bartsch SM, Mui Y, Haidari LA, Spiker ML, Gittelsohn J. A systems approach to obesity. *Nutr Rev.* 2017;75(suppl 1):94–106. doi:10.1093/nutrit/nuw049
5. Rabin BA, Brownson RC. Terminology for dissemination and implementation research. In: Brownson RC, Colditz GA, Proctor EK, eds. *Dissemination and Implementation Research in Health: Translating Science to Practice.* 2nd ed. Oxford University Press; 2017:19–45.
6. Wolfenden L, Reilly K, Kingsland M, et al. Identifying opportunities to develop the science of implementation for community-based non-communicable disease prevention: a review of implementation trials. *Prev Med.* Jan 2019;118:279–285. doi:10.1016/j.ypmed.2018.11.014
7. McLeroy KR, Bibeau D, Steckler A, Glanz K. An ecological perspective on health promotion programs. *Health Educ Q.* 1988;15(4):351–377.
8. Clarke AR, Goddu AP, Nocon RS, et al. Thirty years of disparities intervention research: what are we doing to close racial and ethnic gaps in health care? *Med Care.* 2013;51(11):1020–1026. doi:10.1097/MLR.0b013e3182a97ba3
9. Giles-Corti B, Vernez-Moudon A, Reis R, et al. City planning and population health: a global challenge. *Lancet.* 2016;388(10062):2912–2924. doi:10.1016/S0140-6736(16)30066-6
10. Arredondo EM, Haughton J, Ayala GX, et al. Fe en Accion/Faith in Action: design and implementation of a church-based randomized trial to promote physical activity and cancer screening among churchgoing Latinas. *Contemp Clin Trials.* Nov 2015;45(pt B):404–415. doi:10.1016/j.cct.2015.09.008
11. Finch EA, Kelly MS, Marrero DG, Ackermann RT. Training YMCA wellness instructors to deliver an adapted version of the diabetes prevention program lifestyle intervention. *Diabetes Educ.* 2009;35(2):224–232. doi:10.1177/0145721709331420
12. Campbell MK, Hudson MA, Resnicow K, Blakeney N, Paxton A, Baskin M. Church-based health promotion interventions: evidence and lessons learned. *Annu Rev Public Health.* 2007;28:213–234. doi:10.1146/annurev.publhealth.28.021406.144016
13. Levin J. Partnerships between the faith-based and medical sectors: implications for preventive medicine and public health. *Prev Med Rep.* 2016;4:344–350. doi:10.1016/j.pmedr.2016.07.009
14. Bowen DJ, Beresford SA, Vu T, et al. Baseline data and design for a randomized intervention study of dietary change in religious organizations. *Prev Med.* Sep 2004;39(3):602–611.
15. Sauaia A, Min S-J, Lack D, et al. Church-based breast cancer screening education: impact of two approaches on Latinas enrolled in public and private health insurance plans. *Prev Chronic Dis.* 2007;4(4):A99.
16. Thrasher JF, Campbell MK, Oates V. Behavior-specific social support for healthy behaviors among African American church members: applying optimal matching theory. *Health Educ Behav.* Apr 2004;31(2):193–205.
17. Welsh AL, Sauaia A, Jacobellis J, Min S-J, Byers T. The effect of two church-based interventions on breast cancer screening rates among Medicaid-insured Latinas. *Prev Chronic Dis.* 2005;2(4):A07.
18. Kong BW. Community-based hypertension control programs that work. *J Health Care Poor Underserved.* Nov 1997;8(4):409–415.
19. Bonner G, Williams S, Wilkie D, Hart A, Burnett G, Peacock G. Trust building recruitment strategies for researchers conducting studies in African American (AA) churches: lessons learned. *Am J Hosp Palliat Care.* Dec 2017;34(10):912–917. doi:10.1177/1049909116666799
20. Rai KK, Dogra SA, Barber S, Adab P, Summerbell C; on behalf of the Childhood Obesity Prevention in Islamic Religious Settings' Programme Management Group. A scoping

review and systematic mapping of health promotion interventions associated with obesity in Islamic religious settings in the UK. *Obes Rev.* 2019;20(9):1231–1261. doi:10.1111/obr.12874

21. Williams MV, Palar K, Derose KP. Congregation-based programs to address HIV/AIDS: elements of successful implementation. *J Urban Health.* 2011;88(3):517–532. doi:10.1007/s11524-010-9526-5
22. Fazli GS, Creatore MI, Matheson FI, et al. Identifying mechanisms for facilitating knowledge to action strategies targeting the built environment. *BMC Public Health.* 2017;17(1):1–9. doi:10.1186/s12889-016-3954-4
23. The Public Health National Center for Innovations. The 10 Essential Public Health Services. 2020. https://phnci.org/uploads/resource-files/EPHS-English.pdf
24. Federal Grant and Cooperative Agreement Act, Pub. L. No. 95–224 (1978).
25. Turnock B. *Public Health: What It Is and How It Works.* 5th ed. Jones & Bartlett Learning; 2012.
26. Woolf SH, Purnell JQ, Simon SM, et al. Translating evidence into population health improvement: strategies and barriers. *Annu Rev Public Health.* Mar 18 2015;36:463–482. doi:10.1146/annurev-publhealth-082214-110901
27. Parks RG, Tabak RG, Allen P, et al. Enhancing evidence-based diabetes and chronic disease control among local health departments: a multi-phase dissemination study with a stepped-wedge cluster randomized trial component. *Implement Sci.* 2017;12(1):122. doi:10.1186/s13012-017-0650-4
28. Truman BI, Smith-Akin CK, Hinman AR, et al. Developing the Guide to Community Preventive Services—overview and rationale. The Task Force on Community Preventive Services. *Am J Prev Med.* Jan 2000;18(1)(suppl):18–26. doi:10.1016/s0749-3797(99)00124-5
29. Mercer SL, Banks SM, Verma P, Fisher JS, Corso LC, Carlson V. Guiding the way to public health improvement: exploring the connections between The Community Guide's evidence-based interventions and health department accreditation standards. *J Public Health Manag Pract.* Jan–Feb 2014;20(1):104–110. doi:10.1097/PHH.0b013e3182aa444c
30. Mullen PD, Ramírez G. The promise and pitfalls of systematic reviews. *Annu Rev Public Health.* 2006;27:81–102. doi:10.1146/annurev.publhealth.27.021405.102239
31. Zaza S, Briss PA, Harris KW. *The Guide to Community Preventive Services: What Works to Promote Health?* Oxford University Press; 2005.
32. Substance Abuse and Mental Health Services Administration (SAMHSA). Evidence-Based Practices Resource Center. 2018. Accessed December 30, 2021. https://www.samhsa.gov/resource-search/ebp
33. National Cancer Institute. Evidence-based cancer control programs. 2020. Accessed December 30, 2021. https://ebccp.cancercontrol.cancer.gov/index.do
34. Centers for Disease Control and Prevention (CDC). Compendium of evidence-based interventions and best practices for HIV prevention. 1995. Accessed December 30, 2021. https://www.cdc.gov/hiv/research/interventionresearch/compendium/index.html
35. Lee E, Dobbins M, DeCorby K, McRae L, Tirilis D, Husson H. An optimal search filter for retrieving systematic reviews and meta-analyses. *BMC Med Res Methodol.* 2012;12(1):51. doi:10.1186/1471-2288-12-51
36. The Community Guide. Home page. 1996. Accessed December 15, 2021. https://www.thecommunityguide.org/
37. Substance Abuse and Mental Health Services Administration (SAMHSA). SAMHSA launches Evidence-Based Practices Resource Center to equip clinicians, strengthen communities. April 5, 2018. Accessed December 30, 2021. https://www.samhsa.gov/newsroom/press-announcements/201804050230
38. Centers for Disease Control and Prevention (CDC). HIV. Effective Interventions. 2022. Accessed December 30, 2021. https://www.cdc.gov/hiv/capacity-building-assistance/index.html
39. Brownson RC, Baker EA, Deshpande AD, Gillespie KN. *Evidence-Based Public Health.* Oxford University Press; 2017.
40. Brownson RC, Gurney JG, Land GH. Evidence-based decision making in public health. *J Public Health Manag Pract.* Sep 1999;5(5):86–97.
41. Brownson RC, Allen P, Jacob RR, et al. Controlling chronic diseases through evidence-based decision making: a group-randomized trial. *Prev Chronic Dis.* Nov 30 2017;14:E121. doi:10.5888/pcd14.170326
42. Dodson EA, Baker EA, Brownson RC. Use of evidence-based interventions in state health departments: a qualitative assessment of barriers and solutions. *J Public Health Manag Pract.* Nov–Dec 2010;16(6):E9–E15. doi:10.1097/PHH.0b013e3181d1f1e2
43. Jacobs JA, Dodson EA, Baker EA, Deshpande AD, Brownson RC. Barriers to evidence-based decision making in public health: a national survey of chronic disease practitioners. *Public*

Health Rep. Sep–Oct 2010;125(5):736–742. doi:10.1177/003335491012500516

44. Jacobs JA, Jones E, Gabella BA, Spring B, Brownson RC. Tools for implementing an evidence-based approach in public health practice. *Prev Chronic Dis.* Jun 2012;9110324. doi:10.5888/pcd9.110324
45. Maylahn C, Fleming D, Birkhead G. Health departments in a brave new world. *Prev Chronic Dis.* Mar 2013;10:130003. doi:10.5888/pcd10.130003
46. Brownson RC, Fielding JE, Green LW. Building capacity for evidence-based public health: reconciling the pulls of practice and the push of research. *Annu Rev Public Health.* Apr 1 2018;39:27–53. doi:10.1146/annurev-publhealth-040617-014746
47. Brownson RC, Reis RS, Allen P, et al. Understanding administrative evidence-based practices: findings from a survey of local health department leaders. *Am J Prev Med.* 2014;46(1):49–57. doi:10.1016/j.amepre.2013.08.013
48. Mazzucca S, Parks RG, Tabak RG, et al. Assessing organizational supports for evidence-based decision making in local public health departments in the United States: development and psychometric properties of a new measure. *J Public Health Manag Pract.* Sep/Oct 2019;25(5):454–463. doi:10.1097/phh.0000000000000952
49. Allen P, Sequeira S, Jacob RR, et al. Promoting state health department evidence-based cancer and chronic disease prevention: a multi-phase dissemination study with a cluster randomized trial component. *Implement Sci.* 2013;8:141. doi:10.1186/1748-5908-8-141
50. Dobbins M, Greco L, Yost J, Traynor R, Decorby-Watson K, Yousefi-Nooraie R. A description of a tailored knowledge translation intervention delivered by knowledge brokers within public health departments in Canada. *Health Res Policy Syst.* Jun 20 2019;17(1):63. doi:10.1186/s12961-019-0460-z
51. Armstrong R, Waters E, Dobbins M, et al. Knowledge translation strategies to improve the use of evidence in public health decision making in local government: intervention design and implementation plan. *Implement Sci.* 2013;8:121. doi:10.1186/1748-5908-8-121
52. Armstrong R, Waters E, Moore L, et al. Understanding evidence: a statewide survey to explore evidence-informed public health decision-making in a local government setting. *Implement Sci.* 2014;9:188. doi:10.1186/s13012-014-0188-7
53. Serrano N, Diem G, Grabauskas V, et al. Building the capacity—examining the impact of evidence-based public health trainings in Europe: a mixed methods approach. *Glob Health Promot.* 2019;27(2):1757975918811102. doi:10.1177/1757975918811102
54. Waters E, Armstrong R, Swinburn B, et al. An exploratory cluster randomised controlled trial of knowledge translation strategies to support evidence-informed decision-making in local governments (the KT4LG study). *BMC Public Health.* 2011;11:34. doi:10.1186/1471-2458-11-34
55. Pettman TL, Armstrong R, Jones K, Waters E, Doyle J. Cochrane update: building capacity in evidence-informed decision-making to improve public health. *J Public Health (Oxf).* 2013;35(4):624–627. doi:10.1093/pubmed/fdt119
56. Yousefi Nooraie R, Marin A, Hanneman R, Lohfeld L, Dobbins M. Implementation of evidence-informed practice through central network actors; a case study of three public health units in Canada. *BMC Health Serv Res.* 2017;17(1):208. doi:10.1186/s12913-017-2147-x
57. Diem G, Brownson RC, Grabauskas V, Shatchkute A, Stachenko S. Prevention and control of noncommunicable diseases through evidence-based public health: implementing the NCD 2020 action plan. *Glob Health Promot.* 2016;23(3):5–13. doi:10.1177/1757975914567513
58. Peirson L, Ciliska D, Dobbins M, Mowat D. Building capacity for evidence informed decision making in public health: a case study of organizational change. *BMC Public Health.* 2012;12:137. doi:10.1186/1471-2458-12-137
59. Aarons GA, Ehrhart MG, Farahnak LR, Sklar M. Aligning leadership across systems and organizations to develop a strategic climate for evidence-based practice implementation. *Annu Rev Public Health.* 2014;35:255–274. doi:10.1146/annurev-publhealth-032013-182447
60. Chreim S, Williams BE, Coller KE. Radical change in healthcare organization: mapping transition between templates, enabling factors, and implementation processes. *J Health Organ Manag.* 2012;26(2):215–236. doi:10.1108/14777261211230781
61. Birken S, Clary A, Tabriz AA, et al. Middle managers' role in implementing evidence-based practices in healthcare: a systematic review. *Implement Sci.* Dec 12 2018;13(1):149. doi:10.1186/s13012-018-0843-5
62. Simon PA, Fielding JE. Public health and business: a partnership that makes cents. *Health Aff (Millwood).* 2006;25(4):1029–1039.
63. Keck CW. Lessons learned from an academic health department. *J Public Health Manag Pract.* 2000;6(1):47–52.

64. Council on Education for Public Health. Accreditation criteria and procedures. 2021. Accessed July 9, 2020. https://ceph.org/about/org-info/criteria-procedures-documents/criteria-procedures/
65. Public Health Accreditation Board. Standards and measures for initial accreditation. 2013. Accessed July 9, 2020. https://phaboard.org/wp-content/uploads/PHABSM_WEB_LR1-1.pdf
66. Gordon AK, Chung K, Handler A, Turnock BJ, Schieve LA, Ippoliti P. Final report on public health practice linkages between schools of public health and state health agencies: 1992–1996. *J Public Health Manag Pract.* May 1999;5(3):25–34. doi:10.1097/00124784-199905000-00006
67. Erwin PC, Keck CW. The academic health department: the process of maturation. *J Public Health Manag Pract.* May–Jun 2014;20(3):270–277. doi:10.1097/PHH.0000000000000016
68. Erwin PC, Parks RG, Mazzucca S, et al. Evidence-based public health provided through local health departments: importance of academic-practice partnerships. *Am J Public Health.* 2019;109(5):739–747. doi:10.2105/AJPH.2019.304958
69. Erwin PC, Brownson RC, Livingood WC, Keck CW, Amos K. Development of a research agenda focused on academic health departments. *Am J Public Health.* 2017;107(9):1369–1375. doi:10.2105/AJPH.2017.303847
70. Brownson RC, Allen P, Jacob RR, et al. Understanding mis-implementation in public health practice. *Am J Prev Med.* May 2015;48(5):543–551. doi:10.1016/j.amepre.2014.11.015
71. Padek MM, Mazzucca S, Allen P, et al. Patterns and correlates of mis-implementation in state chronic disease public health practice in the United States. *BMC Public Health.* Jan 28 2021;21(1):101. doi:10.1186/s12889-020-10101-z
72. Allen P, Jacob RR, Parks RG, et al. Perspectives on program mis-implementation among US local public health departments. *BMC Health Serv Res.* Mar 30 2020;20(1):258. doi:10.1186/s12913-020-05141-5
73. Furtado KS, Budd EL, Armstrong R, et al. A cross-country study of mis-implementation in public health practice. *BMC Public Health.* 2019;19(1):270. doi:10.1186/s12889-019-6591-x
74. Moreland-Russell S, Farah Saliba L, Rodriguez Weno E, Smith R, Padek M, Brownson RC. Leading the way: competencies of leadership to prevent mis-implementation of public health programs. *Health Educ Res.* 2022 Sep 23;37(5):279–291. doi:10.1093/her/cyac021. PMID: 36069114; PMCID: PMC9502849.
75. Padek M, Allen P, Erwin PC, et al. Toward optimal implementation of cancer prevention and control programs in public health: a study protocol on mis-implementation. *Implement Sci.* Mar 23 2018;13(1):49. doi:10.1186/s13012-018-0742-9
76. Gelius P, Messing S, Goodwin L, Schow D, Abu-Omar K. What are effective policies for promoting physical activity? A systematic review of reviews. *Prev Med Rep.* 2020;18:101095. doi:10.1016/j.pmedr.2020.101095. PMID: 32346500; PMCID: PMC7182760.
77. Northridge ME, Freeman L. Urban planning and health equity. *J Urban Health.* 2011;88(3):582–597. doi:10.1007/s11524-011-9558-5
78. Carmichael L, Townshend TG, Fischer TB, et al. Urban planning as an enabler of urban health: challenges and good practice in England following the 2012 planning and public health reforms. *Land Use Policy.* 2019;84:154–162. doi:10.1016/j.landusepol.2019.02.043
79. Guglielmin M, Muntaner C, O'Campo P, Shankardass K. A scoping review of the implementation of health in all policies at the local level. *Health Policy.* 2018;122(3):284–292. doi:10.1016/j.healthpol.2017.12.005
80. Sallis JF, Bull F, Burdett R, et al. Use of science to guide city planning policy and practice: how to achieve healthy and sustainable future cities. *Lancet.* Dec 10 2016;388(10062):2936–2947. doi:10.1016/s0140-6736(16)30068-x
81. Pineo H, Zimmermann N, Davies M. Integrating health into the complex urban planning policy and decision-making context: a systems thinking analysis. *Palgrave Commun.* 2020;6(1):21. doi:10.1057/s41599-020-0398-3
82. Braveman P, Egerter S, Williams DR. The social determinants of health: coming of age. *Annu Rev Public Health.* 2011;32(1):381–398. doi:10.1146/annurev-publhealth-031210-101218
83. Sarmiento OL, Díaz del Castillo A, Triana CA, Acevedo MJ, Gonzalez SA, Pratt M. Reclaiming the streets for people: insights from Ciclovías Recreativas in Latin America. *Prev Med.* 2017;103:S34–S40. doi:10.1016/j.ypmed.2016.07.028
84. World Health Organization. The Helsinki statement on Health in All Policies. 2013. Accessed February 26, 2020. https://www.who.int/publications/i/item/9789241506908
85. Shankardass K, Muntaner C, Kokkinen L, et al. The implementation of Health in All Policies initiatives: a systems framework for government action. *Health Res Policy Syst.* 2018;16(1):26. doi:10.1186/s12961-018-0295-z
86. Van Vliet-Brown CE, Shahram S, Oelke ND. Health in All Policies utilization by municipal

governments: scoping review. *Health Promot Int.* 2017;33(4):713–722. doi:10.1093/heapro/dax008

87. Resnicow K, Jackson A, Blissett D, et al. Results of the healthy body healthy spirit trial. *Health Psychol.* 2005;24(4):339–348.
88. Resnicow K, Campbell MK, Carr C, et al. Body and soul. A dietary intervention conducted through African-American churches. *Am J Prev Med.* Aug 2004;27(2):97–105.
89. Lancaster KJ, Carter-Edwards L, Grilo S, Shen C, Schoenthaler AM. Obesity interventions in African American faith-based organizations: a systematic review. *Obes Rev.* 2014;15)(suppl 4):159–176. doi:10.1111/obr.12207
90. Tristão Parra M, Porfírio GJM, Arredondo EM, Atallah Á N. Physical activity interventions in faith-based organizations: a systematic review. *Am J Health Promot.* Mar 2018;32(3):677–690. doi:10.1177/0890117116688107
91. Pinsker EA, Enzler AW, Hoffman MC, et al. A community-driven implementation of the Body and Soul Program in churches in the Twin Cities, Minnesota, 2011–2014. *Prev Chronic Dis.* 2017;14:E26–E26. doi:10.5888/pcd14.160386
92. Allicock M, Campbell MK, Valle CG, Carr C, Resnicow K, Gizlice Z. Evaluating the dissemination of Body & Soul, an evidence-based fruit and vegetable intake intervention: challenges for dissemination and implementation research. *J Nutr Educ Behav.* Nov–Dec 2012;44(6):530–538. doi:10.1016/j.jneb.2011.09.002
93. Allicock M, Johnson LS, Leone L, et al. Promoting fruit and vegetable consumption among members of black churches, Michigan and North Carolina, 2008–2010. *Prev Chronic Dis.* 2013;10:E33. doi:10.5888/pcd10.120161
94. Beard M, Chuang E, Haughton J, Arredondo EM. Determinants of implementation effectiveness in a physical activity program for church-going Latinas. *Fam Community Health.* Oct–Dec 2016;39(4):225–233. doi:10.1097/fch.0000000000000122
95. Maxwell AE, Danao LL, Cayetano RT, Crespi CM, Bastani R. Implementation of an evidence-based intervention to promote colorectal cancer screening in community organizations: a cluster randomized trial. *Transl Behav Med.* Jun 2016;6(2):295–305. doi:10.1007/s13142-015-0349-5
96. Klein KJ, Sorra JS. The challenge of innovation implementation. *Acad Manage Rev.* 1996;21(4):1055–1080. doi:10.2307/259164
97. Cherrington A, Ayala GX, Elder JP, Arredondo EM, Fouad M, Scarinci I. Recognizing the diverse roles of community health workers in the elimination of health disparities: from paid staff to volunteers. *Ethn Dis.* Spring 2010;20(2):189–194.
98. Maxwell AE, Lucas-Wright A, Santifer RE, Vargas C, Gatson J, Chang LC. Promoting cancer screening in partnership with health ministries in 9 African American churches in south Los Angeles: an implementation pilot study. *Prev Chronic Dis.* Sep 19 2019;16:E128. doi:10.5888/pcd16.190135
99. Holt CL, Tagai EK, Santos SLZ, et al. Web-based versus in-person methods for training lay community health advisors to implement health promotion workshops: participant outcomes from a cluster-randomized trial. *Transl Behav Med.* 2018;9(4):573–582. doi:10.1093/tbm/iby065
100. Arredondo EM, Elder JP, Haughton J, et al. Fe en Acción: promoting physical activity among churchgoing Latinas. *Am J Public Health.* Jul 2017;107(7):1109–1115. doi:10.2105/ajph.2017.303785
101. Arredondo EM, Haughton J, Montanez J. Scaling up and disseminating faith in action: discoveries from the sprint training. Symposium title: Transforming innovations into market-ready products: an entrepreneurial approach to D&I science. Proceedings from the 12th Annual Conference on the Science of Dissemination and Implementation. *Implement Sci.* 2020;15(1):25. doi:10.1186/s13012-020-00985-1
102. Alva ML, Hoerger TJ, Jeyaraman R, Amico P, Rojas-Smith L. Impact of the YMCA of the USA diabetes prevention program on Medicare spending and utilization. *Health Aff (Millwood).* 2017;36(3):417–424. doi:10.1377/hlthaff.2016.1307
103. Whittemore R. A systematic review of the translational research on the Diabetes Prevention Program. *Transl Behav Med.* 2011;1(3):480–491. doi:10.1007/s13142-011-0062-y
104. Haire-Joshu D, Hill-Briggs F. The next generation of diabetes translation: a path to health equity. *Annu Rev Public Health.* Apr 1 2019;40:391–410. doi:10.1146/annurev-publhealth-040218-044158
105. Economos CD, Anzman-Frasca S, Koomas AH, et al. Dissemination of healthy kids out of school principles for obesity prevention: a RE-AIM analysis. *Prev Med.* Feb 2019;119:37–43. doi:10.1016/j.ypmed.2018.12.007
106. National Association of County and City Health Officials. 2019 national profile of local health departments. 2020. Accessed August 23, 2020. https://www.naccho.org/uploads/downloadable-resources/Programs/Public-Health-Infrastructure/NACCHO_2019_Profile_final.pdf
107. Brownson RC, Fielding JE, Maylahn CM. Evidence-based public health: a fundamental

concept for public health practice. *Annu Rev Public Health.* Apr 21 2009;30:175–201. doi:10.1146/annurev.publhealth.031308.100134

108. Yancey AK, Fielding JE, Flores GR, Sallis JF, McCarthy WJ, Breslow L. Creating a robust public health infrastructure for physical activity promotion. *Am J Prev Med.* Jan 2007;32(1):68–78. doi:10.1016/j.amepre.2006.08.029
109. Leider JP, Coronado F, Beck AJ, Harper E. Reconciling supply and demand for state and local public health staff in an era of retiring baby boomers. *Am J Prev Med.* 2018;54(3):334–340. doi:10.1016/j.amepre.2017.10.026
110. Eyler AA, Valko C, Ramadas R, Macchi M, Fershteyn Z, Brownson RC. Administrative evidence-based practices in state chronic disease practitioners. *Am J Prev Med.* 2018;54(2):275–283. 10.1016/j.amepre.2017.09.006
111. Roussos ST, Fawcett SB. A review of collaborative partnerships as a strategy for improving community health. *Annu Rev Public Health.* 2000;21:369–402. doi:10.1146/annurev.publhealth.21.1.369
112. Ortiz K, Nash J, Shea L, et al. Partnerships, processes, and outcomes: a health equity-focused scoping meta-review of community-engaged scholarship. *Annu Rev Public Health.* Apr 2 2020;41:177–199. doi:10.1146/annurev-publhealth-040119-094220
113. Rabin BA, Glasgow RE, Kerner JF, Klump MP, Brownson RC. Dissemination and implementation research on community-based cancer prevention: a systematic review. *Am J Prev Med.* Apr 2010;38(4):443–456. doi:10.1016/j.amepre.2009.12.035
114. McNulty M, Smith JD, Villamar J, et al. Implementation research methodologies for achieving scientific equity and health equity. *Ethn Dis.* 2019;29(suppl 1):83–92. doi:10.18865/ed.29.S1.83
115. Corbin JH, Jones J, Barry MM. What makes intersectoral partnerships for health promotion work? A review of the international literature. *Health Promot Int.* 2018;33(1):4–26.
116. Brownson RC, Kumanyika SK, Kreuter MW, Haire-Joshu D. Implementation science should give higher priority to health equity. *Implement Sci.* 2021;16(1):28. doi:10.1186/s13012-021-01097-0
117. McLoughlin GM, Wiedenman EM, Gehlert S, Brownson RC. Looking beyond the lamppost: population-level primary prevention of breast cancer. *Int J Environ Res Public Health.* 2020;17(23):8720.
118. Woodward EN, Singh RS, Ndebele-Ngwenya P, Melgar Castillo A, Dickson KS, Kirchner JE. A more practical guide to incorporating health equity domains in implementation determinant frameworks. *Implement Sci Commun.* 2021;2(1):61. doi:10.1186/s43058-021-00146-5
119. Knott CL, Bowie J, Mullins CD, et al. An approach to adapting a community-based cancer control intervention to organizational context. *Health Promot Pract.* Mar 2020;21(2):168–171. doi:10.1177/1524839919898209
120. Santos SL, Tagai EK, Scheirer MA, et al. Adoption, reach, and implementation of a cancer education intervention in African American churches. *Implement Sci.* Mar 14 2017;12(1):36. doi:10.1186/s13012-017-0566-z
121. Knott CL, Chen C, Bowie JV, et al. Cluster-randomized trial comparing organizationally tailored versus standard approach for integrating an evidence-based cancer control intervention into African American churches. *Transl Behav Med.* 2022 May;12(5):673–682.
122. Williams RM, Zhang J, Woodard N, Slade J, Santos SLZ, Knott CL. Development and validation of an instrument to assess institutionalization of health promotion in faith-based organizations. *Eval Program Plann.* Apr 2020;79:101781. doi:10.1016/j.evalprogplan.2020.101781
123. Scheirer MA, Santos SL, Tagai EK, et al. Dimensions of sustainability for a health communication intervention in African American churches: a multi-methods study. *Implement Sci.* Mar 28 2017;12(1):43. doi:10.1186/s13012-017-0576-x
124. Knott CL, Miech EJ, Slade J, Woodard N, Robinson-Shaneman BJ, Huq M. Evaluation of organizational capacity in the implementation of a church-based cancer education program. *Glob Implement Res Appl.* Mar 2022;2(1):22–33. doi:10.1007/s43477-021-00033-0
125. Mazzucca S, Arredondo EM, Hoelscher DM, et al. Expanding implementation research to prevent chronic diseases in community settings. *Annu Rev Public Health.* Apr 1 2021;42:135–158. doi:10.1146/annurev-publhealth-090419-102547
126. Kerner J, Elwood J, Sutcliffe S. Integrating science with service in cancer control: closing the gap between discovery and delivery. *Cancer Control.* 2010:85–100.

20

Dissemination and Implementation in Social Service Settings

ALICIA C. BUNGER, LISA A. JUCKETT, REBECCA LENGNICK-HALL, DANIELLE R. ADAMS, AND J. CURTIS MCMILLEN

INTRODUCTION

Social service systems are uniquely positioned to disseminate and implement (D&I) health prevention and intervention protocols given their mission to support vulnerable populations. Social service organizations deliver nonmedical services designed to improve social well-being, including the following:

- child maltreatment investigations and remediation efforts, including foster care, residential services, and adoption;
- juvenile justice services (delinquency prevention, services to offending children, juvenile detention, residential services);
- some adult justice services, such as probation, parole, and decarceration;
- economic empowerment or income transfer programs for the poor, such as (in the United States), Temporary Aid for Needy Families and the Supplemental Nutritional Assistance Program;
- some housing programs;
- home- and community-based services for older adults to keep older adults living in the community and out of institutionalized care facilities;
- services for victims of interpersonal violence;
- community-based behavioral health services for those with mental health and/or substance use challenges (private practice psychiatric and counseling services are often excluded).

Besides great diversity in services delivered and populations served, social service organizations also operate in different sectors (i.e., public, nonprofit, for profit). Historically, public governmental agencies delivered social services. However, in the 1970s and 1980s, responsibility for delivering public social services was devolved to private, nongovernmental organizations (NGOs) under the assumption that local organizations can serve their communities better than bureaucratic public agencies.[1] As a result, today's public social service agencies (e.g., child protection) typically contract with private social service organizations to provide services (serving funding and regulatory roles). Although most private social service organizations are not for profit, for-profit social service organizations are also increasing.[2] Therefore, social service organizations represent public, not-for-profit, and for-profit organizations, which often work together in regionalized networks.

Because of this mix of organizations, many interests, agendas, and stakeholders must be managed during implementation. At the same time, social service organizations are often underresourced. These complexities and constraints make it challenging to implement health prevention and intervention models that are not core to social service organizations' mission despite their potential to reach vulnerable groups. Therefore, work in this setting provides important lessons about implementing in some of the most challenging conditions. In this chapter, we discuss (1) why implementing health interventions in social

Alicia C. Bunger, Lisa A. Juckett, Rebecca Lengnick-Hall, Danielle R. Adams, and J. Curtis McMillen, *Dissemination and Implementation in Social Service Settings* In: *Dissemination and Implementation Research in Health.* Edited by: Ross C. Brownson, Graham A. Colditz, and Enola K. Proctor, Oxford University Press. © Oxford University Press 2023. DOI: 10.1093/oso/9780197660690.003.0020 service organizations can lead to improvements in community health, (2) the types of health interventions that can be implemented in social services, (3) the unique context of these organizations, and (4) the multifaceted strategies that are likely necessary for successful D&I. We illustrate these points with two case studies and conclude with future directions.

THE POTENTIAL OF DISSEMINATION AND IMPLEMENTATION OF HEALTH INTERVENTIONS IN SOCIAL SERVICES

Social service organizations provide health-related evidence-based practices (EBPs) or interventions to vulnerable populations in the communities where they live. These organizations typically reach groups impacted by poverty, racism, and other forms of oppression that are linked to disproportionately poor healthcare access and outcomes. Implementing high-quality health interventions in this setting can optimize the delivery of equitable care, particularly if interventions are tailored to the needs and preferences of groups who are highly susceptible to health disparities. Plus, providing evidence-based interventions that improve clients' health outcomes aligns with the missions of many social service systems.

Another Primary Care

For many people deeply involved in social services, the professional most primary to them—chief in importance, most frequently encountered, and first seen in a sequence of help-seeking behaviors—is a social service caseworker. In some instances, the social services case manager serves as the official gatekeeper to other services, including medical care.[3] In these settings, social services case managers can be thought of as a primary care provider, a term usually reserved for a patient's first-line physician. The combination of frequent contact and high levels of client impairment gives social services case managers roles with strong influence. Ideally, these workers know their clients and the contexts in which they live and often serve clients who may not access care without social service workers' assistance.

High Need

Social service clients often possess attributes that put them at high risk for health problems that could be addressed within or outside of the social service system. Decades of research on the social determinants of health suggest that low-income/social position and early life adversity often interact to impact health problems. Health improves incrementally as income/social position rises, and health decreases incrementally as the number of adversities experienced increases.[4] Especially for groups that have been historically marginalized and structurally excluded, these health issues are compounded.[5] Social service sectors are often tasked with remediating or preventing determinants of poor health.

The interplay between socioeconomic indicators, adversity, and health is complex, dynamic, and interactive.[6,7] Both adversity and low-income/social position can affect diet, sleep, unfavorable work conditions for the employed, and acceptance of risky behaviors such as smoking, firearm possession, and heavy substance use. Cumulatively, these risk factors contribute to what many researchers call the biological "wear and tear" of chronic stress on the body, as evidenced by a raft of indicators with health consequences, including pro-inflammation responses,[8] high blood pressure,[9] problematic cholesterol profiles,[10] insulin resistance,[11] obesity,[12,13] gut biome issues,[14] and shortened telomere length,[15] a marker of cellular aging. Each of these processes, pathways, and markers is a potential target for clinical intervention within and external to social service systems of care.

Literature on social service clients' health needs is underdeveloped, segmented by service system, and largely hidden from traditional literature searches in government reports. However, literature on older youth in foster care and older adults receiving home- and community-based services (e.g., home-delivered meals, personal care assistance) might be exemplary. Estimates are that 35% of these youth are obese[16]; cigarette smoking is twice as common as among other teens,[17] and rates of past-year major depression for foster youth[18] are three times as high as that of other youth.[19] Further, compared to the general older adult population, significantly higher proportions of home- and community-based service recipients report feeling depressed (14% vs. 28%),[20] have a history of falling (25% vs. 41%),[21] and live in unsafe housing conditions (10% vs. 24%).[20] Though applicable to only two distinct subgroups of social service clients, these statistics portray the high need for evidence-based interventions that should be implemented to reduce health disparities in the social service setting.

Alignment

Health is generally not the primary reason social service sectors exist. Still, the D&I of evidence-supported health interventions might help social service agencies fulfill their functions. The ways health concerns and service organizational mission align will differ for each system. We offer several examples. Income assistance programs help clients budget their meager means to last through the month. Therefore, they may want to help their clients stop smoking so that provided financial assistance goes further. A program that prevents falls aligns with the mission of an agency that provides in-home services to prevent the need for more costly, institutionalized care. Juvenile justice programs might be deeply invested in substance abuse prevention.

For social service organizations to adopt health-related EBPs, they may also need to be convinced that funding schemes align with their interests and mission, with service sectors preferring to cost shift when possible. Medicaid, an entitled benefit, often becomes the preferred funder to avoid local or state battles over who should pay for a service that benefits social service consumers. Much of child welfare, mental health, and substance use services, for example, are billed to Medicaid.[22] This is less of an option in juvenile justice, however, where a federal inmate exclusion clause does not allow Medicaid dollars to go to services for incarcerated youth.[23] Programs for older adults will want to cost shift to Medicare.

POTENTIAL INTERVENTIONS TO IMPLEMENT IN SOCIAL SERVICE SETTINGS

There is untapped potential to expand the reach of evidence-based health interventions to highly vulnerable groups and potentially improve equity by implementing them in social service organizations. These EBPs might target physical activity levels, healthy eating, food security, housing and transportation, the cessation or prevention of tobacco use, recidivism, safety, and chronic disease management.[24–26] To date, many health interventions implemented in social services involve complex protocols for multifaceted, difficult-to-treat conditions. Substance abuse, conduct disorder, depression, and post-traumatic stress disorder are common targets.[27] Given the position of social service organizations to reach populations with diverse and ever-changing needs, a first step is identifying innovations that *should* be implemented in social service contexts.

Some entities have established intervention repositories to increase awareness of known, health EBPs for social service organizations (Table 20.1). Many of these repositories have a system for rating the strength of the research evidence for each intervention to inform administrators and consumers about programs that may market themselves as evidence based when they are not. To date, these repositories have focused on interventions for use in juvenile justice, child welfare, mental health, and community long-term care services for older adults. Professionals working in other social service systems (e.g., housing, transportation) might need to rely on compilations of EBPs that can be adapted for their contexts and the unique needs of their communities. Recommendations for adaptation can be found in chapter 8 of this book.

THE UNIQUE CONTEXT OF SOCIAL SERVICE SETTINGS

Social service organizations deliver complex services, with scarce resources, under significant external pressure from communities, funders, and regulatory bodies.[28,29] We draw on Damschroder and colleagues' Consolidated Framework for Implementation Research (CFIR)[30] to discuss how outer and inner settings, individual (worker) characteristics, and intervention characteristics should be considered during implementation.

The Outer and Inner Settings

Social service organizations experience intense pressures from the "outer" policy, regulatory, funding, and community environments that influence the structure, processes, culture, and leadership in the "inner" setting of the organization. For instance, in a study of leaders from private social service organizations, Collins-Camargo and her colleagues identified over 500 unique external pressures.[31] Successful implementation in social services likely requires a deep understanding of how

TABLE 20.1 INTERVENTION REPOSITORIES FOR SOCIAL SERVICE ORGANIZATIONS

Repository Name	Intervention Types	Rating Systems
	General Social Services	
Social Programs That Work (https://evidencebasedprograms.org/)	Early childhood, unemployment, chronic health conditions, behavioral health, violence prevention, homelessness, education	Programs that have been shown in RCT studies to produce sizable, sustained benefits. It identifies programs as "top tier," "near top tier," and "suggestive tier" based on their level of evidence.
	Child Welfare	
California Evidence-Based Clearinghouse for Child Welfare (CEBC; http://www.cebc4cw.org)	Child welfare services, parent training, behavioral health, maltreatment prevention, support services	Rates the strength of the research evidence (on a 1–5 scale) and relevance to child welfare; includes programs that are not yet able to be rated.
Title IV-E Prevention Services Clearinghouse (https://preventionservices.abtsites.com/)	Behavioral health and parenting programs to prevent foster care placements	Categorizes interventions as well supported, supported, promising, or does not currently meet criteria based on study number and rigor.
	Home and Community-Based Care for Older Adults	
National Council on Aging (NCOA) (https://www.ncoa.org/evidence-based-programs)	Health promotion and disease prevention interventions for older adults	Includes if programs are demonstrated effective in at least one experimental or quasi-experimental study, have results published in a peer-reviewed journal, have been successfully implemented in at least one nonresearch site, and include dissemination products that are available to the public.
	Juvenile Justice	
Blueprints for Healthy Youth Development (https://www.blueprintsprograms.org/)	Programs that reduce youth antisocial behavior and promote a positive developmental pathway	Categorizes a small number of rigorously tested programs into "model" or "model plus" (with demonstrated efficacy and appropriate for large-scale implementation), and "promising" (requires further empirical evidence before they should be widely implemented).
U.S. Office of Juvenile Justice and Delinquency Prevention (https://www.ojjdp.gov/mpg/)	Juvenile justice, delinquency prevention, child protection and safety	Effective (supported by one or more studies), promising, or not effective.

these external pressures impose significant organizational constraints, the critical bridging factors that must be considered or could be leveraged to account for these outer and inner connections,[32,33] and implementation strategies tailored to this context.[34,35]

Funding and contract expectations influence the resources social service organizations have for implementation. Private social service organizations rely on contracts from public agencies that rarely cover the full cost of services and impose additional unfunded expectations.[36] Funding might also come from private foundation grants and philanthropy; however, these sources are usually time limited and focused on a particular program, which limits sustainability.[37] Most also restrict the amount of money organizations can use for overhead or administrative costs (including quality management, training, electronic case records system, and other implementation supports).[38] These limitations affect how organizations can invest in implementation.[39] While implementers might not be able to modify the funding environment,[40] funders could support the actual costs of implementation. Considering how social service organizations tend to receive less public and private funding when they are located in communities of color and with high poverty,[41,42] funders might also consider directing funds more strategically to target health disparities.

Regulatory pressures impose specific demands for how services are delivered, documented, and staffed.[31] For example, in the United States, the Family First Prevention Services Act permits child welfare agencies to use funding to implement behavioral health and parenting programs, but only those preapproved by the Prevention Services Clearinghouse. This policy is expected to increase implementation among child welfare agencies. However, as Mosley and her colleagues argued, linking policies and funding to the implementation of preapproved interventions could have unintended consequences.[35] Preferencing specific interventions could stifle locally developed interventions (without rigorous evaluation) and disadvantage small social service organizations with fewer resources. Considering how small social service organizations and locally developed programs often target culturally specific and historically oppressed groups, it could be argued that these regulations may widen service inequities. System-level approaches (used by policymakers, funders, accreditors, etc.) to implement and scale-up evidence-based interventions should consider these potential consequences and work locally to align with social service missions and values.[43]

Social service organizations also experience intense demands from the community. Many people use social services—while some are temporary clients, others are more long term and could benefit from evidence-based health interventions. Some social service consumers may also have less competence in daily living and organizational skills than some health protocols require. These clients might have fewer resources and have more comorbid health problems, making implementation more difficult. For instance, will a weight loss program work for a client on psychotropic medications known to lead to weight gain? Will a smoking cessation program work for a person with poor emotion regulation? Will a chronic disease management program work for a client who is homeless for weeks at a time? These complexities may require substantial program adaptations, like adding assessments for readiness or motivational interviewing to intervention protocols, using materials that need less literacy, or parsing the intervention into less complicated processes. Since social service organizations serve diverse racial and ethnic communities, health interventions might also need to be linguistically and culturally adapted to enhance their acceptability, appropriateness, and effectiveness. Some of the adaptations might be uncovered through input from engaged clients and providers who represent the groups (e.g., racial/ethnic, geographic) being targeted as part of intervention implementation.[44]

Considering how social service organizations deliver services within networks, interorganizational relationships also shape implementation (referred to as *cosmopolitanism* in CFIR). These relationships are conduits for new evidence-based interventions and implementation support and may even exert "peer pressure" to adopt innovations.[45,46] Social service organizations might need to collaborate to implement an EBP, particularly those that link services across systems or specialties.[47–49] Because interorganizational relationships can increase pressure and provide implementation support, strategies that build or leverage these relationships could be useful in social service settings. Building relationships with culturally specific organizations (which meet the needs of a particular ethnic or cultural group), or those physically located in communities of color might also have the potential to expand the reach of evidence-based health interventions into diverse communities. These organizations tend to have close connections and trust with groups that are marginalized, but are often not well connected or integrated into local health and human service networks.[50,51]

Social service organizations respond to these complex pressures in many ways, and the outer and inner settings can vary on every possible dimension. Social service organizations tend to be high-stress environments and might not prioritize health intervention implementation as highly if they are not aligned with their mission.[52] Without strong leadership and supervision, it might be challenging to generate a strong culture and climate for implementation among front-line professionals.[53] Strategies that build buy-in, leadership capacity, supervisory skills, and technical assistance (TA) are important.

Individual (Worker) Characteristics

Social service professionals' training, skills, and experiences vary widely. Some positions require doctoral-level training, while others are open to those without a secondary school diploma. Staff might not have prior healthcare training, so implementing health interventions likely requires trainings and materials that meet a range of educational needs.[54] Staff turnover in social service organizations due to high caseloads, occupational stress, and low wages is common and can threaten implementation and sustainment. Social service caseworkers who are overworked might not be good candidates for implementation. However, some evidence suggests that training in EBPs, when combined with supportive coaching and monitoring, may reduce staff turnover.[55] This suggests that implementation strategies that improve workplace conditions might help social service organizations implement successfully; yet, just as health interventions should be tailored to the needs and preferences of target populations, strategies to support intervention implementation could be tailored to their target providers as well. Involving individuals who are representative of the social service provider workforce should be a key component of implementation strategy development in the social service system.[56] Developing implementation strategies that are responsive to the needs of social service providers can optimize strategy effectiveness and build providers' capacity for delivering evidence-based interventions, thereby improving the quality of social services provided to high-risk groups.

Intervention Characteristics

Rogers's diffusion of innovation theory proposed that innovations with greater *relative advantage*, *compatibility*, *trialability*, and *observability*, along with less *complexity*, will be adopted over innovations that do not.[57] Interventions implemented in social services tend to be complex, challenging the most robust implementation strategies. *Treatment Foster Care–Oregon*, for example, is an intervention that is delivered 24 hours per day, 7 days per week, and 365 days per year in teams of six program staff, plus foster parents, serving 10 clients at a time. These interventions require intense training and substantial consultation. The trialability of this kind of intervention is exceptionally low. The compatibility of a protocol with social service agency settings and mission may be just as important in the adoption decision.[58] Considering how social service organizations often reach marginalized communities with unique needs, the interventions might need to be further adapted to be more compatible with cultural practices or beliefs.

These interventions and the multifaceted implementation strategies can be costly since ongoing training and quality assurance are typically required. For organizations that successfully implement these interventions, mounting less complex protocols, like smoking cessation programs, might be easier than for other organizations. However, organizations that attempt implementation and fail might be hesitant to implement a less complex protocol.

Complex, expensive interventions that are difficult to trial require substantial competitive advantage and high observability for adoption. Right now, organizations might experience a substantial competitive advantage just by advertising their EBP,[46] considering low uptake among other organizations. Over time, however, documented improved outcomes will likely be required to sustain these programs.

APPROACHES TO IMPLEMENTATION IN SOCIAL SERVICE ORGANIZATIONS

Approaches to program implementation vary widely in social service organizations given their diversity and complexity. Strong support and multifaceted strategies are often needed. Below, we provide examples of common implementation approaches (e.g., strategies) that might be useful for social service organizations considering their complex contextual constraints.

Intermediary and Purveyor Organizations

Intermediary and purveyor organizations (IPOs) help support implementation by introducing needed external support, technical knowledge, and expertise. Broadly defined, IPOs disseminate and/or implement specific EBPs by engaging in consultation activities, training, quality improvement, outcome evaluation, and policy development.[59] While some programs have an IPO available to support program implementation (especially in behavioral healthcare) (e.g., Children and Family Futures is the purveyor for the sobriety treatment and recovery teams, START model), this is not the case for many other evidence-based health interventions. Moreover, it remains unclear which specific IPO activities (e.g., consultation; training) are most effective for improving implementation outcomes.[60] Nonetheless, since social service organizations might not have the in-house technical knowledge or infrastructure to support implementation, bringing in external support from an IPO could support implementation in this setting, although it likely comes with a cost.

Technical Assistance Tools and Resources

Some groups have developed TA tools and resources to support implementation in social service organizations. The Administration for Community Living (ACL) is a federal organization that provides leadership and support to its network of professionals who serve older adults and individuals living with disabilities. The ACL funds resource centers that provide TA to individual professionals and organizations implementing evidence-based innovations. Tools and assistance include its national clearinghouse for EBP (e.g., chronic disease management programs), training for providers on program delivery, and support for service/program development. While the ACL's resource centers are available to the public, some were developed to support organizations funded through the ACL's competitive grant programs. Systematic evaluations are needed to determine the association between ACL resources and measurable improvements in implementation and sustainment. However, providing public (and free) tools and resources could be a useful, practical, and cost-efficient way to support social service organizations exploring new interventions and preparing for implementation.

Community-Based Learning Collaboratives

Learning collaboratives are commonly used to train and support systems and/or organizations as they learn, implement, and sustain EBPs. Learning collaboratives bring multidisciplinary organizational teams together (comprising front-line providers, supervisors, and leaders) to foster shared learning through learning sessions, small tests of change, and expert coaching.[61–63] Community-based learning collaboratives (CBLCs) include other agencies, municipalities, and/or neighborhoods collaborating with social service organizations to deliver care. CBLCs are purposely structured to foster interprofessional collaboration, shared trust, and information sharing among members, who include clinicians, leaders, and brokers (i.e., ones who make referrals to necessary services).[64] CBLCs have been successful in increasing social service agencies' completion of training programs, leading to improvements in clinicians' implementation of EBPs, particularly in agencies providing trauma-specific services to children and families.[65] Learning collaboratives and CBLCs are time and resource intensive, but have the potential to support intervention scale-up within regional systems and engage partners that social service organizations depend on to deliver care.

CASE STUDIES

Next, we present two case studies that illustrate implementation challenges and strategies in social service organizations. The first case describes implementation of Safe Care, a parent training program, in community based family service organizations.

The second case describes implementation of The Stopping Elderly Accidents, Deaths, and Injuries (STEADI) algorithm, a tool for identifying older adults at risk of falls, in home and community-based service organizations. These cases vary by social service system setting, intervention complexity, implementation determinants, strategies, and the degree to which the interventions are currently disseminated.

Case Study 20.1: Implementing Safe Care in Community-Based Family Service Organizations

Background. About 1 billion children globally have experienced some form of child maltreatment (physical abuse, sexual abuse, emotional abuse, neglect).[66] Child maltreatment can lead to serious immediate and long-term health conditions. Effective parent training interventions have potential to reduce child maltreatment and improve children's long-term well-being since problematic parenting behavior is one of the most common risks for maltreatment.[67]

Health Intervention. SafeCare© is an evidence-based parent training program for parents of children ages 0 to 5. SafeCare providers work with families in their homes, but this can be modified for delivery in a community or virtual setting if needed (e.g., the family is experiencing homelessness; pandemic restrictions). There are three structured modules. In the parent-child/parent-infant interaction module, caregivers learn how to create safe and stable relationships with their children. This includes developing skills to engage in enriching daily activities with their children, minimize difficult child behaviors, and increase positive interactions. In the safety module, caregivers create a safe physical environment by childproofing their homes and learning how to appropriately supervise their children. The health module equips caregivers with the knowledge and skills to identify and address common childhood illnesses and injuries. Typically, the modules are completed in 18 one-hour sessions. SafeCare can be integrated with other services, such as case management, substance use treatment, and more. The length, frequency, and order of the sessions depend on the needs and preferences of the family, but weekly sessions are recommended. Caregivers must meet skill-based criteria before moving on to the next module.[68]

The intervention providers are individuals who have been trained and maintained certification in SafeCare. There are no specific educational requirements, although typical providers are bachelor's degrees trained with some child welfare or social service experience. Initial training is a 4-day, classroom-based or virtual workshop. Afterward, providers are matched with SafeCare coaches, who review and rate audio-recorded client sessions for fidelity. Providers must achieve 85% session fidelity to pass. This fidelity monitoring continues monthly for 2 years, then decreases to quarterly. SafeCare coaches and trainers also go through a training and certification process that is tailored to those roles. SafeCare training, adaptation, and site-level accreditation are currently housed within the National SafeCare Training and Research Center (NSTRC), which is part of the Mark Chaffin Center for Child Development at Georgia State University's School of Public Health (Atlanta, GA, USA).

Implementation Determinants. One key facilitator for SafeCare implementation is the significant amount of published research evidence supporting its effectiveness. Over 40 years, SafeCare has been tested using multiple designs (e.g., randomized controlled trials [RCTs], single-case research, and mixed-methods implementation designs).[69] Notably, most quasi-experimental and RCTs on SafeCare have been conducted with families involved with child protective services. A large, empirical evidence base can be a critical factor in resource-constrained social service settings where policymakers and organizational leaders must justify funding decisions and provide a compelling rationale for choosing a particular EBP. Another key facilitator is SafeCare's adaptability. SafeCare has been adapted in many ways: the way it is delivered (e.g., using virtual delivery during the COVID-19 pandemic),[70] module content and structure,[71] cultural adaptations,[72,73] systematic braiding with other interventions,[74] and use in new geographic areas (e.g., Australia[75]). The adaptability of an intervention may be particularly important in social service settings given the diversity of organizational, provider, and client needs. A third facilitator is having SafeCare guidance, training, and monitoring at the NSTRC. The NSTRC is the international hub for SafeCare providers and disseminates information and SafeCare updates (e.g., curriculum changes) across sites. Finally, NSTRC's implementation model allows agency and site-level trainers to train new staff, which enables agencies and sites to sustain and expand SafeCare independently. Several large successful implementations have been running for years under this model (Oklahoma; San Diego County, CA; Colorado).

SafeCare implementation faces several barriers, including the time it takes (which is likely not billable) for home visitors, coaches, and trainers to achieve and maintain certification. The structure of SafeCare modules may also be an obstacle for providers who are less familiar with structured EBPs or EBPs in general. A third barrier may be the cost and administrative effort associated with SafeCare site-level accreditation, discussed next. Additional costs or unbillable hours can be challenging for social service organizations that rely on tight, time-limited, and regulated funding streams.

Implementation Strategies. Site-level accreditation may be viewed as an implementation and scale-up strategy. Accreditation allows program developers to track and preserve implementation quality across sites over time and allows funders to have confidence that agencies are delivering a model with fidelity. To achieve site-level accreditation, eligible agencies must demonstrate compliance with SafeCare implementation standards that are reviewed and approved annually by the NSTRC. As part of the accreditation process, the NSTRC offers access to data systems, curricular updates, SafeCare publications, marketing materials, and the opportunity for consultation. The cost for accreditation varies by agency size but starts at $2,000 per agency. Sites with many agencies supported by a common implementation center are often bundled together for a discount.

Two other implementation strategies that have been studied in the context of SafeCare implementation are the dynamic adaptation process (DAP) and the interagency collaborative teams (ICT) model. With DAP, implementation resource teams were created to guide SafeCare adaptations in a planned way that preserves model fidelity.[73,76] In the ICT model, an interagency "seed team" was created, and it members became experts in SafeCare; this seed team trained and supported additional interagency implementation teams.[77]

Outcomes. Clinical, implementation, and service outcomes have been evaluated for SafeCare. Clinical outcomes include family behavior changes like those related to safety hazards at home,[78] parenting stress,[79] and caregiver mental health symptoms.[80] Key implementation outcomes studied in relation to SafeCare are adoption, fidelity, and sustainment.[81,82] Other outcomes include whether the benefits outweigh the costs, child welfare recidivism, permanency (children are safely maintained in their homes whenever possible), and job turnover.[83,84]

Case Study 20.2: Implementing the STEADI Toolkit

Background. Falls are the leading cause of injury and injury-related death among older adults in the United States.[85,86] While effective fall prevention programs and interventions are supported by nearly three decades of high-quality research,[87–89] falls continue to impact nearly 13 million older adults—age 65 and over—each year.[90] One group with an extremely high prevalence of fall risk factors includes adults who receive home- and community-based services (HCBSs).[21,91] HCBSs are health and/or social services that delay or prevent the need for hospitalization or institutionalized care. HCBSs are coordinated through local social service agencies, and common services include home-delivered meals, personal care assistance, nutrition counseling, transportation assistance, and homemaking services. Despite the prevalent nature of fall risk factors among HCBS recipients, HCBS agencies are seldom involved in fall prevention care,[92] underscoring a missed opportunity for HCBS staff to evaluate the fall risk needs of clients and assist with coordinating referrals to fall prevention interventions.

Health Intervention. The Stopping Elderly Accidents, Deaths, and Injuries (STEADI) algorithm[93,94] is a decision-support tool to assist care providers in identifying older adults at risk for falling and establishing a fall prevention care plan. The STEADI algorithm was originally developed by the Centers for Disease Control and Prevention (CDC) and is the only federally endorsed fall prevention decision-support tool in the United States. It consists of three components: (1) fall risk screening, (2) in-depth fall risk assessment, and (3) fall prevention interventions or referrals. Though initially developed for use in primary care, the STEADI algorithm has also been adapted and implemented in emergency departments,[95] inpatient care facilities,[96] and community pharmacies,[97] but has yet to be adopted in the HCBS setting.

Implementation Determinants and Strategies. Despite the potential value of using the STEADI algorithm in the HCBS setting, there are factors at every level of the system that influence implementation.[98] One large HCBS agency in the Midwest region of the United States was interested in implementing the STEADI algorithm. Staff, administrators, and research partners from this agency identified several determinants that they would need to address. First, they would need to identify available resources and address frontline workers' knowledge and beliefs about falls. The CDC's curated collection of publicly available tools and resources (https://www.cdc.gov/steadi/index.html) addresses both of these issues. These resources include printable handouts and brochures, training videos, screening tools, and customizable care plans. For instance, publicly available fall risk screening tools may overcome challenges HCBS staff face when trying to identify low-cost screens that are appropriate to implement with older adults. Further, training videos and educational materials/handouts may improve staff's knowledge and beliefs toward implementing fall risk screens, assessments, and interventions with HCBS clients. Second, fall risk screens used to identify HCBS clients at risk for falling would need to be compatible with the resources of the agency and the skills of HCBS staff. To address this challenge, HCBS leaders established a community-research partnership with a local university, identified a list of valid and reliable fall risk screening tools, and selected the one tool perceived to be most compatible with agency resources as perceived by staff. Third, clients identified as a "fall risk" would need to be connected to a fall prevention intervention or service that a client could feasibly access (requiring interorganizational collaborations). By partnering with the state Fall Prevention Coalition, agency staff were able to identify local fall prevention resources and services designed to attenuate fall risk. Last, as there are currently few incentives for HCBS agencies to implement the STEADI algorithm, additional funding lines would help support implementation efforts, prompting the HCBS agency to apply for a 3-year program grant through the Administration for Community Living, which is the federal agency that oversees evidence-based programming implemented with HCBS reicpients.

Outcomes and Future Directions. The staff and administrators at the HCBS agency used these strategies to implement components of the STEADI algorithm. As of June 2020, agency staff implemented standardized fall risk screening questions with 67% of eligible clients. In cases where screens were not implemented with clients, agency staff reported challenges reaching clients via phone (as all in-home screening encounters were restricted given COVID-19 protocols). Additionally, in late 2021, agency staff secured funding from their state Unit on Aging and received reimbursement for every fall risk screen completed with an HCBS client. Going forward, the agency has identified two evidence-based fall prevention programs—endorsed by the National Council on Aging—they plan to implement directly in clients' homes to offset challenges with accessing other fall prevention programs only available in community-based spaces (e.g., senior centers, health clinics).

DIRECTIONS FOR FUTURE RESEARCH

Implementing health interventions in social service organizations has the potential to reach some of the most vulnerable populations. However, five critical questions remain unanswered. First, *to what degree are health interventions delivered by social service organizations?* What types of interventions are implemented? Does implementing health interventions in social service organizations enhance healthcare availability and accessibility? Second, *how compatible are health intervention and prevention protocols with social service settings?* Given the competing demands in health work in the social services, how acceptable are these interventions to social service stakeholders? How are health concerns prioritized among other demands, including behavioral health? Are adoption and uptake rates of these interventions like those found in other settings? What motivates social service organizations to implement health interventions? How do different funding streams, regulations, mandates, and incentives impact the implementation of health interventions in these settings?

Third, *are intervention and prevention protocols designed for other settings effective when implemented in social service settings?* How feasible is it to implement health programs in social service settings? (This question underscores the need for research studies with hybrid designs that examine implementation and effectiveness; see chapter 14). What adaptations are needed to improve fit in social services? With the unique needs of the communities served? Does implementing health interventions in social services impact the outcomes of most interest to social service administrators? How might interventions need to be adapted to promote the implementation of equitable care for vulnerable communities? Does implementing health interventions in this setting reduce health inequities?

Fourth, given the complexity of the context, *what implementation strategies are most effective in social service organizations, and what are the active ingredients*? Given some of the difficulties of bringing complex interventions into resource-constrained settings, social services' implementation strategies tend to be multifaceted, multiphased efforts. The resource scarcity of social service settings makes it all the more important to know what components of these interventions are the most important for successful implementation. Are these strategies effective for implementing in other systems? Can the lessons learned about achieving fidelity to the STEADI algorithm in home visiting settings be applied to medical settings?

Fifth, *how are social service agencies funding the delivery and implementation of evidence-supported health interventions*? How do organizational leaders consider the costs amid the demand for an intervention (e.g., market viability)?[99] What funding streams are being used? Are they negotiating for new billing codes from Medicaid? Are they sustaining grant-funded efforts after the initial funding period? How are social service agencies funding the planning, training, and implementation supports needed to mount and sustain these complex interventions?

SUMMARY

Social service organizations are highly diverse and complex. This requires careful consideration in designing D&I strategies. However, social services' ability to access vulnerable populations with health problems may prove vital in improving the health status of many of our citizens and reducing health disparities. While several well-developed, blended implementation strategies are being used in social services, they all require additional documentation, research, and field experience. Nonetheless, the lessons learned in the social services may help organizations in other systems better implement health interventions with complex consumers in complex settings.

ACKNOWLEDGMENTS

We are grateful to Dr. Daniel Whitaker and Dr. Shannon Self-Brown, National SafeCare Training and Research Center co-directors.

SUGGESTED READINGS AND WEBSITES

Readings

Administration and Policy in Mental Health and Mental Health Services Research. 2016:43(6). Special Issue: System-level implementation of evidence-based practice. Special issue editors: Byron J. Powell and Rinad S. Beidas.

This special issue provides insight into how implementation science is applied in social services across a range of topic areas and contexts.

Human Service Organizations: Management, Leadership, & Governance. 2019:43(4). Special Issue: The future of human service organizational & management research. Special issue editors: Bowen McBeath and Karen Hopkin.

This special issue provides an overview of critical organizational and management practice challenges within social service agencies and needed future research emphases.

Human Service Organizations: Management, Leadership, & Governance.

Ongoing Section: Points of view from human service leaders. Section editors: Karen Hopkins and Bowen McBeath.

This Q&A provides an essential space for prominent organizational leaders to reflect on their experiences, leadership and civic efforts, and thoughts about the future of human services—including the impact of COVID-19 on leadership behaviors.

Selected Theories

Consolidated Framework for Implementation Research (CFIR).

Damschroder LJ, Aron DC, Keith RE, Kirsh SR, Alesander JA Lowery JC. Fostering implementation of health services research findings into practice: a consolidated framework for advancing implementation science. *Implement Sci.* 2009;4:50–65.

This influential integrative article provides practitioners and researchers a useful framework for thinking through some of the issues they might confront when taking on a D&I project in social services.

To view an example of how the CFIR can be applied to a social service setting, see Van Deinse TB, Bunger A, Burgin S, Wilson AB, Cuddeback GS. Using the consolidated framework for implementation research to examine implementation determinants of specialty mental health probation. *Health & Justice.* 2019;7(1):1–12.

The Policy Ecology Framework.

Raghavan R, Bright CL, Shadoin AL. Toward a policy ecology of implementation of evidence-based practices in public mental health settings. *Implement Sci.* 2008;3(1):1–9.

The Policy Ecology Framework expands on the CFIR's "outer context" domain proposing four levels that comprise the broader context of EBP implementation: organizational context, regulatory or purchaser agency, political context, and social context.

To view an example of how the Policy Ecology Framework can be applied to a social service system, see Powell BJ, Beidas RS, Rubin RM, et al. Applying the policy ecology framework to Philadelphia's behavioral health transformation efforts. *Admin Policy Ment Health Ment Health Serv Res.* 2016;43(6):909–926.

Organizational Theory

Birken SA, Bunger AC, Powell BJ, et al. Organizational theory for dissemination and implementation research. *Implement Sci.* 2017;12(1):1–5.

Organizational theories can help researchers describe, explain, and predict implementation within social service agencies and strengthen implementation studies by addressing the complex interactions between organizations and their environment.

To view an example of how four organizational theories can be applied to an intervention (SafeCare) deployed in a social service setting, see the Birken et al. article above.

Selected Websites and Tools

Blueprints for Healthy Youth Development. http://www.colorado.edu/cspv/blueprints

Blueprints for Healthy Youth Development is a project of the Center for the Study and Prevention of Violence at the University of Colorado and serves as a resource for violence and drug prevention programs designed to reduce youth antisocial behavior and promote a positive developmental pathway. It promotes the use of specific model programs with detailed program descriptions, introductory videos, and contact information.

California Evidence-Based Clearinghouse for Child Welfare. http://www.cebc4cw.org

The California Evidence-Based Clearinghouse for Child Welfare provides professionals access to information about the research evidence for programs being used or marketed. It rates programs on the strength of their evidence and their relevancy to child welfare populations and categorizes programs by content area.

Community Tool Box. http://ctb.ku.edu

The Community Tool Box was created by the Center for Community Health and Development at the University of Kansas; it is a well-organized website that offers numerous tools for community development activities, including participatory community assessment and evaluation. Find resources for assessing community needs and resources, addressing social determinants of health, engaging stakeholders, action planning, building leadership, improving cultural competency, planning an evaluation, and sustaining your efforts over time.

Evidence-Based Practices Resource Center. https://www.samhsa.gov/resource-search/ebp

The Evidence-Based Practices Resource Center is operated by SAMHSA and aims to provide communities, clinicians, policymakers, and others in the field with the information and tools they need to incorporate EBPs into their communities or clinical settings. The resource center contains a collection of scientifically based resources for a broad range of audiences, including treatment improvement protocols, toolkits, resource guides, clinical practice guidelines, and other science-based resources.

National American Indian and Alaska Native Mental Health Technology Transfer Center Network. https://mhttcnetwork.org/centers/national-american-indian-and-alaska-native-mhttc/home

The National American Indian and Alaska Native Mental Health Technology Transfer Center Network works with organizations and treatment practitioners involved in the delivery of mental health services to American Indian and Alaska Native (AI/AN) individuals, families and tribal and urban Indian communities to strengthen their capacity to deliver effective EBPs. It contains a repository of evidence-based mental health programs and practices found to be effective with AI/AN school-aged children and youth who experience adverse childhood experiences, including violence and trauma, that contribute to mental health problems.

National Implementation Research Network website. https://nirn.fpg.unc.edu/

The National Implementation Research Network website is designed to contribute to the best practices and science of implementation, organization change, and system reinvention to improve outcomes across the spectrum of human services. It provides a primer on implementation, topical reviews, and guidance on a range of implementation topics.

US Office of Juvenile Justice and Delinquency Prevention Model Programs Guide. https://www.ojjdp.gov/mpg/

The US Office of Juvenile Justice and Delinquency Prevention maintains a Model Programs Guide. It is designed as a resource for practitioners and communities about what works, what is promising, and what does not work in juvenile justice, delinquency prevention, and child protection and safety.

REFERENCES

1. Page S. What's new about the new public management? Administrative change in the human services. *Public Adm Rev.* 2005;65(6):713–727.
2. Mosley JE. Social Service nonprofits: navigating conflicting demands. In: Powell WW, Bromley P, eds. *The Nonprofit Sector: A Research Handbook.* 3rd ed. Stanford University Press; 2020:251–270.
3. Stiffman AR, Pescosolido B, Cabassa LJ. Building a model to understand youth service access: the gateway provider model. *Ment Health Serv Res.* 2004;6(4):189–198.
4. Hughes K, Bellis MA, Hardcastle KA, et al. The effect of multiple adverse childhood experiences on health: a systematic review and meta-analysis. *Lancet Public Health.* 2017;2(8):e356–e366. doi:10.1016/S2468-2667(17)30118-4
5. Williams DR, Lawrence JA, Davis BA. Racism and health: evidence and needed research. *Annu Rev Public Health.* 2019;40:105–125. doi:10.1146/annurev-publhealth-040218-043750
6. Braveman P, Gottlieb L. The social determinants of health: it's time to consider the causes of the causes. *Public Health Rep.* 2014;129(suppl 2):19–31. doi:10.1177/00333549141291S206
7. Shonkoff JP, Slopen N, Williams DR. Early childhood adversity, toxic stress, and the impacts of racism on the foundations of health. *Annu Rev Public Health.* 2021;42:115–134. doi:10.1146/ANNUREV-PUBLHEALTH-090419-101940
8. Baldwin JR, Arseneault L, Caspi A, et al. Childhood victimization and inflammation in young adulthood: a genetically sensitive cohort study. *Brain Behav Immun.* 2018;67:211–217. doi:10.1016/j.bbi.2017.08.025
9. Brummett BH, Babyak MA, Jiang R, et al. Systolic blood pressure and socioeconomic status in a large multi-study population. *SSM Popul Health.* 2019;9. doi:10.1016/j.ssmph.2019.100498
10. McClain AC, Gallo LC, Mattei J. Subjective social status and cardiometabolic risk markers by intersectionality of race/ethnicity and sex among US young adults. *Ann Behav Med.* May 2021;56(5):442–460. doi:10.1093/ABM/KAAB025
11. Subramanyam MA, Diez-Roux AV, Hickson DMA, et al. Subjective social status and psychosocial and metabolic risk factors for cardiovascular disease among African Americans in the Jackson Heart Study. *Soc Sci Med.* 2012;74(8):1146. doi:10.1016/J.SOCSCIMED.2011.12.042
12. Balasooriya NN, Bandara JS, Rohde N. The intergenerational effects of socioeconomic inequality on unhealthy bodyweight. *Health Econ.* 2021;30(4):729–747. doi:10.1002/HEC.4216
13. O'Neill A, Beck K, Chae D, Dyer T, He X, Lee S. The pathway from childhood maltreatment to adulthood obesity: the role of mediation by adolescent depressive symptoms and BMI. *J Adolesc.* 2018;67:22–30. doi:10.1016/J.ADOLESCENCE.2018.05.010
14. O'Mahony SM, Clarke G, Dinan TG, Cryan JF. Early-life adversity and brain development: is the microbiome a missing piece of the puzzle? *Neuroscience.* 2017;342:37–54. doi:10.1016/J.NEUROSCIENCE.2015.09.068
15. Price LH, Kao HT, Burgers DE, Carpenter LL, Tyrka AR. Telomeres and early-life stress: an overview. *Biol Psychiatry.* 2013;73(1):15. doi:10.1016/J.BIOPSYCH.2012.06.025
16. Steele JS, Buchi KF. Medical and mental health of children entering the Utah foster care system. *Pediatrics.* 2008;122(3):e703–709. doi:10.1542/PEDS.2008-0360
17. Vaughn MG, Ollie MT, McMillen JC, Scott L, Munson M. Substance use and abuse among older youth in foster care. *Addict Behav.* 2007;32(9):1929. doi:10.1016/J.ADDBEH.2006.12.012
18. McMillen JC, Zima BT, Scott LD, et al. Prevalence of psychiatric disorders among older youths in the foster care system. *J Am Acad Child Adolesc Psychiatry.* 2005;44(1):88–95. doi:10.1097/01.chi.0000145806.24274.d2
19. Reinherz HZ, Giaconia RM, Lefkowitz ES, Pakiz B, Frost AK. Prevalence of psychiatric disorders in a community population of older adolescents. *J Am Acad Child Adolesc Psychiatry.* 1993;32(2):369–377. doi:10.1097/00004583-199303000-00019
20. Thomas KS, Akobundu U, Dosa D. More than a meal? A randomized control trial comparing the effects of home-delivered meals programs on participants' feelings of loneliness. *J Gerontol B Psychol Sci Soc Sci.* 2016;71(6):1049–1058. doi:10.1093/GERONB/GBV111

21. Choi NG, Sullivan JE, Marti CN. Low-income homebound older adults receiving home-delivered meals: physical and mental health conditions, incidence of falls and hospitalisations. *Health Soc Care Community.* 2019;27(4):e406–e416. doi:10.1111/hsc.12741
22. Raghavan R, Inkelas M, Franke T, Halfon N. Administrative barriers to the adoption of high-quality mental health services for children in foster care: a national study. *Adm Policy Ment Health Ment Health Serv Res.* 2007;34(3):191–201. doi:10.1007/s10488-006-0095-6
23. Acoca L, Stephens J, van Vleet A. *Health Coverage and Care for Youth in the Juvenile Justic System: The Role of Medicaid and CHIP.* 2014. https://www.kff.org/medicaid/issue-brief/health-coverage-and-care-for-youth-in-the-juvenile-justice-system-the-role-of-medicaid-and-chip/
24. Ethier A, Carrier A. A scoping review of the implementation of local health and social services for older adults. *Healthc Policy.* 2021;17(2):105. doi:10.12927/HCPOL.2021.26654
25. Administration for Community Living. National resource centers. 2022. Accessed April 2, 2022. https://acl.gov/programs/strengthening-aging-and-disability-networks/national-resource-centers
26. Kinsky S, Maulsby CH, Jain KM, Charles V, Riordan M, Holtgrave DR. Barriers and facilitators to implementing access to HIV care interventions: a qualitative analysis of the positive charge initiative. *AIDS Educ Prev.* 2015;27(5):391–404. doi:10.1521/aeap.2015.27.5.391
27. Team AVE-BP. Evidence-based programs. https://www.arnoldventures.org/work/evidence-based-policy
28. Despard MR. Challenges in implementing evidence-based practices and programs in nonprofit human service organizations. *J Evid Inf Soc Work.* 2016;13(6):505–522. doi:10.1080/23761407.2015.1086719
29. Proctor E, Bunger A. Implementation science. *Encycl Soc Work.* July 2020. doi:10.1093/ACREFORE/9780199975839.013.1338
30. Damschroder LJ, Aron DC, Keith RE, Kirsh SR, Alexander JA, Lowery JC. Fostering implementation of health services research findings into practice: a consolidated framework for advancing implementation science. *Implement Sci.* 2009;4:50. doi:10.1186/1748-5908-4-50
31. Collins-Camargo C, Chuang E, McBeath B, Mak S. Staying afloat amidst the tempest: external pressures facing private child and family serving agencies and managerial strategies employed to address them. *Hum Serv Organ Manag Leadersh Gov.* 2019;43(2):125–145. doi:10.1080/23303131.2019.1606870
32. Lengnick-Hall R, Willging C, Hurlburt M, Fenwick K, Aarons GA, Aarons GA. Contracting as a bridging factor linking outer and inner contexts during EBP implementation and sustainment: a prospective study across multiple US public sector service systems. *Implement Sci.* 2020;15(1):1–16. doi:10.1186/s13012-020-00999-9
33. Lengnick-Hall R, Willging C, Hurlburt M, et al. Contracting as a bridging factor linking outer and inner contexts during EBP implementation and sustainment: a prospective study across multiple U.S. public sector service systems. *Implementation Sci.* 2020;15:43. https://doi.org/10.1186/s13012-020-00999-9
34. Bunger AC, Lengnick-Hall R. Implementation science and human service organizations research: opportunities and challenges for building on complementary strengths. *Hum Serv Organ Manag Leadersh Gov.* 2019;43(4, SI):258–268. doi:10.1080/23303131.2019.1666765
35. Mosley JE, Marwell NP, Ybarra M. How the "what works" movement is failing human service organizations, and what social work can do to fix it. *Hum Serv Organ Manag Leadersh Gov.* 2019;43(4):326–335. doi:10.1080/23303131.2019.1672598
36. Marwell NP, Calabrese T. A deficit model of collaborative governance: government-nonprofit fiscal relations in the provision of child welfare services. *J Public Adm Res Theory.* 2015;25(4):1031–1058. doi:10.1093/jopart/muu047
37. Rooney P, Frederick H. *Paying for Overhead: A Study of the Impact of Foundations' Overhead Payment Policies on Educational and Human Service Organizations.* 2007. Center on Philanthropy at Indiana University.
38. Gregory AG, Howard D. The nonprofit starvation cycle. *Stanford Soc Innov Rev.* 2009;7(4):49–53.
39. Bunger AC, Despard M, Lee M, Cao Y. The cost of quality: organizational financial health and program quality. *J Evid Inf Soc Work.* 2019;16(1):18–35. doi:10.1080/23761407.2018.1536575
40. Bruns EJ, Parker EM, Hensley S, et al. The role of the outer setting in implementation: associations between state demographic, fiscal, and policy factors and use of evidence-based treatments in mental healthcare. *Implement Sci.* 2019;14(1):1–13. doi:10.1186/s13012-019-0944-9
41. Garrow EE. Does race matter in government funding of nonprofit human service organizations? The interaction of neighborhood poverty and race. *J Public Adm Res Theory.* 2014;24(2):381–405. doi:10.1093/jopart/mus061
42. Paarlberg LE, McGinnis Johnson J, Hannibal B. Race and the public foundation grants marketplace: the differential effect of network status in communities of colour. *Public Manag Rev.*

2020;22(10):1443–1463. doi:10.1080/14719037.2019.1635192

43. Birken SA, Bunger AC, Powell BJ, et al. Organizational theory for dissemination and implementation research. *Implement Sci.* 2017;12(1):62. doi:10.1186/s13012-017-0592-x
44. Hasche LK, Lenze S, Brown T, et al. Adapting collaborative depression care for public community long-term care: using research-practice partnerships. doi:10.1007/s10488-013-0519-z
45. Valente TW. *Network Models of the Diffusion of Innovation.* Hampton Press; 1995. https://www.amazon.com/Diffusion-Innovations-Quantitative-Communication-Subseries/dp/1881303225
46. Proctor EK, Knudsen KJ, Fedoravicius N, Hovmand P, Rosen A, Perron B. Implementation of evidence-based practice in community behavioral health: agency director perspectives. *Adm Policy Ment Heal Ment Heal Serv Res.* 2007;34(5):479–488.
47. Bunger AC, Chuang E, Girth A, et al. Establishing cross-systems collaborations for implementation: protocol for a longitudinal mixed methods study. *Implement Sci.* 2020;15(1):55. doi:10.1186/s13012-020-01016-9
48. Gopalan G, Kerns SEU, Horen MJ, Lowe J. Partnering for success: factors impacting implementation of a cross-systems collaborative model between behavioral health and child welfare. *Adm Policy Ment Health Ment Health Serv Res.* 2021;48(5):839–856. doi:10.1007/S10488-021-01135-5/TABLES/1
49. Van Deinse TB, Bunger A, Burgin S, Wilson AB, Cuddeback GS. Using the Consolidated Framework for Implementation Research to examine implementation determinants of specialty mental health probation. *Health Justice.* 2019;7(1):17. doi:10.1186/s40352-019-0098-5
50. Maleku A, Kagotho N, Baaklini V, Filbrun C, Karandikar S, Mengo C. The human service landscape in the midwestern USA: a mixed methods study of human service equity among the new American population. *Br J Soc Work.* 2020;50(1):195–221. doi:10.1093/bjsw/bcz126
51. Brownson RC, Kumanyika SK, Kreuter MW, Haire-Joshu D. Implementation science should give higher priority to health equity. *Implement Sci.* 2021;16(1):1–16. doi:10.1186/s13012-021-01097-0
52. Wolk CB, Arnold KT, Proctor EK. Implementing evidence-based practices in nonspecialty mental health settings. *Fam Syst Heal.* January 2022;40(2):274–282. doi:10.1037/fsh0000506
53. Bunger AC, Birken SA, Hoffman JA, MacDowell H, Choy-Brown M, Magier E. Elucidating the influence of supervisors' roles on implementation climate. *Implement Sci.* 2019;14(1):1–12. doi:10.1186/s13012-019-0939-6
54. Cunningham N, Cowie J, Watchman K, Methven K. Understanding the training and education needs of homecare workers supporting people with dementia and cancer: a systematic review of reviews. *Dementia.* 2020;19(8):2780–2803. doi:10.1177/1471301219859781
55. Aarons GA, Sommerfeld DH, Hecht DB, Silovsky JF, Chaffin MJ. The impact of evidence-based practice implementation and fidelity monitoring on staff turnover: evidence for a protective effect. *J Consult Clin Psychol.* 2009;77(2):270–280.
56. Juckett LA, Bunck L, Thomas KS. The Older Americans Act 2020 reauthorization: overcoming barriers to service and program implementation. *Public Policy Aging Rep.* 2022;32(1):25–30. doi:10.1093/PPAR/PRAB032
57. Rogers E. *Diffusion of Innovations.* 4th ed. Free Press; 2010.
58. Beidas RS, Stewart RE, Adams DR, et al. A multilevel examination of stakeholder perspectives of implementation of evidence-based practices in a large urban publicly-funded mental health system. *Adm Policy Ment Health.* 2016;43(6):893–908. doi:10.1007/S10488-015-0705-2
59. Franks RP, Bory CT. Who supports the successful implementation and sustainability of evidence-based practices? Defining and understanding the roles of intermediary and purveyor organizations. *New Dir Child Adolesc Dev.* 2015;2015(149):41–56. doi:10.1002/CAD.20112
60. Proctor E, Hooley C, Morse A, McCrary S, Kim H, Kohl PL. Intermediary/purveyor organizations for evidence-based interventions in the US child mental health: characteristics and implementation strategies. *Implement Sci.* 2019;14(1):1–14. doi:10.1186/S13012-018-0845-3/TABLES/3
61. Bunger AC, Doogan N, Hanson RF, Birken SA. Advice-seeking during implementation: a network study of clinicians participating in a learning collaborative. *Implement Sci.* 2018;13(1):101. doi:10.1186/s13012-018-0797-7
62. Bunger AC, Hanson RF, Doogan NJ, Powell BJ, Cao Y, Dunn J. Can learning collaboratives support implementation by rewiring professional networks? *Adm Policy Ment Health.* 2016;43(1):79–92. doi:10.1007/s10488-014-0621-x
63. Nadeem E, Olin SS, Hill LC, Hoagwood KE, Horwitz SM. Understanding the components of quality improvement collaboratives: a systematic literature review. *Milbank Q.* 2013;91(2):354–394. doi:10.1111/milq.12016
64. Helseth SA, Peer SO, Are F, et al. Sustainment of trauma-focused and evidence-based practices

following learning collaborative implementation. *Adm Policy Ment Health Ment Health Serv Res.* 2020;47(4):569–580. doi:10.1007/s10488-020-01024-3
65. Hanson RF, Saunders BE, Ralston E, Moreland AD, Peer SO, Fitzgerald MM. Statewide implementation of child trauma-focused practices using the community-based learning collaborative model. *Psychol Serv.* 2019;16(1):170–181. doi:10.1037/ser0000319
66. Hillis S, Mercy J, Amobi A, Kress H. Global prevalence of past-year violence against children: a systematic review and minimum estimates. *Pediatrics.* 2016;137(3):e20154079. doi:10.1542/peds.2015-4079
67. Chen M, Chan KL. Effects of parenting programs onchildmaltreatmentprevention:ameta-analysis. *Trauma Violence Abuse.* 2016;17(1):88–104. doi:10.1177/1524838014566718
68. National SafeCare Training and Research Center. SafeCare model. February 7, 2022. Accessed February 7, 2022. https://safecare.publichealth.gsu.edu/safecare-curriculum/
69. Guastaferro K, Lutzker JR. A methodological review of SafeCare ®. *J Child Fam Stud.* 2019;28:3268–3285. doi:10.1007/s10826-019-01531-4
70. Self-Brown S, Reuben K, Perry EW, et al. The impact of COVID-19 on the delivery of an evidence-based child maltreatment prevention program: understanding the perspectives of SafeCare® providers. *J Fam Violence.* 2020:37:825–835. doi:10.1007/S10896-020-00217-6
71. Self-Brown S, Osborne MC, Lai BS, De Veauuse Brown N, Glasheen TL, Adams MC. Initial findings from a feasibility trial examining the SafeCare Dad to Kids program with marginalized fathers. *J Fam Violence.* 2017;32(8):751–766. doi:10.1007/S10896-017-9940-5
72. Mills AL, Lopez Mader L, Burke Lefever J, et al. Effects of a brief parenting intervention on latinx mothers and their children. *Fam Process.* December 2021;61(4):1437–1455. doi:10.1111/FAMP.12738
73. Whitaker DJ, Self-Brown S, Weeks EA, et al. Adaptation and implementation of a parenting curriculum in a refugee/immigrant community using a task-shifting approach: a study protocol. *BMC Public Health.* 2021;21(1):1–13. doi:10.1186/S12889-021-11148-2/PEER-REVIEW
74. Guastaferro K, Miller K, Lai BS, et al. Modification to a systematically braided parent-support curriculum: results from a feasibility pilot. *J Child Fam Stud.* 2019;28(7):1780–1789. doi:10.1007/S10826-019-01369-W
75. Albers B, Hateley-Browne J, Steele T, Rose V, Shlonsky A, Mildon R. The early implementation of FFT-CW®, MST-Psychiatric®, and SafeCare® in Australia. *Res Soc Work Pract.* 2020;30(6):658–677. doi:10.1177/1049731520908326
76. Aarons GA, Green AE, Palinkas LA, et al. Dynamic adaptation process to implement an evidence-based child maltreatment intervention. *Implement Sci.* 2012;7(1):1–9. doi:10.1186/1748-5908-7-32/FIGURES/1
77. Hurlburt M, Aarons GA, Fettes D, Willging C, Gunderson L, Chaffin MJ. Interagency collaborative team model for capacity building to scale-up evidence-based practice. *Child Youth Serv Rev.* 2014;39:160–168. doi:10.1016/j.childyouth.2013.10.005
78. Rogers-Brown JS, Self-Brown S, Romano E, Weeks E, Thompson WW, Whitaker DJ. Behavior change across implementations of the SafeCare model in real world settings. *Child Youth Serv Rev.* 2020;117(C):105284. doi:10.1016/J.CHILDYOUTH.2020.105284
79. Whitaker DJ, Self-Brown S, Hayat MJ, et al. Effect of the SafeCare© intervention on parenting outcomes among parents in child welfare systems: a cluster randomized trial. *Prev Med (Baltim).* 2020;138:106167. doi:10.1016/J.YPMED.2020.106167
80. Romano E, Gallitto E, Firth K, Whitaker D. Does the SafeCare parenting program impact caregiver mental health? *J Child Fam Stud.* 2020;29(9):2653–2665. doi:10.1007/S10826-020-01774-6/TABLES/5
81. Chaffin M, Hecht D, Aarons G, Fettes D, Hurlburt M, Ledesma K. EBT fidelity trajectories across training cohorts using the interagency collaborative team strategy. *Adm Policy Ment Health Ment Health Serv Res.* 2016;43(2):144–156. doi:10.1007/s10488-015-0627-z
82. Aarons GA, Green AE, Trott E, et al. The roles of system and organizational leadership in system-wide evidence-based intervention sustainment: a mixed-method study. *Adm Policy Ment Health Ment Health Serv Res.* 2016;43(6):991–1008. doi:10.1007/S10488-016-0751-4/TABLES/7
83. Whitaker DJ, Lyons M, Weeks EA, Hayat MJ, Self-Brown S, Zahidi R. Does adoption of an evidence-based practice lead to job turnover? Results from a randomized trial. *J Community Psychol.* 2020;48(4):1258–1272. doi:10.1002/JCOP.22305/
84. Chaffin M, Hecht D, Bard D, Silovsky JF, Beasley WH. A statewide trial of the SafeCare home-based services model with parents in child protective services. *Pediatrics.* 2012;129(3):509–515. doi:10.1542/PEDS.2011-1840

85. Bergen G, Stevens MR, Burns ER. Falls and fall injuries among adults aged ≥65 years—United States, 2014. *MMWR Morb Mortal Wkly Rep.* 2016;65(37):993–998. doi:10.15585/MMWR.MM6537A2
86. Florence CS, Bergen G, Atherly A, Burns E, Stevens J, Drake C. Medical costs of fatal and nonfatal falls in older adults. *J Am Geriatr Soc.* 2018;66(4):693–698. doi:10.1111/JGS.15304
87. Cheng P, Tan L, Ning P, et al. Comparative effectiveness of published interventions for elderly fall prevention: a systematic review and network meta-analysis. *Int J Environ Res Public Health.* 2018;15(3):498. doi:10.3390/IJERPH15030498
88. Choi M, Hector M. Effectiveness of intervention programs in preventing falls: a systematic review of recent 10 years and meta-analysis. *J Am Med Dir Assoc.* 2012;13(2):188.e13–188.e21. doi:10.1016/J.JAMDA.2011.04.022
89. Petridou ET, Manti EG, Ntinapogias AG, Negri E, Szczerbińska K. What works better for community-dwelling older people at risk to fall? A meta-analysis of multifactorial versus physical exercise-alone interventions. *J Aging Health.* 2009;21(5):713–729. doi:10.1177/0898264309338298
90. Haddad YK, Bergen G, Florence CS. Estimating the economic burden related to older adult falls by state. *J Public Health Manag Pract.* 2019;25(2):E17. doi:10.1097/PHH.0000000000000816
91. Casteel C, Jones J, Gildner P, Bowling JM, Blalock SJ. Falls risks and prevention behaviors among community-dwelling homebound and non-homebound older adults. *J Appl Gerontol.* 2018;37(9):1085–1106. doi:10.1177/0733464816672043
92. Juckett LA, Bunger AC, Bunck L, Balog EJ. Evaluating the implementation of fall risk management practices within home-delivered meal organizations. *J Gerontol Soc Work.* 2021;64(4):372–387. doi:10.1080/01634372.2021.1894521
93. Stevens JA. The STEADI Tool Kit: a fall prevention resource for health care providers. *IHS Prim Care Provid.* 2013;39(9):162.
94. Stevens JA, Phelan EA. Development of STEADI: a fall prevention resource for health care providers. *Health Promot Pract.* 2013;14(5):706–714. doi:10.1177/1524839912463576
95. Greenberg MR, Goodheart V, Jacoby JL, et al. Emergency Department Stopping Elderly Accidents, Deaths and Injuries (ED STEADI) program. *J Emerg Med.* 2020;59(1):1–11. doi:10.1016/J.JEMERMED.2020.04.019
96. Rogers S, Haddad YK, Legha JK, Stannard D, Auerbach A, Eckstrom E. CDC STEADI: Best Practices for Developing an Inpatient Program to Prevent Older Adult Falls after Discharge. Centers for Disease Control and Prevention; National Center for Injury Prevention and Control; 2021:1–39. Accessed January 13, 2023. https://www.cdc.gov/steadi/pdf/steadi-inpatient-guide-508.pdf
97. Blalock SJ, Ferreri SP, Renfro CP, et al. Impact of STEADI-Rx: a community pharmacy-based fall prevention intervention. *J Am Geriatr Soc.* 2020;68(8):1778–1786. doi:10.1111/JGS.16459
98. Bobitt J, Schwingel A. Evidence-based programs for older adults: a disconnect between US national strategy and local senior center implementation. *J Aging Soc Policy.* 2016;29(1):3–19. doi:10.1080/08959420.2016.1186465
99. Proctor EK, Toker E, Tabak R, McKay VR, Hooley C, Evanoff B. Market viability: a neglected concept in implementation science. *Implement Sci.* 2021;16(1):1–8. doi:10.1186/s13012-021-01168-2

21

Implementation Science in Healthcare

ALISON B. HAMILTON AND ARLEEN BROWN

INTRODUCTION

For over two decades, healthcare implementation science as a distinct field has contributed many advances in clinical care, as well as valuable theories and approaches to addressing important conceptual and methodological challenges. It has also stimulated policy and practice and facilitated the field's evolving transformation into a coherent, integrated body of research encompassing multiple disciplines and clinical areas. Many clinical specialties have recently called for more attention to and integration of implementation science, including but not limited to primary care,[1,2] critical care,[3,4] surgery,[5,6] mental health,[7] nursing,[8] oncology,[9,10] cardiology,[11] pharmacy,[12] social work,[13] genomics,[14] complementary medicine,[15] pediatrics, periodontology,[16] and medical education.[17] This chapter briefly reviews key stages in the evolution and development of implementation science in healthcare, describes the design of implementation strategies and programs in varied health settings and systems, and examines implementation barriers, gaps, and future directions in the field. A case study describing an integrated program of implementation research illustrates many of the ideas discussed in the chapter.

EVIDENCE BASE AND THEORY DEVELOPMENT

The field of implementation science in healthcare comprises a rich body of literature, much of which developed through separate streams of activity before its coalescence in the 2000s into a more unified whole. (A thorough history of the field can be found in the previous volume with this chapter.[18]) A host of what are now termed implementation strategies, particularly related to changing physician behavior, were studied in the 1980s and 1990s to address variations and quality gaps in practice. Decades later, reviews of reviews pointed clearly to effective strategies and the promise of combining strategies,[19,20] and extensive research has now been conducted on the range of strategies that have been used,[21,22] along with their mechanisms of action.[23]

The release of the Institute of Medicine's *Crossing the Quality Chasm*[24] prompted extensive attention to quality and intensified promotion of evidence-based medicine. In addition, focus on changing individual physician behavior shifted to organizational change, much of which had roots in quality improvement. The development and application of theories and conceptual frameworks guiding implementation strategies, and research evaluating specific techniques for changing behavior, evolved together with this shift toward organizational change. Implementation scientists began to explore—and measure—organizational "readiness for change," using theories of how individuals change to conceptualize how programs change.[25,26] As the field of implementation science took shape, so did an abundance of theories, models, and frameworks meant to orient implementation research with regard to study design, process, context, determinants, mechanisms, and outcomes.[27–29]

The streams of research activity discussed above represent only a portion of the overall body of activity comprising implementation science in healthcare. Rich portfolios of health-related implementation research have developed within related fields, such as nursing research, health psychology and health promotion, research on substance use disorders,

Alison B. Hamilton and Arleen Brown, *Implementation Science in Healthcare* In: *Dissemination and Implementation Research in Health.* Edited by: Ross C. Brownson, Graham A. Colditz, and Enola K. Proctor, Oxford University Press.
DOI: 10.1093/oso/9780197660690.003.0021

patient safety, health equity and disparities, and others. Historically, this research appeared under labels such as "research utilization" (common in nursing research), "technology transfer" (common in substance use disorders research), and "operations research" (common in research in global health and improvement of health systems). Overlapping bodies of research captured by the labels "dissemination and implementation research in health" in the United States, "knowledge translation" (largely in Canada), and related labels in Europe and elsewhere embody theories, research approaches, and empirical studies closely related to work labeled "quality improvement research in health" and "improvement science" or "quality improvement science."[30] In the United States, the labels "quality improvement research," "patient safety research," and "improvement science" tend to be more common in studies funded by the Agency for Healthcare Research and Quality and by several foundations (e.g., Robert Wood Johnson Foundation, Commonwealth Fund), whereas "dissemination and implementation research" is more commonly seen in studies supported by the US National Institutes of Health and the US Department of Veterans Affairs. NIH and VA studies generally differ from improvement science in their focus on implementation of evidence-based practices to overcome what were termed "translational blocks" almost two decades ago.[31] Thus, despite some differences in their motivations and goals, improvement science and implementation science in health share many common theories, research approaches, and methods and pursue similar aims, questions, and hypotheses, and many have called for, and demonstrated, their integration.[32–35]

DESIGNING DISSEMINATION AND IMPLEMENTATION PROGRAMS AND STRATEGIES IN HEALTH SETTINGS AND SYSTEMS

Robust activity in implementation science in health has produced rich guidance for selecting and designing implementation strategies in healthcare (also see chapter 6). The range of potential implementation strategies and combinations of strategies is limitless, with growing recognition that implementation strategies must be selected on the basis of identified, diagnosed causes of quality and implementation gaps and thorough assessment of barriers and facilitators to practice change. Furthermore, because most implementation or quality gaps have multiple causes and involve multiple barriers to change, implementation programs must generally include multiple components delivered at multiple levels.[36,37] New approaches for diagnosing implementation gaps to identify specific root causes and barriers and facilitators to change, to select and apply relevant theories, and to select and adapt a combination of implementation strategies to local needs and contextual factors continue to emerge.[38–40]

Work to better understand and guide adaptation to respond to the extreme heterogeneity of implementation problems and settings is particularly promising.[41–43] Maintaining the core purpose, or function, of an intervention and/or an implementation strategy while adapting its format, or form, to local circumstances is a promising strategy for maintaining fidelity to the core functions while adapting features and details of its operationalization to conform to local circumstances.[44]

The work of designing programs and strategies has increasingly been contextualized within systems, particularly learning health systems (LHSs) (i.e., healthcare delivery systems that combine research, data science, and quality improvement and that involve the co-production of healthcare and continuous learning).[45] Implementation science has been posited as key to the realization of LHS,[46–48] with an emphasis on organizational learning that accounts for multilevel influences and cross-system contexts.[49] Implementation science has been conceptualized as a "catalyst"[48] for system reform and a "bridge" (e.g., between precision medicine and LHS).[50]

IMPLEMENTATION BARRIERS

Recognition of the importance of identifying and overcoming barriers to implementation in healthcare is well established: Many of the key frameworks for planning and conducting implementation research in healthcare include specific research phases and activities in which barriers are explicitly assessed. Numerous empirical studies in recent decades have documented and classified barriers to implementation. For example, a systematic review found that research barriers, lack of resources, lack of time, inadequate skills, inadequate access, lack of knowledge, and financial barriers were common barriers to evidence-based medicine.[51] Accordingly, core competencies in evidence-based practice[52] and in LHS[53] have been developed.

Although specific barriers vary across the range of healthcare delivery settings (e.g., small physician practices, hospitals), most result from a common set of fundamental characteristics of healthcare. In the previous edition of this volume, Hamilton and Mittman identified three key characteristics that underlie many barriers: (1) high levels of uncertainty in diagnostic and treatment decision-making and in identifying causal links between treatment activities and outcomes, (2) the resulting dominance of professionals and professional norms and culture in healthcare delivery, and (3) the diverse range of constraints and multilevel influences on healthcare practices. These characteristics remain barriers but have shifted and evolved conceptually. For example, uncertainty has been theorized as a component of complexity, as an expected phenomenon to be "embraced"[54] or "tolerated"[55] in order to foster change.[56,57] Professional norms are typically highly stable and not easily influenced by outsiders. Traditional norms of professionalism have tended to favor individual professional judgment over standardized, codified policies and procedures such as clinical practice guidelines. However, there is increasing recognition that implementation science can improve uptake of such guidelines.[58]

Finally, implementation can be impacted by influences at multiple levels, often simultaneously and sometimes unexpectedly. Healthcare practices are influenced by a broad range of factors operating at the level of the individual patient and patient-clinician dyad; at the level of clinical microsystems, clinics, and larger organizations; within professional communities and regions; and at the national policy level. Individual implementation efforts typically involve behavior change strategies aimed at one or two levels (e.g., patients and clinicians). Implementation researchers, clinical leaders, and others attempting to change clinical practices may lack sufficient leverage and authority to influence the full range of factors constraining and influencing the target practices. The need for multilevel, coordinated approaches to implementation is increasingly recognized and pursued.[59–61]

IMPLEMENTATION RESEARCH CASE STUDY

Frameworks guiding the design and conduct of implementation studies and portfolios of implementation research and texts offering broad overviews of implementation science in health describe a series of desirable research activities and study features important for achieving success in identifying, diagnosing, and closing quality and implementation gaps.[62–64] Table 21.1 summarizes much of this guidance by listing key research activities and selected features of these activities. Frameworks are covered in more detail in chapter 4.

Many of the recommended features of implementation research in healthcare are illustrated by a hybrid type II implementation-effectiveness study[79] conducted by Gail Wyatt and colleagues based at the University of California Los Angeles (UCLA). The fundamental motivation for this research was to move an efficacious, culturally tailored intervention (called Eban)[80] into community-based service organizations in order to increase its accessibility and impacts among the target population—African American HIV serodiscordant heterosexual couples—and in the organizations themselves, with a goal of sustainability of expanded organizational capacity and reduced seroconversion.[81] The original cluster randomized trial had found significant reductions in HIV risk behaviors among couples,[80] indicating that community-based implementation would be warranted. Wyatt was an investigator in the original trial, and invited Hamilton to serve as the implementation scientist for the implementation trial.

Designed before the proliferation of implementation science theories, models, and frameworks, the team selected the Program Change Model[26] to guide the study because it offered a phased and theoretically grounded approach to organizational change, a defined set of constructs to evaluate using mixed methods, measures that had strong psychometric properties, and implementation outcomes. A hybrid type II design (one of the first R01 hybrids funded by the National Institute of Mental Health (NIMH)) was selected because the evidence for the efficacy of the intervention was strong, but

TABLE 21.1 KEY FEATURES OF A COMPREHENSIVE IMPLEMENTATION RESEARCH PORTFOLIO AND FEATURES OF INDIVIDUAL STUDIES[a]

Research Activity	Desirable Features and Comments
	Preimplementation Studies
Clinical effectiveness research to develop evidence-based, innovative practices	Research design, methods, sampling, and other features should maximize external validity and policy/practice relevance to increase acceptability to target clinicians and leaders.[65]
Development of evidence-based clinical practice guidelines	Guideline development processes should follow published recommendations for appropriate use of evidence, involvement of key stakeholder groups, sponsorship, etc.[58]
Development of other innovations	Innovation characteristics should facilitate adoption, incorporating features identified by research on the diffusion of innovations.[66,67]
Development of methods and measures for implementation studies	Important research tools include validated, case mix-adjusted measures of implementation outcomes and appropriate data sources; study designs for quantitative impact evaluation with adequate external validity; and research approaches and methods for formative and summative evaluation.[62,68,69]
Documentation of current practices and their determinants	Observational studies to understand current clinical practices and their influences incorporating quantitative and qualitative methods.[70,71]
Measurement and diagnosis of quality or implementation gaps	Observational studies to compare current practices to desired practices and to identify determinants or "root causes" of quality and implementation gaps.[72]
	Observational Implementation Studies
Studies of naturally occurring (policy- and practice-led) implementation processes	Observational studies maximize external validity, avoid artificial elements of researcher-led implementation trials, and offer opportunities to develop insights into barriers, facilitators, and key influences on routine implementation processes and success. Strong research designs are needed to achieve adequate internal validity.[73]
	Interventional Implementation Studies
Phase 1 pilot studies of implementation programs	Pilot studies offer opportunities to develop initial evidence regarding the feasibility, acceptability, and potential effectiveness of implementation strategies and to begin to identify key contextual influences and other factors influencing effectiveness. Emphasis on formative evaluation to modify the implementation program based on frequent measurement of impact and operation.[74]
Phase 2 efficacy-oriented, small-scale trials of implementation programs	Trials of implementation programs under idealized (efficacy-oriented) conditions, such as active research team facilitation and support for participating sites and grant funding for added costs, permit assessment of implementation program effectiveness under best-case conditions. Phase 2 studies feature initial formative evaluation to refine an implementation program followed by emphasis on fidelity (with site-level adaptation guided by a predeveloped adaptation protocol).[75]

(continued)

TABLE 21.1 CONTINUED

Research Activity	Desirable Features and Comments
Phase 3 effectiveness-oriented large trials of implementation programs	Larger trials of implementation programs under routine conditions (e.g., limited or no research team technical assistance or grant support to participating sites) permit assessment of implementation program effectiveness when deployed under real-world conditions. Phase 3 studies feature site-level adaptation guided by a predeveloped adaptation protocol and measurement of sustainment, scale-up/spread potential, costs and cost-effectiveness, and a broad range of outcomes (implementation outcomes and, where feasible, system-level as well as clinical and patient outcomes [clinical, functional, quality of life, etc.]).[76,77]
Phase 4 "postmarketing" study of implementation program	Research-led monitoring and evaluation of policy/practice-led scale-up and spread of an effective implementation program. Phase 4 studies generate feedback to policy/practice leaders to guide their management of an implementation and spread effort.[78]

[a]Adapted with permission from Hamilton and Mittman.[18]

knowledge of its implementation beyond the constraints of a trial was limited. To evaluate effectiveness, a wait-list control design was used to ensure that all eligible clients would eventually receive the intervention. To evaluate implementation, the Program Change Model phases guided the mixed-methods approach, which included surveys and qualitative interviews with key stakeholders across 10 community-based organizations (CBOs) in California, where HIV rates were the third highest in the United States at the time. The counties where Eban was implemented—Los Angeles and Alameda—had the highest proportion of African American HIV cases, motivating the selection of the sites and aligning with the culturally tailored intervention. Implementation strategies and tools were also selected to correspond to the Program Change Model, with different strategies deployed in different phases. An exploratory cost evaluation aim was also proposed.

Prior to this implementation study, most of Hamilton's experience as an implementation scientist had been in the Veterans Health Administration (VA), where much of the early development of the field took place. Community-based implementation (i.e., implementation outside of an integrated healthcare system) was somewhat of a new frontier, though she had some experience with exploring uptake of evidence-based practices in community-based substance use treatment settings.[82,83] Despite strong buy-in from the CBOs, which had not previously provided services to couples, favorable attitudes toward evidence-based practices and low burnout among staff, and strong organizational readiness, implementation was challenging. Several adaptations were made to the intervention in order to make it fit within CBO constraints; for example, the intervention was designed to be delivered by a male-female dyad (to model communication), but the CBOs did not always have a dyad available, so in some cases only one person delivered the intervention, or a "floating" male facilitator (on the UCLA research team) delivered the intervention across several CBOs, thereby potentially limiting its sustainability.

External contextual barriers to implementation were substantial. The team decided to apply constructs from the external context domain of the Consolidated Framework for Implementation Research,[84] discovering that barriers included client needs as a manifestation of social determinants of poverty, community agency resources, and local and national policy changes.[85] Participating CBOs were destabilized by changing federal and state policies, and the research team had to recognize and come to terms with the uncertainties that these changes introduced, including changes to our implementation plans, including our wait-list control design, which was not ultimately viable given the precarity of the CBO clients' lives.

In the main outcomes paper, published in a special issue of *American Psychologist* on advancing psychological science through implementation science,[7] the team reported on results related to condom use and retention, highlighting that challenges with basic resources complicated clients' participation and therefore implementation. In light of couples' vulnerabilities, the team constructed a composite score of "critical vulnerability" and found that depression was persistently related to critical vulnerability and that retention was lower among those with more vulnerability.[86] Despite these challenges, those who did engage in the intervention were satisfied with it, expressing the value of the "cultural stuff" and the techniques they learned for communication.[87] The team also calculated cost, cost-saving, and cost-effectiveness thresholds for the intervention, finding that sites had achievable cost-saving thresholds.[88] Implementation lessons learned from this complex study were applied to the development of another implementation study, funded by the National Heart, Lung, and Blood Institute, focused on increasing individual and organizational capacity to address cardiovascular risk among Black and Latino people living with HIV and histories of trauma, again using a culturally tailored intervention and privileging the needs and experiences of marginalized populations.[89]

RESEARCH GAPS AND DIRECTIONS FOR FUTURE RESEARCH

Continued growth in research interest, activity, and funding in healthcare implementation science offers considerable promise for continued progress in addressing the field's key challenges. Expanded activity and contributions from researchers trained in diverse disciplines and employing a broader range of research approaches and methods will continue to enrich the methodological toolkit, the range of theoretical perspectives, and the breadth of research epistemologies applied to the field's key questions, simultaneously expanding the volume of empirical evidence and insights and the range of implementation problems and settings studied.

Future activity in the field is likely to help address several identified gaps, advance a number of key debates regarding the future of the field, and apply implementation science frameworks and insights to emerging areas of clinical research and innovation, such as precision medicine.[14,50] Important gaps include (1) the limited amount of research attention to barriers and strategies for achieving sustainment and routine scale-up and spread of effective practices following their initial adoption; (2) the need for increased research examining naturally occurring implementation processes (vs. investigator-led implementation); (3) greater attention to implementation processes and mechanisms via approaches such as process evaluation and theory-based evaluation, to complement and help understand and interpret the results of impact-oriented research; (4) the need for more thorough attention to and understanding of de-implementation; and (5) the urgent need to center equity in implementation science. Key challenges to progress in addressing these research gaps include ongoing debates regarding the need for research to inventory, classify, and guide the selection and effective use of theory; debates regarding research approaches and the nature of evidence required to better understand and guide implementation processes and evaluate the effectiveness of alternative implementation strategies and programs; and the need for improved and innovative methods, particularly to address and ameliorate health disparities.

Sustainment, scale-up, and spread. Interest in barriers and facilitators to sustainment and scale-up and spread has increased recently, based on recognition that successful implementation of effective practices through short-term research-led efforts (typically targeting a limited number of research sites) does not naturally lead to sustained adoption in the participating sites or broader adoption in additional sites (see chapter 29). Studies measuring long-term sustainment of resulting practice changes after withdrawal of these resources continue to be rare, particularly in studies in low-income countries.[90] A systematic review of public health interventions in schools found that no interventions were sustained in their entirety, and there was no relationship between evidence of intervention effectiveness and sustainability.[91] Diverse approaches to sustainability continue to pose conceptual challenges, though recent work has consolidated constructs in an effort to achieve greater coherence for the field.[92] A similar need exists for increased attention to scale-up and spread constructs, barriers, processes, and strategies. A range of factors limits the external validity and transferability of the findings from interventional implementation studies assessing effectiveness of an investigator-led implementation program in a small number of sites. Research to understand barriers and facilitators to routine scale-up and spread and to develop effective scale-up strategies is beginning to identify and characterize these and other limitations of current approaches to implementation research and will help develop new guidance for successful scale-up and spread.[93,94] Community engagement is increasingly viewed as critical to scale up of evidence-based interventions,[95] with a growing number of examples from the field.[96]

Observational studies. Increased research attention to sustainment and scale-up and spread processes will help stimulate growth in observational research examining naturally occurring spread as well as phased implementation research programs involving progression from small-scale, efficacy-oriented implementation trials (involving high levels of researcher technical assistance and support for participating sites) to larger-scale, effectiveness-oriented trials and observational studies in which researchers have little or no role in facilitating implementation but serve mainly to evaluate the implementation process. Researcher-led implementation efforts are often highly artificial, addressing quality and implementation gaps viewed as important by researchers but not necessarily by participating sites and involving a range of practice change strategies led by an external research team rather than internal staff. Insights into barriers and facilitators to practice change from research-led implementation efforts have limited external validity, but there is potential for greater application of such insights, such as by engaging practitioners more intentionally in the implementation research endeavor,[97] and by creating more opportunities for implementation research in practice-based research networks (PBRNs), which are also well suited to address health equity issues (see below).[98]

Impact versus process and mechanism focus. Much of the research examining implementation in healthcare has pursued questions of implementation strategy effectiveness and has employed well-established experimental and quasi-experimental research approaches for assessing the effectiveness of various implementation strategies. Researchers are increasingly recognizing that effectiveness of implementation strategies is often highly dependent on contextual factors and the ways in which implementation strategies are delivered and managed.[22] As a result, the main effect of an implementation strategy is often weak and dominated by multiple contextual and delivery factors, limiting the ability of standard evaluation approaches to estimate effectiveness of the core implementation program.[99] In extreme (although arguably common) situations in which outcomes of implementation efforts are driven almost entirely by contextual factors and the manner in which implementation strategies are delivered, with essentially no detectable main effect of the implementation strategy, implementation research efforts must focus on developing insights into the processes and mechanisms of action, pursuing questions such as how, when, where, and why an implementation strategy is effective.[100] Research efforts to develop appropriate methods and approaches for these questions, including theory-based evaluation and realist evaluation, will help broaden the portfolio of such research and increase the likelihood that valid, useful insights and guidance will emerge and better contribute to ongoing efforts to enhance the performance and beneficial impacts of healthcare delivery and health services.

De-implementation. The past decade of implementation science has seen increased attention to de-implementation, that is, stopping current services or practices that are ineffective, harmful, or inappropriate (see chapter 12).[101,102] Given unique challenges associated with de-implementation, some new conceptualizations of outcomes[103] and theories, models, and frameworks[104] have been generated, while potential distinctions between implementation and de-implementation continue to be explored.[105]

Centering equity. Perhaps the most robust (and necessary) recent development in implementation science in healthcare has been an increased emphasis on the critical importance of addressing inequities in healthcare delivery[106,107] and coming to terms with addressing core challenges such as structural racism.[108,109] Guidance on how to study inequities and achieve equity is proliferating, including but not limited to transdisciplinary, community-engaged, and theoretical and conceptual approaches.[110–115] Implementation science leaders in the field have asserted that implementation science can increase the impact of health disparities research,[116] and that an equity lens needs to be integrated in implementation research "from the outset"[117] and should be part of every implementation science project.[118]

SUMMARY

Implementation science in healthcare comprises over 30 years of rich and varied activity that has developed, refined, and applied implementation science concepts, theories, and research approaches. This body of activity has produced valuable empirical findings and has contributed to the continued development of the broader field of implementation science. This chapter briefly describes the development and evolution of implementation science in healthcare. It discusses designing programs and strategies for health settings and systems and examines key barriers, gaps, and future directions in implementation research.

Continued growth in healthcare implementation science will require expanded attention to sustainment and scale-up and spread of effective healthcare practices and attention to the study of routine, naturally occurring implementation processes in addition to experimental evaluation of investigator-led implementation. Progress will also require systematic attention to implementation processes and mechanisms of action, supplementing current interest in measuring the impacts and outcomes of implementation strategies. Implementation strategies are complex, characterized by high levels of heterogeneity and complexity. Research approaches suitable for studying such complexity are needed to generate valuable guidance for decision makers interested in effective implementation in their unique settings, requiring careful selection and adaptation of implementation strategies and active management of implementation settings and processes. An equity lens at the heart of these efforts will ensure that implementation science lives up to its promise of improving health and healthcare for all.

SUGGESTED READINGS AND WEBSITES

Readings

Brownson RC, Kumanyika SK, Kreuter MW, Haire-Joshu D. Implementation science should give higher priority to health equity. Implement Sci. 2021 Dec;16(1):1–6.

This article asserts that every implementation science project should include an equity focus; it lays out recommendations to address implementation research challenges related to centering equity-focused principles.

Kilbourne AM, Glasgow RE, Chambers DA. What can implementation science do for you? Key success stories from the field. J Gen Intern Med. 2020 Nov;35(2):783–787.

This work describes implementation science success stories illustrating the impact of implementation science across broad population groups.

Rudd BN, Davis M, Beidas RS. Integrating implementation science in clinical research to maximize public health impact: a call for the reporting and alignment of implementation strategy use with implementation outcomes in clinical research. Implement Sci. 2020 Dec;15(1):1–1.

This article calls for comprehensive reporting of implementation strategy use and alignment of strategies with implementation outcomes within clinical research.

Shelton RC, Lee M, Brotzman LE, Wolfenden L, Nathan N, Wainberg ML. What is dissemination and implementation science? An introduction and opportunities to advance behavioral medicine and public health globally. Int J Behav Med. 2020 Feb;27(1):3–20.

An overview of dissemination and implementation (D&I) science is provided, highlighting examples of D&I research globally.

Selected Websites and Tools

Society for Implementation Research Collaboration. https://societyforimplementationresearchcollaboration.org/

The Society for Implementation Research Collaboration is a professional society supporting enhanced collaboration among researchers, policy, and practice leaders to strengthen implementation research and its successful application. Key activities include a biennial conference, the SIRC Instrument Review Project, and activities to facilitate networking and mentorship.

National Cancer Institute. https://cancercontrol.cancer.gov/IS/

The National Cancer Institute implementation science website offers an array of resources for implementation researchers, including links to funding opportunities, webinars, training programs, conferences, and sample grant proposals.

14th to 15th Annual Conference on the Science of Dissemination and Implementation in Health | Academy Health
https://academyhealth.org/events/2022-12/15th-annual-conference-science-dissemination-and-implementation-health

The Annual NIH Conference on the Science of Dissemination and Implementation represents the largest annual gathering of dissemination and implementation researchers and research activity in the United States and internationally. The website for each year's conference offers copies of the agenda, participant lists, presentations, and selected session summaries and videos.

Quality Enhancement Research Initiative (QUERI). https://www.queri.research.va.gov/default.cfm

The US Department of Veterans Affairs' Quality Enhancement Research Initiative (QUERI) website provides links to QUERI activities and outputs, including QUERI programs, implementation tools, QUERI webinars, and the QUERI Implementation Guide.

Global Implementation Conference. https://gic.globalimplementation.org/

The Global Implementation Conference "aims to promote implementation practice, science and policy and their active application in human services in order to contribute to demonstrable and socially significant benefits to people and society."

European Implementation Collaborative. https://implementation.eu/events/

The European Implementation Collaborative "aims to build a connected European community of practitioners, researchers, and policy makers with contemporary implementation skills and expertise, improving the quality of life for all people."

Dissemination and Implementation Models in Health. https://dissemination-implementation.org

This website provides users with tools for selecting dissemination and implementation models in health research and practice.

ACKNOWLEDGMENTS

We would like to acknowledge Dr. Brian Mittman's contributions to this chapter's content. Dr. Hamilton is supported by a VA Health Services Research and Development Research Career Scientist Award (RCS 21-135). The Eban II study was funded by the National Institute of Mental Health (MH093230; PI, Wyatt). Drs. Hamilton and Brown are supported by the National Heart, Lung, and Blood Institute (U01 HL142109).

REFERENCES

1. Holtrop JS, Rabin BA, Glasgow RE. Dissemination and implementation science in primary care research and practice: contributions and opportunities. *J Am Board Fam Med.* 2018;31(3):466–478.
2. Prathivadi P, Buckingham P, Chakraborty S, et al. Implementation science: an introduction for primary care. *Fam Pract.* 2021;39(1):219–221. doi:10.1093/fampra/cmab125
3. Barr J, Paulson SS, Kamdar B, et al. The coming of age of implementation science and research in critical care medicine. *Crit Care Med.* Aug 1 2021;49(8):1254–1275. doi:10.1097/ccm.0000000000005131
4. Weiss CH, Krishnan JA, Au DH, et al. An official American Thoracic Society research statement: implementation science in pulmonary, critical care, and sleep medicine. *Am J Respir Crit Care Med.* 2016;194(8):1015–1025.
5. Lane-Fall MB, Cobb BT, Cené CW, Beidas RS. Implementation science in perioperative care. *Anesthesiol Clin.* 2018;36(1):1–15.
6. Hull L, Athanasiou T, Russ S. Implementation science: a neglected opportunity to accelerate improvements in the safety and quality of surgical care. *Ann Surg.* 2017;265(6):1104–1112.
7. Wiltsey Stirman S, Beidas RS. Expanding the reach of psychological science through implementation science: introduction to the special issue. *Am Psychol.* 2020;75(8):1033.
8. Zullig LL, Deschodt M, De Geest S. Embracing implementation science: a paradigm shift for nursing research. *J Nurs Scholarsh.* 2019;52(1): 3–5.
9. Mitchell SA, Chambers DA. Leveraging implementation science to improve cancer care delivery and patient outcomes. *J Oncol Pract.* 2017;13(8):523.
10. Emmons KM, Colditz GA. Realizing the potential of cancer prevention—the role of implementation science. *N Engl J Med.* 2017;376(10):986.
11. Galaviz KI, Barnes GD. Implementation science opportunities in cardiovascular medicine. *Circ Cardiovasc Qual Outcomes.* Jul 2021;14(7):e008109. doi:10.1161/circoutcomes.121.008109
12. Smith MA, Blanchard CM, Vuernick E. The intersection of implementation science and pharmacy practice transformation. *Ann Pharmacother.* 2020;54(1):75–81.
13. Cabassa LJ. Implementation science: why it matters for the future of social work. *J Soc Work Educ.* 2016;52(suppl):S38–S50.

14. Williams JK, Feero WG, Leonard DG, Coleman B. Implementation science, genomic precision medicine, and improved health: a new path forward? *Nurs Outlook*. 2017;65(1):36–40.
15. Steel A, Rapport F, Adams J. Towards an implementation science of complementary health care: some initial considerations for guiding safe, effective clinical decision-making. *Adv Integr Med*. 2018;5(1):5–8.
16. Frantsve-Hawley J, Kumar SS, Rindal DB, Weyant RJ. Implementation science and periodontal practice: translation of evidence into periodontology. *Periodontology 2000*. 2020;84(1):188–201.
17. Thomas DC, Berry A, Djuricich AM, et al. What is implementation science and what forces are driving a change in medical education? *Am J Med Qual*. 2017;32(4):438–444.
18. Hamilton A, Mittman BS. Implementation science in health care. In Brownson R, Colditz G, Proctor E, eds. *Dissemination and Implementation Research in Health: Translating Science to Practice*. Oxford University Press; 2018:385–400.
19. Johnson MJ, May CR. Promoting professional behaviour change in healthcare: what interventions work, and why? A theory-led overview of systematic reviews. *BMJ Open*. Sep 30 2015;5(9):e008592. doi:10.1136/bmjopen-2015-008592
20. Mostofian F, Ruban C, Simunovic N, Bhandari M. Changing physician behavior: what works? *Am J Manag Care*. Jan 2015;21(1):75–84.
21. Leeman J, Birken SA, Powell BJ, Rohweder C, Shea CM. Beyond "implementation strategies": classifying the full range of strategies used in implementation science and practice. *Implement Sci*. Nov 3 2017;12(1):125. doi:10.1186/s13012-017-0657-x
22. Kirchner JE, Smith JL, Powell BJ, Waltz TJ, Proctor EK. Getting a clinical innovation into practice: an introduction to implementation strategies. *Psychiatry Res*. Jan 2020;283:112467. doi:10.1016/j.psychres.2019.06.042
23. Geng EH, Baumann AA, Powell BJ. Mechanism mapping to advance research on implementation strategies. *PLoS Med*. Feb 2022;19(2):e1003918. doi:10.1371/journal.pmed.1003918
24. Institute of Medicine Committee on Quality of Health Care. *Crossing the Quality Chasm: A New Health System for the 21st Century*. National Academies Press; 2001.
25. Weiner BJ. A theory of organizational readiness for change. *Implement Sci*. Oct 19 2009;4:67. doi:10.1186/1748-5908-4-67
26. Simpson DD, Flynn PM. Moving innovations into treatment: a stage-based approach to program change. *J Subst Abuse Treat*. 2007;33(2):111–120.
27. Nilsen P. Making sense of implementation theories, models and frameworks. *Implement Sci*. Apr 21 2015;10:53. doi:10.1186/s13012-015-0242-0
28. Tabak RG, Khoong EC, Chambers DA, Brownson RC. Bridging research and practice: models for dissemination and implementation research. *Am J Prev Med*. Sep 2012;43(3):337–350. doi:10.1016/j.amepre.2012.05.024
29. Damschroder LJ. Clarity out of chaos: use of theory in implementation research. *Psychiatry Res*. Jan 2020;283:112461. doi:10.1016/j.psychres.2019.06.036
30. Reed JE, Davey N, Woodcock T. The foundations of quality improvement science. *Future Hosp J*. 2016;3(3):199.
31. Sung NS, Crowley WF Jr, Genel M, et al. Central challenges facing the national clinical research enterprise. *JAMA*. 2003;289(10):1278–1287.
32. Leeman J, Rohweder C, Lee M, et al. Aligning implementation science with improvement practice: a call to action. *Implement Sci Commun*. Sep 8 2021;2(1):99. doi:10.1186/s43058-021-00201-1
33. Melder A, Robinson T, McLoughlin I, Iedema R, Teede H. Integrating the complexity of healthcare improvement with implementation science: a longitudinal qualitative case study. *BMC Health Serv Res*. Feb 19 2022;22(1):234. doi:10.1186/s12913-022-07505-5
34. Tyler A, Glasgow RE. Implementing improvements: opportunities to integrate quality improvement and implementation science. *Hosp Pediatr*. May 2021;11(5):536–545. doi:10.1542/hpeds.2020-002246
35. Nilsen P, Thor J, Bender M, Leeman J, Andersson-Gäre B, Sevdalis N. Bridging the silos: a comparative analysis of implementation science and improvement science. *Front Health Serv*. 2022:18. https://doi.org/10.3389/frhs.2021.817750
36. Hall KL, Oh A, Perez LG, et al. The ecology of multilevel intervention research. *Transl Behav Med*. Nov 21 2018;8(6):968–978. doi:10.1093/tbm/iby102
37. Yano EM, Green LW, Glanz K, et al. Implementation and spread of interventions into the multilevel context of routine practice and policy: implications for the cancer care continuum. *J Natl Cancer Inst Monogr*. May 2012;2012(44):86–99. doi:10.1093/jncimonographs/lgs004
38. Powell BJ, Beidas RS, Lewis CC, et al. Methods to improve the selection and tailoring of implementation strategies. *J Behav Health Serv Res*. Apr 2017;44(2):177–194. doi:10.1007/s11414-015-9475-6
39. Huynh AK, Hamilton AB, Farmer MM, et al. A pragmatic approach to guide implementation evaluation research: strategy mapping for

complex interventions. *Front Public Health.* 2018;6:134. doi:10.3389/fpubh.2018.00134

40. Ibekwe LN, Walker TJ, Ebunlomo E, et al. Using implementation mapping to develop implementation strategies for the delivery of a cancer prevention and control phone navigation program: a collaboration with 2-1-1. *Health Promot Pract.* Jan 2022;23(1):86–97. doi:10.1177/1524839920957979
41. Kirk MA, Moore JE, Wiltsey Stirman S, Birken SA. Towards a comprehensive model for understanding adaptations' impact: the model for adaptation design and impact (MADI). *Implement Sci.* Jul 20 2020;15(1):56. doi:10.1186/s13012-020-01021-y
42. Miller CJ, Barnett ML, Baumann AA, Gutner CA, Wiltsey-Stirman S. The FRAME-IS: a framework for documenting modifications to implementation strategies in healthcare. *Implement Sci.* Apr 7 2021;16(1):36. doi:10.1186/s13012-021-01105-3
43. Wiltsey Stirman S, Baumann AA, Miller CJ. The FRAME: an expanded framework for reporting adaptations and modifications to evidence-based interventions. *Implement Sci.* Jun 6 2019;14(1):58. doi:10.1186/s13012-019-0898-y
44. Perez Jolles M, Lengnick-Hall R, Mittman BS. Core functions and forms of complex health interventions: a patient-centered medical home illustration. *J Gen Intern Med.* Jun 2019;34(6):1032–1038. doi:10.1007/s11606-018-4818-7
45. Smith M, Saunders R, Stuckhardt L, McGinnis JM, eds. *Best Care at Lower Cost: The Path to Continuously Learning Health Care in America.* National Academies Press; 2013.
46. Jackson GL, Cutrona SL, Kilbourne A, White BS, Everett C, Damschroder LJ. Implementation science: helping healthcare systems improve. *J Am Acad Physician Assist.* 2020;33(1):51–53.
47. Kilbourne AM, Evans E, Atkins D. Learning health systems: driving real-world impact in mental health and substance use disorder research. *FASEB Bioadv.* Aug 2021;3(8):626–638. doi:10.1096/fba.2020-00124
48. Fisher ES, Shortell SM, Savitz LA. Implementation science: a potential catalyst for delivery system reform. *JAMA.* 2016;315(4):339–340.
49. Harrison MI, Shortell SM. Multi-level analysis of the learning health system: integrating contributions from research on organizations and implementation. *Learn Health Syst.* Apr 2021;5(2):e10226. doi:10.1002/lrh2.10226
50. Chambers DA, Feero WG, Khoury MJ. Convergence of implementation science, precision medicine, and the learning health care system: a new model for biomedical research. *JAMA.* 2016;315(18):1941–1942.
51. Sadeghi-Bazargani H, Tabrizi JS, Azami-Aghdash S. Barriers to evidence-based medicine: a systematic review. *J Eval Clin Pract.* Dec 2014;20(6):793–802. doi:10.1111/jep.12222
52. Albarqouni L, Hoffmann T, Straus S, et al. Core competencies in evidence-based practice for health professionals: consensus statement based on a systematic review and Delphi survey. *JAMA Netw Open.* Jun 1 2018;1(2):e180281. doi:10.1001/jamanetworkopen.2018.0281
53. Forrest CB, Chesley FD Jr, Tregear ML, Mistry KB. Development of the learning health system researcher core competencies. *Health Serv Res.* 2018;53(4):2615–2632.
54. Beckett K, Farr M, Kothari A, Wye L, le May A. Embracing complexity and uncertainty to create impact: exploring the processes and transformative potential of co-produced research through development of a social impact model. *Health Res Policy Syst.* Dec 11 2018;16(1):118. doi:10.1186/s12961-018-0375-0
55. Hillen MA, Gutheil CM, Strout TD, Smets EMA, Han PKJ. Tolerance of uncertainty: conceptual analysis, integrative model, and implications for healthcare. *Soc Sci Med.* May 2017;180:62–75. doi:10.1016/j.socscimed.2017.03.024
56. Braithwaite J, Churruca K, Long JC, Ellis LA, Herkes J. When complexity science meets implementation science: a theoretical and empirical analysis of systems change. *BMC Med.* Apr 30 2018;16(1):63. doi:10.1186/s12916-018-1057-z
57. Pomare C, Churruca K, Ellis LA, Long JC, Braithwaite J. A revised model of uncertainty in complex healthcare settings: a scoping review. *J Eval Clin Pract.* Apr 2019;25(2):176–182. doi:10.1111/jep.13079
58. Sarkies MN, Jones LK, Gidding SS, Watts GF. Improving clinical practice guidelines with implementation science. *Nat Rev Cardiol.* 2022;19(1):3–4.
59. Williams NJ. Multilevel mechanisms of implementation strategies in mental health: integrating theory, research, and practice. *Adm Policy Ment Health.* Sep 2016;43(5):783–798. doi:10.1007/s10488-015-0693-2
60. Rabin BA, Nehl E, Elliott T, Deshpande AD, Brownson RC, Glanz K. Individual and setting level predictors of the implementation of a skin cancer prevention program: a multilevel analysis. *Implement Sci.* May 31 2010;5:40. doi:10.1186/1748-5908-5-40
61. Oishi SM, Marshall N, Hamilton AB, Yano EM, Lerner B, Scheuner MT. Assessing multilevel determinants of adoption and implementation of genomic medicine: an organizational mixed-methods approach. *Genet Med.* 2015;17(11):919–926.

62. Brown CH, Curran G, Palinkas LA, et al. An overview of research and evaluation designs for dissemination and implementation. *Ann Rev Public Health*. 2017;38:1–22.
63. Bauer MS, Kirchner J. Implementation science: what is it and why should I care? *Psychiatry Res*. 2020;283:112376.
64. Bauer MS, Damschroder L, Hagedorn H, Smith J, Kilbourne AM. An introduction to implementation science for the non-specialist. *BMC Psychol*. 2015;3(1):1–12.
65. Huebschmann AG, Leavitt IM, Glasgow RE. Making health research matter: a call to increase attention to external validity. *Ann Rev Public Health*. 2019;40:45–63.
66. Dearing JW, Cox JG. Diffusion of innovations theory, principles, and practice. *Health Aff*. 2018;37(2):183–190.
67. Greenhalgh T, Robert G, Macfarlane F, Bate P, Kyriakidou O. Diffusion of innovations in service organizations: systematic review and recommendations. *Milbank Q*. 2004;82(4):581–629. doi:10.1111/j.0887-378X.2004.00325.x
68. Elwy AR, Wasan AD, Gillman AG, et al. Using formative evaluation methods to improve clinical implementation efforts: description and an example. *Psychiatry Res*. 2020;283:112532.
69. Hamilton AB, Finley EP. Qualitative methods in implementation research: an introduction. *Psychiatry Res*. 2019;280:112516.
70. Hamilton AB, Wiltsey-Stirman S, Finley EP, et al. Usual care among providers treating women veterans: managing complexity and multimorbidity in the era of evidence-based practice. *Adm Policy Ment Health*. Mar 2020;47(2):244–253. doi:10.1007/s10488-019-00961-y
71. Garland AF, Bickman L, Chorpita BF. Change what? Identifying quality improvement targets by investigating usual mental health care. *Adm Policy Ment Health*. Mar 2010;37(1–2):15–26. doi:10.1007/s10488-010-0279-y
72. Patel MM, Brown JD, Croake S, et al. The current state of behavioral health quality measures: where are the gaps? *Psychiatr Serv*. Aug 1 2015;66(8):865–871. doi:10.1176/appi.ps.201400589
73. Lui JHL, Brookman-Frazee L, Vázquez AL, et al. Patterns of child mental health service utilization within a multiple EBP system of care. *Adm Policy Ment Health*. 2022;49:506–520. https://doi.org/10.1007/s10488-021-01179-7
74. Zarrett N, Abraczinskas M, Cook BS, Wilson D, Roberts A. Formative process evaluation of the "Connect" Physical Activity Feasibility Trial for adolescents. *Clin Med Insights Pediatr*. 2020;14:1179556520918902. doi:10.1177/1179556520918902
75. Armistead L, Marelich WD, Murphy DA, Schulte MT, Goodrum N, Kim SJ. Implementing a multisite efficacy trial to facilitate maternal disclosure to children: the TRACK HIV Disclosure Intervention. *Transl Behav Med*. 2022 May;12(5):630–641.
76. Young AS, Cohen AN, Chang ET, et al. A clustered controlled trial of the implementation and effectiveness of a medical home to improve health care of people with serious mental illness: study protocol. *BMC Health Serv Res*. Jun 7 2018;18(1):428. doi:10.1186/s12913-018-3237-0
77. Hamilton AB, Farmer MM, Moin T, et al. Enhancing Mental and Physical Health of Women through Engagement and Retention (EMPOWER): a protocol for a program of research. *Implement Sci*. Nov 7 2017;12(1):127. doi:10.1186/s13012-017-0658-9
78. Elwy AR, Maguire EM, McCullough M, et al. From implementation to sustainment: a large-scale adverse event disclosure support program generated through embedded research in the Veterans Health Administration. *Healthcare*. Jun 2021;8(suppl 1):100496. doi:10.1016/j.hjdsi.2020.100496
79. Curran GM, Bauer M, Mittman B, Pyne JM, Stetler C. Effectiveness-implementation hybrid designs: combining elements of clinical effectiveness and implementation research to enhance public health impact. *Medical Care*. 2012;50(3):217.
80. El-Bassel N, Jemmott JB, Landis JR, et al. National Institute of Mental Health multisite Eban HIV/STD prevention intervention for African American HIV serodiscordant couples: a cluster randomized trial. *Arch Iintern Med*. 2010;170(17):1594–1601.
81. Hamilton AB, Mittman BS, Williams JK, et al. Community-based implementation and effectiveness in a randomized trial of a risk reduction intervention for HIV-serodiscordant couples: study protocol. *Implementation Science*. 2014;9(1):1–12.
82. Hamilton Brown A. Integrating research and practice in the CSAT Methamphetamine Treatment Project. *J Subst Abuse Treat*. Mar 2004;26(2):103–108. doi:10.1016/s0740-5472(03)00163-6
83. Obert JL, Brown AH, Zweben J, et al. When treatment meets research: clinical perspectives from the CSAT Methamphetamine Treatment Project. *J Subst Abuse Treat*. Apr 2005;28(3):231–237. doi:10.1016/j.jsat.2004.12.008
84. Damschroder LJ, Aron DC, Keith RE, Kirsh SR, Alexander JA, Lowery JC. Fostering implementation of health services research findings into practice: a consolidated framework for advancing

implementation science. *Implement Sci.* 2009 Dec;4(1):1–15. doi:10.1186/1748-5908-4-50

85. Hamilton AB, Mittman BS, Campbell D, et al. Understanding the impact of external context on community-based implementation of an evidence-based HIV risk reduction intervention. *BMC Health Serv Res.* 2018;18(1):1–10.
86. Wyatt GE, Hamilton AB, Loeb TB, Moss NJ, Zhang M, Liu H. A hybrid effectiveness/implementation trial of an evidence-based intervention for HIV-serodiscordant African American couples. *Am Psychol.* 2020;75(8):1146.
87. Mthembu J, Hamilton AB, Milburn NG, et al. "It had a lot of cultural stuff in it": HIV-serodiscordant African American couples' experiences of a culturally congruent sexual health intervention. *Ethn Dis.* Spring 2020;30(2):269–276. doi:10.18865/ed.30.2.269
88. Maulsby CH, Holtgrave DR, Hamilton AB, Campbell D, Liu H, Wyatt GE. A cost and cost-threshold analysis of implementation of an evidence-based intervention for HIV-serodiscordant couples. *AIDS Behav.* Sep 2019;23(9):2486–2489. doi:10.1007/s10461-019-02558-w
89. Hamilton AB, Brown A, Loeb T, et al. Enhancing patient and organizational readiness for cardiovascular risk reduction among Black and Latinx patients living with HIV: study protocol. *Prog Cardiovasc Dis.* 2020;63(2):101–108.
90. Hailemariam M, Bustos T, Montgomery B, Barajas R, Evans LB, Drahota A. Evidence-based intervention sustainability strategies: a systematic review. *Implement Sci.* 2019;14(1):1–12.
91. Herlitz L, MacIntyre H, Osborn T, Bonell C. The sustainability of public health interventions in schools: a systematic review. *Implement Sci.* 2020;15(1):1–28.
92. Lennox L, Maher L, Reed J. Navigating the sustainability landscape: a systematic review of sustainability approaches in healthcare. *Implement Sci.* 2018;13(1):1–17.
93. Norton WE, McCannon CJ, Schall MW, Mittman BS. A stakeholder-driven agenda for advancing the science and practice of scale-up and spread in health. *Implement Sci.* 2012;7(1):1–6.
94. Côté-Boileau É, Denis J-L, Callery B, Sabean M. The unpredictable journeys of spreading, sustaining and scaling healthcare innovations: a scoping review. *Health Res Policy Syst.* 2019;17(1):1–26.
95. Fagan AA, Bumbarger BK, Barth RP, et al. Scaling up evidence-based interventions in US public systems to prevent behavioral health problems: challenges and opportunities. *Prev Sci.* 2019;20(8):1147–1168.
96. Jones LP, Slade JL, Davenport F, Santos SLZ, Knott CL. Planning for community scale-up of Project HEAL: insights from the SPRINT Initiative. *Health Promot Pract.* 2020;21(6):944–951.
97. Hursting LM, Chambers DA. Practitioner engagement in implementation science: initiatives and opportunities. *J Public Health Manag Pract.* 2021;27(2):102–104.
98. Westfall JM, Roper R, Gaglioti A, Nease DE Jr. Practice-based research networks: strategic opportunities to advance implementation research for health equity. *EthnDis.* 2019;29(suppl 1):113.
99. McCormack B, Rycroft-Malone J, DeCorby K, et al. A realist review of interventions and strategies to promote evidence-informed healthcare: a focus on change agency. *Implement Sci.* 2013;8(1):1–12.
100. Powell BJ, Fernandez ME, Williams NJ, et al. Enhancing the impact of implementation strategies in healthcare: a research agenda. *Front Public Health.* 2019:7:3. doi:10.3389/fpubh.2019.00003. PMID: 30723713; PMCID: PMC6350272.
101. Prasad V, Ioannidis J. *Evidence-Based De-implementation for Contradicted, Unproven, and Aspiring Healthcare Practices.* Springer; 2014:1–5.
102. Norton WE, Kennedy AE, Chambers DA. Studying de-implementation in health: an analysis of funded research grants. *Implement Sci.* 2017;12(1):1–13.
103. Prusaczyk B, Swindle T, Curran G. Defining and conceptualizing outcomes for de-implementation: key distinctions from implementation outcomes. *Implement Sci Commun.* 2020;1(1):1–10.
104. Nilsen P, Ingvarsson S, Hasson H, von Thiele Schwarz U, Augustsson H. Theories, models, and frameworks for de-implementation of low-value care: a scoping review of the literature. *Implement Res Pract.* 2020;1:2633489520953762.
105. Patey AM, Hurt CS, Grimshaw JM, Francis JJ. Changing behaviour "more or less"—do theories of behaviour inform strategies for implementation and de-implementation? A critical interpretive synthesis. *Implement Sci.* 2018;13(1):1–13.
106. Baumann AA, Cabassa LJ. Reframing implementation science to address inequities in healthcare delivery. *BMC Health Serv Res.* 2020;20(1):1–9.
107. Odeny B. Closing the health equity gap: a role for implementation science? *PLoS Med.* 2021;18(9):e1003762.

108. Shelton RC, Adsul P, Oh A. Recommendations for addressing structural racism in implementation science: a call to the field. *Ethn Disease.* 2021;31(suppl 1):357.
109. Shelton RC, Adsul P, Oh A, Moise N, Griffith DM. Application of an antiracism lens in the field of implementation science (IS): recommendations for reframing implementation research with a focus on justice and racial equity. *Implement Res Pract.* 2021;2:26334895211049482.
110. Pyra M, Motley D, Bouris A. Moving toward equity: fostering transdisciplinary research between the social and behavioral sciences and implementation science to end the HIV epidemic. *Curr Opin HIV AIDS.* 2022;17(2):89–99.
111. Snell-Rood C, Jaramillo ET, Hamilton AB, Raskin SE, Nicosia FM, Willging C. Advancing health equity through a theoretically critical implementation science. *Transl Behav Med.* Aug 13 2021;11(8):1617–1625. doi:10.1093/tbm/ibab008
112. Eslava-Schmalbach J, Garzón-Orjuela N, Elias V, Reveiz L, Tran N, Langlois E. Conceptual framework of equity-focused implementation research for health programs (EquIR). *Int J Equity Health.* 2019;18(1):1–11.
113. McNulty M, Smith J, Villamar J, et al. Implementation research methodologies for achieving scientific equity and health equity. *Ethn Dis.* 2019;29(suppl 1):83.
114. Woodward EN, Singh RS, Ndebele-Ngwenya P, Melgar Castillo A, Dickson KS, Kirchner JE. A more practical guide to incorporating health equity domains in implementation determinant frameworks. *Implement Sci Commun.* 2021;2(1):1–16.
115. Shelton RC, Chambers DA, Glasgow RE. An extension of RE-AIM to enhance sustainability: addressing dynamic context and promoting health equity over time. *Front Public Health.* 2020;8:134.
116. Chinman M, Woodward EN, Curran GM, Hausmann LR. Harnessing implementation science to increase the impact of health disparity research. *Med Care.* 2017;55(suppl 9 2):S16.
117. Kerkhoff AD, Farrand E, Marquez C, Cattamanchi A, Handley MA. Addressing health disparities through implementation science—a need to integrate an equity lens from the outset. *Implement Sci.* 2022;17(1):1–4.
118. Brownson RC, Kumanyika SK, Kreuter MW, Haire-Joshu D. Implementation science should give higher priority to health equity. *Implement Sci.* 2021;16(1):1–16.

22

Health Dissemination and Implementation Within Schools

REBEKKA M. LEE, ANDRIA B. EISMAN, AND STEVEN L. GORTMAKER

INTRODUCTION

Schools hold great promise for the promotion of health. In much of the world, individuals spend the majority of their formative years within school settings. Thus, schools are ideal places to initiate healthy behaviors early on to promote lifelong health. A healthy school environment can promote norms about foods and beverages children consume, physical activity participation, and appropriate social behaviors. These healthy environments can be created by local school practices or mandated by top-down policies. In addition to providing healthy environmental defaults and cues, schools are optimal settings for disseminating health education messages discouraging risk-taking behaviors (e.g., smoking, drinking, drug use, or unprotected sex) and can be an important place for delivering basic preventive services (e.g., vaccines, vision screening, behavioral health assessments). Elementary, middle, and high schools as well as preschools and after-school programs are fundamental settings for establishing healthy habits early on for optimal prevention of childhood health risks as well as chronic disease later in life. With sound implementation, schools have the potential for tremendous reach and impact.

Careful implementation and dissemination research is necessary to ensure that the full promise of schools for health promotion is achieved, considering the important public health objectives of improving population health and simultaneously narrowing health disparities. With hundreds of potential health programs, practices, and policies available, schools may find it difficult to discern which interventions should be adopted. Throughout this chapter, we highlight several interventions with strong evidence for effectiveness—such as the Healthy Hunger Free Kids Act, COVID-19 vaccination, and the Michigan Model for Health—that administrators and teachers can prioritize for implementation.

Education, in and of itself, has been targeted as a key factor for future health and poverty reduction across the globe. In fact, the United Nations named universal primary education as one of their eight Millennium Development Goals, achieving an increase in enrollment from 83% in 2000 to 91% in 2015.[1] Furthermore, they recently adopted the 2030 Agenda for Sustainable Development, which includes the goal of "inclusive and equitable quality education and lifelong learning opportunities for all."[2(p17)] The World Health Organization has identified the school setting as particularly important for promoting intersectoral action to address child and adolescent health.[3] Their Health Promoting Schools Framework—a holistic approach that includes a health education curriculum, school environments that promote health, and school engagement with communities and families—has been taken up by countries throughout the world over the past three decades. These efforts have demonstrated modest effects, with the potential for wide population reach in addressing health outcomes such as physical inactivity, smoking, bullying, and excess body mass index.[4]

In the United States, education has been considered a public good since it became mandatory in all states at the close of World War I.

Rebekka M. Lee, Andria B. Eisman, and Steven L. Gortmaker, *Health Dissemination and Implementation Within Schools* In: *Dissemination and Implementation Research in Health.* Edited by: Ross C. Brownson, Graham A. Colditz, and Enola K. Proctor, Oxford University Press.
 DOI: 10.1093/oso/9780197660690.003.0022

While deliberate health promotion by the state has been encouraged since the 1800s, countries today vary dramatically in their role as provider of health services and preventive programs to their citizens—some providing universal healthcare as a similar public good to education, while others like the United States providing a patchwork healthcare system that does not grant health as a human right and is responsible for persistent health inequities.[5,6] By weaving health promotion, above and beyond the delivery of health services, into the public school agenda, there is the opportunity to reach the whole population, including underserved groups (e.g., rural, low income, people of color), with health messages and services that other settings may miss. Moreover, the amount of time that children spend in school is incomparable to other settings, such as primary care. Consider, for instance, the difference between the 30 minutes a doctor might spend with a child at an annual well visit exam compared with the roughly 75,600 minutes (7 hours/day over 180 days) children spend within school walls each year, not including the preschool years. In the United States, this opportunity for education can be expanded further by funding early education—with plenty of evidence successful implementation can cost-effectively improve life outcomes for children.[7] Thus, promoting health within schools has the potential to reinforce the messages of health professionals in a sustained manner, changing norms and everyday behaviors with accumulating effects across the early years of life (Table 22.1).

However, there is a flip side to this potential. Roughly half of funding for schools in the United States comes from local sources.[8,9] Globally, the sources of school funding vary widely: from countries like New Zealand and Mexico supporting education almost exclusively through national funds and countries like Sweden and the United Kingdom getting the majority of school funds locally.[9] This local funding can translate into differences in public school resources and quality. Without careful planning and attention to issues of implementation and dissemination, situating health promotion efforts in schools could actually exacerbate health inequities because communities with fewer resources may not be able to afford to implement health interventions. In this vein, increased attention should be paid toward selecting low-cost solutions for schools and families that will be most acceptable and feasible for dissemination and ensure equitable health behaviors and outcomes across schools with varying resources.

There is still much to be learned about which interventions (e.g., policies, practices, services, and curricula) are best to implement and disseminate within schools, as well as by whom, when, and how. These issues have been highlighted during the COVID-19 pandemic, as the science concerning effective and feasible school-based strategies to mitigate and control infection changed dramatically, sometimes rapidly, over periods of months. This chapter seeks to review the school-based dissemination and implementation evidence base and discuss the specific challenges that schools face in their quest to promote health.

EVIDENCE BASE AND THEORY

Current State of School-Based Health Intervention Evidence

Identifying evidence-based interventions (EBIs) is a crucial first step for accelerating implementation and dissemination of programs most likely to impact population health. Fortunately, intervention development and efficacy research for school-based universal (i.e., Tier 1) prevention and health promotion interventions, as well as selected (i.e., Tier 2) and indicated (i.e., Tier 3) interventions/treatment services,[10] have generated a substantial number of evidence-based options[11]; researchers have developed efficacious school-based interventions to address a range of conditions, including mental health,[12] substance use prevention,[13–15] violence,[16] physical activity and nutrition,[17,18] as well as for developmental conditions (e.g., autism) across the prevention-intervention spectrum.[19] A range of policies, environmental change strategies, curricula, and services within schools have been shown to be effective in improving health. However, with hundreds of potential health programs, practices, and policies available, schools may find it difficult to discern which interventions should be prioritized for implementation. Below we describe several interventions with strong evidence for effectiveness and some helpful resources for finding EBIs to address the health needs of schools.

Health education may be the most common type of health intervention in schools.

TABLE 22.1 TYPOLOGY OF HEALTH INTERVENTIONS IMPLEMENTED AND DISSEMINATED WITHIN SCHOOLS

Type	Definition	Examples
Health-promoting policies	Regulations implemented at the national, state, district, or school level intended to promote children's health in schools	• District wellness policies • State laws mandating physical activity time • Healthy Hunger Free Kids Act: National mandate for improved school meals, access to free potable water, and Smart Snacks nutrition standards for competitive foods • State laws mandating vaccination
Environmental change strategies	School practices that are intended to create healthy environments for children	• Active recess • Clean drinking water access • Classroom-based social skills development (e.g., Responsive Classroom) • Ventilation and filtration for healthy air quality
Health education messages	Health lessons and messages designed to lay the foundation for lifelong health	• Physical education • Sexual health education • Classroom-based curricula (e.g., Planet Health, Michigan Model for Health) • Healthy messaging directed toward students, staff, and parents on posters and in newsletters
Health program and services	Delivery of prevention and clinical care within school setting	• Vision, hearing, and scoliosis screening • Mental health assessment and counseling (e.g., cognitive behavioral therapy) • Contraceptive and pregnancy care

However, the evidence base for curricula varies widely in the sea of current options available to schools. Comprehensive sexual health education[20] and health education curricula targeting multiple interrelated risk factors, such as the Michigan Model for Health™ (MMH),[21,22] are two recommended exemplars. One environmental intervention in schools to highlight is the installation of chilled drinking water dispensers in cafeterias,[18] which has shown effectiveness in improved nutrition among children. School-based health policies, like the federal Healthy, Hunger-Free Kids Act[23] and state vaccine mandates to enter school,[24] have also shown evidence for effectiveness. Schools are also an important setting for delivering prevention and clinical services such as psychosocial treatments such as cognitive behavioral therapy,[25,26] social and emotional learning,[27,28] and substance use prevention.[15,29]

The COVID-19 pandemic has highlighted the importance of strategies to control the spread of infectious disease in schools. One strategy that has proven very cost–effective in the past is vaccination.[30] There are vaccine requirements for school entry in all states of the United States, as well as a national funding program for removing the financial barriers to child vaccines. As a consequence, vaccination rates are quite high.[31] Other strategies, such as improved school ventilation, are still being studied for their impact on improved health.[32]

While there is much research on the efficacy of specific school-based health interventions and numerous web-based resources for identifying EBIs, too few interventions have been replicated or implemented at scale. The Centers for Disease Control and Prevention (CDC) has set forth guidance for how schools can best create healthy school environments and integrate health promotion services, education, and programs for children.[33] It also hosts the Guide to Community Preventive Services online resource, which publishes systematic reviews and recommendations for public use along with supporting materials and considerations for implementation.[34] The National Institutes of Health has funded web initiatives, such as the Evidence-Based Cancer Control Programs database, which scores the evidence base and helps ease implementation of prevention programs with tailored searches for school-based programs.[35] For identifying evidence-based programs that target behavioral health, the Blueprints for Healthy Youth Development website[36] allows users to search for ratings of school-based programs and reviews the benefits and costs of implementation; the What Works Clearinghouse from the Institute of Education Sciences provides evidence reviews and ratings.[37] CASEL (the Collaborative for Academic and Social and Emotional Learning),[38] and the SAMHSA (Substance Abuse and Mental Health Services Administration) Evidence-Based Practice Resource Center[39] are also useful repositories.

Implementation and Dissemination Quality Gap

A large gap remains between the programs, policies, curricula, and services that are suggested as best practices and those that are currently being implemented within schools. In 2016, the School Health Programs and Policies Study (SHPPS) estimated the following: 74% of elementary and 71% of middle schools had specified time requirements for physical education, but only about 20% required the school use a particular physical education curriculum. Most districts require students entering school for the first time to have hearing (80%) and vision (83%) screening, yet 50% of high schools are prohibited from making condoms available to students.[40] We have noted how vaccine requirements for school in all states of the United States, as well as a national funding program, have led to high coverage rates for multiple vaccines in young children and adolescents.[41] For example, in 2020, an estimated 92% of adolescents were vaccinated for measles, mumps, and rubella (MMR), with similar rates by income level.[24] In contrast, effective vaccines were developed for COVID-19 and tested widely and approved for ages 5 and above in 2021. Unfortunately, use of these vaccines quickly became highly politicized, and initial implementation has been poor, with some states barring vaccine requirements.

The broad adoption of programs like DARE (Drug Abuse Resistance Education) over more effective prevention programs is an illustration of how the dissemination and implementation gap can work in reverse. Although this program showed little to no efficacy for preventing substance use behavior, it was the only curriculum endorsed in the 1986 Drug-Free Schools and Communities Act and has been disseminated to over half of US school districts, costing at least $1 billion each year.[42,43] Further underscoring this issue, a 2016 national survey on obesity prevention and wellness found that less than 3% of schools were implementing evidence-based programs, and schools were conducting initiatives like weight loss competitions and calorie counting, which may unintentionally exacerbate student weight stigma in their place.[44] Follow-up qualitative interviews with school administrators revealed that decisions to adopt these (and other) health-related school programs did not include considerations for the evidence base and were typically driven by enthusiastic teachers or parents.[45] Research also showed that formal sexual health education in the United States has declined in recent years.[20] While one step toward creating schools that promote health is to continue to build the evidence base for efficacy of new interventions, addressing the dissemination gap and identifying strategies for de-implementation of ineffective and potentially harmful health initiatives are essential for future public health research.

Organizations Accelerating Implementation and Dissemination in Schools

National and regional organizations throughout the world, such as the CDC and Schools for Health in Europe, provide leadership in promoting evidence-based health programming within schools as well as resources to support delivery. The CDC and the Association for Supervision and Curriculum Development recommend the whole school, whole community, whole child approach as a means for systematically achieving better health for students, consisting of 10 components: health education, physical education and physical activity, health services, nutrition environment and services, counseling and psychological services, social and emotional climate, physical environment, employee wellness, family engagement, and community involvement.[46] The CDC also helps schools implement and disseminate effective programming with their school guidance documents for topics such as chronic disease management for asthma, oral health, and diabetes; health behavior promotion for sleep, social and emotional learning, healthy eating, and physical activity; as well as self-assessment tools (e.g., School Health Index and Health Education Curriculum Analysis Tool).[33]

Similar school-based health guidance, implementation tools, and assessments are promoted by the Schools for Health in Europe network.[47,48] The Schools for Health in Europe network takes a similar whole school approach to the United States, encompassing school policy, school physical environment, school social environment, individual health skills and actions, and community links and health services. Within their recently released standards and indicators, they established that "School Health Promotion strategies, interventions, and evaluation are evidence-based" (p18). The network focuses on health literacy, healthy eating, physical activity, and mental health and provides a rapid assessment tool schools can use to identify current strengths and areas needing improvement.[48]

Theory Base

School-based implementation and dissemination health research has grown significantly in the past decade. Two common implementation models—the RE-AIM (Reach, Effectiveness, Adoption, Implementation, and Maintenance) evaluation framework and the Consolidated Framework for Implementation Research (CFIR) determinants framework—have been successfully applied to dissemination and implementation research within schools.[49–51] Following these implementation frameworks ensures that schools are intentional in planning, taking into account efficacy of interventions as well as the factors that contribute to feasibility and ultimately successful real-world implementation.

The RE-AIM framework has been effectively used as a guide for evaluating implementation within the school context.[49,52–55] RE-AIM identifies five elements that are key for measuring the success of interventions in real-world settings: reach, efficacy, adoption, implementation, and maintenance.[49] In the context of school-based health promotion, reach would refer to the number of children who are served water or fruits and vegetables every day in the school cafeteria as a result of the Healthy, Hunger-Free Kids Act or how many children participate in an active physical education class. Efficacy would refer to changes in children's behavior that can be attributable to a given school-based intervention, such as their fruit and vegetable consumption or physical activity level. Adoption would refer to the number of schools that order chilled drinking water dispensers to promote water consumption, change their lunch menus in alignment with Healthy, Hunger-Free Kids Act policy, or schedule more hours of physical education. Implementation, although closely linked to adoption, refers specifically to whether planned changes in practice or policy are translated into action. For example, implementation studies would assess if foods and beverages served match those on menus, or if scheduled physical activity blocks run successfully. Finally, maintenance refers to the degree to which initiatives like more nutritious offerings at lunch and improved physical education continue over time.

The CFIR has also been applied to the school setting.[50,56–62] The CFIR brings together a variety of theories and frameworks to comprehensively consider the contextual influences on implementation. These domains of influence include the "outer" setting, characteristics of the individual(s) implementing the intervention, characteristics of the intervention, the "inner" setting (in this case, factors related to the school, e.g., the climate and leadership), and processes of implementation such as approaches to planning and engagement of teachers, parents, and students.[50] The framework has been used to understand barriers and facilitators to creating an expanded medical home by connecting primary care with school-based health centers,[57] implementing a school-based vaccination policy,[60] and implementing school-based nutrition and physical activity interventions.[56,61] Recently, this framework has been adapted using a "rac(ism)-conscious" lens, which can help researchers and practitioners improve understanding of how structural racism interacts with intervention uptake in the school setting.[58]

DISSEMINATION AND IMPLEMENTATION CHALLENGES SPECIFIC TO SCHOOL SETTINGS

Adapting Interventions to Diverse School Settings and Student Populations

As researchers choose their targets for implementation and dissemination research within schools, it is essential that the research is designed with enough flexibility so it can adapt to have local relevance and account for the norms and culture within schools. Examples of adaptations to diverse communities include considering regional differences in the availability of fruits and vegetables, inaccessibility to drinking fountains due to lead in school water in low-income communities, or differences in weather and facilities that would impact physical education curricula or policy changes. Interventions that explicitly seek to identify and change local norms about children's food preferences, the safety of drinking water, or the importance of physical activity will also have a greater chance to be implemented and sustained as they will be more relevant to teachers, children, parents, and members of the community. This focus on equity should also be considered within a given school setting: for instance, using comprehensive sexual health education curricula and contraceptive services that are inclusive of gay and transgender youth; tailoring school-based environmental and policy interventions to consider contextual factors identified by communities, such as the availability of healthy foods to ensure equity for low-income students and students of color; and considering how student and parent experiences of discrimination within the school context in leaders' plans for implementation of EBIs.[58,63] While school priorities and cultures will vary across space and time, one key factor to keep in mind as researchers and practitioners develop, implement, and disseminate school-based interventions is the importance of aligning with the primary mission of learning. Thus, all policies, environmental change strategies, health education, programs, and services should be designed to fit easily into current school practices and, if possible, aim to promote academic as well as health objectives.

Considering Economic Cost and Impacts Beyond Health

School-based health promotion research has seldom explicitly applied economic concepts to investigate issues of dissemination and implementation. Cost is a major factor that influences implementation (see chapter 11), especially within public schools, where budgets are tight and resources have to be allocated carefully. Although Levin started to apply cost-effectiveness within education in the 1970s and 1980s, few studies have applied the strategy to compare the relative costs and effects of interventions in schools.[64–66] Cost-effectiveness guidelines have been developed to inform resource distribution decisions,[67] and recent cost-effectiveness research has begun to be applied to health promotion within the school setting. The Childhood Obesity Intervention Cost-Effectiveness Study (CHOICES) project has identified aspects of the Healthy, Hunger-Free Kids Act of 2010—including Smart Snacks—as particularly cost-effective dietary policy interventions[23]; a recent cost-effectiveness assessment of physical activity interventions identified some of the most cost-effective approaches to increasing child physical activity in schools.[68] This cost-effectiveness approach costs out all resources used in providing an intervention, including personnel (e.g., wages and additional time for teachers, administrators, and volunteers); equipment (e.g., curriculum, chilled water dispensers, parent newsletters); and travel. These costs are partitioned out in terms of costs to the health sector, costs to government sectors (in this case, education), and costs incurred by children, families, and staff.[68] Finding cost-effective strategies is particularly important for making health promotion appealing to education leaders, teachers, policymakers, and taxpayers.

A report designed to direct available resources in Australia ranked 160 health interventions and found that policies that have a broad reach and make use of existing personnel and infrastructure can be particularly cost effective and may even be cost saving in the long run.[69] Providing evidence for cost-effectiveness and benefits beyond health can be important for achieving buy-in and continuing support since academics are the number one priority for schools. Policies and practices that do not require extra staff and limited training and equipment are appealing to administrators as they keep costs down and can be more easily maintained once a research project is complete. Planet Health, for instance, was able to keep costs low by incorporating the curriculum into existing class time, requiring just one book per teacher, and calling for minimal extra materials in lessons (see Planet Health case study, next, for more details).[70]

PLANET HEALTH CASE STUDY

Background

The prevalence of childhood obesity in the United States has increased rapidly to historically high levels over recent decades and has only begun to plateau among children aged 2 to 5 and in some communities and states.[71] Moreover, higher rates of obesity persist among minority and economically disadvantaged youth.[72] Obesity is associated with significant health problems in early life, including high cholesterol and hypertension, and is a significant risk factor for adult morbidity and mortality.[73]

Context

Planet Health, conducted in the mid-1990s, was the first field trial of a middle school-based obesity prevention program.[70] It aimed to move beyond the evidence for efficacy of obesity prevention interventions to show effectiveness within a real-world context. Moreover, process evaluations of Planet Health helped to investigate how the program was implemented and disseminated within schools.[74,75] The intervention had a group randomized design with 10 middle schools matched on area characteristics (e.g., school system) and then randomized to receive the intervention.[70] The communities in the sample had a mean income similar to the US average, and the intervention followed boys and girls in grades 6 to 8 over 2 school years. The primary endpoint for the intervention was obesity prevalence. Secondary endpoints included moderate and vigorous physical activity; TV viewing; dietary intake of fat, fruits, and vegetables; and total energy intake. The interdisciplinary curriculum took a population approach to disease prevention and was guided by behavioral choice and social cognitive theories. Intervention components included staff trainings, classroom lesson plans, and materials for physical education teachers, staff wellness sessions, and small funds to put toward fitness improvements.

Findings and Lessons Learned

Intervention Effectiveness

The 2-year Planet Health intervention was effective across a range of outcomes. It reduced TV watching among boys and girl, as well as decreased obesity prevalence, decreased daily calories consumed, and increased fruit and vegetable intake among girls.[70] Girls in the intervention were also less likely to report weight control behavior disorders.[76]

Evidence for Successful Dissemination and Implementation

After the program was shown to be effective, the Boston Public Schools expressed interest in disseminating Planet Health. In a process evaluation of this dissemination effort, teachers delivered the program at intended levels, indicating that Planet Health can be implemented at the intended dose over three school years.[74] Despite reported challenges of planning time and conflicts with school meals programs, vending machines, and home environments, over 75% of teachers planned to continue teaching Planet Health the next year, and self-reported feasibility and acceptability were high.[74] Collecting theory-based process measures of feasibility, acceptability, and sustainability in the dissemination phase of Planet Health helped to show the promise of how similar interventions can be implemented and sustained within a school system.[74] Following this successful dissemination effort, by 2010, more than 10,000 copies of Planet Health had been purchased in all 50 states and more than 20 countries. Moreover, the program has been shown to be cost-effective for reducing obesity in middle school-aged youth and has been recommended by Cancer Control P.L.A.N.E.T. and the Guide to Community Preventive Services as an effective intervention for reducing screen time and improving weight-related outcomes.[77] When Planet Health was part of a multicomponent community-based intervention in 45 middle schools, there was evidence for increases in fruit and vegetable consumption as well as physical activity, decreases in television viewing, as well as decreases in the proportion of overweight and obese children over 3 years.[78] One change implemented in the most recent Planet Health edition was a focus on healthier beverages, reducing sugary beverage intake and promoting water. The original Planet Health study resulted in the first article documenting the impact of increased sugary beverages on unhealthy weight in adolescents.[79]

Lesson 1: School Context Is Challenging for Study Design and Measurement

The Planet Health intervention faced numerous research challenges due to the unique context of the school setting. First, like many school-based interventions, measurement of health behaviors was limited to self-report.[70] This strategy is often more feasible for a field trial, but has limited reliability and validity, especially among children. Evaluation of school-based programs is also complicated due to the difficulty of tracking changes over time. Planet Health investigators were careful to select a sample of students that would be relatively stable over time and chose implementation measures that would withstand any school or personnel changes over a 2-year time period. Although the study did face these design challenges, the benefits of evaluating the intervention for effectiveness in a real-world setting outweigh these limitations.

Lesson 2: Benefits of Adapting Interventions to Diverse School Settings

Considering the various competing demands within school was important to ensure that the curriculum appealed to teachers and administrators and was implemented as intended. Accordingly, lesson evaluations and focus groups were conducted with teachers during the development of the units.[70] One finding from this formative research was that teachers preferred textbooks to web-based materials. Producing a curriculum that teachers are likely to perceive as advantageous and easy to utilize may seem like an obvious step; however, most research does not build in time to discover these implementation preferences and could miss similar factors and end up developing a program that would not be readily adopted by schools and teachers.

Researchers also spent years building authentic school and community partnerships that help to explain the effectiveness of the intervention in a middle school setting and the positive process evaluation finding. The importance of developing partnerships and working within a community-based participatory research (CBPR) framework also stands out as crucial for moving Planet Health beyond a field trial to dissemination throughout the state and across the country.[74]

Lesson 3: Benefits of Considering Economic Cost and Impacts Beyond Health

Researchers took an interdisciplinary approach that incorporates subject and grade-specific learning objectives in the development of Planet Health. The design of the intervention also considered the limited resources available to schools for health promotion. Its low-cost, population approach weaves nutrition and physical activity messaging into math, English, science, and social studies material with existing classroom teachers.[70,77] Each lesson is designed to promote literacy, and the curriculum aligns with the Massachusetts Department of Education Curriculum Frameworks, which is consistent with learning standards in many other states.[80] A research study in two communities also found that training approaches can considerably impact the cost of Planet Health intervention; training costs were considerably lower when a small number of health teachers were trained to implement the curriculum throughout the school rather than all middle school classroom teachers.[81] In addition to the curriculum, the intervention provided small Fitness Funds to purchase items that would help to sustain changes beyond the study period.[70] By designing a curriculum that was inexpensive and supported the school's primary objective, researchers made the curriculum more appealing to teachers and administrators and likely aided initial implementation, maintenance, and dissemination.

Conclusion

The findings from Planet Health hold several key implications for teachers, policymakers, and researchers. First, the importance of building partnerships with schools cannot be overstated. If researchers want to develop programs that will outlive their evaluation, they must collaborate with the people who will be responsible for delivery down the road from the onset. Specific factors that are likely to carry over to other school-based programs are those that are low cost and easy to integrate into existing classroom practices. These principles have also been adopted in the development of the Harvard T. H. Chan School of Public Health Prevention Research Center Food & Fun Afterschool curriculum and Out-of-School Nutrition and Physical Activity Initiative. Developed and scaled up in collaboration with the largest provider of afterschool programming, the YMCA of the United States, these nutrition and physical activity interventions are designed to be easily integrated into a variety of out-of-school time programs and are available free of charge (http://www.foodandfun.org and https://www.osnap.org).

In the realm of school health services, while all interventions may seem beneficial on the surface, they could vary greatly in their cost-effectiveness. For example, vision and hearing screenings in schools may largely duplicate efforts and end up being cost inefficient.[82] A nutrition curriculum that includes grade- and subject-specific academic lessons, a physical activity program that provides 10-minute classroom activity breaks, or a water campaign that combines messages about environmental responsibility are a few examples of innovative approaches that consider the multitude of priorities within the school setting.

MULTILEVEL INFLUENCES ON IMPLEMENTATION AND DISSEMINATION OF HEALTH INTERVENTIONS IN SCHOOL SETTINGS

The gap between determining intervention efficacy in highly controlled research studies with their focus on internal validity and effectiveness under real-world conditions is substantial, including within schools; both education and health fields continue to struggle in efforts to successfully apply research evidence "at any level of scale"[19] and achieve desired health objectives.[19,83,84] Implementation strategies, methods to enhance the uptake, implementation, and sustainment of EBIs,[84] are urgently needed to address this gap, but a key first step is understanding and identifying determinants that are central to implementation success.[83] Determinants, also referred to as implementation barriers or facilitators, are factors that are believed to, or have been empirically demonstrated to, influence implementation outcomes such as uptake or fidelity.[85]

Researchers have made progress in identifying determinants related to school-based implementation. Determinant frameworks, such as the CFIR, are useful in identifying factors that may influence EBI implementation in schools.[85] While an exhaustive discussion of determinants is beyond the scope of this chapter, here we use CFIR 2.0[86] to guide a brief discussion of determinants across multiple levels and build on a recent summary provided by Lyon and Bruns (2019) of factors that potentially influence the success of intervention implementation within schools.[19]

The outer setting includes the larger context in which implementation occurs; this can also be referred to as the macro level and includes influences of the wider environment, such as educational and health policies, guidelines, mandates or directives, and funding availability. We can consider the outer setting the level of the school district and beyond (e.g., regional school service agency, state- and national-level agencies).[85] Researchers found evidence to support the role of outer setting factors in influencing implementation success and sustainment.[57,87,88] For example, a systematic review of school-based interventions found that sociopolitical context (e.g., policies, mandates, directives) and funding environment and funding availability were the most frequently mentioned outer setting determinants across studies.[89] Examples could include degree to which national or state funding is available to support implementation for health-related initiatives such as HIV prevention or active physical education. Other examples include legislation or mandates to provide prevention (e.g., health education curriculum, vaccination) or treatment services (e.g., mental health treatment).

The inner setting in schools is often considered at the building level[90] and can include various characteristics, such as organizational capacity, size, support from principals and superintendents, competing demands, and resources such as space and equipment.[19,90] Factors such as school priorities, for example, prioritizing education over health, school climate, and leadership support are potentially important inner setting determinants.[91] Researchers also posit that factors more specific to implementation, including the organizational implementation context, may be especially relevant in the success of EBI implementation in schools.[90] The organizational implementation context includes implementation leadership,[92] implementation climate or perceptions of organizational support for EBI implementation,[93] and implementation citizenship behavior (i.e., a demonstrated ongoing commitment to the EBI).[94] Despite consensus that determinants related to the inner setting are highly influential for implementation and intervention objectives, we have a dearth of research investigating these factors and little consensus on which factors or combination of factors may be most critical to implementation success.[19] Future research focusing on the inner setting (i.e., at the school level) will aid in identifying key determinants of implementation and how these inner setting determinants may be similar or different from clinical settings.

Characteristics of implementation team members (e.g., deliverers or teachers)[86] in schools such as age, years of experience, expectations, and attitudes about a given intervention, self-efficacy, intention to implement, and others also may influence effective implementation and sustainment of EBIs within schools.[87,91,95,96] Other factors such as knowledge, experience, motivation, and confidence may also influence school-based EBI implementation.[62,97–99] The research exploring individual-level factors has expanded notably in recent years and across a wide range of prevention and treatment interventions; some of this research is also grounded in well-established health behavior theories such as the theory of planned behavior[100] and the health belief model.[101] One reason this level is of interest is that individual determinants are more proximal and may be easier to change than setting-related factors; importantly, however, individual characteristics are undoubtedly influenced by the context in which they occur.[102]

Characteristics of the interventions themselves have also been investigated as they relate to real-world effectiveness in schools. These attributes can include intervention complexity, evidence base, and the cost and time associated with the deploying it. Intervention adaptability, including cultural tailoring, and the perceived usefulness and acceptability to parents, teachers, school nurses, and students are also important for successful implementation and dissemination.[56,103] The design and usability of an intervention, informed by the field of human-centered design, has also emerged as an important factor influencing implementation success.[104] Researchers and practitioners have developed various tools to assess intervention usability and fit with the context, including school contexts, to promote implementation success and increase the likelihood of achieving desired outcomes.[105]

Although research focused on multilevel determinants of EBI implementation in schools has expanded in recent years, there is also notable heterogeneity in how these determinants are conceptualized and operationalized. This heterogeneity poses challenges to providing clear guidance on what determinants are key and when, and it is likely that multiple levels of determinants will need to be addressed.[106] Currently, researchers recommend engaging with school stakeholders and decision makers as partners in assessing determinants across multiple levels and identifying which determinants are most influential to implementation success to design suitable implementation strategies to address them.[106]

OVERCOMING SCHOOL-BASED CHALLENGES

Designing and Deploying Implementation Strategies

Researchers have long acknowledged the central role of implementation strategies in achieving desired public health outcomes of EBIs.[11] The application of implementation strategies in schools, generally, has lagged behind clinical settings[106]; researchers are increasingly designing and deploying them to address key barriers of effective school-based health intervention implementation.[107,108] Although the primary objective of implementation strategies is to enhance intervention delivery to ultimately improve participant (i.e., student) outcomes, a substantial proportion of implementation efforts fail with little or no impact on behavioral or clinical outcomes; the limited success of earlier research investigating strategies has prompted the recognition that strategies must be designed and tailored to address key barriers (i.e., determinants) within a given school context.[109]

Implementation strategies can be single, discrete strategies or multicomponent "bundled" strategies. As with other implementation science settings, advancing the application of implementation strategies in schools has faced conceptual and methodological challenges due to varied classification taxonomies, measures, participants, and heterogeneity in the implementation strategies deployed[106]; as a result, the current evidence base is limited. Studies are underway, however, to begin addressing these gaps and improve the evidence base.

Cook and colleagues have proposed an implementation strategy taxonomy for school settings adapted from the ERIC (Expert Recommendations for Implementing Change)[83] taxonomy called SISTER (School Implementation Strategies, Translating ERIC Resources).[110] This taxonomy supports more consistent terminology and identification of strategies and investigations into the mechanisms by which these strategies work to produce change.[111] While some of the SISTER strategies originally identified in the ERIC project underwent little change, others underwent significant changes or were omitted altogether as they were deemed not relevant to the school setting. A consistent taxonomy will support comparing and synthesizing results across studies in educational settings.

Researchers are also using more systematic approaches to designing implementation strategies to address key determinants in schools and childcare settings.[112–116] These studies use a variety of designs, address a wide range of health issues and developmental stages of children and youth, and focus on different tiers of prevention (i.e., Tier 1, Tier 2) and levels of implementation determinants. For example, the Adaptive School-Based Implementation of CBT (Cognitive Behavioral Therapy) (ASIC) study tests an adaptive implementation strategy using a sequential multiple assignment, randomized trial (SMART) design to deliver a school-based mental health treatment intervention.[113] In this study, school professionals with training in social work, counseling, or psychology receive different implementation strategies to support uptake and fidelity of the CBT intervention. The implementation strategy deployment begins with low-level, low-intensity, and low-cost replicating effective programs (REP)—a theory-based implementation strategy bundle that includes an intervention package, large-group training, and ongoing technical assistance.[117–119] School professionals who do not deliver CBT with fidelity are randomized to receive different types and levels of implementation supports, including coaching and facilitation. Coaching and facilitation have been demonstrated valuable strategies and target different barriers, but the mechanisms by which they enhance fidelity and uptake remain unknown; thus, the study also focuses on elucidating mechanisms of implementation success to inform future deployment of these strategies.[113] This study, and many others currently underway, will help advance school-based implementation strategy deployment by helping us understand what strategies are effective when and how the strategies generate impact to promote their effectiveness and cost-effectiveness.

Cost is a key consideration in optimizing and sustaining implementation efforts. Resource limitations are a frequently cited barrier to the implementation and sustainment of EBIs within schools.[91,120,121] Most economic evaluations have focused on intervention costs and *not* the costs of implementation strategies required to deploy and sustain them (see chapter 11). Decision makers will be reluctant to invest in implementation strategies without knowing what it will cost them, particularly in the context of competing demands and scarce resources.[122] Thus, systematic examination of costs for achieving program outcomes using implementation strategies is vital for EBI sustainability in educational settings. To achieve and sustain public health objectives, pragmatic costing approaches of implementation strategies and understanding the value of these efforts, that is, conducting economic evaluations of implementation, are vital to informing decisions about resource allocation for EBI *and* their implementation.

Methods and Measures to Support Implementation Science

Developing partnerships with teachers and administrators via CBPR strategies is essential for developing initial buy-in for interventions, institutionalizing new school policies, sustaining curricula usage, or maintaining healthy school environments.[123,124] Employing CBPR means including key stakeholders in all stages of the research process—the development of research questions, the choice of intervention strategies and measurement decisions, as well as the review of findings in a manner that can be useful for future planning and intervention. By engaging classroom teachers, superintendents, physical education teachers, counselors, school food service personnel, children, and their families, school-based health interventions are likely to be implemented with greater attention to the real-world barriers to change within schools and be better sustained once any formal study of the intervention is complete.

Care should be taken to develop reliable and valid measures of implementation processes and health outcomes, regardless of study design (see chapter 15).[125] There are benefits and drawbacks to the variety of measurement strategies that are currently utilized in school-based implementation research. Whenever possible, it is beneficial to collect data on the implementation process prospectively to avoid collecting retrospective data that could be influenced by the experience of the participation in the intervention. Most school implementation studies to date rely on self-reports of implementation barriers and facilitators via questionnaire to determine the factors that influence successful change. These self-reports can provide insight into the perceptions of those who are responsible for implementing the interventions, but could be subject to bias; recent research, for example, indicated little problem with water access when reported by school officials, but half of schools were found to have access problems when measured objectively.[126] Researchers should consider who they are collecting reports from when they develop questionnaires to ensure they understand the realities of implementation within the school. For instance, classroom teachers and principals may have differing perspectives of the barriers they face in implementation of a nutrition curriculum—teachers may emphasize resistance from students, while administrators focus more on budget constraints. Observations and in-depth interviews may lend important information to measurement in implementation for future studies.[127] The stages or levels of implementation are also generally self-reported, although they could also come from more objective sources, such as purchasing reports for curricula, attendance at trainings, online reporting systems, or purchases made through school food service. Finally, the measurement of costs has great potential for prioritizing school-based health solutions; however, more research is needed to assess the validity and reliability of these measurement strategies.

RESEARCH GAPS AND DIRECTIONS FOR THE FUTURE

There is much need for more research in the field of school-based implementation and dissemination for health. While there is solid evidence for the efficacy of interventions, from Tier 1 curricula to policies, that are designed to promote health in schools, many have not been translated from "best practice" to "routine practice." More research is needed to identify effective strategies for implementing and disseminating EBIs in schools and understanding how to de-implement current practices that are ineffective or even harmful to child health. Central to this is investigating the *key* determinants or factors that influence the implementation and dissemination of efficacious interventions into real-world settings. A growing number of school-based studies have attempted to tease out the different influences of personnel, setting, and intervention features on intervention effectiveness; this research suffers from inconsistencies in how these factors are conceptualized and operationalized. The field would benefit from measures that can be applied across school settings, including organizational-level implementation measures[90] (e.g., implementation climate and leadership) and health policy implementation measures[128] to continue building the evidence base. Future research should expand the evidence base of implementation mechanism within schools, linking context to implementation strategies and considering the unique context of schools and teachers as implementers in contrast to much of implementation science research that sits within clinical settings. Similar to the inconsistent measurement of implementation and dissemination processes, these moderating factors that make or break the success of an intervention within schools are infrequently measured. When assessed, they vary considerably in how they are operationalized within studies. One major step toward addressing this research gap is for investigators to broaden the traditional intervention effectiveness study that narrowly focuses on short-term behavioral and attitudinal outcomes to include more rigorous study of the intervention implementation process and the factors that positively and negatively affect uptake at each stage. These studies should be rooted in comprehensive theories or frameworks, such as the CFIR and RE-AIM, and employ strong study designs. School-based studies should also continue to build the evidence base on cost and cost-effectiveness. Finally, in order to take advantage of the potential schools have as settings for narrowing health disparities and advancing health equity, research should focus on developing strong school and community partnerships and emphasize the importance of cost-effective strategies for health promotion.

SUMMARY

This chapter began by emphasizing the enormous potential schools hold for impacting population health. Considering the constant presence of school in children's lives for over 12 years, it is important to conduct research and plan programs that can work together across the life course to promote health and seek to understand how schools can help to link children to services beyond the school walls. A large gap between the evidence for effectiveness of school-based health interventions and the types of programs, policies, and services that currently influence the lives of children must be addressed. While school settings offer an unparalleled opportunity to reach large populations of youth with evidence-based public health interventions, the excitement of translating research findings into practice need be balanced by the realities of the educational system and the implementation barriers and facilitators specific to schools. Future school-based dissemination and implementation research cannot overestimate the importance of developing strategies that are compatible with the primary aims of schools: promoting learning through reading, writing, math, and more. Equally important is considering policy and environmental change strategies at the national, state, and district levels to promote health within schools. Policies that make use of existing personnel and infrastructure can be particularly cost-effective. Research within schools should investigate the determinants that influence quality of implementation and assess the impact of interventions and implementation strategies that have been adapted to local contexts and to accommodate real-world barriers.

SUGGESTED READINGS AND WEBSITES

Readings

Allen M, Wilhelm A, Ortega LE, Pergament S, Bates N, Cunningham B. Applying a race(ism)-conscious adaptation of the CFIR framework to understand implementation of a school-based equity-oriented intervention. *Ethn Dis.* 2021;31(suppl 1):375–388.

This article describes a qualitative analysis from a school-based effectiveness-implementation hybrid study. It demonstrates how the Consolidated Framework for Implementation Research can be adapted to explicitly assess how structural racism influences implementation within schools.

Cook CR, Lyon AR, Locke J, Waltz T, Powell BJ. Adapting a compilation of implementation strategies to advance school-based implementation research and practice. *Prev Sci.* 2019;20(6):914–935.

The study of implementation strategies within schools settings has advanced in recent years. This article describes how the Expert Recommendations for Implementing Change (ERIC) menu of implementation strategies originally developed for clinical settings was adapted to the education sector.

Gortmaker SL, Wang YC, Long MW, et al. Three interventions that reduce childhood obesity are projected to save more than they cost to implement. *Health Aff (Millwood).* 2015;34(11):1932–1939.

This article describes the CHOICES modeling approach used to assess the cost-effectiveness of dietary intervention, including policy changes within school settings due to the Healthy Hunger Free Kids Act. It examines impact on cost-effectiveness metrics, total costs, and population health outcomes.

Selected Websites and Tools

Blueprints for Healthy Youth Development. http://www.blueprintsprograms.com

The Blueprints website provides a database of evidence-based programs for positive youth development. Practitioners interested in school-based interventions can narrow their search using the program selector by setting. The site provides ratings of evidence as well as information about costs and funding strategies.

ChangeLab Solutions: Childcare & Schools—Supporting Children's Health. https://www.changelabsolutions.org/child-care-schools

ChangeLab Solutions provides community-based solutions for America's most common and preventable diseases. Their Child Care and Schools page provides practical tools that can support school-based implementation, such as a fact sheet on school drinking water access and model policy language for Safe Routes to School.

Evidence-Based Cancer Control Programs (EBCCP). https://ebccp.cancercontrol.cancer.gov

This is a database of evidence-based interventions and program materials designed for cancer prevention. School-based practitioners can search by setting to identify program materials, ratings provided by external experts, and assessments of implementation metrics according to the RE-AIM framework.

Centers for Disease Control and Prevention: Healthy Schools. https://www.cdc.gov/healthyschools/

The CDC Healthy Schools page provides links to data and statistics, training opportunities, state programs, and tools for promoting health within the school setting. There are specific areas devoted to nutrition, physical activity, obesity prevention, chronic health conditions, and wellness policies.

Harvard T. H. Chan School of Public Health Prevention Research Center (HPRC). https://www.hsph.harvard.edu/prc/

The Harvard School of Public Health Prevention Research Center website includes links to sample lessons from Planet Health and Eat Well and Keep Moving (a similar curriculum designed for elementary grades). The HPRC Food and Fun Afterschool and OSNAP materials also include planning tools designed to improve implementation of nutrition and physical activity changes in resource-tight settings.

Schools for Health in Europe. https://www.schoolsforhealth.org/

Schools for Health in Europe aims to support organizations and professionals to further develop and sustain school health promotion by providing the European platform for school health promotion. The network is coordinated by the Netherlands Institute for Health Promotion as a WHO Collaborating Center for School Health Promotion.

REFERENCES

1. United Nations. Millennium goals.2002. Accessed January 31, 2022. https://www.un.org/millenniumgoals/
2. United Nations. Transforming our world: the 2030 Agenda for Sustainable Development 2015. https://documents-dds-ny.un.org/doc/UNDOC/GEN/N15/291/89/PDF/N1529189.pdf?OpenElement
3. World Health Organization (WHO). *European Strategy for Child and Adolescent Health and Development.* WHO Regional Office for Europe; 2008.
4. Langford R, Bonell C, Jones H, et al. The World Health Organization's Health Promoting Schools framework: a Cochrane systematic review and meta-analysis. *BMC Public Health.* Feb 12 2015;15:130. doi:10.1186/s12889-015-1360-y
5. Young I. Health promotion in schools—a historical perspective. *Promot Educ.* 2005;12(3–4):112–117, 184–190, 205–211.
6. Chadwick E. *Report of the Sanitary Conditions of the Labouring Population of Great Britain.* 1842. London: W. Clowes and Sons.
7. Cannon JS, Kilburn MR, Karoly LA, Mattox T, Muchow AN, Buenaventura M. Investing early: taking stock of outcomes and economic returns from early childhood programs. *Rand Health Q.* Mar 2018;7(4):6.
8. National Center for Education Statistics. *Public School Revenue Sources. Condition of Education.* U.S. Department of Education, Institute of Education Sciences. 2022. Retrieved January 16, 2023, from https://nces.ed.gov/programs/coe/indicator/cma
9. Organization for Economic Cooperation and Development (OECD). *Education at a Glance 2018: OECD Indicators.* OECD Publishing; 2018.
10. August GJ, Piehler TF, Miller FG. Getting "SMART" about implementing multi-tiered systems of support to promote school mental health. *J Sch Psychol.* 2018;66:85–96. doi:10.1016/j.jsp.2017.10.001
11. Inman DD, van Bakergem KM, Larosa AC, Garr DR. Evidence-based health promotion programs for schools and communities. *Am J Prev Med.* Feb 2011;40(2):207–219. doi:10.1016/j.amepre.2010.10.031
12. Dray J, Bowman J, Campbell E, et al. Systematic review of universal resilience-focused interventions targeting child and adolescent mental health in the school setting. *J Am Acad Child Adolesc Psychiatry.* Oct 2017;56(10):813–824. doi:10.1016/j.jaac.2017.07.780
13. Thomas RE, McLellan J, Perera R. School-based programmes for preventing smoking. *Cochrane Database Syst Rev.* 2013;2013(4):CD001293.
14. Faggiano F, Vigna-Taglianti FD, Versino E, Zambon A, Borraccino A, Lemma P. School-based prevention for illicit drugs' use. *The Cochrane Database Syst Rev.* 2005;8(4):CD003020.
15. Hodder RK, Freund M, Wolfenden L, et al. Systematic review of universal school-based "resilience" interventions targeting adolescent tobacco, alcohol or illicit substance use: a meta-analysis. *Prev Med.* Jul 2017;100:248–268. doi:10.1016/j.ypmed.2017.04.003
16. Mytton JA, DiGuiseppi C, Gough D, Taylor RS, Logan S. School-based secondary prevention programmes for preventing violence. *Cochrane Database Syst Rev.* 2006;2006(3):CD004606.
17. Dobbins M DK, Robeson P, Husson H, Tirilis D. School-based physical activity programs for promoting physical activity and fitness in children and adolescents aged 6–18. *Cochrane Database Syst Rev.* 2009 Jan 21;(1):CD007651. doi:10.1002/14651858.CD007651
18. Kenney EL, Cradock AL, Long MW, et al. Cost-effectiveness of water promotion strategies in schools for preventing childhood obesity and increasing water intake. *Obesity (Silver Spring).* 2019;27(12):2037–2045. doi:10.1002/oby.22615
19. Lyon AR, Bruns EJ. From evidence to impact: joining our best school mental health practices with our best implementation strategies. *School Ment Health.* Mar 2019;11(1):106–114. doi:10.1007/s12310-018-09306-w
20. Goldfarb ES, Lieberman LD. Three decades of research: the case for comprehensive sex education. *J Adolesc Health.* 2021;68(1):13–27. doi:10.1016/j.jadohealth.2020.07.036

21. MacArthur G, Caldwell DM, Redmore J, et al. Individual-, family-, and school-level interventions targeting multiple risk behaviours in young people. *Cochrane Database Syst Rev.* 2018;10:CD009927. doi:10.1002/14651858.CD009927.pub2
22. O'neill JM, Clark JK, Jones JA. Promoting mental health and preventing substance abuse and violence in elementary students: a randomized control study of the Michigan Model for Health. *J Sch Health.* Jun 2011;81(6):320–330. doi:10.1111/j.1746-1561.2011.00597.x
23. Gortmaker SL, Wang YC, Long MW, et al. Three interventions that reduce childhood obesity are projected to save more than they cost to implement. *Health Aff (Millwood).* Nov 2015;34(11):1932–1939. doi:10.1377/hlthaff.2015.0631
24. Pingali C, Yankey D, Elam-Evans LD, et al. National, regional, state, and selected local area vaccination coverage among adolescents aged 13–17 years—United States, 2020. *MMWR Morb Mortal Wkly Rep.* Sep 03 2021;70(35):1183–1190. doi:10.15585/mmwr.mm7035a1
25. Caldwell DM, Davies SR, Hetrick SE, et al. School-based interventions to prevent anxiety and depression in children and young people: a systematic review and network meta-analysis. *Lancet Psychiatry.* 2019;6(12):1011–1020. doi:10.1016/S2215-0366(19)30403-1
26. Hetrick SE, Cox GR, Witt KG, Bir JJ, Merry SN. Cognitive behavioural therapy (CBT), third-wave CBT and interpersonal therapy (IPT) based interventions for preventing depression in children and adolescents. *Cochrane Database Syst Rev.* Aug 09 2016;(8):CD003380. doi:10.1002/14651858.CD003380.pub4
27. Durlak JA, Weissberg RP, Dymnicki AB, Taylor RD, Schellinger KB. The impact of enhancing students' social and emotional learning: a meta-analysis of school-based universal interventions. *Child Dev.* Jan–Feb 2011;82(1):405–432. doi:10.1111/j.1467-8624.2010.01564.x
28. Fenwick-Smith A, Dahlberg EE, Thompson SC. Systematic review of resilience-enhancing, universal, primary school-based mental health promotion programs. *BMC Psychol.* Jul 05 2018;6(1):30. doi:10.1186/s40359-018-0242-3
29. Das JK, Salam RA, Arshad A, Finkelstein Y, Bhutta ZA. Interventions for adolescent substance abuse: an overview of systematic reviews. *J Adolesc Health.* Oct 2016;59(4S):S61–S75. doi:10.1016/j.jadohealth.2016.06.021
30. Zhou F, Shefer A, Wenger J, et al. Economic evaluation of the routine childhood immunization program in the United States, 2009. *Pediatrics.* Apr 2014;133(4):577–585. doi:10.1542/peds.2013-0698
31. Walsh B, Doherty E, O'Neill C. Since the start of the vaccines for children program, uptake has increased, and most disparities have decreased. *Health Aff (Millwood).* Feb 2016;35(2):356–364. doi:10.1377/hlthaff.2015.1019
32. Jones E, Young A, Clevenger K, et al. Schools for health: risk reduction strategies for reopening schools. Harvard T. H. Chan School of Public Health Healthy Buildings program. 2020. Accessed January 31, 2022. https://schools.forhealth.org/risk-reduction-strategies-for-reopening-schools/
33. Prevention CfDCa. CDC Healthy Schools. Division of Population Health, National Center for Chronic Disease Prevention and Health Promotion. Accessed January 16, 2023. https://www.cdc.gov/healthyschools/
34. Community Preventive Services Task Force. The Community Guide. Accessed 2022, January 31. https://www.thecommunityguide.org/content/guide-clinical-preventive-services-0
35. Institute National Cancer Institute. Evidence-Based Cancer Control Programs home page. Accessed January 31, 2022. https://ebccp.cancercontrol.cancer.gov
36. Science University of Colorado Boulder, Institute of Behavioral Science. Blueprints for Healthy Youth Development home page. Accessed January 31, 2022. https://www.blueprintsprograms.org/
37. Assistance Institute for Education Sciences, U.S. Department of Education. What Works Clearinghouse. Accessed January 31, 2022. https://ies.ed.gov/ncee/wwc/
38. Collaborative for Academic, Social, and Emotional Learning (CASEL). Home page. Accessed January 31, 2022. https://casel.org/systemic-implementation/
39. Substance Abuse and Mental Health Services Administration (SAMHSA). Evidence-Based Practices Resource Center home page. Accessed January 31, 2022. https://www.samhsa.gov/resource-search/ebp
40. Centers for Disease Control and Prevention (CDC). Results from the School Health Policies and Practices Study. 2016. https://www.cdc.gov/healthyyouth/data/shpps/pdf/shpps-results_2016.pdf
41. Center for State, Tribal, Local, and Territorial Support, Centers for Disease Control and Prevention. State school immunization requirements and vaccine exemption laws. https://www.cdc.gov/phlp/docs/school-vaccinations.pdf
42. Ennett ST, Tobler NS, Ringwalt CL, Flewelling RL. How effective is drug abuse resistance

education? A meta-analysis of Project DARE outcome evaluations. *Am J Public Health.* September 1 1994;84(9):1394–1401. doi:10.2105/ajph.84.9.1394
43. Shepard EM. *The Economic Costs of D.AR.E.* 2001. Syracuse, NY: Institution of Industrial Relations. https://usiraq.procon.org/sourcefiles/2001EconCosts.pdf
44. Kenney EL, Wintner S, Lee RM, Austin SB. Obesity prevention interventions in US public schools: are schools using programs that promote weight stigma? *Prev Chronic Dis.* 2017;14:E142. doi:10.5888/pcd14.160605
45. Lee R, Plummer R, Gordon A, Brion-Meisels G, Kenney E. A qualitative exploration of factors influencing implementation of stigmatizing programs in schools: Setting the groundwork for de-implementation. Presented at: Conference of the Science of Dissemination and Implementation in Health; 2021. Washington DC.
46. Lewallen TC, Hunt H, Potts-Datema W, Zaza S, Giles W. The whole school, whole community, whole child model: a new approach for improving educational attainment and healthy development for students. *J Sch Health.* Nov 2015;85(11):729–739. doi:10.1111/josh.12310
47. Burgher MS, Rasmussen VB, Rivett D. *The European Network of Health Promoting Schools: The Alliance of Education and Health.* 1999. https://www.euro.who.int/__data/assets/pdf_file/0004/252391/E62361.pdf
48. Schools for Health in Europe. Accessed July 14, 2010. https://www.schoolsforhealth.org/sites/default/files/editor/standards_and_indicators_2.pdf
49. Glasgow RE, Vogt TM, Boles SM. Evaluating the public health impact of health promotion interventions: the RE-AIM framework. *Am J Public Health.* 1999;89(9):1322–1327.
50. Damschroder LJ, Aron DC, Keith RE, Kirsh SR, Alexander JA, Lowery JC. Fostering implementation of health services research findings into practice: a consolidated framework for advancing implementation science. *Implement Sci.* Aug 07 2009;4:50. doi:10.1186/1748-5908-4-50
51. Nilsen P. Making sense of implementation theories, models and frameworks. *Implement Sci.* Apr 21 2015;10(53). doi:10.1186/s13012-015-0242-0. https://implementationscience.biomedcentral.com/articles/10.1186/s13012-015-0242-0#citeas
52. McGoey T, Root Z, Bruner MW, Law B. Evaluation of physical activity interventions in youth via the Reach, Efficacy/Effectiveness, Adoption, Implementation, and Maintenance (RE-AIM) framework: a systematic review of randomised and non-randomised trials. *Prev Med.* Jul 2015;76:58–67. doi:10.1016/j.ypmed.2015.04.006
53. Marhefka SL, Noble CA, Walsh-Buhi ER, et al. Key considerations and recommended strategies for conducting a school-based longitudinal RE-AIM evaluation: insights from a 28-school cluster randomized trial. *Health Promot Pract.* Oct 04 2021;24(1):15248399211042339. doi:10.1177/15248399211042339
54. Natale RA, Kolomeyer E, Robleto A, Jaffery Z, Spector R. Utilizing the RE-AIM framework to determine effectiveness of a preschool intervention program on social-emotional outcomes. *Eval Program Plann.* 2020;79:101773. doi:10.1016/j.evalprogplan.2019.101773
55. Bastos PO, Cavalcante ASP, Pereira WMG, et al. Health promoting school interventions in Latin America: a systematic review protocol on the dimensions of the RE-AIM framework. *Int J Environ Res Public Health.* 2020;17(15):5558. https://www.mdpi.com/1660-4601/17/15/5558
56. Norman Å, Nyberg G, Elinder LS, Berlin A. One size does not fit all-qualitative process evaluation of the Healthy School Start parental support programme to prevent overweight and obesity among children in disadvantaged areas in Sweden. *BMC Public Health.* Jan 14 2016;16(37). https://www.ncbi.nlm.nih.gov/pmc/articles/PMC4712479/
57. Riley M, Laurie AR, Plegue MA, Richarson CR. The adolescent "expanded medical home": school-based health centers partner with a primary care clinic to improve population health and mitigate social determinants of health. *J Am Board Fam Med.* May–Jun 2016;29(3):339–347. doi:10.3122/jabfm.2016.03.150303
58. Allen M, Wilhelm A, Ortega LE, Pergament S, Bates N, Cunningham B. Applying a race(ism)-conscious adaptation of the CFIR framework to understand implementation of a school-based equity-oriented intervention. *Ethn Dis.* 2021;31(suppl 1):375–388. doi:10.18865/ed.31.S1.375
59. Hudson KG, Lawton R, Hugh-Jones S. Factors affecting the implementation of a whole school mindfulness program: a qualitative study using the consolidated framework for implementation research. *BMC Health Serv Res.* Feb 22 2020;20(1):133. doi:10.1186/s12913-020-4942-z
60. Colón-López V, Soto-Abreu R, Medina-Laabes DT, et al. Implementation of the human papillomavirus school-entry requirement in Puerto Rico: barriers and facilitators using the consolidated framework for implementation research. *Hum Vaccin Immunother.* 2021;17(11):4423–4432. doi:10.1080/21645515.2021.1955609

61. McLoughlin GM, Candal P, Vazou S, et al. Evaluating the implementation of the SWITCH® school wellness intervention and capacity-building process through multiple methods. *Int J Behav Nutr Phys Act.* 2020;17(1):162. doi:10.1186/s12966-020-01070-y
62. Leung E, Wanner KJ, Senter L, Brown A, Middleton D. What will it take? Using an implementation research framework to identify facilitators and barriers in implementing a school-based referral system for sexual health services. *BMC Health Serv Res.* Apr 07 2020;20(1):292. doi:10.1186/s12913-020-05147-z
63. Kumanyika SK, Swank M, Stachecki J, Whitt-Glover MC, Brennan LK. Examining the evidence for policy and environmental strategies to prevent childhood obesity in black communities: new directions and next steps. *Obes Rev.* Oct 2014;15(suppl 4):177–203. doi:10.1111/obr.12206
64. Levin HM. Waiting for Godot: cost-effectiveness analysis in education. *New Dir Eval.* 2001;90:55–68.
65. Levin HM, Glass GV, Meister GR. Cost-effectiveness of computer-assisted instruction. *Eval Rev.* 1987;11(1):50–72.
66. Hummel-Rossi B, Ashdown J. The state of cost-benefit and cost-effectiveness analyses in education. *Rev Educ Res.* 2002;72(1):1–30.
67. Weinstein MC, Siegel JE, Gold MR, Kamlet MS, Russell LB. Recommendations of the Panel on Cost-Effectiveness in Health and Medicine. *JAMA.* Oct 16 1996;276(15):1253–1258.
68. Cradock AL, Barrett JL, Kenney EL, et al. Using cost-effectiveness analysis to prioritize policy and programmatic approaches to physical activity promotion and obesity prevention in childhood. *Prev Med.* 2017;95(suppl): S17–S27. doi:10.1016/j.ypmed.2016.10.017
69. Vos T, Carter R, Barendregt J, Mihalopoulos C, Veerman JL, Magnus A, Cobiac L, Bertram MY, Wallace AL, ACE–Prevention Team (2010). Assessing Cost-Effectiveness in Prevention (ACE–Prevention): Final Report. University of Queensland, Brisbane and Deakin University, Melbourne.
70. Gortmaker SL, Peterson K, Wiecha J, et al. Reducing obesity via a school-based interdisciplinary intervention among youth: Planet Health. *Arch Pediatr Adolesc Med.* Apr 1999;153(4):409–418.
71. Ogden CL, Carroll MD, Lawman HG, et al. Trends in obesity prevalence among children and adolescents in the United States, 1988–1994 through 2013–2014. *JAMA.* Jun 07 2016;315(21):2292–2299. doi:10.1001/jama.2016.6361
72. Ogden CL, Fryar CD, Martin CB, et al. Trends in obesity prevalence by race and Hispanic origin—1999–2000 to 2017–2018. *JAMA.* Sep 22 2020;324(12):1208–1210. doi:10.1001/jama.2020.14590
73. Freedman DS, Dietz WH, Srinivasan SR, Berenson GS. The relation of overweight to cardiovascular risk factors among children and adolescents: the Bogalusa Heart Study. *Pediatrics.* Jun 1999;103(6 pt 1):1175–1182.
74. Wiecha JL, El Ayadi AM, Fuemmeler BF, et al. Diffusion of an integrated health education program in an urban school system: Planet Health. *J Pediatr Psychol.* Sep 2004;29(6):467–474.
75. Franks A, Kelder SH, Dino GA, et al. School-based programs: lessons learned from CATCH, Planet Health, and Not-on-Tobacco. *Prev Chronic Dis.* April 2007;4(2). Available from: http://www.cdc.gov/pcd/issues/2007/apr/06_0105.htm
76. Austin SB, Field AE, Wiecha J, Peterson KE, Gortmaker SL. The impact of a school-based obesity prevention trial on disordered weight-control behaviors in early adolescent girls. *Arch Pediatr Adolesc Med.* Mar 2005;159(3):225–230.
77. Wang LY, Yang Q, Lowry R, Wechsler H. Economic analysis of a school-based obesity prevention program. *Obes Res.* 2003;11(11):1313–1324.
78. Peterson KE, Spadano-Gasbarro JL, Greaney ML, et al. Three-year improvements in weight status and weight-related behaviors in middle school students: the Healthy Choices Study. *PLoS One.* 2015;10(8):e0134470. doi:10.1371/journal.pone.0134470
79. Ludwig DS, Peterson KE, Gortmaker SL. Relation between consumption of sugar-sweetened drinks and childhood obesity: a prospective, observational analysis. *Lancet.* 2001;357(9255):505–508.
80. Carter J, Wiecha JL, Peterson KE, Nobrega S, Gortmaker SL. *Planet Health: An Interdisciplinary Curriculum for Teaching Middle School Nutrition and Physical Activity.* 2nd ed. Human Kinetics; 2007.
81. Blaine RE, Franckle RL, Ganter C, et al. Using school staff members to implement a childhood obesity prevention intervention in low-income school districts: the Massachusetts Childhood Obesity Research Demonstration (MA-CORD Project), 2012–2014. *Prev Chronic Dis.* 2017;14:E03. doi:10.5888/pcd14.160381
82. Deuson RR, Hoekstra EJ, Sedjo R, et al. The Denver school-based adolescent hepatitis B vaccination program: a cost analysis with risk simulation. *Am J Public Health.* Nov 1999;89(11):1722–1727.
83. Powell BJ, Waltz TJ, Chinman MJ, et al. A refined compilation of implementation strategies: results from the Expert Recommendations for Implementing Change (ERIC) project.

Implement Sci. Feb 12 2015;10:21. doi:10.1186/s13012-015-0209-1
84. Proctor EK, Powell BJ, McMillen JC. Implementation strategies: recommendations for specifying and reporting. *Implement Sci.* Dec 01 2013;8:139. doi:10.1186/1748-5908-8-139
85. Nilsen P, Bernhardsson S. Context matters in implementation science: a scoping review of determinant frameworks that describe contextual determinants for implementation outcomes. *BMC Health Serv Res.* Mar 25 2019;19(1):189. doi:10.1186/s12913-019-4015-3
86. Damschroder LJ, Reardon CM, Widerquist MAO, et al. The updated Consolidated Framework for Implementation Research based on user feedback. *Implementation Sci.* 2022;17:75. https://doi.org/10.1186/s13012-022-01245-0.
87. Lee RM, Okechukwu C, Emmons KM, Gortmaker SL. Impact of implementation factors on children's water consumption in the Out-of-School Nutrition and Physical Activity group-randomized trial. *New Dir Youth Dev.* 2014;2014(143):79–101. doi:10.1002/yd.20105
88. Hastmann TJ, Bopp M, Fallon EA, Rosenkranz RR, Dzewaltowski DA. Factors influencing the implementation of organized physical activity and fruit and vegetable snacks in the HOP'N after-school obesity prevention program. *J Nutr Educ Behav.* Jan–Feb 2013;45(1):60–68. doi:10.1016/j.jneb.2012.06.005
89. Shoesmith A, Hall A, Wolfenden L, et al. Barriers and facilitators influencing the sustainment of health behaviour interventions in schools and childcare services: a systematic review. *Implement Sci.* 2021;16(1):62. doi:10.1186/s13012-021-01134-y
90. Lyon AR, Cook CR, Brown EC, et al. Assessing organizational implementation context in the education sector: confirmatory factor analysis of measures of implementation leadership, climate, and citizenship. *Implement Sci.* 2018;13(1):5. doi:10.1186/s13012-017-0705-6
91. Herlitz L, MacIntyre H, Osborn T, Bonell C. The sustainability of public health interventions in schools: a systematic review. *Implement Sci.* 2020;15(1):4. doi:10.1186/s13012-019-0961-8
92. Aarons GA, Ehrhart MG, Farahnak LR, Sklar M. Aligning leadership across systems and organizations to develop a strategic climate for evidence-based practice implementation. *Annu Rev Public Health.* 2014;35:255–274. doi:10.1146/annurev-publhealth-032013-182447
93. Ehrhart MG, Aarons GA, Farahnak LR. Assessing the organizational context for EBP implementation: the development and validity testing of the Implementation Climate Scale (ICS). *Implement Sci.* Oct 23 2014;9:157. doi:10.1186/s13012-014-0157-1
94. Ehrhart MG, Aarons GA, Farahnak LR. Going above and beyond for implementation: the development and validity testing of the Implementation Citizenship Behavior Scale (ICBS). *Implement Sci.* May 07 2015;10:65. doi:10.1186/s13012-015-0255-8
95. Harris BR, Shaw BA, Sherman BR, Lawson HA. Screening, brief intervention, and referral to treatment for adolescents: attitudes, perceptions, and practice of New York school-based health center providers. *Subst Abus.* 2016;37(1):161–167. doi:10.1080/08897077.2015.1015703
96. Domitrovich CE, Pas ET, Bradshaw CP, et al. Individual and School organizational factors that influence implementation of the PAX Good Behavior Game Intervention. *Prev Sci.* Nov 2015;16(8):1064–1074. doi:10.1007/s11121-015-0557-8
97. Eisman AB, Kilbourne AM, Greene D, Walton M, Cunningham R. The user-program interaction: how teacher experience shapes the relationship between intervention packaging and fidelity to a state-adopted health curriculum. *Prev Sci.* 2020;21(6):820–829. doi:10.1007/s11121-020-01120-8
98. Leeman J, Wiecha JL, Vu M, et al. School health implementation tools: a mixed methods evaluation of factors influencing their use. *Implement Sci.* 2018;13(1):48. doi:10.1186/s13012-018-0738-5
99. Locke J, Kang-Yi C, Frederick L, Mandell DS. Individual and organizational characteristics predicting intervention use for children with autism in schools. *Autism.* 2020;24(5):1152–1163. doi:10.1177/1362361319895923
100. Ajzen I. From intentions to actions: a theory of planned behavior. In: Kuhl J, Beckmann J, eds. *Action Control.* SSP Springer Series in Social Psychology; 1985:11–39.
101. Hochbaum G. *Public Participation in Medical Screening Programs: A Socio-Psychological Study.* US Department of Health, Education, and Welfare; 1958.
102. Lyon AR, Pullmann MD, Dorsey S, et al. Protocol for a hybrid type 2 cluster randomized trial of trauma-focused cognitive behavioral therapy and a pragmatic individual-level implementation strategy. *Implement Sci.* 2021;16(1):3. doi:10.1186/s13012-020-01064-1
103. Alhassan S, Greever C, Nwaokelemeh O, Mendoza A, Barr-Anderson DJ. Facilitators, barriers, and components of a culturally tailored afterschool physical activity program in

preadolescent African American girls and their mothers. *Ethn Dis.* 2014;24(1):8–13.

104. Lyon AR, Koerner K. User-centered design for psychosocial intervention development and implementation. *Clin Psychol (New York).* Jun 2016;23(2):180–200. doi:10.1111/cpsp.12154
105. Blase K, Kiser L, Van Dyke M. *The Hexagon Tool: Exploring Context.* National Implementation Research Network, FPG Child Development Institute, University of North Carolina at Chapel Hill; 2013.
106. Wolfenden L, Nathan NK, Sutherland R, et al. Strategies for enhancing the implementation of school-based policies or practices targeting risk factors for chronic disease. *Cochrane Database Syst Rev.* 2017;11:CD011677. doi:10.1002/14651858.CD011677.pub2
107. Lyon AR, Cook CR, Locke J, Davis C, Powell BJ, Waltz TJ. Importance and feasibility of an adapted set of implementation strategies in schools. *J Sch Psychol.* 2019;76:66–77. doi:10.1016/j.jsp.2019.07.014
108. Hagermoser Sanetti LM, Collier-Meek MA. Increasing implementation science literacy to address the research-to-practice gap in school psychology. *J Sch Psychol.* Oct 2019;76:33–47. doi:10.1016/j.jsp.2019.07.008
109. Powell BJ, Fernandez ME, Williams NJ, et al. Enhancing the impact of implementation strategies in healthcare: a research agenda. *Front Public Health.* 2019;7:3. doi:10.3389/fpubh.2019.00003
110. Cook CR, Lyon AR, Locke J, Waltz T, Powell BJ. Adapting a compilation of implementation strategies to advance school-based implementation research and practice. *Prev Sci.* 2019;20(6):914–935. doi:10.1007/s11121-019-01017-1
111. Lewis CC, Klasnja P, Powell BJ, et al. From classification to causality: advancing understanding of mechanisms of change in implementation science. *Front Public Health.* 2018;6:136. doi:10.3389/fpubh.2018.00136
112. Lyon AR, Munson SA, Renn BN, et al. Use of human-centered design to improve implementation of evidence-based psychotherapies in low-resource communities: protocol for studies applying a framework to assess usability. *JMIR Res Protoc.* Oct 09 2019;8(10):e14990. doi:10.2196/14990
113. Kilbourne AM, Smith SN, Choi SY, et al. Adaptive School-based Implementation of CBT (ASIC): clustered-SMART for building an optimized adaptive implementation intervention to improve uptake of mental health interventions in schools. *Implement Sci.* 2018;13(1):119. doi:10.1186/s13012-018-0808-8
114. Swindle T, Johnson SL, Whiteside-Mansell L, Curran GM. A mixed methods protocol for developing and testing implementation strategies for evidence-based obesity prevention in childcare: a cluster randomized hybrid type III trial. *Implement Sci.* 2017;12(1):90. doi:10.1186/s13012-017-0624-6
115. Sutherland R, Campbell E, Nathan N, et al. A cluster randomised trial of an intervention to increase the implementation of physical activity practices in secondary schools: study protocol for scaling up the Physical Activity 4 Everyone (PA4E1) program. *BMC Public Health.* Jul 04 2019;19(1):883. doi:10.1186/s12889-019-6965-0
116. Eisman AB, Heinze J, Kilbourne AM, Franzen S, Melde C, McGarrell E. Comprehensive approaches to addressing mental health needs and enhancing school security: a hybrid type II cluster randomized trial. *Health Justice.* Jan 14 2020;8(1):2. doi:10.1186/s40352-020-0104-y
117. Kilbourne AM, Goodrich DE, Lai Z, et al. Reengaging veterans with serious mental illness into care: preliminary results from a national randomized trial. *Psychiatr Serv.* Jan 01 2015;66(1):90–93. doi:10.1176/appi.ps.201300497
118. Eisman AB, Hutton DW, Prosser LA, Smith SN, Kilbourne AM. Cost-effectiveness of the Adaptive Implementation of Effective Programs Trial (ADEPT): approaches to adopting implementation strategies. *Implement Sci.* 2020;15(1):109. doi:10.1186/s13012-020-01069-w
119. Kelly JA, Heckman TG, Stevenson LY, et al. Transfer of research-based HIV prevention interventions to community service providers: fidelity and adaptation. *AIDS Educ Prev.* 2000;12(5)(suppl):87–98.
120. Bond GR, Drake RE, McHugo GJ, Peterson AE, Jones AM, Williams J. Long-term sustainability of evidence-based practices in community mental health agencies. *Adm Policy Ment Health.* Mar 2014;41(2):228–236. doi:10.1007/s10488-012-0461-5
121. Roundfield KD, Lang JM. Costs to community mental health agencies to sustain an evidence-based practice. *Psychiatr Serv.* Sep 01 2017;68(9):876–882. doi:10.1176/appi.ps.201600193
122. Eisman AB, Kilbourne AM, Dopp AR, Saldana L, Eisenberg D. Economic evaluation in implementation science: making the business case for implementation strategies. *Psychiatry Res.* 2020;283:112433. doi:10.1016/j.psychres.2019.06.008
123. Israel BA, Schulz AJ, Parker EA, Becker AB. Review of community-based research: assessing partnership approaches to improve

public health. *Annu Rev Public Health.* 1998;19:173–202.

124. Leung MW, Yen IH, Minkler M. Community based participatory research: a promising approach for increasing epidemiology's relevance in the 21st century. *Int J Epidemiol.* Jun 2004;33(3):499–506.
125. Shadish WR, Cook TD, Campbell DT. *Experimental and Quasi-Experimental Designs for Generalized Causal Inference.* Houghton Mifflin; 2002.
126. Kenney EL, Gortmaker SL, Cohen JF, Rimm EB, Cradock AL. Limited school drinking water access for youth. *J Adolesc Health.* 2016;59(1):24–29. doi:10.1016/j.jadohealth.2016.03.010
127. Resnicow K, Davis M, Smith M, et al. How best to measure implementation of school health curricula: a comparison of three measures. *Health Educ Res.* Jun 1998;13(2): 239–250.
128. McLoughlin GM, Allen P, Walsh-Bailey C, Brownson RC. A systematic review of school health policy measurement tools: implementation determinants and outcomes. *Implement Sci Commun.* Jun 26 2021;2(1):67. doi:10.1186/s43058-021-00169-y

23

Dissemination and Implementation Research in the Workplace*

PEGGY A. HANNON, REBECCA J. GUERIN, CHRISTINE M. KAVA, AND JEFFREY R. HARRIS

Acronyms

OSH: occupational safety and health
TWH: Total Worker Health
WHP: workplace health promotion

INTRODUCTION

Work is increasingly recognized as a powerful social determinant of health,[1] and the workplace environment impacts employed adults' access to health promotion and health and safety protection. We use the term workplace health promotion (WHP) to refer to a variety of benefit, communication, policy, and program approaches that encompass primary prevention though lifestyle behaviors (e.g., healthy eating and engaging in physical activity) and vaccinations, early detection of disease through screening, and treatment and management of chronic illness. Occupational safety and health (OSH) is defined as the science of the anticipation, recognition, evaluation, and control of workplace-related hazards that could harm the health, safety, and well-being of workers.[2] OSH has traditionally focused on activities that prevent occupational injury, illness, and disease ("health protection"); these include workplace redesigns to eliminate known hazards, equipment safety enhancements, safety training, and provision and use of personal protective equipment.[3] WHP and OSH have traditionally operated in independent silos, with separate administrators and organizational reporting structures.[3] For this reason, we discuss WHP and OSH separately for most of this chapter. In recent decades, recognizing synergies and potential costs savings, employers, researchers, safety professionals, and others in the OSH and WHP communities have promoted the "integration" of the workplace protection and health promotion domains.[3] Toward the end of the chapter, we discuss the National Institute for Occupational Safety and Health (NIOSH) *Total Worker Health*® approach in the United States that combines OSH and WHP.

We use two models to show the different levels of influence that employers may use to address WHP and OSH. The socioecological model states that health behavior is influenced by intrapersonal, interpersonal, institutional, community, and public policy-level factors[4] and is useful for considering WHP (Figure 23.1). The workplace shapes the daily environment in which health-related choices are made and interpersonal interactions occur. In the United States, most adults under the age of 65 obtain health insurance through an employer (their own or a family member's), so the workplace also impacts access to healthcare. Employers may have an incentive to address health behavior and safety across levels of the socioecological model in order to increase the health and productivity of their workforce. Using physical activity as an example, Table 23.1 shows examples of how the workplace

* Disclaimer: The findings and conclusions in this report are those of the author(s) and do not necessarily represent the official position of the National Institute for Occupational Safety and Health, Centers for Disease Control and Prevention.

Peggy A. Hannon, Rebecca J. Guerin, Christine M. Kava, and Jeffrey R. Harris, *Dissemination and Implementation Research in the Workplace* In: *Dissemination and Implementation Research in Health.* Edited by: Ross C. Brownson, Graham A. Colditz, and Enola K. Proctor, Oxford University Press.
 DOI: 10.1093/oso/9780197660690.003.0023

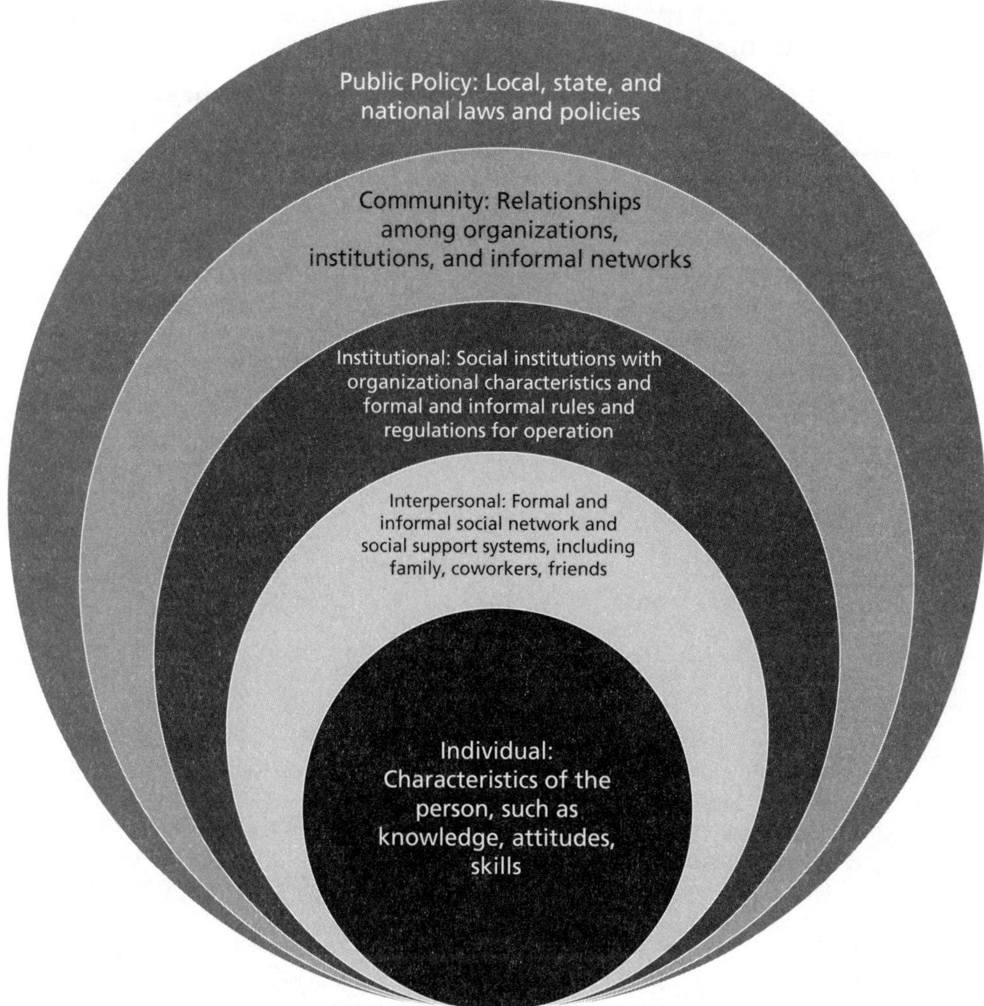

FIGURE 23.1 Socioecological model levels and definitions.

can impact health across different levels of the socioecological model.

Employers and practitioners' OSH efforts are also most effective when they are considered within a multilevel framework.[6] The hierarchy of controls (HOC; see Figure 23.2) is an effective framework for guiding the design of OSH interventions.[6] The hazard control methods at the top of the HOC graphic are more effective and protective than those at the bottom.[6] These methods range from elimination of the hazard to the use of personal protective equipment (PPE)—the least effective strategy, which potentially shifts the burden of protection to the worker.[7,8] Table 23.1 shows hearing loss prevention strategies at each level of the HOC.

Workplaces are not all created equal in their willingness, capacity, and resources to implement WHP and voluntary OSH programs. Thus, there is tremendous variation in the effectiveness of programs and policies they implement. These differences are often driven in part by the resources available, such that employers in small businesses and employers in low-wage industries may offer fewer WHP and OSH opportunities to their workers.[9,10] For example, in a recent employer survey, only 40% of employers with 10–24 workers offered any type of WHP program, compared with 92% of employers with 500 or more workers.[11] Differences in health opportunities for these workers have the potential to exacerbate existing health disparities. We refer to research

TABLE 23.1 WHP AND OSH INTERVENTION EXAMPLES ACROSS SOCIOECOLOGICAL MODEL AND HIERARCHY OF CONTROL LEVELS

Socioecological Model Level	Example: Physical Activity	Hierarchy of Controls Level	Example: Hearing Loss Prevention[5]
Public policy	Incentives to be physically active/ discounts on health insurance premiums allowed under the Affordable Care Act	**Elimination**	Require that noise reduction be factored into building design standards
Community	Workplace promotes and holds events at nearby community parks, YMCAs, or other locations that support physical activity	**Substitution**	Substitute loud for quieter equipment
Institutional	Workplace offers on-site physical activity facilities and/ or subsidized gym memberships	**Engineering controls**	Redesign equipment to eliminate noise sources and construct barriers that prevent noise from reaching a worker
Interpersonal	Workplace sponsors team physical activity program or challenge	**Administrative controls**	Schedule shifts to minimize noise exposure and provide quiet and convenient lunch and break areas
Individual	Workplace provides information about physical activity guidelines	**Personal protective equipment (PPE)**	Provide hearing protection devices, such as earplugs or earmuffs to workers, at no cost, so that workers are exposed to noise levels lower than established occupational exposure limits

Note. The intent of this table is to provide examples of each level of the SEM and the HOC, not to compare the two models.

with small businesses throughout the chapter; business size and industry are often the best available indicators of workers at risk for health disparities. Effective dissemination and implementation of WHP and OSH evidence-based programs will be key to addressing health equity in the workplace.

In this chapter, we first address the current state of WHP and OSH practice and research. We describe how current WHP and OSH programs are structured, which employers are most likely to offer such programs, whether the programs are evidence based, and who the key players are. We then provide an overview of dissemination and implementation research in WHP and OSH, including challenges and gaps in the field. We close with two case studies, one focused on a large employer's adoption of the *Total Worker Health*® ("TWH") approach, and the other focused on disseminating evidence-based WHP interventions to small workplaces.

To aid readers, we define employers, workplaces, and worksites. *Employers* are organizations, public or private, with workers (workers include employees as well as temporary workers, contractors, etc.). A *workplace* includes not only the physical location of work, but also the social, cultural, and policy environment created by an employer. We deliberately differentiate more broadly defined workplaces, often with multiple locations, from more narrowly defined physical *worksites*, the locations where workers actually work. Given the different

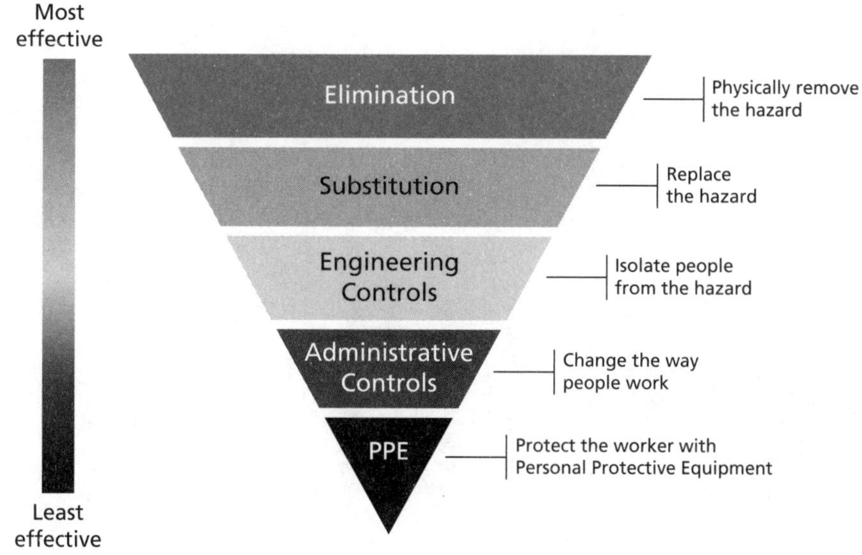

FIGURE 23.2 Hierarchy of controls.

Source: Reprinted with permission from the National Institute for Occupational Safety and Health (NIOSH). Hierarchy of controls. 2015. Accessed Feb 7, 2022. https://www.cdc.gov/niosh/topics/hierarchy/default.html

definitions used to define workplace size, we share the size definition used for small workplaces (when relevant) in the research we cite.

CURRENT STATE OF WORKPLACE HEALTH PROMOTION AND OCCUPATIONAL SAFETY AND HEALTH

Workplace Health Promotion

WHP Program Structures and Evidence Base

CDC workplace health model. The Workplace Health Model from the Centers for Disease Control and Prevention (CDC) (Figure 23.3) offers a comprehensive, systematic, and stepwise framework for WHP programs and has four components: assessment, planning and management, implementation, and evaluation.[12] The assessment component measures the workplace's current state at three socioecological levels: individual, organizational, and community. The planning and management component ensures readiness for implementation by addressing five infrastructural needs: leadership support, management, a plan for workplace health improvement, dedicated resources, and communications. The implementation component includes health-promoting processes in four areas: programs, policies, benefits, and environmental support. The evaluation component measures outcomes in four areas: worker productivity, healthcare costs, improved health outcomes, and organizational change, or the "culture of health." The Workplace Health Model is widely used, as discussed below. The importance of organizational climate and culture is covered in depth in chapter 9.

Who administers WHP programs? The Kaiser Family Foundation and the Health Research and Educational Trust (KFF/HRET) conduct an annual survey of employers. In 2017, but not since, the KFF/HRET survey asked employers who administered their health screening programs, defined as biometric screening, health risk assessment (HRA), or both.[13] The survey found that employers rely heavily on their health plans, and that reliance on health plans is inversely related to employer size. Among employers offering health insurance, 88% of small employers (from 3 to 199 workers) said that their programs are provided by their health insurer or third-party administrator, as did 70% of large employers (≥200 workers); 9% and 12%, respectively, provided the programs themselves (percentages do not add to 100% because different types of programs have different administrators).

WORKPLACE
HEALTH
MODEL

1 ASSESSMENT

INDIVIDUAL
(e.g. demographics, health risks, use of services)

ORGANIZATIONAL
(e.g. current practices, work environment, infrastructure)

COMMUNITY
(e.g. transportation, food and retail, parks and recreation)

2 PLANNING & MANAGEMENT

LEADERSHIP SUPPORT
(e.g. role models and champions)

MANAGEMENT
(e.g. workplace health coordinator, committee)

WORKPLACE HEALTH IMPROVEMENT PLAN
(e.g. goals and strategies)

DEDICATED RESOURCES
(e.g. costs, partners/vendors, staffing)

COMMUNICATIONS
(e.g. marketing, messages, systems)

1 ASSESSMENT
2 PLANNING & MANAGEMENT
3 IMPLEMENTATION
4 EVALATION

CONTEXTUAL FACTORS
(e.g. company size, company sector, capacity, geography)

4 EVALATION

WORKER PRODUCTIVITY
(e.g. absenteeism, presenteeism)

HEALTHCARE COSTS
(e.g. quality of care, performance standards)

IMPROVED HEALTH OUTCOMES
(e.g. reduced disease and disability)

ORGANIZATIONAL CHANGE, "CULTURE OF HEALTH"
(e.g. morale, recruitment/retention, alignment of health and business objectives)

3 IMPLEMENTATION

PROGRAMS
(e.g. education and counseling)

POLICIES
(e.g. organizational rules)

BENEFITS
(e.g. insurance, incentives)

ENVIRONMENTAL SUPPORT
(e.g. access points, opportunities, physical/social)

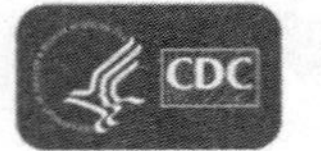

FIGURE 23.3 CDC workplace health model.

The other administrators of WHP programs are vendors. In the 2017 KFF/HRET survey, 28% of small and 48% of large employers said third-party vendors provided their programs.[13] A growing workplace wellness industry includes vendors ranging from those offering a full range of services to those that are highly specialized, for example, those conducting HRAs only or those offering HRAs along with web-based lifestyle management tools.[14] The vendors serving large employers are relatively few in number and often serve a national market. The vendors serving small and midsize employers serve more local markets.[15] One potential advantage of external administration of WHP programs is reducing employees' concerns about privacy. A recent national survey of large health plans and vendors offering WHP revealed three trends.[16] First, the workplace wellness industry is becoming more diverse and competitive. Second, there is an increased focus on affecting worker health by modifying workplace culture. Third, employers are increasingly interested in assessing broad measures of program value beyond reduction of healthcare costs; these measures include worker retention, job satisfaction, and productivity.

Employers usually purchase WHP and other insurance services via intermediaries.[17] The intermediaries used most commonly by large employers are consulting firms.[17] The intermediaries used most commonly by small and midsize employers are insurance brokers.[18] These brokers often sell WHP programs along with other services, such as health and other insurance products.[18] Small and midsize employers also commonly purchase health insurance in groups via aggregators, such as chambers of commerce and trade associations.[19]

Which employers have WHP programs? WHP offerings and comprehensiveness vary by employer size and industry. In 2021, the KFF/HRET survey[20] found that, among employers offering health insurance benefits, large employers were more likely than small employers to offer smoking cessation programs (69% vs. 42%, large vs. small); weight loss programs (63% vs. 44%); and lifestyle/behavioral coaching (71% vs. 48%). The 2020 version of the KFF/HRET survey[21] found large variation in offerings by industry, with state and local government most likely to offer WHP programs and retail employers least likely.

Further information comes from the Workplace Health in America survey, a national survey conducted by the US Department of Health and Human Services. This survey counts WHP programs as "comprehensive" if they offer all of five elements: health education, integration with the organization's structure, linkage to related programs, supportive social and physical environment, and worksite screening.[11] In 2017, 17% of employers of all sizes offered comprehensive programs. Those that had a person assigned to WHP, had an annual budget for WHP, and had health program experience for longer than 5 years were, respectively, 19.5 times, 38.2 times, and 8.4 times more likely to offer comprehensive programs than those that did not (all P values $< .001$).

Which workers participate in WHP programs? The 2020 KFF/HRET survey found that 44% and 45%, respectively, of workers in large companies completed health-risk assessments and biometric screening (small companies were not asked this question).[21] Determinants of participation have been studied at both individual and organizational levels. At the individual level, a recent literature review found that workers were more likely to participate in WHP programs if they were older, female, in good health, and had a supervisor supportive of participation.[22] Higher wage levels were also associated with higher participation.[23] At the organizational level, participation was associated with organizational and leadership support and incentives.[24]

WHP impact, and disparities in impact, on health behaviors and health outcomes. The question of effectiveness continues to vex WHP practitioners and researchers.[25] For each of the four health-promoting processes (policies, programs, benefits, and environmental supports) laid out by the CDC workplace health model, there are good examples of effective interventions that can and are being delivered in workplace settings. For example, smoke-free workplace policies have been shown to aid cessation and protect against exposure to secondhand smoke. Similarly, environmental supports, such as workplace walking trails and gym facilities in or near workplaces, have been shown to increase physical activity. Both the CDC's Guide to Community Preventive Services (https://www.thecommunityguide.org) and the Cochrane Collaboration (https://www.

cochrane.org) list other effective workplace-based interventions.

The question is whether such interventions are effective when combined into multifaceted WHP programs and implemented by employers and their insurers and vendors in real-world workplaces. Several studies of comprehensive programs over the years have shown effectiveness, but these studies, usually with voluntary participation, have been criticized for their potential for selection bias.[25] Recently, two randomized controlled trials of WHP programs, one in a large US warehouse retail company[26] and the other at the University of Illinois,[27] showed only modest effects on a small number of health behaviors and no effects on more distal health and financial outcomes. Participation rates in both these studies were low, 35% and 27%, respectively, and their offerings were not comprehensive.[28]

Factors influencing program effectiveness. In addition to the recent review of determinants of worker participation in WHP programs,[22] two older reviews assessed key factors associated with program effectiveness. A 2013 RAND review commissioned by the federal government listed five factors: (1) use of existing resources and relationships, (2) leadership engagement at all levels, (3) effective communication strategies, (4) opportunity for workers to engage, and (5) continuous evaluation.[29] In another recent review, Goetzel cited the importance of a "culture of health," defined as "one in which individuals and their organizations are able to make healthy life choices within a larger social environment that values, provides, and promotes options that are capable of producing health and well-being for everyone regardless of background or environment."[30] The CDC workplace health model also stresses the importance of evaluating an employer's culture of health.[12]

Role of Industry Organizations, Governmental Agencies, and Regulators in WHP

The US workplace wellness industry was estimated to generate $10 billion in annual revenue in 2019,[31] but it is loosely organized and largely unregulated. There is no national trade association of vendors, though there is a small professional association, the International Association for Worksite Health Promotion (https://www.iawhp.org). The National Committee for Quality Assurance, a private nonprofit organization, developed a Wellness and Health Promotion Accreditation.[32] To be accredited, insurers and vendors must pay a fee, so the number of accredited organizations is small and largely limited to those serving national employers.

Government and industry organizations sponsor publicly available scorecards that guide employers in assessing their WHP programs. Developed in 2012, the free CDC Worksite Health Scorecard has rapidly gained prominence.[33] As of 2019, more than 2,800 employers from 48 states had completed the scorecard.[33] CDC has also developed and delivered Work@Health, a companion WHP training program for employers, delivered via in-person, online, and hybrid formats.[34] Other commonly used scorecards[35] include the American Heart Association's Workplace Health Achievement Index,[36] the Health Enhancement Research Organization's Health and Well-Being Best Practices Scorecard,[37] and the Wellness Council of America's Well Workplace Checklist.[38]

Occupational Safety and Health

OSH Program Structures and Evidence Base

Who administers OSH? Under the Occupational Safety and Health Act of 1970, employers are responsible for providing safe and healthful workplaces for their workers. The OSH Act also created the Occupational Safety and Health Administration (OSHA) within the US Department of Labor. OSHA's mission is to ensure that workers work in a safe and healthful environment by setting and enforcing standards, authorizing the secretary of labor to assess civil monetary penalties for noncompliance,[39] and providing training, outreach, education, and assistance. Employers must comply with all applicable OSHA standards and with the General Duty Clause of the OSH Act, which requires employers to keep their workplace free of serious recognized hazards. Despite its importance, the OSH Act has faced challenges, including that state and local public sector workers are not covered by federal OSHA, and the law may not be equipped to address working conditions and worker-employer relationships that are radically different from those that existed more than 50 years ago when it was enacted.[40]

The OSH Act also established the National Institute for Occupational Safety and Health (NIOSH), within the Department of Health and Human Services.[41] NIOSH produces research, including developing exposure criteria for toxic materials and harmful physical agents, that can support OSHA's formulation of safety and health standards.[41] NIOSH provides the only dedicated federal investment for a wide range of research activities to prevent the societal cost of work-related fatalities, injuries, and illnesses in the United States and has issued guidance documents on newer and emerging issues, such as workplace violence and occupational exposure to nanoparticles such as nanosilver used in the manufacture of electronics and textiles.[39,41,42] Research in or directly relevant to the OSH field is carried out in government laboratories (including at NIOSH), universities, the private sector, and in institutions affiliated with organized labor.[43]

Which employers have OSH in place? Which workers benefit from OSH protections? Under the OSH Act, most US employers have the responsibility for administering OSH programs in workplaces. Larger businesses may have dedicated OSH professionals on staff and/or safety committees with representation from management, safety professionals, and workers. Core OSH professions (occupational safety, industrial hygiene, occupational medicine, and occupational health nursing) focus on different aspects of OSH activities, but share a common goal of identifying hazards in the workplace and assisting employers and workers in eliminating or mitigating the attendant risks.[43] Many of these professionals work on a contractual basis or as consultants.[42] Workers in smaller businesses may rarely encounter one of these OSH professionals.[43] For several reasons, including a lack of resources, peer networks, and motivation to engage in non-production-related activities, smaller businesses with fewer than 250 workers have been shown to engage in fewer safety activities than larger businesses and may benefit from assistance with OSH activities from external organizations (intermediaries),[10] such as insurance companies, healthcare providers, and trade and professional associations.

OSHA recommends practices to provide employers, workers, and worker representatives (including labor unions or religious or community groups) with a flexible framework for addressing safety and health issues in diverse workplaces. These recommendations include seven core elements for a safety and health program: management leadership; worker participation; hazard identification and assessment; hazard prevention and control; education and training; program evaluation and improvement; and communication and coordination for host employers, contractors, and staffing agencies.[44] OSHA recognizes that, for health and safety programs to succeed, workers (and if applicable, their representatives) must participate in developing and implementing every program component. The OSHA recommended practices also align with voluntary, international, and national consensus standards, such as ANSI/ASSP Z10-2019. This national consensus standard (from the American National Standards Institute [ANSI] and the American Society of Safety Professionals [ASSP]) defines the minimum requirements for an occupational health and safety management system using a "systems-thinking" approach that recognizes that an organization's processes are dynamic and interrelated, and that worker participation plays a critical role in successful implementation of voluntary standards.[45]

OSH impact, and disparities in impact, on safety and health injury/disability outcomes. Since enactment of the OSH Act, worker deaths in the United States are down, from about 38 worker deaths a day in 1970 to 15 a day in 2019. Worker injuries and illnesses have declined, from 10.9 incidents per 100 workers in 1972 to 2.8 per 100 in 2019.[46] Previous studies indicated that OSHA standards are effective in preventing occupational injuries and illnesses.[40,47]

Despite this progress, the challenge for preventing work-related injuries, illnesses, and deaths remains substantial, as millions of U.S. workers are injured annually, and thousands are killed.[40] Work-related morbidity and mortality risks are especially high in certain industries, including manufacturing, agriculture, and healthcare[40,48] and among certain worker populations, where declines in worker illnesses and injuries have not been evenly distributed.[1]

For example, young workers ages 15–24 years in the United States experience a disproportionate burden of work-related injury compared to adult workers, and these injuries can have lifelong physical, social, and emotional impacts.[49] Older workers also face disproportionate risks. Although older US workers (≥55 years) have experienced similar or lower rates of work-related injuries and illnesses compared with younger workers, older workers face a greater risk of being killed at work than workers as a whole.[50]

In 2020, approximately 17% of the US civilian labor force was foreign born.[51] Research indicates that workers from racial/ethnic minority groups and immigrants experience a disproportionate burden of negative OSH outcomes. These groups are overrepresented in dangerous occupations[52] and have limited access to worker protection resources.[53] Many workers in "precarious" job arrangements are hesitant to refuse hazardous work or to report hazards for fear of retribution.[1,40]

Workers may also be members of multiple groups at disproportionate risk for injury and illness and therefore experience overlapping structural inequities.[1] For example, women and workers from racial and ethnic minority groups make up a disproportionate share of the low-wage workforce in some temporary occupations, including security guards, home healthcare, hospitality, and logistics.[54] Immigrant workers and those of lower socioeconomic status are frequently employed in higher risk occupations (e.g., construction and agriculture), which are often subject to outdoor extreme weather conditions exacerbated by climate change.[55] Therefore, the increased health and safety risks associated with temporary and contingent work arrangements accrue to workers already experiencing increased injury and fatality rates.[1,54,55]

Factors influencing program effectiveness. Many effective OSH interventions improve worker safety, health, and well-being. Positive effects range from preventing occupational injuries and hearing loss to reducing musculoskeletal, skin, and lung diseases[7,56] and reducing work-related stress.[57] Many OSH interventions have proven to be effective under controlled conditions, but their implementation in practice is often difficult. Interventions may not work as expected, especially in small businesses.[10]

Costs may affect employers' ability or willingness to implement effective OSH interventions. A review by Keefe et al.[7] identified the enforcement of the OSHA Noise Standard as a control technology not being used to maximal benefit to reduce exposure at the source and protect workers from hearing loss. Affordability was cited as the main reason why employers (particularly those in small and medium-size enterprises where some exposures occur at the highest levels) rely on less costly and potentially less protective solutions (e.g., PPE) rather than on expensive retrofits to buildings and structures.[7]

OVERVIEW OF DISSEMINATION AND IMPLEMENTATION RESEARCH IN WORKPLACE SETTINGS

There are far fewer studies specific to disseminating and implementing evidence-based WHP and OSH programs than studies investigating the effectiveness of new programs. Drawing from key constructs in the dissemination and implementation literature, we cover several factors that may influence dissemination and implementation of effective WHP/OSH programs. These factors include employers' and workers' motivations to adopt health promotion programs; workplace readiness and capacity to implement programs; the extent to which effective programs can be adapted to fit the workplace context and workers' needs; and the extent to which effective programs are sustained.

Workplace Health Promotion

Employer and worker motivations to adopt WHP programs. Employers and workers may have different motivations and interests in WHP programs. One of employers' primary motivations to adopt these programs is containing healthcare costs.[58] Much of the controversy about WHP effectiveness hinges on healthcare cost return on investment as *the* metric of WHP success. Additional motivations for WHP found in our work with employers and in other studies include recruitment and retention of workers, improving worker productivity, improving morale, and reducing worker turnover.[59,60] Some also cite altruistic motives, wishing to implement WHP programs to help improve workers' health or believing it's the right thing to do.[61]

Worker participation in WHP programs is often low; in a large-scale trial evaluating a multicomponent workplace wellness program, participation rates ranged from 34% to 45%.[26] A common strategy to increase participation is to deliver incentives for participation.

However, discovering whether workers see programs as relevant to their needs may be a more beneficial first step. The topics most wellness programs address align with behaviors that workers need to change, want to change, and are actively trying to change. These behaviors include healthy eating, physical activity, weight management, smoking cessation, and stress management.[62–64]

The nature of job activities may impact the health interests of employers and workers. For example, employers with workers in sedentary jobs may be interested in physical activity and/or weight management; in contrast, employers with workers in physically active and demanding jobs often display little interest in increasing their workers' physical activity. Employers who retain workers long term and have an aging workforce are more likely to prioritize chronic disease prevention and management.

Readiness and capacity to implement effective WHP programs. Readiness at the organizational level is characterized in Weiner's theory of organizational readiness to change.[65] The theory identifies two facets of readiness for change: change commitment (a shared resolve among organizational members to implement a change) and change efficacy (a shared belief among organizational members that they have a collective capability to implement a change). Change commitment and change efficacy are influenced by change valence (how much organizational members value the proposed change) and informational assessment (organizational members' perceptions of the tasks and resources needed to implement the change). Change valence and informational assessment are predicted by contextual factors, such as the organizational culture, resources, and past experiences with change. Change commitment and change efficacy predict change-related effort, which in turn predicts implementation success (see Figure 23.4).

Many employers face readiness and capacity challenges to adopting and implementing WHP programs, including lack of financial resources, competing demands, and lack of management support.[66] Additional logistical challenges include lack of space for programming, workers spread across multiple worksites and shifts, workers without access to computers at work, and workers with limited English proficiency.[63,66] Small and medium-size worksites exhibit less readiness and capacity for WHP than large worksites[9,61,67]; we also see differences by industry (e.g., employers in industries such as education show more readiness and capacity than employers in accommodation and food services).[68] There are limited tools to measure readiness and capacity for WHP.

Adapting WHP programs to fit different workplace contexts and worker populations. Workers who work night shifts, less than 20 hours a week, receive hourly pay, are temporary or contract workers, and are in blue-collar jobs are less likely to participate in WHP programs.[69] To meet the needs of underserved worker groups, effective WHP programs need

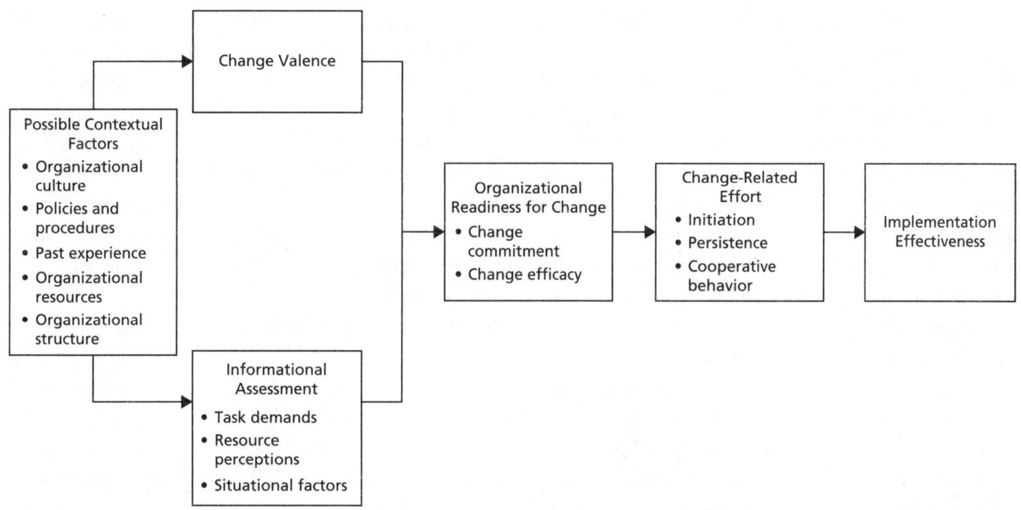

FIGURE 23.4 Theory of organizational readiness to change (Weiner, 2009).[65]

to be adapted to fit various workplace populations and contexts. Recent calls have been made for employers to systematically collect information on the health preferences and social needs of various worker groups to create more inclusive and equitable WHP programming (and this step would fit into the needs assessment described above).[70]

Translation of evidence-based interventions into practice within diverse settings and populations is gaining increasing attention.[71] Many programs are tested via rigorous randomized controlled trials that have strict participation criteria; workplaces willing to participate in such trials are often not representative of workplaces in general.[72] In a scoping review of frameworks to guide adaptations of evidence-based public health interventions, the authors identified key steps to the adaptation process, including assess community capacity, determinants, and needs; review and select evidence-based interventions; consult with content experts and partners; decide on and make intervention adaptations; train implementers; pretest adapted materials; and implement and evaluate the adapted intervention.[73] One study used a framework[74] to help guide adaptations to a weight management intervention for low-wage workers.[75] Tabak and colleagues conducted formative research with key partners and beneficiaries (e.g., food service workers) to inform intervention adaptations, for example, replacing interactive voice response with text messages to enhance reach. This study showed how adaptation frameworks can guide effective adaption and marketing of an intervention for dissemination to a different audience from the original testing audience.

Sustainability of WHP programs. Sustainability is a key aspect of successful implementation. Moore and colleagues[76] defined sustainability as (a) the continued delivery of a program, clinical intervention, and/or implementation strategies and (b) maintenance of individual behavior change, noting that program and behavioral changes may evolve or adapt over time while continuing to offer benefits at the individual and systems level. Multiple barriers and facilitators can influence whether an evidence-based intervention is sustained, and calls have been made to test and document use of sustainability frameworks and intervention adaptations to enhance sustainability in order to advance our knowledge in this area.[77,78]

There is an increasing focus on measuring long-term outcomes in studies evaluating the effectiveness of WHP programs. One study examined the sustainability of a WHP program that incorporated gamification principles and found significant, clinical improvements on several clinical outcomes (e.g., blood pressure) at both 1 and 2 years after the intervention began.[79] In contrast, a WHP program designed for blue-collar workers in the construction industry demonstrated significant intervention effects on body weight, waist circumference, physical activity, and intake of sugar-sweetened beverages at 6 months, but these changes were no longer significant at 12 months.[80] Additional research is needed to help us understand which programs are sustainable and which conditions promote sustainability of WHP programs.

Occupational Safety and Health

Employer and worker motivations to adopt OSH measures. Legal compliance with OSH safety laws and regulations (and the risk of sanctions for noncompliance) are important motivators for employers to adopt OSH measures. For example, OSHA's 1991 blood-borne pathogens standard, enacted in response to the US HIV/AIDS crisis, has contributed to a substantial decline in healthcare worker risk for blood-borne diseases.[40,81] However, some noted challenges with the current regulatory environment[40] have potentially placed an increased reliance on employers to monitor their own compliance with OSH laws and to provide worker protections.[82]

A business case for OSH advances the premise that the economic advantages to organizations (in terms of reducing Workers' Compensation rates, worker presenteeism and absenteeism, and increasing worker productivity) outweigh the costs of implementing voluntary OSH programs.[82] However, ethical arguments about OSH being the "right thing to do"[83] and the fear of loss of corporate credibility and reputational damage[84] are cited as other, important motivators for employers to adopt and implement OSH programs and activities. Contextual factors as experienced by business owners and managers, including access to resources; characteristics of the manager, including their own personal estimation of the extent of work-related safety and health risks and the need for OSH precautions if these risks are underestimated or perceived to be beyond their control[10]; and the workplace culture have also been shown to influence their motivation for adoption of participatory OSH programs.[85]

Readiness and capacity to implement effective OSH measures. When considering uptake of some voluntary OSH strategies, business enterprises engage in a complex cost-benefit analysis regarding the risks and advantages of change. When making adoption decisions, partners and beneficiaries may prioritize factors such as compatibility with existing programs, cost-effectiveness, the values and culture of the organization, and relative advantage over other programs.[86] An assessment of organizational readiness for change[65] is an important precursor to the successful implementation of participatory OSH programs.[87] Both managers' and workers' ability to envision future improvement and their shared interest in WHP and OSH have been demonstrated to be key to new program adoption.[87]

An organizational readiness for change tool was developed to help prepare for implementation of a participatory OSH program based on TWH principles in eight domains: (1) current safety/health/well-being programs; (2) current organizational approaches to safety/health/well-being; (3) resources available for safety/health/well-being; (4) resources and readiness for change initiatives to improve safety/health/well-being; (5) resources and readiness for use of teams in programmatic initiatives; (6) teamwork; (7) resources and readiness for worker participation; and (8) management communication about safety/health/well-being.[88] This tool has been used prospectively to assess potential facilitators and barriers to implementing a participatory TWH program in five public healthcare facilities, allowing program implementers to be proactive in tailoring aspects of the implementation to better fit the needs of the organization.[89]

Adapting OSH approaches to fit different workplace contexts and worker populations. Successful OSH efforts require implementing programs that are both evidence based and fit the needs of the organization and its workers.[90] For example, it is generally necessary to tailor interventions to the specific needs and context of small businesses, and several facilitators and drivers have been identified that can be used to adapt participatory OSH programs to meet the needs of end users.[91] Given that, to be effective, OSH interventions should be tailored to specific organizational contexts, generalizing and transferring them to other organizations presents substantial challenges.[92] Contextual fit is especially relevant for organizational-level interventions (typical of OSH), requiring participation from multiple parties and new practices and procedures to support worker engagement.[89]

Balancing fidelity and adaptation has been explored extensively in the dissemination and implementation literature, but only to a limited degree in OSH.[90] While intervention adaptation is inevitable, and even desirable, to meet the local needs and constraints of end users, the value of adaptation (and fidelity to the original program design) when implementing a voluntary OSH program may be different for various program providers and recipients, and recommendations have been proposed for reconciling respective roles.[90]

Intervention adaptation is especially important in addressing occupational health equity concerns, where one-size-fits-all approaches are likely to be ineffective for workers and employers from diverse populations. For example, PPE, which has been critical for healthcare workers during the COVID-19 pandemic[6] and in other high-risk industries like construction, has not traditionally been designed for women and racial/ethnic minorities. Ill-fitting equipment may decrease effectiveness, increase exposure risks, and deter workers from using it.[93] PPE are being adapted to account for a wider range of body shapes and sizes, ensuring that it is accessible and effective for all workers.[55] Research has also been conducted on the need to adapt OSH training programs to meet the needs of workers who experience several languages and/or who work in settings that put them at increased risk of exposure to hazards.[53]

Sustainability of OSH measures/programs. Intervention maintenance and long-term sustainability have been shown to be more likely when such programs are aligned with the organizational mission and values and enjoy the support and involvement of several key groups and individuals (e.g., senior managers, policymakers, community leaders, and workers).[92] Adequate resources, breadth of worker participation, and management support have been shown to be important preconditions for program sustainability.[92,94] Research has demonstrated barriers to OSH program sustainability include communication among workers, staff turnover and overreliance on individual champions, inconsistent management commitment, and lack of a reward system for participation.[94]

Including worker input at every step of program design and implementation improves the ability to identify the presence and causes of workplace hazards, creates a sense of program ownership among workers, enhances their understanding of how the program works, and helps sustain the program over time.[44]

RESEARCH GAPS AND FUTURE DIRECTIONS

Limited Application of Implementation Science Theories and Frameworks

There are over 60 published dissemination and implementation frameworks and models,[95] yet there remains a gap in the application of these frameworks to address WHP/OSH.[96] Some WHP/OSH studies have used frameworks like the Consolidated Framework for Implementation Research (CFIR) and RE-AIM (Reach, Effectiveness, Adoption, Implementation, and Maintenance) to understand contextual factors that influence implementation and to inform program evaluation. These and other frameworks could also be used to inform engagement among partners and beneficiaries during WHP/OSH program implementation, develop logic models for implementation, and select and adapt implementation strategies.[97] In recent years, several dissemination and implementation frameworks have been developed, revised, and extended to explicitly focus on health equity; examples include an extension of the RE-AIM framework,[98] the application of an intersectionality lens to the Theoretical Domains Framework,[99] and a race(ism)-conscious adaptation of the CFIR.[100] Future research should apply equity-focused dissemination and implementation frameworks to address health disparities when implementing WHP/OSH programs.

Limited Study of Workplace Contextual Factors

Few WHP or OSH studies to date have identified contextual factors that could have played a role in influencing intervention effectiveness.[90,101] Randomized controlled trials, considered the gold standard in WHP and OSH research, aim to minimize variance, effectively "controlling out" context rather than assessing it.[90] A systematic review of TWH studies[102] identified only a limited number of interventions focusing on multilevel contextual factors (e.g., work organization, union membership, health insurance status, management support, and worker stress related to company downsizing). Variation in intervention effectiveness by individual, worksite, organizational, or community factors was not assessed in any of the identified studies.[102]

Research is needed that takes a systems-level approach to consider factors beyond the workplace that have direct and indirect effects on worker health.[55,82,101] This requires understanding the importance of broad social, economic, and political factors that affect workers directly and indirectly by influencing the adoption of WHP and OSH policies, practices, and programs by employers and other organizational decision makers.[82] Understanding the forces shaping the future of work is critical for anticipating the outcomes associated with changes in the conditions of employment.[55,82] This will in turn inform decision-making on interventions that protect and promote worker safety, health, and well-being.[82]

Limited Integration of WHP and OSH

As mentioned previously in this chapter, recognizing the benefits of the "integration" of the workplace protection and health promotion domains,[3,103] NIOSH developed the TWH approach in 2011.[104] TWH is defined as policies, programs, and practices that integrate protection from work-related safety and health hazards with promotion of efforts to advance worker well-being.[41,104] Growing evidence indicates that integrated health interventions are successful in addressing a wide range of OSH and well-being outcomes,[105] suggesting the need for wider adoption of this approach. The TWH paradigm acknowledges the interaction of work and nonwork factors,[55] such as social determinants of health,[1] that affect OSH outcomes. Although TWH efforts and activities have increased in recent years, it is still an emerging area with opportunities to study dissemination and implementation research questions[101] (e.g., whether and why different types of employers may find an integrated approach more or less acceptable and feasible than separate WHP and OSH programs).

COVID-19 and the Future of Work

Most research cited in this chapter pre-dates the COVID-19 pandemic, which exerted multiple and extensive impacts on work and the workplace in the United States. COVID-related restrictions limited business operations and revenue, with small businesses disproportionately likely to close, lay off staff, and/or lose revenue.[106] The risk of COVID-19 is closely tied to employment patterns,[107] as workers deemed essential are disproportionately racial or ethnic minorities, are paid low wages, and labor in jobs that cannot currently be done from home.[107,108] They work in both healthcare and nonhealthcare occupations,[107] such as in food preparation, construction, transportation, corrections, and first response.[88,108] In one survey, more than half of essential workers reported they leaned on unhealthy habits to get through the pandemic; 80% said their sleep was affected, and almost 40% said they were drinking more to cope with stress. Fifty percent said they gained weight (median 20 pounds).[109] The COVID-19 crisis also highlights the urgent need to focus on the mental health aspects of occupational health, including among the nation's public health and healthcare workers,[110] and the impact of job loss and decreased work hours on mental health outcomes during the pandemic.[111] For other workers who teleworked throughout the pandemic, the future of work may look very different and provide more flexibility around where and when work happens.[82] Workers are voicing more desire for a broader range of wellness benefits, such as mental health support and flexible scheduling,[112] and some employers are responding. The 2021 KFF/HRET survey[20] found that large employers were more likely than small employers to have changed offerings in response to the COVID-19 pandemic: 34% versus 17% expanded or modified existing programs to better address the needs of people working from home; 58% versus 38% provided or expanded online counseling for emotional and financial distress. New awareness of health and risk disparities in our workforce coupled with increased worker leverage during staffing shortages may create opportunities for OSH and WHP researchers to partner with employers, workers, and dissemination partners to determine new priorities and needs and how best to address them.

CASE STUDY 23.1: DOW CHEMICAL COMPANY AND TOTAL WORKER HEALTH

Background

The Dow Chemical Company was created in 1897 and is a global manufacturer of plastics, chemicals, and agricultural products (https://corporate.dow.com). It operates worldwide and had 35,700 full-time workers at the end of 2020.[113]

History

Dow has had an occupational health program for more than 100 years and a WHP program for more than 30 years.[114] In 2015, it merged these programs to create a TWH program and made its implementation part of its 2025 Sustainability Goals. Dow's TWH strategy has three interdependent elements: Healthy Culture, Healthy Workplace, and Healthy People.

The Healthy Culture Index is based on the CDC Worksite Health Scorecard with its major components: organizational support, tobacco control, nutrition, lactation support, physical activity, and stress management. In addition, it includes industrial hygiene practices, workplace exposure assessment, access to healthy options, and worker health culture.[115]

The Healthy Workplace element identifies workplace health risks and prioritizes and reduces them utilizing an HOC approach (preferring engineering controls to reduce risk rather than relying on PPE; https://www.cdc.gov/niosh/twh/guidelines.html). This element also relies on free worksite health clinics operated at 58 sites globally.[116] Other components of the Healthy Workplace include an integrated well-being strategy, with resources aimed at physical, mental, community, and financial well-being, along with a worker-assistance program; case management for those with chronic illness; traditional health insurance; and well-being champions on-site and available via social media.

The Healthy People element integrates traditional measures of both occupational health and health promotion. For example, it measures occupational injuries and illnesses. Safety measures are published annually.[114] It also measures the American Heart Association's "Life's Simple 7," which include blood pressure, cholesterol, blood sugar, physical activity, healthy eating, weight management, and tobacco avoidance or cessation.[117]

Examples of Dow's integrated TWH approach include smoking cessation programs as part of training for respirator wearers; installation of sit/stand and walking workstations for office workers, along with management of personal safety risks inherent in these stations; and physical activity programs aimed at reducing ergonomic risks to minimize injuries.[115] The 2020 Dow Sustainability Report[114] profiles selected results of the program. These include improvements in safety metrics as well as implementation of distancing and other approaches to minimizing COVID-19 transmission in the workplace. NIOSH also highlights the program as part of its "Promising Practices" website.[118]

Implications for Practitioners, Policymakers, and Researchers

Dow provides an example of a large multinational company with many potential workplace hazards. It has long been active in both occupational health and health promotion but integrated those approaches only recently. Historically, Dow has conducted and published health promotion research[119] and is a promising site for practical and research insights into TWH implementation in the future.

CASE STUDY 23.2: DISSEMINATING EVIDENCE-BASED PROGRAMS TO SMALL WORKSITES VIA CONNECT TO WELLNESS

Background

Small employers face two major barriers in adopting and implementing evidence-based programs for their workers: (1) lack of information needed to find, choose, and adapt programs and (2) lack of resources required to implement programs.[120] Small employers need help in selecting programs, and they need programs that are low cost or free and take little time to implement.

The Community Guide (https://www.thecommunityguide.org) lists evidence-based strategies for cancer screening, healthy eating, physical activity, and tobacco cessation that worksites of all sizes can adopt and implement. In addition, all 50 states provide breast and cervical cancer screening and treatment free of charge for low-income and uninsured women, as well as free telephone quit lines for tobacco cessation for smokers. Very few small worksites promote these services, even though they are most likely to have workers that are eligible for their services.[121,122]

Connect to Wellness Intervention and Research

The Health Promotion Research Center (HPRC) at the University of Washington collaborated with the American Cancer Society to develop and test an intervention, *Connect to Wellness*,[†] to disseminate evidence-based programs to small employers (20–250 workers) in low-wage industries. The HPRC Dissemination and Implementation Framework[123] guides our intervention and dissemination research activities. Employers participating in Connect to Wellness complete activities with the assistance of a trained interventionist. In the assessment phase, the interventionist measures current worksite implementation of cancer screening, nutrition, physical activity, and tobacco cessation programs. In the recommendations phase, the interventionist creates a tailored *Recommendations Report* and delivers the report in a face-to-face meeting with the employer. At the Recommendations Report meeting, the interventionist provides *implementation toolkits* for each of the recommended programs. During the implementation phase, the employer begins adopting the recommended programs and promoting them to workers. The interventionist contacts worksites monthly by email or telephone during this phase to offer implementation assistance.

We conducted three studies to develop and test Connect to Wellness, including a randomized controlled trial.[124,125] The primary outcome

[†] *Connect to Wellness* was originally called HealthLinks, and early papers about the program use the HealthLinks name. We discovered that a different workplace health promotion program was using the same name, so we rebranded the program as *Connect to Wellness* in 2020.

was worksite-level adoption and implementation of evidence-based programs. We measured programs by asking several questions about each one and then using a scoring algorithm to calculate a score ranging from 0% to 100% implementation for each program. In each study, total worksite implementation increased at least 20% (absolute) from baseline to follow-up.[121,125]

Lessons Learned

One of the most challenging aspects of Connect to Wellness, as with many similar programs, is recruiting employers to participate. It is especially difficult to recruit employers in some of the lowest-wage industries we prioritize due to their risk profile, such as accommodation and food services and retail trade. Two reasons for this include very limited staff time and budget for wellness at these workplaces and perception that chronic disease prevention is irrelevant for their (comparatively) young, high-turnover workforce.[126] Recruiting employers via warm referral from their health insurance provider is very effective,[127] but this strategy only reaches employers that offer health insurance. Recently, we added new toolkits with interventions to manage stress and address COVID-19 risk and vaccination. These topics may be of more universal interest than chronic disease prevention. Adapting and tailoring the menu of evidence-based interventions to fit audience capacity and needs will likely be key to Connect to Wellness future reach and impact.

One of the core elements of Connect to Wellness is assistance from a trained interventionist. Connect to Wellness is offered as a free service, and this assistance component makes scale-up challenging. We pilot tested a training model in which we distance-trained local health department staff (e.g., health educators and public health nurses) in several counties in Washington State to deliver Connect to Wellness to worksites in their communities, and this was successful.[122] We are currently attempting to scale up this model to local health departments in other states. Two key challenges to engaging health departments currently include the shift in CDC funding for health departments from disease prevention to disease management[128] and the COVID-19 pandemic. In light of these challenges, we opened recruitment to state health departments, many of whom are already doing some level of WHP activity.[129]

Implications for Practitioners, Policymakers, and Researchers

Small businesses face unique challenges to adopting and implementing health promotion programs. Connect to Wellness disseminates a simple, three-step process of implementing evidence-based interventions and provides free in-person assistance from a trained interventionist. One of the key challenges for practice and research is to match the level of assistance given with the level needed for employers to be successful in implementing programs. Our use of a specific dissemination and implementation framework[123] helped us build a program of research around small worksites in low-wage industries; the program includes formative research with these employers and their workers, efficacy testing of Connect to Wellness, building out and testing additional implementation strategies such as wellness committees, and new partnerships to attempt scale-up.

SUMMARY

The workplace gives us an opportunity to reach more than 60% of noninstitutionalized adults in the United States (https://data.census.gov/cedsci/all?q=employment). A substantial body of evidence demonstrates the effectiveness of a range of WHP and OSH programs, but comparatively little research focuses on disseminating and implementing effective WHP and OSH programs. WHP and OSH traditionally operate in distinct silos; TWH is an integrated approach that is gaining popularity, but far from universal adoption. Partnerships between academic researchers, employers, governmental organizations, and for-profit and not-for-profit vendors are needed to identify (and create) effective WHP, OSH, and TWH programs; tailor them to meet the needs and capacities of employers and workers across size and industry categories; market them effectively; provide appropriate levels of implementation assistance; and evaluate impact and use the results to improve the programs and increase their reach.[123,130]

SUGGESTED READINGS AND WEBSITES

Selected Readings

Tamers SL, Chosewood LC, Streit J (Eds.). Worker safety, health, and well-being in the USA. *Int J Environ Res Public Health.* 2021;19(3) Special Issue. Accessed January 10, 2022. https://www.mdpi.com/journal/ijerph/special_issues/worker_health

Articles in this special issue address topics related to the future of work in the United States, work as an important social determinant of health, and implications for worker safety, health, and well-being. Included are articles with a dissemination and implementation perspective and that apply a Total Worker Health approach.

Kaiser Family Foundation and Health Research & Educational Trust. *Employer Health Benefits: 2021 Annual Survey.* Kaiser Family Foundation and Health Research & Educational Trust; 2021. Accessed December 12, 2021. https://www.kff.org/health-costs/report/2021-employer-health-benefits-survey/

This report summarizes the 2021 KFF/HRET survey of employer health benefits. This report, from a US employer survey conducted annually for the past 24 years, highlights changes employers have made in response to the COVID-19 pandemic. Survey reports and resources from prior KFF/HRET surveys (1998–2021) are also available at the link.

Rothstein MA (Ed.) The Occupational Safety and Health Act at 50, 1970–2020. *Am J Public Health.* 2020;110(5, special section):621–647. Accessed January 15, 2022. https://ajph.aphapublications.org/toc/ajph/110/5

This special section of the American Journal of Public Health *commemorates the 50th anniversary of the Occupational Safety and Health Act by including views from a range of experts on important issues—past, present, and future—in the areas of occupational safety and health regulation and beyond.*

Pollack Porter KM, Campbell L, Carson A, et al. Driving health equity in the workplace. American Heart Association CEO Roundtable; 2021. https://www.heart.org/en/about-us/office-of-health-equity/driving-health-equity-in-the-workplace

This report, written by a diverse group of WHP experts in academia and industry, lays out 20 actions that employers can take today to increase health equity in their workplaces. The 20 actions, with supporting evidence, are divided into 15 internal actions that workers can take within their own organizations and 5 external actions that lie in the realm of public policy for which employers should advocate. An example of an internal action is offering paid family and medical leave; an external example is advocating for high-quality, accessible, and affordable early care and education for children.

Hudson HL, Nigam JAS, Sauter SL, Chosewood C, Schill AL, Howard J, eds. Total Worker Health. American Psychological Association; 2019.

This volume presents approaches for implementing integrative prevention programs to address policies, programs, and practices that address risks arising from both the physical and organizational work environment and that extend beyond the workplace. These include applications for diverse worker occupations and industries. Evidence of program effectiveness is also discussed.

Selected Websites and Tools

Centers for Disease Control and Prevention, Workplace Health Promotion. https://www.cdc.gov/workplacehealthpromotion/index.htmlAccessed November 20, 2021. Published March 8, 2019.

This website provides information on CDC's workplace health promotion activities and tools. It includes their Workplace Health Model and Workplace Health Scorecard, both cited in this review, as well as links to evidence-based policies, programs, and communications; data and surveillance; and other tools and resources to support workplace health promotion practitioners and researchers.

Cochrane Database of Systematic Reviews. http://www.cochranelibrary.com/cochrane-database-of-systematic-reviews/index.html. Accessed November 13, 2021.

This searchable database of systematic reviews uses literature from global sources, including both high-income and lower- and-middle-income countries. At the time of writing of this chapter, there were eight reviews on primary and secondary prevention in workplace settings.

The Cochrane Database also includes a specific focus on occupational safety and health at https://work.cochrane.org/cochrane-reviews-about-occupational-safety-and-health.Accessed November 13, 2021.

The Community Guide, Worksite Health. https://www.thecommunityguide.org/topic/worksite-health.Accessed December 5, 2021.

This website summarizes the recommendations and systematic reviews related to workplace health promotion from CDC's Community Guide. Links are provided to stories from the field and other resources. It is worth exploring other topics on the Community Guide's website as evidence-based strategies in other topic areas are often relevant to workplace health promotion. For example, several strategies for cancer screening (distributing small media or home test kits) can be implemented in the workplace.

Total Worker Health Planning, Assessment, and Evaluation Tools. https://www.cdc.gov/niosh/twh/tools.html January 11, 2023.

This site provides a list of free, publicly available resources that can support the planning, assessment, and evaluation of programs, policies, and practices aligned with a TWH approach.

REFERENCES

1. Flynn MA, Check P, Steege AL, Siven JM, Syron LN. Health equity and a paradigm shift in occupational safety and health. *Int J Environ Res Public Health.* 2021;19(1):349.
2. Alli BO. *Fundamental Principles of Occupational Health and Safety.* 2nd ed. International Labour Office; 2008.
3. Loeppke RR, Hohn T, Baase C, et al. Integrating health and safety in the workplace: how closely aligning health and safety strategies can yield measurable benefits. *J Occup Environ Med.* 2015;57(5):585–597.
4. McLeroy KR, Bibeau D, Steckler A, Glanz K. An ecological perspective on health promotion programs. *Health Educ Q.* 1988;15(4):351–377.
5. National Institute for Occupational Safety and Health (NIOSH). Reducing noise exposure: noise controls. 2018. Accessed February 7, 2022. https://www.cdc.gov/niosh/topics/noise/reducenoiseexposure/noisecontrols.html
6. National Institute for Occupational Safety and Health (NIOSH). Hierarchy of controls. 2015. Accessed February 7, 2022. https://www.cdc.gov/niosh/topics/hierarchy/default.html
7. Janson DJ, Clift BC, Dhokia V. PPE fit of healthcare workers during the COVID-19 pandemic. *Appl Ergon.* 2022;99:103610.
8. Keefe AR, Demers PA, Neis B, et al. A scoping review to identify strategies that work to prevent four important occupational diseases. *Am J Ind Med.* 2020;63(6):490–516.
9. Harris JR, Hannon PA, Beresford SA, Linnan LA, McLellan DL. Health promotion in smaller workplaces in the United States. *Annu Rev Public Health.* 2014;35:327–342.
10. Sinclair RC, Cunningham TR. Safety activities in small businesses. *Saf Sci.* 2014;64:32–38.
11. Linnan LA, Cluff L, Lang JE, Penne M, Leff MS. Results of the Workplace Health in America survey. *Am J Health Promot.* 2019;33(5):652–665.
12. Centers for Disease Control and Prevention. Workplace health model. 2021. Accessed Dec 6, 2021. https://www.cdc.gov/workplacehealthpromotion/model/index.html
13. Kaiser Family Foundation and Health Research & Educational Trust. Employer *Health Benefits: 2017 Annual Survey.* Kaiser Family Foundation and Health Research & Educational Trust; 2017.
14. Society for Human Resource Management. Wellness programs—compare and research wellness programs companies and businesses. 2022. Accessed February 7, 2022. https://vendordirectory.shrm.org/category/benefits-health-welfare/wellness-programs
15. Rooke L. *An Analysis of Services Offered by Comprehensive Wellness Vendors in Washington State.* Masters thesis. Health Services, University of Washington; 2015.
16. Abraham J, White KM. Tracking the changing landscape of corporate wellness companies. *Health Aff (Millwood).* 2017;36(2):222–228.
17. Marquis MS, Long SH. Who helps employers design their health insurance benefits? *Health Aff (Millwood).* 2000;19(1):133–138.
18. Thornton M, Hammerback K, Abraham JM, Brosseau L, Harris JR, Linnan LA. Using a social capital framework to explore a broker's role in small employer wellness program uptake and implementation. *Am J Health Promot.* 2021;35(2):214–225.
19. Harris JR, Hammerback KR, Hannon PA, et al. Group purchasing of workplace health promotion services for small employers. *J Occup Environ Med.* 2014;56(7):765–770.
20. Kaiser Family Foundation and Health Research & Educational Trust. *Employer Health Benefits: 2021 Annual Survey.* Kaiser Family Foundation and Health Research & Educational Trust; 2021.
21. Kaiser Family Foundation and Health Research & Educational Trust. *Employer Health Benefits: 2020 Annual Survey.* Kaiser Family Foundation and Health Research & Educational Trust; 2020.
22. Smidt MN, Jimmieson NL, Bradley LM. Predicting employee participation in, and satisfaction with, wellness programs: the role of employee, supervisor, and organizational support. *J Occup Environ Med.* 2021;63(12):1005–1018.
23. Sherman BW, Addy C. Association of wage with employee participation in health assessments and biometric screening. *Am J Health Promot.* 2018;32(2):440–445.
24. Grossmeier J, Castle PH, Pitts JS, et al. Workplace well-being factors that predict employee participation, health and medical cost impact, and perceived support. *Am J Health Promot.* 2020;34(4):349–358.
25. Abraham JM. Employer wellness programs—a work in progress. *JAMA.* 2019;321(15):1462–1463.
26. Song Z, Baicker K. Effect of a workplace wellness program on employee health and economic outcomes: a randomized clinical trial. *JAMA.* 2019;321(15):1491–1501.
27. Jones D, Molitor D, Reif J. What do workplace wellness programs do? Evidence from the Illinois Workplace Wellness Study. *Q J Econ.* 2019;134(4):1747–1791.
28. Goetzel RZ. Commentary on the Study: "What Do Workplace Wellness Programs Do? Evidence

From the Illinois Workplace Wellness Study." *Am J Health Promot.* 2020;34(4):440–444.

29. Mattke S, Liu H, Caloyeras JP, et al. *Workplace Wellness Programs Study: Final Report.* RAND Corporation. 2013. RR-254-DOL. Accessed December 16, 2021. https://www.rand.org/t/RR254
30. Goetzel RZ, Henke RM, Tabrizi M, et al. Do workplace health promotion (wellness) programs work? *J Occup Environ Med.* 2014;56(9):927–934.
31. Research and Markets. US corporate wellness market—industry outlook and forecast 2021–2026. February 2021. Accessed December 16, 2021. https://www.researchandmarkets.com/reports/5239809
32. National Committee for Quality Assurance (NCQA). Wellness and health promotion accreditation/certification. 2022. Accessed February 7, 2022. https://www.ncqa.org/programs/health-plans/wellness-and-health-promotion-whp/
33. Lang JE, Mummert A, Roemer EC, Kent KB, Koffman DM, Goetzel RZ. The CDC Worksite Health ScoreCard: an assessment tool to promote employee health and well-being. *Am J Health Promot.* 2020;34(3):319–321.
34. Cluff LA, Lang JE, Rineer JR, Jones-Jack NH, Strazza KM. Training employers to implement health promotion programs: results from the CDC Work@Health(R) program. *Am J Health Promot.* 2018;32(4):1062–1069.
35. Grossmeier J. Updated employer tools identify practices associated with population health outcomes. *Am J Health Promot.* 2020;34(3):316–317.
36. Calitz C, Pham K. American Heart Association's Workplace Health Achievement Index. *Am J Health Promot.* 2020;34(3):317–318.
37. Rosenbaum E, Grossmeier J, Imboden M, Noeldner S. The HERO Health and Well-Being Best Practices Scorecard in collaboration with Mercer (HERO Scorecard). *Am J Health Promot.* 2020;34(3):321–323.
38. Martin S, Picarella R, Pitts JS. Measuring a whole systems approach to wellness with the Well Workplace Checklist. *Am J Health Promot.* 2020;34(3):323–326.
39. Rothstein MA. The Occupational Safety and Health Act at 50: Introduction to the Special Section. *Am J Public Health.* 2020;110(5):613–614.
40. Michaels D, Barab J. The Occupational Safety and Health Administration at 50: Protecting Workers in a Changing Economy. *Am J Public Health.* 2020;110(5):631–635.
41. Howard J. NIOSH: a short history. *Am J Public Health.* 2020;110(5):629–630.
42. Kuempel E, Roberts JR, Roth G, et al. Current Intelligence Bulletin *70: Health Effects of Occupational Exposure to Silver Nanomaterials.* Centers for Disease Control and Prevention, National Institute for Occupational Safety and Health; 2021.
43. Institute of Medicine. *Safe Work in the 21st Century: Education and Training Needs for the Next Decade's Occupational Safety and Health Personnel.* National Academies Press; 2000.
44. Occupational Safety and Health Administration (OSHA). Recommended practices for safety and health. 2016. Accessed February 7, 2022. https://www.osha.gov/sites/default/files/publications/OSHA3885.pdf
45. Occupational Health and Safety Management Systems. *American National Standards Institute (ANSI) Z10-2019 Standard.* 2019. American Society of Safety Professionals, Secretariat.
46. US Department of Labor—Occupational Safety and Health Administration (OSHA). Commonly used statistics. 2021. Accessed February 7, 2022. https://www.osha.gov/data/commonstats
47. Levine DI, Toffel MW, Johnson MS. Randomized government safety inspections reduce worker injuries with no detectable job loss. *Science.* 2012;336(6083):907–911.
48. US Department of Labor, Bureau of Labor Statistics. Employer-reported workplace injuries and illnesses—2020. 2021. Accessed February 7, 2022. https://www.bls.gov/news.release/pdf/osh.pdf
49. Guerin RJ, Reichard AA, Derk S, Hendricks KJ, Menger-Ogle LM, Okun AH. Nonfatal occupational injuries to younger workers—United States, 2012–2018. *MMWR Morb Mortal Wkly Rep.* 2020;69(35):1204–1209.
50. US Department of Labor, Bureau of Labor Statistics. 25 years of worker injury, illness, and fatality case data. 2019. Accessed Feb 7, 2022. https://www.bls.gov/spotlight/2019/25-years-of-worker-injury-illness-and-fatality-case-data/pdf/25-years-of-worker-injury-illness-and-fatality-case-data.pdf
51. US Department of Labor, Bureau of Labor Statistics. Foreign-born workers: labor force characteristics—2020. May 18, 2021. Accessed February 7, 2022. https://www.bls.gov/news.release/pdf/forbrn.pdf
52. Steege AL, Baron S, Marsh SM, Menendez CC, Meyers JR. Examining occupational health and safety disparities using national data: a cause for continuing concern. *Am J Ind Med.* 2014;57:527–538.
53. Cunningham TR, Guerin RJ, Keller BM, Flynn MA, Salgado C, Hudson D. Differences in safety training among smaller and larger construction firms with non-native workers:

evidence of overlapping vulnerabilities. *Saf Sci.* 2018;103:62–69.
54. Weil D. The future of Occupational Safety and Health protection in a fissured economy. *Am J Public Health.* 2020;110(5):640–641.
55. Tamers SL, Streit J, Pana-Cryan R, et al. Envisioning the future of work to safeguard the safety, health, and well-being of the workforce: a perspective from the CDC's National Institute for Occupational Safety and Health. *Am J Ind Med.* 2020;63(12):1065–1084.
56. Teufer B, Ebenberger A, Affengruber L, et al. Evidence-based occupational health and safety interventions: a comprehensive overview of reviews. *BMJ Open.* 2019;9(12):e032528.
57. Richardson KM, Rothstein HR. Effects of occupational stress management intervention programs: a meta-analysis. *J Occup Health Psychol.* 2008;13(1):69–93.
58. Abraham JM. Taking stock of employer wellness program effectiveness—where should employers invest? *JAMA Intern Med.* 2020;180(7):960–961.
59. Pescud M, Teal R, Shilton T, et al. Employers' views on the promotion of workplace health and wellbeing: a qualitative study. *BMC Public Health.* 2015;15:642.
60. Passey DG, Hammerback K, Huff A, Harris JR, Hannon PA. The role of managers in employee wellness programs: a mixed-methods study. *Am J Health Promot.* 2018;32(8):1697–1705.
61. Pfeffer J, Vilendrer S, Joseph G, Kim J, Singer SJ. Employers' role in employee health: why they do what they do. *J Occup Environ Med.* 2020;62(11):e601–e610.
62. McCleary K, Goetzel RZ, Roemer EC, Berko J, Kent K, Torre H. Employer and employee opinions about workplace health promotion (wellness) programs: results of the 2015 Harris Poll Nielsen Survey. *J Occup Environ Med.* 2017;59(3):256–263.
63. Parrish AT, Hammerback K, Hannon PA, Mason C, Wilkie MN, Harris JR. Supporting the health of low socioeconomic status employees: qualitative perspectives from employees and large companies. *J Occup Environ Med.* 2018;60(7):577–583.
64. Dale AM, Enke C, Buckner-Petty S, et al. Availability and use of workplace supports for health promotion among employees of small and large businesses. *Am J Health Promot.* 2019;33(1):30–38.
65. Weiner BJ. A theory of organizational readiness for change. *Implement Sci.* 2009;4:67.
66. Weinstein M, Cheddie K. Adoption and implementation barriers for worksite health programs in the United States. *Int J Environ Res Public Health.* 2021;18(22):12030.
67. Stiehl E, Shivaprakash N, Thatcher E, et al. Worksite health promotion for low-wage workers: a scoping literature review. *Am J Health Promot.* 2018;32(2):359–373.
68. Hannon PA, Garson G, Harris JR, Hammerback K, Sopher CJ, Clegg-Thorp C. Workplace health promotion implementation, readiness, and capacity among midsize employers in low-wage industries: a national survey. *J Occup Environ Med.* 2012;54(11):1337–1343.
69. Tsai R, Alterman T, Grosch JW, Luckhaupt SE. Availability of and participation in workplace health promotion programs by sociodemographic, occupation, and work organization characteristics in US workers. *Am J Health Promot.* 2019;33(7):1028–1038.
70. Sherman BW, Kelly RK, Payne-Foster P. Integrating workforce health into employer diversity, equity and inclusion efforts. *Am J Health Promot.* 2021;35(5):609–612.
71. Castro FG, Yasui M. Advances in EBI development for diverse populations: towards a science of intervention adaptation. *Prev Sci.* 2017;18(6):623–629.
72. Monti S, Grosso V, Todoerti M, Caporali R. Randomized controlled trials and real-world data: differences and similarities to untangle literature data. *Rheumatology (Oxford).* 2018;57(57)(suppl 7):vii54–vii58.
73. Escoffery C, Lebow-Skelley E, Udelson H, et al. A scoping study of frameworks for adapting public health evidence-based interventions. *Transl Behav Med.* 2019;9(1):1–10.
74. Baumann AA, Cabassa LJ, Stirman SW. Adaptation in dissemination and implementation science. In: Brownson RC, Colditz GA, Proctor EK, eds. *Dissemination and Implementation Research in Health: Translating Science to Practice.* 2nd ed. Oxford University Press; 2017:285–300.
75. Tabak RG, Strickland JR, Stein RI, et al. Development of a scalable weight loss intervention for low-income workers through adaptation of interactive obesity treatment approach (iOTA). *BMC Public Health.* 2018;18(1):1265.
76. Moore JE, Mascarenhas A, Bain J, Straus SE. Developing a comprehensive definition of sustainability. *Implement Sci.* 2017;12(1):110.
77. Hailemariam M, Bustos T, Montgomery B, Barajas R, Evans LB, Drahota A. Evidence-based intervention sustainability strategies: a systematic review. *Implement Sci.* 2019;14(1):57.
78. Shelton RC, Lee M. Sustaining evidence-based interventions and policies: recent innovations and future directions in implementation science. *Am J Public Health.* 2019;109(S2):S132–S134.

79. Lowensteyn I, Berberian V, Berger C, Da Costa D, Joseph L, Grover SA. The sustainability of a workplace wellness program that incorporates gamification principles: participant engagement and health benefits after 2 years. *Am J Health Promot.* 2019;33(6):850–858.
80. Viester L, Verhagen E, Bongers PM, van der Beek AJ. Effectiveness of a worksite intervention for male construction workers on dietary and physical activity behaviors, body mass index, and health outcomes: results of a randomized controlled trial. *Am J Health Promot.* 2018;32(3):795–805.
81. Phillips EK, Conaway MR, Jagger JC. Percutaneous injuries before and after the Needlestick Safety and Prevention Act. *N Engl J Med.* 2012;366(7):670–671.
82. Sorensen G, Dennerlein JT, Peters SE, Sabbath EL, Kelly EL, Wagner GR. The future of research on work, safety, health and wellbeing: a guiding conceptual framework. *Soc Sci Med.* 2021;269:113593.
83. Miller P, Haslam C. Why employers spend money on employee health: interviews with occupational health and safety professionals from British industry. *Saf Sci.* 2009;47(2):163–169.
84. Verbeek J. The economic dimension of occupational health and safety. *Scand J Work Environ Health.* 2009;35(6):401–402.
85. Kvorning LV, Hasle P, Christensen U. Motivational factors influencing small construction and auto repair enterprises to participate in occupational health and safety programmes. *Saf Sci.* 2015;71:253–263.
86. Schulte PA, Cunningham TR, Nickels L, et al. Translation research in occupational safety and health: a proposed framework. *Am J Ind Med.* 2017;60(12):1011–1022.
87. Zhang Y, Flum M, West C, Punnett L. Assessing organizational readiness for a participatory occupational health/health promotion intervention in skilled nursing facilities. *Health Promot Pract.* 2015;16(5):724–732.
88. Robertson MM, Tubbs D, Henning RA, Nobrega S, Calvo A, Murphy LA. Assessment of organizational readiness for participatory occupational safety, health and well-being programs. *Work.* 2021;69(4):1317–1342.
89. Nobrega SM, Morocho C, Robertson MM, et al. Using a mixed method approach to tailor the implementation of a participatory Total Worker Health® program in public healthcare facilities. *Preprint, Dec 30, Research Square.* 2020. doi:https://doi.org/10.21203/rs.3.rs-135537/v1
90. von Thiele Schwarz U, Hasson H, Lindfors P. Applying a fidelity framework to understand adaptations in an occupational health intervention. *Work.* 2015;51(2):195–203.
91. Cagno E, Masi D, Leao CP. Drivers for OSH interventions in small and medium-sized enterprises. *Int J Occup Saf Ergon.* 2016;22(1):102–115.
92. Herrera-Sanchez IM, Leon-Perez JM, Leon-Rubio JM. Steps to ensure a successful implementation of Occupational Health and Safety interventions at an organizational level. *Front Psychol.* 2017;8:2135.
93. Flynn MA, Keller B, DeLaney SC. Promotion of alternative-sized personal protective equipment. *J Safety Res.* 2017;63:43–46.
94. Kotejoshyer R, Zhang Y, Flum M, Fleishman J, Punnett L. Prospective evaluation of fidelity, impact and sustainability of participatory workplace health teams in skilled nursing facilities. *Int J Environ Res Public Health.* 2019;16(9):1494.
95. Tabak RG, Khoong EC, Chambers DA, Brownson RC. Bridging research and practice: models for dissemination and implementation research. *Am J Prev Med.* 2012;43(3):337–350.
96. Guerin RJ, Glasgow RE, Tyler A, Rabin BA, Huebschmann AG. Methods to improve the translation of evidence-based interventions: a primer on dissemination and implementation science for occupational safety and health researchers and practitioners. *Saf Sci.* 2022;152.
97. Moullin JC, Dickson KS, Stadnick NA, et al. Ten recommendations for using implementation frameworks in research and practice. *Implement Sci Commun.* 2020;1(1):42.
98. Shelton RC, Chambers DA, Glasgow RE. An extension of RE-AIM to enhance sustainability: addressing dynamic context and promoting health equity over time. *Front Public Health.* 2020;8:134.
99. Etherington C, Rodrigues IB, Giangregorio L, et al. Applying an intersectionality lens to the theoretical domains framework: a tool for thinking about how intersecting social identities and structures of power influence behaviour. *BMC Med Res Methodol.* 2020;20(1):169.
100. Allen M, Wilhelm A, Ortega LE, Pergament S, Bates N, Cunningham B. Applying a race(ism)-conscious adaptation of the CFIR framework to understand implementation of a school-based equity-oriented intervention. *Ethn Dis.* 2021;31(suppl 1):375–388.
101. Guerin RJ, Harden SM, Rabin BA, et al. Dissemination and implementation science approaches for occupational safety and health research: implications for advancing Total

Worker Health. *Int J Environ Res Public Health.* 2021;18(21):11050.
102. Feltner C, Peterson K, Palmieri Weber R, et al. The effectiveness of Total Worker Health interventions: a systematic review for a National Institutes of Health Pathways to Prevention Workshop. *Ann Intern Med.* 2016;165(4):262–269.
103. Punnett L, Cavallari JM, Henning RA, Nobrega S, Dugan AG, Cherniack MG. Defining "integration" for Total Worker Health®: a new proposal. *Ann Work Expo Health.* 2020;64(3):223–235.
104. Tamers SL, Chosewood LC, Childress A, Hudson H, Nigam J, Chang CC. Total Worker Health® 2014–2018: the novel approach to worker safety, health, and well-being evolves. *Int J Environ Res Public Health.* 2019;16(3):321.
105. Anger WK, Elliot DL, Bodner T, et al. Effectiveness of total worker health interventions. *J Occup Health Psychol.* 2015;20(2):226–247.
106. Katare B, Marshall MI, Valdivia CB. Bend or break? Small business survival and strategies during the COVID-19 shock. *Int J Disaster Risk Reduct.* 2021;61:102332.
107. Michaels D, Wagner GR. Occupational Safety and Health Administration (OSHA) and worker safety during the COVID-19 pandemic. *JAMA.* 2020;324(14):1389–1390.
108. Do DP, Frank R. US frontline workers and COVID-19 inequities. *Prev Med.* 2021;153:106833.
109. *Stress in America: One Year Later, a New Wave of Pandemic Health Concerns* [Press release]. American Psychological Association; March 2021.
110. Bryant-Genevier J, Rao CY, Lopes-Cardozo B, et al. Symptoms of depression, anxiety, post-traumatic stress disorder, and suicidal ideation among state, tribal, local, and territorial public health workers during the COVID-19 pandemic—United States, March–April 2021. *MMWR Morb Mortal Wkly Rep.* 2021;70(48):1680–1685.
111. Guerin RJ, Barile JP, Thompson WW, McKnight-Eily L, Okun AH. Investigating the impact of job loss and decreased work hours on physical and mental health outcomes among US adults during the COVID-19 pandemic. *J Occup Environ Med.* 2021;63(9):e571–e579.
112. Childress R. New data shows how COVID-19 has changed the workplace. *Associations Now.* September 22, 2021. Accessed January 28, 2022. https://associationsnow.com/2021/09/new-data-shows-how-covid-19-has-changed-the-workplace/
113. US Securities and Exchange Commission. Form 10-K, Dow Chemical Company. 2020. Accessed January 24, 2022. https://www.sec.gov/Archives/edgar/data/29915/000175178821000010/dow-20201231.htm
114. Dow Chemical Company. Intersections, 2020 environmental, social and governance report. 2020. Accessed Jan 24, 2022. https://corporate.dow.com/en-us/esg/report.html
115. American Heart Association. Workplace health playbook: the Dow Chemical Company—Total Worker Health. 2021. Accessed December 17, 2021. https://playbook.heart.org/the-dow-chemical-company-total-worker-health
116. Dow Chemical Company. Employee health and wellness. 2022. Accessed Feb 7, 2022. https://corporate.dow.com/en-us/esg/report/health-and-safety/employee-wellness.html
117. American Heart Association. My Life Check—Life's Simple 7. 2022. Accessed February 7, 2022. https://www.heart.org/en/healthy-living/healthy-lifestyle/my-life-check--lifes-simple-7
118. National Institute for Occupational Safety and Health (NIOSH). Total Worker Health in action: December 2017—creating value at Dow Chemical through Total Worker Health initiatives. December 2017. Accessed February 7, 2022. https://www.cdc.gov/niosh/twh/newsletter/twhnewsv6n4.html#Promising
119. Aikens KA, Astin J, Pelletier KR, et al. Mindfulness goes to work: impact of an online workplace intervention. *J Occup Environ Med.* 2014;56(7):721–731.
120. Hannon PA, Helfrich CD, Chan KG, et al. Development and pilot test of the workplace readiness questionnaire, a theory-based instrument to measure small workplaces' readiness to implement wellness programs. *Am J Health Promot.* 2017;31(1):67–75.
121. Hannon PA, Hammerback K, Kohn MJ, et al. Disseminating evidence-based interventions in small, low-wage worksites: a randomized controlled trial in King County, Washington (2014–2017). *Am J Public Health.* 2019;109(12):1739–1746.
122. Harris JR, Hammerback K, Brown M, et al. Local health jurisdiction staff deliver health promotion to small worksites, Washington. *J Public Health Manag Pract.* 2021;27(2):117–124.
123. Harris JR, Cheadle A, Hannon PA, et al. A framework for disseminating evidence-based health promotion practices. *Prev Chronic Dis.* 2012;9:E22.
124. Hannon PA, Hammerback K, Allen CL, et al. HealthLinks randomized controlled trial:

design and baseline results. *Contemp Clin Trials.* 2016;48:1–11.

125. Laing SS, Hannon PA, Talburt A, Kimpe S, Williams B, Harris JR. Increasing evidence-based workplace health promotion best practices in small and low-wage companies, Mason County, Washington, 2009. *Prev Chronic Dis.* 2012;9:E83.
126. Allen CL, Hammerback K, Harris JR, Hannon PA, Parrish AT. Feasibility of workplace health promotion for restaurant workers, Seattle, 2012. *Prev Chronic Dis.* 2015;12:E172.
127. Hammerback K, Hannon PA, Parrish AT, Allen C, Kohn MJ, Harris JR. Comparing strategies for recruiting small, low-wage worksites for community-based health promotion research. *Health Educ Behav.* 2018;45(5):690–696.
128. Brown MC, Kava C, Bekemeier B, et al. Local health departments' capacity for workplace health promotion programs to prevent chronic disease: comparison of rural, micropolitan, and urban contexts. *J Public Health Manag Pract.* 2021;27(5):E183–E188.
129. Linnan LA, Leff MS, Martini MC, et al. Workplace health promotion and safety in state and territorial health departments in the United States: a national mixed-methods study of activity, capacity, and growth opportunities. *BMC Public Health.* 2019;19(1):291.
130. Steensma JT, Kreuter MW, Casey CM, Bernhardt JM. Enhancing dissemination through marketing and distribution systems: a vision for public health. In: Brownson RC, Colditz GA, Proctor EK, eds. *Dissemination and Implementation Research in Health: Translating Science to Practice.* 2nd ed. Oxford University Press; 2018:191–200.

24

Policy Dissemination and Implementation Research

JONATHAN PURTLE, ERIKA L. CRABLE, GRACELYN CRUDEN, MATTHEW LEE, REBECCA LENGNICK-HALL, DIANA SILVER, AND RAMESH RAGHAVAN

INTRODUCTION

Public policies shape the structure of societies. They influence distribution of wealth, power, prestige, and opportunities for health within them. Inequitable polices are a root cause of health disparities.[1,2] For these reasons, a wide range of actors—spanning from corporate lobbyists and foreign governments to advocacy organizations and concerned citizens—expends considerable resources to influence the policymaking and implementation process. For those of us in the field of implementation science in health, we engage in policy-focused work to promote the passage and implementation of policies that are aligned with evidence about "what works" to improve population health and health equity. To this end, *policy dissemination research* seeks to understand how research evidence can be most effectively communicated to policymakers and integrated into policymaking processes, and *policy implementation research* seeks to understanding how the rollout of polices can be optimized to maximize health benefits.[3] Examples of policies that could be the focus of a dissemination and implementation (D&I) study include those that directly improve population health (e.g., clean indoor air laws) and those that increase the reach, fidelity, and thus impact of an evidence-based clinical intervention (e.g., insurance coverage laws).

Despite the fundamental role of policies in shaping population health and in determining the impact of evidence-based interventions (EBIs), policy-focused research has historically been underrepresented the field of implementation science in health. For example, a review of D&I research funded by the National Institutes of Health (NIH) between 2007 and 2014 found that only 12 projects (less than 10%) examined policy issues, with most considering policy as a contextual factor—not the primary focus of inquiry.[4] However, policy is receiving increasing attention in the field.[3,5–10]

Scholars of D&I have recently published calls for a greater emphasis on policy,[3,5–9] recent reviews have cataloged measures and strategies for policy-focused D&I research,[11–13] and randomized controlled trials have tested policy-focused D&I strategies.[14–22] Entire journals (e.g., *Evidence & Policy, Health Research Policy and Systems*) are dedicated to policy-focused evidence translation, and funders such as the National Science Foundation and William T. Grant Foundation have issued calls for policy translation research. Initiatives in the United States (e.g., the US Commission on Evidence-Based Policymaking) and globally (e.g., the World Health Organization Evidence-Informed Policy Network,[23] the Global Commission on Evidence to Address Societal Challenges) have been launched to bridge evidence-to-policy gaps.

Against this backdrop, this chapter provides an overview of policy-focused D&I research. It should be noted that the chapter is focused on *research*. Other reviews provide overviews of issues related to the *practice* of research-to-policy translation and barriers to evidence-informed policymaking.[6,24–26] It should also be

Jonathan Purtle, Erika L. Crable, Gracelyn Cruden, Matthew Lee, Rebecca Lengnick-Hall, Diana Silver, and Ramesh Raghavan, *Policy Dissemination and Implementation Research* In: *Dissemination and Implementation Research in Health.* Edited by: Ross C. Brownson, Graham A. Colditz, and Enola K. Proctor, Oxford University Press. © Oxford University Press 2023. DOI: 10.1093/oso/9780197660690.003.0024 emphasized that the chapter focuses on "big P policies" enacted by government entities (e.g., laws, administrative rules) as opposed to "little p policies," which are adopted by organizations (e.g., funding priorities, professional guidelines). Frameworks, constructs, measures, and methods developed for D&I research in organizational settings (chapter 4) are often appropriate for studying little p policies. Last, the chapter largely draws from studies conducted in the United States, but the guidance provided is likely to be applicable to health policy research in most developed countries. Policy-focused D&I research in low- and middle-income countries is an important area for future research.

CONCEPTUALIZING POLICY IN D&I RESEARCH

Given that the field of implementation science in health has primarily focused on clinical, organizational, and community-based interventions, it can be challenging for D&I researchers to grasp how to approach policy in their work. Figure 24.1 offers a simplistic schematic to illustrate three broad ways to conceptualize policy in D&I research.

In Box A, the focus is on policymaking before a policy is enacted, with the goal of promoting the passage of policies that are aligned with high-quality evidence and promoting health equity. Policy dissemination research can help achieve this goal.[6] In Box C, the focus is on policy implementation, after the policy is enacted, with the goal of optimizing the rollout of policies to maximize health benefits and health equity. Policy implementation research can help achieve this goal.[27] Ideally, there is a feedback loop in which findings from policy implementation research subsequently inform policymaking processes so that policies are designed to proactively address implementation challenges and equity concerns. In Boxes A and C, a specific policy is "the thing," per Geoffrey Curran's implementation science teaching terminology.[28] In Box B, a clinical, organizational, or community-based intervention is the thing, and the focus is on understanding how policy functions as a contextual factor and affects implementation success and health equity. Here, policy can be conceptualized as a "bridging factor"—a construct from the exploration, preparation, implementation, sustainment (EPIS) framework—that connects outer- and inner-context (e.g., a policy related to contracting requirements for an EBI affects an organization's implementation climate).[29]

As Crable and colleagues described,[30] there are key elements to specify in policy D&I research. These include, but are not limited to the following:

- the specific policy of focus and its key attributes (e.g., regulatory requirements, fiscal dimensions, dates related to enactment, implementation, and reporting);
- the key types of policymakers, implementers, and other stakeholders and how their roles change over

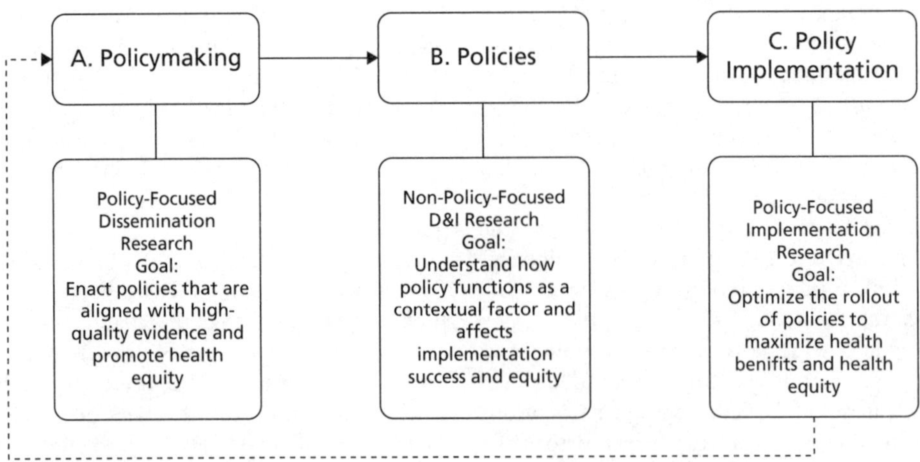

FIGURE 24.1 Conceptualizing policy in D&I research.

TABLE 24.1 KEY DIFFERENCES BETWEEN ELECTED AND ADMINISTRATIVE POLICYMAKERS THAT ARE RELEVANT TO DISSEMINATION RESEARCH

Domain	Elected Policymakers[a]	Administrative Policymakers
Content expertise about health issues	Unlikely to have content expertise in specific health issues	Likely to have content expertise in at least one specific health issue, with most policymakers having advanced degrees in the health sciences (e.g., MD, PhD, MPH)
Primary sources of accountability	Constituents, political party	Governor, senior leadership within agencies, state legislature
Scope	Very broad; health is one of dozens of domains of issues that elected officials address	Narrowly focused on health issues, often one specific area of health issues (e.g., chronic disease, mental health)
Primary roles in policy process	Policy development	Policy implementation, as well as policy development

[a]The staff of elected policymakers are also an important group to consider that often have more content expertise on health issues and a narrower scope than elected officials but share the same sources of accountability. In the United States, the extent to which elected officials have dedicated staff varies dramatically (see National Conference of State Legislatures: https://www.ncsl.org/research/about-state-legislatures/full-and-part-time-legislatures.aspx).

time through policymaking and implementation processes; and
- which outer- and inner-context constructs may be especially important for the success of policy D&I efforts.

In terms of specifying the policymakers that are the target audience in dissemination research, it is often helpful to differentiate between elected policymakers (e.g., state legislators, county council officials, mayors) and nonelected administrative policymakers (e.g., agency directors).[6] Table 24.1 summarizes key differences between these two types of policymakers.

HEALTH EQUITY IN POLICY D&I RESEARCH

Failure to consider issues related to equity in policy-focused D&I research can lead to the production of knowledge that either maintains or exacerbates health inequities. However, policy D&I research also has great potential to advance health equity by targeting policies, as well as the uneven implementation of policies, that can produce and perpetuate health inequities.[31] There are *at least* three equity-related dimensions to consider in policy-focused D&I research. The first relates to the policies that are selected to be the focus of a policy D&I study. Caution should be exercised when focusing on policies that are intended to increase the reach of EBIs because such spread often inadvertently increases the magnitude of persistent health inequities.[32,33] The potential of policy D&I research to reduce health inequities is likely maximized when studies focus on the adoption and implementation of social and economic policies (e.g., across domains, e.g., housing, education, and criminal justice) that shape the structural determinants of health and dismantle policies that reinforce structural racism and other systems of oppression.[34] For example, there would be potential health equity benefits to studying policies that foster permanent supportive housing in policy D&I research. These policies are recommended by the US Community Preventive Services Task Force as an evidence-based approach to promoting health equity.[35]

A second equity consideration for policy-focused D&I research is recognizing that many policymakers—and members of the general public—are not knowledgeable about the existence of health inequities or their causes.[36] For example, a survey of city policymakers in the United States found that only 42% of mayors strongly agreed that health disparities existed in their city; the proportion was only 18% among socially conservative mayors.[37,38] Policy D&I researchers should be cognizant of the fact that limited policymaker and public knowledge about health inequities is a characteristic of the sociopolitical context in which policy is made and implemented. Another consideration relates to the fact that many policymakers, like the general public, have implicit biases and negative attitudes toward racial and ethnic minority populations and other groups that experience health inequities.[39] Because of this, disseminating poorly framed messages about health equity can have unintended, or "boomerang," effects among some audiences in which these messages reduce support for evidence-based policies that would promote health equity.[40,41] This evidence underscores the importance of message tailoring and thoughtful dissemination about health equity issues.[42]

Third, it is critical to measure how the policy implementation process and outcomes vary across social groups within a population and to assess the implications of uneven policy implementation and enforcement. Studies have shown that issues such as the targeted enforcement of punitive policies within some communities, along with a failed reach of health-promoting and other beneficial policies within communities, and altogether failing to consider the cultural context and social and economic circumstances of communities in policy implementation lead to inequities in implementation processes and outcomes.[27,43–46] Examples of inequity in policy implementation include polices related to child welfare[47,48] and tobacco control.[27]

POLICY DISSEMINATION RESEARCH

Dissemination research is defined by the NIH as "the scientific study of targeted distribution of information and intervention materials to a specific public health or clinical practice audience." In policy-focused dissemination research, policymakers are the audience of focus. Questions related to how research evidence can be most effectively communicated to policymakers, how policymakers' use of research evidence can be enhanced, and what influences the adoption of evidence-informed policies are core to policy dissemination research. Writing this chapter in 2022, there are reasons why one might be skeptical about the idea that evidence-informed policymaking can be improved. Policymakers, and the public, are forced to continuously navigate a turbulent sea of disinformation, misinformation, and credible evidence within climates of scientific uncertainty.[49,50] Indeed, it would be naïve to believe that the mere dissemination of research evidence alone—even if delivered with optimal precision—could dramatically influence a policymaker's behavior.[24,51]

Although dissemination is not a panacea to the challenges of evidence-informed policymaking, dissemination activities can improve the alignment of policymaking processes with evidence if the right message is delivered to the right policymaker from the right source at the right time. This notion is supported by research from fields such as consumer psychology, communication science, and dissemination research, which showed that the strategic packaging of information can affect knowledge, attitudes, and behavior.[52]

Historical Context of Policy Dissemination Research

Although policy-focused dissemination research has been understudied within the field of implementation science in health,[4] social scientists have been exploring issues related to research use in policymaking since at least the 1960s in the United States. A foundational early contribution is the work of Carol Wiess, who developed a typology of how research is used in policymaking.[53–55] Four of these purposes have been the focus of extensive study. *Conceptual* (i.e., "enlightenment") research use relates to that which broadly shapes how a policymaker thinks about an issue. *Instrumental* (i.e., "problem-solving") research use relates to that in which research directly informs a policy decision. *Tactical* (i.e., "political" or "symbolic") research use relates to that in which research is used persuade someone to support a policy position. Finally, *imposed* research use relates to that which is carried out to satisfy mandates for research use, often with the goal of encouraging instrumental research use. Another key contribution from this era is Caplan's two-communities theory, which posits that a fundamental barrier to research-to-policy translation is that "social scientists and policy makers live in separate worlds with different and often conflicting values, different reward systems, and different languages."[56(p459)] (Brownson et al. applied this theory to health policy and contemporary contexts in a 2006 review.[57])

By the 1980s, the language and concept of "dissemination" had entered literature about research use in policymaking. For example, in the early 1980s two community psychologists conducted a randomized controlled trial to determine whether mailing Illinois state senators an evidence summary about child motor vehicle safety affected their voting behavior on the issue (it did).[58] The prominent public administration scholar Eugene Bardach published an article, "The Dissemination of Policy Research to Policymakers" in 1984 that described conditions that foster research-to-policy translation.[57,59] Concerns about policymaker-focused dissemination efforts were also published around this time. For instance, an article, "If Dissemination Is the Solution, What Is the Problem?" thoughtfully critiqued the idea that disseminating research findings to policymakers was an answer to social problems,[60] and a commentary by an NIH official discussed the risks of research evidence being misinterpreted and misused by policymakers.[61]

Types of Health Policy Dissemination Research Studies

Policy dissemination research can be thought of spanning at least five types of (sometimes overlapping) studies: formative audience research studies, audience segmentation studies, dissemination effectiveness studies, studies of research use in policymaking, and policy diffusion studies.

Formative Audience Research Studies

Formative audience research seeks to describe the attributes of policymakers with the aims of providing an empirical foundation to inform the design and distribution of dissemination materials.[62] Survey and interview methods are used in these studies. Achieving reasonable response rates can be a challenge in policymaker surveys, especially with elected officials. Luckily, information is often available to compare respondents and nonrespondents on demographic variables. Nonresponse weights can also be developed and applied in analyses.

A formative audience research study may assess the *sources that policymakers turn to for research evidence*. This information has utility for dissemination practice because it can identify the types of knowledge brokers and intermediaries that are optimally positioned to provide research evidence to policymakers.[63] Numerous studies have surveyed elected and administrative policymakers using items such as, "If you were going to seek out [insert health issue] research to make a policy decision, who would you turn to?" and instructing respondents to select up to three sources from a list of eight.

Studies may also characterize what policymakers perceive as the *most important features of disseminated evidence*. This information can inform the selection of evidence that is included in policy briefs and other dissemination materials to help ensure that materials are perceived as relevant, are engaged with, and are cognitively processed.[52,64] Surveys have presented policymakers with lists of features that could be included in dissemination materials (e.g., economic evidence, narratives, local data) and instructed them to rate "How important would it be that the research have each of the following characteristics?" on Likert scales. These studies can also assess policymaker preferences for receiving evidence via synchronous modes of dissemination, such as legislative testimony.[65]

Finally, formative studies can shed light on policymakers' knowledge and attitudes about specific policies, interventions, and health issues. Surveys have assessed the extent to which policymakers agree with factual statements about health issues and interventions (to assess knowledge),[66] support for evidence-based policies,[20,67–69] and perceptions of the relative importance and different health policy issues.[70–72] Analyses can estimate the prevalence and correlates of knowledge and attitudes to inform decisions about how evidence is framed for different policymaker audiences.

Constructs related to "attributes of innovations" (e.g., "relative advantage," "compatibility," "complexity") from Everett Rogers's theory of the diffusion of innovations can also be assessed in formative audience research.[73] For example, a survey assessed these constructs among state mental health agency policymakers to examine associations between attitudes toward policies that incentivize the use of EBIs and agency adoption of these policies.[74] Content analyses of textual artifacts from policymaking (e.g., bills, policymakers' social media posts) can also shed light on policymakers' knowledge and attitudes and avoid challenges related to low survey response rates. For example, analyses of state legislators' Twitter posts have assessed trends in the prevalence and correlates of attitudes related to COVID-19 and opioids.[75–77]

Audience Segmentation Studies

Audience segmentation studies seek to understand how dissemination materials might be tailored for different types of policymakers. Segments of policymakers may vary in terms of preferences for dissemination materials or knowledge and attitudes about a health issue.[61] Dissemination materials that are tailored to account for such variations are generally more effective than "one-size-fits-all" materials.[52,78] There are two general approaches to audience segmentation.

Demographic separation approaches involve stratifying a population of policymakers according to demographic variables and assessing differences in dissemination preferences, knowledge, attitudes, and behaviors across strata. Studies using this approach have segmented policymakers such as state legislators and city mayors according to variables, including ideology, political party affiliation, and prioritization of different health issues (e.g., cancer control,[79,80] behavioral health[81]). A benefit of demographic separation is that segmenting variables are readily observable, which facilitates the delivery of tailored dissemination materials to the larger population of policymakers beyond the survey sample.

Empirical clustering approaches to audience segmentation use statistical techniques such as latent class analysis and k-means clustering to identify patterns in relationships between multiple, and typically nondemographic, variables. These variables may include dissemination preferences, knowledge, attitudes, and behaviors. Statistical models identify "classes" of clustered variables and indicate the class to which each policymaker has the highest probability of belonging. Subsequent analyses then assess associations between nonlatent demographic variables and class (i.e., segment) membership.

This approach has been used with survey data from state legislators to identify audience segments that vary in terms of dissemination preferences[82] and conceptualizations of behavioral health policy issues.[83] A recent study emailed dissemination materials to state legislators and used email to view data and latent class analysis to identify audience segments of legislators based on email engagement behavior.[84] A benefit to empirical clustering is that it can produce highly nuanced segment profiles within a population of policymakers.

Dissemination Effectiveness Studies

Dissemination effectiveness studies may involve the prospective randomization of policymakers to experimental conditions, deploying dissemination strategies, and assessing outcomes. A major purpose of these studies is to determinate which dissemination strategies are most effective. Outcomes in policymaker-focused dissemination effectiveness studies may include engagement with dissemination materials (assessed by email views, policy brief link clicks, or requests for expert consultation); uses of the research evidence (assessed by analyzing textual artifacts of policymaking processes or surveys); and knowledge and attitudes (assessed via surveys).[52] Dissemination effectiveness studies conducted with policymakers have manipulated features of dissemination materials such as email subject lines,[16] the body text of emails,[17] statistical maps and narratives,[18-20] the geographic level of epidemiologic data,[21] economic data,[22] and indicators of public opinion.[85]

Given that policymakers share information with each other during policymaking processes, cluster randomized designs—in which geopolitical units, such as states, are randomized instead of individual policymakers—are typically appropriate to avoid contamination across study conditions. It is also important to prespecify and assess how variables such as political party affiliation and ideology might moderate the effects of dissemination materials. For example, a recent dissemination effectiveness experiment found that the inclusion of economic evidence increased engagement with dissemination materials among Democrat but not Republican state legislators[22]; another experiment with state legislators that found inclusion of narratives increased support for evidence-based child care policies among Democrats, but decreased support among Republicans.[20]

Studies of Research Use in Policymaking

The concept of "evidence-based practice" is core to implementation science, but it is not directly transferable from clinical to policy contexts.[51] Clinical evidence on the effectiveness of an EBI is most often rated in quality based on a hierarchy of evidence, with the randomized trial at the top of the evidence pyramid.[86] Given that it is generally not feasible or ethical to randomize populations to policy exposures, policy can at best be evidence informed. Measures of the *use of research evidence* in policymaking have become accepted indicators of evidence-informed policymaking with the (untested)[24] assumption that more evidence use results in more evidence-informed policymaking.

Research use in policymaking has been quantitively and qualitatively[87–93] studied for over half a century. Measures of research use in policymaking are typically treated as dependent variables, and individual-, organization-, and policy-level determinants of research use serve as independent variables. Research use can be measured across different timescales (e.g., past year, during a specific phases of the policy process) and in reference to use for different purposes (e.g., conceptual, instrumental).[94] There are numerous self-report measures of research use in policymaking,[95] many of which have been psychometrically validated. Table 24.2 summarizes key information about some of these measures.

In addition to self-report measures, artifacts of policymaking processes can be coded to describe uses of research in policymaking. For example, Gollust and colleagues coded bills, reports, and news media articles to illustrate how research evidence was used in childhood obesity policymaking in Minnesota.[103] More recently, Yanovitzky and Weber developed an instrument to code artifacts of policymaking processes according Weiss's typology of research use for different purposes.[104] Crowley and colleagues used a similar approach to code for research use in child-focused bills introduced in the US Congress, using this measure as an outcome in a policymaker-focused evidence translation experiment.[14]

Policy Diffusion Studies

A complement to studies focused on the uses of research evidence at the policymaker level, policy diffusion studies seek to understand how policy adoption (i.e., the enactment of a specific policy) spreads across geopolitical units (e.g., states). Policy diffusion studies have been conducted since the 1960s in the United States. In these studies, the dependent variable is state-level policy adoption (typically yes/no), and independent variables are state-level characteristics (e.g., population demographics, political leadership, economic indicators, interest group pressure) internal, as well as external, to states. Event history analysis methods—a suite of quantitative, quasi-experimental approaches[105]—are typically used to model these relationships.

Policy diffusion research has identified factors that affect policy adoption, all of which are worth considering in policy-focused dissemination studies. One factor is *economic competition* between states, which has been shown to affect the diffusion of policies related to welfare programs and lotteries.[106,107] Studies have also demonstrated how policy diffusion can function as a *social learning* process.[108] Thus, rather than adopting policies to compete with other states, states may look to those with similar economies,[109] in close proximity,[110] or with similar ideologies[111] to select policy responses to problems. Policy diffusion can also be influenced by *pressure from interest groups*.[112] Studies have documented how professional organizations and policy entrepreneurs facilitate the diffusion of policies across states with a focus on how state legislators' uses professional associations[113] and how interest groups may be successful in campaigning for policy adoption.[114]

Theories and Frameworks for Policy Dissemination Research

Because dissemination is, at its core, communication, theories of persuasive communication from fields such as social and consumer psychology can be useful in policymaker-focused dissemination research.[52] Such theories include the elaboration likelihood model, the persuasion knowledge model, and the theory of planned behavior. Brownson and colleagues' model of dissemination research[115] also has utility, as does Rogers's theory of the diffusion of innovations. Because policymaker-focused dissemination research seeks to infuse research evidence into policymaking, classical theories of policymaking are also relevant.[116] Below we highlight two frameworks that are useful for policy dissemination research.

Multiple-Streams Framework

Developed by John Kingdon, multiple streams is a political science framework that is widely used in the social sciences.[117] Multiple streams is founded on the premise that countless issues are constantly competing for policymakers' attention and posits that three "streams" influence if and how issues are addressed: (1) a problem stream, consisting of issues that are

TABLE 24.2 EXAMPLES OF MEASURES OF RESEARCH USE IN POLICYMAKING

Instrument Name	Country Developed	Year Published	Items	Psychometric Properties Reported
Legislative Use of Research Survey[96]	United States	2021	• Total scale: 35 items • Reported used of research evidence subscale: 7 items • Value of research evidence for policy work subscale: 8 items • Interaction with researchers subscale: 8 items • General information sources subscale: 5 items • Research information subscale: 7 items	Internal consistency (Cronbach α): • Total scale: Not reported • Reported use of research evidence subscale: 0.89 • Value of research evidence for policy work subscale: 0.85 • Interaction with researchers subscale: 0.89 • General information sources subscale: 0.64 • Research information subscale: 0.68
Standard Interview for Evidence Use (SIEU)[97]	United States	2016	• Total scale: 45 items • Input subscale: 17 items • Process subscale: 16 items • Output substance: 12 items	Internal consistency (Cronbach α): • Total SIEU scale: 0.88 • Input subscale: 0.70–0.86 • Process subscale: 0.71–0.88 • Output subscale: 0.71–0.88
Staff Assessment of EnGagement With Evidence (SAGE) structured interview[98]	Australia	2016	• Structured qualitative interview questions: 22 • Checklist: 66 items	• Face validity and interview question clarity were vetted with and refined based on feedback from a convenience sample of policymakers and researchers • Group of researchers and policymakers engaged in a consensus process to identify checklist items
Organizational Research Access, Culture, and Leadership (ORACLe) measure of organizational capacity for research use in policymaking[99]	Australia	2015	• Structured qualitative interview questions: 23	• Not reported

Evidence Utilization in Policymaking Measurement Tool (EUPMT)[100]	Iran	2017	• Total scale: 40 items that cover five constructs: behavior, intention, attitude, subjective norm, and perceived behavioral control	Content validity: 83% Face validity: 67% Internal consistency (Cronbach α): between subscales 0.70–0.90 Intraclass correlation coefficient: between subscales 0.75–0.87; 0.89 for total scale
Theory of Planned Behavior instrument to assess intentions to use research in policy in the future[101]	Canada	2011	• Total scale: 15 items across 12 questions	Internal consistency (Cronbach α): • Behavioral intention subscale: 0.89 • Attitude subscale: 0.73 • Subjective norm subscale: 0.79 • Perceived behavioral control subscale: 0.68
Bogenschneider's measures of research use in policymaking[102]	United States	2011	Total scale: 33 items • Value of research subscale: 5 items • Research-seeking subscale: 6 items • Use of research subscale: 3 items • Research presentation presences subscale: 4 items • Priority placed on unbiased research subscale: 1 item • Action orientation of research subscale: 3 items • Conceptual research use subscale: 4 items • Research quality subscale: 1 item • Research timing subscale: 1 item • Political framing subscale: 4 items	Internal consistency (Cronbach α): • Value of research subscale: 0.83–0.89 • Research-seeking subscale: 0.65–0.82 • Use of research subscale: 0.61–0.84 • Research presentation presences subscale: 0.65–0.80 • Priority placed on unbiased research subscale: n/a • Action orientation of research subscale: 0.61–0.77 • Conceptual research use subscale: 0.72–0.77 • Research quality subscale: n/a • Research timing subscale: n/a • Political framing subscale: 0.64–0.70

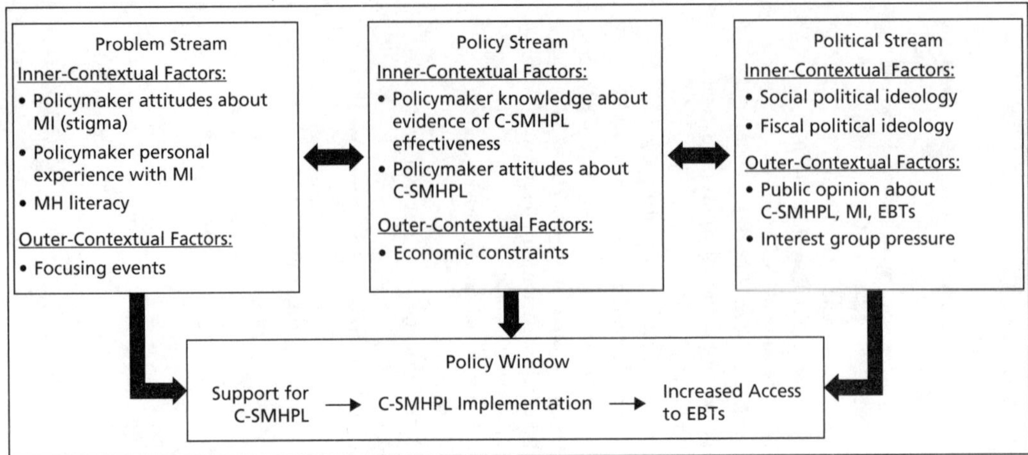

FIGURE 24.2 Conceptual framework for an audience research study to disseminate evidence about comprehensive state mental health parity legislation to state legislators.

Source: Reprinted with permission from Purtle et al.[118]

perceived by policymakers and the public as needing to be addressed; (2) a policy stream, consisting of potential solutions to these problems; and (3) a political stream, consisting of public opinion and the broader sociopolitical context surrounding policymaking. When these three streams converge around an issue, a "policy window" opens and "policy entrepreneurs" (e.g., advocates, researchers) can advance their policy proposals. The multiple streams framework was not created with the intent of structuring D&I research and thus might require adaptation. An example of such adaptation was provided by Purtle and colleagues, who modified the multiple streams framework for an audience research study focused on disseminating evidence about comprehensive state mental health parity legislation to state legislators (Figure 24.2).[118]

The SPIRIT Action Framework

The SPIRIT action framework is focused on the determinants of research use in policymaking. The framework is the product of a literature review, interviews with policymakers, and an interactive framework development process.[119] The SPIRIT action and multiple streams frameworks are similar in that they both emphasize the importance of considering sociopolitical context when disseminating research evidence to policymakers. However, whereas multiple streams is primarily a *descriptive framework* designed to characterize the policymaking process, the SPIRIT action framework is a *predictive framework* designed to identify factors that can be modified to promote evidence-informed policymaking. As Redman and colleagues described, the SPIRIT action framework was developed with the explicit purpose "to guide the development and testing of strategies to increase the use of research in policy."[119(p153)] The framework has since informed the development of measures,[94] study designs,[120,121] and interventions[15] to improve the use of research evidence among administrative policymakers in health agencies.

POLICY-FOCUSED IMPLEMENTATION RESEARCH

Implementation research is defined by the NIH as "the scientific study of the use of strategies to adopt and integrate evidence-based health interventions into clinical and community settings to improve individual outcomes and benefit population health." When applied to policy-focused work, policies are analogous to the "intervention" and "adopt[ion]" and "integrat[ion]" and relate to the extent to which policies are executed to maximize benefits for population health. Policy implementation studies may have goals, such as understanding the extent to which a policy has been enforced and the determinants of enforcement, understanding how interactions between policies at different levels (e.g., federal, state, local) affect implementation outcomes, and identifying strategies that can be used to improve policy implementation outcomes.

Historical Context of Policy Implementation Research

Policy implementation has been the focus of studies in fields such as public administration and management research and political science since at least the 1970s.[122,123] Initial work in these fields characterized policy implementation as relating to the question of, What happens after a bill becomes a law?[124] As the fields evolved, the central question became, How do governments put policies into effect?[125]

Early policy implementation research was largely exploratory and documented cases of implementation failure using a "top-down" approach that primarily focused on the perspectives of policymakers. A foundational contribution was the 1973 publication of Pressman and Wildavsky's book *Implementation*, which described the failed implementation of a federal economic development program in Oakland, California.[126] The case study found that policy implementation was hindered by issues such as ambiguous policy language and objectives, insufficient resources, poor policy compliance, and community opposition. As the authors described, these challenges led to a process of "dual implementation" where: "There are, then, two implementation processes. One is the initially perceived, formally defined, prospectively expected set of causal links required to result in a desired outcome; the other is the unexpected nexus of causality that actually evolves during implementation" (p. 217).

In response to early top-down policy implementation research, critics contended that there was too much emphasis on implementation failures and factors at the policymaker level. A more "bottom-up" approach emerged in the 1980s that placed greater emphasis on the role of front-line staff involved with policy implementation. This generation of research shifted the focus away from classifying policy implementation as a success or a failure and focused on the implementation decisions of those who interpret and translate policies into action. These studies made a strong distinction between those who make formal policy decisions and those who are tasked with carrying out, monitoring, and evaluating those policies.[127] Sometimes referred to as "street-level bureaucrats," these stakeholders are frequently confronted with uncertainty and ambiguity and are forced to make interpretations and adaptations during the policy implementation process—which in turn affect implementation outcomes.[128] Fierce polarization between the top-down and bottom-up scholars led to a schism in policy implementation research, with a third generation of studies emerging in the late 1980s that synthesized the two approaches and promoted more rigorous methodologies, including longitudinal designs and comparative multiple-case studies.[122]

Types of Health Policy Implementation Research Studies

Hoagwood and colleagues identified two broad categories of policy implementation research studies: *policy process implementation studies* and *policy impact implementation studies.*[3] The outcomes assessed in these studies varied according to the policy of focus, but a 2020 systematic review identified several instruments to measure health policy implementation outcomes.[12]

Policy Process Implementation Studies

There are two types of studies within the policy process implementation studies category. First, a policy process implementation study might simply describe the process through which a policy was implemented. Such studies can document what actions were performed by which stakeholders to execute policy implementation. For example, Purtle and colleagues coded open-ended survey response data from state mental health agency officials to implementation strategies listed in the Expert Recommendations for Implementing Change (ERIC) compendium with the aim of describing interagency strategies that these policymakers used to support implementation of a federal behavioral health law.[129]

Studies in this category could also assess stakeholders' perceptions of barriers and facilitators to policy implementation, the acceptability and feasibility of strategies that could enhance policy implementation, and the extent to which a policy had been enforced. For example, Crable and colleagues assessed barriers, facilitators, and strategies related to implementation of a Medicaid section 1115 waiver policy intended to provide reimbursement for evidence-based substance use disorder services.[130] The EPIS framework and ERIC compendium guided thematic analysis of interview data. Quantitative measures of acceptability, appropriateness, and feasibility can also be used in surveys to identify strategies that might be used to improve policy implementation processes.[131] The case study from Lee and colleagues below also provides an example of a policy process implementations study focused on health equity and policy sustainability.

Case Study 24.1: Operationalizing Equity to Study Policy Sustainability: A Mixed-Methods Case Study Evaluating the Implementation and Sustainment of Tobacco Control Policies in Asian American Communities in New York City

Little is known about how to plan for sustainability and track adaptations to policy implementation, as well as the ways that key sustainability factors and strategies relate to the equitable delivery of policies on the ground and in community settings. The purpose of this mixed-methods case study,[27] led by Matthew Lee and colleagues, was to explore the long-term sustainability and equity of tobacco control policies in New York City (NYC) to understand and contextualize their reach and impact on persistent smoking and tobacco-related health disparities in underserved communities, particularly among Asian Americans and other immigrant communities.

Within the tobacco control landscape, NYC is widely considered to be an early adopter, innovator, and champion of tobacco policies. The city currently has some of the most comprehensive smoke-free air laws in the country and excise taxes that are more than double the national average, and other municipalities often look to NYC before making their own tobacco control policy decisions.[132–135] Literature reviews have examined the uneven passage of smoke-free laws and policies and their effects on health equity in the United States. This body of literature indicates that uneven policy adoption and implementation across settings has exacerbated tobacco-related health disparities, particularly among people with low incomes, people with substance use and other mental health disorders, and rural residents.[136] In one review, across 117 relevant studies the only policy approach with the clearest and most consistent evidence of having a positive equity impact was increasing the purchase prices of cigarettes.[137] However, because the review only examined equity impacts in regard to socioeconomic status, their findings do not extend to other dimensions, including racial and gender equity.

The limited impacts of tobacco control policies on Asian Americans is another wrinkle in the tobacco control success story. Despite substantial successes in the broader tobacco control movement, persistent smoking- and tobacco-related disparities suggest that underserved populations, particularly Asian Americans and immigrant communities, are not being reached by broad "one-size-fits-all" policies and approaches in tobacco control.[133,137,138] Using a single, in-depth, convergent-parallel, mixed-methods case study, Lee and colleagues explored why tobacco control policies in NYC have failed to address smoking-related health inequities, particularly among Asian Americans. Data were collected and analyzed across five key primary and secondary sources:

1. *Policymaking documents*: text of key tobacco bills and statutes, as well as transcripts and testimonials from when they were first proposed, amended, debated, and adopted.
2. *Local newspaper coverage*: articles from a database of 29 major newspapers in NYC covering the policies and their impacts on local communities and businesses over time.
3. *Key informant interviews*: conducted with community members and community leaders at local health and advocacy organizations in NYC that primarily serve immigrant and Asian American communities ($n = 21$).
4. *Direct observation periods*: conducted within and around the health and advocacy organizations, as well as in majority Asian neighborhoods and Asian ethnic enclaves ($n = 15$).
5. *Community health survey (2012–2017)*: conducted annually by the NYC Department of Health and Mental Hygiene.

The findings point to the importance of understanding policy sustainability not as a static end goal, but rather as a dynamic set of processes and outcomes that impact health and health equity. Findings clustered across three key themes. First, since the initial adoption of comprehensive local tobacco control measures in NYC in 2002, broad "one-size-fits-all" approaches to policy implementation and monitoring have been sustained, which have had and continue to have limited reach and impact within underserved Asian American and immigrant communities. Second, two delayed adaptation efforts were made by policymakers during the sustainability phase, one in 2012 and another in 2018; these were intended to improve on prior uneven implementation to better reach Chinese-speaking communities. Third, community-based organizations have played a direct role in functioning as not only key stakeholders but also key implementers to ensure that tobacco and other health policies are reaching communities that the designated or official implementers cannot reach. This suggests the need for further study of *unofficial implementers* in policy-focused implementation science—those who have not been formally designated as the ones responsible for ensuring that implementation takes place, but are still delivering implementation strategies to ensure adoption, integration, and sustainment.

Informed by these themes and findings, a working operational definition of policy sustainability was developed and refined that will be applied in future equity-focused research. Tentatively, policy sustainability is

- After a sufficient period of **time** after the policy has achieved full initial implementation;
- The evidence-supported policy and its implementation strategies continue to be **delivered evenly** across communities; and
- The policy **monitoring and enforcement** are maintained; with the recognition that
- The policy will likely **evolve or adapt** in response to changes in the evidence base and in the inner and outer context, while
- Continuing to meet dynamic population and community needs and priorities, and producing **equitable benefits** for individuals and systems.

Overall, this case study points to the potential for policy sustainability research to advance health and health equity by identifying factors and mechanisms that can be improved to maximize and sustain the equitable reach and impact of public policies. By focusing on dynamic contextual factors and sustainability as a set of processes and outcomes, the findings from this case study raise critical questions about the criteria typically used to evaluate whether policy interventions are evidence based and effective by asking: (1) effective for whom? (2) based on what evidence? and (3) what happens as dynamic populations and contexts change over time? These questions highlight how the tobacco control success story was largely constructed around broad population-wide benefits while overlooking underserved Asian American and immigrant communities, who continue to bear the brunt of smoking and tobacco-related health disparities.

Policy Impact Implementation Studies

Studies within this category use experimental or quasi-experimental designs to assess the main effect of a policy on implementation outcomes, the moderating effect of policy implementation outcomes on policy effectiveness outcomes, or the main effect of policy implementation strategies on policy implementation and/or effectiveness outcomes. For example, McGinty and colleagues used a quasi-experimental design to understand how the implementation of state medical cannabis laws affect treatment for chronic noncancer pain (implementation outcomes) and adverse opioid outcomes (effectiveness outcomes).[139] Dopp and colleagues used a quasi-experimental design to compare the effects of two different policy approaches to financing an evidence-based treatment on implementation outcomes.[140] There is a need for research that experimentally tests the effects of policy implementation strategies on policy implementation and effectiveness outcomes.

Theories and Frameworks for Policy Implementation Research

Many theories of policy implementation from the field of public administration and management research can be useful for policy-focused implementation science studies. These include Sabatier and Mazmanian's policy implementation framework[141] and Lipsky's theory of street-level bureaucracy,[128] both published in 1980. Below we highlight two more recent frameworks from the field of implementation science in health.

Policy Ecology Framework

The policy ecology framework (PEF)[142] was designed for a specific purpose: to help policymakers in local and state administrative units (i.e., departments or divisions of mental health, child welfare, Medicaid, and juvenile justice) identify and deploy policy strategies to improve access to, and the quality of, services for children exposed to psychological trauma. Because the goal of the PEF was to enhance utilization of these strategies (conceptualized as "policy levers"), the framework was constructed around an enumeration of such tools. The PEF conceptualizes policy levers as falling within a set of four nested contexts.

At the provider organization level, policymakers can deploy tools such as enhancing the reimbursement rate for EBIs. At the state or local agency level, policymakers can structure their bidding and contracting procedures in ways that promote access and quality. At the political level, loan forgiveness programs can enhance a workforce capable of delivering high-quality interventions. At the societal level, policymakers can support social marketing efforts to reduce mental illness stigma. It is not expected that a single state or local agency will engage in all of these actions. Instead, this enumeration provides a set of choices that state and local policymakers can consider.

The PEF has been used to inform state and local policy implementation efforts within the United States. At the local level, Powell and colleagues used the framework to describe efforts taken by the city of Philadelphia to transform its behavioral health system.[143] At the state level, Stone and colleagues used the PEF to identify policy levers that can support EBIs within the Maryland Medicaid Health Home Program,[144] and Aby applied the PEF to examine how Minnesota's Cultural and Ethnic Minority Infrastructure Grant program can enhance equity for cultural and ethnic minority persons in the state.[145]

Integrated Framework of Policy Implementation

Bullock and colleagues' integrated framework of policy implementation was created through a critical interpretive synthesis of research in the fields of implementation science in health, public policy, and knowledge translation.[146] Policy is central to the framework. Situating policy at the center of the framework is a departure from how it is typically conceptualized in implementation science research: as an outer-contextual factor distilled to the focus of the implementation effort. The integrated framework consists of two related models: one that focuses on the implementation process and one that focuses on determinants of implementation success.

DIRECTIONS FOR FUTURE RESEARCH

Policy D&I research has a rich history in the fields of public administration and management research and political science but is still an emerging area in the contemporary field of implementation science in health. Here, we highlight five areas that we perceive as priorities for future research.

Understanding and Minimizing the Impact of Misinformation and Disinformation on Policymaking

Given that misinformation and disinformation has become commonplace in public and political discourses, there is a critical need for policy dissemination researchers to understand—and ideally help minimize—the spread and effects of misinformation and disinformation in health policymaking.[49,50] Research in fields such as communication science and political science has studied these issues extensively, and there would be benefit to integrating key findings and methods into policy-focused dissemination research. There could also be value in adapting and testing "debunking" interventions (which are reactive) and "prebunking" interventions (which are preventive) to minimize the effects of misinformation and disinformation on health policymaking.[147] Policy dissemination researchers should also be cautious of "boomerang effects," in which a message has an effect opposite to that intended (e.g., an attempt to correct misinformation or disinformation results in a stronger belief in falsehoods).

Using Social Media Data in Policy-Focused D&I Research

Social media platforms—such as Facebook and Twitter—play an influential role in politics and policymaking, but have not yet been a substantive focus of policy D&I research. A 2014 study found that almost all US Congresspersons on federal health committees had Twitter accounts and used the platform to engage in dialogue with their constituents about health issues.[148] Studies have used natural language processing methods to analyze policymakers' social media posts about health issues[75–77] and also used posts as outcomes in dissemination experiments with policymakers.[22] However, methods for using policymaker social media data in D&I research remain underdeveloped and are an area for future work. As noted above, a practical advantage to using social media data is that they are publicly available and negate challenges related to nonresponse bias in policymaker surveys.

Measuring Outer Context in Policy-Focused D&I Research

Given that implementation science research in health has largely focused on clinical, organizational, and community-based interventions, policy has typically been conceptualized as an outer-context factor distant from an EBI that is central to the study. However, in policy-focused D&I research, policy is central. This raises questions about what are important outer-context constructs for policy-focused D&I research and how they can be measured. Research from the field of political science indicated that constructs related to public opinion, news media coverage, and corporate pressure all affect policymaking and implementation processes[149] and should thus be considered as outer-contextual factors in policy-focused implementation science research. Established methods for measuring these constructs exist (e.g., public opinion surveys, content analysis of news and social media). There is a need to integrate these methods into policy-focused D&I research and analyze the mechanism through which they might affect implementation outcomes and moderate implementation strategy effects.

Using Decision Science and Systems Science Methods in Policy-Focused D&I Research

Decision science is an interdisciplinary field that has been largely untapped in policy D&I research. Decision science focuses on individual and group processes and behaviors that shape decision makers' preferences and decisions and uses methods to help decision makers make an optimal decision given available information. Decision science methods could also help elicit preferences and values to elucidate the extent to which policymakers assign importance to different dimensions of a decision. These methods include discrete choice experiments, best-worst scaling, and analytic hierarchy processes. For example, Mackie and colleagues used a best-worst scaling experiment to identify which claims-based outcomes related to antipsychotic monitoring were of highest priority to policymakers and other policy stakeholders.[150]

Also, while systems science methods are becoming commonplace in implementation science research (chapter 13), their application to policy-focused D&I research questions remains underdeveloped. Specific opportunities for integrating system science methods include a group model-building process in which policymakers and other policy stakeholder share knowledge and experiences to develop a solution to a policy implementation problem, agent-based models to explore the dynamics through which evidence-supported policies are adopted under different scenarios,[151] and social network analyses to characterize policymaking networks.[152,153]

Enhancing Policy Implementation Research Methods

Although there is substantive theory to inform policy implementation research, there is a need for methods development and refinement in the area of health policy implementation science. Priorities in this area include, but are not limited to,

- establishing consensus definitions for policy implementation strategies and articulating the mechanisms through which they may affect policy implementation outcomes;
- expanding methods for studying the causal effects of policy implementation strategies using nonexperimental designs;
- establishing consensus definitions for a core set of policy implementation outcomes, developing/refining psychometrically strong measures to

assess them and standards for rigor in policy-focused D&I research;
- determining the types of quantitative analysis techniques that are best suited for policy implementation research;
- developing methods to assess the moderating effects of outer-context variables on policy implementation outcomes; and
- Expanding the research methods for fully integrating health equity in policy D&I research.

SUMMARY

In policy-focused D&I research, a policy is "the thing"[28] that is central to the investigation. Policy can also be studied as a contextual factor non-policy-focused work in which the D&I of an EBI is the central concern. *Policy dissemination research* seeks to understand how research evidence can be most effectively communicated to policymakers and integrated into policymaking processes. These studies may aim to describe attributes of a population of policymakers, identify discrete audience segments of policymakers, test the effects of dissemination strategies, characterize the use of research evidence in policymaking, and identify factors associated with the diffusion of policies across jurisdictions. *Policy implementation research* seeks to understand how the rollout of polices can be optimized to maximize health benefits. Such studies may aim to describe the process through which a policy was implemented, assess stakeholders' perceptions of implementation and appetite for implementation strategies, and determine the effect of a policy on implementation outcomes, the moderating effect of policy implementation outcomes on policy effectiveness outcomes, or the main effect of policy implementation strategies on policy implementation and/or effectiveness outcomes. Future directions for policy D&I research include studying misinformation and disinformation in policymaking, using social media data from policymakers, measuring outer-context variables, using decision science and systems science methods, and methodological development in the area of policy implementation research.

The study of evidence-to-policy translation and policy implementation has a rich history but is still an emerging area in the field of D&I science in health. Developing policy D&I research is critical to maximizing the public health impact of the field of implementation science and also has potential to improve population health and enhance health equity. Policy-focused D&I research is also important for developing effective strategies to combat the effects of actors who seek to influence policies in ways that are diametrically opposed to the goals of public health and health equity.

SUGGESTED READINGS AND WEBSITES

Readings

Allen P, Pilar M, Walsh-Bailey C, et al. Quantitative measures of health policy implementation determinants and outcomes: a systematic review. *Implement Sci.* 2020;15(1):1–17.

This article is a systematic review of measures used in policy implementation research.

Ashcraft LE, Quinn DA, Brownson RC. Strategies for effective dissemination of research to United States policymakers: a systematic review. *Implement Sci.* 2020;15(1):1–7.

This article is a review of dissemination strategies to communicate research evidence to policymakers in the United States.

Brownson RC, Kumanyika SK, Kreuter MW, Haire-Joshu D. Implementation science should give higher priority to health equity. *Implementation Science.* 2021;16(1):1–16.

This conceptual article provides guidance to sharpen the focus on health equity in implementation science research, with sections dedicated to policy-focused D&I research.

Combs T, Nelson KL, Luke D, et al. Simulating the role of knowledge brokers in policy making in state agencies: an agent-based model. *Health Serv Res.* 2022 Jun;57 Suppl 1(Suppl 1):122–136. doi:10.1111/1475-6773.13916. Epub 2022 Mar 4.

An example is provided of a multimethod study using survey, interview, and systems science methods to study the use of research evidence in policymaking.

Doucet F. *Centering the Margins: (Re)defining Useful Research Evidence Through Critical Perspectives.* William T Grant Foundation; 2019.

This book is a thought-provoking review that illustrates the imperative of incorporating critical race theory and other critical perspectives into the study of the use of research evidence in policymaking.

Haynes A, Rowbotham SJ, Redman S, Brennan S, Williamson A, Moore G. What can we learn from interventions that aim to increase policy-makers' capacity to use research? A realist scoping review. *Health Res Policy Syst.* 2018;16(1):1–27.

An informative review is provided of strategies to increase policymakers' capacity to use research evidence in policymaking.

Hoagwood KE, Purtle J, Spandorfer J, Peth-Pierce R, Horwitz SM. Aligning dissemination and implementation science with health policies to improve children's mental health. *Am Psychol.* 2020;75(8):1130.

This is a conceptual article that provides a typology of policy-focused dissemination and implementation studies.

Nilsen P, Ståhl C, Roback K, Cairney P. Never the twain shall meet? A comparison of implementation science and policy implementation research. *Implement Sci.* 2013;8:63.

A foundational article is provided that compares how policy implementation is conceptualized and studied in two related fields: public administration research and implementation science in health.

Oliver K, Lorenc T, Innvær S. New directions in evidence-based policy research: a critical analysis of the literature. *Health Res Policy Syst.* 2014;12(1):34.

A thoughtful review is provided of barriers to the use of research evidence in policymaking, and a summary of priorities for future research and theory development is given.

Weiss CH. The many meanings of research utilization. *Public Admin Rev.* 1979;39(5):426–431.

This foundation article describes the many different ways that research evidence can be used in policymaking.

Selected Websites and Tools

Global Commission on Evidence to Address Social Change. https://www.mcmasterforum.org/networks/evidence-commission

This website and report adopts a global perspective and outlines key challenges to evidence-based policymaking and strategies to address them.

Research-to-Policy Collaboration. https://research2policy.org/

This site is an example of an ongoing intervention and practice initiative aimed at improving the use of research evidence in policymaking in the US Congress.

The Use of Research Evidence: A Methods Repository. https://uremethods.org/methods-resources/

Provided on this website is a database and repository of methods to study the use of research of evidence in policymaking.

REFERENCES

1. Williams DR. Miles to go before we sleep: racial inequities in health. *J Health Soc Behav.* 2012 Sep;53(3):279–295.
2. Galea S, Tracy M, Hoggatt KJ, DiMaggio C, Karpati A. Estimated deaths attributable to social factors in the United States. *Am J Public Health.* 2011 Aug;101(8):1456–1465.
3. Hoagwood KE, Purtle J, Spandorfer J, Peth-Pierce R, Horwitz SM. Aligning dissemination and implementation science with health policies to improve children's mental health. *Am Psychol.* 2020 Nov;75(8):1130.
4. Purtle J, Peters R, Brownson RC. A review of policy dissemination and implementation research funded by the National Institutes of Health, 2007–2014. *Implement Sci.* 2015;11(1):1–8.
5. Emmons KM, Gandelman E. Translating behavioral medicine evidence to public policy. *J Behav Med.* 2019;42(1):84–94.
6. Purtle J, Nelson KL, Bruns EJ, Hoagwood KE. Dissemination Strategies to Accelerate the Policy Impact of Children's Mental Health Services Research. *Psychiatr Serv.* 2020:appi. ps. 201900527.
7. Emmons KM, Chambers DA. Policy implementation science–an unexplored strategy to address social determinants of health. *Ethn Dis.* 2021;31(1):133.
8. Emmons KM, Chambers D, Abazeed A. Embracing policy implementation science to ensure translation of evidence to cancer control policy. *Transl Behav Med.* 2021 Nov;11(11):1972–1979.
9. Oh A, Abazeed A, Chambers DA. Policy implementation science to advance population health: the potential for learning health policy systems. *Front Public Health.* 2021;9:681602.
10. Brownson RC, Shelton RC, Geng EH, Glasgow RE. Revisiting concepts of evidence in implementation science. *Implement Sci.* 2022 Dec;17(1):1–25.
11. Ashcraft LE, Quinn DA, Brownson RC. Strategies for effective dissemination of research to United States policymakers: a systematic review. *Implement Sci.* 2020 Dec;15(1):1–7.
12. Allen P, Pilar M, Walsh-Bailey C, et al. Quantitative measures of health policy implementation determinants and outcomes: a systematic review. *Implement Sci.* 2020;15(1):1–17.
13. McHugh S, Dorsey CN, Mettert K, Purtle J, Bruns E, Lewis CC. Measures of outer setting constructs for implementation research: a systematic review and analysis of psychometric quality. *Implement Res Pract.* 2020 Jul;1:2633489520940022.
14. Crowley DM, Scott JT, Long EC, et al. Lawmakers' use of scientific evidence can be improved. *Proc Natl Acad Sci U S A.* 2021;118(9).
15. Williamson A, Barker D, Green S, et al. Increasing the capacity of policy agencies to use

research findings: a stepped-wedge trial. *Health Res Policy Syst.* 2019;17(1):1–16.

16. Long EC, Pugel J, Scott JT, et al. Rapid-cycle experimentation with state and federal policymakers for optimizing the reach of racial equity research. *Am J Public Health.* 2021(0):e1–e4.
17. Levine AS. Single conversations expand practitioners' use of research: evidence from a field experiment. *PS Polit Sci Polit.* 2021:1–6.
18. Niederdeppe J, Winett LB, Xu Y, Fowler EF, Gollust SE. Evidence-based message strategies to increase public support for state investment in early childhood education: results from a longitudinal panel experiment. *Milbank Q.* 2021.
19. Niederdeppe J, Roh S, Dreisbach C. How narrative focus and a statistical map shape health policy support among state legislators. *Health Commun.* 2016;31(2):242–255.
20. Winett LB, Niederdeppe J, Xu Y, Gollust SE, Fowler EF. When "Tried and True" Advocacy Strategies Backfire: Narrative Messages Can Undermine State Legislator Support for Early Childcare Policies. *J Public Interest Commun.* 2021;5(1):45–45.
21. Brownson RC, Dodson EA, Stamatakis KA, et al. Communicating evidence-based information on cancer prevention to state-level policy makers. *J Natl Cancer Inst.* 2011;103(4):306–316.
22. Purtle J, Nelson KL, Gebrekristos L, Lê-Scherban F, Gollust SE. Partisan differences in the effects of economic evidence and local data on legislator engagement with dissemination materials about behavioral health: a dissemination trial. *Implement Sci.* 2022;17(1):1–15.
23. Lester L, Haby MM, Chapman E, Kuchenmüller T. Evaluation of the performance and achievements of the WHO Evidence-informed Policy Network (EVIPNet) Europe. *Health Res Policy Syst.* 2020 Dec;18(1):1–9.
24. Oliver K, Lorenc T, Innvær S. New directions in evidence-based policy research: a critical analysis of the literature. *Health Res Policy Syst.* 2014;12(1):34.
25. Oliver K, Innvar S, Lorenc T, Woodman J, Thomas J. A systematic review of barriers to and facilitators of the use of evidence by policymakers. *BMC Health Serv Res.* 2014;14(1):2.
26. Weiner BJ, Lewis CC, Sherr K, editors. *Practical Implementation Science: Moving Evidence into Action.* Springer Publishing Company; 2022 Mar 18.
27. Lee M, Kwon SC, Russo R, Purtle J, Shelton RC. Policy sustainability research to advance health equity: findings from a mixed methods case study of the implementation and sustainability of tobacco control policies in New York City. Paper presented at: "Best of D&I" conference session at the 13th Annual Conference on the Science of Dissemination and Implementation in Health; 2020. Washington, D.C., December 14–16, 2020.
28. Curran GM. Implementation science made too simple: a teaching tool. *Implement Sci Commun.* 2020 Dec;1(1):1–3.
29. Lengnick-Hall R, Stadnick NA, Dickson KS, Moullin JC, Aarons GA. Forms and functions of bridging factors: specifying the dynamic links between outer and inner contexts during implementation and sustainment. *Implement Sci.* 2021 Dec;16(1):1–3.
30. Crable EL, Lengnick-Hall R, Stadnick NA, Moullin JC, Aarons GA. Where is "policy" in dissemination and implementation science? Recommendations to advance theories, models, and frameworks: EPIS as a case example. *Implement Sci.* 2022;17(1):1–14.
31. Brownson RC, Kumanyika SK, Kreuter MW, Haire-Joshu D. Implementation science should give higher priority to health equity. *Implement Sci.* 2021 Dec;16(1):1–6.
32. Lorenc T, Petticrew M, Welch V, Tugwell P. What types of interventions generate inequalities? Evidence from systematic reviews. *J Epidemiol Community Health.* 2013 Feb 1;67(2):190–193.
33. Thomson K, Hillier-Brown F, Todd A, McNamara C, Huijts T, Bambra C. The effects of public health policies on health inequalities in high-income countries: an umbrella review. *BMC Public Health.* 2018 Dec;18(1):1–21.
34. Brownson RC, Shelton RC, Geng EH, Glasgow RE. Revisiting concepts of evidence in implementation science. *Implement Sci.* 2022 Dec;17(1):1–25.
35. U.S. Community Preventive Services Taskforce. Health Equity: Permanent Supportive Housing with Housing First (Housing First Programs. Available at: https://www.thecommunityguide.org/findings/health-equity-housing-first-programs#:~:text=The%20Community%20Preventive%20Services%20Task ahadc.
36. Gollust SE, Vogel RI, Rothman A, Yzer M, Fowler EF, Nagler RH. Americans' perceptions of disparities in COVID-19 mortality: results from a nationally-representative survey. *Prev Med.* 2020 Dec 1;141:106278.
37. Purtle J, Henson RM, Carroll-Scott A, Kolker J, Joshi R, Diez Roux AV. US mayors' and health commissioners' opinions about health disparities in their cities. *Am J Public Health.* 2018 May;108(5):634–641.
38. Purtle J, Joshi R, Lê-Scherban F, Henson RM, Diez Roux AV. Linking Data on constituent health with elected officials' opinions: associations

between urban health disparities and mayoral officials' beliefs about health disparities in their cities. *Milbank Q.* 2021 Sep;99(3):794–827.

39. Farrer L, Marinetti C, Cavaco YK, Costongs C. Advocacy for health equity: a synthesis review. *Milbank Q.* 2015 Jun;93(2):392–437.
40. Gollust SE, Nelson KL, Purtle J. Selecting evidence to frame the consequences of adverse childhood experiences: testing effects on public support for policy action, multi-sector responsibility, and stigma. *Prev Med.* 2022 Jan 1;154:106912.
41. Winett LB, Niederdeppe J, Xu Y, Gollust SE, Fowler EF. When "Tried and True" advocacy strategies backfire: narrative messages can undermine state legislator support for early childcare policies. *J Public Interest Comm.* 2021 Jul 13;5(1):45.
42. Bye L, Ghirardelli A, Fontes A. Promoting health equity and population health: how Americans' views differ. *Health Aff.* 2016 Nov 1;35(11):1982–1990.
43. Asada Y, Hughes A, Chriqui J. Insights on the intersection of health equity and school nutrition policy implementation: an exploratory qualitative secondary analysis. *Health Educ Behav.* 2017 Oct;44(5):685–695.
44. Richardson DM, Steeves-Reece A, Martin A, Hurtado DA, Dumet LM, Goodman JM. Employee experiences with a newly adopted paid parental leave policy: equity considerations for policy implementation. *Health Aff.* 2019 Apr 10;3(1):117–123.
45. Davidovitz M, Cohen N. Politicians' involvement in street-level policy implementation: implications for social equity. *Public Policy Adm.* 2021 Jun 23:09520767211024033.
46. Shelton RC, Lee M. Sustaining evidence-based interventions and policies: recent innovations and future directions in implementation science. *Am J Public Health.* 2019 Feb;109(S2):S132–134.
47. Dettlaff AJ, Boyd R. Racial disproportionality and disparities in the child welfare system: why do they exist, and what can be done to address them? *Ann Am Acad Pol Soc Sci.* 2020 Nov;692(1):253–274.
48. Anyon Y. Reducing racial disparities and disproportionalities in the child welfare system: Policy perspectives about how to serve the best interests of African American youth. *Child Youth Serv Rev.* 2011 Feb 1;33(2):242–253.
49. Iyengar S, Massey DS. Scientific communication in a post-truth society. *Proc Natl Acad Sci U S A.* 2019;116(16):7656–7661.
50. Scheufele DA, Krause NM. Science audiences, misinformation, and fake news. *Proc Natl Acad Sci U S A.* 2019;116(16):7662–7669.
51. Cairney P, Oliver K. Evidence-based policymaking is not like evidence-based medicine, so how far should you go to bridge the divide between evidence and policy? *Health Res Policy Syst.* 2017;15(1):1–11.
52. Purtle J, Marzalik J, Halfond R, Bufka L, Teachman B, Aarons G. Towards the Data-Driven Dissemination of Findings from Psychological Science. *Am Psychol.* 2020.
53. Weiss CH. Research for policy's sake: The enlightenment function of social research. *Policy Anal.* 1977:531–545.
54. Weiss CH. The many meanings of research utilization. *Public Adm Rev.* 1979;39(5):426–431.
55. Weiss CH, Murphy-Graham E, Birkeland S. An alternate route to policy influence: How evaluations affect DARE. *Am J Eval.* 2005;26(1):12–30.
56. Caplan N. The two-communities theory and knowledge utilization. *Am Behav Sci.* 1979 Jan;22(3):459–470.
57. Brownson RC, Royer C, Ewing R, McBride TD. Researchers and policymakers: travelers in parallel universes. *Am J Prev Med.* 2006 Feb 1;30(2):164–172.
58. Jason LA, Rose T. Influencing the passage of child passenger restraint legislation. *Am J Community Psychol.* 1984;12(4):485–494.
59. Bardach E. The dissemination of policy research to policymakers. *Knowledge.* 1984;6(2):125–144.
60. Knott J, Wildavsky A. If dissemination is the solution, what is the problem? *Knowledge.* 1980 Jun;1(4):537–78.
61. Parloff MB. Can psychotherapy research guide the policymaker? A little knowledge may be a dangerous thing. *Am Psychol.* 1979 Apr;34(4):296.
62. Slater MD. Theory and method in health audience segmentation. *J Health Commun.* 1996;1(3):267–284.
63. Brownson RC, Eyler AA, Harris JK, Moore JB, Tabak RG. Research full report: getting the word out: new approaches for disseminating public health science. *J Public Health Manag Pract.* 2018;24(2):102.
64. Petty RE, Cacioppo JT. The elaboration likelihood model of persuasion. In: *Communication and Persuasion.* Springer; 1986:1–24.
65. Moreland-Russell S, Barbero C, Andersen S, Geary N, Dodson EA, Brownson RC. "Hearing from all sides" How legislative testimony influences state level policy-makers in the United States. *Int J Health Policy Manag.* 2015 Feb;4(2):91.
66. Purtle J, Lê-Scherban F, Wang X, Brown E, Chilton M. State legislators' opinions about adverse childhood experiences as risk factors for adult behavioral health conditions. *Psychiatr Serv.* 2019 Oct 1;70(10):894–900.

67. Welch PJ, Dake JA, Price JH, Thompson AJ, Ubokudom SE. State legislators' support for evidence-based obesity reduction policies. *Prev Med.* 2012;55(5):427–429.
68. Nelson KL, Purtle J. Factors associated with state legislators' support for opioid use disorder parity laws. *Int J Drug Policy.* 2020 Aug 1;82:102792.
69. Purtle J, Lê-Scherban FÉ, Wang XI, Shattuck PT, Proctor EK, Brownson RC. State legislators' support for behavioral health parity laws: the influence of mutable and fixed factors at multiple levels. *Milbank Q.* 2019 Dec;97(4):1200–1232.
70. Clement DM. Factors influencing Georgia legislators' decision-making on nurse practitioner scope of practice. *Policy Polit Nurs Pract.* 2018 Nov;19(3-4):91–99.
71. Godinez Puig L, Lusk K, Glick D, Einstein KL, Palmer M, Fox S, Wang ML. Perceptions of public health priorities and accountability among US mayors. *Public Health Rep.* 2021 Mar;136(2):161–171.
72. Purtle J, Nelson KL, Henson RM, Horwitz SM, McKay MM, Hoagwood KE. Policy makers' priorities for addressing youth substance use and factors that influence priorities. *Psychiatr Serv.* 2021 Aug 13:appi–ps.
73. Rogers EM. *Diffusion of Innovations.* Simon and Schuster; 2010.
74. Stewart RE, Marcus SC, Hadley TR, Hepburn BM, Mandell DS. State adoption of incentives to promote evidence-based practices in behavioral health systems. *Psychiatr Serv.* 2018 Jun 1;69(6):685–688.
75. Engel-Rebitzer E, Stokes DC, Buttenheim A, Purtle J, Meisel ZF. Changes in legislator vaccine-engagement on Twitter before and after the arrival of the COVID-19 pandemic. *Hum Vaccines Immunother.* 2021:1–5.
76. Guntuku SC, Purtle J, Meisel ZF, Merchant RM, Agarwal A. Partisan differences in Twitter language among US legislators during the COVID-19 pandemic: cross-sectional Study. *J Medical Internet Res.* 2021;23(6):e27300.
77. Stokes DC, Purtle J, Meisel ZF, Agarwal AK. State legislators' divergent social media response to the opioid epidemic from 2014 to 2019: longitudinal topic modeling analysis. *J Gen Intern Med.* 2021:1–10.
78. Noar SM, Benac CN, Harris MS. Does tailoring matter? Meta-analytic review of tailored print health behavior change interventions. *Psychol Bull.* 2007;133(4):673.
79. Brownson RC, Dodson EA, Kerner JF, Moreland-Russell S. Framing research for state policymakers who place a priority on cancer. *Cancer Causes & Control.* 2016 Aug;27(8):1035–1041.
80. Morshed AB, Dodson EA, Tabak RG, Brownson RC. Comparison of research framing preferences and information use of State legislators and advocates involved in cancer control, United States, 2012–2013. *Prev Chronic Dis.* 2017;14.
81. Purtle J, Dodson EA, Brownson RC. Uses of research evidence by State legislators who prioritize behavioral health issues. *Psychiatr Serv.* 2016 Dec 1;67(12):1355–1361.
82. Smith NR, Mazzucca S, Hall MG, Hassmiller Lich K, Brownson RC, Frerichs L. Opportunities to improve policy dissemination by tailoring communication materials to the research priorities of legislators. *Implement Sci Commun.* 2022 Dec;3(1):1–9.
83. Purtle J, Lê-Scherban F, Wang X, Shattuck PT, Proctor EK, Brownson RC. Audience segmentation to disseminate behavioral health evidence to legislators: an empirical clustering analysis. *Implement Sci.* 2018;13(1):121.
84. Pugel J, Long EC, Fernandes MA, Cruz K, Giray C, Crowley DM, Scott JT. Who is listening? Profiles of policymaker engagement with scientific communication. *Policy & Internet.* 2022 Mar;14(1):186–201.
85. Butler DM, Nickerson DW. Can learning constituency opinion affect how legislators vote? Results from a field experiment. *Q J Polit Sci.* 2011;6(1):55–83.
86. Akobeng AK. Understanding randomised controlled trials. *Arch Dis Child.* 2005 Aug 1;90(8):840–844.
87. Purtle J, Peters R, Kolker J, Diez Roux AV. Uses of population health rankings in local policy contexts: a multisite case study. *Med Care Res Rev.* 2019;76(4):478–496.
88. Haynes AS, Gillespie JA, Derrick GE, et al. Galvanizers, guides, champions, and shields: the many ways that policymakers use public health researchers. *Milbank Q.* 2011;89(4):564–598.
89. Jack S, Dobbins M, Tonmyr L, Dudding P, Brooks S, Kennedy B. Research evidence utilization in policy development by child welfare administrators. *Child Welfare.* 2010;89(4).
90. Hyde JK, Mackie TI, Palinkas LA, Niemi E, Leslie LK. Evidence use in mental health policy making for children in foster care. *Adm Policy Ment Health Ment Health Serv Res.* 2016;43(1):52–66.
91. Waddell C, Lavis JN, Abelson J, et al. Research use in children's mental health policy in Canada: maintaining vigilance amid ambiguity. *Soc Sci Med.* 2005;61(8):1649–1657.
92. Jewell CJ, Bero LA. "Developing good taste in evidence": facilitators of and hindrances to evidence-informed health policymaking in state government. *Milbank Q.* 2008;86(2):177–208.

93. Meisel ZF, Mitchell J, Polsky D, et al. Strengthening partnerships between substance use researchers and policy makers to take advantage of a window of opportunity. *Subst Abuse Treat Prev Policy.* 2019;14(1):12.
94. Purtle J, Nelson KL, Horwitz SM, McKay MM, Hoagwood KE. Determinants of using children's mental health research in policymaking: variation by type of research use and phase of policy process. *Implement Sci.* 2021 Dec;16(1):1–5.
95. Asgharzadeh A, Shabaninejad H, Aryankhesal A, Majdzadeh R. Instruments for assessing organisational capacity for use of evidence in health sector policy making: a systematic scoping review. *Evid Policy.* 2021 Feb 1;17(1):29–57.
96. Long EC, Smith RL, Scott JT, Gay B, Giray C, Storace R, Guillot-Wright S, Crowley DM. A new measure to understand the role of science in US Congress: lessons learned from the Legislative Use of Research Survey (LURS). *Evid Policy.* 2021 Nov 1;17(4):689–707.
97. Palinkas LA, Garcia AR, Aarons GA, Finno-Velasquez M, Holloway IW, Mackie TI, Leslie LK, Chamberlain P. Measuring use of research evidence: the structured interview for evidence use. *Res Soc Work Pract.* 2016 Sep;26(5):550–564.
98. Makkar SR, Brennan S, Turner T, Williamson A, Redman S, Green S. The development of SAGE: a tool to evaluate how policymakers' engage with and use research in health policymaking. *Res Eval.* 2016:rvv044.
99. Makkar SR, Turner T, Williamson A, Louviere J, Redman S, Haynes A, Green S, Brennan S. The development of ORACLe: a measure of an organisation's capacity to engage in evidence-informed health policy. *Health Res Policy Syst.* 2015 Dec;14(1):1–8.
100. Imani-Nasab MH, Yazdizadeh B, Salehi M, Seyedin H, Majdzadeh R. Validity and reliability of the evidence utilisation in policymaking measurement tool (EUPMT). *Health Res Policy Syst.* 2017 Dec;15(1):1–1.
101. Boyko JA, Lavis JN, Dobbins M, Souza NM. Reliability of a tool for measuring theory of planned behaviour constructs for use in evaluating research use in policymaking. *Health Res Policy Syst.* 2011;9(1):1.
102. Bogenschneider K, Corbett TJ. *Evidence-based Policymaking: Insights from Policy-minded Researchers and Research-minded Policymakers.* Routledge; 2011.
103. Gollust SE, Kite HA, Benning SJ, Callanan RA, Weisman SR, Nanney MS. Use of research evidence in state policymaking for childhood obesity prevention in Minnesota. *Am J Public Health.* 2014;104(10):1894–1900.
104. Yanovitzky I, Weber M. analysing use of evidence in public policymaking processes: a theory-grounded content analysis methodology. *Evid Policy.* 2020;16(1):65–82.
105. Yamaguchi K. *Event History Analysis.* Sage; 1991.
106. Baybeck B, Berry WD, Siegel DA. A strategic theory of policy diffusion via intergovernmental competition. *J Polit.* 2011;73(1):232–247.
107. Volden C. The politics of competitive federalism: a race to the bottom in welfare benefits? *Am J Polit Sci.* 2002;46(2):352–363.
108. Volden C, Ting MM, Carpenter DP. A formal model of learning and policy diffusion. *Am Polit Sci Rev.* 2008;102(3):319–332.
109. Volden C. States as policy laboratories: emulating success in the children's health insurance program. *Am J Polit Sci.* 2006;50(2):294–312.
110. Case AC, Rosen HS, Hines JR. Budget spillovers and fiscal policy interdependence: Evidence from the states. *J Public Econ.* 1993;52(3):285–307.
111. Grossback LJ, Nicholson-Crotty S, Peterson DAM. Ideology and learning in policy diffusion. *Am Polit Res.* 2004;32(5):521–545.
112. Mintrom M. Policy entrepreneurs and the diffusion of innovation. *Am J Polit Sci.* 1997;41(3):738–770.
113. Pomeranz JL, Silver D. State legislative strategies to pass, enhance, and obscure preemption of local public health policy-making. *Am J Prev Med.* 2020;59(3):333–342.
114. Pomeranz JL, Silver D, Lieff SA. State gun-control, gun-rights, and preemptive firearm-related laws across 50 US states for 2009–2018. *Am J Public Health.* 2021;111(7):1273–1280.
115. Brownson RC, Eyler AA, Harris JK, Moore JB, Tabak RG. Getting the word out. *J Public Health Manag Pract.* 2018;24(2):102–111.
116. Weible CM, Sabatier PA. *Theories of the Policy Process.* Routledge; 2018.
117. Kingdon JW. *Agendas, Alternatives, and Public Policies.* New York: Addison-Wesley Educational Publishers, Inc.; 2003.
118. Purtle J, Lê-Scherban F, Shattuck P, Proctor EK, Brownson RC. An audience research study to disseminate evidence about comprehensive state mental health parity legislation to US State policymakers: protocol. *Implement Sci.* 2017 Dec;12(1):1–3.
119. Redman S, Turner T, Davies H, et al. The SPIRIT action framework: a structured approach to selecting and testing strategies to increase the use of research in policy. *Soc Sci Med.* 2015;136:147–155.
120. Cipher Investigators. Supporting policy in health with research: an intervention trial

(SPIRIT)—protocol for a stepped wedge trial. *BMJ Open.* 2014 Jul 1;4(7):e005293.

121. Haynes A, Brennan S, Carter S, O'Connor D, Schneider CH, Turner T, Gallego G. Protocol for the process evaluation of a complex intervention designed to increase the use of research in health policy and program organisations (the SPIRIT study). *Implement Sci.* 2014 Dec;9(1):1–2.
122. Nilsen P, Ståhl C, Roback K, Cairney P. Never the twain shall meet?—a comparison of implementation science and policy implementation research. *Implement Sci.* 2013 Dec;8(1):1–2.
123. Mugambwa J, Nabeta N, Ngoma M, Rudaheranwa N, Kaberuka W, Munene J. Policy implementation: conceptual foundations, accumulated wisdom and new directions. *J Public Adm Res Theory.* 2018;8:211–232.
124. Bardach E. *The Implementation Game: What Happens After a Bill Becomes a Law.* Cambridge, MA: MIT Press; 1977.
125. Winter W. Implementation. In: Peters B, Pierre J, eds. *Handbook of Public Policy.* London: Sage Publications; 2006:151–166.
126. Pressman J, Wildavsky A. *Implementation: How great expectations in Washington are dashed in Oakland; Or why it's amazing that federal programs work at all expanded,* 3rd ed. Berkeley and Los Angeles, CA: University of California Press; 1984.
127. Nakamura R, Smallwood F. *Politics of Policy Implementation.* New York: St. Martin's Press; 1980.
128. Lipsky M. *Street-Level Bureaucracy: Dilemmas of the Individual in Public Services.* New York: Russell Sage Foundation; 1980.
129. Purtle J, Borchers B, Clement T, Mauri A. Inter-agency strategies used by state mental health agencies to assist with federal behavioral health parity implementation. *J Behav Health Serv Res.* 2018 Jul;45(3):516–526.
130. Crable EL, Benintendi A, Jones DK, Walley AY, Hicks JM, Drainoni ML. Translating Medicaid policy into practice: policy implementation strategies from three US states' experiences enhancing substance use disorder treatment. *Implement Sci.* 2022 Dec;17(1):1–4.
131. Weiner BJ, Lewis CC, Stanick C, Powell BJ, Dorsey CN, Clary AS, Boynton MH, Halko H. Psychometric assessment of three newly developed implementation outcome measures. *Implement Sci.* 2017 Dec;12(1):1–2.
132. Weiner BJ, Lewis CC, Stanick C, Powell BJ, Dorsey CN, Clary AS, Boynton MH, Halko H. Psychometric assessment of three newly developed implementation outcome measures. *Implement Sci.* 2017 Dec;12(1):1–2.
133. Li SJ, Kwon SC, Weerasinghe I, Rey MJ, Trinh-Shevrin C. Smoking among Asian Americans: acculturation and gender in the context of tobacco control policies in New York City. *Health Promot Pract.* 2013;14(5):18s–28s.
134. Chang C, Leighton J, Mostashari F, McCord C, Frieden TR. The New York City Smoke-Free Air Act: second-hand smoke as a worker health and safety issue. *Am J Ind Med.* 2004 Aug;46(2):188–195.
135. Moreland-Russell S, Combs T, Schroth K, Luke D. Success in the city: the road to implementation of Tobacco 21 and Sensible Tobacco Enforcement in New York City. *Tob Control.* 2016 Oct 1;25(suppl 1):i6–i9.
136. Hafez AY, Gonzalez M, Kulik MC, Vijayaraghavan M, Glantz SA. Uneven access to smoke-free laws and policies and its effect on health equity in the United States: 2000–2019. *Am J Public Health.* 2019 Nov;109(11):1568–1575.
137. Brown T, Platt S, Amos A. Equity impact of population-level interventions and policies to reduce smoking in adults: a systematic review. *Drug Alcohol Depend.* 2014;138:7–16.
138. Lew R, Chen WW. Promising practices to eliminate tobacco disparities among Asian American, Native Hawaiian and Pacific Islander communities. *Health Promot Pract.* 2013;14(5 suppl):6S–9S.
139. McGinty EE, Tormohlen KN, Barry CL, Bicket MC, Rutkow L, Stuart EA. Protocol: mixed-methods study of how implementation of US state medical cannabis laws affects treatment of chronic non-cancer pain and adverse opioid outcomes. *Implement Sci.* 2021 Dec;16(1):1–3.
140. Dopp AR, Hunter SB, Godley MD, et al. Comparing two federal financing strategies on penetration and sustainment of the adolescent community reinforcement approach for substance use disorders: protocol for a mixed-method study. *Implement Sci Commun.* 2022;3(1):1–17.
141. Sabatier P, Mazmanian D. The implementation of public policy: a framework of analysis. *Policy Stud J.* 1980;8(4):538–560.
142. Raghavan R, Bright CL, Shadoin A. Toward a policy ecology of implementation of mental health interventions. *Implement Sci.* 2008;3:26.
143. Powell BJ, Beidas RS, Rubin RM, et al. Applying the policy ecology framework to Philadelphia's behavioral health transformation efforts. *Administration and Policy in Mental Health.* 2016;43(6):909–926.
144. Stone EM, Daumit GL, Kennedy-Hendricks A, McGinty EE. The policy ecology of behavioral health homes: case study of Maryland's

Medicaid Health Home program. *Adm Policy Ment Health Ment Health Serv Res.* 2020;47(1):60–72.

145. Aby MJ. Race and equity in statewide implementation programs: an application of the policy ecology of implementation framework. *Adm Policy Ment Health Ment Health Serv Res.* 2020;47(6):946–960.
146. Bullock HL, Lavis JN, Wilson MG, Mulvale G, Miatello A. Understanding the implementation of evidence-informed policies and practices from a policy perspective: a critical interpretive synthesis. *Implement Sci.* 2021 Dec;16(1):1–24.
147. Ecker UK, Lewandowsky S, Cook J, et al. The psychological drivers of misinformation belief and its resistance to correction. *Nat. Rev. Psychol.* 2022 Jan;1(1):13–29.
148. Kapp JM, Hensel B, Schnoring KT. Is Twitter a forum for disseminating research to health policy makers? *Ann Epidemiol.* 2015;25(12):883–887.
149. Burstein P. The determinants of public policy: what matters and how much. *Policy Stud J.* 2020 Feb;48(1):87–110.
150. Mackie TI, Kovacs KM, Simmel C, Crystal S, Neese-Todd S, Akincigil A. A best-worst scaling experiment to identify patient-centered claims-based outcomes for evaluation of pediatric anti-psychotic monitoring programs. *Health Serv Res.* 2021 Jun;56(3):418–431.
151. Combs T, Nelson KL, Luke D, et al. Simulating the role of knowledge brokers in policy making in state agencies: an agent-based model. *Health Serv Res.* 2022 Mar 4.
152. McGee ZA, Jones BD. Reconceptualizing the policy subsystem: integration with complexity theory and social network analysis. *Policy Stud J.* 2019 May;47:S138–S158.
153. Varone F, Ingold K, Jourdain C, Schneider V. Studying policy advocacy through social network analysis. *Eur Political Sci.* 2017 Sep;16:322–336.

25

Health Equity in Dissemination and Implementation Science

STEPHANIE L. FITZPATRICK, BETH A. GLENN, O. KENRIK DURU, AND CHANDRA L. FORD

INTRODUCTION

The events of 2020—COVID-19 pandemic, racial reckoning, and climate change—shined a spotlight on persistent and striking racial, ethnic, and socioeconomic disparities in health and healthcare in the United States.[1–3] Although the health of the overall US population has improved substantially over the last 100 years, as evidenced by a 30-year increase in average life expectancy,[4] racial and ethnic marginalized populations continue to lag behind the general population on many health metrics, including incidence, prevalence, morbidity, and mortality rates for most chronic conditions; life expectancy; and quality-of-life indicators.[5,6] The root causes of these disparities include avoidable, unjust inequities in the social determinants of health, defined by the World Health Organization as conditions in which people are born, grow, live, work and age.[7] Historical injustices, like structural racism, can influence present-day disease patterns. For instance, discriminatory laws, which historically restricted Black/African Americans' access to basic goods and services, including healthcare, arguably continue to impose a burden on the health of this population.[8–10] They help explain how Black/African Americans came to reside in underresourced neighborhoods and why distrust of providers remains a challenge. Similarly, American Indian populations were subjected to discrimination and genocide and have historically lagged behind on multiple health indices.[11–14] Immigration trends since the passage of the 1965 Hart-Celler Immigration and Nationality Act have also helped shape the health of the US population.[15] In the past, "selective migration" prevailed such that US emigres included skilled workers and were healthier than their nonimmigrant counterparts; however, more recent immigrants have substantially poorer access to healthcare, particularly preventive services, and they may be more likely to reside in health-compromising neighborhoods.[16–18]

With the recent exacerbation of inequities in social determinants of health among already vulnerable, marginalized populations, efforts to advance health equity have become even more urgent.[19] The concept of health equity is not new, with seminal papers and studies published as early as the 1800s.[20] Unfortunately, the term *health equity* is often thought to mean the same as "equality." Equality means to give everyone the same exact resources, access, and opportunities to achieve good health. However, equality is not sufficient as it ignores the contextual/historical factors and underlying structural determinants (e.g., racism) that impact health and may actually further widen the health disparities gap. In contrast, health equity "implies that everyone should have a *fair opportunity* to attain their full health potential, and none should be disadvantaged from achieving this potential, if it can be avoided."[21(p433)] Health and healthcare disparities refer to measurable differences in health outcomes and healthcare access and utilization between socially and economically disadvantaged and advantaged groups.[22] Health equity involves recognizing and rectifying historical injustices and providing resources according

Stephanie L. Fitzpatrick, Beth A. Glenn, O. Kenrik Duru, and Chandra L. Ford, *Health Equity in Dissemination and Implementation Science* In: *Dissemination and Implementation Research in Health.* Edited by: Ross C. Brownson, Graham A. Colditz, and Enola K. Proctor, Oxford University Press.
 DOI: 10.1093/oso/9780197660690.003.0025

to need to improve the health and healthcare of the socially and economically disadvantaged while not making it worse for the socially and economically advantaged.[23] In other words, by working toward greater health equity we are reducing health and healthcare disparities while improving population health overall.[22]

The concept of health equity is highly relevant to dissemination and implementation (D&I) science because there is a need for "evidence-based interventions" (EBIs) that can be implemented successfully and sustained in the communities most impacted by inequities. Though increasingly considered foundational for the field, health equity is not always acknowledged and integrated explicitly in D&I research or the interventions that are developed and evaluated with an eye toward scale-up or widespread implementation. Thus, most current EBIs are limited in terms of advancing health equity. For instance, numerous EBIs address a risk factor for chronic disease (e.g., obesity), but very few address the upstream causes of chronic disease, such as certain policies and land development plans (e.g., redlining)[24] that promote residential segregation and limit access to healthy food or safe neighborhoods to regularly engage in physical activity among primarily racial and ethnic marginalized and socioeconomically disadvantaged groups.[9] Further, an intervention to promote physical activity that is effective in a randomized trial conducted primarily among affluent, non-Latino/a/x Whites may not yield the same results when implemented in a community setting or among members of a diverse population. Part of the challenge is that intervention strategies and messages developed for mainstream populations that have the favorable circumstances to benefit from the intervention may be less relevant, effective, and/or adopted among racial and ethnic marginalized communities, thus the persistence or widening of health disparities.

There is a need to reexamine current D&I interventions, strategies, measures, methods, and frameworks through a *health equity lens*, which Kumanyika defined as "a set of field glasses that allows one to see both overt and subtle injustices at work, including the historical, social, political, and environmental contexts that may interfere with or facilitate a person being able to reach their full health potential."[25(p1354)] To do this means going beyond language translation to culturally adapt existing interventions for use in new settings and populations; identifying strategies to equitably disseminate, implement, and sustain interventions or emerging technologies that have the potential to be equally effective across diverse populations; and considering the various contextual systems and policies at the community and health system levels that may perpetuate or exacerbate inequities.[26]

This chapter provides a focused, narrative review of D&I efforts, considerations, and issues in the context of advancing health equity. The chapter begins with a discussion of challenges to promoting health equity in D&I research. It goes on to discuss models and frameworks that can be used to conceptualize and guide the D&I process with a health equity lens. The chapter continues with an overview of D&I research with a health equity lens in four prevention areas (physical activity/obesity/ nutrition, cancer screening, HIV/sexually transmitted infections [STIs], and vaccinations). Finally, it presents a case study of D&I from a health equity perspective related to diabetes prevention, future directions to move the field forward, and a list of useful resources. While this chapter focuses primarily on health equity issues in the United States, it draws on literature from other countries. In addition, health equity issues in other countries (chapter 26) and settings (chapters 19–24) are covered elsewhere.

CHALLENGES IN DISSEMINATION AND IMPLEMENTATION RESEARCH TO PROMOTE HEALTH EQUITY

Traditionally, EBIs have been applied inequitably across different communities and settings, which predictably skews the application of best practices toward population groups and organizations with higher capacity and resources.[27] When this occurs, innovations can be slow to reach populations who are underserved based on marginalized status related to race and ethnicity, gender, sexual orientation, socioeconomic status, and other demographic factors.[28] As a result, these marginalized populations continue to experience avoidable health inequities. In the following sections, we describe challenges to D&I research to promote health equity. These include an inadequate consideration of the external context (e.g., structural racism), traditional emphasis on individual-level EBIs, a dearth of equity-relevant metrics and measures, and lack of diversity in settings and participants (Box 25.1).

BOX 25.1

CHALLENGES IN D&I RESEARCH TO PROMOTE HEALTH EQUITY

ACKNOWLEDGMENT OF CONTEXTS AND UNDERLYING STRUCTURAL FACTORS

- EBIs do not adequately address upstream factors such as social determinants of health
- Importance of systemic racism in the adoption, acceptability, appropriateness, fidelity, and reach of EBIs may be downplayed

RIGOROUS MULTILEVEL APPROACH FOR EVIDENCE-BASED INTERVENTIONS

- Sample sizes of multilevel EBI studies are often inadequate
- Statistical approaches may not account for complexity of data across levels (e.g., individual, community, health system) or potential interactions between levels
- Some study designs do not facilitate disentangling which components affect which outcomes and in which combinations[29,30]

METRICS AND MEASURES

- There is a need for equity-based implementation science measures in D&I research
- Potential inequities in the feasibility, fidelity, penetration, acceptability, sustainability, uptake, and cost of EBIs are rarely explored when implemented in routine practice settings serving marginalized populations[31]

INCLUSION OF DIVERSE SETTINGS AND STUDY POPULATIONS

- Socioeconomically marginalized groups are underrepresented in D&I research and may not respond to audiovisual and print health promotion materials and messages targeting "general" audiences
- Lack of representation of marginalized communities in the development and implementation of EBIs limits its external validity

Lack of Acknowledgment of Contexts and Underlying Structural Factors, Including Racism

Many risk factors for disease and illness are shaped by adverse social determinants of health and long-standing societal injustices. However, most EBIs are organized around downstream diseases and risk factors (e.g., type 2 diabetes and related complications), with inadequate attention to upstream factors and solutions relevant to marginalized populations (e.g., low-cost diabetes prevention programs that are accessible to individuals working hourly jobs with little work flexibility). This failure to account for the broader context in which participants grow, live, work, and play limits the applicability and generalizability of EBIs across populations, settings, and time periods.[26] Furthermore, existing D&I research often deflects attention from the role of health systems caring for marginalized populations in unintentionally creating or maintaining disparities. Systemic challenges such as lack of leadership, inadequate data systems, or a scattered organizational climate can inadvertently worsen disparities in care and health outcomes.[28]

For example, the US Preventive Services Task Force recently updated the recommendation on hypertension screening in adults to include two approaches to measure blood pressure outside of the clinic (i.e., ambulatory and home-based blood pressure monitoring).[32] Implementation of this recommendation could potentially decrease disparities in hypertension screening by circumventing barriers for patients from marginalized backgrounds to be screened in the clinic (e.g., inflexible work schedules, lack of transportation to get to the clinic, and limited clinic hours or appointment slots). On the other hand, ambulatory and home-based blood pressure monitors are not covered by most payers[33]; they require digital literacy and numeracy for accurate use, and few clinical workflows and electronic health record systems are set up to document home blood pressure readings. Thus, without a multilevel approach addressing these barriers to implementation, benefits of this recommendation may be limited to the socioeconomically advantaged, thereby worsening disparities.

In addition, D&I research has not always typically, or explicitly, considered the role of structural racism in health behaviors and outcomes, although the need for such consideration has become increasingly clear with the racial awakening of 2020.[34] Structural racism has been defined as race-based oppression deeply embedded in and throughout systems, laws, written or unwritten policies, entrenched practices, and established beliefs and attitudes that produce, condone, and perpetuate widespread unfair treatment of people of racial and ethnic marginalized backgrounds.[35] Systemic and structural racism can function as contextual factors that may influence adoption, acceptability, appropriateness, fidelity, and reach of EBIs as well as implementation and sustainability of EBIs across levels.[36] For instance, the criteria that private and public insurers require patients to meet to cover diabetes technology (e.g., insulin pump or continuous glucose monitor) as a medical necessity, such as quarterly face-to-face visits with a provider or demonstration of good glycemic control, systematically disadvantages patients from low-income, racial, and ethnic marginalized backgrounds.[37] This systemic form of racism is often further perpetuated during clinical encounters as providers are often seen as the "gatekeepers" to accessing these devices.[38,39] Without considering the pervasive effects of structural racism in D&I research, well-meaning efforts may actually reinforce or exacerbate disparities.[36]

Lack of a Multilevel, Multisystem Approach for EBIs

Historically, many EBIs have been developed, implemented, and evaluated at the individual level, without regard for how they might promote health equity or affect existing group-level disparities. Multilevel interventions, developed with consideration of the broader societal context, including existing policies, communities, and organizations, are more likely to address and advance health equity (also see chapter 4).[36] Multilevel interventions require targeting two or more levels of influence at the same time or in close temporal proximity. Assessing both the direct and interactive effect across levels of influence can help identify the different multilevel and systemic factors affecting marginalized populations. Agurs-Collins and colleagues (2019)[29] provided a helpful illustration of a multilevel intervention to address the multilevel risk factors for smoking among Black/African American men. For example, at the social conditions and policy level, a potential risk factor is living in a state with low tax and greater production of tobacco, so a possible intervention could be increasing the tobacco tax. To address risk factors at the individual level, such as smoking menthol cigarettes, men could be offered smoking cessation counseling.

Inadequate Metrics and Measures

Comprehensive literature reviews of D&I research have shown that few studies explicitly focus on health equity as a key implementation outcome.[26] There is a need for both measures of social determinants of health and specific equity-based implementation science measures that can be used in research studies.[26] As part of a contextual assessment, these measures should be included in D&I frameworks together with better measures of structural racism, which extend beyond interpersonal racism. Such an approach that includes social and structural determinants may allow researchers to identify and test potential mechanisms of inequities and specifically whether well-designed EBIs can reduce different forms of racism.[36]

Inclusion of Underserved Populations and Lack of Diversity in Settings

Relatively little D&I research has been conducted in settings with large proportions of racial and ethnic marginalized and other underserved populations.[40,41] Racial and ethnic, lower-income, rural, aged, and other socioeconomically marginalized population groups have generally been considered "hard to reach" by researchers. This may be due to conscious nonparticipation by group members; lack of capacity or infrastructure to absorb opportunity or transactional costs among organizations or settings that serve disadvantaged populations; investigators' failure to engage these populations or settings; or use of research methods that are not culturally appropriate.

There are significant concerns about the external validity of EBIs that have limited representation of marginalized communities; these studies are often "retrofitted" for different settings rather than being designed specifically with racially, ethnically, and socioeconomically diverse populations in mind.[26] These EBIs often neglect the unique needs and context of these communities and may reinforce or exacerbate disparities in outcomes.[31,36]

In summary, in order to promote health equity in D&I research, researchers and practitioners should consider the challenges described above in the planning phases. Multilevel EBIs designed with health equity in mind; with the involvement of marginalized populations and key community partners; using equity-focused methods and metrics; and considering the role of structural racism in contributing to health disparities are needed. This work should be guided by models and frameworks that have an explicit equity focus, as described further below.

MODELS AND FRAMEWORKS TO CONCEPTUALIZE, MEASURE, AND ADDRESS HEALTH EQUITY IN D&I RESEARCH

A small but growing number of models and frameworks explicitly focus on health equity to guide D&I research.[26] As described below, several existing and emerging models can be used to conceptualize D&I processes, determinants, and outcomes through a health equity lens. These heuristics differ from other implementation frameworks as they aid researchers in considering the historical, cultural, economic, and political forces that created and reinforce health inequities as well as the contextual factors across all levels of a socioecological framework (i.e., individual, interpersonal, organizational, community, policy) that may facilitate or limit implementation of an EBI designed to advance health equity.[42] They also inform the level(s) at which to intervene (e.g., at the individual, health system, and/or community level) and provide points of entry of when to assess if the intervention is reducing health disparities.[43,44] The summaries below illustrate potential applications of these models to advance health equity, but they do not attempt to evaluate the models based on empirical evidence. Although work to empirically test some of these models and frameworks is underway, there is still an opportunity and a need for greater application and refinement of these models and frameworks to EBIs for various chronic conditions and populations to elevate the importance of health equity in D&I science.[30,31,45,46]

Expanding Established Models Using a Health Equity Lens

Equity-Dissemination & Implementation (EQ-DI) Framework

Although it can be considered an emerging framework, the EQ-DI framework proposes an approach to "sensitize" existing D&I models and frameworks using a health equity lens while using established D&I science to "operationalize" the D&I of EBIs designed to advance health equity.[42] By applying a health equity lens to sensitize D&I models and frameworks, determinants of social and health inequities are acknowledged throughout D&I planning, execution, and evaluation. Adaptation of evidence-based, multilevel interventions and implementation strategies to address health inequities are informed by the socioecological contexts in which individuals interact with each other, the community, and various systems. Furthermore, evaluation of implementation with an equity lens aims to examine the persistence or reduction of health disparities. For example, sensitizing the established Reach, Effectiveness, Adoption, Implementation, and Maintenance (RE-AIM) framework[47] from a health equity lens may involve assessing inequities in access to the intervention across different populations (reach); examining differences in outcomes accounting for context (effectiveness); tracking and enhancing uptake of the intervention among low-resource settings (adoption); monitoring the delivery of the intervention to diverse communities (implementation); and assessing the long-term impact on health disparities given the potential change or evolution of contexts (e.g., at the community and health system levels) over time (maintenance). See Shelton and colleagues (2021)[48] for additional discussion on extending the RE-AIM framework to enhance sustainability from a health equity perspective.

The EQ-DI approach also emphasizes that the established D&I models and frameworks can be used to provide a roadmap for disseminating and implementing a health-equity-focused EBI. The toolkits, methodologies, and evaluation plans provided by established D&I models can be used to inform knowledge-to-action processes to operationalize implementation. As the evidence for more health equity-focused interventions grows, D&I will be key in the planning and evaluation of these interventions for sustainability and scalability.

Transcreation Framework

The transcreation framework for community-engaged behavioral interventions to reduce health disparities provides a framework for designing and delivering interventions in underserved, underresourced communities to reduce health disparities.[49] Grounded in community-based participatory research (CBPR),[50] the framework emphasizes that the intervention resonates with the community, engages communities from the very beginning, community members serve as interventionists, and the intervention is tested in community settings.

The transcreation framework consists of seven steps that may be followed sequentially or iteratively. The first is to identify community infrastructure and engage partners. This step involves identifying community settings with the necessary infrastructure for delivering the intervention and are convenient for the population of interest. In addition, this first step consists of forming an academic-community partnership based on CBPR principles (i.e., trust, shared decision-making, and valuing community knowledge). The second step is to specify a theoretical framework that acknowledges multilevel determinants of the health inequity(ies) in the community and, in partnership with community members, identify one or more theories of behavior change relevant to the population of interest. The third step involves review of the literature and conducting a formative evaluation in partnership with community members to inform design of the intervention. This formative work also includes identifying cultural, practical, organizational, and contextual factors that may impact intervention design, effectiveness, and sustainability. The fourth step is designing the intervention that (a) addresses hypothesized mechanisms of action; (b) is appropriate and accessible to the population of interest; and (c) can be delivered using existing resources or incorporates a plan for capacity building. This step also involves deciding on the intervention delivery format, intervention mapping to ensure there is rationale for each component, key stakeholder review, and development of an intervention manual to ensure fidelity.

Steps 5–7 of the transcreation framework focus on establishing intervention effectiveness and implementation processes. Specifically, step 5 consists of designing a study to test the intervention, including determining methods for recruitment and data collection as well as outcome measures. Step 6 is building community capacity to deliver the intervention by providing resources (e.g., funding) to enhance community infrastructure or training the community interventionists. Finally, step 7 is creating and implementing methods for ongoing monitoring and assessment of the intervention and implementation processes, including providing ongoing technical assistance. Despite the number of steps in the transcreation framework, the focus on genuine community partnerships and engagement throughout the design and implementation process enhances the probability of uptake and sustainability in communities most impacted by health inequities.

Emerging Models

Explicit considerations of health equity throughout the whole implementation process as well as measurement of health disparities and determinants of health inequities as part of contextual assessments prior to implementation efforts are common themes among the emerging models. This section summarizes the Health Equity Implementation Framework, Health Equity Measurement Framework (HEMF), and the Conceptual Framework for Equity-Focused Implementation Research (EquIR). The Health Equity Implementation Framework[44] provides guidance on assessing and addressing health equity and determinants of implementation simultaneously; the HEMF[51] showcases the mechanisms by which social determinants of health and other factors drive healthcare utilization and health outcomes to provide direction for more empirical work related to health equity; and the EquIR[43] emphasizes assessment of health equity before, during, and after implementation.

Health Equity Implementation Framework

The Health Equity Implementation Framework (Figure 25.1) is based on the integration of two established D&I models: the integrated Promoting Action on Research Implementation in Health Services (i-PARIHS)[52] and the Health Care Disparities Framework.[53] Based on i-PARIHS, the Health Equity Implementation Framework focuses on three levels of determinants of implementation: (1) health system-level

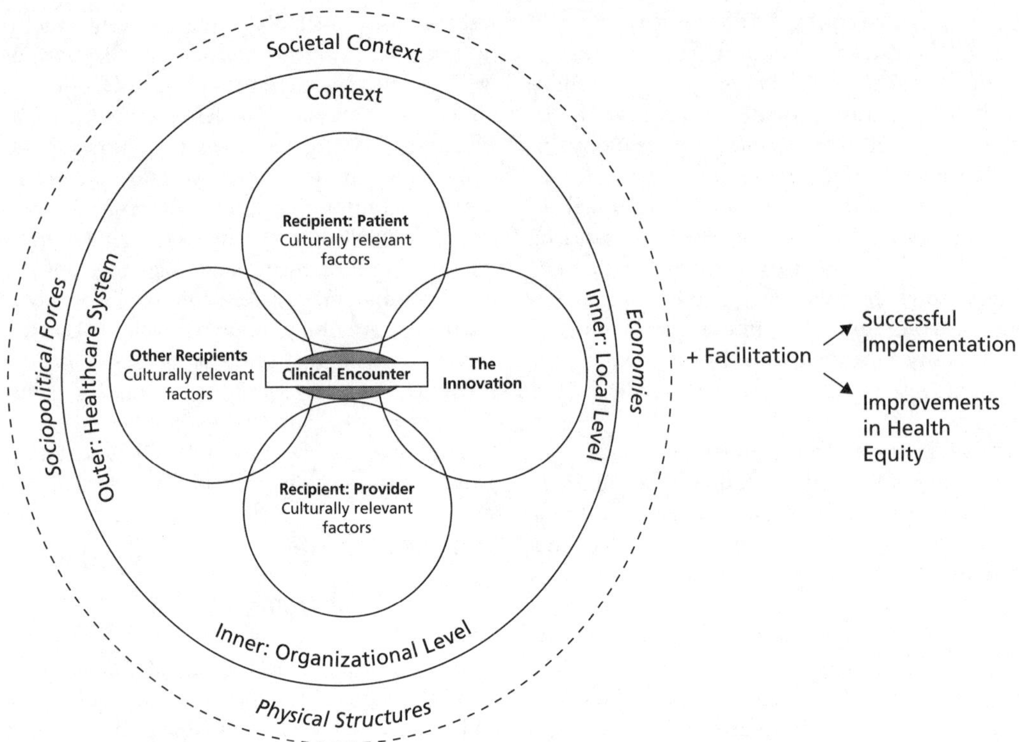

FIGURE 25.1 Health equity implementation framework, which showcases three equity domains (clinical encounter, culturally relevant factors of recipients, and societal context) adapted to an existing determinant and process framework, the integrated Promoting Action on Research Implementation in Health Services (i-PARIHS). Source: Reprinted with permission from Woodward EN, Matthieu MM, Uchendu US, Rogal S, Kirchner JE. The health equity implementation framework: proposal and preliminary study of hepatitis C virus treatment. *Implement Sci.* 2019;14(1):26.

context, such as leadership support and system structure (inner context) or state- or federal-level mandates and incentives (outer context); (2) recipients, such as the patients and providers; and (3) characteristics of the EBI, new program, or policy. The framework also involves assessing determinants of health and healthcare disparities among vulnerable populations, borrowing from the Health Care Disparities Framework. These determinants include patient (e.g., health beliefs, medical mistrust) and provider (e.g., time burden, biases based on patient background) factors; the patient-provider interaction during a clinical encounter; and the healthcare system's culture or readiness concerning reducing disparities.

By combining these two models, the Health Equity Implementation Framework focuses on multilevel factors that affect implementation and health equity, including those unique to marginalized populations (e.g., structural racism) and the complex nature of healthcare systems. Furthermore, this framework acknowledges the overarching societal influence, such as sociopolitical forces in which patients are trying to be healthy and providers are providing healthcare. In practice, the Health Equity Implementation Framework provides researchers the ability to adapt either the EBI or the implementation strategies or both for marginalized populations to advance health equity. By simultaneously addressing health equity and determinants of implementation, the time to equitably disseminate the EBI to all populations in need of it may be significantly shortened.[44,54]

Health Equity Measurement Framework

The HEMF was initially developed based on a synthesis of existing social determinants of health and health system utilization frameworks and then expanded based on literature review and consultation with key stakeholders. Based on these various sources, the HEMF provides a diagram of the various causal pathways among several concepts that affect health. The concepts covered in the HEMF are socioeconomic, cultural, and political context; health policy context; social stratification; social location; material and social circumstances; environment; biological factors; health-related behaviors; beliefs; stress; quality of care; and healthcare utilization.[51] Below are some examples of existing measures that may be used to directly or indirectly assess some of these concepts.

Researchers can use the HEMF to guide measurement and monitoring of health equity as well as inform policymaking. For instance, although functioning at a broader level, the socioeconomic, cultural, and political context concept has major implications for an individual's opportunity to be healthy, such as determining access to good quality healthcare, safe neighborhoods, and healthy, affordable food. Capturing the socioeconomic, cultural, and political context may involve qualitative interviews to understand the history of current policies and how they exacerbate health inequities and to assess cultural norms.

The socioeconomic, cultural, and political context concept influences a number of the other concepts, including the social stratification and environment concepts. Social stratification refers to how society is hierarchically structured based on systematic inequities in power and resources and can be used to determine an individual's social location (i.e., their sociocultural and economic position in the hierarchy). This social structure indirectly impacts who is more likely to be vulnerable to certain chronic conditions, quality of care received, and likelihood of medical complications. Researchers may consider using the one-item MacArthur Subjective Social Status Scale[55] to measure an individual's perceived social rank or position relative to others in their group to assess social location.

The concept of material circumstances is related to the financial means to live a healthy life. Social risks, or adverse social conditions, are the result of inequities in social determinants of health and include food and housing insecurity, lack of transportation, poor or nonexistent health coverage for medical care and supplies, social isolation, and overall financial hardships.[56] The relationship between limited material circumstances or social risks and poor health, including increased risk for diabetes and cardiovascular disease, have been well established in the literature.[57,58] There are a number of measurement tools now available to assess social risks including: (a) the Centers for Medicare and Medicaid Services (CMS) Accountable Health Communities Health-Related Social Needs Screening Tool[59]; (b) Protocol for Responding to and Assessing Patients' Assets, Risks, and Experiences (PRAPARE) assessment tool[60]; (c) USDA (US Department of Agriculture) six-item Household Food Security Survey[61]; and (d) the two-item Hunger Vital Sign.[62] See Henrikson et al., 2019, for a systematic review of the psychometric and pragmatic properties of existing social risk screening tools.[63]

Related to the material circumstances concept, the environment concept, which covers the physical and social features of where the individual lives, works, and plays, can also be a source of health inequities. Although there are some neighborhood scales available, there has been much development in the use of geographic information system (GIS) mapping[64] to objectively understand the physical and social features of a community. Use of this methodology also informs calculations of indexes, such as the neighborhood[65] and social[66] deprivation indexes as well as the social vulnerability index.[67] Last, depending on the health system, the electronic health record (EHR) is a good source to extract data related to material circumstances, environment (based on patient addresses), and healthcare utilization concepts within the HEMF. The EHR-based data could be used to help inform implementation efforts as well as determine effectiveness of implementation strategies. See Casey and colleagues (2016) for a review on using the EHR for population health.[68]

Conceptual Framework for Equity-Focused Implementation Research

Equity-focused implementation research (EquIR) is an approach to evaluate the effect of a health policy, program, or intervention on equity during and after implementation and informs how to intervene to improve implementation.[43] The EquIR conceptual framework was developed in three phases: (1) systematic review; (2) stakeholder interviews and analysis; and (3) assessment of the face validity of the framework via key expert and stakeholder interviews. Figure 25.2 shows the EquIR framework, which should be followed clockwise starting with "population health status." More specifically, the first step in using the EquIR framework is to identify the health status of the population of interest for the health program or intervention as well as the general population in order to get a sense of disparities and possible subpopulations to include. In the second step, which is focused on "planning the program," relevant research questions, measures used to quantify the disparities to be addressed, and the equity-focused program or intervention (preferably evidence based or evidence informed) should be identified.

The third step, "designing EquIR" is focused on identifying implementers of the health program or intervention as well as any potential barriers and facilitators to implementation, especially equitable implementation. In the "implementing EquIR" phase (fourth step), strategies to overcome barriers, including resources and incentives to support implementation, are identified. Furthermore, strategies for monitoring and evaluating outcomes as

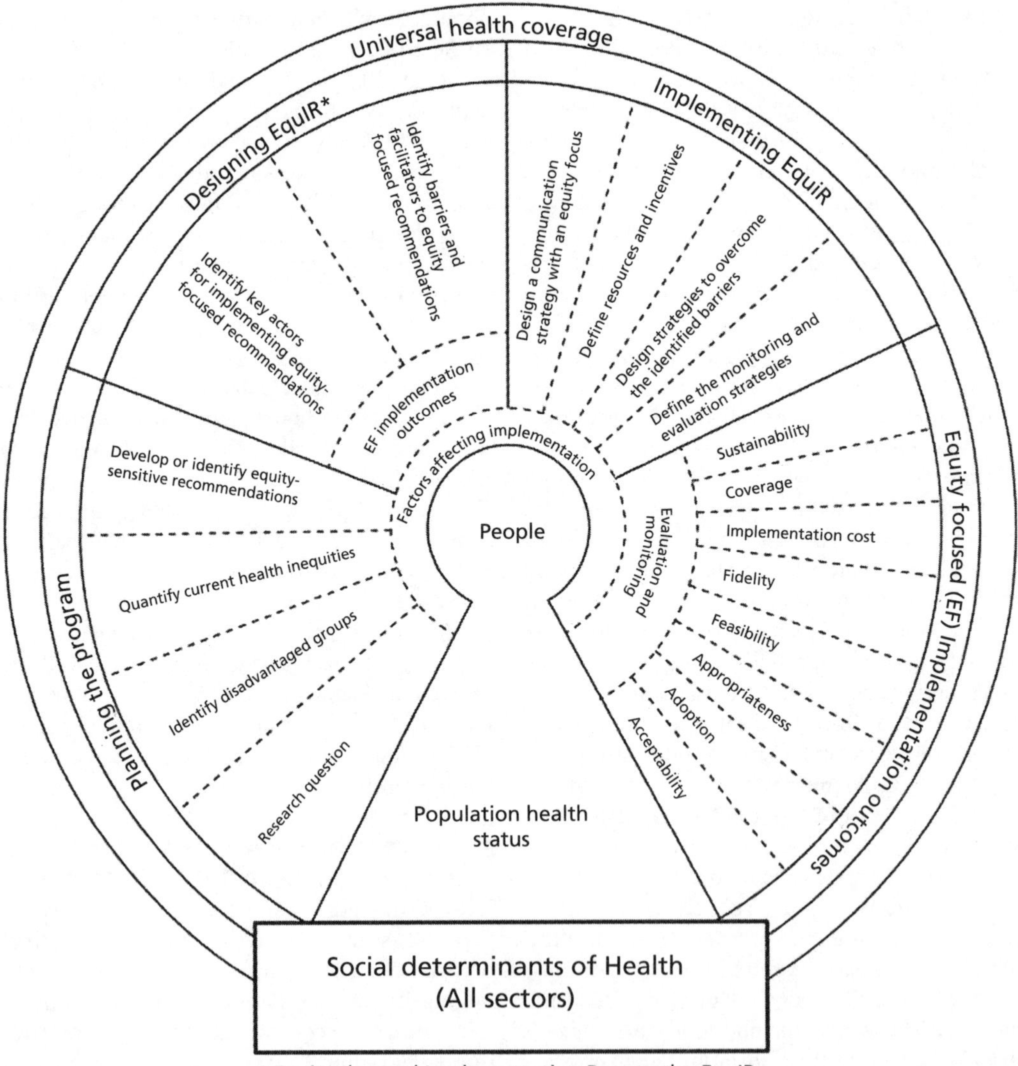

FIGURE 25.2 Conceptual framework of equity-focused implementation research (EquIR).

Source: Reprinted with permission from Eslava-Schmalbach J, Garzon-Orjuela N, Elias V, Reveiz L, Tran N, Langlois EV. Conceptual framework of equity-focused implementation research for health programs (EquIR). *Int J Equity Health.* 2019;18(1):80.

well as strategies to disseminate are defined during this step.

Throughout the implementation, equity-focused implementation outcomes should be assessed (i.e., step 5) among the advantaged and disadvantaged groups: (a) acceptability; (b) adoption; (c) appropriateness; (d) feasibility; (e) fidelity; (f) implementation cost; (g) coverage; and (h) sustainability. The sixth step actually goes back to the first step, which is to examine the population health status to see if the program or intervention reduced disparities. However, depending on the disparity being addressed, it could be a long time before any impact is seen. Therefore, the EquIR framework suggests focusing on the short-term implementation outcomes listed above as the progress or lack thereof in these outcomes will indicate if the population health status will be improved or not in the long term.

In summary, as the evidence base for health equity-focused D&I research expands, existing models will continue to be refined and new models will emerge, including those with a particular focus on how structural racism shapes inequitable implementation as well as antiracism frameworks.[69,70] D&I researchers should also seek to expand ways in which existing models not specifically developed to address health equity can better serve these purposes.

OVERVIEW AND SYNTHESIS OF EMPIRICAL DISSEMINATION AND IMPLEMENTATION RESEARCH WITH HEALTH EQUITY IMPLICATIONS

A growing number of D&I studies have been conducted in low-resource settings, often with a specific focus on racial and ethnic marginalized populations.[71] In this section, clinic and community-based D&I efforts are summarized in four prevention areas (cancer screening, physical activity/nutrition/obesity, HIV/STIs, and vaccinations) with a specific focus on describing work within racial and ethnic marginalized communities. The goal is to provide a snapshot of documented efforts in this small but rapidly expanding literature rather than to critique individual studies.

Cancer Screening

One of the most developed subfields of D&I equity-focused research has been in the area of cancer screening promotion. At the time D&I research began its rapid expansion in the mid-2000s, there was a robust evidence base from effectiveness studies for the promotion of breast and cervical cancer screening, conducted in both clinical and community settings, including numerous projects in low-resource settings.[72] Since that time, a substantial number of studies have also identified EBIs to promote colorectal cancer screening.[73]

The body of literature evaluating the effectiveness of the National Breast and Cervical Cancer Early Detection Program (NBCCEDP) funded by the Centers for Disease Control and Prevention (CDC) and the Colorectal Cancer Control Program (CRCCP) screening initiatives has expanded in recent years. Studies have found that the NBCCEDP program is cost-effective and associated with improvements in a number of health outcomes[74–76]; however, only a small fraction of eligible women participate in the program, estimated at around 15% for breast cancer screening and 7% for cervical cancer screening.[77] Evaluations of the CRCCP also suggest that the program is effective in improving colorectal cancer (CRC) screening uptake in vulnerable groups, including a number of initiatives within Federally Qualified Health Centers (FQHCs).[78,79] In fact, early success of the CRCCP program led the NBCCEDP to focus its efforts on clinical settings serving high-need patients (e.g., FQHCs) and ensure that grantees implement EBIs that have been used successfully in racial and ethnic marginalized communities (e.g., community health worker model, patient navigation) whenever possible.

These initiatives have collectively narrowed disparities in cervical, breast, and colorectal cancer screening, though disparities in screening by race and ethnicity, insurance status, English proficiency, and nativity still persist.[80] In addition, challenges to follow-up after abnormal cancer screening findings remain, particularly with regards to CRC screening.[81,82] Last, interventions to address upstream factors (medical mistrust, transportation barriers, unmet child-care needs, and discrimination) that may serve as barriers to receipt of any healthcare, including cancer screening, are urgently needed.

Physical Activity, Nutrition, and Obesity Prevention and Control

Over the past several decades, substantial efforts have sought to identify effective obesity prevention and control programs and policies that can be implemented across the population and have the potential to be scalable and sustainable.[83] A large number of obesity-focused initiatives have been set in public schools given the number of hours children spend in school each day, the proportion of calories consumed during school hours, and the potential for schools as a setting to reach socially and economically disadvantaged youth.[84–86] Although systematic reviews have demonstrated the effectiveness of multicomponent school-based interventions in increasing physical activity, the effect sizes are typically small, particularly when the outcome is objectively measured physical activity (vs. self-report) and in effectiveness (vs. efficacy) studies given substantial variation in implementation.[87–90]

A recent systematic review by Kennedy and colleagues (2020) investigated the extent to which school-based physical activity intervention studies (n = 14) reported data on RE-AIM dimensions.[86] Although all studies reported on the number of students reached with the intervention, few reported the sociodemographic characteristics or the representativeness of those reached. Most studies reported the rate of participation, but few reported on the characteristics of adopters versus nonadopters. These omissions pose major challenges to practitioners and policymakers seeking to implement EBIs, particularly in low-resource settings and for youth with racial and ethnic marginalized backgrounds.

A systematic review by Cassar and colleagues (2019) examined application of implementation models to plan study protocols or interventions or as a guide to interpret study results.[91] Although implementation models were commonly applied in the 17 unique studies included in the review, most focused on result interpretation and were not utilized to guide program planning, which may contribute to well-documented failures to translate research findings to real-world practice. Furthermore, despite the potential for school-based initiatives to reach socioeconomically disadvantaged children, who may be at increased risk for obesity, studies have found that school-based programs are not equitably implemented and, if so, may end up exacerbating disparities.[92,93]

A growing number of D&I initiatives have targeted the afterschool setting. In 2011, the YMCA of the United States adopted the Healthy Eating and Physical Activity Standards (HEPA) for all of their afterschool programs (ASPs).[94] The goal of the standards related to physical activity was to ensure that children accumulated 30 minutes of moderate-to-vigorous physical activity (MVPA) daily during the ASP, 50% of recommended physical activity minutes. The standards also sought to ensure that ASPs served a fruit or vegetable and water daily while eliminating fried foods, sugar-sweetened food and beverages, and trans fat. YMCA ASPs are located in more than 10,000 communities across the country, serving over 9 million youth, including a substantial number of low-income and racial and ethnic marginalized children; thus, effective implementation of these standards could have a substantial positive influence on childhood obesity. In 2015 YMCA ASPs in South Carolina decided to use a coordinated statewide training framework to enhance adoption of standards. In an evaluation of the first year of the program, Weaver and colleagues (2017) did not observe overall improvements in nutrition and physical activity outcomes.[95] However, improvements in some outcomes (physical activity minutes in girls, frequency of serving fruits/vegetables, dessert avoidance) were associated with greater program implementation. A 2-year evaluation of the initiative observed no overall effect of the program on MVPA, but substantially greater MVPA among children attending ASPs with greater adoption of physical activity elements and incorporation of physical activity supportive practices.[96]

Despite some advancements in D&I research to increase physical activity and reduce obesity prevalence particularly in school and community-based settings, there is greater need for implementation studies with an explicit focus on health equity. Based on Kumanyika's Getting to Equity in Obesity Prevention Framework,[25] multilevel (e.g., family, school, community), multisector, and multisystem (e.g., education, social services, local businesses) interventions that promote policy and systems changes while supporting individual and community capacity to engage in health behavior change may be more effective in preventing or reducing the prevalence of obesity in marginalized communities by doing the following: (1) increasing healthy options; (2) reducing deterrents (e.g., promotion of unhealthy products, discrimination); (3) improving social and economic resources; and (4) building on community capacity.

HIV/Sexually Transmitted Infections

National HIV prevention and treatment efforts, including highly active antiretroviral therapy (HAART) have taken us from a peak of 130,000 HIV infections annually in the mid-1980s to approximately 34,800 in 2019.[97] However, the HIV epidemic continues to hit marginalized populations hardest, disproportionately affecting men who have sex with men (MSM) and transgender, Black/African American, Latino/a/x, low-income, and rural communities.[98]

Research has shown that individual-level HIV risk behavior does not vary significantly by race,[99,100] and there are other factors at play that are linked to the continued high prevalence of HIV among marginalized populations. HIV transmission is tightly linked to structural factors, stigma, and ongoing social exclusion based on sexual orientation, housing segregation, poverty, poor healthcare, and racially skewed mass incarceration.[101] These factors lead to HIV "hotspots" where individuals are more likely to come in contact with the disease and less likely to have the resources to obtain comprehensive treatment for it. There has been an increasing recognition over the past several decades of the complex interactions underlying the HIV epidemic, with corresponding efforts to incorporate multilevel approaches in both large-scale national policy, targeted investments in prevention and testing in high-prevalence communities,[102] and D&I research that aims to promote health equity in HIV prevention and treatment.

Several important D&I research studies tailored to local context, including multilevel interventions, have identified potentially effective strategies to reduce disparities in HIV prevention and treatment in marginalized communities. The AIDS Initiative for Minority Men (AIMM) targeted young Black/African American men aged 18–29 living in Louisiana who had HIV or were at risk for HIV, including both MSM and heterosexual men.[103] AIMM implemented a multilevel approach to HIV prevention with a focus on testing, building self-efficacy, treatment adherence, and service connectivity. The intervention implemented health and social service navigation, education, job coordination, stigma reduction, and safe space creation. Findings included linkage of 62% of HIV-positive participants to HIV care within 3 months and 43% of unemployed individuals finding work through the program. AIMM also identified housing discrimination in over one-third of housing vacancies when callers identified themselves as Black/African American and/or MSM as compared to White and heterosexual and was able to educate program participants about the signs of housing discrimination, legal rights to fair housing, and any legal recourse available to them in the event of a fair housing violation.

The Linking Inmates to Care in Los Angeles (LINK-LA) intervention connected HIV-positive men and transgender women inmates with peer navigation to connect them with ongoing HIV treatment and sustain viral suppression on release from incarceration.[104] Most LINK-LA participants were either Black/African American or Latino/a/x, and the majority had substance use issues. Peer navigators met with participants for 12 weeks to model retention and adherence behaviors, starting when they were still in jail and accompanying the participant to two scheduled HIV medical appointments after release. Intervention participants were more likely to maintain viral suppression at 12 months compared to control participants, who did not have access to the peer navigator.

The numbers of new HIV cases and deaths from HIV/AIDS in the United States have declined significantly over the past two decades due to ongoing efforts to increase rates of treatment with HAART and use of preexposure prophylaxis (PrEP) in order to prevent HIV transmission. However, addressing HIV disparities for marginalized groups will require D&I research that directly targets HIV-related stigma and related societal barriers, particularly in communities without a history of HIV-related activism.

Child and Adolescent Vaccination

Universal coverage programs for childhood vaccinations have been in place since the 1940s in the United States.[105] Coverage rates have increased over time and have generally remained quite high, with rates of recommended childhood vaccinations at 24 months ranging between 80% and 90%.[106] Uptake of vaccines mandated for kindergarten entry is even higher, hovering at around 95%.[107] This high level of vaccine coverage was achieved through a combination of activities, primarily at the policy level, including coordinated efforts at the federal, state, and local levels to promote vaccination, CDC's Vaccines for Children program, state-based immunization registries, recommendations from professional organizations regarding importance of vaccination, systematic collection of data to measure coverage, prioritization of immunizations by governmental and professional bodies, and school vaccine mandates.[105]

However, gaps in immunization rates between non-Latino/a/x White and racial and ethnic marginalized children were first identified in the 1970s and continue to persist today, although they have narrowed over time.[108] Insurance status is one of the factors that underlie persistent racial and ethnic disparities in vaccination, with substantial gaps in vaccine uptake between insured versus uninsured children. Although disparities in vaccine uptake between public and privately insured children and by poverty level persist, these differences tend to be small. These findings highlight the need to ensure that families are aware of the nearly universal accessibility of low-cost or free vaccines through the federally funded Vaccines for Children program.

Although the Advisory Committee on Immunization Practices introduced the "adolescent vaccine platform" in 1997, it was not until the mid-2000s that the platform included the three currently recommended vaccines: Tdap, meningococcal, and human papillomavirus (HPV). Rates of uptake for Tdap (mandated for school entry in most states) and the first dose of the meningoccocal vaccine are relatively high, nearing 80%, with no meaningful disparities by race and ethnicity or poverty status.[109] Rates of uptake among uninsured adolescents are lower than privately insured patients (10 percentage points difference in rates or less), but no meaningful disparities were observed between publically and privately insured adolescents in recent population-based data. Uptake for the HPV vaccine has stalled, with less than 50% of adolescents "up to date" with the recommended HPV vaccine schedule. Rates of HPV vaccine uptake are lower in uninsured adolescents compared to those with public or private insurance, but minimal racial and ethnic disparities are documented in national data. In fact, the National Immunization Survey–Teen (NIS-Teen) data from 2019, the last year before the onset of the COVID-19 pandemic, revealed that HPV vaccine up-to-date rates were slightly higher for Black/African American and Latino/a/x adolescents compared to non-Latino/a/x White adolescents.[109] The relative lack of racial and ethnic disparities in adolescent vaccination can be considered a success story. Factors that have likely contributed include the ability to leverage the strong existing vaccine infrastructure developed for childhood vaccinations, the availability of the Vaccines for Children program from the start (vs. the 50-year lag between introduction of childhood vaccines and formation of Vaccines for Children in 1994) and, in the case of Tdap, school mandates.

Despite being considered one of the most valuable public health interventions in history, the success of efforts to ensure equitable uptake of vaccinations in children is increasingly threatened. Although the prevalence of strong antivaccination attitudes is relatively rare, population-based data suggest it has grown over the past decade, as reflected in the proportion of children receiving no vaccines and requests for exemptions from school vaccine mandates.[110,111] Furthermore, the field has acknowledged the growth of vaccine hesitancy, which may not deter vaccination altogether but likely represents a significant barrier to vaccine promotion efforts.[112] Although antivaccination beliefs were once considered more of an issue among non-Latino/a/x White parents embracing a "natural" lifestyle, racial and ethnic marginalized, particularly Black/African American and Latino/a/x communities, have had some of the highest levels of concern about the COVID-19 vaccine.[113,114] It is not yet clear how the onset of the COVID-19 pandemic and development of the COVID-19 vaccine will ultimately affect youth vaccination rates overall. Although public health efforts to disseminate the COVID-19 vaccine purposely incorporated evidence-based vaccine promotion strategies for racial and ethnic marginalized and low-income communities (e.g., locating vaccine sites in underserved areas, partnering with trusted community institutions), racial and ethnic disparities in COVID-19 have been documented in vaccine uptake.[114] Research and surveillance efforts are needed to monitor the long-term impact of the COVID-19 pandemic on youth vaccination rates and, ultimately, vaccine-preventable disease in children and adults.

CASE STUDY 25.1: DIABETES PREVENTION PROGRAM

Background

In addition to D&I-related advancements in cancer, over the past few years there has been substantial momentum in national efforts to prevent or delay type 2 diabetes. There are 88 million adults in the United States living with prediabetes,[115] of whom 5%–10% will develop diabetes in the next year.[116] Adults from low-socioeconomic and/or racial and ethnic marginalized groups are disproportionately burdened by prediabetes,[115] are at higher risk for developing diabetes,[117] and once diagnosed, are more likely to experience complications from diabetes compared to White adults and those of higher socioeconomic status.[118]

In the late 1990s, the seminal Diabetes Prevention Program (DPP) randomized clinical trial conclusively demonstrated that participation in an intensive behavioral lifestyle intervention consisting of nutrition, physical activity, and behavioral counseling was more effective in reducing the incidence of type 2 diabetes (i.e., a reduction of 58%) and producing clinically significant weight loss (i.e., ≥ 7% loss of initial weight) than were metformin or placebo among a large, racially and ethnically diverse study population.[119] Since the original trial, several translational studies have established the effectiveness of the DPP lifestyle intervention delivered in both clinical and community-based settings; by different providers (e.g., clinicians, health coaches, and community health workers)[120–123]; and among specific underserved populations. such as the successful Special Diabetes Program for Indians Diabetes Prevention Program demonstration project.[124]

Context

In 2010, the CDC established the National Diabetes Prevention Program (NDPP). A key component of NDPP is the lifestyle change program, which is modeled after the original trial's lifestyle intervention arm and consists of a standard curriculum that is delivered over a 12-month period. As part of the NDPP Diabetes Prevention Recognition Program, organizations can apply to be recognized by the CDC as providers of NDPP by meeting a set of criteria, including having at least 60% of program completers achieve 5% weight loss, a combination of 4% weight loss and ≥ 150 minutes of physical activity per week on average, or a 0.2% reduction in hemoglobin A_{1C}.[125]

Given the demonstration of real-world effectiveness of NDPP across different settings and populations, especially among older adults,[120] in 2018 the CMS began to reimburse CDC-recognized clinical and community-based providers to deliver the NDPP curriculum in an in-person group format to Medicare beneficiaries as well as Medicaid recipients in some states. Although based on the NDPP curriculum, because sites must go through additional criteria to be recognized as a Medicare provider, the CMS-funded program is often referred to as Medicare DPP (MDPP). Initially, MDPP was designed as a 24-month program with a performance-based payment model in which suppliers are reimbursed based on participant session attendance and achieving 5% weight loss.

Findings

Equitable D&I of both NDPP and MDPP has been challenging. In an evaluation of the early implementation of NDPP lifestyle program (i.e., 2012–2016), there were approximately 14,700 eligible participants enrolled across the 220 organizations recognized by the CDC to deliver NDPP at the time.[126] Despite clinically significant weight loss, overall, on average, Black/African American participants were significantly less likely to achieve ≥ 5% weight loss compared to non-Latino/a/x White participants (27% vs. 43%). Also, both Black/African American (median of 13 sessions) and Latino/a/x (median of 11 sessions) participants attended fewer sessions than White participants (median of 16 sessions). Several other studies have also suggested limited reach and effectiveness of NDPP in low-income and marginalized communities.[127,128] Uptake of MDPP has particularly been suboptimal, especially in racial and ethnic marginalized communities. As of March 2021, there were 940 MDPP suppliers in the United States[129]; however, about 38 states did not have an MDPP program site, had less than one site per 100,000 Medicare beneficiaries, and/or the program was limited to a single municipality.[130] Between 2018 and 2021, only 3,300 beneficiaries of the estimated

50,000 eligible, had enrolled, 72% of whom were White women.[130]

Applying a health equity lens to the RE-AIM framework (an example of the EQ-DI[42] approach described previously in this chapter), economic, social, and environmental contexts need to be considered to understand and address the inequities in program reach, effectiveness, adoption, implementation, and maintenance.[131] The presence of social risk factors such as lack of transportation, poor access to healthcare, and childcare needs are all possible barriers to optimal engagement in NDPP, including regular session attendance or being able to travel to the clinic and/or afford the required lab tests to determine program eligibility (e.g., fasting blood glucose or hemoglobin A_{1C}). Furthermore, low-income, racial, and ethnic marginalized individuals tend to live in underresourced neighborhoods with poor access to healthy, affordable food or safe spaces to engage in physical activity.[132] Given these contextual and structural barriers to health behavior change, achieving clinically significant weight loss of 5% or greater can be particularly challenging among low-income and racial and ethnic marginalized communities.[128] Thus, basing reimbursement on participant attendance and achieving 5% weight loss is a deterrent and may explain the poor adoption among potential MDPP suppliers who predominantly serve members of marginalized communities,[128,130]

Lessons Learned

To date, there are now over 2,000 CDC-recognized NDPP sites across the United States, and there have been over 300,000 participants.[133] Sites include healthcare settings, community-based organizations, universities, and public health departments. Since early implementation, the CDC and its partners have developed national awareness campaigns and enhanced technical assistance by making toolkits and other resources available on the website as well as creating a customer service center to support current NDPP providers. In addition to in-person groups, organizations can also deliver NDPP as an online/digital program, distance learning (i.e., via videoconferencing), or a combination of these delivery modalities, which has expanded reach. Furthermore, there has been increased effort to train Spanish-speaking lifestyle coaches, and there was a recent update to the Latino/a/x culturally tailored version of the curriculum (see website in list of suggested readings and websites below). Thus, with time, the reach, adoption, and strategies to implement NDPP have improved. However, there is a need for continued D&I research with a health equity lens to examine if these changes are actually reducing diabetes-related disparities.

On the other hand, there have been minimal changes with MDPP. Some positive changes include that it is now being reimbursed as a 1-year instead of a 2-year program, which creates less burden and quicker payment for suppliers.[134] Also, the majority of MDPP sites are supplied by community-based organizations, which may enhance reach, especially in underserved, marginalized communities.[130] However, the payment model is still based on performance, and the program has to be delivered in an in-person group format to be reimbursed. During the COVID-19 pandemic emergency period, CMS did allow for sites to offer the program via telehealth, but this change was temporary and still did not include reimbursement for digital DPP providers. CMS should consider a risk-adjusted payment model to account for inequities in social determinants of health and expand coverage to include online and digital delivery of MDPP to enhance reach and adoption.[131] Of course, evaluation of these strategies would be needed to determine the effect on health and healthcare disparities.

DIRECTIONS FOR FUTURE RESEARCH

Although there has been an acceleration in equity-focused D&I research over the past several years, much remains to be studied to advance health equity at a population level. Future D&I research should include measurement of social determinants of health (at the community and individual level) to link to health outcomes, which will aid in identifying mechanisms of health inequities and inform intervention design.[26] Furthermore, there is a need for greater integration of equity in implementation models and frameworks as well as implementation strategies and outcomes.[26,54,135] By applying an equity lens throughout the intervention development and implementation process, EBIs may be more effective in actually addressing health inequities and reducing disparities. There is also growing

TABLE 25.1 RECOMMENDATIONS TO ADVANCE HEALTH EQUITY WITHIN D&I SCIENCE[a]

Domain	Recommendation	Core Elements
Evidence base	1. Link social determinants of health with health outcomes 2. Build equity into all policies	• Identify opportunities to address social risk in primary care • Describe the role of social determinants (including structural racism) as moderators of behavior change • Incorporate health and equity consideration in policy decisions across sectors • Analyze barriers to change with an equity focus
Methods and measures	3. Use equity-relevant metrics 4. Study what is already happening 5. Integrate equity into models 6. Design and tailor implementation strategies	• Expand macro-level metrics to focus on upstream indicators to measure progress toward equity in communities • Identify new metrics in studies to address context and historical disadvantage • Work with practitioners and policymakers to conduct natural experiments • Enhance the role of equity in tailored implementation • Identify methods for fully integrating equity into existing models • Enhance the explicit focus on equity among implementation strategies
Context	7. Connect systems and sectors outside of health 8. Engage organizations (including community-based organizations), internally and externally	• Establish the premise that justice across societal sectors is essential (antiracism approach) • Evaluate existing programs and policies regarding their equity impacts • Externally, bring on new equity partners, share power and decision-making, and break down funding silos
Cross-cutting issues	9. Build capacity for equity 10. Focus on equity in dissemination efforts	• Develop and fund health equity-focused D&I training programs • Increase engagement of persons in trainings from historically underrepresented backgrounds • Engage with equity-focused partners early and often in the research process

[a] Adapted with permission from Brownson and colleagues, 2021.[26]

opportunity to evaluate implementation strategies to improve adoption of health equity-focused interventions in healthcare and community-based settings.[30,31] Applying antiracism approaches to future D&I research, including examining and addressing the impact of structural racism on health, may inform not only equitable implementation, but also de-implementation of inequitable policies, practices, and programs.[36,70] While antiracism processes can help explain pathways by which racism contributes to specific health inequities, they are more necessary for their usefulness in challenging the norms and structures of institutions, including those of institutions advancing D&I research. There is also a great need for additional health equity-focused D&I research in other marginalized groups and communities, including lesbian, gay, bisexual, transgender and/or gender expansive, queer and/or questioning, intersex, asexual, and two-spirit, and queer/questioning (LGBTQIA2S+), immigrants and refugees, and rural residents.[45] Last, ensuring the availability of ongoing high-quality training opportunities in health equity-focused D&I science is essential to pursue these future directions and advance health equity. See Table 25.1, which is adapted from Brownson and colleagues (2021),[26] which provides recommendations to promote health equity in D&I Science.

SUMMARY

Throughout this chapter we have demonstrated not only the relevance, but also the necessity of applying an equity lens to D&I science to advance health equity. There are several challenges to promoting health equity in D&I research, including possible inadvertent exacerbation of health and healthcare disparities; lack of acknowledgment of contexts and other underlying structural factors such as racism; limited use of a multilevel, multisector, and/or multisystems approach for EBIs; inadequate use of equity-relevant metrics and methods; and lack of inclusion of low-resource settings or marginalized populations in efficacy, effectiveness, and implementation studies. However, applying a health equity lens to established D&I models and frameworks (EQ-DI; transcreation framework) or increased use of health equity-focused emerging models and frameworks (e.g., Health Equity Implementation Framework or EquIR) can help alleviate these challenges. There is growing application of health equity-focused D&I research in multiple areas, including cancer screening, obesity prevention, HIV/STIs, and vaccinations, with promising findings in reducing health disparities. Despite these advancements, there is much work to be done to prioritize health equity in D&I research, from considering social determinants of health in the study design to intentionally involving community partners throughout the intervention development and implementation process (also see chapter 10). To truly advance health equity at the population level, an equity lens must be applied to enhance EBI effectiveness and relevance as well as to strategies to implement, sustain, and scale EBIs across diverse communities and settings.

ACKNOWLEDGMENTS

We dedicate this chapter to the memory of our close friend and colleague Dr. Toni Yancey, who spearheaded the original version of this chapter. Toni was a force of nature who was passionate about promoting physical activity, mentoring the next generation of health equity scholars, and improving the health of marginalized communities. In addition to being a physician and professor in the UCLA Fielding School of Public Health, Toni was a former model and Division 1 basketball player and a poet and spoken word artist. Although her accolades are too numerous to detail here, two that she was particularly proud of include her creation of "Instant Recess," an award-winning program to integrate 10-minute bouts of physical activity into organizational routine, and her appointment to the board of directors of the Partnership for a Healthier America, the nonprofit that guided first lady Michelle Obama's Let's Move campaign. We lost Toni far too soon, but know that her memory continues to inspire countless individuals and organizations in their efforts to achieve health equity.

We also acknowledge Drs. Shiriki Kumanyika and Rachel Shelton for their wisdom and support in updating this important, timely chapter.

SUGGESTED READINGS AND WEBSITES

Readings

Bailey ZD, Krieger N, Agenor M, Graves J, Linos N, Bassett MT. Structural racism and health inequities in the USA: evidence and interventions. *Lancet.* 2017;389(10077):1453–1463.

This is a comprehensive review of how structural racism is the root cause of health inequities and provides considerations for future research.

Braveman P. What are health disparities and health equity? We need to be clear. *Public Health Rep.* 2014;129(suppl 2):5–8.

This article defines and distinguishes the terms health disparities *and* health equity.

Brownson RC, Kumanyika SK, Kreuter MW, Haire-Joshu D. Implementation science should give higher priority to health equity. *Implement Sci.* 2021;16(1):28.

This article describes implementation research challenges in promoting health equity as well as recommendations and ideas to address these challenges.

Eslava-Schmalbach J, Garzon-Orjuela N, Elias V, Reveiz L, Tran N, Langlois EV. Conceptual framework of equity-focused implementation research for health programs (EquIR). *Int J Equity Health*. 2019;18(1):80.

This article describes the EquIR framework and provides examples of application to evaluate public health programs and policies in Latin American countries.

Ford CL, Griffith DM, Bruce M, Gilbert K, eds. *Racism: Science and Tools for the Public Health Professional*. American Public Health Association Press; 2019.

This edited book provides concrete guidance to understand and address racism among diverse populations, and it offers resources (definitions, examples, etc.) for doing so.

Kumanyika SK. A framework for increasing equity impact in obesity prevention. *Am J Public Health*. 2019;109(10):1350–1357.

This article describes a framework for designing multilevel, multisector, and multisystem interventions with an equity lens to reduce health disparities.

Napoles AM, Stewart AL. Transcreation: an implementation science framework for community-engaged behavioral interventions to reduce health disparities. *BMC Health Serv Res*. 2018;18(1):710.

This article describes the transcreation framework, which can be used to guide community-engaged dissemination and implementation research.

Shelton RC, Adsul P, Oh A, Moise N, Griffith DM. Application of an antiracism lens in the field of implementation science (IS): recommendations for reframing implementation research with a focus on justice and racial equity. *Implement Res Pract*. 2021;2:1–19.

This article provides recommendations on how to address structural racism as a root cause of health inequities by applying an antiracism lens to implementation science frameworks, strategies, measures, and outcomes.

Woodward EN, Matthieu MM, Uchendu US, Rogal S, Kirchner JE. The health equity implementation framework: proposal and preliminary study of hepatitis C virus treatment. *Implement Sci*. 2019;14(1):26.

This article describes the development and components of the Health Equity Implementation Framework along with an example for application.

Selected Websites and Tools

Centers for Disease Control and Prevention (CDC) Compendium of Evidence-Based Interventions and Best Practices for HIV Prevention. https://www.cdc.gov/hiv/research/interventionresearch/compendium/index.html

This website provides information about and access to tested evidence-based interventions and best practices for HIV prevention identified through systematic reviews that were conducted as part of the CDC's Prevention Research Synthesis (PRS) Project.

Centers for Disease Control and Prevention (CDC) National Diabetes Prevention Program and the National Alliance for Hispanic Health Prevent T2 program. https://www.cdc.gov/diabetes/prevention/index.html and https://www.healthyamericas.org/diabetes

These websites describe the National Diabetes Prevention Program and the Prevent T2 program for Hispanic participants, respectively, and both include tools and resources for program adoption.

Centers for Disease Control and Prevention (CDC) on the Social Determinants of Health. https://www.cdc.gov/socialdeterminants/index.htm

This website explains the domains of social determinants of health, sources for social determinant data, and tools/policy resources to address social determinants of health.

National Cancer Institute Division of Cancer Control and Population Sciences Implementation Science. https://cancercontrol.cancer.gov/is

This website is intended for use by planners, program staff, and researchers seeking data and other resources to guide the design, implementation, and evaluation of evidence-based cancer control programs.

National Institutes of Health PhenX Toolkit. https://www.phenxtoolkit.org/

This website consists of a web-based catalogue of recommended measurement protocols selected by experts to include in studies. Further, this website provides measures related to social determinants of health and the COVID-19 pandemic.

World Health Organization Commission on the Social Determinants of Health. http://www.who.int/social_determinants/thecommission/finalreport/en/

This website explains what the social determinants of health are. Further, it provides reports, summaries, and media information to encourage researchers and practitioners to move beyond studying disparities toward addressing their root causes.

REFERENCES

1. Ford CL. Commentary: addressing inequities in the era of COVID-19: the pandemic and the urgent need for critical race theory. *Fam Community Health*. 2020;43(3):184–186.

2. Williams DR, Cooper LA. COVID-19 and health equity—a new kind of "herd immunity." *JAMA.* 2020;323(24):2478–2480.
3. National Academies of Sciences, Engineering, and Medicine. *Communities, Climate Change, and Health Equity: Proceedings of a Workshop in Brief.* Washington, DC: The National Academies Press; 2022. https://doi.org/10.17226/26435
4. National Center for Health Statistics (US). *Health, United States, 2004: With Chartbook on Trends in the Health of Americans.* Centers for Disease Control and Prevention; 2004.
5. Harper S, MacLehose RF, Kaufman JS. Trends in the black-white life expectancy gap among US states, 1990–2009. *Health Aff (Millwood).* 2014;33(8):1375–1382.
6. National Center for Health Statistics (US). *Health, United States, 2019.* Centers for Disease Control and Prevention; 2021.
7. Marmot M, Commission on Social Determinants of Health. Achieving health equity: from root causes to fair outcomes. *Lancet.* 2007;370(9593):1153–1163.
8. Ford CL, Harawa NT. A new conceptualization of ethnicity for social epidemiologic and health equity research. *Soc Sci Med.* 2010;71(2):251–258.
9. Bailey ZD, Krieger N, Agenor M, Graves J, Linos N, Bassett MT. Structural racism and health inequities in the USA: evidence and interventions. *Lancet.* 2017;389(10077):1453–1463.
10. Bailey ZD, Feldman JM, Bassett MT. How structural racism works—racist policies as a root cause of US racial health inequities. *N Engl J Med.* 2021;384(8):768–773.
11. Warne D, Frizzell LB. American Indian health policy: historical trends and contemporary issues. *Am J Public Health.* 2014;104(suppl 3):S263–S267.
12. Hutchinson RN, Shin S. Systematic review of health disparities for cardiovascular diseases and associated factors among American Indian and Alaska Native populations. *PLoS One.* 2014;9(1):e80973.
13. Jacobs-Wingo JL, Espey DK, Groom AV, Phillips LE, Haverkamp DS, Stanley SL. Causes and disparities in death rates among urban American Indian and Alaska Native populations, 1999–2009. *Am J Public Health.* 2016;106(5):906–914.
14. Warne DL, D. American Indian health disparities: psychosocial influences. *Soc Personal Psychol Compass.* 2015;9(10):567–579.
15. Gee GC, Ford CL. Structural racism and health inequities: old issues, new directions. *Du Bois Rev.* 2011;8(1):115–132.
16. Chang CD. Social determinants of health and health disparities among immigrants and their children. *Curr Probl Pediatr Adolesc Health Care.* 2019;49(1):23–30.
17. Hall E, Cuellar NG. Immigrant health in the United States: a trajectory toward change. *J Transcult Nurs.* 2016;27(6):611–626.
18. Singh GK, Rodriguez-Lainz A, Kogan MD. Immigrant health inequalities in the United States: use of eight major national data systems. *Sci World J.* 2013;2013:512313.
19. Kumanyika SK. Health equity is the issue we have been waiting for. *J Public Health Manag Pract.* 2016;22(suppl 1):S8–S10.
20. Yao Q, Li X, Luo F, Yang L, Liu C, Sun J. The historical roots and seminal research on health equity: a referenced publication year spectroscopy (RPYS) analysis. *Int J Equity Health.* 2019;18(1):152.
21. Whitehead M. The concepts and principles of equity and health. *Int J Health Serv.* 1992;22(3):429–445.
22. Braveman P. What are health disparities and health equity? We need to be clear. *Public Health Rep.* 2014;129(suppl 2):5–8.
23. Jones CP. Systems of power, axes of inequity: parallels, intersections, braiding the strands. *Med Care.* 2014;52(10)(suppl 3):S71–S75.
24. Li M, Yuan F. Historical redlining and food environments: a study of 102 urban areas in the United States. *Health Place.* 2022;75:102775.
25. Kumanyika SK. A framework for increasing equity impact in obesity prevention. *Am J Public Health.* 2019;109(10):1350–1357.
26. Brownson RC, Kumanyika SK, Kreuter MW, Haire-Joshu D. Implementation science should give higher priority to health equity. *Implement Sci.* 2021;16(1):28.
27. McNulty M, Smith JD, Villamar J, et al. Implementation research methodologies for achieving scientific equity and health equity. *Ethn Dis.* 2019;29(suppl 1):83–92.
28. Chinman M, Woodward EN, Curran GM, Hausmann LRM. Harnessing implementation science to increase the impact of health equity research. *Med Care.* 2017;55(suppl 9 suppl 2):S16–S23.
29. Agurs-Collins T, Persky S, Paskett ED, et al. Designing and assessing multilevel interventions to improve minority health and reduce health disparities. *Am J Public Health.* 2019;109(S1):S86–S93.
30. Galaviz KI, Breland JY, Sanders M, et al. Implementation science to address health disparities during the coronavirus pandemic. *Health Equity.* 2020;4(1):463–467.
31. Baumann AA, Cabassa LJ. Reframing implementation science to address inequities in healthcare delivery. *BMC Health Serv Res.* 2020;20(1):190.

32. US Preventive Services Task Force, Krist AH, Davidson KW, et al. Screening for hypertension in Adults: US Preventive Services Task Force reaffirmation recommendation statement. *JAMA*. 2021;325(16):1650–1656.
33. Ferdinand KC, Brown AL. Will the 2021 USPSTF hypertension screening recommendation decrease or worsen racial/ethnic disparities in blood pressure control? *JAMA Netw Open*. 2021;4(4):e213718.
34. Braveman PA, Arkin E, Proctor D, Kauh T, Holm N. Systemic and structural racism: definitions, examples, health damages, and approaches to dismantling. *Health Aff (Millwood)*. 2022;41(2):171–178.
35. Bonilla-Silva E. Rethinking racism: toward a structural interpretation. *Am Sociol Rev*. 1997;62(3):465–480.
36. Shelton RC, Adsul P, Oh A. Recommendations for addressing structural racism in implementation science: a call to the field. *Ethn Dis*. 2021;31(Suppl 1):357–364.
37. Fantasia KL, Wirunsawanya K, Lee C, Rizo I. Racial disparities in diabetes technology use and outcomes in type 1 diabetes in a safety-net hospital. *J Diabetes Sci Technol*. 2021;15(5):1010–1017.
38. Addala A, Hanes S, Naranjo D, Maahs DM, Hood KK. Provider implicit bias impacts pediatric type 1 diabetes technology recommendations in the United States: findings from the Gatekeeper Study. *J Diabetes Sci Technol*. 2021;15(5):1027–1033.
39. Agarwal S, Crespo-Ramos G, Long JA, Miller VA. "I didn't really have a choice": qualitative analysis of racial-ethnic disparities in diabetes technology use among young adults with type 1 diabetes. *Diabetes Technol Ther*. 2021;23(9):616–622.
40. Rabin BA, Glasgow RE, Kerner JF, Klump MP, Brownson RC. Dissemination and implementation research on community-based cancer prevention: a systematic review. *Am J Prev Med*. 2010;38(4):443–456.
41. Whitt-Glover MC, Kumanyika SK. Systematic review of interventions to increase physical activity and physical fitness in African-Americans. *Am J Health Promot*. 2009;23(6):S33–S56.
42. Yousefi Nooraie R, Kwan BM, Cohn E, et al. Advancing health equity through CTSA programs: opportunities for interaction between health equity, dissemination and implementation, and translational science. *J Clin Transl Sci*. 2020;4(3):168–175.
43. Eslava-Schmalbach J, Garzon-Orjuela N, Elias V, Reveiz L, Tran N, Langlois EV. Conceptual framework of equity-focused implementation research for health programs (EquIR). *Int J Equity Health*. 2019;18(1):80.
44. Woodward EN, Matthieu MM, Uchendu US, Rogal S, Kirchner JE. The health equity implementation framework: proposal and preliminary study of hepatitis C virus treatment. *Implement Sci*. 2019;14(1):26.
45. Sterling MR, Echeverria SE, Commodore-Mensah Y, Breland JY, Nunez-Smith M. Health equity and implementation science in heart, lung, blood, and sleep-related research: emerging themes from the 2018 Saunders-Watkins Leadership Workshop. *Circ Cardiovasc Qual Outcomes*. 2019;12(10):e005586.
46. Haire-Joshu D, Hill-Briggs F. The next generation of diabetes translation: a path to health equity. *Annu Rev Public Health*. 2019;40 : 391–410.
47. Glasgow RE, Vogt TM, Boles SM. Evaluating the public health impact of health promotion interventions: the RE-AIM framework. *Am J Public Health*. 1999;89(9):1322–1327.
48. Shelton RC, Chambers DA, Glasgow RE. An extension of RE-AIM to enhance sustainability: addressing dynamic context and promoting health equity over time. *Front Public Health*. 2020;8:134.
49. Napoles AM, Stewart AL. Transcreation: an implementation science framework for community-engaged behavioral interventions to reduce health disparities. *BMC Health Serv Res*. 2018;18(1):710.
50. Israel BA, Schulz AJ, Parker EA, Becker AB. Review of community-based research: assessing partnership approaches to improve public health. *Annu Rev Public Health*. 1998;19:173–202.
51. Dover DC, Belon AP. The health equity measurement framework: a comprehensive model to measure social inequities in health. *Int J Equity Health*. 2019;18(1):36.
52. Harvey G, Kitson A. PARIHS revisited: from heuristic to integrated framework for the successful implementation of knowledge into practice. *Implement Sci*. 2016;11:33.
53. Kilbourne AM, Switzer G, Hyman K, Crowley-Matoka M, Fine MJ. Advancing health disparities research within the health care system: a conceptual framework. *Am J Public Health*. 2006;96(12):2113–2121.
54. Woodward EN, Singh RS, Ndebele-Ngwenya P, Melgar Castillo A, Dickson KS, Kirchner JE. A more practical guide to incorporating health equity domains in implementation determinant frameworks. *Implement Sci Commun*. 2021;2(1):61.
55. Operario D, Adler NE, Williams DR. Subjective social status: reliability and predictive utility for global health. *Psychol Health*. 2004;19(2):237–246.

56. Alderwick H, Gottlieb LM. Meanings and misunderstandings: a social determinants of health lexicon for health care systems. *Milbank Q.* 2019;97(2):407–419.
57. Hill-Briggs F, Adler NE, Berkowitz SA, et al. Social determinants of health and diabetes: a scientific review. *Diabetes Care.* 2020;44(1):258–279.
58. Berkowitz SA, Berkowitz TSZ, Meigs JB, Wexler DJ. Trends in food insecurity for adults with cardiometabolic disease in the United States: 2005–2012. *PLoS One.* 2017;12(6):e0179172.
59. Alley DE, Asomugha CN, Conway PH, Sanghavi DM. Accountable health communities—addressing social needs through Medicare and Medicaid. *N Engl J Med.* 2016;374(1):8–11.
60. National Association of Community Health Centers. Protocol for Responding to and Assessing Patients' Assets, Risks, and Experiences (PRAPARE). 2020. Accessed March 31, 2022. https://www.nachc.org/research-and-data/prapare/prapare_one_pager_sept_2016-2/
61. Blumberg SJ, Bialostosky K, Hamilton WL, Briefel RR. The effectiveness of a short form of the Household Food Security Scale. *Am J Public Health.* 1999;89(8):1231–1234.
62. Hager ER, Quigg AM, Black MM, et al. Development and validity of a 2-item screen to identify families at risk for food insecurity. *Pediatrics.* 2010;126(1):e26–e32.
63. Henrikson NB, Blasi PR, Dorsey CN, et al. Psychometric and pragmatic properties of social risk screening tools: a systematic review. *Am J Prev Med.* 2019;57(6)(suppl 1):S13–S24.
64. Soret S, McCleary KJ, Rivers PA, Montgomery SB. Understanding health disparities through geographic information systems. In: Khan O, Skinner R, ed. *Geographic Information Systems and Health Applications.* Idea Group Publishing; 2003:12–42.
65. Andrews MR, Tamura K, Claudel SE, et al. Geospatial analysis of Neighborhood Deprivation Index (NDI) for the United States by county. *J Maps.* 2020;16(1):101–112.
66. Butler DC, Petterson S, Phillips RL, Bazemore AW. Measures of social deprivation that predict health care access and need within a rational area of primary care service delivery. *Health Serv Res.* 2013;48(2 Pt 1):539–559.
67. Cutter SLB, Boruff BJ; Shirley W.L. Social vulnerability to environmental hazards. *Soc Sci Q.* 2003;84(2):242–261.
68. Casey JA, Schwartz BS, Stewart WF, Adler NE. Using electronic health records for population health research: a review of methods and applications. *Ann Rev Public Health.* 2016;37: 61–81.
69. Allen M, Wilhelm A, Ortega LE, Pergament S, Bates N, Cunningham B. Applying a race(ism)-conscious adaptation of the CFIR framework to understand implementation of a school-based equity-oriented intervention. *Ethn Dis.* 2021;31(suppl 1):375–388.
70. Shelton RC, Adsul P, Oh A, Moise N, Griffith DM. Application of an antiracism lens in the field of implementation science (IS): recommendations for reframing implementation research with a focus on justice and racial equity. *Implement Res Pract.* 2021;2:1–19.
71. Neta G, Clyne M, Chambers DA. Dissemination and implementation research at the National Cancer Institute: a review of funded studies (2006–2019) and opportunities to advance the field. *Cancer Epidemiol Biomarkers Prev.* 2021;30(2):260–267.
72. Sabatino SA, Lawrence B, Elder R, et al. Effectiveness of interventions to increase screening for breast, cervical, and colorectal cancers: nine updated systematic reviews for the guide to community preventive services. *Am J Prev Med.* 2012;43(1):97–118.
73. Dougherty MK, Brenner AT, Crockett SD, et al. Evaluation of interventions intended to increase colorectal cancer screening rates in the United States: a systematic review and meta-analysis. *JAMA Intern Med.* 2018;178(12):1645–1658.
74. Rim SH, Allaire BT, Ekwueme DU, et al. Cost-effectiveness of breast cancer screening in the National Breast and Cervical Cancer Early Detection Program. *Cancer Causes Control.* 2019;30(8):819–826.
75. Pollack LM, Ekwueme DU, Hung MC, Miller JW, Chang SH. Estimating the impact of increasing cervical cancer screening in the National Breast and Cervical Cancer Early Detection Program among low-income women in the USA. *Cancer Causes Control.* 2020;31(7):691–702.
76. Khushalani JS, Trogdon JG, Ekwueme DU, Yabroff KR. Economics of public health programs for underserved populations: a review of economic analysis of the National Breast and Cervical Cancer Early Detection Program. *Cancer Causes Control.* 2019;30(12):1351–1363.
77. Tangka F, Kenny K, Miller J, Howard DH. The eligibility and reach of the National Breast and Cervical Cancer Early Detection Program after implementation of the Affordable Care Act. *Cancer Causes Control.* 2020;31(5):473–489.
78. Bitler MP, Carpenter CS, Horn D. Effects of the Colorectal Cancer Control Program. *Health Econ.* 2021;30(11):2667–2685.
79. Tangka FKL, Subramanian S, Hoover S, et al. Identifying optimal approaches to scale up

colorectal cancer screening: an overview of the Centers for Disease Control and Prevention (CDC)'s learning laboratory. *Cancer Causes Control.* 2019;30(2):169–175.

80. Tong M, Hill L, Artiga S. Racial disparities in cancer outcomes, screening, and treatment. Kaiser Family Foundation. 2022. Accessed March 31, 2022. https://www.kff.org/racial-equity-and-health-policy/issue-brief/racial-disparities-in-cancer-outcomes-screening-and-treatment/.
81. Green BB, Baldwin LM, West II, Schwartz M, Coronado GD. Low rates of colonoscopy follow-up after a positive fecal immunochemical test in a Medicaid health plan delivered mailed colorectal cancer screening program. *J Prim Care Community Health.* 2020;11:2150132720958525.
82. Cooper GS, Grimes A, Werner J, Cao S, Fu P, Stange KC. Barriers to follow-up colonoscopy after positive FIT or multitarget stool DNA testing. *J Am Board Fam Med.* 2021;34(1):61–69.
83. Gortmaker SL, Swinburn BA, Levy D, et al. Changing the future of obesity: science, policy, and action. *Lancet.* 2011;378(9793):838–847.
84. Gortmaker SL, Wang YC, Long MW, et al. Three interventions that reduce childhood obesity are projected to save more than they cost to implement. *Health Aff (Millwood).* 2015;34(11):1932–1939.
85. Yuksel HS, Sahin FN, Maksimovic N, Drid P, Bianco A. School-based intervention programs for preventing obesity and promoting physical activity and fitness: a systematic review. *Int J Environ Res Public Health.* 2020;17(1):347–368.
86. Kennedy SG, McKay HA, Naylor PJ, Lubans DR. Implementation and scale-up of school-based physical activity interventions. In: Brusseau TA, Fairclough SJ, Lubans DR, eds. *The Routledge Handbook of Youth Physical Activity.* Routledge; 2020:438–460.
87. Dobbins M, Husson H, DeCorby K, LaRocca RL. School-based physical activity programs for promoting physical activity and fitness in children and adolescents aged 6 to 18. *Cochrane Database Syst Rev.* 2013;(2):CD007651.
88. Kriemler S, Meyer U, Martin E, van Sluijs EM, Andersen LB, Martin BW. Effect of school-based interventions on physical activity and fitness in children and adolescents: a review of reviews and systematic update. *Br J Sports Med.* 2011;45(11):923–930.
89. Love R, Adams J, van Sluijs EMF. Are school-based physical activity interventions effective and equitable? A meta-analysis of cluster randomized controlled trials with accelerometer-assessed activity. *Obes Rev.* 2019;20(6):859–870.
90. Sutherland RL, Jackson JK, Lane C, et al. A systematic review of adaptations and effectiveness of scaled-up nutrition interventions. *Nutr Rev.* 2022;80(4):962–979.
91. Cassar S, Salmon J, Timperio A, et al. Adoption, implementation and sustainability of school-based physical activity and sedentary behaviour interventions in real-world settings: a systematic review. *Int J Behav Nutr Phys Act.* 2019;16(1):120.
92. Love RE, Adams J, van Sluijs EMF. Equity effects of children's physical activity interventions: a systematic scoping review. *Int J Behav Nutr Phys Act.* 2017;14(1):134.
93. Hartwig TB, Sanders T, Vasconcellos D, et al. School-based interventions modestly increase physical activity and cardiorespiratory fitness but are least effective for youth who need them most: an individual participant pooled analysis of 20 controlled trials. *Br J Sports Med.* 2021;55:721–729.
94. Vinluan MH, Hofman J. Transforming out-of-school time environments: the Y's commitment to healthy eating and physical activity standards. *Am J Health Promotion.* 2014;28(3)(suppl):S116–S118.
95. Weaver RG, Moore JB, Turner-McGrievy B, et al. Identifying strategies programs adopt to meet healthy eating and physical activity standards in afterschool programs. *Health Educ Behav.* 2017;44(4):536–547.
96. Beets MW, Glenn Weaver R, Brazendale K, et al. Statewide dissemination and implementation of physical activity standards in afterschool programs: two-year results. *BMC Public Health.* 2018;18(1):819.
97. HIV.gov. US statistics. October 27, 2022. Accessed March 31, 2022. https://www.hiv.gov/hiv-basics/overview/data-and-trends/statistics
98. Centers for Disease Control and Prevention. HIV basic statistics. Updated October 1, 2021. Accessed March 31, 2022. https://www.cdc.gov/hiv/basics/statistics.html
99. Millett GA, Peterson JL, Flores SA, et al. Comparisons of disparities and risks of HIV infection in Black and other men who have sex with men in Canada, UK, and USA: a meta-analysis. *Lancet.* 2012;380(9839):341–348.
100. Adimora AA, Schoenbach VJ, Taylor EM, Khan MR, Schwartz RJ. Concurrent partnerships, nonmonogamous partners, and substance use among women in the United States. *Am J Public Health.* 2011;101(1):128–136.
101. Robinson R, Moodie-Mills AC. HIV/AIDS inequality: structural barriers to prevention, treatment, and care in communities of color. Center for American Progress, Berkeley Law University of California. 2012. Accessed March

31, 2022. https://cdn.americanprogress.org/wp-content/uploads/issues/2012/07/pdf/hiv_community_of_color.pdf?_ga=2.77363669.1158113109.1648791092-674681517.1648791091

102. Hutchinson AB, Farnham PG, Duffy N, et al. Return on public health investment: CDC's expanded HIV testing initiative. *J Acquir Immune Defic Syndr.* 2012;59(3):281–286.
103. Brewer R, Daunis C, Ebaady S, et al. Implementation of a socio-structural demonstration project to improve HIV outcomes among young Black men in the Deep South. *J Racial Ethn Health Disparities.* 2019;6(4):775–789.
104. Cunningham WE, Weiss RE, Nakazono T, et al. Effectiveness of a peer navigation intervention to sustain viral suppression among HIV-positive men and transgender women released from jail: the LINK LA Randomized Clinical Trial. *JAMA Intern Med.* 2018;178(4):542–553.
105. Hinman AR, Orenstein WA, Schuchat A. Vaccine-preventable diseases, immunizations, and the Epidemic Intelligence Service. *Am J Epidemiol.* 2011;174(11)(suppl):S16–S22.
106. Hill HA, Singleton JA, Yankey D, Elam-Evans LD, Pingali SC, Kang Y. Vaccination coverage by age 24 months among children born in 2015 and 2016—National Immunization Survey–Child, United States, 2016–2018. *MMWR Morb Mortal Wkly Rep.* 2019;68(41):913–918.
107. Seither R, McGill MT, Kriss JL, et al. Vaccination coverage with selected vaccines and exemption rates among children in kindergarten—United States, 2019–20 school year. *MMWR Morb Mortal Wkly Rep.* 2021;70(3):75–82.
108. Centers for Disease Control and Prevention. ChildVaxView. Updated November 3, 2017. Accessed March 31, 2022. https://www.cdc.gov/vaccines/imz-managers/coverage/childvaxview/index.html
109. Centers for Disease Control and Prevention. TeenVaxView. August 24, 2017. Accessed March 31, 2022. https://www.cdc.gov/vaccines/imz-managers/coverage/teenvaxview/index.html
110. Hill HA, Elam-Evans LD, Yankey D, Singleton JA, Kang Y. Vaccination coverage among children aged 19–35 months—United States, 2017. *MMWR Morb Mortal Wkly Rep.* 2018;67(40):1123–1128.
111. Bednarczyk RA, King AR, Lahijani A, Omer SB. Current landscape of nonmedical vaccination exemptions in the United States: impact of policy changes. *Expert Rev Vaccines.* 2019;18(2):175–190.
112. Dube E, Ward JK, Verger P, MacDonald NE. Vaccine hesitancy, acceptance, and anti-vaccination: trends and future prospects for public health. *Ann Rev Public Health.* 2021;42:175–191.
113. Kricorian K, Turner K. COVID-19 vaccine acceptance and beliefs among Black and Hispanic Americans. *PLoS One.* 2021;16(8):e0256122.
114. Ndugga N, Hill L, Artiga S, Haldar S. Latest data on COVID-19 vaccinations by race/ethnicity. Kaiser Family Foundation. 2022. Accessed March 31, 2022. https://www.kff.org/coronavirus-covid-19/issue-brief/latest-data-on-covid-19-vaccinations-by-race-ethnicity/
115. Centers for Disease Control and Prevention. *National Diabetes Statistics Report, 2017.* Centers for Disease Control and Prevention, US Department of Health and Human Services. 2017. Accessed July 26, 2019. https://www.cdc.gov/diabetes/data/statistics/statistics-report.html
116. Gerstein HC, Santaguida P, Raina P, et al. Annual incidence and relative risk of diabetes in people with various categories of dysglycemia: a systematic overview and meta-analysis of prospective studies. *Diabetes Res Clin Pract.* 2007;78(3):305–312.
117. Benoit SR, Hora I, Albright AL, Gregg EW. New directions in incidence and prevalence of diagnosed diabetes in the USA. *BMJ Open Diabetes Res Care.* 2019;7(1):e000657.
118. Spanakis EK, Golden SH. Race/ethnic difference in diabetes and diabetic complications. *Curr Diab Rep.* 2013;13(6):814–823.
119. Knowler WC, Barrett-Connor E, Fowler SE, et al. Reduction in the incidence of type 2 diabetes with lifestyle intervention or metformin. *New Engl J Med.* 2002;346(6):393–403.
120. Hinnant L, Razi S, Lewis R, et al. Evaluation of the Health Care Innovation Awards: community resource planning, prevention, and monitoring annual report 2015. Awardee-Level Findings. YMCA of the USA. October 2015. Accessed November 9, 2016. https://innovation.cms.gov/Files/reports/hcia-ymcadpp-evalrpt.pdf
121. Dunkley AJ, Bodicoat DH, Greaves CJ, et al. Diabetes prevention in the real world: effectiveness of pragmatic lifestyle interventions for the prevention of type 2 diabetes and of the impact of adherence to guideline recommendations: a systematic review and meta-analysis. *Diabetes Care.* 2014;37(4):922–933.
122. Mudaliar U, Zabetian A, Goodman M, et al. Cardiometabolic risk factor changes observed in diabetes prevention programs in US settings: a systematic review and meta-analysis. *PLoS Med.* 2016;13(7):e1002095.

123. Whittemore R. A systematic review of the translational research on the Diabetes Prevention Program. *Transl Behav Med.* 2011;1(3):480–491.
124. Jiang L, Johnson A, Pratte K, et al. Long-term outcomes of lifestyle intervention to prevent diabetes in American Indian and Alaska Native communities: the Special Diabetes Program for Indians Diabetes Prevention Program. *Diabetes Care.* 2018;41(7):1462–1470.
125. Centers for Disease Control and Prevention. Centers for Disease Control and Prevention Diabetes Prevention Recognition Program: standards and operating procedures. Centers for Disease Control and Prevention, US Department of Health and Human Services. March 1, 2018. Accessed June 24, 2019. https://www.cdc.gov/diabetes/prevention/pdf/dprp-standards.pdf
126. Ely EK, Gruss SM, Luman ET, et al. A National Effort to Prevent Type 2 Diabetes: Participant-Level Evaluation of CDC's National Diabetes Prevention Program. *Diabetes Care.* 2017;40(10):1331–1341.
127. Ritchie ND, Christoe-Frazier L, McFann KK, Havranek EP, Pereira RI. Effect of the National Diabetes Prevention Program on weight loss for English- and Spanish-speaking Latinos. *Am J Health Promot.* 2018;32(3):812–815.
128. Ritchie ND, Gritz RM. New Medicare diabetes prevention coverage may limit beneficiary access and widen health disparities. *Med Care.* 2018;56(11):908–911.
129. Yan A, Chen Z, Wang M, Mendez CE, Egede LE. Accessibility of Medicare diabetes prevention programs and variation by state, race, and ethnicity. *JAMA Netw Open.* 2021;4(10):e2128797.
130. Ritchie ND, Sauder KA, Gritz RM. Medicare Diabetes Prevention Program: where are the suppliers? *Am J Manag Care.* 2020;26(6):e198–e201.
131. Formagini T, Brooks JV, Jacobson LT, Roberts AW. Reimbursement Policies for Diabetes Prevention Program (DPP): implications for racial and ethnic health disparities. *Kans J Med.* 2021;14:234–237.
132. Larson NI, Story MT, Nelson MC. Neighborhood environments: disparities in access to healthy foods in the U.S. *Am J Prev Med.* 2009;36(1):74–81.
133. Ritchie ND, Baucom KJW, Sauder KA. Current perspectives on the impact of the national Diabetes Prevention Program: building on successes and overcoming challenges. *Diabetes Metab Syndr Obes.* 2020;13:2949–2957.
134. Savage LC, Sanghavi D. The Medicare Diabetes Prevention Program: why hasn't its promise been fulfilled? 2021. Accessed March 31, 2022. https://www.healthaffairs.org/do/10.1377/forefront.20211118.578433
135. Gaias LM, Arnold KT, Liu FF, Pullmann MD, Duong MT, Lyon AR. Adapting Strategies to Promote Implementation Reach and Equity (ASPIRE) in school mental health services. *Psychology Sch.* 2022;59(12):2471–2485.

26

Implementation Science in the Global Context

Novel Applications and Bidirectional Opportunities

ELVIN H. GENG, MOSA MOSHABELA, AND OLAKUNLE ALONGE

INTRODUCTION: OPPORTUNITIES FOR IMPLEMENTATION SCIENCE IN GLOBAL CONTEXT

The growth of implementation research globally has created two synergistic opportunities. First, over the last 30 years, national health systems in many lower- and middle-income countries (LMICs) have grown markedly[1] and now have much stronger basic health system capabilities (e.g., workforce, infrastructure, essential commodities) than even a few decades ago. These foundations imply that the primary focus for public health and healthcare has grown from building health systems to now include design and use of implementation strategies—or the planned, purposeful activities to enhance use of evidence-based interventions (EBIs). At the same time, these emerging health systems continue to have gaps that both constrain and shape strategies for implementation. At present, for example, most countries procure essential diagnostics, medications, and other health commodities, but they have national supply chains that are not rapid and consistent and often fail to reach the "last mile" to populations in need. Likewise, most LMICs have expanding training programs for healthcare workers (HCWs), but the right skill mix, adequate management, acceptable renumeration (particularly in a global labor market), and quality of services remain challenges. The development of health systems, in short, both enables and constrains implementation and, by implication, shapes issues for implementation science.

The growth of implementation research globally, however, also presents a complementary opportunity, which is to use the global context to grow the maturing corpus of methods and perspectives in the field of implementation science itself. Even though the field continues to evolve, certain ideas are increasingly recognized as anchoring the field. Conceptualizing activities to implement systematically as *implementation strategies* has facilitated their categorization, identification of effects, and further scrutiny of their mechanisms.[2,3] Another core concept in implementation research is *implementation outcomes*—the immediate effects of implementation strategies such as appropriateness and acceptability.[2] In addition, a host of frameworks and theories (e.g., normalization process theory, the Consolidated Framework for Implementation Research [CFIR]) offer shared hermeneutical or interpretative scaffolding that enables a coherent scientific discourse.[4–6] These ideas (and others) now undergird dedicated scientific journals, academic and practice meetings, textbooks, proposed competencies, as well as academic departments.[4] How does this current body of ideas stand up where health systems as well as larger socioeconomic settings differ markedly? Use of ideas from implementation science in a global context has and will continue to confront contextual variation that can potentially broaden considerations and provoke insights. To be concrete, the per capita number of physicians is 6.5 per 1,000 in France, but 0.83 in Peru and 0.04 in Malawi.[7] Examining the implementation of EBIs in these vastly different settings will help the field to "pressure

Elvin H. Geng, Mosa Moshabela, and Olakunle Alonge, *Implementation Science in the Global Context* In: *Dissemination and Implementation Research in Health.* Edited by: Ross C. Brownson, Graham A. Colditz, and Enola K. Proctor, Oxford University Press. © Oxford University Press 2023.
DOI: 10.1093/oso/9780197660690.003.0026

test" and revisit, reinvent, retire, or reify certain concepts and perspectives and holds the promise of strengthening the field.

In this chapter we attempt to advance both application of emerging knowledge in a global context and reflect on considerations in these global contexts for implementation science. To do so, we illustrate potential contributions of implementation science to applied problems in global settings. To keep the health systems front and center, we use an adaptation of the World Health Organization Health System Building Blocks (HSBB) framework[8] as an organizing lens. We also describe key strategies used to address implementation in a global context and how these strategies can optimize services within health system constraints. Finally, we also call attention to opportunities for problems in global settings to provoke insights about implementation. The chapter seeks to present implementation science in the global context as a dialectic that advances both applied and methodological insights in both LMICs as well as HIC (i.e., globally).

RISING GLOBAL WEALTH AND HEALTH AS THE OUTER CONTEXT

The past 30 years have been marked by both rising wealth and improving health around the world, even if progress has been uneven. In 1978, governments from around the world gathered to plan the future of the health sector; this led to the Alma Ata Declaration,[9] a call for universal primary care as an explicit goal for governments everywhere.[10] The need for a system that provides basic health services for all calls for investments in the foundational pillars of a health system: developing the workforce, procuring essential medications, providing buildings and infrastructures, and providing insurance and financing, among others. Universal primary care is also a firm foundation for a science of implementation of specific EBIs.

While not the only factor, rising wealth has fueled the growth of health services and improved health over the last 30 years. Using World Bank classifications, of 51 countries classified as low income in 1990 (gross national income [GNI] of less than $610 per capita), 25 had risen to lower-middle income status by 2020 (i.e., $1,006 to $3,975 per capita), and 4 became upper-middle income countries (i.e., $3,976 to $12,275 per capita). Overall in 1990, there were 39 countries classified as high income, while by 2020, there were 80 countries classified as high income. Conversely, 51 countries were lower income in 1990, but that number fell to 27 by 2020 (Figure 26.1).

During the last 30 years, however, governmental investments in health have in general grown faster than income. A landmark 1993 World Bank analysis suggested that health itself increases wealth (rather than that wealth begets health), which stimulated financing for the health sector.[11] Overall, national health budgets in LMICS grew approximately 30% faster than total rise in incomes.[12] Donor and development aid targeting health has also expanded, rising from $1 to $40 billion a year between 1990 and 2010. While donor funding represents a small fraction of health spending globally, it plays an important role in some countries and for some disease conditions. For instance, donor funding made up 27% of all health expenditures in countries classified as lower income in 2020. Up to half of national health budgets in some countries supported by the US President's Emergency Fund for AIDS Relief (PEPFAR) come from donor HIV programs. In Zambia, approximately 50% of the overall $400 million health budget in 2020 came from the PEPFAR.[13]

These investments in health have yielded dividends. According to the World Bank, life expectancy in Peru has risen by 10 years and in Kenya by 9 years (compared to 4 years in the United States) over the last 30 years. This optimism is reflected in the 2018 Lancet Global Health Commission projection that by 2035 the world could see a "Grand Convergence"[14] where important indicators of health (e.g., under 5 mortality, maternal mortality, deaths from infectious diseases) could reach similar levels between HICs and LMICs even without a broader convergence of wealth globally.[15]

Nevertheless, even as progress overall has been clear, disparities within LMICs have become a growing concern. While on average life expectancy has grown by 10 years in much of Africa and Asia over the last 30 years, the growth has been far lower among the poorest 10%, where it has remained stagnant.[16] Furthermore, whether progress in population health will be resilient enough to

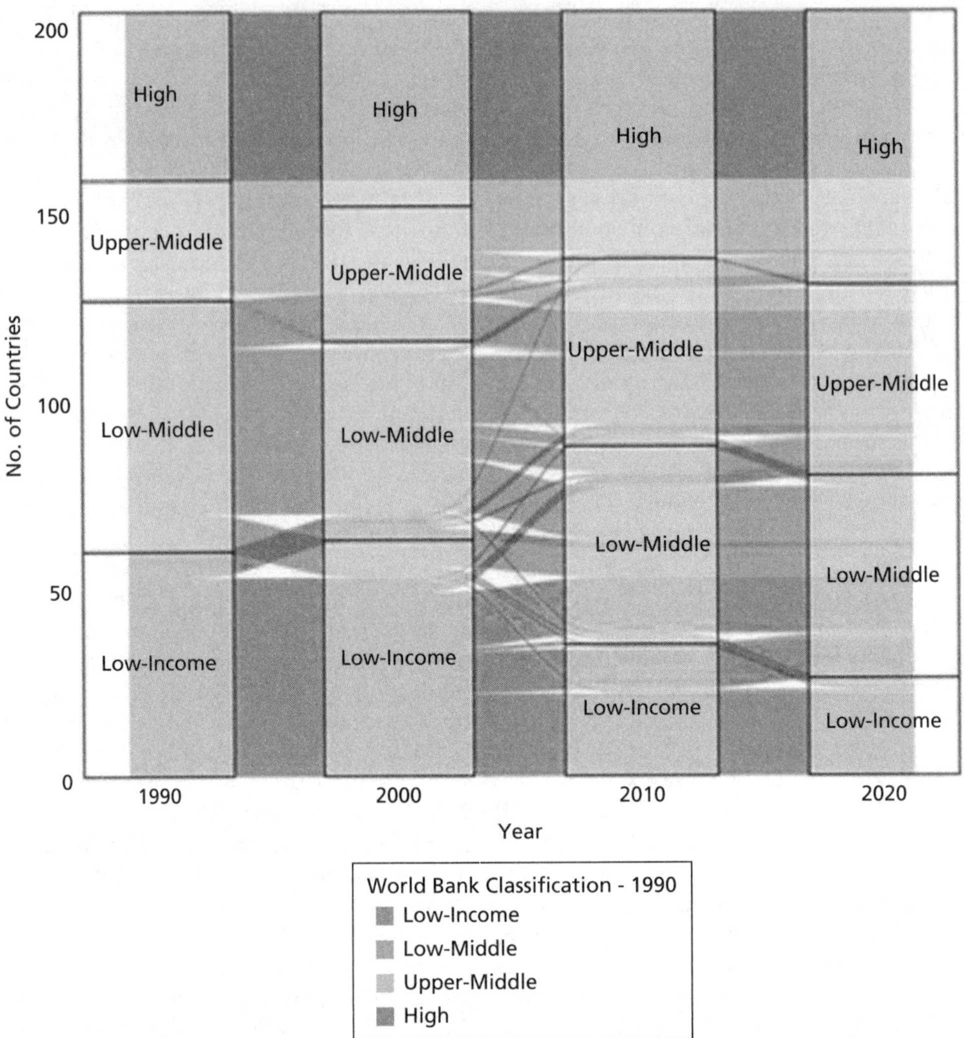

FIGURE 26.1 Alluvial plot showing classification of countries by World Bank income level using the atlas method. Income thresholds for income classifications were not static over time in this method. Countries qualified as "low income" in 1990 if per capita income was less than $610 per year, whereas the threshold for low income was $1,045 per year in 2020. Overall, the total proportion of countries in the low income and lower middle categories fell, while countries in the upper middle and high categories rose.

Image credit: Aaloke Mody, MD.

continue in the face of a global COVID-19 pandemic remains to be seen. Recent estimates suggested that disruptions to tuberculosis (TB) programs due to COVID-19 could result in as many as 20 million additional lives lost over the coming 10 years.[17] The COVID-19 pandemic has also driven 500 million persons into dire poverty, which has predictable effects on health. A final assessment of whether the world has the political will to both address COVID-19 itself (including vaccines and emerging treatments) and secure progress to date across a range of health conditions remains to be seen.

HEALTH SYSTEMS AS THE IMMEDIATE CONTEXT FOR IMPLEMENTATION

The growth of health systems around the world has now made the purposeful, coordinated, organized activities—implementation—increasing the center of attention in public health and global health sciences. After all, if no health systems are present, there are no mechanisms with which to implement most EBIs. But the presence of health system capabilities does not automatically imply effective, equitable, sustainable utilization of EBIs. Health system capabilities (and their gaps in any particular setting) can be used as a lens to organize fundamental constraints imposed by health systems on implementation strategies and their acceptability, appropriateness, fit, and effects. Our discussion of implementation science in the global context therefore begins with a grounding in the immediate context of implementation: health systems in LMICs.

We use an adapted version of the WHO HSBB framework (Table 26.1) as a heuristic for linking implementation strategies to health syste4ms—something that current frameworks touch on, but do not center. The WHO defines a health system as "all the organizations, institutions, resources and people whose primary purpose is to improve health,"[18(pvi)] and the HSBB framework conceives of this system as composed of six domains (Table 26.1): service delivery, workforce, essential medications, information systems, financing, and governance.[18] To address criticisms[19,20] that the original framework lacked a community pillar, we place communities at the center (Figure 26.2). We see implementation as the activities that link a health system to people and communities.

TABLE 26.1 FOUNDATIONS OF IMPLEMENTATION STRATEGIES LINKED WITH WHO HEALTH SYSTEMS BUILDING BLOCKS[a]

Building Block	Description	Potential Measures
Service delivery infrastructure	Health care infrastructure; models and architecture of the delivery system	• Number and distribution of health facilities per 10,000 population • General service readiness score for health facilities • Health facility assessments • Proportion of health facilities offering specific services • Number and distribution of health facilities offering specific services per 10,000 population
Human resources for health	Number and quality of workforce; performance	• Number of health workers per 10,000 population • Distribution of health workers by occupation/ specialization, region, place of work and sex
Information systems	Surveillance; health records; reporting	• Monitoring of key vital statistics • Extent of electronic medical records
Product, vaccine, medications, technologies	Present availability and affordability of goods and services	• Average availability of 14 selected essential medicines in public and private health facilities • Median consumer price ratio of 14 selected essential medicines in public and private health facilities
Financing	National financing; insurance and social protections; costs	• General government expenditure on health as a proportion of general government expenditure (GGHE/GGE) • The ratio of household out-of-pocket payments for health to total expenditure on health
Leadership and governance	Oversight and regulation of health system at regional and local levels	• Rules based: ownership arrangements, decentralization, stakeholder participation, • Existence of an up-to-date national health strategy linked to national needs and priorities • Existence of key health sector documents that are disseminated regularly (e.g., budget documents, annual performance reviews and health indicators)

[a]Adapted with permission World Health Organization. Everybody's Business: Strengthening Health Systems to Improve Health Outcomes, WHO's Framework for Action; 2007.

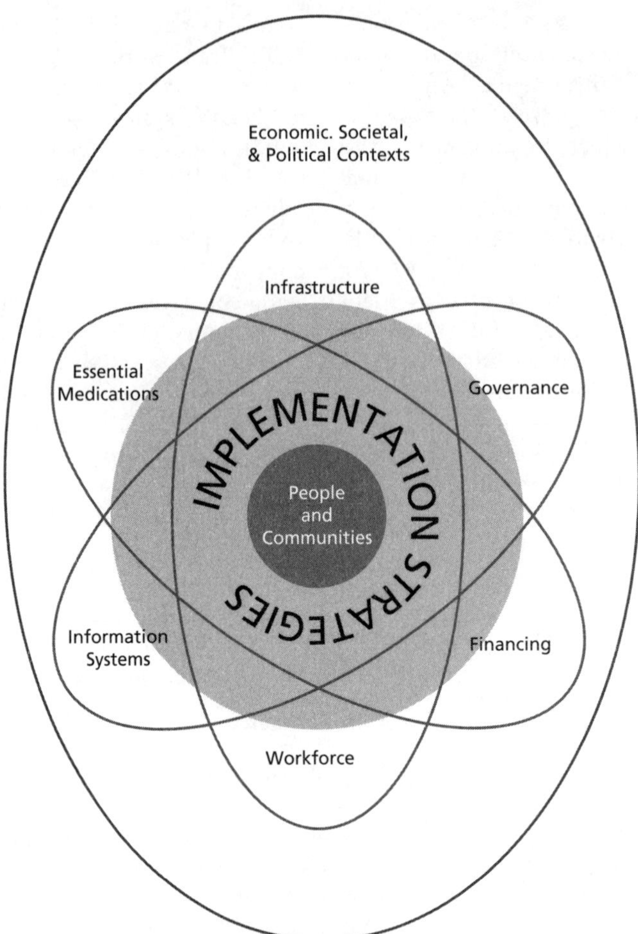

FIGURE 26.2 The "atomic" framework places implementation strategies within health systems building blocks, which act as the local set of constraints that both determine which strategies are relevant as well as influence their effects. HSBB gaps take on different configurations in different locations, implying that context is variable. By extension, this implies that appropriate implementation strategies differ across settings. This figure also places implementation strategies between systems and communities, indicating that strategies are the means by which structures can be translated into services and eventually health benefits for populations. The largest circle is the economic, societal, and political context, including investments in health, which generate the local HSBB.

Implementation efforts optimize services within those constraints.

Health System Building Blocks determine the potential utility and effects of any given implementation strategy. For example, the shortage of HCWs (workforce pillar) is an acute issue in many LMICs across Africa, South America, and Asia, and this constraint defines usability and utility of any particular implementation strategy. In 2019, Norway had 4.4 doctors per 1,000 persons, while Rwanda had 0.1, Laos 0.2, and Kenya 0.4,[15] which drives strategies. In a study on maternal child health in Zambia, researchers documented that women avoided facility delivery (an EBI championed in global health) because staffing shortfalls mean the only birth attendant at the facility was male, which women in the community found unacceptable.[21] In this setting, the constraints created by an inadequate workforce mean that strategies to improve HCW performance (e.g., "audit and feedback") might be less helpful than methods to increase staffing through "task shifting" or use of female community health workers. The effects of HSBB configuration on prioritization of strategies are often more subtle than in this example, but in principle similar.

Conceptualizing implementation strategies between HSBB (the immediate context) and communities or people (the target) also helps to bound implementation research. In this conceptual schema, research on approaches to improving the HSBB themselves (e.g., labor market for HCWs) falls into the category of health systems research (Figure 26.1). On the other hand, research on populations and communities that is unlike from health systems fits poorly with this conceptualization of implementation research. For example, much research on malaria is centered in LMIC settings where the prevalence of malaria is highest, but the efficacy or effectiveness of bed nets in the abstract, outside of any delivery or engagement approaches, does not in and of itself inform implementation.

The emphasis on HSBB also cautions against research meant to inform implementation strategies that are disconnected from health systems gaps. For example, directly observed therapy, which has been widely used for TB treatment (in which a HCW observes the patient swallowing a pill) was tested for HIV treatment in Africa in several randomized trials. While yielding an effect in studies, the prospect of directly observed therapy for the millions of persons on HIV treatment in Africa is misaligned with the crises in HCWs. Of note, implementation researchers in HICs have also called for greater attention to health systems and structures in studies of implementation.[22]

APPLICATION OF IMPLEMENTATION SCIENCE IN THE GLOBAL CONTEXT

Implementation research's focus on strategies to advance use of EBIs in the global context complements and leverages the existing research discourses. First, a large body of research to improve health in global contexts has focused on the major economic, social, and policy drivers of health, seeking primarily to inform policymakers. This work seeks to examine cross-country burden of disease (e.g., work from the Institute for Health Metrics and Evaluation) or macroscopic drivers of health systems[23] and comprises the core of "global health competencies." While understanding these macroscopic issues are absolutely necessary, implementation science's focus on strategies to use interventions force us to systematically examine the behavior of health systems vis-à-vis a particular intervention. A second thread in global health has also focused on efficacy of interventions that address high-burden issues in global contexts but has limited consideration of how these interventions should be used. A Cochrane review identified only three methods of distribution and use, specifically whether people were given insecticide-treated bed nets free or could buy them at a subsidized price or full market price.[24] To date, few studies on community engagement, social marketing, social networks, social influence, or other methods of adherence counseling, monitoring, or other methods have been done. Advancing the distribution, adoption, and sustained use of bed nets is an area ripe for implementation science. Finally, much operations research in the global context is focused on the performance of a particular program or setting. As Remme and colleagues suggested, implementation science seeks to create generalizable insights and can complement existing operations research.

Implementation science can help advance health research by providing theories and frameworks for understanding the implementation problem systematically. The Theoretical Domains Framework maps out drivers of HCW behavior that have been broadly applied in HICs but which present opportunities in LMICs as well. Efforts to design health promotion, such as the PRECEDE (*p*redisposing, *r*einforcing, and *e*nabling *c*onstructs in *e*ducational/*e*cological *d*iagnosis and *e*valuation) PROCEDE (*p*olicy, *r*egulatory, and *o*rganizational *c*onstructs in *e*ducation and *e*nvironmental *d*evelopment) model or intervention mapping are broadly resonant in LMICs, with principles that are particularly relevant when stakeholder engagement is important. In addition, the notion that change is driven by mutually reinforcing "predisposing, enabling, and reinforcing" factors is widely applicable where multiple barriers to health system performance may require redress across several domains. For example, this framework was used to design a multicomponent strategy that increased the rate of HIV treatment initiation by threefold in a stepped-wedge cluster randomized trial in western Uganda. Frameworks such as RE-AIM (Reach, Effectiveness, Adoption, Implementation, and Maintenance; which can help shape evaluation questions) have made explicit that efficacy is not sufficient. SMS messages to HCWs to influence clinical behavior, for example, may have a far smaller effect than practice facilitation, but have the potential to touch far more HCWs (given the ubiquity of cell networks and the fact that HCWs almost invariably have cell phones) and cost less than organizing, delivering, and monitoring practice facilitation. Frameworks in implementation research help bring systematic consideration of context as well as multilevel considerations regarding health systems into view when considering an EBI. This is an especially important consideration in settings where the constraints imposed by the outer setting on the inner (as depicted in the CFIR), and in turn by the inner on the implementation processes, are so prominent. Central constructs in implementation science (e.g., CFIR) call attention to a systematic understanding of what works, how to consider the role of strategies, and how to call out problems as well as insights.

IMPLEMENTATION STRATEGIES IN A GLOBAL CONTEXT

The growth of implementation science in the global context has also been accompanied by awareness that strategies of high relevance in LMICs may be distinct from those in HICs (see chapter 6). For example, in HICs, practice facilitation and audit and feedback are prevalent methods, but in the global context gaps in HSBBs may make these strategies useful in fewer settings while other strategies may take on more importance. In addition, while we treat existing taxonomies of strategies (e.g., Expert Recommendations for Implementing Change [ERIC],[25] Effective Practice and Organization of Care [EPOC],[26] or others) as general guides on how to group strategies whenever possible in order to avoid unneeded duplication of categories, we also recognize the diversity of strategies used in the global context, even if not formalized in current taxonomies, that represent a wide array of activities that can be formalized and bounded. In this chapter, we present a nonsystematic summary of implementation strategies that are prevalent in LMICs and organize them according to the HSBB gaps within which they seek to optimize service delivery (Figure 26.2).

Implementation Strategies to Overcome Workforce Shortages

Overall, both absolute shortages of HCWs and misalignment of skills with population health needs are widespread in LMICs (as well as in many HIC settings). Estimates suggest that there will be a global shortage of 15 million HCWs in 2030.[27] Kenya, for example, has 160 operating orthopedic surgeons in the country (communication from Kenya Medical Research Institute 2022). The workforce shortage is exacerbated by "brain drain" from LMICs: Some studies suggest that 10% of physicians trained in Africa, South Asia, and the Caribbean work in Europe, North America, or Australia.[28] Similar estimates suggest that in many countries in Africa more than 20% of all nurses trained in Africa work outside of the African continent.[29] Simultaneously, tasks that are assigned to HCWs specific cadres may not match the labor needs. Even in Latin America, where most countries have a larger healthcare and public health workforce, significant skills-needs imbalances persist (e.g., by specialty, geography). Some donor programs have emphasized training (e.g., PEPFAR),[30] and clinical and professional education has become a top policy concern.

Even as efforts to build the healthcare labor force grow, innovative implementation strategies have emerged to optimize reach, quality, quantity, and services within these constraints—strategies highlighted in this section (Table 26.2). One approach to optimization in many settings is to fine-tune the alignment between the available healthcare workforce and the tasks needed to deliver health services. This can be done through delegating tasks traditionally reserved for doctors to nurses (or from nurses to other cadres) when the original cadres are in limited supply. Task shifting has been endorsed by one of the major policy summits,[31] which has called for creation of policies and mechanisms to optimize skills-needs mix. A related set of strategies creates roles for lay workers to offset labor deficits. Community health workers are individuals who often lack formal training in healthcare but leverage knowledge of local social and geographical information to advance the delivery of services. Community health workers have been studied in HIV service delivery,[32] treatment for mental health,[33] maternal child health,[34] and even surgical specialties[35] and in general have

TABLE 26.2 NONSYSTEMATIC COLLECTION OF IMPLEMENTATION STRATEGIES USED IN MANY LOWER- AND MIDDLE-INCOME COUNTRIES AND REGIONS[a]

Implementation Strategies Under Workforce Constraints			
Strategy and Description	Rationale	Evidence for Strategy	Research Questions
Strategy: Role revision and task shifting/sharing. **Description**: Task shifting is the rational redistribution of tasks among healthcare teams to better match workforce activities with population health needs. Often tasks are shifted from more trained healthcare workers (who are fewer in number) to those with less training.	• Shortages of higher-trained cadres make task shifting a common approach to increase workforce efficiency. • Adjustment of tasks can optimize the fit between skills available and tasks needed for population health. • By reorganizing the workforce, task shifting can make more efficient use of existing human resources.	• Task shifting is been supported by high-level policy initiatives (e.g., in the Addis Ababa Declaration) • Empirical studies in Asia, Africa, and South America suggest redistribution of tasks lead to equivalent clinical outcomes for many conditions.[2] • For example, in Mozambique, assistant medical officers produced surgical outcomes similar to those of physicians.[35] • In Uganda, nonphysician clinicians and physicians agreed in HIV/AIDS patient assessments of clinical stage, risk for TB, and treatment.[36]	• Not all data support effectiveness. Some studies of task shifting did not produce anticipated effects (including in a cluster randomized trial in South Africa, which trained nurses to prescribe HIV treatment, but initiations did not increase). • Although high-level policy declarations call for governments to create an enabling policy environment for training and accreditation, research is needed to identify how to revise roles and shift tasks and measure effects.
Strategy: Incorporation of informal or lay workers into service delivery. **Description**: Often, persons without official or professional degrees are hired by the health system to carry out both facility-based and community-based tasks, including • Patient follow-up, • Administrative tasks, and • Less technical activities that do not require specialized training.	• Including lay health workers in the health system when the formal healthcare workforce is limited can extend a region's services through two mechanisms: • A given budget can be extended reach because general lay health workers are less costly than doctors, nurses, and pharmacists. • Community-based lay health workers have particular social and geographic knowledge that enables engagement with populations more effectively in some cases.	• Evidence to date suggest equivalent outcomes in many settings between lay and traditional cadres. • A study in Kenya found no clinical differences between clinic-based and community-based treatment for people living with HIV/AIDS with digital decision support.[32] • Mental health has made use of lay health workers with positive effects.[37] • A Cochrane review of 50 studies found CHWs improved immunizations and screening.[38]	• More data on acceptability and quality may be needed. • In a recent trial of community-based HIV treatment initiation in Swaziland, nearly half of patients reported they did not "trust" healthcare workers, [41] and a choice experiment in Kenya suggested that patients prefer professionals to lay healthcare workers,[42] all else being equal. • Evidence about the specific tasks LHWs can contribute most to is needed.[38]

(continued)

TABLE 26.2 CONTINUED

Implementation Strategies Under Workforce Constraints

Strategy and Description	Rationale	Evidence for Strategy	Research Questions
		• A meta-analysis from Bangladesh, India, Nepal, Pakistan, the Philippines, and Tanzania demonstrated CHW reduced pneumonia-specific mortality by 36% in children.[39,40]	
Strategy: Crowdsourcing design of health services. **Description**: Drawing the public and end users into design and delivery of services.	• Drawing from sociology as well as modern design thinking, the notion that communities contain wisdom for solving problems has become well established. • Approaches bring laypersons or end users into the creation of services (to enhance appropriateness and acceptability) or delivery of services (to extend reach and efficiency). • These approaches may have particular promise for health services targeting groups that are outside of the mainstream and who may be marginalized.	• Crowdsourcing has been found in randomized trials to be effective in a range of activities from promoting HIV prevention to HIV and STI testing in China and Nigeria.[43] • Offering incentives for community members to identify and refer individuals with chronic cough in a randomized trial led to rises in TB diagnoses.[44] • "Treatment observatories" are the systematic and regular collection of quantitative data across the HIV prevention, care, and treatment cascade in HIV by persons living with HIV, thus making monitoring a public or crowdsourced activity	• At what stage and how to use different segments of communities remain research questions. • How to adjudicate in a balanced way the perspectives of different segments of the "crowd" remain active topics of investigation.

Implementation Strategies Under Infrastructural Constraints			
Strategy and Description	Rationale	Evidence and Research Examples	Issues and Questions
Strategy: Creating mobile or community-based service delivery points. **Description**: In order to reach a greater percentage of particularly rural populations, programs have tested and deployed nontraditional means of delivery of a range of services outside of traditional facility-based mechanisms using, for example, mobile vans, community pharmacies, or community-based patient groups.	• When the reach of existing infrastructure is limited and larger investments to build additional facilities are not available, mobile health units or temporary community-based service and drug delivery sites are used in some settings.	• A wide swath of literature examines these models. Patients receiving HIV treatment in Africa who visited community drug distribution points for refills exhibited excellent retention. • Community-based hypertension and diabetes management have been attempted in many settings,[45] including in Mexico[46,47]	• Quality of services remains a concern for community-based service delivery. • The costs of community-based services may also be high. • Integration of different chronic conditions remains a challenge. For example, the recent effort to push HIV therapy into the community complicates efforts to layer on new services such as hypertension screening.
Strategy: Differentiated services delivery (DSD). **Description**: These methods alter the timing, frequency, nature, and location of interactions with the health facility in order to minimize opportunity costs for patients receiving chronic care.	• DSD models grew out of early scale-up in HIV services that were based on standardized visit intervals at high-volume facilities. • In order to treat the number of people needing ART, DSD models were developed to allow stable patients fewer visits and sicker patients access to acute care.	• Community adherence groups were originally described in Mozambique,[48] where individuals in a group take turns picking up medications at the facility and distributing them to others in the community. • Other models include community drug distribution points where a mobile pharmacy visits certain locations at given time intervals. • In fast-track models, the facility prepares medication refills ahead of time, allowing patients to pick up medicines more quickly.	• Research on the right mix of differentiated service delivery options in a region are needed.

(continued)

TABLE 26.2 CONTINUED

Implementation Strategies Under Infrastructural Constraints			
Strategy and Description	Rationale	Evidence and Research Examples	Issues and Questions
		• Urban adherence groups bring relatively large numbers of people into monthly meetings to pick up medicines and for social and/or instrumental support. Such services have been most widely used for HIV, but are also being tested for noncommunicable disease, TB, childhood diseases, and primary care.	
Strategy: Incorporation of informal health sector into the formal health sector. **Description**: Incorporating traditional and religious healers into health systems to serve as connection or access points for patients.	• In many countries, traditional healers remain the first point of contact for many rural populations. • Increasingly, the policy environment seeks to include rather than exclude traditional healers. • Recent implementation strategies seek to leverage the connections they have with the communities to extend healthcare, effectively expanding the reach of the health system automatically.	• In a trial in a district of Uganda, Sundararajan et al. found that the offer of HIV testing by traditional healers increased HIV testing markedly.[49]	• These approaches face policy barriers, with some perspectives that nontraditional healers should be kept out of the formal medical sector because of their adherence to non-evidence-based treatments.

Implementation Strategies Where Livelihood Demands and Limited Financial Protections Are Prominent			
Strategy and Description Rationale	Rationale	Selected Evidence	Outstanding Issues
Strategy: Pay-it-forward mechanisms[50] **Description**: People who are helped or supported will in turn help or support someone else who they don't necessarily know. • People are contacted when a community-based organization or agency offers to pay voluntarily for a needed service. • After receipt of the service people are asked to donate into a pool to allow others to also receive the service.	• Approach is based on the observation that people tend to have a "reflex" for reciprocity, originally shown by experiments where tips increased after a waiter gave "free" mints to customers.[51] • Used to mobilize individual resources for preventive healthcare in middle-income countries where individuals have access to preventive health services but are unlikely to pay out of pocket. • Payments for services can be sustained even though individuals will often not pay for the services themselves, and norms related to services may also be altered.	• To increase STI testing for MSM in China, men were told that someone from a community-based organization paid for them to get a free STI test, and testing increased from 18% to 56%. In addition, when those receiving testing were asked to pay into the system, 95% agreed, and they agreed to pay 36% of the costs of a subsequent test.[52]	• Theoretical issues in the social and psychological mechanisms remain unknown.[50]
Strategy: Economic incentives conditional on receipt of a health service. **Description**: Conditional cash transfers (CCTs) for completion of a health-related behavior [53] are the most common, but food or other goods in lieu of cash as well as lotteries are related strategies.	CCTs aim to alleviate intergenerational poverty while also addressing challenges that contribute to poverty in the present. • One tactic is to change the price point of an activity (making a clinic visit that has $10 of opportunity costs less attractive than making a clinic visit where a CCT reduces the opportunity costs) or by acting on intertemporal inconsistency, where people intend to go to medical care but defer or delay it, often indefinitely, because other more immediate needs prevail.	• When costs are a barrier, conditional cash has been found to have effects on HIV testing and retrieval of HIV test results; adherence to HIV medications; retention; and viral load; as well as other health-related behaviors. • In Tanzania, a randomized trial of CCT for appointment adherence after starting HIV treatment improved retention and suppression by 10% at 6 months after starting HIV treatment.[54]	• While in some settings CCTs have been widely adopted, including for consistent healthcare in Mexico as well as for making clinic appointments in Brazil; they have also been criticized as unrealistic or inequitable if given for one condition (e.g., HIV). • Are incentives of food instead of cash equally effective?

(continued)

TABLE 26.2 CONTINUED

Implementation Strategies to Bolster Governance and Management			
Strategy	Rationale	Evidence	Discussion
Strategy: Community or stakeholder oversight for use of EBIs. **Description**: Making healthcare performance data available to community oversight boards. • Health facility committees give healthcare workers or community representatives the ability to collect, review, and respond to patient grievances and also provide feedback to communities.[55]	• In addition to empowering community members to take action, making activities at health facilities visible—something that is normally opaque—may increase the motivation and responsiveness of healthcare workers, who might not only exert more effort but also undertake activities to improve a range of activities, including patient processes and flow.	• Many of these are covered in an excellent review by Baptise et al.[56] • In an important paper from Uganda, which was widely heralded but not replicated, a community oversight board was created, quality oversight meetings were held, and under 5 mortality was reduced by 33%.[57] • A separate cluster-randomized trial in Malawi found that Community Score Cards increased service utilization across several domains.[58,59]	• Research is needed on how to incorporate community oversight into health systems, as well as enhancing measurement approaches.
Strategy: Performance-based financing (PBF) focused on use of EBIs. **Description**: One approach used to advance EBIs is to use payment dependent on performance or use of evidence-based practice. Payment is sometimes targeting facilities, but is also used to supplement salaries of healthcare workers in LMICs.	• Recent years have seen an ascendancy of market-based approaches in public health. These approaches assume that some of the mechanisms that promote drug competition in the marketplace can also enhance performance in the public sector.	• A randomized trial impact evaluation conducted in Rwanda in parallel with a national performance-based financing rollout for maternal child health found 23% increased institutional deliveries as well as an overall increase in the quality of care.[57,60] • A similar evaluation in Burundi found an increase of 22% in facility deliveries. • Research suggests that reputational incentives, rather than payment, can motivate health services in Zambia.[61]	• Questions remain about the mechanisms of performance-based financing. • They have not worked in all settings but remain an important implementation strategy where management and governance are weak.

Strategy: Enhancing organizational function through management training and systems improvement. **Description**: A set of management practices that standardize processes and structure to reduce variation in performance, achieve predictable results, and improve outcomes for patients. • Usually based on specific metrics of performance as well as a suite of improvement techniques. • Closely aligned with quality improvement, practice facilitation, or coaching, they have been widely used to enhance the use of EBIs in LMICs.	• The delivery of healthcare is a complicated task but one that in some cases requires consistency for high quality. • Some of the managerial approaches used for manufacturing have been applied to healthcare delivery in a variety of settings to improve systems performance.	• Quality improvement methods based on performance data, application of root cause analyses (using tools such as fishbone diagrams), and small tests of change have been widely used in many settings and have been applied with LMICs to improve maternal child health, malaria treatment, HIV testing, and other programs.[62] • In a three-country cluster randomized trial, the system analysis and improvement approach (SAIA) reduced drop-offs in the Prevent Mother-to-Child Transmission (PMTCT) cascade and improved HIV early infant diagnosis and HIV treatment in Kenya and in Mozambique.[63]	• Data on the conditions needed to implement quality improvement program successfully are needed. • Quality improvement may have effects on systems performance outside of the specific metrics targeted, and research into such effects is warranted.

(continued)

TABLE 26.2 CONTINUED

Information and Technology			
Strategy	Rationale	Evidence	Questions
Strategy: Digital decision support to advance use of EBIs. **Description**: SMS messages to target patient behavior can support EBIs, including prevention, testing, and treatment adherence. Messages can also be delivered to HCWs to advance engagement, training, and decision support.	• Many healthcare workers operate in lower-level health facilities where contact with continuing medical education as well as other healthcare workers is limited, and therefore the spread of new practices or decision support is limited. • Patient access to specialists or higher-level facilities is often very attenuated, and many lower-level health delivery points of services are inconstantly connected by internet or other digital connections.	• SMS messages have been used to enhance HIV treatment in Uganda and in randomized trials have improved both measures of adherence to HIV medications as well as clinical outcomes such as viral load. • To enhance guideline-concordant malaria treatment in Kenya, a cluster randomized trial successfully provided decision support.[64]	• Debate exists about the mechanisms of effect, but some see it acting through reminders (e.g., a cue to action), as well as creating a sense of connectivity and care with the facility, through encouragement and relationship building.
Strategy: Automated or semiautomated digital communication and engagement in services. **Description**: The widespread adoption and familiarity across many populations with mobile technology and corresponding applications allow people to engage with health and public health systems conveniently as they live their lives.	• The recent COVID-19 pandemic has highlighted the ways in which technology can magnify traditional public health activities. • Contact tracing, quarantine, and isolation are well-established means of controlling infectious diseases, such as HIV, STIs, and tuberculosis, and were ripe for digital engagement strategies. • The ubiquity of cell phone and mobility data has allowed contacts to be identified nearly instantly at scale.	• SMS messages as appointment reminder use a light touch and are widely used, including at some level of scale for maternal child health in South Africa (e.g., MomConnect); Kenya (e.g., Ushauari); and many countries in Asia and Latin America. • During the pandemic many of these technologies were used to accelerate contact tracing and case identification, particularly in Korea, Taiwan, and other locations in Asia.[65]	• While such technological solutions require societal buy-in not feasible in many Western counties, other settings, including democratic societies, implemented such technology-based solutions.

[a]The strategies are organized by the WHO Health Systems Building Blocks (e.g., workforce, infrastructure, governance), which create the constraints that define the relevance of implementation strategies as well as their effects in advancing the use of EBIs. The table describes each strategy, its rationale, and contains some notes on evidence and pending research questions.

been found to deliver comparable quality of care when adequately trained, supervised, and enumerated.

Further innovations to optimize efforts in support of health services are to engage the public or specific communities in service delivery. Innovative studies have demonstrated that people who have more contact with the health system can often be used to extend the reach of the health system into their social networks. In Pakistan, a study incentivizing members of the community to identify individuals with chronic cough successfully increased diagnosis of tuberculosis.[66] Crowdsourcing using open competitions and other methods have been shown to improve design and uptake of sexually transmitted infection (STI) testing, HIV testing, and vaccination efforts in research from Asia and Africa.[67] The advent of HIV self-testing technology, for example, created possibilities in this regard. Several studies sought to understand whether sex workers could distribute HIV tests to partners and other sex workers in their social networks[68] or pregnant women who are accessing antenatal care would deliver self-test kits to their male partners who were not in contact with the health system.[69] In each of these settings, HIV testing rates improved.

Research questions around optimization of the workforce remain. Not all studies of task sharing or shifting demonstrate anticipated effects on increasing service delivery. A trial in South Africa to demonstrate that training nurses to prescribe HIV medication would increase the number of patients started on treatment found no such effect even though nurses were successfully trained.[70] In a recent randomized trial where individuals were offered HIV treatment initiation in the community, a substantial fraction of patients refused, citing they did not "trust" the lay HCWs.[70] Discrete choice experiments in Kenya have found that even though patients would like to minimize contact with the health system, all things being equal they would rather interact with professional HCWs than with lay HCWs.[71]

Strategies Addressing Service Delivery and Infrastructure Gaps

To deliver services, many health systems must overcome shortages in the number of clinics and hospitals. Many prominent implementation strategies therefore seek to improve the accessibility of services even when the physical accessibility of facilities cannot be immediately changed. A recent study using a variety of geospatial and demographic public data sources found that 8.9% of the global population (646 million people) cannot reach a healthcare facility within 1 hour if they have access to motorized transport, and 43.3% (3.16 billion people) cannot reach a healthcare facility by foot within 1 hour, illustrating the relevance and need for these strategies.[72]

A range of delivery models to improve HIV care gained prominence and have been collectively referred to as differentiated service delivery (DSD), which also has implications for other noncommunicable, chronic conditions in the global context. DSD models alter the timing, nature, and location of health services away from traditional facility-based care to enhance accessibility and ease; many models also exist.[73] At a time when supply chains were limited and patients needed to make monthly visits to pick up medications, community adherence groups existed in which six patients formed a group and patients took turns making the monthly journey to the clinic in order to pick up medication for the entire group (one patient made two trips per year).[74] Other models include vans that distribute medication at specific points in the community on specific days of the week—essentially offering a mobile pharmacy—or use of lockers in in urban areas where medications are stored by a pharmacist and patients use a code to access medication at a time of their choosing.

Another way to extend the infrastructure for healthcare service delivery is to engage institutions and structures that traditionally have not been fully incorporated into the health system. Religious institutions or churches command the attention of many people, and recent work has sought to identify opportunities to extend delivery of health services to this sector. In many cases, public health seeks to leverage influence with the community through opinion leaders in these institutions (e.g., pastors), while in other cases these institutions are used as infrastructure for healthcare (e.g., using a church for a vaccination or testing site). For example, while traditional healers in Africa and Asia are sometimes thought by the mainstream biomedical public health system to provide unsound advice and therefore represent a problem, recent innovative solutions have sought to engage traditional healers, who are often the first point of contact, for a range of activities. Randomized trials have shown this approach to increasing HIV testing in Uganda and other outcomes.[49] In other work, pastors were able to promote voluntary adult male circumcision for HIV prevention in Tanzania, where circumcision in adults is not a traditional practice.[75]

Strategies Addressing Limited Financial Protections and Livelihood Constraints

The limited ability of people to afford the direct and indirect (i.e., opportunity) costs of illness is a prominent feature motivating implementation research in the global context. Even free medications, as in the case of HIV treatment in much of the world, incurs substantial opportunity costs (time, lost wages) that those living with relatively few livelihood cushions can afford. Costs that may not be prohibitive can still represent important barriers to access for people who meet livelihood needs precariously. A 2017 report estimated that 100 million individuals a year are pushed into extreme poverty due to healthcare costs, and that number rose as much as five-fold during COVID.[76]

While there is much research at the policy and financing level (e.g., creation of health service coverage), an emerging class of implementation strategies seeks to enable greater use of EBIs even within constraints imposed by costs. In many middle-income countries, prevention modalities are available and generally not cost prohibitive but nevertheless demand an out-of-pocket cost. These costs can lead to delays or temporal discounting. The HPV vaccine is widely available in China, but current estimates show fewer than 10% of eligible women have accessed it, mostly because of the cost ($37), which is a major barrier. A novel strategy exploits the psychological reflex of reciprocity (the tendency of humans naturally to return generosity).[77] In recent research, investigators paid for preventive health interventions for individuals, and after receipt of other service, individuals were asked to donate for someone else to receive the vaccine.[50] This approach paid for increased uptake of preventive health services (e.g., STI testing, vaccination) in China.[52]

CASE STUDY 26.1: REVOLVING PHARMACY FUNDS (RPF) TO INCREASE SUCCESSFUL DELIVERY OF MEDICATIONS FOR HYPERTENSION AND DIABETES OVER THE LAST MILE TO POPULATIONS IN NEED, WITH RPF MOTIVATED BY LIMITATIONS IN THE SUPPLY CHAIN INFRASTRUCTURE

Background: In many middle- or lower-income countries even though essential medications are approved, available, and affordable in some urban settings, they are frequently unavailable in rural settings, thus precluding access to EBIs for a notable segment of the population. One example of this are antihypertensive medications, which cost as little as $5 for a year's supply, making them affordable to most people in countries like India, Zambia, Kenya, and other places. Given that hypertension is extremely prevalent (as high as 30% in individuals over 50) and there is a rising tide of morbidity related to hypertension, creating a supply chain for the last mile to make affordable medications accessible is critical.

Strategy: One creative implementation strategy that has been used to extend supply chains to the last mile are "revolving pharmacy funds" (RPF). In this schema, inventory at a local a "micropharmacy" is created through a single donation from a governmental or nongovernmental organization. Medication stock is procured, and the medications are sold at a markup, thus enabling a local pharmacist to make a profit, order more medication from suppliers, and replenish the medication supply. Essentially, by overcoming initial capital requirements, such schema can create and extend the supply chain to critical needed areas. In Kenya, a group of investigators documented the use and scale up of RPF and found that this model, with several adaptations, was able to sustain a supply chain to target communities. The study details use of RFPs in 72 pharmacies in rural western Kenya over 10 years and found it consistently supplied 22 categories of cardiovascular disease (CVD) medicines and increased availability of essential CVD medications from less than 30% to more than 90% of the time. Medications available included thiazide diuretics, beta-blockers, insulin, statins, and other key CVD medications to patients in western Kenya. The estimated programmed running cost was US$6.5–$25 per patient.[79]

Lessons Learned: This case study provides several lessons for implementation strategies in a global context. First, important strategies for optimizing implementation of EBIs occur within local constraints created by realities in the health system building blocks. In other words, the potential contribution of any particular strategy is contextually enabled and bounded by health system building blocks. Second, in addition, this creative strategy in this case targeted financing mechanism and supply chains to advance health system functionality—demonstrating a creative way to optimize even without resolving larger health system problems. For policymakers, such micro approaches might represent efficient investments. Additional research is needed to examine the long-term sustainability and effects as well as policies to enhance further scale up.

A wide variety of research addresses the use of conditional cash transfers for preventive healthcare, childhood immunizations, HIV services. Conditional cash can operate through both changing the price point of accessing healthcare, and also — given the theory of "present bias" in behavioral economics — counteracting our natural tendency to exaggerated devaluing of benefits that will accrue in the future (as preventive health generally does).[78]

Governance and Management

One feature of health systems and public systems in general in the global context is that additional strengthening of governance and management capacity may be needed at not only the national but also the regional, local, and facility levels—again also a challenge in HIC. A number of implementation strategies seek to enhance the use of EBIs through enhancing accountability and responsiveness of healthcare and public health through governance and management approaches.[80–82]

In order to increase accountability, some strategies seek to bring health facility performance into community and public view. Early studies that instituted community oversight boards to monitor performance were in some cases able to document improvements.[83] Additional approaches included treatment observatories where patients themselves act in a monitoring capacity. For example, reporting stockouts or other failures at the health system creates greater accountability. To start, strategies include promoting the assessment of patient experience or satisfaction through surveys or exit interviews in numerous settings; faculty boards made up of community members who review facility performance in Africa and Asia; scorecards or report cards that are public ally available, or things like "citizen juries" tested in Thailand. While these strategies differ in form, they in general seek to increase visibility and build organizational and institutional mechanisms for consumers to exert influence and power over delivery systems.

Another major thread of strategies involves management efforts within the facility using quality improvement methods for organizational improvement based originally on approaches derived from manufacturing.[84] These have been widely used and in many cases have shown success. These approaches are varied in form, but all make use of two pillars: one is to collect data about service delivery performance, and the second is to use that information to direct improvement efforts. HCWs typically receive training on understanding processes and conducting root cause analyses (e.g., use of fishbone diagrams) in order to identify and solve problems. Improvement efforts have been used to advance a variety of medical conditions, including HIV, childhood diarrhea, surgeries, and procedural specialties. A recent meta-analysis from 15 countries suggested that improvement efforts with first responders resulted in an overall decrease in mortality close to 50% (relative risk [RR] 0.47, 95% CI 0.28 to 0.78).[85] The heterogeneity of effects, however, is a notable limitation to the use of these strategies at scale, and future research directions on ownership, ensuring ownership of improvement efforts, and identifying "core" elements of improvement methods.[86]

DATA AND TECHNOLOGY

The rise of global technological infrastructure can be leveraged for improvement in health services. As of 2019, 95% of Asia was reachable by cell signal, and 75% of Africa had access to 3G networks. This infrastructure has led to revolutions across a range of societal and economic functions, including the rise of mobile banking.[87] Application of emerging technologies to advance the implementation of EBIs holds great promise in systems under a variety of constraints. These strategies have worked through improved communications, supply chain management, HCW information, and patient and community engagement. For example, SMS technology has been widely used to engage patients in care, through medication reminders, appointment reminders, or test results. The "WelTel" trial reported in the *Lancet* in 2010 suggested that weekly text messages to persons living with HIV improved clinical outcomes,[88] and this intervention has also demonstrated effects in other chronic conditions.[89] Since that time numerous studies have repeatedly shown SMS to have some effects. In addition, digital and cellular technologies have also been used to engage HCWs and encourage them to use EBIs. It has long been known that guidelines for malaria treatment are not often followed. In a cluster randomized trial in Kenya published in 2011, HCWs who were sent text messages reminding them of guideline practices improved their guideline concordant care, defined by a composite of diagnostic and management practices, by 24%.[90] Given the ubiquity of SMS coverage and the fact that almost all HCWs have cell phones, this strategy has the potential to improve the delivery of evidence-based care in regions of the world where healthcare facilities are often remote and not connecting on a day-to-day basis with other systems.[90]

LEARNING FROM GLOBAL CONTEXTS

Implementation science also stands to grow as a field through the growing discourse in global contexts. First, innovation and spread often occur more rapidly in global contexts than in HICs,[91] which may offer lessons for the field more generally. For example, soon after efficacy studies found that in persons with both HIV and TB, rapid treatment initiation for HIV after starting TB therapy (as opposed to the traditional practice of waiting 2 or more months) improved clinical outcomes, a study in Uganda found that practice had changed rapidly in day-to-day care.[92] Experts have also called attention to terrain ripe for innovations in implementation created by constraints in many global settings that must be unpacked for generalizable lessons.[91]

Second, it is worth noting that many of the implementation issues in LMICs are remarkably similar in HICs. In many US states where public health services are relatively underfunded, healthcare agencies and community organizations can apply for federal funding to address specific issues of public health. A clinic might receive a grant from the Centers for Disease Control and Prevention or from the Health Resources and Services Administration for expanding STI testing, while another clinic in the region might apply for funding to improve treatment for HIV. Because no local public health agency oversees both of these projects, fragmentation can sometime develop. This resembles closely the situation in some countries that are funded by PEPFAR, in both funding mechanism and the resulting fragmented health system. These health systems similarities provide opportunities for synergistic and cross -cutting insights for implementation science.

Implementation Outcomes in a Global Context

Implementation outcomes, or the extent to which the intentions of the implementation activities have occurred (formally defined as "effects of deliberate and purposive actions to implement new treatments, practices, and services")[93(p65)] are a critical element of implementation science with broad relevance in global contexts. Conceiving of and measuring implementation outcomes in research allows a clear examination of the immediate effects of implementation strategies, as well as how they occur and help interpretation of downstream service delivery and clinical outcomes (see chapter 15). Proctor proposed eight implementation outcomes, including the following: acceptability (perception among implementation stakeholders that a given treatment, service, practice, or innovation is agreeable, palatable, or satisfactory); appropriateness (the perceived fit, relevance, or compatibility of the innovation or evidence-based practice for a given practice setting, provider, or consumer); penetration (the integration of a practice within a service setting and its subsystems); and others.[93] The global context, however, brings attention to additional domains of the outcomes of implementation worth considering.

Acceptability and Preferences

Research in global contexts has often used acceptability in trials and other designs to anticipate user uptake, but these studies have consistently found that high acceptability in research studies does not translate into desirability for use in practice.[94] Over the last 20 years, in HIV prevention research conducted in Africa, several highly promising female-controlled methods of prevention (e.g., tenofovir vaginal gel), as well as for voluntary adult male circumcision for HIV prevention, demonstrated high levels of self-reported "acceptability" in trial participants, but poor subsequent uptake.[95] In malaria control, many studies have found the use of bed nets to be effective (including costs) for preventing malaria, but in practice people often do not use the bed nets even when freely distributed and in some cases use them as fishing nets.[96] These failures have pushed researchers to deepen our understanding of user behavior, including increasing adoption of deeper ethnographic work, as well as user-centered design methods,[97] and the increasing incorporation of novel marketing methods—a field entirely focused on understanding how to deliver products that people want and will use (or in fact buy)—such as discrete choice experiments and best-worst scaling.[98–100]

Feasibility

A second outcome that has been widely used in implementation science in global contexts is feasibility ("defined as the extent to which an EBI can be successfully used or carried out within a given agency or setting").[93(p69)] In global contexts, many technologically based projects to introduce innovations fail in part because the feasibility has not been adequately considered. For example, goal-directed aggressive fluid resuscitation for sepsis yielded important mortality benefits in HICs but has had limited reproducibility in many global contexts because of both the equipment and training required to carry it out. Global contexts, however, have also demonstrated that feasibility is a moving target and can be used as an excuse to not invest in progress. In 2004, HIV treatment was widely considered "not feasible" in the global setting given the absence of longitudinal healthcare; workforce shortages; and weak financial management. Yet by 2006 the confluence of political will, funding, and strategic advocacy led to a global scale-up of HIV treatment. Whether something is not feasible or whether there is inadequate commitment may be two sides of the same coin, and poor feasibility may not be adequate justification against implementation activities.

Implementation Outcomes

The HSBB gaps in global contexts also mean additional implementation outcomes may be useful. Several useful domains are worth exploring in greater depth in global context:

- *"Robustness."* Given the fact that health systems generally have a range of EBIs to take up, one important consideration for any strategy that is implemented is whether it can be leveraged for one or multiple EBIs. For example, in HIV programs, whether quality improvement methods funded to improve use of one EBI could also have "lift-all-boats" effects and improve use of other EBIs would be an important dimension to consider. Certain strategies might have narrow effects (an incentive to improve one EBI may only improve the use of that one EBI), while others may have broader effects (quality improvement directed at one EBI could have skills transferable to other EBIs).

- "*Butterfly Effects.*" Another implementation outcome of value could be unintended effects, which could be negative or positive outcomes.[101,102] There is much enthusiasm in Africa for addressing noncommunicable diseases such as hypertension in HIV clinics and a push to introduce screening through "task shifting" where lay health workers take on activities normally done by nurses in order to overcome healthcare workforce shortages. For example, asking lay health workers already employed by HIV clinics (who currently carry out adherence counseling and administrative tasks) in Zambia to take blood pressure measurements may well increase the screening for hypertension (an EBI), but at the same time might then compromise the quality or quantity of counseling. On the other hand, enhancing capacities of the workforce may also improve other unanticipated functionality. By definition, many of these can only be ascertained in retrospect, but their presence may also push investigators to anticipate a wider array of potential effects and prepare research to understand and manage them.
- "*Alignment.*" Stakeholders in some settings include a diversity of actors, which along with national governments include multilateral mechanisms (e.g., the Global Fund) as well as unilateral mechanisms (e.g., PEPFAR), that leads to fractured health systems at the systems level, the organizational level, and the HCW level, creating a difficult pathway for individuals to navigate systems and their inefficiencies. Coordination and linkages between actors in the health systems represent a particularly important consideration in the global context, where vertical health services (focused on one health condition), limited healthcare infrastructure, and sometimes decentralized systems with a mix of private and public actors means that thinking about how the pieces fit together is requisite to understanding use of EBIs. Indeed, excessive attention on the use of one EBI runs the risk of "stealing from Peter to pay Paul." A 2009 WHO report on health systems noted: "Every intervention, from the simplest to the most complex, has an effect on the overall system, and the overall system has an effect on every intervention."[103(p19)]

CONCLUSIONS

Knowledge Production and Epistemic Justice

The production of knowledge designed to generalize, particularly in the context of global health, must grapple with the current epistemic discussion about equity and justice. Emerging critiques suggest that current framing and explanations adopt a foreign gaze that unfairly elevates certain points of view and discounts others, not because of their inherent worth, but because of who presents them.[104] In addition, critiques have also pointed to "hermeneutical injustice" where interpretative frameworks for discourse are situated and in service existing power dynamics.[105] Global health, it is argued, must generate a more balanced view of problems and solutions, incorporate more voices from the South, and value regional and local as well as epistemically balanced ways of knowing.

A knowledge generation approach that values local and regional perspectives is particularly important for implementation science in the global context. The field's focus on the contextual nature of implementation strategies naturally elevates regional, local, and contextual expertise (whether across social divides within regions or between). While it is true that many of the barriers to implementation are shared, the importance of the particular and local implies the importance of local and particular perspectives in solutions. In other words, if implementation science seeks the right balance of universalizing insights and contextualized knowledge, the methods and the workforce producing this knowledge need to reflect these layers of expertise to create an epistemically balanced approach to science.

For example, delays in connecting with healthcare seeking among persons with TB is widely considered an important challenge in public health. While hyperbolic temporal discounting leading to delays in healthcare seeking may be a universal human cognitive bias (as identified by behavioral economists), the cognitive bias may have a relatively small overall effect in a setting where delays are also driven by livelihood demands, difficult-to-access healthcare services, or limited financial protections. These factors—often obvious to local investigators seeking to change outcomes—likely influence outcomes in addition to, and perhaps more than, a universal "cognitive bias." Insights that combine localizing and universalizing insights are aligned with the goals of implementation science.

SUMMARY

While the health of the world has improved over the last decades, much progress is still needed—progress that implementation science can contribute to if deployed appropriately. In a global context, the health system plays an important role in deciding which strategies will fit, as well as influencing the effects of those strategies. Research on implementation therefore must be attuned to formal and scientific ways to examine that context. Strategies that optimize implementation within workforce shortages (e.g., task shifting); restricted infrastructure (e.g., home-based care); governance (e.g., social accountability strategies); financing (e.g., social insurance schema); and others represent important approaches to optimize the use of EBIs for health and population health outcomes, especially in LMICs. At the same time, the application in new settings also allows us to conceptualize domains of implementation outcomes relevant where HSBBs are weak. Some of these concepts, such as ripple effects, unintended consequences, simultaneity, and robustness, have implications in many settings throughout the world and could enrich implementation science more generally.

ACKNOWLEDGMENTS

We thank Anne Trolard and Brittney Sandler for help with editing and Ashley Sturm and Aaloke Mody for creating figures.

SUGGESTED READINGS AND WEBSITES

Readings

Amanyire G, Semitala FC, Namusobya J, et al. Effects of a multicomponent intervention to streamline initiation of antiretroviral therapy in Africa: a stepped-wedge cluster-randomised trial. *Lancet HIV.* 2016 Nov 1;3(11):e539–e548.

This article addresses the use of a traditional implementation science framework for the design of a multilevel intervention in Uganda.

Baptiste S, Manouan A, Garcia P, Etya'ale H, Swan T, Jallow W. Community-led monitoring: When community data drives implementation strategies. *Curr HIV/AIDS Rep.* 2020 Oct;17(5):415–421.

Although focused on HIV, this review presents a compelling summary of strategies to alter governance mechanisms of health systems and put end users into the system itself.

de Walque D. The use of financial incentives to prevent unhealthy behaviors: a review. *Soc Sci Med.* 2020 Sep 1;261:113236.

This article reviews the use of economic incentives for a variety of health conditions outside of HIV.

Downs JA, Mwakisole AH, Chandika AB, et al. Educating religious leaders to promote uptake of male circumcision in Tanzania: a cluster randomized trial. *Lancet.* 2017 Mar 18;389(10074):1124–1132.

An example is provided of partnering with religious leaders to influence community norms and change uptake of health interventions in Tanzania.

Hogan DR, Stevens GA, Hosseinpoor AR, Boerma T. Monitoring universal health coverage within the sustainable development goals: development and baseline data for an index of essential health services. *Lancet Glob Health.* 2018 Feb 1;6(2):e152–e168.

This article provides an important summary of progress in universal health coverage around the world.

Khan AJ, Khowaja S, Khan FS, et al. Engaging the private sector to increase tuberculosis case detection: an impact evaluation study. *Lancet Infect Dis.* 2012;12(8):608–616.

Discussed in this article is leveraging community and crowd-based referral networks to diagnose TB.

Roy M, Bolton Moore C, Sikazwe I, Holmes CB. A review of differentiated service delivery for HIV treatment: effectiveness, mechanisms, targeting, and scale. *Curr HIV/AIDS Rep.* 2019 Aug;16(4):324–334.

The article provides a review of the family of implementation strategies used to advance HIV treatment in Africa, Asia, and beyond. The article illustrates the nuances and variation in service delivery models for HIV treatment and also their proposed mechanisms.

Yang F, Zhang TP, Tang W, et al. Pay-it-forward gonorrhea and chlamydia testing among men who have sex with men in China: a randomized controlled trial. *Lancet Infect Dis.* 2020 Aug 1;20(8):976–782.

A randomized trial showing the effects of a novel implementation strategy to encourage uptake of preventive health services in settings where preventive services have significant out-of-pocket costs.

Zuora D, Sudoi RK, Akhwale WS, et al. The effect of mobile phone text-message reminders on Kenyan health workers' adherence to malaria treatment guidelines: a cluster randomized trial. *Lancet.* 2011 Aug 27;378(9793):795–803.

The article demonstrates the use of digital technologies to enhance healthcare worker capability and evidence-based decision-making through malaria treatment.

Selected Websites and Tools

Global Health Competencies Toolkit, 2018.
Accessed August 23, 2022
https://www.cugh.org/online-tools/competencies-toolkit/

This website provides a review of competencies and global health.

Global Burden of Disease (GBD), 2022
Accessed August 23, 2022
https://www.healthdata.org/gbd/2019

The link provides widely used resources to visualize the global burden of disease, which can inform implementation efforts.

WHO Implementation Research Resources
Published 2022
Accessed August 23, 2022
https://implementationscience-gacd.org/who-ir/

Provided at this site is a synopsis of tools and resources focused on global health and implementation science.

REFERENCES

1. Ravishankar N, Gubbins P, Cooley RJ, et al. Financing of global health: tracking development assistance for health from 1990 to 2007. *Lancet.* 2009;373(9681):2113–2124. doi:10.1016/S0140-6736(09)60881-3
2. Proctor E, Silmere H, Raghavan R, et al. Outcomes for implementation research: conceptual distinctions, measurement challenges, and research agenda. *Adm Policy Ment Health Ment Health Serv Res.* 2011;38(2):65–76.
3. Proctor EK, Powell BJ, McMillen JC. Implementation strategies: recommendations for specifying and reporting. *Implement Sci.* 2013;8(1):1–11.
4. Armstrong R, Sales A. Welcome to implementation science communications. *Implement Sci Commun.* 2020;1(1):1–3.
5. Birken SA, Powell BJ, Presseau J, et al. Combined use of the Consolidated Framework for Implementation Research (CFIR) and the Theoretical Domains Framework (TDF): a systematic review. *Implement Sci.* 2017;12(1):1–14.
6. May CR, Mair F, Finch T, et al. Development of a theory of implementation and integration: Normalization Process Theory. *Implement Sci.* 2009;4(1):1–9.
7. World Bank. Physicians (per 1,000 people). World Health Organization Global Health Workforce Statistics. Accessed April 25, 2022. https://data.worldbank.org/indicator/SH.MED.PHYS.ZS
8. World Health Organization. *Everybody's Business: Strengthening Health Systems to Improve Health Outcomes, WHO's Framework for Action.* Geneva: WHO; 2007.
9. World Health Organization. *Declaration of alma-ata.* No. WHO/EURO: 1978-3938-43697-61471. World Health Organization. Regional Office for Europe; 1978. https://cdn.who.int/media/docs/default-source/documents/almaata-declaration-en.pdf?sfvrsn=7b3c2167_2
10. Watkins DA, Yamey G, Schäferhoff M, et al. Alma-Ata at 40 years: reflections from the Lancet Commission on Investing in Health. *Lancet.* 2018;392(10156):1434–1460. doi:10.1016/S0140-6736(18)32389-4
11. World Bank. *World Development Report 1993.* Oxford University Press; 1993. doi:10.1596/0-1952-0890-0
12. Ravishankar N, Gubbins P, Cooley RJ, et al. Financing of global health: tracking development assistance for health from 1990 to 2007. *Lancet.* 2009;373(9681):2113–2124.
13. Grépin KA, Pinkstaff CB, Shroff ZC, Ghaffar A. Donor funding health policy and systems research in low- and middle-income countries: how much, from where and to whom. *Health Res Policy Syst.* 2017;15(1):1–8. doi:10.1186/S12961-017-0224-6/FIGURES/3
14. Jamison DT, Summers LH, Alleyne G, et al. Global health 2035: a world converging within a generation. *Lancet.* 2013;382(9908):1898–1955. doi:10.1016/S0140-6736(13)62105-4
15. Hogan DR, Stevens GA, Hosseinpoor AR, Boerma T. Monitoring universal health coverage within the Sustainable Development Goals: development and baseline data for an index of essential health services. *Lancet Glob Health.* 2018;6(2):e152–e168. doi:10.1016/S2214-109X(17)30472-2
16. Wang H, Naghavi M, Allen C, et al. Global, regional, and national life expectancy, all-cause mortality, and cause-specific mortality for 249 causes of death, 1980–2015: a systematic analysis for the Global Burden of Disease Study 2015. *Lancet.* 2016;388(10053):1459–1544. doi:10.1016/S0140-6736(16)31012-1
17. Pai M, Kasaeva T, Swaminathan S. Covid-19's devastating effect on tuberculosis care—a path to recovery. *N Engl J Med.* 2022 Apr 21;386(16):1490–1493. doi:10.1056/NEJMP2118145/SUPPL_FILE/NEJMP2118145_DISCLOSURES.PDF

18. Indicators AH. *Monitoring the Building Blocks of Health Systems.* WHO Document Production Services, Geneva, Switzerland; 2010.
19. Sacks E, Morrow M, Story WT, et al. Beyond the building blocks: integrating community roles into health systems frameworks to achieve health for all. *BMJ Glob Health.* 2019;3(suppl 3):e001384. doi:10.1136/bmjgh-2018-001384
20. Mounier-Jack S, Griffiths UK, Closser S, Burchett H, Marchal B. Measuring the health systems impact of disease control programmes: a critical reflection on the WHO building blocks framework. *BMC Public Health.* 2014;14:278. doi:10.1186/1471-2458-14-278
21. Mutale W, Bond V, Mwanamwenge MT, et al. Systems thinking in practice: the current status of the six WHO building blocks for health system strengthening in three BHOMA intervention districts of Zambia: a baseline qualitative study. *BMC Health Serv Res.* 2013;13(1):291. doi:10.1186/1472-6963-13-291
22. Stewart RE, Mandell DS, Beidas RS. Lessons from Maslow: prioritizing funding to improve the quality of community mental health and substance use services. *Psychiatr Serv.* 2021;72(10):1219–1221. doi:10.1176/appi.ps.202000209
23. Sawleshwarkar S, Negin J. A review of global health competencies for postgraduate public health education. *Front Public Health.* 2017;5(Mar):46. doi:10.3389/FPUBH.2017.00046
24. Polec LA, Petkovic J, Welch V, et al. Strategies to increase the ownership and use of insecticide-treated bednets to prevent malaria. *Cochrane Database Syst.* 2015;11(1):1–27.
25. Powell BJ, Waltz TJ, Chinman MJ, et al. A refined compilation of implementation strategies: results from the Expert Recommendations for Implementing Change (ERIC) project. *Implement Sci.* 2015;10(1):1–14. doi:10.1186/S13012-015-0209-1/TABLES/3
26. Effective Practice and Organisation of Care (EPOC). EPOC Taxonomy; 2015. epoc.cochrane.org/epoc-taxonomy (accessed August 23, 2022).
27. Liu JX, Goryakin Y, Maeda A, Bruckner T, Scheffler R. Global health workforce labor market projections for 2030. *Hum Res Health.* 2017;15(1):1–12. doi:10.1186/S12960-017-0187-2/FIGURES/2
28. Mullan F. The metrics of the physician brain drain. *N Engl J Med.* 2009;353(17):1810–1818. doi:10.1056/NEJMSA050004
29. Clemens MA, Pettersson Gelander G. A new database of health professional emigration from Africa. Center for Global Development Working Paper No. 95. 2006. Center for Global Development, Washington, DC.
30. Collins FS, Glass RI, Whitescarver J, Wakefield M, Goosby EP. Developing health workforce capacity in Africa. *Science (New York, NY).* 2010;330(6009):1324. doi:10.1126/SCIENCE.1199930
31. Organization WH. *Task Shifting: Rational Redistribution of Tasks Among Health Workforce Teams: Global Recommendations and Guidelines.* WHO Document Production Services; 2008.
32. Selke HM, Kimaiyo S, Sidle JE, et al. Task-shifting of antiretroviral delivery from health care workers to persons living with HIV/AIDS: clinical outcomes of a community-based program in Kenya. *J Acquir Immune Defic Syndr.* 2010;55(4):483–490.
33. Patel V, Weiss HA, Chowdhary N, et al. Effectiveness of an intervention led by lay health counsellors for depressive and anxiety disorders in primary care in Goa, India (MANAS): a cluster randomised controlled trial. *Lancet.* 2010;376(9758):2086–2095.
34. Rahman A, Malik A, Sikander S, Roberts C, Creed F. Cognitive behaviour therapy-based intervention by community health workers for mothers with depression and their infants in rural Pakistan: a cluster-randomised controlled trial. *Lancet.* 2008;372(9642):902–909.
35. Pereira C, Bugalho A, Bergström S, Vaz F, Cotiro M. A comparative study of caesarean deliveries by assistant medical officers and obstetricians in Mozambique. *BJOG.* 1996;103(6):508–512.
36. Vasan A, Kenya-Mugisha N, Seung KJ, et al. Agreement between physicians and non-physician clinicians in starting antiretroviral therapy in rural Uganda. *Hum Resour Health.* 2009;7(1):75. doi:10.1186/1478-4491-7-75
37. Patel V, Weiss HA, Chowdhary N, et al. Effectiveness of an intervention led by lay health counsellors for depressive and anxiety disorders in primary care in Goa, India (MANAS): a cluster randomised controlled trial. *Lancet.* 2010;376(9758):2086–2095.
38. Lipp A. Lay health workers in primary and community health care for maternal and child health and the management of infectious diseases: a review synopsis. *Public Health Nurs.* 2011 May;28(3):243–245.
39. Wollinka O, Keeley E, Burkhalter BR, Bashir N. Hearth Nutrition Model: Applications in Haiti, Vietnam, and Bangladesh. Arlington, Va., USA: BASICS. 1997.
40. Sazawal S, Black RE. Effect of pneumonia case management on mortality in neonates, infants, and preschool children: a

meta-analysis of community-based trials. *Lancet Infect Dis.* 2003;3(9):547–556. doi:10.1016/S1473-3099(03)00737-0

41. Amstutz A, Lejone TI, Khesa L, et al. VIBRA trial–effect of village-based refill of ART following home-based same-day ART initiation vs. clinic-based ART refill on viral suppression among individuals living with HIV: protocol of a cluster-randomized clinical trial in rural Lesotho. *Trials.* 2019;20(1):1–14.
42. Dommaraju S, Hagey J, Odeny TA, et al. Preferences of people living with HIV for differentiated care models in Kenya: a discrete choice experiment. *PLoS One.* 2021;16(8):e0255650.
43. Tang W, Mao J, Liu C, et al. Crowdsourcing health communication about condom use in men who have sex with men in China: a randomised controlled trial. *Lancet.* 2016;388:S73.
44. Khan AJ, Khowaja S, Khan FS, et al. Engaging the private sector to increase tuberculosis case detection: an impact evaluation study. *Lancet Infect Dis.* 2012;12(8):608–616.
45. Flor LS, Wilson S, Bhatt P, et al. Community-based interventions for detection and management of diabetes and hypertension in underserved communities: a mixed-methods evaluation in Brazil, India, South Africa and the USA. *BMJ Glob Health.* 2020;5(6):e001959. doi:10.1136/BMJGH-2019-001959
46. Farzadfar F, Murray CJL, Gakidou E, et al. Effectiveness of diabetes and hypertension management by rural primary health-care workers (Behvarz workers) in Iran: a nationally representative observational study. *Lancet.* 2012;379(9810):47–54. doi:10.1016/S0140-6736(11)61349-4
47. Liang X, Chen J, Liu Y, He C, Li T. The effect of hypertension and diabetes management in southwest China: a before- and after-intervention study. *PLoS One.* 2014;9(3):e91801. doi:10.1371/JOURNAL.PONE.0091801
48. Decroo T, Koole O, Remartinez D, et al. Four-year retention and risk factors for attrition among members of community ART groups in Tete, Mozambique. *Trop Med Int Health.* 2014;19(5):514–521. doi:10.1111/TMI.12278
49. Sundararajan R, Ponticiello M, Lee MH, et al. Traditional healer-delivered point-of-care HIV testing versus referral to clinical facilities for adults of unknown serostatus in rural Uganda: a mixed-methods, cluster-randomised trial. *Lancet Glob Health.* 2021;9(11):e1579–e1588. doi:10.1016/S2214-109X(21)00366-1
50. Tang W, Wu D, Yang F, et al. How kindness can be contagious in healthcare. *Nat Med.* 2021;27(7):1142–1144.
51. Cialdini RB, Kallgren CA, Reno RR. A focus theory of normative conduct: a theoretical refinement and reevaluation of the role of norms in human behavior. *Adv Exp Soc Psychol.* 1991;24(C):201–234. doi:10.1016/S0065-2601(08)60330-5
52. Yang F, Zhang TP, Tang W, et al. Pay-it-forward gonorrhoea and chlamydia testing among men who have sex with men in China: a randomised controlled trial. *Lancet Infect Dis.* 2020;20(8):976–982.
53. de Walque D. The use of financial incentives to prevent unhealthy behaviors: a review. *Soc Sci Med.* 2020;261:113236.
54. Fahey CA, Njau PF, Katabaro E, et al. Financial incentives to promote retention in care and viral suppression in adults with HIV initiating antiretroviral therapy in Tanzania: a three-arm randomised controlled trial. *Lancet HIV.* 2020;7(11):e762–e771.
55. McCoy DC, Hall JA, Ridge M. A systematic review of the literature for evidence on health facility committees in low-and middle-income countries. *Health Policy Plann.* 2012;27(6):449–466.
56. Baptiste S, Manouan A, Garcia P, Etya'ale H, Swan T, Jallow W. Community-led monitoring: when community data drives implementation strategies. *Curr HIV/AIDS Rep.* 2020;17(5):415–421.
57. Björkman M, Svensson J. Power to the people: evidence from a randomized field experiment on community-based monitoring in Uganda. *Q J Econ.* 2009;124(2):735–769. doi:10.1162/QJEC.2009.124.2.735
58. Blake C, Annorbah-Sarpei NA, Bailey C, et al. Scorecards and social accountability for improved maternal and newborn health services: a pilot in the Ashanti and Volta regions of Ghana. *Int J Gynecol Obstet.* 2016;135(3):372–379.
59. Gullo S, Galavotti C, Sebert Kuhlmann A, Msiska T, Hastings P, Marti CN. Effects of a social accountability approach, CARE's Community Score Card, on reproductive health-related outcomes in Malawi: a cluster-randomized controlled evaluation. *PLoS One.* 2017;12(2):e0171316.
60. Basinga P, Gertler PJ, Binagwaho A, Soucat ALB, Sturdy J, Vermeersch CMJ. Effect on maternal and child health services in Rwanda of payment to primary health-care providers for performance: an impact evaluation. *Lancet.* 2011;377(9775):1421–1428.
61. Ashraf N, Bandiera O, Jack BK. No margin, no mission? A field experiment on incentives for public service delivery. *J Public Econ.* 2014;120:1–17.
62. Sollecito WA, Johnson JK. The global evolution of continuous quality improvement: from Japanese

manufacturing to global health services. *McLaughlin and Kaluzny's Continuous Quality Improvement in Health Care*. 2013;3–48. http://samples.jblearning.com/9781284126594/9781284126594_CH01_Pass05.pdf
63. Rustagi AS, Gimbel S, Nduati R, et al. Health facility factors and quality of services to prevent mother-to-child HIV transmission in Côte d'Ivoire, Kenya, and Mozambique. *Int J STD AIDS*. 2017;28(8):788–799.
64. Zurovac D, Sudoi RK, Akhwale WS, et al. The effect of mobile phone text-message reminders on Kenyan health workers' adherence to malaria treatment guidelines: a cluster randomised trial. *Lancet*. 2011;378(9793):795–803.
65. Kleinman RA, Merkel C. Digital contact tracing for COVID-19. *CMAJ*. 2020;192(24):E653–E656.
66. Khan AJ, Khowaja S, Khan FS, et al. Engaging the private sector to increase tuberculosis case detection: an impact evaluation study. *Lancet Infect Dis*. 2012;12(8):608–616.
67. Tang W, Mao J, Liu C, et al. Crowdsourcing health communication about condom use in men who have sex with men in China: a randomised controlled trial. *Lancet*. 2016;388:S73.
68. Napierala S, Desmond NA, Kumwenda MK, et al. HIV self-testing services for female sex workers, Malawi and Zimbabwe. *Bull World Health Organ*. 2019;97(11):764. doi:10.2471/BLT.18.223560
69. Thirumurthy H, Masters SH, Mavedzenge SN, Maman S, Omanga E, Agot K. Promoting male partner HIV testing and safer sexual decision making through secondary distribution of self-tests by HIV-negative female sex workers and women receiving antenatal and post-partum care in Kenya: a cohort study. *Lancet HIV*. 2016;3(6):e266–e274. doi:10.1016/S2352-3018(16)00041-2
70. Fairall LR, Folb N, Timmerman V, et al. Educational outreach with an integrated clinical tool for nurse-led non-communicable chronic disease management in primary care in South Africa: a pragmatic cluster randomised controlled trial. *PLoS Med*. 2016;13(11):e1002178. doi:10.1371/JOURNAL.PMED.1002178
71. Dommaraju S, Hagey J, Odeny TA, et al. Preferences of people living with HIV for differentiated care models in Kenya: a discrete choice experiment. *PLoS One*. 2021;16(8):e0255650.
72. Weiss DJ, Nelson A, Vargas-Ruiz CA, et al. Global maps of travel time to healthcare facilities. *Nat Med*. 2020;26(12):1835–1838. doi:10.1038/s41591-020-1059-1
73. Roy M, Moore CB, Sikazwe I, Holmes CB. A review of differentiated service delivery for HIV treatment: effectiveness, mechanisms, targeting, and scale. *Curr HIV/AIDS Rep*. 2019;16(4):324–334.
74. Decroo T, Telfer B, Biot M, et al. Distribution of antiretroviral treatment through self-forming groups of patients in Tete Province, Mozambique. *J Acquir Immune Defic Syndr*. 2011;56(2):e39–e44. doi:10.1097/QAI.0b013e3182055138
75. Downs JA, Fuunay LD, Fuunay M, et al. "The body we leave behind": a qualitative study of obstacles and opportunities for increasing uptake of male circumcision among Tanzanian Christians. *BMJ Open*. 2013;3(5):e002802. doi:10.1136/BMJOPEN-2013-002802
76. World Bank. *Tracking Universal Health Coverage: 2017 Global Monitoring Report*. World Bank Group. 2017. Accessed April 25, 2022. https://documents.worldbank.org/en/publication/documents-reports/documentdetail/640121513095868125/tracking-universal-health-coverage-2017-global-monitoring-report
77. Cialdini RB. The science of persuasion. *Sci Am*. 2001;284:76–81. Accessed April 25, 2022. https://www.jstor.org/stable/26059056?casa_token=YZOs06QbjcAAAAAA%3ANbttKCmlbg2U0BgpojQYnkc7zZTUysl06m_vmbeAw1NSY_FoUMLv5xpDrHEHaZcQQB5gYAKBjlkbC2_-z-kqq3u6iJ2JP5IiTJp_qbxzhS23dcRmZYHI&seq=1
78. Galárraga O, Sosa-Rubí SG. Conditional economic incentives to improve HIV prevention and treatment in low-income and middle-income countries. *Lancet HIV*. 2019;6(10):e705–e714.
79. Tran DN, Manji I, Njuguna B, et al. Solving the problem of access to cardiovascular medicines: revolving fund pharmacy models in rural western Kenya. *BMJ Glob Health*. 2020;5:3116. doi:10.1136/bmjgh-2020-003116
80. Shrivastava SR, Shrivastava PS, Ramasamy J. Community monitoring: a strategy to watch out for. *Gateways*. 2013;6:170–177.
81. Gurung G, Derrett S, Gauld R, Hill PC. Why service users do not complain or have "voice": a mixed-methods study from Nepal's rural primary health care system. *BMC Health Serv Res*. 2017;17(1):1–10. doi:10.1186/S12913-017-2034-5/TABLES/1
82. Falisse JB, Meessen B, Ndayishimiye J, Bossuyt M. Community participation and voice mechanisms under performance-based financing schemes in Burundi. *Trop Med Int Health*. 2012;17(5):674–682. doi:10.1111/J.1365-3156.2012.02973.X
83. Baptiste S, Manouan A, Garcia P, Etya'ale H, Swan T, Jallow W. Community-led monitoring: when community data drives implementation strategies. *Curr HIV/AIDS Reps*. 2020 Oct;17(5):415–421.

84. Leatherman S, Ferris TG, Berwick D, Omaswa F, Crisp N. The role of quality improvement in strengthening health systems in developing countries. *Int J Qual Health Care*. 2010;22(4): 237–243.
85. Jin J, Akau'ola S, Yip CH, et al. Effectiveness of quality improvement processes, interventions, and structure in trauma systems in low- and middle-income countries: a systematic review and meta-analysis. *World J Surg*. 2021;45(7):1982–1998. doi:10.1007/S00268-021-06065-9/FIGURES/4
86. Wagenaar BH, Hirschhorn LR, Henley C, et al. Data-driven quality improvement in low- and middle-income country health systems: lessons from seven years of implementation experience across Mozambique, Rwanda, and Zambia. *BMC Health Serv Res*. 2017 Dec;17(suppl 3):65–75.
87. Jack W, Suri T. Risk sharing and transactions costs: evidence from Kenya's mobile money revolution. *Am Econ Rev*. 2014;104(1):183–223. doi:10.1257/AER.104.1.183
88. Lester RT, Ritvo P, Mills EJ, et al. Effects of a mobile phone short message service on antiretroviral treatment adherence in Kenya (WelTel Kenya1): a randomised trial. *Lancet*. 2010;376(9755):1838–1845. doi:10.1016/S0140-6736(10)61997-6
89. Krishna S, Boren SA. Diabetes self-management care via cell phone: a systematic review. *J Diabetes Sci Technol*. 2008;2(3):509–517. doi:10.1177/193229680800200324
90. Zurovac D, Sudoi RK, Akhwale WS, et al. The effect of mobile phone text-message reminders on Kenyan health workers' adherence to malaria treatment guidelines: a cluster randomised trial. *Lancet*. 2011;378(9793):795–803.
91. Yapa HM, Bärnighausen T. Implementation science in resource-poor countries and communities. *Implement Sci*. 2018;13(1):154. doi:10.1186/s13012-018-0847-1
92. Vijayan T, Semitala FC, Matsiko N, et al. Changes in the timing of antiretroviral therapy initiation in HIV-infected patients with tuberculosis in Uganda: a study of the diffusion of evidence into practice in the global response to HIV/AIDS. *Clin Infect Dis*. 2013;57(12):1766–1772.
93. Proctor E, Silmere H, Raghavan R, et al. Outcomes for implementation research: conceptual distinctions, measurement challenges, and research agenda. *Adm Policy Ment Health*. 2011;38(2):65–76. doi:10.1007/S10488-010-0319-7
94. Amico KR, Bekker LG. Global PrEP roll-out: recommendations for programmatic success. *Lancet HIV*. 2019;6(2):e137–e140.
95. Geng EH, Glidden D v, Padian N. Strengthening HIV-prevention trials: a dose of implementation science? *Lancet Infect Dis*. 2018;18(11):1166–1168.
96. McLean KA, Byanaku A, Kubikonse A, Tshowe V, Katensi S, Lehman AG. Fishing with bed nets on Lake Tanganyika: a randomized survey. *Malar J*. 2014;13(1):1–5.
97. Beres LK, Simbeza S, Holmes CB, et al. Human-centered design lessons for implementation science: improving the implementation of a patient-centered care intervention. *J Acquir Immune Defic Syndr (1999)*. 2019;82(3):S230. doi:10.1097/QAI.0000000000002216
98. Eshun-Wilson I, Kim HY, Schwartz S, Conte M, Glidden D V, Geng EH. Exploring relative preferences for HIV service features using discrete choice experiments: a synthetic review. *Curr HIV/AIDS Rep*. 2020;17(5):467–477. doi:10.1007/S11904-020-00520-3/FIGURES/1
99. Griffin JB, Ridgeway K, Montgomery E, et al. Vaginal ring acceptability and related preferences among women in low- and middle-income countries: a systematic review and narrative synthesis. *PLoS One*. 2019;14(11):e0224898. doi:10.1371/JOURNAL.PONE.0224898
100. Zanolini A, Sikombe K, Sikazwe I, et al. Understanding preferences for HIV care and treatment in Zambia: evidence from a discrete choice experiment among patients who have been lost to follow-up. *PLoS Med*. 2018;15(8):e1002636. doi:10.1371/JOURNAL.PMED.1002636
101. Gleick J. *Chaos: Making a New Science*. Penguin; 2008.
102. Lorenz EN. Deterministic nonperiodic flow. *J Atmos Sci*. 1963;20(2):130–141.
103. World Health Organization. *The World Health Report: 2000: Health Systems: Improving Performance*. World Health Organization; 2000. Accessed March 27, 2022. https://apps.who.int/iris/handle/10665/42281
104. Büyüm AM, Kenney C, Koris A, Mkumba L, Raveendran Y. Decolonising global health: if not now, when? *BMJ Glob Health*. 2020;5(8):e003394. doi:10.1136/BMJGH-2020-003394
105. Bhakuni H, Abimbola S. Epistemic injustice in academic global health. *Lancet Glob Health*. 2021;9(10):e1465–e1470. doi:10.1016/S2214-109X(21)00301-6

SECTION 6

Dissemination and Scale-Up

27

Designing for Dissemination and Sustainability

Principles, Methods, and Frameworks for Ensuring Fit to Context

BETHANY M. KWAN, DOUGLAS A. LUKE, PRAJAKTA ADSUL, HARRIET KOORTS, ELAINE H. MORRATO, AND RUSSELL E. GLASGOW

INTRODUCTION

Over the last 20 years, the field of dissemination and implementation (D&I) science has emerged as part of a collective commitment to accelerate and improve translation of evidence into practice.[1] Barriers to dissemination, sustainability, and health impacts of translating evidence to practice in health and healthcare range from poor fit between evidence-based innovations and the context in which such innovations are meant to be used to cultures and systems that fail to incentivize and support active dissemination and translation of evidence into practice.[2–4] Within D&I science, the concepts of *designing for dissemination*—and more recently, *designing for sustainability*—refer to principles and methods for addressing the need for innovation "fit to context" as well as early and active dissemination and sustainability planning. Designing for dissemination and sustainability (D4DS) approaches may enhance the equitable and sustainable impact of evidence-based innovations on health and well-being of populations. D4DS is recognized as a key competency for D&I researchers.[5]

Traditionally, research paradigms used to develop and test innovations for translation into practice have been grounded in a sequential pipeline approach. This approach does not adequately incorporate early planning activities and stakeholder engagement necessary for innovation adoption, integration, and sustainment in real-world settings or the systems and structures that can help or hinder the process. The extent to which academics engage in research designed to translate to practice is linked to factors embedded in the academic system structure, such as current performance models and funding and publishing criteria.[6] Greater focus on advancing the science of ensuring fit to context is warranted to ensure health innovations will achieve broad and equitable adoption, sustainability, and impact on health.[7]

In this chapter, we define and describe the rationale for adopting a D4DS approach to research and describe products, principles, systems, and methods useful for D4DS. We introduce the fit-to-context framework (F2C) for designing for dissemination and sustainability, a process framework encompassing four stages for a long-term research endeavor. We provide case examples of research endeavors representative of D4DS principles and impact. In addition, we discuss approaches to D4DS with a health equity focus, both in the processes undertaken when employing such an approach and as an expected outcome of the processes undertaken. We anticipate that designing with consideration of research structures and distribution systems will enhance adoption and sustainment as well as mitigate inequities in access to health innovations.

RATIONALE FOR A D4DS APPROACH

There is a well-documented chasm between how researchers disseminate their findings and how

Bethany M. Kwan, Douglas A. Luke, Prajakta Adsul, Harriet Koorts, Elaine H. Morrato, and Russell E. Glasgow, *Designing for Dissemination and Sustainability* In: *Dissemination and Implementation Research in Health.* Edited by: Ross C. Brownson, Graham A. Colditz, and Enola K. Proctor, Oxford University Press. © Oxford University Press 2023. DOI: 10.1093/oso/9780197660690.003.0027 communities, practitioners, and policymakers learn about and use the latest evidence.[8] Passive diffusion of evidence-based interventions is ineffective, resulting in only small changes in the uptake of new practices.[9,10] According to the *push-pull* capacity model,[11] successful dissemination requires a basis in science and technology (the push), a demand from organizations or the populations being served (the pull), and the delivery ability of community, public health and healthcare systems (capacity). Dissemination strategies have often focused too much on the push side of this model, while lacking creative approaches and resources to address pull and capacity. The push-pull disconnect between researchers and practitioners was illustrated in a 2002 *Designing for Dissemination* workshop sponsored by the US National Cancer Institute.[12] A key workshop insight was the endorsement of the importance of active dissemination of the evidence—but neither researchers nor practitioners assumed the responsibility for dissemination activities. When leadership and ownership for dissemination are absent or when capacity is lacking, dissemination often sinks to a low priority in already overstressed systems.[13,14]

A D4DS perspective situates the responsibility for active dissemination within the research enterprise (i.e., researchers and research partners, research institutions, funders, scientific publishing, and communication platforms), with appropriate supportive systems, processes, and policies. Guidance on frameworks and necessary systems and processes have previously been proposed, such as Nutbeam's 1996 ideas on how to enhance dissemination beyond traditional journal article publications, incentives to reward researchers for translational research, and expanded practitioner training.[15] In 2006, Bauman and colleagues[16] proposed a six-step dissemination framework, which highlights the need to (1) describe the innovation; (2) identify the target audience, the sequence, timing, and format for dissemination; (3) define the communication channels; (4) determine the role of key policymakers and partnerships; (5) identify the barriers and facilitators for dissemination; and (6) evaluate the dissemination process. More recently, the PRACTIS (PRACTical planning for Implementation and Scale-up) guide assists researchers, practitioners, and policymakers to characterize the intended implementation context and identify potential adopters and decision makers within the system(s) that influence, and are influenced by, innovation and implementation processes.[17]

While there has been progress in advancing the D4DS perspective, there remain substantial gaps in researcher self-reported adoption of foundational D4DS activities, such as stakeholder engagement and planning for active dissemination. A 2012 study of US public health researchers showed only half of respondents (53%) had personnel dedicated to dissemination to nonresearch audiences.[13] Only 17% used a model to plan their dissemination activities, and 34% always or usually involved stakeholders in the research process. A similar 2018 survey of US and Canadian researchers found some improvement in stakeholder engagement in D4DS processes relative to the 2012 report, yet also identified a continuing misalignment between which dissemination methods impact a researcher's career and the methods that impact practice and policy.[18] Note the term *stakeholder* is increasingly seen as a remnant of colonialism; henceforth, we use terms such as "partner," "adopter," "decision maker," or other precise descriptors of those with a vested interest in a research initiative unless directly referencing another source.

While theories, methods, and outcomes of evidence-based adoption and implementation have been widely studied,[19,20] less attention has been paid to factors related to successful sustainability of programs and practices postimplementation.[21] Programs and practices need to be sustained over time to achieve their desired health impacts and associated outcomes.[22] Sustainable impact may also require that innovations become embedded in systems for population-level health improvement.[23] Many evidence-based programs and policies are not sustained after initial implementation, wasting large amounts of financial, organizational, and social capital.[24] For instance, a minority of efficacious health behavior innovations become embedded in systems at scale.[23] More recently, new work has made the case for more systematic study of sustainability, including conceptual development,[25] methods development,[26–28] and applications to a wide variety of health disciplines, including public health, mental health, and healthcare delivery systems.[29,30] Thus, planning for dissemination and sustainability needs to be more highly prioritized in the conduct of clinical and translational research and ideally earlier in the development and evidence-generation process.

ESSENTIAL COMPONENTS OF A D4DS APPROACH

When using D4DS in health research, there are three essential components: the research product itself, the dissemination plan needed to promote initial adoption and use, and the sustainability plan supporting sustained program delivery or innovation use over time.

Component 1: Designing a Research Product With the End in Mind

The **research product** is the health innovation to be disseminated. It can be an intervention, program, treatment, device, service model, policy, guideline, or implementation strategy resulting from clinical and translational research. To illustrate, Table 27.1 provides examples of research products found in a case example of designing for diabetes care.

A central principle in D4DS is *beginning with the end in mind*, meaning to plan for active dissemination and sustainability at the outset of a research effort.[31] That is, in adopting a D4DS perspective, scientists should start by considering who will ultimately benefit from uptake and use of the research product—and who may not and if expected benefits are likely to be equitable. Consider who will need to change practice or policy, who will need to invest resources, and who will need to develop new skills or apply skills in new ways. A second D4DS principle—*ensuring product-context fit*—refers to when the products of research are developed in ways that match the needs, resources, workflows, and contextual characteristics of the target audience and setting.[1] That is, D4DS means ensuring research products fit the context of intended use, at both the outset and over time. Note, we consider similar terms—such as "problem-solution fit" and "innovation-context fit"—part of the broad product-context fit concept.

TABLE 27.1 RESEARCH PRODUCT TYPES, DEFINITIONS, AND DESIGNING FOR DIABETES CARE CASE EXAMPLE

Research Product Type	Product Type Definition	Case Example: Designing for Diabetes Care117–119
Evidence	The generalizable knowledge resulting from the conduct of research and evaluation	People with diabetes benefit from diabetes self-management education and support (DSMS/E).
Programs, interventions, and services	Health promotion and/or disease prevention or educational programs, interventions, initiatives, treatments, or services	Diabetes shared medical appointments (SMAs) are an effective, efficient DSMS/E service model.
Technology and equipment	Devices, software, hardware, web-based, and other tools and equipment for disease prevention or management, research, evaluation, or educational purposes	Telehealth platforms can be used to deliver DSMS/E via diabetes SMAs virtually.
Dissemination and implementation strategies	Methods, approaches, guides, or materials for dissemination, implementation, and sustainment of effective, equitable, and efficient public health and healthcare practices in real-world settings	The Enhanced Replicating Effective Programs framework with external practice facilitation can be used to guide implementation of diabetes SMAs.
Policy, recommendations, and guidelines	Local and/or national public health and healthcare guidelines, practice or implementation standards, and policies emerging from the evidence base	Diabetes care guidelines recommend DSMS/E in primary care settings and inform practice priorities.
Methods	Research and evaluation techniques, instruments, tools, models, measures, and/or equipment	Validated measures of diabetes distress and self-care can be used to assess patient-centered outcomes for DSMS/E.

Poor innovation-context fit can arise very early in the research process, such that the research evidence prioritized by investigators or funders may or may not align with community needs or perspectives and the evidence required by the target audience to promote adoption.[6] The innovation-context fit is relevant when considering the wider multisector systems in which organizations are situated (e.g., health, transport, and education systems). An innovation designed for fit to organizational context will align with organizational goals and capacity for change, thus enhancing receptiveness of the organization to investing in adoption of the innovation. For example, the innovation-system fit relates to system readiness for change,[32] such that a system's capacity for change is an integral component for successful scale-up of health innovations.[33] System readiness and capacity for change are concepts that could be addressed during early planning and phases for scale-up, which may be achievable by adopting a systems perspective on scaling innovations for sustainable implementation.[34] More on scale-up of effective interventions is found in chapter 29.

Organizational support for innovations is essential for innovation uptake. Such support can be challenging to achieve even in contexts where the setting goals and innovation outcomes are highly congruent[35]; however, in contexts where goals and outcomes do not align, organizational systems and structures can have an increasingly dominant role in determining the innovation-context fit.[36]

Component 2: A Systems Approach to Planning for Active Dissemination

A third principle in D4DS is *planning for active dissemination.* Active dissemination refers to "an active approach of spreading evidence-based interventions to the target audience via determined channels using planned strategies."[37(p22)] A dissemination plan includes messaging about the relative advantages of the innovation for a specific target audience; how that message is packaged given communication preferences of the audience; and the communication channel by which that message is delivered to reach the intended audience. Consideration of the broader systems and structures in which a research product is meant to be used should inform product messaging, packaging, and communication channels. Messaging the value of a product in ways that align with the needs and perspectives of decision makers within larger systems is critical to adoption.

There are public health, delivery, education, and health policy systems and structures that are needed to support local and national policy change, workforce development, and change management. Planning for active dissemination requires understanding the characteristics of systems, organizations, and delivery settings in which research products are to be adopted and used, such as physical infrastructure or organizational culture.[13,38] Innovations intended for scale-up are often planned without an understanding of the prospective context and setting for use, the partnerships required, the role of potential adopters and decision makers in dissemination, or the scale-up resources needed.[17] Active dissemination should build and leverage existing system capacity and structures for marketing and distribution of research products (e.g., community dissemination pathways).[39] For instance, knowledge brokers acting between academic and practice settings and embedded researcher-practitioner partnerships and joint appointments between universities and government/nongovernment organizations can support an integrated process of D4DS.[40]

Component 3: Planning for Sustainability

A sustainability plan addresses the systems, resources, and value proposition that will support continued use of the research product in the real world. Particularly important for sustainability planning is engagement of those who make decisions at both local or organizational levels ("small p policy") and national or international levels ("big P policy") about how and by whom public health and healthcare should be delivered and financed.[41] Designing research products such that they address a policy need that can be effectively communicated to policy- and system-level decision maker audiences helps to ensure long-term and sustained impacts of innovation.[42]

CASE EXAMPLE

The Hunter New England Population Health (HNEPH) research-practice partnership is a government-funded population health unit in partnership with the School of Medicine and Public Health at the University of Newcastle,

Australia.[40] University researchers are embedded within the HNEPH unit, collocated to work alongside service delivery staff. A single-integrated governance structure oversees both service delivery and research initiatives, with senior researchers holding service delivery roles and health service managers leading research initiatives. This integrated research-practice partnership has optimized the coproduction of research so that it aligns with policy needs and enhanced active dissemination of research evidence as outputs are readily available for end users and decision makers, and it has streamlined the use of resources to achieve scientific and service delivery objectives.

FRAMEWORKS AND MODELS FOR D4DS

Process, evaluation, and determinants frameworks provide structure to the D4DS process and include a variety of approaches from D&I science. Several specific frameworks have been demonstrated as useful for D4DS. For instance, the IDEAS (Integrate, DEsign, Assess, and Share) Framework describes a step-by-step process for design of digital health interventions based in design thinking, behavioral theory, user-centered design, and dissemination approaches.[43] The research lifecycle framework from the US Department of Veterans Affairs Office of Research and Development Research-to-Real-World Workgroup explicitly incorporates scale-up, spread, and sustain phases of research, depicting the need for a research business plan, common impact metrics, and a sustainability plan as critical steps in translation of research innovations into routine practice.[44] Among other D&I frameworks with implementation or planning phases ideal for D4DS are the exploration, preparation, implementation, and sustainment (EPIS) framework,[45] the integrated Promoting Action on Research Implementation in Health Services (i-PARIHS) framework,[46] and the World Health Organization ExpandNet framework for scaling up.[47]

The D&I context and determinants frameworks such as diffusion of innovation theory[48] and the PRISM (practical, robust implementation and sustainability model) expansion of Reach, Effectiveness, Adoption, Implementation, and Maintenance (RE-AIM)[49] can also guide consideration of multilevel factors known to influence dissemination, impact, and sustainability during the design process, informing product features that address barriers and facilitators.[50] To enable effective planning for D4DS, Klesges and colleagues illustrated the usefulness of the RE-AIM framework for designing studies with a higher likelihood of future dissemination.[51]

Also, D&I science has contributed methodology and frameworks for planning for adaptation to ensure sustained fit to context.[52] For instance, the dynamic sustainability framework describes the need to expect and plan for pivots and iteration of the innovation and implementation process over time given anticipated dynamic context and changes in effectiveness on scale-up.[25] Although still an emerging area, guiding adaptations in a way that maintains the core functions or principles of a program, but adapts the form or specifics of how the program is delivered in ways that fit local context are promising directions.[53,54]

THE FIT-TO-CONTEXT FRAMEWORK: A NEW ITERATIVE APPROACH TO DESIGNING FOR DISSEMINATION AND SUSTAINABILITY

While the frameworks and models noted above are all relevant to D4DS, there is no single model that explicitly considers design of a research product and dissemination and sustainability plans from the perspective of ensuring fit to context. Fit to context—the fundamental concept in D4DS—serves as the basis of the process framework we present here (Figure 27.1). This F2C framework for D4DS was informed by and expands on previous work to define processes, products, and system changes needed to support D4DS efforts, push-pull-capacity concepts, and logic models in D&I.[13,55] The framework is represented as an iterative logic model depicting four phases in D4DS in ways that enhance the likelihood of research product adoption, sustainment, and ultimately more equitable impact on health. The conceptualization of D4DS as ensuring *fit to context* recognizes that the products being designed are culturally appropriate, feasible for use in resource-limited settings, align with the strengths and assets of the intended audience and setting, and impact outcomes that matter to communities and partners.[56,57]

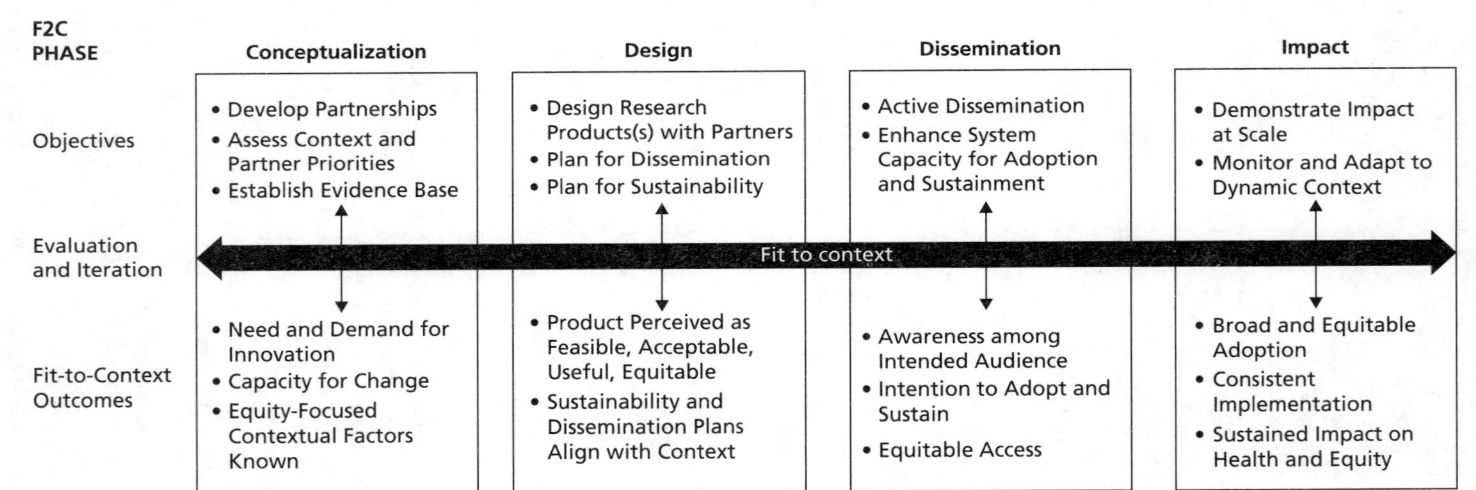

FIGURE 27.1 The fit-to-context (F2C) framework for designing for dissemination and sustainability.

The research product is informed by an initial conceptualization phase and product design phase. The *conceptualization phase* determines the need and demand for a solution to a health problem (the "pull") and draws on an evidence base of effective strategies for addressing the health problem. To effectively disseminate the evidence in response to the demand, a D4DS approach then considers a *product design phase* (determining the "research product" to be disseminated, how the product will be packaged and delivered, and how it would be sustained in real-world settings). The design phase of D4DS involves an active process of developing a research product and planning for its dissemination, scale-up, and sustainment as well as evaluating and iteratively improving design phase outcomes relevant to ensuring fit to context.

Research product design and the resulting dissemination plan is followed by an active *dissemination phase* (making use of systems and infrastructure [the "capacity"] to distribute the product package with broad reach to intended audiences [the "push"]). The final *impact phase* considers research product adoption, sustainment, and ultimate impact on health and health equity at the population level.

Evaluation occurs at every D4DS phase and is ideally iterative and ongoing to ensure continued fit to context and equitable reach, adoption, sustainment, and health impact over time. Various research and design methods, study designs, and outcome assessments are relevant across phases. Conceptualization and design phases are generally consistent with developmental/exploratory phases of research, including pilot and feasibility testing of health innovations. Dissemination and impact phases are consistent with full-scale randomized controlled trials, pragmatic and hybrid implementation-effectiveness trials, demonstration projects, quality improvement, and health system embedded research. Other D&I frameworks—especially those for informing approaches to community and partner engagement, assessment of contextual factors, and situation-specific determinants of dissemination and sustainability and measuring design phase outcomes and impact—are seen as complementary and are integrated into the F2C framework phases.

Fit-to-Context Decision Points Across the D4DS Phases

Each F2C framework phase includes an assessment of the extent to which phase-specific questions about fit to context have been answered before moving to the next D4DS phase versus continued iteration within the current phase (Table 27.2, "key question and phase outcome").

- In the conceptualization phase, the goal is to develop partnerships and assess the context in which a research product would be used and determine key partners' level of satisfaction with the current state, the demand for change, and a relevant evidence base. A context analysis can include identifying the characteristics of the recipients, the delivery setting, and implementation and sustainability infrastructure,[49] which can inform the design, dissemination, and impact phases. On demonstrating need, demand, and capacity for change (e.g., partners agree that a new approach is needed in a particular context), the next phase is to design a research product that addresses that demand and fits the expected context for use.
- During the product design phase, the objective is to co-design research product(s) and dissemination and sustainability plans with partners. Assessment of F2C design phase outcomes involves evaluation of perceived acceptability, appropriateness, and feasibility[58]; implementability[59]; costs, resources, and sustainability at the setting level[60]; and usability, usefulness, and user satisfaction at the user level.[61] Other design phase outcomes may include needed adaptations to fit changes in context over time or when translating a product for use in a new setting.[25] Evaluation and research methods of design phase outcomes range from user testing (e.g., system usability, user satisfaction, and engagement)[62] to pilot/feasibility studies and other research designs appropriate for testing D&I strategies[63] and can use quantitative and/or qualitative methods. Ideally, design phase outcomes are assessed rapidly and

TABLE 27.2 THE FIT-TO-CONTEXT (F2C) FRAMEWORK FOR DESIGNING FOR DISSEMINATION AND SUSTAINABILITY

F2C Phase Questions and Outcomes	F2C Phase Objectives	F2C Phase Exemplar Methods	F2C Phase Research Approach
Key questions to be answered and ***outcomes*** *to be assessed at each F2C phase*	*Actions to be taken by the research team and partners at each F2C phase*	*Research methods particularly relevant to co-design research products and evaluate and iterate "fit-to-context" outcomes at each F2C phase*	*Research approaches particularly relevant at each F2C phase*
		F2C Conceptualization Phase	
Based on evidence and partner input, to what extent is there a ***need, demand, and capacity*** *for a new approach, product, or change in practice or policy in the context for intended use? To what extent are* ***contextual factors*** *relevant to* ***equitable impact known****?*	Develop partnerships to address a priority health problem with an established evidence base. Assess the context (the characteristics of the recipients, the delivery setting, systems of communication and influence, and implementation and sustainability infrastructure) for which an innovative and equity-focused research product will be used.	• Literature review • Community-based participatory research • Partner and community engagement • Customer discovery • Situation/SWOT analysis • Process evaluation • Context analysis • Determinants analysis • Systems mapping and modeling • Social network analysis • Market research • Logic models • Needs assessment	• Partnership development • Partner engagement in research conceptualization and planning • Formative research • Baseline evaluation • Developmental/exploratory research
		F2CF Design Phase	
To what extent is the new approach, device, or change in practice or policy ***perceived as feasible, acceptable, useful, effective, and equitable*** *by the intended audience in the intended setting? How well do* ***plans for active dissemination and sustainability align with context****?*	Co-design research products(s) with partners that meet the needs, demand, and capacity for change established in the conceptualization phase. Create plans for active dissemination that align with the messaging, packaging, and distribution channels best suited for the intended audience and setting.	• Human & user-centered design/user testing • Participatory methods and co-design • Value proposition design • Market viability analysis • Business model generation • Intervention/implementation mapping • Optimization methods	• Developmental/exploratory research • Pilot/feasibility studies • "Proof-of-concept" studies • Small-scale pragmatic trials

	Determine a viable strategy for sustainability of the research product(s) in real-world contexts for intended use.	• Adaptation methods • Logic models • Rapid prototyping • Graphic design and other art forms	
	F2C Dissemination Phase		
How well does the ***active, planned dissemination strategy*** *work to create* ***awareness*** *and* ***intention to adopt and sustain*** *the product? To what extent does the system capacity for adoption and sustainment create* ***equitable access****?*	Enact design phase plans for active dissemination of the research product(s) to intended audiences using appropriate distribution channels and leveraging known systems of communication and influence. Build and leverage system capacity for broad and equitable adoption and sustainment in the intended context.	• Dissemination trial designs • Hybrid implementation/ effectiveness trials • Adaptation frameworks and methods • Logic models	• Larger scale, pragmatic trials • Demonstration projects • Quality improvement • Program evaluation • Learning Health Systems research
	F2C Impact Phase		
To what extent does the product demonstrate ***equitable impact on health*** *and* ***continued fit to context*** *over time in real-world contexts?*	Demonstrate equitable impact of research product(s) and active dissemination and sustainability plans at scale. Monitor and adapt research product(s), dissemination, and sustainment plans to ensure fit to dynamic context in real-world settings and populations.	• Pragmatic trial designs • Real-world evidence/observational methods • Economic and cost analysis • Hybrid implementation/ effectiveness trials • Policy analysis • Fidelity and adaptation methods • De-implementation methods	• Larger scale, pragmatic trials • Demonstration projects • Quality improvement • Public health surveillance • Program evaluation • Learning Health Systems research

iteratively based on successive prototypes or minimum viable products before moving on to distribution and large-scale testing.
- In the dissemination phase, the resulting research product is packaged and made available to users through a variety of platforms with messaging tailored to audience needs and perspectives. It may also include building and leveraging system capacity for broad and equitable adoption of the product. F2C outcomes in the dissemination phase include successfully reaching the intended audience by creating product awareness, enhancing intention to adopt and sustain use of the product in the intended context, and ensuring equitable access to products and services.

Notably, the way a research product is messaged, packaged, and distributed to intended audiences is an aspect of the D4DS approach parallel to, but distinct from, the design of the research product itself. *This step is the most overlooked component of D4DS.*[18] Messages, packaging, and distribution plans should be aligned with how that audience best receives information and should leverage existing and familiar distribution channels, platforms, and systems of communication and influence.[64] While dissemination to academic audiences, through conference presentations and journal articles, is necessary for academic researcher career advancement, dissemination to nonacademic audiences is necessary to achieve broad adoption.[65]

- In the impact phase, research tests the extent to which a research product exerts a sustained impact on health and health equity—the ultimate goal for the effective design and dissemination of research products. The impact phase should consider dynamic context, monitoring outcomes, and the need for adaptation over time. The impact phase may also reveal the need for "de-implementation" of innovations that no longer fit the context due to new, superior innovations or changes in context.

During any F2C phase (Table 27.2), it may become clear that the envisioned dissemination product is not a fit to context or target audience needs—necessitating a pivot or possibly abandoning the idea altogether. This is a valuable outcome as it can prevent continuing to invest resources in a product unlikely to be broadly adopted.[66] Clinicians, healthcare organizations, public health officials, and communities can waste time and resources on adapting and adopting solutions that are ultimately not scalable or financially sustainable, thereby providing a negative-feedback loop and reducing motivation to engage in the implementation of future solutions.[67]

Methods for Designing for Fit to Context Across D4DS Phases

A variety of methods are particularly relevant to each F2C framework D4DS phase, including participatory and co-design methods; context and situation analysis; systems science methods; business and marketing approaches; and methods from the fields of communication and the arts. This is not an exhaustive list, and many more methods from D&I and other disciplines may be appropriate for fulfilling D4DS principles. Several of these topics are covered in detail in chapters 10, 13, and 28.

Participatory and Co-design Methods

Guided by participatory perspectives on D&I,[68] D4DS encourages partnerships among transdisciplinary researchers, practitioners involved in the delivery of an intervention and impacted by the research, and, critically, the individuals and communities impacted by the research. That is, design is done in partnership with the intended audience—a participatory, co-design approach. Many types of partners can be involved at appropriate stages in the design process, from multiple systems, cultures, and socioecological levels, including members of the public, practitioners, policymakers, and payers, in both the health sector and beyond.[69] Community and partner engagement is important in all D4DS phases and is especially valuable during the conceptualization phase, orienting all future research activities to the needs, priorities, assets, and strengths of communities from the outset. Resources are available for selecting engagement methods most appropriate for project, organizational, and implementation team resources and constraints.[70]

Participatory co-design methods include techniques such as brokered or deliberative dialogue,[71] co-design/co-production such as experience-based co-design and behavioral design teams,[72] group model building and concept mapping,[73] consensus approaches such as nominal group technique or Delphi processes,[74] and the double-diamond design approach.[75] Co-design processes benefit from leveraging multisectoral partnerships among academic, industry, health system and community groups.[76] Considering and designing for the consumer perspective—which may include direct marketing to consumers—is an important form of collaborative program development.[77]

Context and Situation Analysis

A critical aspect of D4DS is gaining an in-depth understanding of the context in which a product is intended to be used and sustained. By context we include multilevel influences and factors such as culture, history, relationships, resources, and other factors as well as geographical setting. Methods for assessing context inform tailoring products that fit context[78,79] and adapting to changing context over time.[25,57] Context and situation analysis methods yield insights into the unmet needs and perspectives of the intended audience; the existing networks, systems, processes, and workflows into which the product will be integrated; and the resources available to support sustained use.[80]

Context and situation analysis methods include process mapping, network analysis, needs assessment, ethnography, and discourse analysis.[81,82] Customer discovery and value proposition design methods guide assessment of potential adopters and decision makers' context of intended use of an innovation; this process yields validated message framing about the value of a product on metrics most important for the target audience and in the context of competing alternatives.[83,84] Qualitative and mixed methods such as surveys, key informant interviews, and focus groups designed to assess audience needs, circumstances, and perspectives may be used during product design to understand contextual factors likely to influence dissemination, use, and sustainability.[85]

Systems Science Approaches

Dissemination and sustainability activities are embedded within complex social, health, cultural, organizational, and political systems.[86,87] Systems science approaches such as systems thinking, systems mapping, computational modeling, system dynamics modeling, agent-based modeling, and human factors engineering have all been used in D4DS endeavors.[76,88] These are distinct but related approaches for addressing the interactive and complex adaptive systems issues in dissemination and sustainment. For instance, systems thinking based on complex adaptive systems with system dynamics mapping has been used to inform large-scale change related to guideline implementation in Canada[89] and health services outcomes in the US Veterans Administration system.[90] A review of system dynamics applications in injury prevention research concluded that building capacity for system dynamics can support partner engagement and policy analysis.[91] Others have demonstrated the usefulness of iterative engineering approaches to successful program D&I.[92]

Complexity and systems science approaches focus attention on three specific substantive issues: dynamics, heterogeneity, and interactivity. First, the organizations and communities who are adopting and implementing new evidence-based practices are *dynamic*, not static. Systems perspectives can help focus attention on these dynamics, including feedback loops, indirect effects, and unintended consequences, as well as the need for program adaptation over time.[25] Second and third, these complex systems are made up of *heterogeneous* actors (e.g., patients, healthcare providers, regulatory agencies, commercial businesses, etc.) who *interact* with one another. Systems tools such as social network analysis and system mapping reveal and explore these interactions and thus are useful for dissemination design.[93,94]

Business and Marketing Approaches

Best business practices embrace a multi-stage development process consistent with D4DS principles: (1) problem-solution fit; (2) product-market fit; and (3) business model fit.[95] In the first stage, the developer gathers evidence demonstrating that the innovation is designed to solve an important job to be done, problem, or goal from the adopter's point of view better than competing alternatives will generate sufficient value to promote adoption. In the second stage, the developer validates that the innovation does indeed provide that value and that there is a market of potential adopters. In the last stage, the developer ensures the value proposition is embedded in a financially sustainable and scalable business model.

Communication and the Arts

Methods from the fields of communication, media production, advertising, journalism, and graphic design are useful for design of messaging, packaging, and distribution plans.[96,97] Packaging dissemination products can take multiple forms, such as web-based "knowledge translation platforms,"[98] evidence search and synthesis tools,[99] and professional learning and training platforms.[100] The web and social media are valuable channels for research dissemination and health communication with the public and clinical and public health professional audiences.[101,102] There are opportunities to explore "arts-based knowledge translation"[103]—the process of using "diverse art genres (visual arts, performing arts, creative writing, multimedia including video and photography) to communicate research"[104]—for dissemination to health care and public health audiences. Use of visual graphics can support communication with and translation of complex science concepts to target audiences.[105] Presenting data in engaging, easily understood ways is a hallmark of effective evidence communication to many audiences. End-user preferences for how evidence should be packaged and delivered need to be considered, as preferences can vary by audience.[106]

Packaging Dissemination Products Case Example

The MOVE! Weight-Management Program for Veterans in the US Veterans Health Administration (VHA) was designed to translate best practice guidance and evidence on weight loss into practice.[107] The program was packaged in the form of a toolkit consisting of patient handouts, promotional brochures, clinical references, and administrative manuals (https://www.move.va.gov/ReferenceTools.asp); marketing materials (e.g., posters, banners, pens); and online discipline-specific training modules about weight management with continuing education credit. All VHA networks and medical centers received the packaged intervention. Established VHA policy and clinical practice guidelines now require weight management programs, with MOVE! recommended.

A Focus on Health Equity Across D4DS Phases

We posit the F2C framework can be useful in designing for equitable reach and impact on health. To do so, the F2C conceptualization phase begins with considerations for individuals and communities with differential access to health interventions based on social, structural, and political determinants of health (i.e., education, economic stability, slavery, racism, health policies, unsafe neighborhoods, among others).[108] During the F2C design phase, researchers should ensure representation from communities for whom inequities may arise without consideration of social, structural, and political determinants. In addition, use of science communication approaches sensitized to cultures and to diversity, equity, and inclusion principles[109] enhances the likelihood that research products will reach historically and systematically marginalized communities.[110]

Critically, we advocate for engagement of population subgroups that have and continue to experience discrimination, trauma, and injustices and settings that perpetuate racism and discrimination. Designing from a F2C perspective builds on priorities for the partners and operates with the purpose of translating research findings into policy, practice, and system changes toward improving health, with an explicit goal of enhancing progress toward health equity.[111] A newer understanding on how to promote social justice within design thinking has been gaining recent traction and includes an explicit focus on the "ways that design reproduces and/or challenges the matrix of domination (e.g., white supremacy, heteropatriarchy, capitalism, ableism, settler colonialism, and other forms of structural inequality)."[112] For example, a "design justice" perspective centers co-design within the voices of the community, incorporates what is already working in the community, and facilitates change as a collaborative process.[112]

SUMMARY

Most health innovations are neither translated into practice nor sustained due to poor product-context fit as well as lack of emphasis on active dissemination and insufficient systems and infrastructure to support scale-up and sustainability. An F2C perspective using a D4DS approach places the responsibility for active dissemination in the scope of work for

TABLE 27.3 SUMMARY OF RECOMMENDED PRINCIPLES, METHODS, AND SYSTEMS FOR FIT TO CONTEXT AND DESIGNING FOR DISSEMINATION AND SUSTAINABILITY

Recommendation	Explanation
Embrace the Principles of Designing for Dissemination and Sustainability (D4DS)	
Recommendation 1: Begin with dissemination, sustainment, and equitable impact in mind.	It is not enough to begin with anticipated health outcomes in mind—begin by asking, who will influence the decision to adopt and sustain an innovation? Who is expected to deliver, benefit from, and pay for services and products? How can we reach the intended audience? How can we ensure equitable impact?
Recommendation 2: Prioritize the needs and perspectives of potential adopters, recipients, and decision makers at every stage of the process.	Involve partners representing multiple perspectives and context levels, including potential adopters and decision makers, to ensure products will fit the context of intended use; keep partners involved throughout the process to improve quality of adaptations.
Recommendation 3: Appreciate the value of a rapid and iterative approach and the need for periodic adaptation.	Anticipate and plan for the need to adapt programs or strategies in response to changes in context over time.
Apply Methods for D4DS	
Recommendation 4. Incorporate team science and systems science principles and practices.	D4DS is a collaborative enterprise and produces products that will influence systems of prevention, care, and health. Team and systems science best practices can help ensure that teams work well together and that they produce better products.
Recommendation 5. Employ strategic communication techniques tailored to the intended audience(s).	Audience segmentation and tailored messaging help ensure messages and materials will align with audience members' values, priorities, and ways of receiving information.
Recommendation 6. Evaluate adoption, equity, and sustainment at scale.	Conduct rigorous evaluation of research product adoption, equity, and sustainment impacts using both randomized and nonrandomized designs.
Develop Systems and Structures to Incentivize D4DS	
Recommendation 7. Establish and promote research training programs that acculturate trainees to the D4DS perspective and teach D4DS skills.	Build capacity for use of D4DS methods through training in partnership development and community engagement, user-centered design, and dissemination and sustainability planning.
Recommendation 8. Provide resources to support programs and policies that inform D4DS and develop pragmatic evidence.	Provide support and funding for systems and infrastructure needed to embrace a D4DS approach.

[a]Adapted with permission from Kwan et al.[113]

the research enterprise and related partners. We offer the F2C framework to D4DS as an iterative process that emphasizes the design phase of developing a research product and corresponding dissemination and sustainability plans. We list a range of methods for design, testing, and adaptation that can be used individually or in combination during each D4DS phase. To advance the science and practice of D4DS, we should reorient toward a mindset of beginning with the end in mind, requiring consideration of the needs of the intended audience and setting for use of research products from the outset.

To accelerate adoption of either our proposed F2C or another D4DS approach, we must have systems and organizational cultures and values that incentivize and facilitate partner engagement, active dissemination, and planning for sustainability.[13] We should equally consider and assess the systems and structures that *impact* and are *impacted by* dissemination efforts.[34] Table 27.3 summarizes key recommendations for embracing the principles of D4DS, skills needed to apply D4DS methods, and systems needed to incentivize a D4DS approach to research.[113] Ultimately, a D4DS approach advocates for transdisciplinary research paradigms (i.e., integrating various disciplines such as health communications, political science, economics, and public health, among others). Such research paradigms, in close engagement and collaborations with implementers and policymakers, have the potential to provide multisectoral solutions and products to achieving broad, sustainable health and health equity impact.[114,115]

ACKNOWLEDGMENT

Parts of this chapter were adapted with permission from the *Annual Review of Public Health*, Volume 43 © 2022 by Annual Reviews www.annualreviews.org.

SUGGESTED READINGS AND RESOURCES

Readings

Koorts H, Eakin E, Estabrooks P, Timperio A, Salmon J, Bauman A. Implementation and scale up of population physical activity interventions for clinical and community settings: the PRACTIS guide. *Int J Behav Nutr Phys Activ.* 2018 Dec;15(1):1–1. https://doi.org/10.1186/s12966-018-0678-0

The PRACTIS guide addresses how to plan for implementation and scale-up during intervention development, testing, and ongoing adaptation. The guide is framed around the principle that prioritizing factors relevant to dissemination, implementation, and scale-up early within the research process will enable potential barriers to be addressed and their impact measured. The guide is aimed at researchers, practitioners, and policymakers, with varying levels of implementation experience and expertise, to navigate the complex considerations and decision-making processes involved in translating evidence-based interventions into practice.

Kwan BM, Brownson RC, Glasgow RE, Morrato EH, Luke DA. Designing for dissemination and sustainability to promote equitable impacts on health. *Annu Rev Public Health.* 2022;43(1):331–353. https://doi.org/10.1146/annurev-publhealth-052220-112457

This narrative review of the literature on designing for dissemination and sustainability served as the basis for this chapter. It provides an in-depth review of the history of designing for dissemination concepts and frameworks. An organizing schema, adapted in this chapter as the F2C framework, was used to guide presentation of designing for dissemination methods and case examples.

Paina L, Peters DH. Understanding pathways for scaling up health services through the lens of complex adaptive systems. *Health Policy Plann.* 2012 Aug 1;27(5):365–373. https://doi.org/10.1093/heapol/czr054

This resource describes how to understand and interpret changes in health systems through a complex adaptive system lens. The article provides examples of how the behaviors of complex adaptive systems influence implementation and scale-up and suggests ways we can use a systems lens in the future to improve implementation efforts.

•Pauwels L, Mannay D. *The SAGE Handbook of Visual Research Methods.* Sage; 2019.

This text describes a visual research technique for public engagement and communication, ranging from visual media production, photovoice, visual ethnography, anthropological filmmaking, multimodal strategies, and making arguments with images.[116]

Selected Websites and Tools

Agency for Healthcare Research and Quality. https://www.ahrq.gov/sites/default/files/wysiwyg/professionals/quality-patient-safety/patient-safety-resources/resources/advances-in-patient-safety/vol4/planningtool.pdf

The Agency for Healthcare Research and Quality supported development of the Dissemination Planning Tool: Exhibit A from Volume 4, as part of efforts in Advances in Patient Safety: From Research to Implementation. The tool guides users through the components of creating a dissemination plan for research findings and products.

Henriksen K, Battles JB, Marks ES, Lewin DI, eds. Advances in patient safety: from research to implementation. Vol. 4, Programs, tools, and products. AHRQ Publication No. 05-0021-4. Rockville, MD: Agency for Healthcare Research and Quality; February 2005.

Clinical Sustainability Assessment Tool and Program Sustainability Assessment Tool. https://sustaintool.org/

Washington University in St. Louis's Clinical Sustainability Assessment Tool and Program Sustainability Assessment Tool aid in assessment of the sustainability capacity of a program or clinical practice to inform sustainability planning.

Communication Handbooks for Clinical Trials. https://communications4clintrials.org/

The Microbicides Media and Communication Initiative, a multipartner collaboration then housed at the Global Campaign for Microbicides at PATH (now coordinated by AVAC), and by Family Health International (now FHI 360) produced the Communication Handbooks for Clinical Trials. The handbook provides guidance on preparing and budgeting for communications, developing a strategic communication plan, developing and using key messages, communicating science clearly, and working with the media.

D&I Design for Dissemination (D4D) tool. https://ictr.wisc.edu/dissemination-implementation-launchpad/di-design-for-dissemination/

The University of Wisconsin-Madison's Institute for Clinical and Translational Research D&I Design for Dissemination (D4D) tool incudes a D4D Introduction Flyer, a D4D Engaging Adopters Booklet, a precall planning sheet, and a letter of support template.

Stakeholder Engagement Navigator. DICEmethods.org

The University of Colorado's Data Science to Patient Value initiative and the Colorado Clinical and Translational Sciences Institute's Stakeholder Engagement Navigator is an educational and interactive web tool for clinical and translational scientists seeking education and strategies for stakeholder engagement in research planning, conduct, and dissemination.

Exchanging Knowledge: A Research Dissemination Toolkit. https://www.american.edu/provost/ogps/graduate-studies/upload/dissemination-toolkit.pdf

The University of Regina's Community Research Unit's "Exchanging Knowledge: A Research Dissemination Toolkit" provides guidance on dissemination planning for community-based research.

The Health Foundation. https://www.health.org.uk/publications/communicating-your-research-a-toolkit

The Health Foundation, a UK-based independent charity, produced the "Communicating Your Research—A Toolkit" to help increase influence and impact in health and healthcare.

IM-Adapt. https://www.imadapt.org/#/

The University of Texas Health Science Center at Houston's IM-Adapt is an online program based on intervention mapping designed to guide identification and adaptation of cancer control interventions that fit the needs of the population and setting.

TDR. Communications and Advocacy. http://adphealth.org/irtoolkit/communications-and-advocacy/

TDR is a program supported by UNICEF, UNDP, World Bank, and the WHO and created the TDR Implementation Research Toolkit. Part of the toolkit includes a section on communications and advocacy to guide policy advocacy and strategic communications to specific stakeholders and audiences.

Translational Sciences Benefits Model. Translating for Impact Toolkit. https://translationalsciencebenefits.wustl.edu/toolkit/

Washington University in St. Louis's Translational Sciences Benefits Model website includes a Translating for Impact Toolkit, useful for mapping stakeholder needs, benefits, products, and impacts and planning for dissemination.

REFERENCES

1. Brownson RC, Colditz GA, Proctor EK. *Dissemination and Implementation Research in Health: Translating Science to Practice.* Oxford University Press; 2018.
2. Fraser I. Organizational research with impact: working backwards. *Worldviews Evid Based Nurs.* 2004;1:S52–S59.
3. Tabak RG, Stamatakis KA, Jacobs JA, Brownson RC. What predicts dissemination efforts among public health researchers in the United States? *Public Health Rep.* 2014;129(4):361–368.
4. Glasgow RE, Estabrooks PE. Pragmatic applications of RE-AIM for health care initiatives in community and clinical settings. *Prev Chronic Dis.* 2018;15:170271. doi:https://doi.org/10.5888/pcd15.170271
5. Padek M, Colditz G, Dobbins M, et al. Developing educational competencies for dissemination and implementation research training programs: an exploratory analysis using card sorts. *Implement Sci.* 2015;10(1):1–9.
6. Koorts H, Naylor P-J, Laws R, Love P, Maple J-L, van Nassau F. What hinders and helps academics to conduct dissemination and implementation (D&I) research in the field of nutrition and physical activity? An international perspective. *Int J Behav Nutr Phy.* 2020;17(1):7.
7. Baumann AA, Cabassa LJ. Reframing implementation science to address inequities in healthcare delivery. *BMC Health Serv Res.* 2020;20(1):1–9.
8. Brownson RC, Fielding JE, Green LW. Building capacity for evidence-based public health:

reconciling the pulls of practice and the push of research. *Annu Rev Public Health.* 2018;39:27–53.

9. Bero LA, Grilli R, Grimshaw JM, Harvey E, Oxman AD, Thomson MA. Closing the gap between research and practice: an overview of systematic reviews of interventions to promote the implementation of research findings. *BMJ.* 1998;317(7156):465–468.
10. Lehoux P, Denis J-L, Tailliez S, Hivon M. Dissemination of health technology assessments: identifying the visions guiding an evolving policy innovation in Canada. *J Health Polit Policy Law.* 2005;30(4):603–642.
11. Farrelly MC, Chaloupka FJ, Berg CJ, et al. Taking stock of tobacco control program and policy science and impact in the United States. *J Addict Behav Ther.* 2017;1(2).
12. National Cancer Institute. Designing for dissemination: conference summary report. In: National Cancer Institute 2002.
13. Brownson RC, Jacobs JA, Tabak RG, Hoehner CM, Stamatakis KA. Designing for dissemination among public health researchers: findings from a national survey in the United States. *Am J Public Health.* 2013;103(9):1693–1699.
14. Kerner J, Rimer B, Emmons K. Introduction to the special section on dissemination: dissemination research and research dissemination: how can we close the gap? *Health Psychol.* 2005;24(5):443.
15. Nutbeam D. Achieving "best practice" in health promotion: improving the fit between research and practice. *Health Educ Res.* 1996;11(3):317–326.
16. Bauman AE, Nelson DE, Pratt M, Matsudo V, Schoeppe S. Dissemination of physical activity evidence, programs, policies, and surveillance in the international public health arena. *Am J Prev Med.* 2006;31(4):57–65.
17. Koorts H, Eakin E, Estabrooks P, Timperio A, Salmon J, Bauman A. Implementation and scale up of population physical activity interventions for clinical and community settings: the PRACTIS guide. *Int J Behav Nutr Phy.* 2018;15(1):51.
18. Knoepke CE, Ingle MP, Matlock DD, Brownson RC, Glasgow RE. Dissemination and stakeholder engagement practices among dissemination & implementation scientists: results from an online survey. *PLoS One.* 2019;14(11):e0216971.
19. Lobb R, Colditz GA. Implementation science and its application to population health. *Annu Rev Public Health.* 2013;34:235–251.
20. Proctor E, Silmere H, Raghavan R, et al. Outcomes for implementation research: conceptual distinctions, measurement challenges, and research agenda. *Adm Policy Ment Health.* 2011;38(2):65–76.
21. Stirman SW, Kimberly J, Cook N, Calloway A, Castro F, Charns M. The sustainability of new programs and innovations: a review of the empirical literature and recommendations for future research. *Implement Sci.* 2012;7(1):1–19.
22. Scheirer MA. Is sustainability possible? A review and commentary on empirical studies of program sustainability. *Am J Eval.* 2005;26(3):320–347.
23. Reis RS, Salvo D, Ogilvie D, Lambert EV, Goenka S, Brownson RC. Scaling up physical activity interventions worldwide: stepping up to larger and smarter approaches to get people moving. *Lancet.* 2016;388(10051):1337–1348.
24. Goodman RM, Steckler A. A model for the institutionalization of health promotion programs. *Fam Community Health.* 1989;11(4):63–78.
25. Chambers DA, Glasgow RE, Stange KC. The dynamic sustainability framework: addressing the paradox of sustainment amid ongoing change. *Implement Sci.* 2013;8(1):1–11.
26. Luke DA, Calhoun A, Robichaux CB, Elliott MB, Moreland-Russell S. The Program Sustainability Assessment Tool: a new instrument for public health programs. *Prev Chronic Dis.* 2014;11:130184. doi:http://dx.doi.org/10.5888/pcd11.130184
27. Palinkas LA, Chou C-P, Spear SE, Mendon SJ, Villamar J, Brown CH. Measurement of sustainment of prevention programs and initiatives: the sustainment measurement system scale. *Implement Sci.* 2020;15(1):1–15.
28. Malone S, Prewitt K, Hackett R, et al. The Clinical Sustainability Assessment Tool: measuring organizational capacity to promote sustainability in healthcare. *Implement Sci Commun.* 2021;2:77.
29. Braithwaite J, Ludlow K, Testa L, et al. Built to last? The sustainability of healthcare system improvements, programmes and interventions: a systematic integrative review. *BMJ Open.* 2020;10(6):e036453.
30. Shelton RC, Lee M. Sustaining evidence-based interventions and policies: recent innovations and future directions in implementation science. *Am J Public Health.* 2019;109(S2):S132–S134.
31. Balis LE, Strayer TE 3rd, Ramalingam N, Harden SM. Beginning with the end in mind: contextual considerations for scaling-out a community-based intervention. *Front Public Health.* 2018;6:357–357.
32. Greenhalgh T, Robert G, Macfarlane F, Bate P, Kyriakidou O. Diffusion of innovations in service organizations: systematic

review and recommendations. *Milbank Q.* 2004;82(4):581–629.

33. Simmons R, Fajans P, Ghiron L. *Scaling Up Health Service Delivery: From Pilot Innovations to Policies and Programmes.* World Health Organization; 2007.
34. Koorts H, Rutter H. A systems approach to scale-up for population health improvement. *Health Res Policy Syst.* 2021;19(1):27.
35. Geerligs L, Rankin NM, Shepherd HL, Butow P. Hospital-based interventions: a systematic review of staff-reported barriers and facilitators to implementation processes. *Implement Sci.* 2018;13(1):36.
36. Leahy AA, Eather N, Smith JJ, et al. School-based physical activity intervention for older adolescents: rationale and study protocol for the Burn 2 Learn cluster randomised controlled trial. *BMJ Open.* 2019;9(5):e026029.
37. Rabin BA, Brownson RC. Terminology for dissemination and implementation research. In: Brownson RC, Colditz GA, Proctor EK, eds. Dissemination and Implementation Research in Health: Translating Science to Practice. Vol. 2. Oxford University Press; 2017:19–45.
38. Birken SA, Bunger AC, Powell BJ, et al. Organizational theory for dissemination and implementation research. *Implement Sci.* 2017;12(1):62.
39. Kreuter MW, Bernhardt JM. Reframing the dissemination challenge: a marketing and distribution perspective. *Am J Public Health.* 2009;99(12):2123–2127.
40. Wolfenden L, Yoong SL, Williams CM, et al. Embedding researchers in health service organizations improves research translation and health service performance: the Australian Hunter New England Population Health example. *J Clin Epidemiol.* 2017;85:3–11.
41. Brownson RC, Chriqui JF, Stamatakis KA. Understanding evidence-based public health policy. *Am J Public Health.* 2009;99(9):1576–1583.
42. Haynes A, Rowbotham SJ, Redman S, Brennan S, Williamson A, Moore G. What can we learn from interventions that aim to increase policy-makers' capacity to use research? A realist scoping review. *Health Res Policy Syst.* 2018;16(1):31.
43. Mummah SA, Robinson TN, King AC, Gardner CD, Sutton S. IDEAS (Integrate, Design, Assess, and Share): a framework and toolkit of strategies for the development of more effective digital interventions to change health behavior. *J Med Internet Res.* 2016;18(12):e317.
44. Kilbourne AM, Braganza MZ, Bowersox NW, et al. Research lifecycle to increase the substantial real-world impact of research: accelerating innovations to application. *Med Care.* 2019;57(10)(suppl 3):S206–S212.
45. Moullin JC, Dickson KS, Stadnick NA, Rabin B, Aarons GA. Systematic review of the exploration, preparation, implementation, sustainment (EPIS) framework. *Implement Sci.* 2019;14(1):1–16.
46. Laycock A, Harvey G, Percival N, et al. Application of the i-PARIHS framework for enhancing understanding of interactive dissemination to achieve wide-scale improvement in Indigenous primary healthcare. *Health Res Policy Syst.* 2018;16(1):1–16.
47. World Health Organization. *Practical Guidance for Scaling Up Health Service Innovations.* World Health Organization; 2009.
48. Dearing JW. Improving the state of health programming by using diffusion theory. *J Health Commun.* 2004;9(S1):21–36.
49. Feldstein AC, Glasgow RE. A practical, robust implementation and sustainability model (PRISM) for integrating research findings into practice. *Jt Comm J Qual Patient Saf.* 2008;34(4):228–243.
50. Bodkin A, Hakimi S. Sustainable by design: a systematic review of factors for health promotion program sustainability. *BMC Public Health.* 2020;20(1):1–16.
51. Klesges LM, Estabrooks PA, Dzewaltowski DA, Bull SS, Glasgow RE. Beginning with the application in mind: designing and planning health behavior change interventions to enhance dissemination. *Ann Behav Med.* 2005;29(2):66–75.
52. Escoffery C, Lebow-Skelley E, Udelson H, et al. A scoping study of frameworks for adapting public health evidence-based interventions. *Transl Behav Med.* 2019;9(1):1–10.
53. Chambers DA, Norton WE. The adaptome: advancing the science of intervention adaptation. *Am J Prev Med.* 2016;51(4):S124–S131.
54. Perez Jolles M, Lengnick-Hall R, Mittman BS. Core functions and forms of complex health interventions: a patient-centered medical home illustration. *J Gen Intern Med.* 2019;34(6):1032–1038.
55. Owen N, Goode A, Sugiyama T, et al. Designing for dissemination in chronic disease prevention and management. In: Brownson RC, Colditz GA, Proctor EK, eds. *Dissemination and Implementation Research in Health: Translating Science to Practice.* Oxford University Press; 2017:107–120.
56. Nooraie RY, Kwan BM, Cohn E, et al. Advancing health equity through CTSA programs: opportunities for interaction between health equity, dissemination and implementation, and translational science. *J Clin Transl Sci.* 2020;4(3):168–175.
57. Shelton RC, Chambers DA, Glasgow RE. An extension of RE-AIM to enhance sustainability:

addressing dynamic context and promoting health equity over time. *Front Public Health.* 2020;8:134.

58. Weiner BJ, Lewis CC, Stanick C, et al. Psychometric assessment of three newly developed implementation outcome measures. *Implement Sci.* 2017;12(1):1–12.
59. Kastner M, Estey E, Hayden L, et al. The development of a guideline implementability tool (GUIDE-IT): a qualitative study of family physician perspectives. *BMC Fam Pract.* 2014;15(1):19.
60. Kastner M, Sayal R, Oliver D, Straus SE, Dolovich L. Sustainability and scalability of a volunteer-based primary care intervention (Health TAPESTRY): a mixed-methods analysis. *BMC Health Serv Res.* 2017;17(1):1–21.
61. Porat T, Marshall IJ, Sadler E, et al. Collaborative design of a decision aid for stroke survivors with multimorbidity: a qualitative study in the UK engaging key stakeholders. *BMJ Open.* 2019;9(8):e030385.
62. Rosenbaum SE, Glenton C, Nylund HK, Oxman AD. User testing and stakeholder feedback contributed to the development of understandable and useful Summary of Findings tables for Cochrane reviews. *J Clin Epidemiol.* 2010;63(6):607–619.
63. Mazzucca S, Tabak RG, Pilar M, et al. Variation in research designs used to test the effectiveness of dissemination and implementation strategies: a review. *Front Public Health.* 2018;6:32.
64. Brownson RC, Eyler AA, Harris JK, Moore JB, Tabak RG. Getting the word out: new approaches for disseminating public health science. *J Public Health Manag Pract.* 2018;24(2):102–111.
65. McNeal DM, Glasgow RE, Brownson RC, et al. Perspectives of scientists on disseminating research findings to non-research audiences. *J Clin Transl Sci.* 2021;5(1):E61. doi:10.1017/cts.2020.563
66. Craven MP, Goodwin R, Rawsthorne M, et al. Try to see it my way: exploring the co-design of visual presentations of wellbeing through a workshop process. *Perspect Public Health.* 2019;139(3):153–161.
67. Hodgkins M, Khoury C, Katz C, Lloyd S, Barron M. Health care industry requires a roadmap to accelerate the impact of digital health innovations. *Health Affairs Blog.* 2018. doi:10.1377/hblog20180606.523635
68. Ramanadhan S, Davis MM, Armstrong R, et al. Participatory implementation science to increase the impact of evidence-based cancer prevention and control. *Cancer Causes Control.* 2018;29(3):363–369.
69. Concannon TW, Fuster M, Saunders T, et al. A systematic review of stakeholder engagement in comparative effectiveness and patient-centered outcomes research. *J Gen Intern Med.* 2014;29(12):1692–1701.
70. Kwan BM, Ytell K, Coors M, et al. A stakeholder engagement method navigator webtool for clinical and translational science. *J Clin Transl Sci.* 2021;5(1):E180. doi:10.1017/cts.2021.850
71. Parsons JA, Lavery JV. Brokered dialogue: a new research method for controversial health and social issues. *BMC Med Res Methodol.* 2012;12(1):92.
72. Robertson T, Darling M, Leifer J, Footer O. Behavioral design teams: the next frontier in clinical delivery innovation? *Issue Brief (Commonwealth Fund).* 2017;2017:1–16.
73. Green AE, Fettes DL, Aarons GA. A concept mapping approach to guide and understand dissemination and implementation. *J Behav Health Serv Res.* 2012;39(4):362–373.
74. Carter N, Lavis JN, MacDonald-Rencz S. Use of modified Delphi to plan knowledge translation for decision makers: an application in the field of advanced practice nursing. *Policy Polit Nurs Pract.* 2014;15(3–4):93–101.
75. Daly-Smith A, Quarmby T, Archbold VSJ, et al. Using a multi-stakeholder experience-based design process to co-develop the Creating Active Schools Framework. *Int J Behav Nutr Phy.* 2020;17(1):13.
76. Robinson K, Elliott SJ, Driedger SM, et al. Using linking systems to build capacity and enhance dissemination in heart health promotion: a Canadian multiple-case study. *Health Educ Res.* 2005;20(5):499–513.
77. Sanders MR, Kirby JN. Consumer engagement and the development, evaluation, and dissemination of evidence-based parenting programs. *Behav Ther.* 2012;43(2):236–250.
78. Pfadenhauer LM, Gerhardus A, Mozygemba K, et al. Making sense of complexity in context and implementation: the context and implementation of complex interventions (CICI) framework. *Implement Sci.* 2017;12(1):1–17.
79. Nilsen P, Bernhardsson S. Context matters in implementation science: a scoping review of determinant frameworks that describe contextual determinants for implementation outcomes. *BMC Health Serv Res.* 2019;19(1):1–21.
80. Bergström A, Dinh H, Duong D, et al. The Context Assessment for Community Health tool—investigating why what works where in low- and middle-income settings. *BMC Health Serv Res.* 2014;14(2):1–2.
81. Evans-Agnew RA, Johnson S, Liu F, Boutain DM. Applying critical discourse analysis in health policy research: case studies in regional,

organizational, and global health. *Policy Polit Nurs Pract.* 2016;17(3):136–146.
82. Luke DA, Harris JK. Network analysis in public health: history, methods, and applications. *Annu Rev Public Health.* 2007;28:69–93.
83. Nearing K, Rainwater J, Morrato E, et al. I-Corps@NCATS: a novel designing-for-dissemination learning laboratory for clinical and translational researchers to increase intervention relevance and speed dissemination. *Implement Sci.* 2020;15(suppl 1):25.
84. Osterwalder A, Pigneur Y, Bernarda G, Smith A. *Value Proposition Design: How to Create Products and Services Customers Want.* John Wiley & Sons; 2014.
85. Salloum RG, Theis RP, Pbert L, et al. Stakeholder engagement in developing an electronic clinical support tool for tobacco prevention in adolescent primary care. *Children.* 2018;5(12):170. https://doi.org/10.3390/children5120170
86. Northridge ME, Metcalf SS. Enhancing implementation science by applying best principles of systems science. *Health Res Policy Syst.* 2016;14(1):1–8.
87. Luke DA, Stamatakis KA. Systems science methods in public health: dynamics, networks, and agents. *Annu Rev Public Health.* 2012;33:357–376.
88. Willis CD, Mitton C, Gordon J, Best A. System tools for system change. *BMJ Qual Saf.* 2012;21(3):250–262.
89. Best A, Berland A, Herbert C, et al. Using systems thinking to support clinical system transformation. *J Health Organ Manag.* 2016;30(3):302–323.
90. Zimmerman L, Lounsbury DW, Rosen CS, Kimerling R, Trafton JA, Lindley SE. Participatory system dynamics modeling: increasing stakeholder engagement and precision to improve implementation planning in systems. *Adm Policy Ment Health.* 2016;43(6):834–849.
91. Naumann RB, Austin AE, Sheble L, Lich KH. System dynamics applications to injury and violence prevention: a systematic review. *Curr Epidemiol Rep.* 2019;6(2):248–262.
92. Quanbeck A, Brown RT, Zgierska AE, Johnson RA, Robinson JM, Jacobson N. Systems consultation: protocol for a novel implementation strategy designed to promote evidence-based practice in primary care. *Health Res Policy Syst.* 2016;14(1):1–10.
93. Valente TW. Network interventions. *Science.* 2012;337(6090):49–53.
94. Luke DA, Wald LM, Carothers BJ, Bach LE, Harris JK. Network influences on dissemination of evidence-based guidelines in state tobacco control programs. *Health Educ Behav.* 2013;40(1)(suppl):33S–42S.
95. Bland DJ, Osterwalder A. *Testing Business Ideas: A Field Guide for Rapid Experimentation.* John Wiley & Sons; 2019.
96. McCormack L, Sheridan S, Lewis M, et al. *Communication and Dissemination Strategies to Facilitate the Use of Health-Related Evidence.* Agency for Healthcare Research and Quality. 2013. Evidence Report/Technology Assessment 213.
97. Botsis T, Fairman JE, Moran MB, Anagnostou V. Visual storytelling enhances knowledge dissemination in biomedical science. *J Biomed Inform.* 2020;107:103458.
98. Berman J, Mitambo C, Matanje-Mwagomba B, et al. Building a knowledge translation platform in Malawi to support evidence-informed health policy. *Health Res Policy Syst.* 2015;13:73.
99. Dobbins M, DeCorby K, Robeson P, Husson H, Tirilis D, Greco L. A knowledge management tool for public health: health-evidence.ca. *BMC Public Health.* 2010;10(1):1–16.
100. Guerry JD. Another way through the two-way mirror: a review of psychotherapy.net. *Cogn Behav Pract.* 2016;23(2):256–261.
101. Chan TM, Dzara K, Dimeo SP, Bhalerao A, Maggio LA. Social media in knowledge translation and education for physicians and trainees: a scoping review. *Perspect Med Educ.* 2020;9(1):20–30.
102. Kapp JM, Hensel B, Schnoring KT. Is Twitter a forum for disseminating research to health policy makers? *Ann Epidemiol.* 2015;25(12):883–887.
103. Archibald MM, Caine V, Scott SD. The development of a classification schema for arts-based approaches to knowledge translation. *Worldviews Evid Based Nurs.* 2014;11(5):316–324.
104. Kukkonen T, Cooper A. An arts-based knowledge translation (ABKT) planning framework for researchers. *Evid Policy.* 2019;15(2):293–311.
105. Ninomiya MEM. More than words: using visual graphics for community-based health research. *Can J Public Health.* 2017;108(1):e91–e94.
106. Turck CJ, Silva MA, Tremblay SR, Sachse SL. A preliminary study of health care professionals' preferences for infographics versus conventional abstracts for communicating the results of clinical research. *J Contin Educ Health Prof.* 2014;34:S36–S38.
107. Kinsinger LS, Jones KR, Kahwati L, et al. Design and dissemination of the MOVE! weight-management program for veterans. *Prev Chronic Dis.* 2009;6(3):A98.
108. Crear-Perry J, Correa-de-Araujo R, Lewis Johnson T, McLemore MR, Neilson E, Wallace M. Social and structural determinants of health

inequities in maternal health. *J Womens Health.* 2021;30(2):230–235.

109. Dutta MJ. Communicating about culture and health: theorizing culture-centered and cultural sensitivity approaches. *Commun Theory.* 2007;17(3):304–328.
110. Canfield KN, Menezes S, Matsuda SB, et al. Science communication demands a critical approach that centers inclusion, equity, and intersectionality. *Front Commun.* 2020;5:2.
111. Wallerstein N, Duran B, Oetzel JG, Minkler M. *Community-Based Participatory Research for Health: Advancing Social and Health Equity.* John Wiley & Sons; 2017.
112. Costanza-Chock S. *Design Justice: Community-Led Practices to Build the Worlds We Need.* MIT Press; 2020.
113. Kwan BM, Brownson RC, Glasgow RE, Morrato EH, Luke DA. Designing for dissemination and sustainability to promote equitable impacts on health. *Annu Rev Public Health.* 2022;43(1):331–353.
114. Alonge O, Frattaroli S, Davey-Rothwell M, Baral S. A trans-disciplinary approach for teaching implementation research and practice in public health. *Pedagogy Health Promot.* 2016;2(2):127–136.
115. National Academies of Sciences, Engineering, and Medicine. Exploring Equity in Multisector Community Health Partnerships: Proceedings of a Workshop. Washington, DC: The National Academies Press; 2018. https://doi.org/10.17226/24786
116. Pauwels L, Mannay D. *The SAGE Handbook of Visual Research Methods.* Sage; 2019.
117. Kwan BM, Dickinson LM, Glasgow RE, et al. The Invested in Diabetes study protocol: a cluster randomized pragmatic trial comparing standardized and patient-driven diabetes shared medical appointments. *Trials.* 2020;21(1):1–14.
118. Kwan BM, Rementer J, Ritchie ND, et al. Adapting diabetes shared medical appointments to fit context for practice-based research (PBR). *J Am Board Fam Med.* 2020;33(5):716–727.
119. Glasgow RE, Gurfinkel D, Waxmonsky J, et al. Protocol refinement for a diabetes pragmatic trial using the PRECIS-2 framework. *BMC Health Serv Res.* 2021;21:1039.

28

Enhancing Dissemination Through Marketing and Distribution Systems

A Vision for Public Health

NIKO VERDECIAS, JOSEPH T. STEENSMA, MATTHEW W. KREUTER, AND JAY M. BERNHARDT

INTRODUCTION

The long lag time between discovery of new knowledge and its application in public health and clinical settings is well documented[1] and described in numerous other chapters in this book. Along this evidence-to-practice cycle, there is no shortage of evidence-based approaches and empirically supported programs to enhance the public's health,[2,3] but there are few *systems* in place to bring these discoveries to the attention of practitioners and into use in practice settings. In business, the process of taking a product or service from the point of development to the point of use by consumers is carried out by a *marketing and distribution system*.[4] In previous work, we have argued that marketing and distribution responsibilities within the broad public health system are largely unassigned, underemphasized, and/or underfunded for disseminating effective public health programs, and without them widespread adoption of evidence-based approaches is unlikely.[5] By understanding and applying fundamentals of marketing, efforts to disseminate public health solutions could be more effective. This chapter builds on our earlier work by (1) providing a framework from which to understand marketing, (2) proposing three specific components of a marketing and distribution system for evidence-based public health practices, and (3) describing how the potential benefits of such a system could be evaluated through dissemination research.

A CASE STUDY

In a classic example, a team of public health researchers in St. Louis, Missouri, created the ABC Immunization Calendar in the late 1990s. It was a simple computer software program designed to help community health centers boost low rates of immunization among babies and toddlers. The program used information from new parents and a digital photograph of their baby to create personalized monthly calendars that were given to the family during their baby's first 2 years of life. The calendars provided health and developmental information matched to the baby's age and reminders of the baby's next appointment in the vaccination series. Each time the parent and baby returned for a required vaccination, the program would take a new picture of the baby and print more months of the calendar (to cover the period leading to the next vaccination).

The program was well received in a pilot study[6] and increased child vaccination rates from 65% to 82% in an efficacy trial.[7] Based on these results, the research team obtained dissemination grant funding and adapted the program for widespread use.[8] A survey was conducted among potential user organizations to determine what computer platform and operating systems they were using. The ABC software was then reprogrammed to maximize compatibility with existing infrastructure. A user's guide was developed to help organizations install and use the program.

Niko Verdecias, Joseph T. Steensma, Matthew W. Kreuter, and Jay M. Bernhardt, *Enhancing Dissemination Through Marketing and Distribution Systems* In: *Dissemination and Implementation Research in Health.* Edited by: Ross C. Brownson, Graham A. Colditz, and Enola K. Proctor, Oxford University Press.
 DOI: 10.1093/oso/9780197660690.003.0028

An implementation guide was developed to help organizations decide how to integrate the program into their standard procedures and implement it. A promotional brochure with sample calendars and published articles was created and distributed at national meetings and to any person or organization that expressed interest. Training was provided, and some computer equipment was made available on loan. These efforts led to four Federally Qualified Health Centers (FQHCs) in the St. Louis area adopting the ABC Immunization Calendar. The program was delivered to thousands of families, and some centers used the program for many years.

Was the ABC Immunization Calendar a dissemination success? The research team adhered closely to conventional wisdom about translating public health science into practice. The intervention was tested for feasibility, acceptability, and efficacy in real-world settings. When positive results were found, the research team identified potential adopters, learned about their practice settings, and adapted the program accordingly. They created instruction manuals to help adopters use the software and to customize an implementation plan for their organization. They provided training and technical assistance. Local organizations adopted and used the program. But there are 7,500 FQHCs in the United States, reaching 17 million Americans. The ABC Immunization Calendar was adopted by four of them. In the grand scheme of things, the program's impact on the public's health was negligible.

Why didn't a program that's fast, easy, cheap, and effective find a home in more FQHCs? What should the research team have done differently to maximize its adoption and use? This story illustrates the limitations of current approaches to disseminating evidence-based programs and the need for marketing and distribution systems to support those efforts. For example, it's not the case that 7,496 FQHCs rejected the ABC Immunization Calendar. Rather, they *never even heard of it.* And if they had heard of it and wanted to adopt it, how would they obtain a copy? Could a small, university-based research team duplicate and distribute software and instruction manuals to hundreds or thousands of potential adopters? Could such a team also provide timely training and technical assistance to a mass of users? Are they trained to do this? Would they know how to set up such an operation? Would they *want* to do it? Would their university reward them for spending time on this? Thus, even well-intentioned, dissemination-minded researchers trying to do the right thing and following recommendations that are nearly universally accepted today will run up against demands that they are not trained to understand or address, lack the capacity to carry out, and are not viewed as central to the mission of the organizations where they work.

FROM SOCIETAL NEEDS TO CUSTOMERS AND EVERYTHING IN BETWEEN

In the example above, the ABC Immunization Calendar program was developed to meet a specific societal need. There was a need to increase childhood vaccination rates, and a solution was developed that appeared to meet this need in an efficient and effective manner. In spite of its advantages, there was not widespread uptake of the solution. To understand why this was the case, it is useful to understand how solutions are developed, marketed, and ultimately adopted by end users.

The old axiom that "necessity is the mother of invention" is accurate: Most great advancements (in public health and otherwise) were made because society had an unmet need, and enough people were impacted by the need to create a viable market for a solution. Unmet needs have costs associated with them, both personal and societal, and innovations bring value when the sum of their costs and benefits exceed the costs of the unmet need.[9]

If a need is big enough, there may be several people or entities trying to innovate around that need. In the academic realm, we often refer to these people as "colleagues"; in business, we call them "the competition." In theory, as more competitors move in to solve a problem, the market becomes more efficient as competitors jostle to have consumers adopt their products or services.[10] This is how markets are born and how they should behave. In a perfect world, the most valuable solutions persist, while less-valuable solutions join laserdiscs and Betamax video tapes in the dustbin of failed innovations.

Note that value and effectiveness are not synonymous. Value is a product of effectiveness and cost. For example, Solution A might have a very low cost and good (but not great) effectiveness, whereas Solution B is slightly more effective, but 10 times the cost. In this example, for most people Solution A is likely to be perceived as providing more value than Solution B. As illustrated in the case of ABC Immunization Calendars, however, even valuable innovations can fail to achieve widespread uptake. Is this evidence that market approaches don't apply in the context of research dissemination, or is there something beyond the value a solution brings to the market that needs to be taken into account?

A Framework for Customer Identification

Researchers have an arsenal of tools, such as community-based participatory research[11–14] (CBPR) that aim to establish partnerships, gain an understanding of a problem(s), and shape evidence-based intervention strategies. Using data, researchers identify a prominent problem, but that only offers one perspective of that problem. The intended partners need a platform to share how that problem manifests in their setting and how it affects their customers. Approaches like CBPR allow partners to join different skills and expertise to address complex problems. However, those efforts are sometimes limited to a particular solution geared to a particular customer, leaving subpopulations without the benefits of an effective solution. Efforts also, at times, skew toward an implementation process focus without broader application to dissemination efforts. We have already established that nearly all innovations start with a need, but how does an innovation go from addressing a "theoretical need" to "widespread adoption" with actual customers? This is the real challenge for a dissemination-oriented scientist: finding customers. It is incorrect to think of potential customers (users, clients) as any person or entity that might benefit from a particular solution. Rather, potential customers are a subset of that population with characteristics that make them amenable to trying a particular solution and have the means to adopt the solution.

Failure to properly identify customers is the undoing of many valuable innovations. These principles are partially grounded in diffusion theory[15] (see chapter 3) and should be applied early in the research process so that innovations (often in the form of evidence-based interventions) can be better designed for dissemination.[16]

To identify a customer, one can ask these five questions (Figure 28.1):

- What is the need/problem?
- Who deals with the need/problem?
- How are they dealing with the need or problem?
- In what ways is your solution better?
- Who would value the ways in which your solution is better?

Although the questions are simple and straightforward, the answers are often complicated. But the answers will reveal critically important information:

- By identifying the problem one has identified the societal need;
- By identifying who deals with the problem, one has identified the market for the solution;
- By identifying the ways in which the market deals with the problem, one has identified the competition for their product or service;
- By identifying in what ways one's product or service is better, one has identified where the value lies, which is called *the value proposition*; and
- If one can identify who would perceive the most benefit from the value proposition, one has identified the potential customers for the solution.

Returning to the ABC Immunization Calendars example, researchers had identified the need, and the market was clearly defined. Further, they understood how the market was dealing with the issue and had a service that was valuable. Researchers often have a deep understanding of the problems they are trying to solve and, at least sometimes, who in society is dealing with the problem. That said, in the ABC Immunization Calendar case the researchers had not articulated a value proposition in the context of other alternatives, and they did not know who would value the ABC Immunization Calendars over alternatives, one of which is maintaining the status quo. In other words, who were their target customers? Is it FQHCs? Public health departments? Social service agencies? New parents? The market for

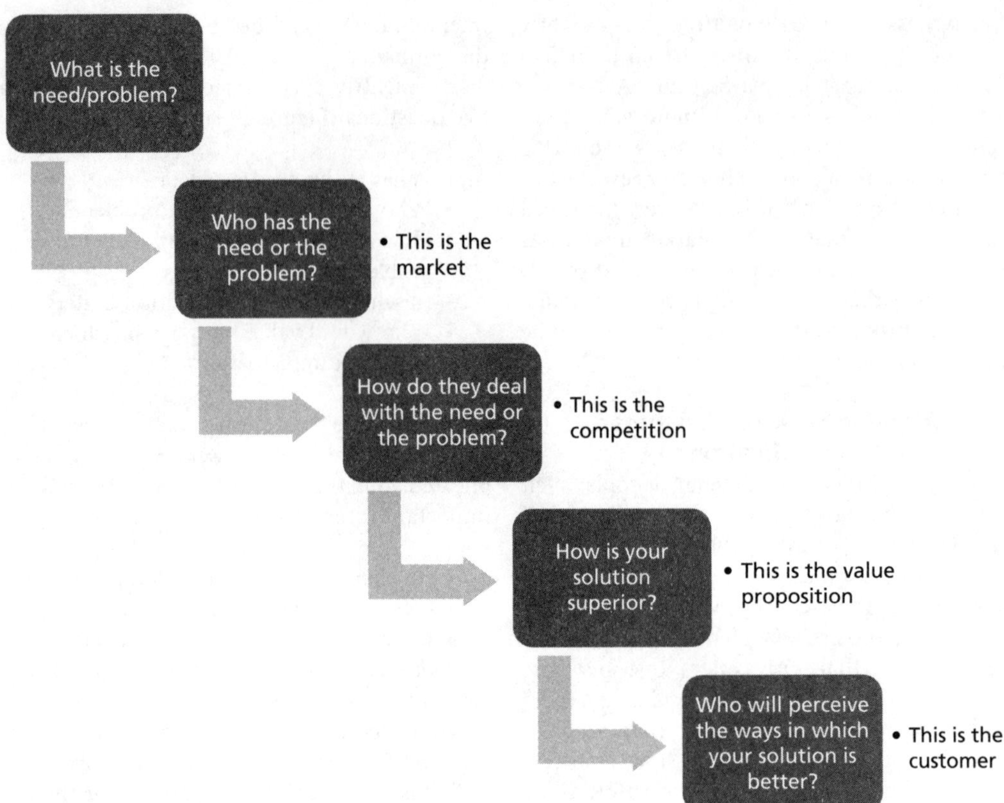

FIGURE 28.1 Five questions to identify customers, competitors, and a value proposition.

the service had been defined, but the customer had not. A better definition of the customer helps identify the proper channel(s) for reaching the customer.

The ABC Immunization Calendar case elucidates common challenges for dissemination-oriented researchers. As challenging as it is to produce, deliver, and support innovations such as the ABC Immunization Calendar, it is equally difficult to understand the competitive landscape and identify which segments of the market represent the best prospects for potential customers. Creating valuable solutions to society's challenges is not enough to garner widespread uptake if those solutions are unknown to those who would value them most and/or the solutions cannot be delivered effectively.

In short, the ABC Immunization Calendar was not lacking in potential value to society; it was lacking in the areas of marketing and distribution. One way to address such deficiencies would be to better prepare individual researchers to think and act as marketers. Alternatively, public health might establish marketing and distribution systems designed to accelerate movement of proven solutions into practice.

A MARKETING AND DISTRIBUTION PERSPECTIVE

Marketing and distribution systems are designed to bring products and services from their point of development to their point of use. This typically occurs through a system of interconnected organizations or intermediaries.[4] Collectively, these intermediaries identify potential users, promote the product to them, provide them with easy access to the product through convenient (and usually local) channels, allow them to see and use the product before acquiring it, help them acquire it, and support the product after purchase if the buyer has questions or problems.[17] Without such systems, every "producer" would have to interact directly with every potential customer or user to promote, distribute, and support a product or program. As illustrated by the previous case example, such interaction would be impractical and inefficient, and in business practice it is rare.

In understanding how a marketing and distribution system might improve dissemination of evidence-based interventions into public health practice, three key characteristics of the business model stand out. First, there is specialization of labor. It is not expected that the person (or organization) that developed a product will be the same one that manufactures it, distributes it, promotes it, sells it, services it, and supports the users that buy it.

Second, each of these responsibilities is assigned. It is the primary responsibility of someone (or some organization) to ensure that its part of the distribution chain is fulfilled. It is someone's job. If it's not carried out, they don't get paid.

Finally, all parts of the process are integrated. Even when carried out by different individuals (or organizations), these efforts are highly coordinated. In public health, most steps in the marketing and distribution process are unassigned, underemphasized, and underfunded. If they are undertaken at all, it is usually only as one of many responsibilities of someone who may lack the training or resources to do it well. And rarely are there financial or other tangible incentives for distributing or adopting evidence-based public health programs and services.

A SYSTEM FOR PUBLIC HEALTH

In the remainder of this chapter, we propose and discuss three parts of a marketing and distribution system to build a dissemination support system that could help bring more evidence-based interventions into public health practice.[18] These are (1) user review panels; (2) design and marketing teams; and (3) dissemination field agents. After each is described, we present a model system that would incorporate all three in an integrated fashion.

User Review Panels

For decades in the United States, popular televised talent competitions like *American Idol* and *America's Got Talent* have employed a voter experience based on combined expert and user reviews. TV shows like these bring competitors together to showcase their talent (e.g., singing, dancing) on a weekly basis. After each performance, contestants are critiqued by celebrity judges, and the TV audience votes for their favorite performer. The contestant that received the fewest votes is eliminated from the competition. This continues until one contestant remains and is declared the winner.

The format of these competitions entails a process and format that illustrates key differences between expert reviews and user reviews. For example, to compete on *American Idol* the most talented 12–18 singers were selected from 10,000+ aspirants who all went through a rigorous audition process. This occurred through an *expert review.* The judges evaluated auditioning singers based on a range of criteria they believe predicted success. This is not unlike the process of systematic evidence reviews in public health, wherein teams of scholars (i.e., experts) evaluate the strength of scientific findings for different types of interventions. Those with strong and consistent supporting evidence are "selected" and recommended for use in practice.

On *American Idol*, expert reviews were also provided after each song performed by a contestant. These critiques provided voters in the TV audience with some additional information on which they might base their decisions. But the viewing audience ultimately determined who won and lost. This is *user review.* Members of the voting audience were "users" because they would be the ones who purchased (or didn't) the music recorded by the winner. In essence, their votes reflect market demand for one singer versus another.

On *American Idol*, it's striking how often this market demand diverged from expert critiques. Why is that? One explanation is that not all viewers value the same things as music experts. Assuming that all of the finalists have a very high level of talent (and therefore a high likelihood of career success), it makes sense to leave this decision to market demand. We can apply the same logic to the process of disseminating evidence-based public health programs and strategies. When expert review has provided a menu of proven solutions, adopters and users (i.e., the market) will determine which, if any, meet their own unique needs and preferences. Knowing this, and in the absence of high cost, in-depth marketing research on intermediaries and end users, we should consider how to integrate formal user review processes into dissemination efforts in order to better identify potential customers/users.

We start with two assumptions: (1) Not all evidence-based interventions will work equally well in real-world practice settings; and (2) there are insufficient resources to develop every successful (i.e., empirically supported) prototype into a program or policy for active dissemination to adopters. Thus, a primary goal of user review panels in public health dissemination would be to identify those evidence-based programs and approaches that adopters really want and believe can be implemented. In other words, identify programs and approaches likely to be in high demand by different market segments. Just like the winner of *American Idol*, this subset of evidence-based interventions would then receive priority treatment and resources to be developed, adapted, and promoted for wider use. Programs and approaches not selected for focused development and marketing could still be adopted and used, but would not benefit from the same attention and resources.

Depending on the nature and type of evidence-based interventions being considered (and therefore the types of organizations—*customers*—likely to adopt a particular program or approach), user review panels might include representatives from community-based organizations, schools, city planners, policymakers, state and local health departments, FQHCs, healthcare systems, primary care providers, health foundations, and other organizations. These panels would review types of evidence-based based interventions (e.g., client reminder systems) as well as specific programs within each type. They could rate each on criteria like ease of use, organizational fit, implementation burden, acceptability to clients or patients, feasibility, as well as classic predictors of adoption, such relative advantage and trialability as described by Rogers (2003).[15] Interventions rated as most promising by a user review panel would be turned over to a design and marketing team to prepare them for widespread use and active promotion.

Design and Marketing Teams

At a 2002 Designing for Dissemination conference of invited researchers, practitioners, and intermediaries from across the United States, researchers were consistently the least likely to believe that translation and dissemination of research findings was their responsibility, felt unprepared in the science of dissemination and communication, and expressed that their interests and strengths were in areas other than translational work.[19] Researchers' interests and skills in translational science have grown in the 20 years since this meeting. However, only 28% of public health scientists report their dissemination efforts as excellent or good,[20] and nearly one-third rated their dissemination efforts as poor.[21] Formal training in disciplines related to the design, marketing, and distribution of public health programs and services is still uncommon, and there are few if any incentives—financial or otherwise—for researchers to actively disseminate their evidence-based public health programs.[20,22]

As noted in chapter 16 in this book and elsewhere,[23–27] greater attention to external validity during research design, analysis, and dissemination can help researchers and practitioners design programs that have higher translational potential. While we agree that greater understanding of these steps would enhance the translational efforts of scientists, we argue that design and marketing functions are sufficiently important and complex, and they require specialized expertise and dedicated personnel.

Although the details may vary case by case, there is a general sequence of actions that design and marketing teams carry out to make a promising product—like an evidence-based intervention—ready for the market. *Market research* is used to learn as much as possible about organizations or individuals that might adopt an intervention. What are their goals? How would this intervention help them achieve those goals? How would they use the intervention? How would it be integrated within their current client flow, operations, systems, and processes? Who within the organization would make the decision whether or not to adopt the intervention? Who would be responsible for implementing it? What are their concerns about the intervention? What would they change about the intervention? How will they sustain the intervention's implementation as needs and resources change?

Responses to questions like these would inform a wide range of design and distribution functions. For example, products routinely undergo *adaptation* or *reformulation* to maximize their appeal to potential users. If market research shows that potential adopters of a particular public health intervention are excited about Feature X or concerned about Feature Y, a smart design team would adapt the intervention accordingly. Also, it is often the case that the version of a program used in research under controlled conditions is not yet ready for use in practice settings. Knowing how, by whom, and for what purposes it will be used will help a design team reshape and package the program for use in specific nonresearch settings. In the world of dissemination, success and failure are not measured in *p* values and effect sizes; they are measured in uptake and satisfaction. To be successful in this context, an intervention must be malleable, and the developers must be willing to continually refine (or even redefine) the intervention to maximize their customers' value.

Using *audience segmentation*, a design team can distinguish between different subgroups of users and create targeted marketing and distribution strategies for each. Audience segments might be defined by organization type (e.g., schools, public health departments, FQHCs), populations served, intended use of the intervention, or any combination of these and other characteristics. What's important is that the characteristics shared within each subgroup, or segment, lead to distinct, actionable strategies for promoting and distributing the evidence-based intervention to specific types of potential customers. For example, different message strategies (e.g., "cost-effective" vs. "clients love it"); messengers (e.g., trusted peers vs. trade associations); and channels (e.g., conferences vs. online communities) might be indicated for different segments.

A design and marketing team would not only create the dissemination strategy, but also execute it. This would include many critical operational functions, including building partnerships, establishing a distribution system, providing training, technical assistance and user support services, coordinating and evaluating the overall process, and creating tangible incentives and rewards for adoption. These and other operational functions of a marketing and distribution system have been described in our previous work.[5] The question is not *whether* these functions are needed to more effectively disseminate evidence-based public health interventions, but rather *who* will perform them.[17] For the most part, they are currently unassigned. We believe it is unrealistic to expect public health researchers to possess the skills and have the time and/or the organizational support that would be needed to do these tasks well. A dedicated public health design and marketing team would have both.

Dissemination Field Agents

What do real estate agents, travel agents, and talent agents have in common? Each has specialized expertise and provides assistance with complex tasks that are often unfamiliar to those who use their services. They do this through direct contact—in person, by phone, and/or electronically—with their clients. These interactions are usually goal directed: buying or selling a house, planning a trip, negotiating a contract.

In public health, a corps of dissemination field agents could operate in a similar fashion, as a kind of evidence-based public health sales force. These specialists would have extensive knowledge of evidence-based interventions and expertise in how to adapt and implement the interventions in different settings and for different populations. They would work closely and proactively with customers to help them understand and choose from available strategies. They could provide detailed information about specific evidence-based programs, approaches, or policies across health topics and practice settings. If an organization decided to try an intervention, dissemination field agents would help them prepare and succeed by providing training and ongoing technical assistance to adapt, implement, and evaluate the evidence-based program, practice, or policy they chose. This provides an opportunity for everyone's investment in the process, therefore helping to move strategies beyond short-lived implementation outcomes toward attaining long-term sustained success.

Additionally, they could provide valuable feedback to the design team about customers and their changing needs and preferences. Such agents would be the "boots on the ground" listening to the voice of the customer and providing needed feedback to the team. These field agents would have similar training and functions as the knowledge brokers described in chapter 2.

Elements of this approach have shown promise. New York City's Public Health Detailing Program, which has been adopted by other state agencies, aims to help primary care providers improve patient care related to key public health challenges like vaccination, cancer screening, opioid misuse, obesity, and HIV testing.[28–32] Program representatives—*agents*, in our terminology—work in three communities with a high burden of poor health. They meet with doctors, physician assistants, nurse practitioners, and administrators to promote clinical preventive services and chronic disease management and to distribute "detailing action kits" that include evidence summaries, patient education materials, other small media, referral forms, chart stickers, community resource guides, and lists of service providers. Other public health efforts like this, modeled after physician detailing by pharmaceutical representatives, have been around for at least 40 years,[33] though mostly on a local level.

Nationally, the National Cancer Institute's (NCI's) Cancer Information Service (CIS) created the Partnership Program to help put cancer control science into practice to eliminate health disparities.[34] The CIS hired and trained 45 partnership coordinators in 35 states. These staff developed relationships with local, regional, and national organizations for the purposes of sharing information and networking, jointly developing cancer control projects using evidence-based approaches in minority and medically underserved populations, and increasing the capacity of partners to move science into practice. With its national scope, emphasis on translating science into practice, and coordination under a single administrative unit (CIS), elements of the Partnership Program could be followed in establishing a corps of dissemination field agents. However, despite a promising start and numerous successes, the program was short-lived and replaced by NCI's National Outreach Network (NON).[35–36] NON expanded the Partnership Program efforts by facilitating linkages between community health educators (akin to our concept of dissemination field agents) and cancer health center hubs across the United States.[36] NON's focus on disseminating cancer-related information and conducting evidence-based outreach using connections to care models that are tailored to the community's needs resulted in an increase in cancer-related awareness, improved health behaviors, and increased likelihood to get colorectal cancer screening among all racial/ethnic groups who participated in NON.[36]

AN INTEGRATED APPROACH

How would these three recommendations—*user review panels, design and marketing teams*, and *dissemination field agents*—come together in a coordinated marketing and distribution system to bring more evidence-based interventions into public health practice? Here's one vision. Imagine a new administrative unit within one of the nation's public health agencies being charged with accelerating the translation of science to practice. A first step would be to identify the universe of evidence-based approaches and practices. This is easier today than it ever has been, with a growing number of inventories of effective programs as well as systematic evidence reviews like the Community Guide.[37]

User review panels would be charged with narrowing this pool of eligible interventions to a smaller set that addresses genuine user demand in ways that are highly appealing to potential adopters. Because the scope of this task would be great, it may be necessary to impose some initial restrictions, like focusing on evidence-based approaches that address leading causes of death and disease or setting up separate panels for specific practice settings and/or health problems. These user reviews would necessarily be ongoing, but would provide periodic priority rankings of which evidence-based interventions were in greatest demand. A major collateral benefit of this process would be that its results, when shared, could redirect the efforts of public health scientists to better meet the needs of practice organizations and even suggest specific partnerships for practice-based research.

These priority rankings would set the agenda for a design and marketing team. Starting with the highest priority interventions, the team would work closely with developers and potential adopters to (1) define specific target audiences most likely to adopt each program; (2) make the programs ready for use in practice by these targeted adopters; and (3) develop strategies to effectively promote the program to these groups. Over time, the number of programs would grow. The result of these efforts would be an ever-expanding menu of evidence-based, high-demand, practice-ready programs. As user demand shifted (e.g., for emerging public health challenges), the items on the menu would expand accordingly.

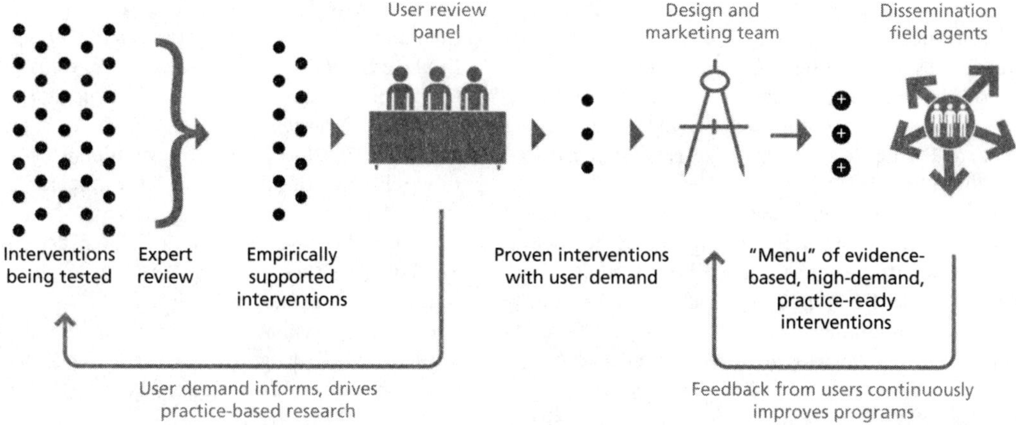

FIGURE 28.2 Integrating user review panels, design and marketing teams, and dissemination field agents in a new system for moving evidence-based programs into public health practice.

This "menu" would establish the parameters of activity for a corps of dissemination field agents. Initially, agents would execute the plans of the design and marketing team. They would seek out organizations identified as potential adopters and share with them the menu of programs designed for their unique practice setting. They would aim to establish positive relationships with organizations, ideally viewed as trusted and competent sources of information about evidence-based public health and prevention programs. When organizations express interest in one or more menu item, agents would shift their focus to providing technical assistance and support for implementation. One of the great advantages of having a field corps is that its members will quickly gain firsthand knowledge of the strengths and limitations of programs in different settings and the challenges and solutions related to implementation. This invaluable information would inform ongoing and iterative activities of the design and marketing team via a formal feedback loop. It would also create a network of agents that could help each other (and each other's clients) by sharing their experiences.

Figure 28.2 illustrates how user review panels, design and marketing teams, and dissemination field agents might be linked in an integrated approach to disseminating evidence-based public health programs.

SUMMARY

We realize that the vision of taking a more market-oriented approach to dissemination likely raises more questions than it answers. Who would build and operate such a system? Who would pay for it? Would researchers who have developed and evaluated public health interventions cooperate in sharing their programs and products? What tangible incentives can be created at each step of the process to encourage dissemination and adoption? What would constitute success for such an effort, and how would we measure it? All are important questions and worthy of thoughtful answers that match their complexity. Doing so is beyond the scope of this chapter, but ongoing in our work. We hope the ideas presented here will stimulate others' thinking about systems and infrastructure to enhance dissemination and welcome critiques, refinement, and additions to our proposed model.

SUGGESTED READINGS AND WEBSITES

Readings

Akbar MB, Garnelo-Gomez I, Ndupu L, Barnes E, Foster C. An analysis of social marketing practice: factors associated with success. *Health Mark Q*. 2021;1–21.

This article describes factors that contribute to successful social marketing practices.

Chichirez CM, Purcărea VL. Health marketing and behavioral change: a review of the literature. *J Med Life*. 2018;11(1):15–19.

The article examines literature focused on various social marketing-relevant theories, models, and strategies utilized to understand and predict behavior.

Dix CF, Brennan L, Reid M, et al. Nutrition meets social marketing: targeting health promotion campaigns to young adults using the Living and Eating for Health Segments. *Nutrients.* 2021;13(9):3151.

This article reports outcomes of a study that used social marketing practices to impact nutrition and health messages targeted toward young adults.

Kotler P, Keller KL. *Marketing Management.* Pearson Education Limited; 2016.

A useful introduction is made by an author with extensive experience in health and social marketing.

Kreuter MW, Bernhardt J. Reframing the dissemination challenge: a marketing and distribution perspective. *Am J Public Health.* 2009;99(12):2123–2127.

Critiques are given about current approaches to disseminating evidence-based public health programs, as are explanations concerning how and why a marketing and distribution system would enhance these efforts.

Williams A, Bowen SA, Murphy M, Costa K, Echavarria C, Knight M. Enhancing the adoption of evidence-based health marketing and promotion strategies in local communities: building a communication dissemination and support system for the national diabetes prevention program. *Health Promot Pract.* 2021;15248399211013817.

The article describes a successful health communication marketing and promotion support system that increases the utilization of effective marketing approaches with targeted messaging.

Woolf SH, Purnell JQ, Simon SM, et al. Translating evidence into population health improvement: strategies and barriers. *Annu Rev Public Health.* 2015;36:463–482.

The four principles for successfully influencing population health are reviewed, citing national and local examples.

Selected Websites and Tools

Diffusion of Effective Behavioral Interventions. http://effectiveinterventions.org/en/home.aspx

Effective Interventions provides an inventory of effective HIV and STD prevention and control programs, as well as information on how to use them.

REFERENCES

1. Green L, Ottoson J, Garcia C, Hiatt R. Diffusion theory and knowledge dissemination, utilization and integration. *Annu Rev Public Health.* 2009;30:151–174.
2. Zaza S, Briss P, Harris K, eds. *The Guide to Community Preventive Services: What Works to Promote Health?* Oxford University Press; 2005.
3. Office of Disease Prevention. *Evidence-Based Practices, Programs, and Resources.* Accessed January 17, 2023. https://prevention.nih.gov/research-priorities/dissemination-implementation/evidence-based-practices-programs
4. Palmatier RW, Sivadas E, Stern LW, Ansary AI. *Marketing Channel Strategy: An Omni-Channel Approach.* 9th ed. Routledge; 2019.
5. Kreuter M, Bernhardt J. Reframing the dissemination challenge: a marketing and distribution perspective. *Am J Public Health.* 2009;99(12):2123–2127.
6. Kreuter M, Vehige E, McGuire A. Using computer-tailored calendars to promote childhood immunization. *Public Health Rep.* 1996;111(2):176–178.
7. Kreuter M, Caburnay C, Chen J, Donlin M. Effectiveness of individually tailored calendars in promoting childhood immunization in urban public health centers. *Am J Public Health.* January 2004;94(1):122–127.
8. Caburnay C, Kreuter M, Donlin M. Disseminating effective health promotion programs from prevention research to community organizations. *J Public Health Manage Pract.* March 2001;7(2):81–89.
9. Porter ME, Kramer MR Creating shared value. In: Lenssen G, Smith N, eds. *Managing Sustainable Business.* Springer; 2019:323–346.
10. Bishop M. *Essential Economics: An A to Z Guide.* Public Affairs; 2016.
11. Israel BA, Parker EA, Rowe Z, et al. Community-based participatory research: lessons learned from the Centers for Children's Environmental Health and Disease Prevention Research. *Environ Health Perspect.* 2005;113(10):1463. doi:10.1289/EHP.7675
12. Israel BA, Schulz AJ, Parker EA, Becker AB. Review of community-based research: assessing partnership approaches to improve public health. *Annu Rev Public Health.* 1998;19:173–202.
13. Minkler M. Linking science and policy through community-based participatory research to study and address health disparities. *Am J Public Health.* 2010;100(suppl 1):S81–S87.
14. Ortiz K, Nash J, Shea L, et al. Partnerships, processes, and outcomes: a health equity-focused scoping meta-review of community-engaged scholarship. *Annu Rev Public Health.* 2020;41:177–199.
15. Rogers EM. *Diffusion of Innovations.* Free Press; 2003.

16. Brownson RC. Bridging research and practice to implement strategic public health science. *Am J Public Health*. 2021;111(8):1389. doi:10.2105/AJPH.2021.306393
17. Kotler P, Keller KL. *Marketing Management*. Pearson; 2014.
18. Kreuter MW, Wang ML. From evidence to impact: recommendations for a dissemination support system. *New Dir Child Adolesc Dev*. 2015;2015(149):11–23. doi:10.1002/CAD.20110
19. Chambers D, Simpson L, Neta G, et al. Proceedings from the 9th annual conference on the science of dissemination and implementation. *Implement Sci*. 2017;12(1):1–55. https://doi.org/10.1186/S13012-017-0575-Y
20. Brownson RC, Eyler AA, Harris JK, Moore JB, Tabak RG. Getting the word out: new approaches for disseminating public health science. *J Public Health Manag Pract*. 2018;24(2):102–111. doi:10.1097/PHH.0000000000000673
21. McNeal DM, Glasgow RE, Brownson RC, et al. Perspectives of scientists on disseminating research findings to non-research audiences. *J Clin Transl Sci*. 2021;5(1):61–62. doi:10.1017/CTS.2020.563
22. Hanneke R, Link JM. The complex nature of research dissemination practices among public health faculty researchers. *J Med Libr Assoc*. 2019;107(3):341. doi:10.5195/JMLA.2019.524
23. Neta G, Glasgow RE, Carpenter CR, et al. A framework for enhancing the value of research for dissemination and implementation. *Am J Public Health*. 2015;105(1):49. doi:10.2105/AJPH.2014.302206
24. Feely M, Seay KD, Lanier P, Auslander W, Kohl PL. Measuring fidelity in research studies: a field guide to developing a comprehensive fidelity measurement system. *Child Adolesc Soc Work J*. 2018;35(3):139–152. doi:10.1007/s10560-017-0512-6
25. Huebschmann AG, Leavitt IM, Glasgow RE. Making health research matter: a call to increase attention to external validity. *Annu Rev Public Health*. 2019;40:45–63.
26. Glasgow RE, Huebschmann AG, Brownson RC. Expanding the CONSORT figure: increasing transparency in reporting on external validity. *Am J Prev Med*. 2018;55(3):422–430.
27. Green LW, Glasgow RE. Evaluating the relevance, generalization, and applicability of research: issues in external validation and translation methodology. *Eval Health Prof*. 2006;29(1):126–153.
28. New York City Department of Health and Mental Hygiene. Public health action kits—NYC health. Accessed January 14, 2023https://www1.nyc.gov/site/doh/providers/resources/public-health-action-kits.page
29. San Francisco Department of Public Health. Rapid ART detailing aid. Accessed January 14, 2023. https://getsfcba.org/resources/rapid-art-detailing-aid/
30. Itzkowitz SH, Winawer SJ, Krauskopf M, et al. New York Citywide Colon Cancer Control Coalition (C5): a public health effort to increase colon cancer screening and address health disparities. *Cancer*. 2016;122(2):269. doi:10.1002/CNCR.29595.
31. Kattan JA, Tuazon E, Paone D, et al. Public health detailing—a successful strategy to promote judicious opioid analgesic prescribing. *Am J Public Health*. 2016;106(8):1430. doi:10.2105/AJPH.2016.303274.
32. Whitaker DE, Snyder FR, San Miguel-Majors SL, Bailey LAO, Springfield SA. Screen to Save: results from NCI's colorectal cancer outreach and screening initiative to promote awareness and knowledge of colorectal cancer in racial/ethnic and rural populations. *Cancer Epidemiol Biomarkers Prev*. 2020;29(5):910–917. doi:10.1158/1055-9965.EPI-19-0972.
33. Butler B, Godfrey Erskine E (1970). Public health detailing: selling ideas to the private practitioner in his office. *Am J Public Health*. 1970;60(10):1996–2002.
34. LaPorta M, Hagood H, Kornfeld J, Treimann J. Partnerships as a means of reaching special populations: evaluating the NCI's CIS Partnership Program. *J Cancer Educ*. 2007;22:S35–S40.
35. Dresser MG, Short L, Wedemeyer L, et al. Public health detailing of primary care providers: New York City's experience, 2003–2010. *Am J Public Health*. 2012;102(suppl 3):S342. doi:10.2105/AJPH.2011.300622
36. National Cancer Institute. National Outreach Network (NON). Accessed January 17, 2023. https://www.cancer.gov/about-nci/organization/crchd/inp/non
37. CDC. The Guide to Community Preventive Services (The Community Guide). Accessed January 14, 2023. https://www.thecommunityguide.org/

29

Scale-up and Sustainment of Effective Interventions

LUKE WOLFENDEN, RACHEL SUTHERLAND, RACHEL C. SHELTON, SZE LIN YOONG, AND NICOLE NATHAN

INTRODUCTION

Widespread and routine use of effective health interventions is the ultimate goal of health and medical research. By "scaling up" the routine adoption and implementation of effective interventions across health services and systems, much of the burden of disease could be alleviated. Yet, even when robust research evidence is generated systematically, from efficacy and effectiveness studies to dissemination and implementation trials, rarely are evidence-based interventions (EBIs) delivered at a scale that could yield population health improvements.[1] One reason for the failure to scaleup effective intervention is what some call the *know-do*" or "*knowledge to practice gap*—the gap between what we know is effective in improving health outcomes and what gets implemented at scale. That is, while significant research investment is applied to the development of new health interventions, there has been very little investment to understand how best to support the large-scale adoption, implementation, and integration of EBIs into health systems. For example, less than 3% of research published in the eight top-ranking nutrition journals were implementation, dissemination, or population-level studies.[2] The lack of evidence to support the effective scale-up of health interventions has impeded equitable and sustainable improvements in population health.

The sustainability of effective health interventions is required if the long-term public health benefits of such interventions that are implemented in practice, including those implemented at scale, are to be realized. Sustainability has been defined as (1) after a defined period of time; (2) the program, clinical intervention, and/or implementation strategies continue to be delivered; (3) individual behavior change (i.e., clinician, patient) is maintained; (4) the program and individual behavior change may evolve or adapt; while (5) continuing to produce benefits for individuals/systems.[3–5] The sustainability of evidence-based programs is acknowledged as one of the "most significant translational research problems of our time".[6] Understanding how best to sustain EBIs, particularly those that have been implemented at scale is an important area of focus within implementation science.

WHAT IS SCALE UP AND WHY IS IT IMPORTANT?

In general terms, scaling up refers to the process to "expand or replicate pilot or small-scale projects to reach more people and/ or broaden the effectiveness of an intervention."[7(pXI)] Once associated with haste, urgency, and haphazard approaches, today scale-up is emerging as a new and complex field of study.[8,9] It is a process that applies a systematic approach to supporting the adoption and implementation of an intervention that has demonstrated an effect at a local level to regional, national, or international levels by addressing the system and infrastructure issues arising during full-scale implementation.[8–10] Referred to by McCoy[11] as an intersection between art and science, scale-up is often the result of collaborations with policy makers, end users, and researchers to take a proven health intervention and enhance its dissemination, adoption, implementation,

Luke Wolfenden, Rachel Sutherland, Rachel C. Shelton, Sze Lin Yoong, and Nicole Nathan, *Scale-up and Sustainment of Effective Interventions*
In: *Dissemination and Implementation Research in Health.* Edited by: Ross C. Brownson, Graham A. Colditz, and Enola K. Proctor, Oxford University Press.
 DOI: 10.1093/oso/9780197660690.003.0029

and sustainability throughout an entire system to achieve greater health impact.[12] The term *intervention* is used broadly to represent the evidence-based practice, policy, service, or technology being scaled up.

KEY DEFINITIONS, SCALE-UP, SPREAD, SCALE-OUT, AND HORIZONTAL AND VERTICAL SCALING

One of the many complexities of scale-up is the minefield of terminology that is emerging to capture nuances of the process. While the terms "spread," "scale-up,", and "diffusion" were often used interchangeably in some implementation science and health literature, key definitions are emerging to support the use of consistent terminology. Key scale-up terms and their definitions are provided in Table 29.1.

THE ORIGINS OF SCALE-UP

While the application of science, including implementation science, to scale-up is in its infancy, scaling up health interventions is not novel.[13] Indeed, the experiences and response of lower-and middle-income countries (LMICs) to outbreaks of communicable disease or efforts to prevent them have occurred for decades and provided much of our current understanding of the process.[8] A narrative review conducted by Milat and colleagues[13] found six of the eight scaling up models or frameworks identified were based on experiences and guidance from communicable disease prevention and control in LMICs. The Framework for Going to Full Scale developed by Barker and colleagues[21] describes four key phases in the scaling up process—(1) *setup*; (2) *developing the scalable unit*; (3) *test of scale-up*; and (4) *go to full Scale*)—has been successfully applied in Ghana to scale up effective maternal and child health programs to more than 80% of public and faith-based hospitals and in South Africa to reduce mother-to-child HIV transmission from 19% in 2005 to less than 5% in 2010. There are also a range of examples of the successful scale-up of chronic disease prevention programs in high-income countries, in particular fiscal interventions targeting tobacco control and population-wide screening initiatives for the prevention and early detection of cancer.[22] One of the most successful, and well researched, examples of scale-up is in the field of diabetes prevention. Effective community-based diabetes prevention programs developed in the United States have been adapted and scaled up across the United States, Finland, Australia, and India over the past 20 years.[23-27] These, however, remain the exception

TABLE 29.1 KEY DEFINITIONS OF COMMON SCALE-UP TERMS AS APPLIED TO HEALTH SYSTEMS/HEALTH INTERVENTIONS

Term	Defined as
Scale up	Deliberate efforts to increase the impact of successfully tested health interventions to benefit more people and to foster policy and program development on a lasting basis.[13,14]
Scaling out	The implementation of evidence-based interventions in either new populations or new delivery systems or both.[15,26]
Scalability	The ability of a health intervention shown to be efficacious on a small scale and/or under controlled conditions to be expanded under real-world conditions to reach a greater proportion of the eligible population, while retaining effectiveness.[17]
Spread	The organic process of diffusion of a local improvement within a health system to replicate (with little modification) an intervention within a health system.[10,18]
Diffusion	The process by which an innovation is communicated through certain channels over time among the members of a social system.[19]
"Vertical" scale-up	The introduction of an intervention across a whole system that results in institutionalization of a change through policy, regulation, financing, or health systems.[20]
"Horizontal" scale-up	The expansion from replication to scale-up ("horizontal" scale-up), which includes the introduction of an intervention across different sites or groups in a phased manner that expands from replication to scale-up.

rather than the rule. In most fields, examples of large-scale implementation of EBIs remain elusive, and research to better understand the scale-up process is nacent.[26,27]

The evolution of our understanding of scale-up has been informed by a range of theoretical perspectives. Implementation science takes a mechanical, structured, and staged based approach to scale-up; complexity science has a more ecological perspective, emphasizing flexibility and adaptive processes to facilitate scale-up within complex systems; while social sciences approaches consider how organizational and broader social forces influence behavior, including that required for the spread and scale-up of programs.[9] Approaches to scale-up may draw on multiple perspectives. In this text, we primarily draw on perspectives of scale-up with roots in implementation science. As these disciplines and others continue to develop, so too will our understanding of scale-up. Greater research in the coming decade will also help elucidate the interventions, strategies, and contexts most amenable for scale-up, and with it, the development of tools to assist with application of these insights to enhance the success of scale-up efforts.

WHERE DOES SCALE-UP FIT IN THE RESEARCH TRANSLATION PROCESS?

Research process models describe ideal stages of progression of research into routine practice. These start from formative evaluation and hypothesis generation, through to testing the effects of interventions, methods to disseminate and implement them, and finally strategies to scale-up, embed, and sustain the intervention into health systems (Figure 29.1). In this context, scaling up a program or innovation is often considered a separate process following earlier testing of the intervention, dissemination, and implementation strategies. However, viewing these stages independently and in sequence may complicate efforts to scale up. The potential to scaleup should be considered:

- while designing the health intervention to ensure complexity and characteristics of scalable interventions are considered[30];
- throughout the effectiveness trial phase to ensure the health intervention fits within the policy context and aligns with stakeholder and end user needs[31]; and
- through the implementation and dissemination research phases to ensure consideration of implementation at scale.

Indeed, early consideration of these factors will address the many complexities of moving a project from pilot to wide-scale uptake.[32] With this in mind, Figure 29.1 shows scale-up as a planned and iterative *process* commencing early in the research process and progressing across the research translation pipeline.

The Process of Scaling-up

A number of frameworks have been developed that describe the process of scale-up and guide actions to facilitate beneficial scale-up outcomes. A systematic review in 2015 identified eight such frameworks;[13] however, a number of others have since been published.[32,33] Perhaps the most influential of these to date has been the World Health Organization's ExpandNet,[30] which describes nine steps to scale-up. While there is variation in the number and actions outlined in these frameworks and an acknowledgment that the scale-up process is often not linear, broadly these included phases related to (1) formative work to prepare for scale-up; (2) executing a scale-up plan and implementing an intervention at scale; (3) evaluation; and (4) monitoring and sustaining scale-up (see Box 29.1).

Considering Scalability in Intervention Development

Many health interventions are developed and tested that are not amenable to implementation at scale.[34] Identifying interventions that are well suited to scale-up in the context in which it is to occur may improve the likelihood that scale-up efforts are successful. To this end, a number of studies have sought to better understand the scalability of an intervention to facilitate both intervention development and selection for scale-up. Scalability is "the ability of a health intervention shown to be efficacious on a small scale and or under controlled conditions to be expanded under real world conditions to reach a greater proportion of the eligible population, while retaining effectiveness."[17(p289)] It is often confused with the ability to increase reach, without consideration of other important dimensions of the definition, that is, capacity for continued effectiveness or impact and the

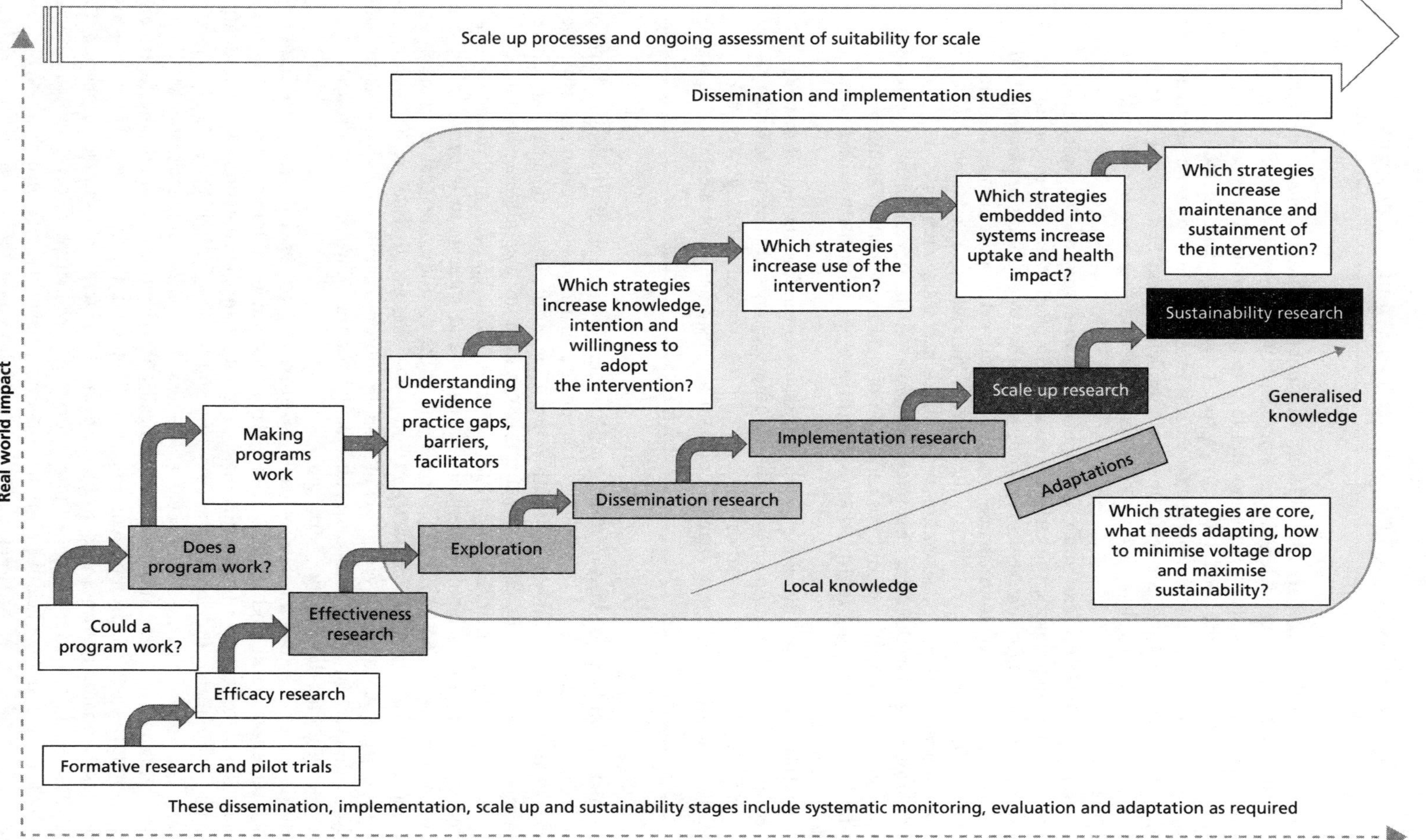

FIGURE 29.1 Summary of the scale-up process.

Source: Adapted with permission from the original figure by Brown and colleagues (2017)[28] and amended version by Deenik.[29]

BOX 29.1

BROAD PHASES INCLUDED IN SCALE-UP FRAMEWORKS

1. **Formative work to prepare for scale-up.** This phase includes undertaking research, engaging relevant stakeholders, identifying attributes of interventions, contexts and stakeholder capacity for scale-up and factors that may facilitate or impede it. This work should be used to develop a specific scale-up plan, including a compelling rationale for scaling-up, the health intervention and strategies to achieve implementation at scale, the scale-up agents/implementers, their specific roles, the systems to support scale-up within routine practice and the resources required for scale up.
2. **Executing a scale-up plan and implementing an intervention "at scale."** This phase encompasses undertaking the tasks of the scale-up plan, including preparing the system for the health intervention, coordinating the execution of implementation strategies via the existing systems, establishing supportive governance, ongoing monitoring, and evaluation. This will require a foundation of stakeholder support and consultation with those authorized to make necessary changes.
3. **Monitoring and evaluation.** This phase encompasses the development of systems for routine data collection and the collection of data to evaluate scale-up processes and impacts, including information to inform strategy refinements and further improvement.
4. **Sustaining scale-up.** This phase involves changes to the functioning of systems required for sustained implementation, including changes in structures (ways of organizing), practice (ways of doing), and culture (ways of thinking). Vertical scale-up strategies are particularly important for sustained implementation at scale.

extent to which it can be embedded in routine health services.[35]

A range of tools has been developed with the intention to support the development or selection of existing interventions that best suited to scale-up.[36] The Intervention Scalability Assessment Tool (ISAT),[37] for example, includes five domains characterizing the context in which the intervention is to be scaled up (description of the problem; the proposed intervention; the broader strategic and political context; evidence of effectiveness; and intervention costs and benefits) and five domains used to assess implementation and scale-up requirements (fidelity and adaptation, reach and acceptability, delivery setting and workforce, implementation infrastructure, and sustainability). The tool prompts consideration of these domains by those responsible for funding, selecting, or undertaking or those impacted by the scale-up of a health program. It assumes the scalability of an intervention is enhanced when the implementation context and capacity are supportive of scale-up. However, a number of challenges have been reported in the use of scalability assessments, including difficulties identifying sufficient information to assess some attributes of the intervention (e.g., cost) and when they should occur,[35] and there is little empirical evidence yet of their validity or that their application improves successful scale-up. Examples of the application of scalability assessments to public health programs are provided elsewhere.[38]

Determinants and Barriers to Scale-up

As is recommended for the design of strategies to improve implementation per se, identifying and understanding barriers and contextual factors that may influence the scale-up of health interventions is important to enhance the likelihood that such efforts will be successful. O'Hara, for example, suggested that formative evaluation for scale-up incorporate methods including evidence synthesis, consultation and qualitative research with the target audience, and situational and environmental analysis of the systems required for scale-up.[39]

TABLE 29.2 BARRIERS AND FACILITATORS IN SCALING-UP OF PUBLIC HEALTH INTERVENTIONS[a]

Barriers	Facilitators
Lack of financial, human, material, and other relevant resources required for scale up	Sufficient advocacy (e.g., involvement of champions at multiple levels to draw attention to the problem, facilitate policy/other changes to support intervention scale-up)
Logistical barriers (existing health service structures, geographical restrictions, lack of supplies)	Political will/political support of the problem/intervention approach
Weak health systems and governance	Alignment with existing policies/guidelines
Lack of intra- and cross-sectoral collaborations at multiple levels	Characteristics of the intervention and available data on relevance, importance, and cost-effectiveness
Lack of research, monitoring, and evaluation	Availability of strategic scale-up plan
Sociocultural environment—incompatible with social and cultural norms and preferences	Training and supervision
Lack of need/demand for the intervention across multiple levels, existence of local innovations	Organizational incentives and rewards
Competing priorities for end users/implementers	

[a]From Bulthuis 2019,[42] Miake-Lye 2019,[43] Troup 2021,[44] Ezezika 2021.[45]

Such methods have been reported to be useful in the successful scale-up of a telephone-based coaching service to improve physical activity and nutrition in Australia.[39] Barriers to scale-up are likely to be dynamic and vary across the scale-up phases. New barriers may arise as stakeholders become more familiar with the intervention or move from planning to executing a scale-up plan—with many of the barriers difficult or indeed impossible to anticipate. The dynamic nature of the processes necessitates flexible approaches to scale-up and processes to facilitate adaptations to scale-up strategies as challenges emerge.[40]

A number of reviews have described the barriers and facilitators to scaleup across a range of health programs and topics. Across different areas, the primary challenges with scaling up include limited resources, including a lack of funding to devote to scaling-up a program, competing priorities, a perceived lack of need for the proposed intervention, and a lack of policy/political support (see Table 29.2 for summary of barriers and facilitators summarized in reviews).[41–45] However, a recent study using systems analysis described a complex web of interrelated factors that may be causally related to the outcomes of scaling up nutrition and physical activity interventions.[41] The study suggested that factors such as intervention reach and cost are related to increased likelihood of scale up in some circumstances, but their presence may not be critical. In a review of the scale-up of interventions in LMICs, building technical and management capacity of stakeholders and community engagement and collaborations appeared to be particularly useful in ensuring sustained implementation at scale; however, factors such as high staff turnover appeared associated with decay.[42]

Adaptation and Scale-up

Adaptations are deliberate alterations to the design or delivery of an intervention to improving its fit or effectiveness in a given context.[46] Adaptations may be particularly common, and indeed necessary, as programs are scaled up to accommodate increasingly diverse population groups and costs and logistical challenges that occur with greater scale. For example, there may be a need to pare back the number or intensity of intervention strategies to reduce delivery costs or ensure program materials and content are appropriate, engaging, and understood for a range of cultural groups in the community. Indeed, reviews across a range of clinical and public health interventions suggested that such adaptations are ubiquitous as part of the scale-up process.[47,48] Descriptions of the nature of adaptations to interventions that have been scaled up have indicated that adaptations to the mode of delivery are most frequently reported, such as changes from face-to-face to telephone or web-based modes of delivery interventions or support of their implementation.[48] Presumably such adaptations are made to enhance scalability through reducing relative costs and improving potential reach. Other frequently reported adaptations are related to changes made to improve the fit of the intervention with the characteristics of the setting in which it is to be delivered and changes to program content.[49]

While adaptations are necessary, they have the potential to influence the effectiveness of interventions particularly if adaptations are made to the "core" components of the intervention responsible for driving intervention effects. For example, reductions in the length, number, or duration of core intervention components in order to facilitate greater program reach or reduce costs could be accompanied by a reduction in the effectiveness of interventions. From a population perspective, the community health impact of a program is a function of its reach and its effectiveness. As such, the widespread implementation of a less effective intervention may yield greater health benefits than a more effective intervention that is only able to be implemented on a small scale.[50] Nonetheless, at any scale, the effect size of an intervention must remain at a level that is therapeutic for it to be beneficial. Reviews of diabetes prevention, obesity, physician activity, and nutrition programs suggested the effectiveness of interventions following scale-up typically reduce by 25%–50% of that reported in efficacy and effectiveness studies.[51,52] This phenomenon of effect reduction at scale is often termed *voltage drop* or the *scale-up penalty*.[47,48,53] An understanding of core intervention and implementation strategy components and an appraisal of the potential impact of the adaptations to these can help those responsible for scaling up interventions ensure the beneficial impacts of interventions to the community are preserved.

Despite implementation science texts describing a number of adaptation frameworks, specific guidance regarding the processes of adaptations for scale-up is limited. Nonetheless, the processes undertaken by a number of are well described elsewhere, including the scale-up physical activity ("Choose to Move"[54] and Physical Activity 4 Everyone [PA4E1][55,56]) and diabetes prevention programs.[24] Miller et al.[57] put forward a decision tree, describing a nonlinear and recursive series of decision points to describe a dynamic process in which adaptations can occur and that has been suggested to be suitable for scale-up. The decision tree includes explicit assessment and consideration of any voltage drop in effect that may occur at scale (see Figure 29.2).

Implementation "At Scale"

Despite it being the goal of scale-up efforts, there remains no agreed definition of what constitutes "at scale." Some authors have operationally and arbitrarily defined it as the delivery of interventions in 50 or more "organizational units," such as a school, childcare service, or workplace. Other conceptualizations of implementation at scale suggest it is related to the delivery of an EBI at a scale capable of producing population-wide improvements in public health.[58] Strategies to implement interventions at scale will depend, in part, on the type of scale-up. Vertical scaling up strategies may place greater emphasis on leveraging existing health systems and structures and funding mechanisms, whereas horizontal scaling efforts may seek to achieve expansion of the intervention across a greater number of sites through modifying delivery modalities and infrastructure. Action Schools! British Columbia (AS!BC), a school-based physical activity intervention, is one of a few examples of successful scale-up of physical activity interventions. It employed both horizontal scale-up strategies such as the establishment of a central support service to provide technical assistance to school personnel to facilitate intervention delivery and vertical scale-up strategies, including embedding the interventions in local schools via local action plans and across the school system via embedding within the Directorate of Agencies for School Health (DASH).[59]

Strategies to improve the implementation of EBIs across a range of settings have typically yielded only modest improvements in program implementation.[60–62] Achieving improvement in implementation at scale, therefore, represents a considerable challenge. Systematic reviews of the effectiveness of strategies to improve implementation of chronic disease prevention

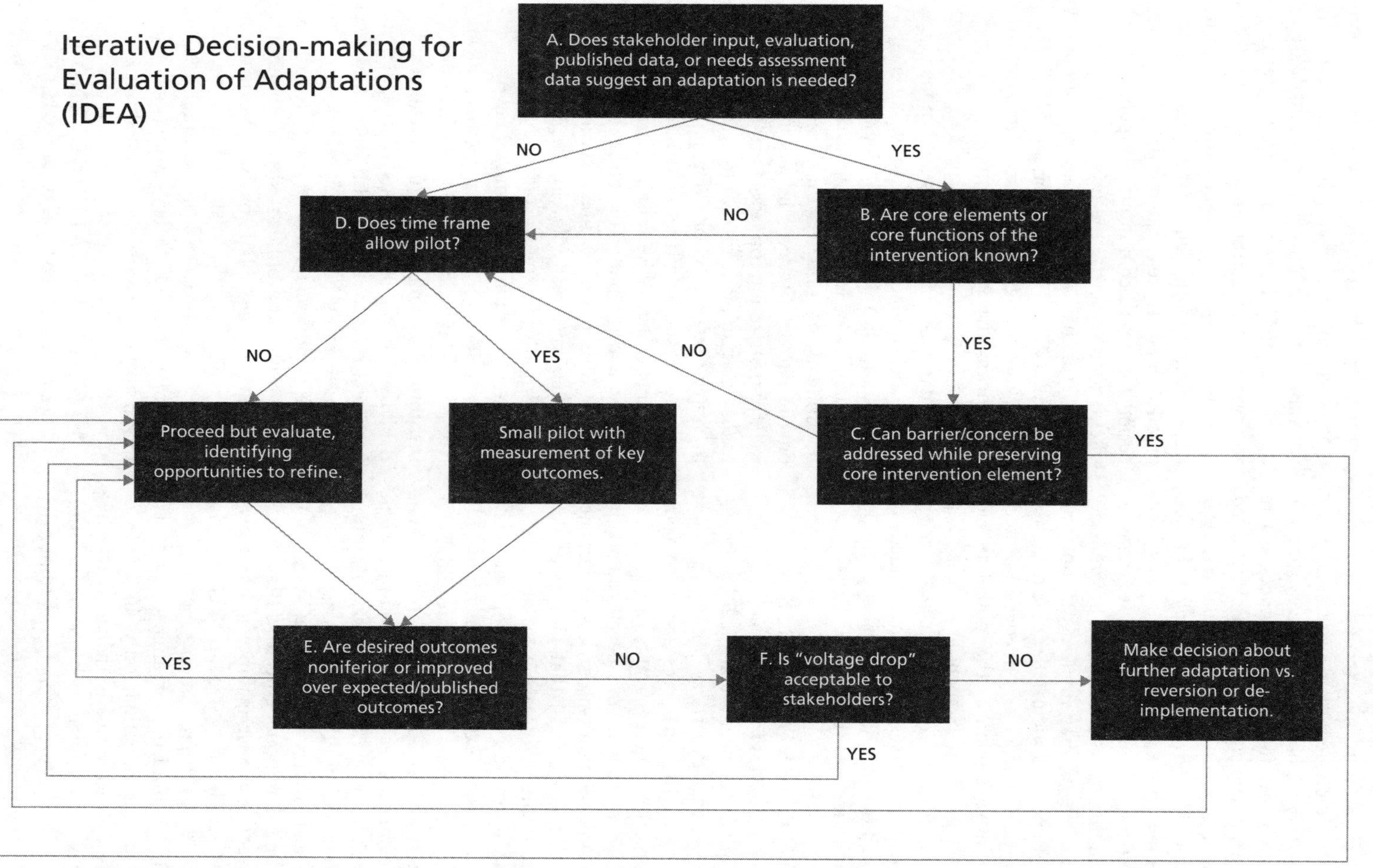

FIGURE 29.2 The Iterative Decision-making for Evaluation of Adaptations (IDEA).

Source: Reprinted with permission from Miller et al.[57]

programs at scale (>50 sites) in community settings identified just eight trials.[63] The effects of strategies tested in these trials on measures of program implementation were mixed.[60–62] Nonetheless, a number of effective examples of scale-up exist, including instances where large-scale implementation has been achieved without a significant "scale-up penalty." These have employed conventional implementation science-based approaches in the development of their strategies to implement programs at scale, including the application of theoretically guided processes to map implementation strategies to overcome anticipated implementation barriers. In the absence of evidence to provide more definitive guidance, the potential success of strategies to implement at scale is likely maximized through comprehensive strategy development processes as recommended by current implementation and scale-up frameworks and guidelines (Box 29.2).[64–66]

WHY SUSTAINABILITY MATTERS

Sustainability has been identified by implementation science experts as "one of the most significant translational research problems of our time."[6(p2)] There have been significant advancements made in the development and testing of interventions, programs, treatments, and practices (e.g., EBIs) that aim to prevent and address chronic disease in communities.[69] Despite this investment in developing, evaluating, and to some extent implementing EBIs, sustaining the routine and widespread delivery of public health and healthcare interventions and their impact over time is a common challenge across a range of settings, organizations, populations, and health issues.[6,70–72]

Empirical studies suggest that only about half of clinical and public health EBIs are sustained over time. Sustainability is likely even more challenging in low-resource contexts.[73] A review of 19 health promotion programs from a portfolio of funded programs found that 1 to 6 years after adoption, only 40%–60% of programs were continually delivered to some extent (e.g., delivering at least one of the original components over time).[74] Additionally, a review by Wiltsey Stirman et al.[75] of 125 research studies further highlighted the challenge of sustaining a range of public health and clinical programs; the authors found that less than 50% of EBIs continued at high levels of fidelity to the original intervention (e.g., not all core components of the original program were delivered). It is important to note that most empirical research in this area has not thoroughly examined the sustainability of policy-oriented EBIs or policy-related settings, an important gap in the existing literature.[76]

There are many reasons why sustaining EBIs matters in implementation research and practice. First, there is often a delay or latency period for many community or public health interventions whereby the impact at the population level may not be apparent until many years after initial delivery of the EBI.[77] Thus, lack of continuing or sustaining programs over time means that the program and its benefits will not fully achieve its impact or potential, particularly among settings and populations that face numerous structural barriers to health and healthcare. Additionally, lack of sustainability of EBIs has implications for lost investments of valuable time and resources on the part of funders and organizations, as well as frustration on the part of administrators and implementers who were involved in implementation efforts for programs that were not sustained. There may also be ethical questions that may be raised by policymakers, funders, and the public of continuing to invest in new EBIs if we are not sustaining existing EBIs that are already developed. Additionally, abandoning or failing to continue programs in clinical or community settings may also create or reinforce negative perceptions and mistrust of research and public health/healthcare institutions among community members, particularly among populations that experience persistent social and health inequities that have historically been marginalized. If we are to apply implementation science to promote health equity and build trust with community partners, it is essential that we prioritize and actively plan for the sustained and equitable delivery and impact of EBIs (see Table 29.3 for a summary table of challenges and opportunities in advancing work on sustainability).

CONCEPTUALIZING AND DEFINING SUSTAINABILITY

There has been much variability in how sustainability has been named, conceptualized, and operationalized across public health, healthcare, and implementation science, which historically has made the literature in this

BOX 29.2

CASE STUDY: IMPROVING ADOLESCENT PHYSICAL ACTIVITY LEVELS VIA STRUCTURE SCALE-UP RESEARCH: THE PHYSICAL ACTIVITY 4 EVERYONE EXPERIENCE

In Australia, 9 in 10 Australian adolescents are considered physically inactive, yet few effective coordinated and comprehensive physical activity programs targeting secondary schools exist. Physical Activity 4 Everyone (PA4E1) was developed to fill this gap, targeting schools located in lower socioeconomic areas. PA4E1 is a comprehensive multicomponent physical activity program consisting of seven physical activity (PA) strategies addressing the curriculum, physical education, school environment, and links with parents and the community. Schools are supported to implement the program over a 24-month period, supporting adolescents to maintain their activity levels in a critical window where activity levels significantly decline. Health promotion practitioners employed by local health districts provide implementation support to teachers. The program was rigorously planned in partnership with key stakeholders, including the Education Department, teachers, and end users to ensure it was contextually relevant, acceptable, and feasible to implement using the available infrastructure.

A randomized controlled trial (RCT) (hybrid type 1 effectiveness implementation trial, 2012–2014) found students attending PA4E1 schools participated in 49 minutes more moderate to vigorous physical activity (MVPA) per week[67] and experienced less unhealthy weight gain (2 kg)[68] than students attending the control schools. The intervention was also found to be cost-effective. On the basis of the trial findings, government stakeholders were interested in making the program more broadly available to benefit more students.

Making use of implementation and scale-up frameworks and in co-production with researchers and end users (principals, teachers, and students), formative evaluation was undertaken to inform the scale of PA4E1 across 49 schools. This included

1. Collection of data on the potential barriers and enablers of implementing PA4E1 practices in secondary schools at scale;
2. Developing targeting implementation strategies based on the Theoretical Domains Framework to address the identified barriers;
3. Consultation with key stakeholders to prioritize the implementation strategies and embed within existing systems; and
4. Formation of an expert advisory group to review the scaled-up intervention.

Informed, in part, by this work, the program sought to retain the core intervention components to retain effectiveness while enabling greater reach. This included replacing (1) face-to-face teacher professional learning with a hybrid online and face-to-face model; (2) project specific learning with accredited education sector courses; (3) verbal prompts and manually generated feedback reports with automated prompts and feedback via an online portal; (4) the external change agent with both an internal (School Champion) and an external (Support Officer) change agent; and (5) paper resources with an online portal. A full description is provided in Figures 29.3 and 29.4. A randomized controlled implementation trial was conducted to evaluate the effectiveness of the scale-up strategies on implementation outcomes (school uptake of school PA practices. At 24-month follow-up, the proportion of schools implementing at least four of the seven physical activity strategies (primary outcome) was significantly higher in the program group (16/23, 69%) than the control group (0/25, 0%) ($P < .001$).[55]

Due to adaptations, the scale-up trial cost A$17,296 per school (A$117.30 per student).[55] Implementation of school PA practices was consistent with the original trial at 12 months; however, a small voltage drop was observed between trials at 24-month follow-up, where PA practice update remained consistent but did not increase. Modifications to the implementation support where documented through the trial using Stirman et al.'s 2019 expanded framework FRAME,[8] indicating they were primarily fidelity consistent.

area disparate and challenging to synthesize. A number of terms have been used to refer to sustainability that capture related but distinct aspects of sustainability, including *routinization, institutionalization, sustainment, durability, maintenance*, and *long-term follow-up/implementation*, as well as terms related to discontinuing programs (e.g., *discontinuation, de-adoption, de-implementation*).[5,72,75,79] Historically there has been a focus on conceptualizing sustainability as *institutionalization* or *routinization* (e.g., maintaining organizational practices, procedures, and policies started during implementation or integrating into existing organizational routines, policies, or budgets).[80] However, increasingly there is consideration that institutionalization may not fully capture all important dimensions of sustainability, and there is increasing consideration of the dynamic nature of sustainability as opposed to a static end goal.[81] Additionally, in early dissemination and implementation frameworks and models, the term *maintenance* was often used to conceptualize notions of sustainability; for example, in the Reach, Effectiveness, Adoption, Implementation, and Maintenance (RE-AIM) model introduced in 1999,[82] Glasgow and colleagues operationalized maintenance to include the longer-term impact of the EBI and continued delivery or institutionalization of program components over time (typically assessed at relatively short-term intervals, e.g., 6 months after initial implementation). Recent extensions of RE-AIM explicitly focus on more dynamic, equitable, and longer-term conceptualizations of sustainability[4] (see chapters 4 and 17 about RE-AIM).

The basic premise of many definitions of sustainability reflects the continued delivery of EBIs over time[4,5] (often referred to as sustainment) with continued health benefits and impact among the population/setting of focus. Recent definitions of sustainability capture more dynamic and multidimensional conceptualizations of sustainability and recognize the importance of adaptations of the EBI over time. Specifically, Moore and colleagues defined sustainability as the following: "(1) after a defined period of time, (2) the program, clinical intervention, and/or implementation strategies continue to be delivered and/or (3) individual behaviour change (i.e., clinician, patient) is maintained; (4) the program and individual behaviour change may evolve or adapt while (5) continuing to produce benefits for individuals/systems."[3(p5)]

It is important for researchers and practitioners to provide a clear definition and conceptualization of sustainability, ideally aligned with existing definitions and conceptualizations; this includes determining what time period will be assessed to meaningfully capture and track sustainability initially and over time. While ideal to comprehensively capture sustainability through the collection of multiple indicators,[83] it is useful to partner and engage with stakeholders to determine which aspects of sustainment or sustainability are feasible and meaningful to capture (e.g., sustained health benefits/impact, continued delivery of the EBI and/or implementation strategies, sustained infrastructure to deliver). This often requires having a detailed sense of what the EBI and its core components are (i.e., the essential functions or key ingredients of the EBI that are necessary to produce the desired outcome, informed by theory or through empirical testing), so they have a clear understanding of how the EBI has evolved or adapted over time.

In some cases researchers have made a distinction between *sustainability* as a process (e.g., planning for sustainability) or a characteristic of an intervention (e.g., extent to which an EBI can continue to be delivered over time), and *sustainment* as an outcome of interest in an implementation science study.[70] However, there has been a lack of clarity in the literature between these terms and their distinction. It is

PA4E1 Physical Activity Practices		
Efficacy Trial (2014–2016)		**Scale-up Trial (2017–2020)**
1: Teaching strategies to maximize students' physical activity in health and PE lessons This included teachers leading two pedometer based lessons per teacher each term. Teachers received training and resources to maximize activity in PE including pedometers (lessons to allow monitoring of activity) and workshop learnings including principles for PE teaching (EAASE – Efficient, Active, Autonomous, Success, Enjoyable).	→	**1: Quality PE Lessons** PE department to use documented principles or guidelines for teachers to maximise PE quality, active learning time and student engagement in PE lessons (Program schools used the SAAFE principles – Supportive, Autonomous, Active, Fair, Enjoyable). Each PE teacher to also participate in peer observation of a practical PE lesson, at least once a year. Desirable – peer observation feedback to be against the department's quality PE principles.
2: Development and monitoring of student physical activity plans within PE lessons This included Grade seven students in year one and Grade eight students in year two developing individual physical activity plans that set goals and actions and recorded progress against timelines, fitness assessments and provision of rewards. Plans were to be reviewed and modified each school term.	→	**2: Student PA plans** All Grade 7 students to develop a personal PA plan which includes i) personal goals to improve or maintain activity or fitness ii) actions and timelines to achieve goals; and iii) progress monitoring. Goals to be reviewed once within year. Desirable – students in Grades 8-10 to also develop a personal PA plan.
3: Enhanced school sport program The practice was for all grade eight students to participate in a 10-week program during school sport. The program was based on the effective 'Program X' and included lessons and fitness activities focused on lifelong physical activity skills and knowledge.	→	**3: Enhanced school sport program** School to deliver a short (10-12 weeks) structured PA Program (i.e. Resistance Training for Teens) designed to target resistance training and improve adolescents' fitness and provide them with knowledge, motivation and skills to engage in a range of lifelong physical activities. The program should be delivered to all students in at least one Grade between 7 and 10 (Program schools delivered the Resistance Training for Teens program to all of Grade 7).
4: Development/modification of school policies Schools were to develop or modify existing school policies that aimed to enhance student physical activity through collaboration between the head PE teacher, in school consultant (support strategy 1), and school executive.	→	**5: School PA policy or procedure** School to develop a policy which included (i) provision of at least 150 minutes per week of moderate to vigorous physical activity during school time for all students in Grade 7-10; and include iii) supportive practices to enhance all students' PA (at least 3 of the PA4E1 practices 1-2, 6-7).
5: Physical activity programs during school breaks Schools were encouraged to offer teacher supervised physical activity at recess and lunchtime on at least 2 days per week.	→	**4: Recess and lunchtime PA** Supervised recess and/or lunchtime PA sessions to be offered to all students in Grades 7-10 at least 3 days per week. PA equipment to be freely available to students at least three days per week at recess and/or lunch. Desirable – at least one organised recess or lunch activity per week should target girls and sessions should be promoted to students at least once per term.
6: Promotion of community physical activity providers (community links) Schools hosted a physical activity exhibition that promoted local physical activity providers to students in Grade 8.	→	**6: Links with community PA providers** School has at least 3 links that go beyond promotion of the provider (e.g. in newsletters) to involve an agreement, connection, partnership (e.g. out of hours sessions on school facilities, presentation by providers at school). Links should be designed to support 'outside of school time' activity. Links to be communicated to students and families at least once per term. Desirable – at least one of the community links is to promote free or low-cost options in the community.
7: Parent engagement Schools were to send information to parents via newsletters and the school website promoting physical activity and local providers, once per term.	→	**7: Communication PA messages to all parents** All parents of students in Grades 7-10 to receive PA messages designed to increase parent knowledge, attitudes and support towards PA, at least once per term. These exclude messages only about school events e.g. carnivals, or school sports timetables or results, or promotion (advertisements for) community PA providers.

FIGURE 29.3 Summary of the physical activity practices in the PA4E1 efficacy trial and the PA4E1 scale-up trial.

Source: Reproduced with permission from McLaughlin et al.[54]

PA4E1 Implementation Support Strategies	
Efficacy Trial (2014–2016)	**Scale-up Trial (2017–2020)**
1: In-School Consultant A trained PE teacher was placed within each school (in school physical activity consultant) for 1 day per week over the intervention period to support intervention implementation. →	**2.Embedded school-staff: in-School Champions** An existing school PE teacher is to be allocated the role of in-School Champion to support implementation. The position is funded by the NSW Department of Health for half a day per week ($350AUD per fortnight).
→	**3: External Implementation Support** A Health Promotion Support Officer (ideally with PE teacher training) is appointed to support schools with the program, co-located within the relevant local health district. Support is offered in the form of face-to-face site visits, phone calls and emails according to a schedule (outlined in detail elsewhere).
2: Leadership and Committee A school committee was established, including school executive, Head PE teacher, community representative, student representative and parent representative, or responsibility was added to an existing committee, to lead and oversee the intervention. Schools executives were asked to sign a partnership agreement. Committee to meet once per term. →	**1: Executive and leadership support** PA4E1 partnership agreement to be signed by school executive. New or existing school committee formed to oversee the program. The school committee should be inclusive of an in-School Champion and school executive to oversee the program and should meet at least once per term.
3: Teacher Training PE teachers were offered three two-hour face-to-face practice learning workshops (all schools together) focused on delivery of lessons to increase students' MVPA. All PE teachers involved in the delivery of the enhanced school sports program were invited to face-to-face training (at least once PE teacher per school to attend- all invited). →	**4: Teacher professional learning** In-School Champions to attend face-to-face training at the start of the program, half-way through (12 months) and prior to finishing the program (24 months). Online videos (6x10minutes) with knowledge check quizzes delivered to in-School Champions and PE Teachers via the program website. Enhanced school training offered to those involved in its delivery. School PA policy training offered to in –School champions of Government schools.
4: Resources Schools were provided with AUD$11,874 worth of resources. This included paper-based, annual outlining all physical activity intervention strategies and associated materials; approximately AUD$6000 of physical activity equipment (e.g. pedometers, resistance devices, games consoles, equipment boxes); and promotional materials for teachers (e.g. shirts/lanyards) and students (e.g. balls, water bottles). →	**5: Resources** Electronic resources delivered via the program website. Limited amounts of equipment and physical resources to be sent to schools, including a $100 AUD equipment voucher, 5 gym sticks and PA4E1 SAAFE posters
5. Prompts An in-school consultant provided prompts to teaching staff to implement the intervention strategies via e-mail, electronic calendar reminders and in face-to-face meetings →	**6: Provision of prompts and reminders** Automated messages to be sent each term to in-School Champions to prompt completion of termly surveys and also professional learning videos. Additionally, contact to be made by Support Officers to in-School Champions according to a schedule (outline in detail elsewhere).
6. Feedback Reports Records kept by the in-school consultant were the basis of quarterly intervention implementation feedback reports (on how was the school progressing with the practices) provided via email and hard copy to Principals and Head of PE →	**7: Implementation performance monitoring and feedback** In-School Champion to complete termly surveys and received an automated feedback report via email, generated from the responses to the termly survey on the program website. This repot also to be sent to school Principals via email.

FIGURE 29.4 Summary of the implementation support strategies offered to schools in the PA4E1 efficacy trial and the PA4E1 scale-up trial.

Source: Reproduced with permission from McLaughlin et al.[54]

important to note that[7] researchers and practitioners often do not think about or plan for sustainability up front, particularly given that it is commonly conceptualized as the last or final stage in the overall life cycle of an EBI. Here, as discussed further in this chapter, we highlight the importance of both planning for sustainability early on and conceptualizing sustainability as a longer-term domain and outcome that is distinct from implementation.

WHAT FACTORS INFLUENCE AND MATTER FOR SUSTAINABILITY?

It is useful to conduct a contextual assessment to better understand the multilevel factors that may influence the long-term delivery and impact of an EBI to inform planning for sustainability and to help address and reduce barriers to sustainability. Historically, there has been much focus on the role of funding as a key determinant that impacts sustainability of EBIs across a range of settings.[84] Funding, financing, and organizational resources to support EBI delivery are often minimal and short term, which limits continuity over the long term without additional investment, support, or evidence of possible return on investment.[74] Ongoing evaluation of implementation rates and outcomes along with feedback loops to funders are crucial to justify investment in program sustainment. However, while funding and resources are certainly important factors,[85] there is growing research to suggest that funding alone is likely insufficient to facilitate sustainability, and other multilevel factors also matter (and in some cases may even be able to compensate for lack of funding or resources).

There is value in using an existing conceptual framework in informing this assessment as an initial starting place to help provide shared grounding and guidance for researchers and practitioners. Conceptual frameworks can help build an evidence base for what factors matter in real-world settings by using shared constructs and terminology and promoting transparency and can greatly enhance planning for sustainability.[70,86,87] There are several conceptual frameworks in the field that may be useful to inform data collection or empirical assessment or testing of the multilevel factors that may impact sustainability.[5,75,88] Broadly speaking, most conceptual frameworks in this area identify determinants of sustainability at multiple levels, with consideration that these categories of domains are likely dynamically related and interact: (1) policy or outer contextual factors; (2) inner contextual or organizational factors; (3) implementation processes; (4) characteristics of the EBIs; and (4) characteristics of implementers and populations.

The Integrated Sustainability Framework is an example of an empirically informed and theoretically grounded framework that identifies multilevel factors that have been commonly associated with sustainability across different settings, contexts, and populations and can be used as a starting place for identifying and refining understanding of factors that are important to consider within a certain setting.[70] Specifically, this framework considers dynamic interactions among outer contextual factors, inner contextual or organizational factors, implementation processes, intervention characteristics, and implementer/population characteristics that operate to impact sustainability. These include outer contextual or policy-related factors (e.g., the broader sociopolitical context, existing policies, funding environment, external partnerships with organizations/stakeholders); inner contextual or organizational-level factors (e.g., resources and internal funding, leadership, presence of program champions, organizational readiness and support, staff stability; alignment of internal practices/policies; EBI culture); implementation processes (e.g., ongoing training, planning for sustainability, stakeholder engagement; coaching/feedback, capacity building); characteristics of the EBIs (e.g., adaptability, benefits, fit with setting and population); characteristics of implementers (e.g., skills, attitudes, motivations, role clarity); and characteristics of populations (e.g., literacy, language, experiences of stigma, mistrust, discrimination, and other social characteristics). (See Shoesmith et al.[84] for a detailed description of domains and constructs within the Integrated Sustainability Framework and Shelton et al.[89] for an example of how to refine and adapt the framework using community engagement to better reflect community contexts and specific settings.)

Additionally, the exploration, preparation, implementation, and sustainment (EPIS) model identifies specific factors related to the outer system and inner organizational context that are relevant to each of these phases, as well as "bridging" factors that reflect the interplay between outer and inner contexts (e.g., bridging organizations or intermediaries).[90] In the sustainment phase, the infrastructure, processes, and supports enable the EBI to continue to be delivered and embedded. Factors in the outer context that are considered to be important in the sustainment phase include leadership, policies, funding, and academic-public partnerships, while organizational characteristics, staffing, fidelity monitoring, and organizational resources are thought to be important determinants in the inner context. Additionally, the Capacity for Sustainability Framework[91] and accompanying the Program Sustainability Assessment Tool (PSAT) and Clinical Sustainability Assessment Tool (CSAT) can also be used to guide contextual assessments, reflection, and planning and are described in more detail under measures (see https://sustaintool.org).[92] It is important to note that some of the determinants of or barriers to implementation may also serve as barriers to sustainability (e.g., how costly and complex the intervention is; how well it fits with organizational context and the population; organizational readiness, support, and resources).[93] Additionally, there may also be sustainability-specific determinants (e.g., issues of staff and leadership turnover and attrition; dynamic policy landscape and shifting organizational priorities).[81,94–96]

SETTING, INTERVENTION, AND EQUITY CONSIDERATIONS

There are some factors that appear important to sustainability across a range of settings. For example, in examining settings that have strong organizational foundations and infrastructure (e.g., schools, clinics, hospitals, and worksites), staff and leadership attrition and turnover have been commonly identified as a challenge to sustainability.[70,88,97] Across state and local health departments in the United States, research suggested that salient reasons for ending effective programs include funding priorities changing or funding ending, changes in leadership or policymaker support, and loss of program champions.[98,99] However, there is also growing consideration that factors that influence sustainability likely differ across settings and contexts, or that certain factors are particularly salient or influential within certain contexts (e.g., in school settings, alignment with educational curricula and priorities may be particularly important).

The importance of factors may also vary depending on the nature of the EBI.[74] For example, for interventions delivered in their entirety by an individual (e.g., clinicians prescribing a new medication or treatment) may be strongly influenced by individual financial factors and the extent to which it continues to be reimbursed or provider motivation to continue the new practice. Broad-scale systems changes, however, may require diverse efforts and investments to achieve change over a longer time period, and environmental contexts (norms, policies, funding) are likely to be especially influential for sustaining changes in broader health systems.[74]

There may be some additional considerations and complexity with respect to sustaining interventions among minority populations or settings that have been historically disadvantaged or have limited resources. For example, there may be differences in the capacity, training, and resources available to providers within organizations and available at the systems level; different learning needs, literacy, and educational levels; and language preferences of the populations being served; as well as additional community experiences of intergenerational trauma and mistrust of public health/medicine based on historical or ongoing experiences of racism.[73,100] It is not surprising that we face substantial challenges to sustaining EBIs, particularly in settings and populations that experience numerous interconnected structural and social barriers to health. It is important to remember that there are some foundational reasons why sustainability is challenging in the context of promoting health equity, as many existing EBIs were not developed or evaluated with equity in mind, and many have not engaged communities experiencing inequities as partners in their development. Thus, in many cases the EBI is not a good fit from the start (e.g., was not developed with/for the community, is not culturally or contextually appropriate, and is not acceptable or feasible in light of limited resources).

Research suggests specific factors may be important to consider when sustaining interventions in settings that have been historically disadvantaged, including LMICs. Iwelunmor et al. (2016) reviewed 41 studies across 26 countries in sub-Saharan Africa and found that

TABLE 29.3 CHALLENGES AND OPPORTUNITIES TO CONSIDER IN ADVANCING THE SUSTAINABILITY OF EBIS

1. Challenge: Sustainability is often conceptualized as the last or final stage in the life cycle of an EBI, and researchers and practitioners do not always think about sustainability up front or plan from it at the outset.	Opportunities: • Consider whether you have a clear sense of "what" you are trying to sustain (e.g., the core components or active ingredients of the evidence-based program you are trying to sustain). If you are involved with EBI development or selection, consider factors that matter for sustainability like cost, complexity, adaptability, and fit with context. Apply guiding principles from "designing for dissemination and sustainability" in the development and refinement of EBIs.[78] • Consider planning tools (e.g., Program Sustainability Assessment Tool or Clinical Sustainability Assessment Tool) or sustainability frameworks that can be applied up front to help advance understanding of context that matters for sustainability and help identify potential barriers and facilitators to consider and address related to sustainability (e.g., Integrated Sustainability Framework, EPIS framework). • Identify and engage key partners early and often in meaningful ways to enhance the likelihood of sustainment, and to facilitate sustainability an equitable way across populations and settings.
2. Challenge: Often we neither work with stakeholders to determine what "counts" as sustainability of the EBI and what is meaningful to partners nor consider adaptations that are made over time in dynamic contexts.	Opportunities: • Working from existing definitions, engage with stakeholders to specify conceptualizations of sustainability, with considerations of pros and cons of evaluation approaches (resources, time feasibility), and strengths and limitations of various conceptualizations. Ideally capture multiple dimensions of sustainability (e.g., sustained use of EBI with fidelity? maintenance of partnerships? continued impact on health behaviors or outcomes?). • Consistent with dynamic conceptualizations of sustainability, consider the extent to which adaptations of EBIs are tracked, to help advance understanding of their impact and how the EBI changes over time based on changing needs, evidence, and context. Existing tools, frameworks, and models for adaptation can guide this process (see chapter 8, adaptation chapter). • Have a clear understanding of the core components of the EBI that are driving the intervention effect. If adaptations to the EBI are needed, for scale or sustainability, ensure that the core components remain or are refined or optimized.
3. Challenge: Often we do not think about, plan for, or have resources dedicated to measuring or assessing or monitoring sustainability over time, and have little information about the long-term value or return on investment of EBIs.	• Consider existing planning or evaluation tools (e.g., RE-AIM model) and determine the time period when sustainability will be assessed (e.g., 6 months after cessation of active implementation support and annually over the next 5 years); if possible, assess using both qualitative and quantitative sources of information. Prioritize understanding the extent to which sustainability is equitable across different subgroups or settings. • Use existing systems or administrative data to track sustainability when available. Consider tracking the costs or cost-effectiveness of the EBI over time to advance understanding of what is needed for sustainability and the long-term return on investment. • Ideally track indicators of sustainability prospectively over time and seek to understand perceptions of sustainability and determinants of sustainability from the perspective of multiple stakeholders.

(*continued*)

TABLE 29.3 CONTINUED

4. Challenge: There are multilevel policy, organizational and contextual factors that may present specific challenges to sustainability of EBIs (e.g., dynamic policy landscape, shifting organizational and funding priorities; limited funding/financing for implementation; implementer attrition and turnover).	• In planning for sustainability or advancing understanding of factors that matter for sustainability, consider applying frameworks that specifically examine or consider determinants of sustainability; consider and evaluate how determinants of sustainability might be similar or different from determinants of implementation. • Think about linking identified determinants or barriers to sustainability with sustainability strategies that could address them. Use a taxonomy or compilation of sustainability strategies that provides sufficient detail of the strategy to enable replication by others. • Develop, refine, and empirically test strategies to enhance sustainability to build an evidence base in the area of effective and equitable sustainability strategies.

community mobilization, engagement, and resources were essential to consider, as well as working with existing resources, providing adaptable interventions that are flexible to local context, and considering the broader societal and political context and upheavals.[101] This review suggested that in low-resource settings, providing opportunities for stakeholder engagement in the beginning may help enhance the likelihood of sustainability by facilitating ownership and ensuring that delivery of and refinements to the intervention occur to reflect local cultural norms and sociopolitical context. Additionally, Hodge and Turner reviewed 28 studies of sustained delivery of evidence-based programs in disadvantaged communities globally and found that program burden, benefits, and perceived competence in ability to deliver the program were distinctively important with respect to program characteristics, whereas staff mobility and turnover, supervision and peer support, and ongoing technical assistance and organizational support were particularly important when implementing programs in settings with complex systems and limited resources.[73]

FIDELITY AND ADAPTATION IN RELATION TO SUSTAINABILITY

It is increasingly recognized that it can be challenging to deliver EBIs with high fidelity when EBPs are being implemented among new populations or settings than where they were originally developed or tested or if the EBI may be a poor fit from the start with the organization or population. Research suggested that adaptations (both planned adaptations and unplanned adaptations) are common during implementation. This is certainly true as well for sustainability of EBIs, and being able to deliver them with high fidelity over time is often unrealistic and may be not be appropriate in light of dynamic contexts in which EBPs are embedded. In the context of sustainability research, few studies have reported which programs continue or not and why, as well as what adaptations were made and their health impact.[102] More detailed coverage of fidelity and adaptation is provided in chapters 7 and 8.

Consistent with these findings, there has been a shift in the field: Rather than conceptualizing sustainability as a static end goal, scholars are recognizing sustainability as more dynamic in nature. This shift allows for capacity building and planned adaptations in response to changing scientific evidence, shifting population needs, and dynamic contexts. This is well aligned with a framework introduced by Chambers and colleagues called the Dynamic Sustainability Framework.[81] This framework revisits assumptions that EBIs will deliver fewer benefits over time as they are sustained (voltage drop) and that benefits will decline when inevitably deviating from strict fidelity protocols (program drift). Instead, the Dynamic Sustainability Framework proposes that EBIs should be tested and refined in the settings in which they are being implemented; this may involve identifying core components of the intervention but using data tracking, continued learning, and evaluation to inform which adaptations may need to be made to enhance fit with new or changing settings, populations, and evidence. An important part of this continued learning and process may be tracking, monitoring, and evaluating what implications these adaptations have on sustainability outcomes, as well as health indicators/outcomes and cost (e.g., to inform understanding of return on investment).

PLANNING TO SUSTAIN EVIDENCE-BASED INTERVENTIONS

In this chapter we have already identified that there is a range of factors that impact the sustainability of an EBI, such as characteristics of the innovation, the context in which it is being implemented, or other macro factors, such as the political environment.[70,88,103] As such, it is essential that these factors are considered when both the EBI and strategies to support its adoption, implementation, and sustainment are being designed or selected.

Sustainability Planning Tools

Researchers and practitioners may find a sustainability planning tool or framework useful to help in this process. A literature review of both published and grey literature tools identified a number of sustainability assessment and planning tools for use in clinical and community settings.[104] Common to all these tools is the involvement of stakeholders (i.e., practitioners, end users, decision makers, funding agencies, researchers) in the sustainability assessment. While all the identified tools have limitations, those that appear to be either most widely used or are more user friendly are described below. It is hoped that as use of these tools grows, their validity and applicability to a broad range of contexts may be enhanced.

- *CSAT and PSAT*: The Center for Public Health Systems Science at Washington University in St. Louis has developed two tools that may help researchers and practitioners plan for sustainability of their EBIs. Applicable to both clinical and public health settings, the *Capacity for Sustainability Framework*[91] and its related measures; the 35-item CSAT[105]; and the 40-item PSAT[106] provide a step-by-step guide that delivery agencies, funders, or stakeholders can use, as a group or as individuals, to evaluate the sustainability capacity of a program. Following this assessment, teams have access to tools and resources to support their development of an action plan; to prioritize the areas where program sustainability capacity needs to be built. These tools are available online (https://sustaintool.org/psat/understand/ and https://sustaintool.org/csat/understand/). Testing of the validity of these tools is still underway, so it is still not clear if they capture all relevant domains of sustainability.
- The *RAND Getting to Outcomes (GTO): Promoting Accountability Through Methods and Tools for Planning, Implementation, and Evaluation*[107] was developed to address a broad range of public health issues, including substance abuse, homelessness, teen pregnancy, and mental health and aims to build the capacity of organizations to effectively choose evidence-based practices and then plan, implement, and sustain those practices.[108]
- Similarly, the *National Health Service (NHS) Sustainability Model and Guide*[109] is a user-friendly tool that helps teams self-assess the likelihood of their practice being sustained. The accompanying NHS Sustainability Guide provides practical advice on how practitioners might increase the likelihood of sustainability of their initiative within their specific context. The tool has been used extensively in clinical practice initiatives[110] and is available online (https://www.england.nhs.uk/improvement-hub/wp-content/uploads/sites/44/2017/11/NHS-Sustainability-Model-2010.pdf).

THE EFFECTIVENESS OF STRATEGIES TO SUSTAIN EVIDENCE-BASED INTERVENTIONS

The evidence of effective strategies for sustaining EBIs is however still an emerging area within the field.[76] A 2019 review by Hailemairam et al.[111] of strategies used to sustain public health interventions within community-based settings identified just six studies that purposefully set out to sustain an EBI. The review identified only nine sustainability strategies, the most frequently used being (1) ongoing funding, (2) booster training, and supervision and feedback. Other, less frequently used, strategies included (1) obtaining organizational leadership and stakeholder support for prioritizing the continued use of the EBI, (2) agency priorities, and/or program needs are aligned with EBI, (3) maintenance or buy-in of staff, (4) accessing new or existing financial support to facilitate sustainment, (5) adaptation of the EBI to increase continued fit/compatibility within the organization, (6) mutual adaptation between the EBI and organization (e.g., adaptation of the EBI to improve fit and alignment of the organizations' procedures), and (7) monitoring EBI effectiveness. However, there was insufficient evidence to determine the effectiveness of any one strategy.

Attempts are however being made to identify strategies that may be most effective in sustaining EBIs. This has been particularly important in LMICs whose health disparities could be improved through sustained implementation of EBIs.[89] For example, a 2015 systematic review of 41 health interventions implemented in 26 countries in sub-Saharan Africa sought to understand what strategies were used by countries who have sustained implementation of EBIs.[101] The review found that community ownership and mobilization strategies were crucial for intervention sustainability. Other naturalistic studies in LMICs[101,112,113] have reported that strategies such as capacity-building and community empowerment, train-the-trainer models, quality assurance checks, and feedback have supported the sustainment of EBIs. Such strategies may also be effective for those working to implement and sustain EBIs in historically marginalized racial/ethnic groups.[114] Community-based participatory research, described in detail in chapter 10, which meaningfully involves communities in decision-making, increases the likelihood of program implementation and sustainability as the process enables contextual factors to be taken into consideration and adapted for as needed.[115] While there are limited published prospective trials that aim to specifically test sustainability strategies, there are a number of published protocols that aim to do so,[116–119] which suggests that these trials are underway, and we could expect study findings in the coming years.

MONITORING AND MEASURING SUSTAINABILITY

Monitoring the implementation of all EBIs, especially those that are using scarce public health funds, is essential if we are to identify which interventions are, and continue to be, effective and cost-effective and therefore are of benefit to the community. This information may be used by policymakers to make informed decisions about whether EBIs should continue or be adapted or de-implemented.

What to Measure

Researchers may consider using Moore et al.'s definition of sustainability to help specify which aspect of sustainability they wish to measure,[3] that is, (1) if the program, clinical intervention, and/or implementation strategies have continued to be delivered (and potentially adapted); and (2) if individual (i.e., clinician, patient) behavior change is maintained and/or evolved. Additionally, others have also highlighted the importance of measuring the extent to which community and organizational infrastructure, capacity, and partnerships to deliver the EBI are maintained.[70] Furthermore, if we are to ensure our efforts to sustain EBIs do not cause further health inequities, researchers will need to embed equity-relevant measures to help identify early on (1) if health disparities occur, and if so (2) diagnose the underlying causes of this. Brownson et al. (2021) have proposed four categories of measurement for equity in implementation science that, at its most comprehensive stage, encourages researchers to measure if equity was sustained (e.g., sustained organizational change).[120]

How to Measure

If we are to ensure the long-term delivery of public health programs in clinical and community settings, a clear understanding of the determinants of the sustainment of these EBIs is needed, which is reliant on reliable, valid, and pragmatic measures.[121] Birken and colleagues found in their 2020 review,[122] despite there being more than 70 sustainability theories and frameworks, few have developed valid and reliable tools for measuring sustainment or sustainability. Findings from other recent reviews[123] suggest that efforts are however being made to address this. A 2020 review by Moullin et al.[124] of the most frequently used, comprehensive and/or validated sustainability measures identified 11 measures, 10 of which measured constructs of sustainment as an outcome, and 9 measured factors that influence sustainability (e.g., determinants). It is important to note that many of these tools have been found to be limited by poorly reported psychometric properties; few have been evaluated outside of the United States, most are only available in English; are too specific to context or intervention; or provide limited instructions on how to score and interpret scores or are too long and not pragmatic for use. These reviews include a summary of each of the tools that researchers may find useful if trying to locate a relevant measure to use in their field.

In the absence of a relevant, valid tool researchers may be able to use sustainability frameworks to help identify how to measure other dimensions of sustainability. For example, the recent extension of the RE-AIM framework to enhance sustainability by Shelton et al. (2020)[4] recommended that the dynamic contextual and equity factors that have implications for sustainability be assessed across RE-AIM dimensions. This framework provides pragmatic guidance for researchers and practitioners to consider as they are transitioning from initial implementation to longer-term sustainability for each of the RE-AIM dimensions and assessments. For example, what adaptations are needed to continue delivering the EBI long term? Is the EBI equitably sustained across populations and settings?

SUMMARY

The widespread and ongoing use of most beneficial health interventions is required to maximize the benefits of the health system to the community. Within implementation science, the fields of scale-up and sustainability have an important role to play in contributing to improving the health system to this end. Diverse and inconsistent use of terminology remains and represents challenges for the advancement of the science of scale-up and sustainability. While conceptual understanding of each continues to evolve, formative research has identified their complexity and documented a range of factors that influence program implementation and sustainability. Perhaps most nascent are experimental studies and other research methods to better understand the factors that are causally related to the scale-up and sustainability of EBIs and, importantly, the effectiveness of strategies in facilitating such outcomes. The conduct of these studies represents a significant opportunity for further research.

SUGGESTED READINGS AND WEBSITES

Readings

Ben Charif A, Zomahoun HT, Gogovor A, et al. Tools for assessing the scalability of innovations in health: a systematic review. *Health Res Policy Syst*. 2022 Dec;20(1):1–20.

This comprehensive systematic review is a useful resource to help identify tools to assess the scalability of health interventions. However, the review notes gaps in the current development process, coverage, and psychometric properties of many tools, identifying an opportunity for future research to advance the field.

Bulthuis SE, Kok MC, Raven J, Dieleman MA. Factors influencing the scale-up of public health interventions in low-and middle-income countries: a qualitative systematic literature review. *Health Policy Plann*. 2020 Mar 1;35(2):219–234.

The study provides a comprehensive and contemporary synthesis of qualitative literature describing multilevel factors that influence the scale-up of public health interventions in low- and middle-income countries. The review focuses on vertical scale-up approaches.

Chambers DA, Glasgow RE, Stange KC. The dynamic sustainability framework: addressing the paradox of sustainment amid ongoing change. *Implement Sci*. 2013 Dec;8(1):1.

This article proposes a shift in how sustainability has evolved from being considered as the endgame of a translational research process to a suggested "adaptation phase" that integrates and institutionalizes interventions within local organizational and cultural contexts. In this article, the authors reflect on traditional assumptions about voltage drop and program drift and propose a dynamic sustainability framework that involves continued learning and problem-solving, ongoing adaptation of interventions with a primary focus on fit between interventions and multilevel contexts, and expectations for ongoing improvement as opposed to diminishing outcomes over time.

Greenhalgh T, Papoutsi C. Spreading and scaling up innovation and improvement. *BMJ*. 2019 May 10;365.

This article provides an overview of the field of scale-up including a discussion of the theoretical perspectives that have contributed to our understanding of the process.

Hailemariam M, Bustos T, Montgomery B, Barajas R, Evans LB, Drahota A. Evidence-based intervention sustainability strategies: a systematic review. *Implement Sci.* 2019 Dec;14(1):1–2.

This systematic review summarizes the various definitions used within the literature for sustainment. It also provides a broad overview of strategies used to sustain evidence-based interventions within public health.

McKay H, Naylor PJ, Lau E, et al. Implementation and scale-up of physical activity and behavioural nutrition interventions: an evaluation roadmap. *Int J Behav Nutr Phys Activ.* 2019 Dec;16(1):1–2.

This article provides identified conceptual frameworks that can be used to support the design and evaluation of scale-up initiatives. It also makes recommendations regarding the relevant outcomes and determinant factors and measures that could be used in such evaluations.

Milat AJ, Bauman A, Redman S. Narrative review of models and success factors for scaling up public health interventions. *Implement Sci.* 2015 Dec;10(1):1.

The review provides focus on the defining and describing frameworks, processes, and methods of scaling up public health initiatives. The review provides insights into how conceptual frameworks can assist both policymakers and researchers to determine the type of research that is most useful at different stages of scaling up processes.

Moullin JC, Sklar M, Green A, et al. Advancing the pragmatic measurement of sustainment: a narrative review of measures. *Implement Sci Commun.* 2020 Dec;1(1):1–8.

This narrative review identified 11 measures of sustainment and sustainability determinants across a broad range of settings. While the review describes a number of limitations with the included measures, it may provide a useful starting point for those wishing to identify a measure for their study. The review provides general guidance about how and in what circumstances each measure could be used.

Scheirer MA, Dearing JW. An agenda for research on the sustainability of public health programs. *Am J Public Health.* 2011 Nov;101(11):2059–2067.

This foundational paper proposes an agenda for improved research and evaluation on the sustainability of public health programs. It provides guidance for researchers, practitioners, and policymakers on the planning, implementation, and evaluation of the sustainability of public health programs.

Shelton RC, Cooper BR, Stirman SW. The sustainability of evidence-based interventions and practices in public health and health care. *Annu Rev Public Health.* 2018 Apr 1;39:55–76.

This review critically examines and discusses conceptual and methodological issues in studying sustainability, identifies key indicators of sustainability, summarizes empirical research and the multilevel factors that have been found to influence the sustainability of interventions in a range of public health and healthcare settings, and highlights key areas for future research. Additionally, this article introduces the integrated sustainability framework and identifies considerations regarding adaptation and evolution of EBIs in the context of sustainability.

Selected Websites and Tools

ExpandNet. Advancing the science and practice of scale up. https://expandnet.net/

ExpandNet is an international network of researchers, policymakers, and others who seek to advance the science and practice of scale-up. The network provides a range of scale-up services and training and has published tools and technical reports, and the website maintains an updated bibliography of scale-up articles.

Sustaintool.org. https://sustaintool.org/

This website provides tools and resources related to conceptualization and measurement of sustainability capacity, as well as measurement tools and resources related to the Program Sustainability Assessment Tool (PSAT) and the Clinical Sustainability Assessment Tool (CSAT).

REFERENCES

1. World Health Organization. *World Health Organization Bridging the "Know–Do" Gap: Meeting on Knowledge Translation in Global Health.* World Health Organization; 2006.
2. Yoong SL, Jackson J, Barnes C, et al. Changing landscape of nutrition and dietetics research? A bibliographic analysis of top-tier published research in 1998 and 2018. *Public Health Nutr.* 2021;24(6):1318–1327.
3. Moore JE, Mascarenhas A, Bain J, Straus SE. Developing a comprehensive definition of sustainability. *Implement Sci.* 2017;12(1):1–8.
4. Shelton RC, Chambers DA, Glasgow RE. An extension of RE-AIM to enhance sustainability: addressing dynamic context and promoting health equity over time. *Front Public Health.* 2020;8(134):1–8.
5. Scheirer MA, Dearing JW. An agenda for research on the sustainability of public health programs. *Am J Public Health.* 2011;101(11):2059–2067.
6. Proctor E, Luke D, Calhoun A, et al. Sustainability of evidence-based healthcare: research agenda, methodological advances, and infrastructure support. *Implement Sci.* 2015;10(1):1–13.
7. World Health Organization. Scaling up projects and initiatives for better health: from concepts to practice. 2016, Geneva:World Health Organization. (https://apps.who.int/iris/bitstr

eam/handle/10665/343809/9789289051552-eng.pdf)
8. Ben Charif A, Zomahoun HTV, LeBlanc A, et al. Effective strategies for scaling up evidence-based practices in primary care: a systematic review. *Implement Sci.* 2017;12(1):1–13.
9. Greenhalgh T, Papoutsi C. Spreading and scaling up innovation and improvement. *BMJ.* 2019;365:I2068.
10. Nelson EC, Batalden PB, Huber TP, et al. Microsystems in health care: part 1. Learning from high-performing front-line clinical units. *Jt Comm J Qual Improv.* 2002;28(9):472–493.
11. McCoy KP. The science, and art, of program dissemination: strategies, successes, and challenges. *New Dir Child Adolesc Dev.* 2015;2015(149):1–10.
12. Zan T. The role of scale-up in strengthening health systems. fhi360. The Science of Improving Lives. 2012. Accessed 23 January 2022. https://www.fhi360.org/sites/default/files/media/documents/resource-scale-up-health-systems-strengthening.pdf
13. Milat AJ, Bauman A, Redman S. Narrative review of models and success factors for scaling up public health interventions. *Implement Sci.* 2015;10(1):1–11.
14. World Health Organization. *Practical Guidance for Scaling Up Health Service Innovations.* World Health Organization; 2009.
15. Aarons GA, Sklar M, Mustanski B, Benbow N, Brown CH. "Scaling-out" evidence-based interventions to new populations or new health care delivery systems. *Implement Sci.* 2017;12(1):111.
16. McLaughlin M, Duff J, Sutherland R, Campbell E, Wolfenden L, Wiggers J. Protocol for a mixed methods process evaluation of a hybrid implementation-effectiveness trial of a scaled-up whole-school physical activity program for adolescents: Physical Activity 4 Everyone (PA4E1). *Trials.* 2020;21(1):268.
17. Milat AJ, King L, Bauman AE, Redman S. The concept of scalability: increasing the scale and potential adoption of health promotion interventions into policy and practice. *Health Promot Int.* 2013;28(3):285–298.
18. Massoud M, Donohue K, McCannon C. *Options for Large-Scale Spread of Simple, High-Impact Interventions.* University Research Co. LLC (URC); 2010.
19. Rogers EM. Diffusion of innovations: an overview. In: Anderson JG, Jay SJ, eds. Use and *Impact of Computers* in *Clinical Medicine.* Springer; 1981:113–131.
20. Hanson K, Ranson MK, Oliveira-Cruz V, Mills A. Expanding access to priority health interventions: a framework for understanding the constraints to scaling-up. *J Int Dev.* 2003;15(1):1–14.
21. Barker PM, Reid A, Schall MW. A framework for scaling up health interventions: lessons from large-scale improvement initiatives in Africa. *Implement Sci.* 2015;11(1):1–11.
22. Gaziano TA, Pagidipati N. Scaling up chronic disease prevention interventions in lower-and middle-income countries. *Annu Rev Public Health.* 2013;34:317–335.
23. Diabetes Prevention Program Research Group. Reduction in the incidence of type 2 diabetes with lifestyle intervention or metformin. *N Engl J Med.* 2002;346(6):393–403.
24. Mathews E, Thomas E, Absetz P, et al. Cultural adaptation of a peer-led lifestyle intervention program for diabetes prevention in India: the Kerala diabetes prevention program (K-DPP). *BMC Public Health.* 2018;17(1):974.
25. Ravindranath R, Oldenburg B, Balachandran S, et al. Scale-up of the Kerala Diabetes Prevention Program (K-DPP) in Kerala, India: implementation evaluation findings. *Transl Behav Med.* 2020;10(1):5–12.
26. Indig D, Lee K, Grunseit A, Milat A, Bauman A. Pathways for scaling up public health interventions. *BMC Public Health.* 2017;18(1):68.
27. Reis RS, Salvo D, Ogilvie D, Lambert EV, Goenka S, Brownson RC. Scaling up physical activity interventions worldwide: stepping up to larger and smarter approaches to get people moving. *Lancet.* 2016;388(10051):1337–1348.
28. Brown CH, Curran G, Palinkas LA, et al. An overview of research and evaluation designs for dissemination and implementation. *Annl Rev Public Health.* 2017;38:1–22.
29. Deenik J, Czosnek L, Teasdale SB, et al. From impact factors to real impact: translating evidence on lifestyle interventions into routine mental health care. *Transl Behav Med.* 2019;10(4):1070–1073.
30. World Health Organization. Beginning with the end in mind: planning pilot projects and other programmatic research for successful scaling up; 2011. France: World Health Organization. (https://apps.who.int/iris/bitstream/handle/10665/44708/9789241502320_eng.pdf?sequence=1&isAllowed=y.)
31. Brownson RC, Jacobs JA, Tabak RG, Hoehner CM, Stamatakis KA. Designing for dissemination among public health researchers: findings from a national survey in the United States. *Am J Public Health.* 2013;103(9):1693–1699.
32. Greenhalgh T, Wherton J, Papoutsi C, et al. Beyond adoption: a new framework for

theorizing and evaluating nonadoption, abandonment, and challenges to the scale-up, spread, and sustainability of health and care technologies. *J Med Internet Res.* 2017;19(11):e367.
33. Nguyen DTK, McLaren L, Oelke ND, McIntyre L. Developing a framework to inform scale-up success for population health interventions: a critical interpretive synthesis of the literature. *Glob Health Res Policy.* 2020;5:18.
34. Weaver C, DeRosier ME. Commentary on scaling-up evidence-based interventions in public systems. *Prev Sci.* 2019;20(8):1178–1188.
35. Zamboni K, Schellenberg J, Hanson C, Betran AP, Dumont A. Assessing scalability of an intervention: why, how and who? *Health Policy Plann.* 2019;34(7):544–552.
36. Ben Charif A, Hassani K, Wong ST, et al. Assessment of scalability of evidence-based innovations in community-based primary health care: a cross-sectional study. *CMAJ Open.* 2018;6(4):E520–E527.
37. Milat A, Lee K, Conte K, et al. Intervention Scalability Assessment Tool: a decision support tool for health policy makers and implementers. *Health Res Policy Syst.* 2020;18(1):1.
38. Lee K, Milat A, Grunseit A, Conte K, Wolfenden L, Bauman A. The Intervention Scalability Assessment Tool: a pilot study assessing five interventions for scalability. *Public Health Res Pract.* 2020;30(2):e3022011.
39. O'Hara BJ, Phongsavan P, King L, et al. "Translational formative evaluation": critical in up-scaling public health programmes. *Health Promot Int.* 2013;29(1):38–46.
40. Spicer N, Bhattacharya D, Dimka R, et al. "Scaling-up is a craft not a science": catalysing scale-up of health innovations in Ethiopia, India and Nigeria. *Soc Sci Med.* 2014;121:30–38.
41. Koorts H, Cassar S, Salmon J, Lawrence M, Salmon P, Dorling H. Mechanisms of scaling up: combining a realist perspective and systems analysis to understand successfully scaled interventions. *Int J Behav Nutr Phys Activ.* 2021;18(1):42.
42. Bulthuis SE, Kok MC, Raven J, Dieleman MA. Factors influencing the scale-up of public health interventions in low- and middle-income countries: a qualitative systematic literature review. *Health Policy Plann.* 2019;35(2):219–234.
43. Miake-Lye IM, Mak SS, Lambert-Kerzner AC, et al. Scaling Beyond Early Adopters: A Systematic Review and Key Informant Perspectives. VA ESP Project #05-226; 2019. Posted final reports are located on the ESP search page. https://www.hsrd.research.va.gov/publications/esp/reports.cfm.
44. Troup J, Fuhr DC, Woodward A, Sondorp E, Roberts B. Barriers and facilitators for scaling up mental health and psychosocial support interventions in low- and middle-income countries for populations affected by humanitarian crises: a systematic review. *Int J Ment Health Syst.* 2021;15(1):5.
45. Ezezika O, Gong J, Abdirahman H, Sellen D. Barriers and facilitators to the implementation of large-scale nutrition interventions in Africa: a scoping review. *Glob Implement Res Appl.* 2021;1(1):38–52.
46. Stirman SW, Baumann AA, Miller CJ. The FRAME: an expanded framework for reporting adaptations and modifications to evidence-based interventions. *Implement Sci.* 2019;14(1):1–10.
47. Lane C, McCrabb S, Nathan N, et al. How effective are physical activity interventions when they are scaled-up: a systematic review. *Int J Behav Nutr Phys Activ.* 2021;18(1):1–11.
48. McCrabb S, Lane C, Hall A, et al. Scaling-up evidence-based obesity interventions: a systematic review assessing intervention adaptations and effectiveness and quantifying the scale-up penalty. *Obes Rev.* 2019;20(7):964–982.
49. Gray SM, McKay HA, Hoy CL, et al. Getting ready for scale-up of an effective older adult physical activity program: characterizing the adaptation process. *Prev Sci.* 2020;21(3):355–365.
50. Martin P, Murray LK, Darnell D, Dorsey S. Transdiagnostic treatment approaches for greater public health impact: implementing principles of evidence-based mental health interventions. *Clin Psychol Sci Pract.* 2018;25(4):e12270.
51. Eriksson J, Lindström J, Valle T, et al. Prevention of type II diabetes in subjects with impaired glucose tolerance: the Diabetes Prevention Study (DPS) in Finland Study design and 1-year interim report on the feasibility of the lifestyle intervention programme. *Diabetologia.* 1999;42(7):793–801.
52. Laatikainen T, Dunbar JA, Chapman A, et al. Prevention of type 2 diabetes by lifestyle intervention in an Australian primary health care setting: Greater Green Triangle (GGT) Diabetes Prevention Project. *BMC Public Health.* 2007;7(1):1–7.
53. Tommeraas T, Ogden T. Is there a scale-up penalty? Testing behavioral change in the scaling up of parent management training in Norway. *Adm Policy Ment Health Ment Health Serv Res.* 2017;44(2):203–216.
54. McLaughlin M, Campbell E, Sutherland R, et al. Extent, type and reasons for adaptation and modification when scaling-up an effective physical activity program: Physical Activity 4 Everyone

(PA4E1). *Front Health Services.* 2021;1:719194. doi:10.3389/frhs.2021.719194

55. Sutherland R, Campbell E, McLaughlin M, et al. Scale-up of the Physical Activity 4 Everyone (PA4E1) intervention in secondary schools: 24-month implementation and cost outcomes from a cluster randomised controlled trial. *Int J Behav Nutr Phys Activ.* 2021;18(1):137.
56. Sutherland R, Campbell E, Nathan N, et al. A cluster randomised trial of an intervention to increase the implementation of physical activity practices in secondary schools: study protocol for scaling up the Physical Activity 4 Everyone (PA4E1) program. *BMC Public Health.* 2019;19(1):883.
57. Miller CJ, Wiltsey-Stirman S, Baumann AA. Iterative Decision-making for Evaluation of Adaptations (IDEA): a decision tree for balancing adaptation, fidelity, and intervention impact. *J Community Psychol.* 2020;48(4):1163–1177.
58. Fagan AA, Bumbarger BK, Barth RP, et al. Scaling up evidence-based interventions in US public systems to prevent behavioral health problems: challenges and opportunities. *Prev Sci.* 2019;20(8):1147–1168.
59. McKay HA, Macdonald HM, Nettlefold L, Masse LC, Day M, Naylor P-J. Action Schools! BC implementation: from efficacy to effectiveness to scale-up. *Br J Sports Med.* 2015;49(4):210.
60. Wolfenden L, McCrabb S, Barnes C, et al. trategies for enhancing the implementation of school-based policies or practices targeting diet, physical activity, obesity, tobacco or alcohol use. *Cochrane Database Syst Rev.* 2022;8(8):CD011677.
61. Wolfenden L, Goldman S, Stacey FG, et al. Strategies to improve the implementation of workplace-based policies or practices targeting tobacco, alcohol, diet, physical activity and obesity. *Cochrane Database Syst Rev.* 2018;11(11):CD012439.
62. Wolfenden L, Barnes C Jones J, et al. Strategies to improve the implementation of healthy eating, physical activity and obesity prevention policies, practices or programmes within childcare services. *Cochrane Database Syst Rev.* 2020;2(2):CD011779.
63. Wolfenden L, Reilly K, Kingsland M, et al. Identifying opportunities to develop the science of implementation for community-based non-communicable disease prevention: a review of implementation trials. *Prev Med.* 2019;118:279–285.
64. Atkins L, Francis J, Islam R, et al. A guide to using the Theoretical Domains Framework of behaviour change to investigate implementation problems. *Implement Sci.* 2017;12(1):77.
65. Koorts H, Eakin E, Estabrooks P, Timperio A, Salmon J, Bauman A. Implementation and scale up of population physical activity interventions for clinical and community settings: the PRACTIS guide. *Int J Behav Nutr Phys Activ.* 2018;15(1):1–11.
66. Milat AJ, Newson R, King L, et al. A guide to scaling up population health interventions. *Public Health Res Pract.* 2016;26(1):e2611604.
67. Hollis JL, Sutherland R, Campbell L, et al. Effects of a "school-based" physical activity intervention on adiposity in adolescents from economically disadvantaged communities: secondary outcomes of the "Physical Activity 4 Everyone" RCT. *Int J Obes.* 2016;40(10):1486–1493.
68. Sutherland RL, Campbell EM, Lubans DR, et al. The Physical Activity 4 Everyone cluster randomized trial: 2-year outcomes of a school physical activity intervention among adolescents. *Am J Prev Med.* 2016;51(2):195–205.
69. Emmons KM, Colditz GA. Realizing the potential of cancer prevention—the role of implementation science. *N Engl J Med.* 2017;376(10):986–990.
70. Shelton RC, Cooper BR, Stirman SW. The sustainability of evidence-based interventions and practices in public health and health care. *Ann Rev Public Health.* 2018;39(1):55–76.
71. Shediac-Rizkallah MC, Bone LR. Planning for the sustainability of community-based health programs: conceptual frameworks and future directions for research, practice and policy. *Health Educ Res.* 1998;13(1):87–108.
72. Braithwaite J, Ludlow K, Testa L, et al. Built to last? The sustainability of healthcare system improvements, programmes and interventions: a systematic integrative review. *BMJ Open.* 2020;10(6):e036453.
73. Hodge LM, Turner KM. Sustained implementation of evidence-based programs in disadvantaged communities: a conceptual framework of supporting factors. *Am J Community Psychol.* 2016;58(1–2):192–210.
74. Scheirer MA. Is sustainability possible? A review and commentary on empirical studies of program sustainability. *Am J Eval.* 2005;26(3):320–347.
75. Wiltsey Stirman S, Kimberly J, Cook N, Calloway A, Castro F, Charns M. The sustainability of new programs and innovations: a review of the empirical literature and recommendations for future research. *Implement Sci.* 2012;7(17):1–19.
76. Shelton RC, Lee M. Sustaining evidence-based interventions and policies: recent innovations and future directions in implementation science. *Am J Public Health.* 2019;109(S2):S132–S134.
77. Walugembe DR, Sibbald S, Le Ber MJ, Kothari A. Sustainability of public health interventions:

where are the gaps? *Health Res Policy Syst.* 2019;17(1):1–7.

78. Kwan BM, Brownson RC, Glasgow RE, Morrato EH, Luke DA. Designing for dissemination and sustainability to promote equitable impacts on health. *Ann Rev Public Health.* 2022;43(1):331–353.
79. Walsh-Bailey C, Tsai E, Tabak RG, et al. A scoping review of de-implementation frameworks and models. *Implement Sci.* 2021;16(1):1–18.
80. Yin RK. Life histories of innovations: how new practices become routinized. *Public Adm Rev.* 1981;41(1):21–28.
81. Chambers DA, Glasgow RE, Stange KC. The dynamic sustainability framework: addressing the paradox of sustainment amid ongoing change. *Implement Sci.* 2013;8(1):117.
82. Glasgow RE, Vogt TM, Boles SM. Evaluating the public health impact of health promotion interventions: the RE-AIM framework. *Am J Public Health.* 1999;89(9):1322–1327.
83. Scheirer MA, Santos SL, Tagai EK, et al. Dimensions of sustainability for a health communication intervention in African American churches: a multi-methods study. *Implement Sci.* 2017;12(43)1–12.
84. Bossert TJ. Can they get along without us? Sustainability of donor-supported health projects in Central America and Africa. *Soc Sci Med.* 1990;30(9):1015–1023.
85. Palinkas LA, Chou C-P, Spear SE, Mendon SJ, Villamar J, Brown CH. Measurement of sustainment of prevention programs and initiatives: the sustainment measurement system scale. *Implement Sci.* 2020;15(1):1–15.
86. Tabak RG, Khoong EC, Chambers DA, Brownson RC. Bridging research and practice: models for dissemination and implementation research. *Am J Prev Med.* 2012;43(3):337–350.
87. Damschroder LJ. Clarity out of chaos: use of theory in implementation research. *Psychiatry Res.* 2020;283:112461.
88. Herlitz L, MacIntyre H, Osborn T, Bonell C. The sustainability of public health interventions in schools: a systematic review. *Implement Sci.* 2020;15(4):1–28.
89. Shelton RC, Charles T-A, Dunston SK, Jandorf L, Erwin DO. Advancing understanding of the sustainability of lay health advisor (LHA) programs for African-American women in community settings. *Transl Behav Med.* 2017;7(3):415–426.
90. Aarons GA, Hurlburt M, Horwitz SM. Advancing a conceptual model of evidence-based practice implementation in public service sectors. *Adm Policy Ment Health.* 2011;38(1):4–23.
91. Schell SF, Luke DA, Schooley MW, et al. Public health program capacity for sustainability: a new framework. *Implement Sci.* 2013;8(1):15.
92. Center for Public Health Systems Science. Rate the sustainability capacity of your program or clinical practice to help plan for its future. 2022. Accessed January 23, 2022. https://sustaintool.org
93. Damschroder LJ, Aron DC, Keith RE, Kirsh SR, Alexander JA, Lowery JC. Fostering implementation of health services research findings into practice: a consolidated framework for advancing implementation science. *Implement Sci.* 2009;4(50):1–15.
94. Scheirer MA. Linking sustainability research to intervention types. *Am J Public Health.* 2013;103(4):e73–e80.
95. Shelton RC, Dunston SK, Leoce N, et al. Predictors of activity level and retention among African American lay health advisors (LHAs) from the National Witness Project: implications for the implementation and sustainability of community-based LHA programs from a longitudinal study. *Implement Sci.* 2016;11(41):1–14.
96. Walkosz BJ, Buller DB, Andersen PA, Scott MD, Cutter GR. The sustainability of an occupational skin cancer prevention program. *J Occup Env Med.* 2015;57(11):1207–1213.
97. Cassar S, Salmon J, Timperio A, et al. Adoption, implementation and sustainability of school-based physical activity and sedentary behaviour interventions in real-world settings: a systematic review. *Int J Behav Nutr Phys Activ.* 2019;16(120):1–13.
98. Brownson RC, Allen P, Jacob RR, et al. Understanding mis-implementation in public health practice. *Am J Prev Med.* 2015;48(5):543–551.
99. Padek MM, Mazzucca S, Allen P, et al. Patterns and correlates of mis-implementation in state chronic disease public health practice in the United States. *BMC Public Health.* 2021;21(101):1–11.
100. Baumann AA, Cabassa LJ. Reframing implementation science to address inequities in healthcare delivery. *BMC Health Serv Res.* 2020;20(1):1–9.
101. Iwelunmor J, Blackstone S, Veira D, et al. Toward the sustainability of health interventions implemented in sub-Saharan Africa: a systematic review and conceptual framework. *Implement Sci.* 2016;11(43):1–27.
102. Wiltsey Stirman S, Calloway A, Toder K, et al. Community mental health provider modifications to cognitive therapy:

implications for sustainability. *Psychiatr Serv.* 2013;64(10):1056–1059.

103. Scudder AT, Taber-Thomas SM, Schaffner K, Pemberton JR, Hunter L, Herschell AD. A mixed-methods study of system-level sustainability of evidence-based practices in 12 large-scale implementation initiatives. *Health Res Policy Syst.* 2017;15(102):1–13.
104. Hutchinson K. *Literature Review of Program Sustainability Assessment Tools.* Community Solutions Planning & Evaluation; 2010.
105. Malone S, Prewitt K, Hacket R, et al. The Clinical Sustainability Assessment Tool: measuring organizational capacity to promote sustainability in healthcare. *Implement Sci Commun.* 2021;2(77):1–12.
106. Calhoun A, Mainor A, Moreland-Russell S, Maier RC, Brossart L, Luke DA. Using the Program Sustainability Assessment Tool to assess and plan for sustainability. *Prev Chronic Dis.* 2014;11:E11.
107. Johnson K, Collins D, Wandersman A. Sustaining innovations in community prevention systems: a data-informed sustainability strategy. *J Community Psychol.* 2013;41(3):322–340.
108. Chinman M, Hunter SB, Ebener P, et al. The getting to outcomes demonstration and evaluation: an illustration of the prevention support system. *Am J Community Psychol.* 2008;41(3–4):206–224.
109. Maher L, Gustafson D, Evans A. *Sustainability Model and Guide.* National Health Service; 2010.
110. Doyle C, Howe C, Woodcock T, et al. Making change last: applying the NHS institute for innovation and improvement sustainability model to healthcare improvement. *Implement Sci.* 2013;8(127):127.
111. Hailemariam M, Bustos T, Montgomery B, Barajas R, Evans LB, Drahota A. Evidence-based intervention sustainability strategies: a systematic review. *Implement Sci.* 2019;14(57):1–12.
112. Llauradó E, Aceves-Martins M, Tarro L, et al. The "Som la Pera" intervention: sustainability capacity evaluation of a peer-led social-marketing intervention to encourage healthy lifestyles among adolescents. *Transl Behav Med.* 2018;8(5):739–744.
113. Vamos S, Mumbi M, Cook R, Chitalu N, Weiss SM, Jones DL. Translation and sustainability of an HIV prevention intervention in Lusaka, Zambia. *Transl Behav Med.* 2014;4(2):141–148.
114. Shelton RC, Adsul P, Oh A. Recommendations for addressing structural racism in implementation science: a call to the field. *Ethn Dis.* 2021;31(suppl 1):357–364.
115. Binagwaho A, Frisch MF, Udoh K, et al. Implementation research: an efficient and effective tool to accelerate universal health coverage. *Int J Health Policy Manag.* 2020;9(5):182–184.
116. Vitale R, Blaine T, Zofkie E, et al. Developing an evidence-based program sustainability training curriculum: a group randomized, multi-phase approach. *Implement Sci.* 2018;13(1):1–12.
117. Kastner M, Sayal R, Oliver D, Straus SE, Dolovich L. Sustainability and scalability of a volunteer-based primary care intervention (Health TAPESTRY): a mixed-methods analysis. *BMC Health Serv Res.* 2017;17(54):1–21.
118. Johnson JE, Wiltsey-Stirman S, Sikorskii A, et al. Protocol for the ROSE sustainment (ROSES) study, a sequential multiple assignment randomized trial to determine the minimum necessary intervention to maintain a postpartum depression prevention program in prenatal clinics serving low-income women. *Implement Sci.* 2018;13(115):1–12.
119. Wiltsey Stirman S, Finley EP, Shields N, et al. Improving and sustaining delivery of CPT for PTSD in mental health systems: a cluster randomized trial. *Implement Sci.* 2017;12(32):1–11.
120. Brownson RC, Kumanyika SK, Kreuter MW, Haire-Joshu D. Implementation science should give higher priority to health equity. *Implement Sci.* 2021;16(1):28.
121. Hall A, Shoesmith A, Shelton RC, Lane C, Wolfenden L, Nathan N. Adaptation and validation of the Program Sustainability Assessment Tool (PSAT) for use in the elementary school setting. *Int J Environ Res Public Health.* 2021;18(21):11414.
122. Birken SA, Haines ER, Hwang S, Chambers DA, Bunger AC, Nilsen P. Advancing understanding and identifying strategies for sustaining evidence-based practices: a review of reviews. *Implement Sci.* 2020;15(88):1–13.
123. Mettert K, Lewis C, Dorsey C, Halko H, Weiner B. Measuring implementation outcomes: an updated systematic review of measures' psychometric properties. *Implement Res Pract.* 2020;1:1–29.
124. Moullin JC, Sklar M, Green A, et al. Advancing the pragmatic measurement of sustainment: a narrative review of measures. *Implement Sci Commun.* 2020;1(76):1–28.

30

Training and Capacity Building in Dissemination and Implementation Science

RACHEL DAVIS, NICK SEVDALIS, AND ANA A. BAUMANN

INTRODUCTION

The field of dissemination and implementation (D&I) science has seen considerable growth over the years.[1,2] Consequentially, the need to build capacity in individuals and institutions conducting D&I-related research has being pushed to the forefront as an emerging area of international priority.[3–7] Capacity building—defined as a process which leads to greater individual, organizational or system capabilities to conduct and implement high-quality research and practice[8–11] can take many forms. Early examples date back to the 1990s when the Veterans Health Administration established (in 1998) the *Quality Enhancement Research Initiative* (QUERI),[12–14] with the aim of better understanding optimal ways to implement research-driven best practices. Numerous academic, government, and commercial centers and departments have since been created (e.g., in the United States,[15,16] Canada,[17] Australia,[18] the United Kingdom,[19] and globally).[20] Increasingly, funding is available for D&I-related faculty positions and research,[1,21] research networks,[22,23] professional societies and groups,[24,25] and scientific conferences and meetings.[26–28] In 2006, *Implementation Science* was established, the flagship journal in the field,[29] followed by several other journals[30,31] (or specialist implementation science "sections" within journals[32] and electronic libraries and databases (e.g., the Cochrane[33]) focusing on D&I-related insights.

One important avenue for building capacity in D&I research (and the focus of this chapter) is through the development and delivery of teaching, mentoring, and training initiatives.[5] Arguably, implementation issues will be more appropriately and efficiently addressed if individuals (teams or organizations) are trained to have the requisite knowledge (i.e., why the research-practice gap occurs) and skillset (i.e., to formulate a plan through the application of D&I methodology). Traditionally, training was (and still is to a large extent) aimed at individuals involved in conducting research (i.e., "researchers"),[5,34–42] though more recently the importance of training those faced with translating evidence into practice (i.e., "implementers"—such as practitioners or policy implementers)[22,43–46] and (to a lesser extent) those tasked with training others in D&I methodologies (e.g., "educators" or "leaders")[47–50] has been emphasized. Some work has been done to identify the unique training needs and required competencies of each one of these groups. For instance, researchers require training more focused on learning about methods, the determinants of implementation process, designs, and the importance of examining the internal and external validity of their work; whereas practitioners need to learn about pragmatic designs and how to optimally implement interventions to achieve high uptake, sustainability, and scale-up. Previously, we have advocated for the importance of cross-teaching researchers and practitioners as this collaboration could advance the science and decrease the current practitioner-researcher gap that seems to have emerged between implementation research and practice activities and roles.[51] However, this literature is still nascent, and much needs to be discussed and

Rachel Davis, Nick Sevdalis, and Ana A. Baumann, *Training and Capacity Building in Dissemination and Implementation Science* In: *Dissemination and Implementation Research in Health.* Edited by: Ross C. Brownson, Graham A. Colditz, and Enola K. Proctor, Oxford University Press.
 DOI: 10.1093/oso/9780197660690.003.0030

evaluated about the unique training required for each of these groups of implementation trainees.

This chapter is organized into five sections. First, we begin with an overview of how training in D&I can be conceptualized, drawing on the key features that training may comprise. Next, we discuss the current state of capacity-building research and highlight some of the methodological challenges of developing and delivering training in relation to these research insights. A discussion of health equity in training is then presented—an important, but often overlooked area.[52] We conclude by summarizing some of the key priorities for future work in capacity building in D&I. We also provide examples of training in D&I currently available (purposefully selected for their difference in scope and structure) by drawing from two initiatives that we are involved in.

CONCEPTUALIZING TRAINING IN D&I

When examining any phenomenon in D&I (whether it be training, an intervention to better implement clinical guidelines, or development and validation of outcome measures to assess implementation effectiveness), conceptualization is an important part of the process, helping to define and make sense of the issue that you are setting out to address.[53] In the same way, in training terms, thinking about how D&I training initiatives can be categorized enables a clearer understanding of the nature and range of training on offer and where the potential gaps for learning may be.[5,7] While it is not possible to delve too deeply into this discussion here, it is important to highlight some of the key features of training initiatives (and thus how they can be conceptualized). Doing this enables those interested in learning about research (on training) and practice (i.e., the delivery of actual training) to make sense of the current training benchmark and, in turn, what should be prioritized in the future.[5] Figure 30.1 illustrates the "who" (audience), "how" (type of training), and "why" (needs and wants) of D&I training initiatives. Box 30.1 takes this one step further, depicting the way in which the different training can be broken down further and conceptualized.

We present two training initiatives that we are involved in the UK Implementation Science Masterclass (ISM)[54] and trainings

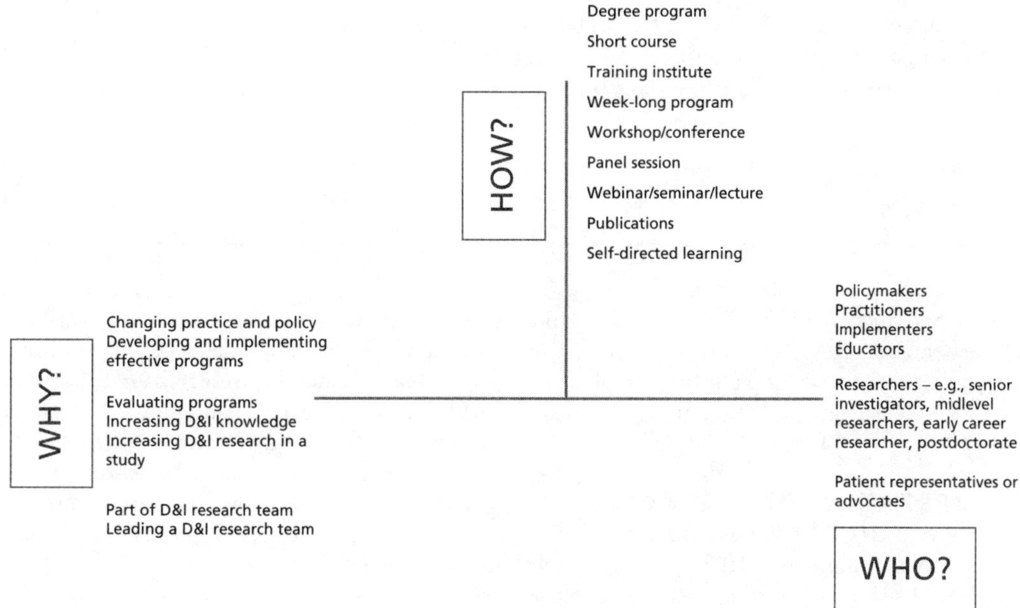

FIGURE 30.1 Multiple axes depicting the "who," "how," and "why" of D&I training programs.

Source: Reproduced with permission from Chambers DA, Proctor EK, Brownson RC, Straus SE. Mapping training needs for dissemination and implementation research: lessons from a synthesis of existing D&I research training programs. *Transl Behav Med*. Sep 2017;7(3):593–601.

BOX 30.1

CONCEPTUALIZING TRAINING IN D&I

- ***Type of training***—how the training is defined (e.g., workshop, webinar, training institute, fellowship program, clerkship, graduate certificate, or course/module that forms part of an academic program).
- ***Frequency***—whether the training is a "one-off," with the intent of catering for a priority identified at that time, versus more frequent occurrences of training, such as a postgraduate program in D&I where a new intake of learners starts each year.
- ***Duration***—when the training is held (e.g., summer, winter) and over what period (e.g., 1 hour/a day/a week/a year or more).
- ***Audience and eligibility***—whether the training is aimed at a specific audience (e.g., researchers or practitioners [or both] or those with experience in a specific D&I methodology [e.g., beginners, intermediate, or advanced learners]) or involves a competitive application processor is open to all.
- ***Capacity***—the number of individuals that can undertake the training at any one time.
- ***Structure***—the components the training comprises, for example, a combination of weekly lessons, phone calls, and a work placement.
- ***Assessment***—whether an approach is undertaken to assess knowledge and/or skill acquisition (e.g., project or field implementation study).
- ***Mode of delivery***—how the training is delivered (e.g., online, face to face, or a "blended" approach).
- ***Topics and context***—whether the training is focused on a specific context (e.g., dementia or mental health) or has wider applicability. Depending on the implementation issue in question, content may provide a general overview of D&I principles or focus on specific topics or aspects of methodology, such as theory (e.g., Reach, Effectiveness, Adoption, Implementation, and Maintenance [RE-AIM]), trials (e.g., hybrid designs), outcome measures (e.g., implementation outcomes).
- ***Ongoing support***—whether any ongoing support (e.g., mentoring, online forum, discussion groups with trainees) is provided after the completion of the training and who provides this support.

Adapted from Davis and D'Lima, 2021.[5]

hosted and related to the Dissemination and Implementation Research Core (DIRC) in the United States,[3] which provide further illustration of this categorization system (see Case Studies 30.1 and 30.2).

RESEARCH ON CAPACITY BUILDING IN D&I

For many paradigms of D&I inquiry, research is often the first (and sometimes only) step to help understand the issue at hand. In this respect, capacity building in D&I is somewhat different. To date, given the relative infancy of the field the focus (and consequentially most of the resource) has been on "upskilling" individuals (teams or organizations), through the development and delivery of training, rather than conducting research or evaluation on the training—which is often a side product (and only if time and funding allow). Despite this, however, studies of D&I training are gaining traction,[7] with an increasing number of experts highlighting that to effectively build capacity in D&I, we first need to understand what training appears to work and what we could be doing better[3,5,49,59–61] and how these extend to a wide range of individuals (implementers, researchers, and educators).[4,7,43,44,62–65] For some training programs, there are now mixed-methods evaluations.[66–68]

CASE STUDY 30.1: IMPLEMENTATION SCIENCE MASTERCLASS

The ISM was originally conceived in 2013 and delivered for the first time in 2014; it has since been delivered annually, either face to face or virtually, with the exception of 2020, when the ISM was cancelled due to the uncertainties and pressures caused by the global COVID-19 pandemic. The ISM was pump primed by research funds, through the National Institute of Health Research (NIHR) in England and their strategic investment in applied health and more recently social care research. This investment has translated into regionally organized applied research collaborations, which aim to bring together academic, health-care provider, public health, and policymaking organizations and experts to identify priority areas for applied health research. These partnerships seek to address evidence gaps and, critically, mobilize evidence into practice to reduce the well-known evidence-practice, or implementation, gaps in health and social care delivery.

As part of this effort, the NIHR supported the development of the ISM with the aim to offer an accessible avenue for capacity building of relevance to scientists and academics, clinicians, health and social care managers, policymakers, and indeed service users. To enhance accessibility, the ISM is focused on methods and concepts and hence aims to be applicable across specialties and professional groups; likewise, the ISM has taken a broad perspective on recruitment, with no prerequisites for attendance. In more recent years, the ISM has implemented a structure to the taught curriculum, such that an introductory and advanced strands are offered to delegates. The ISM is delivered via a combination of taught lectures, workshops, and small-group teaching/interacting activities, all of which are synchronous. (Note that delegates are offered a shortlist of one or two core readings preattendance, which they are encouraged to read; delegates typically approach faculty after the course to seek advice, although this is not offered as a structured educational/mentoring scheme.)

The ISM curriculum covers four main blocks of materials, as follows:

1. *Introduction to implementation science*: rationale and need for the science and its methods; how it compares/contrasts to clinical and other types of research.
2. *Implementation theories and frameworks*: coverage of specific theories and frameworks; approaches and tools to help select theories for study/evaluation purposes; practical examples.
3. *Research and evaluation methods and designs*: hybrid designs; Medical Research Council complex intervention evaluation framework; logic models/theory of change methods; process evaluations; statistical mechanism analyses.
4. *Specialist topics*: comparison of implementation science to related fields (e.g., improvement science); "embedded researcher" applications; stakeholder engagement methods. These are regularly updated to keep the curriculum fresh.

An evaluation of the ISM through self-reported data on training content, delivery, and relevance collected from 323 delegates between 2014 and 2019 showed positive reception of the course and impact on delegates' practices.

For the purpose of this section, we have categorized research and evaluation on training into three areas (which often overlap based on methodological aims and design): (1) needs assessment, relating to examining training needs and/or the evaluation of training initiatives; (2) competency development, including the development of core competencies in D&I and the development and delivery of relevant curricula attached to these competencies; and (3) training opportunities, covering the availability and accessibility of

CASE STUDY 30.2: THE DISSEMINATION AND IMPLEMENTATION RESEARCH CORE AT WASHINGTON UNIVERSITY IN ST. LOUIS

The DIRC is a methods core from the Washington University Institute for Clinical and Translational Science (ICTS) at Washington University in St. Louis (Missouri, United States). DIRC began in 2007 as a pilot program, and since 2009, it has been conceptualized as a core to provide technical assistance to investigators.[3] The DIRC mission is to accelerate the public health impact of clinical and health services research through advancing the D&I science and equipping investigators with D&I research. Currently, it has two codirectors (Drs. Elvin Geng and Ana Baumann), four lead faculty, and a coordinator. The DIRC is further supported by postdoctoral students, alongside PhD and master's level research assistants.

To accomplish their mission, the DIRC codirectors and faculty conduct presentations about D&I at multiple spaces at the university (e.g., training programs, classes, departmental grand rounds) and workshops cosponsored by other centers from the university.[3,55] To investigators with their grants, the DIRC team provides consultations and materials for the investigative team. To support the development of the science, the DIRC team develops toolkits, literature reviews, and papers.[56,57] Additionally, the DIRC team works closely with other clinical and translational science awards nationally.[3]

Training in this model of service is different, therefore, as the ones outlined in this chapter (e.g., Implementation Research Institute [IRI], Mentored Training for Dissemination and Implementation Research in Cancer [MT-DIRC], Training Institute for Dissemination and Implementation Research in Health [TIDIRH]) in several ways: (a) The "mentees" (i.e., those providing DIRC services) do not necessarily go through formal D&I training in the form of courses; (b) the mentees learn "on the job" how to conduct a literature search and how to interpret the literature to make the findings "digestible" for their customers; (c) while traditional trainings are topic oriented, the mentees provide customer support for projects in different topics (e.g., cancer, sickle cell, HIV) and in different areas (e.g., emergency department, primary care setting) in the United States and globally; and (d) the trainings are in all aspects of translational science (e.g., treatment development, support of guideline adherence[58]). The mentees are trained through three processes: (1) overshadowing a faculty lead on the consultation and support of a customer's project; (2) development of specific outcomes (e.g., toolkit) with the supervision of a faculty; and (3) conducting a part of a funded project (e.g., development of interview guide and analysis of qualitative data using D&I lens).

D&I training or training resources. While it is not possible to provide an overview of all the research and evaluation findings to date, in what follows we summarize some of the key studies.

Evaluating D&I Training to Assess Training Needs

Interest in assessing training needs in D&I is growing. To date, most of this research centers on identifying training needs through the evaluation of established training programs (e.g., the ISM[54] and IRI[69,70]; see Case Studies 30.1 and 30.2), though some studies exist that assess training needs more generally.[71,72] In this context, evaluations can take several forms. For example, it could involve an assessment of trainees' knowledge or (less explored) skill acquisition, or it may include reflections on training from the trainees' perspective or (to a lesser extent) the trainers' perspective.[3,5,34,44,54,73]

Evaluative research to date shows that individuals are interested in learning about D&I in a variety of ways (in the way training is both structured and delivered).[5,34,37,38,40,58,69,70,74–80] While training initiatives may differ in merit and focus (i.e., in terms of their key features; see Box 30.1), the need for training, appetite to learn, and interest in D&I concepts and value (in terms of increasing understanding and confidence) are commonly reported benefits across studies.[5,34,37,38,40,69,70,77,78,80] Research on the application of D&I training in practice (i.e., applying knowledge and skills), while sparser, suggests that giving trainees opportunities to apply concepts to their own projects (i.e., demonstrating application of knowledge/skills) as well as exposure to projects at different stages of implementation (through their own and other trainees' projects) reinforces understanding.[77,81,82]

Evaluations have also shown that one component of training that appears to be particularly central to the development of D&I scholars is mentoring.[69,78,83] Benefits to both the trainee and the mentor have been reported, including research productivity, career satisfaction, and career success.[69,83–86] For example, an evaluation of the IRI (see Case Study 30.2) that assessed the benefit of training over the longer term (2-year period) found mentoring was significantly related to collaborations on new research, grant submissions, and scholarly publications.[70] Other training initiatives reported in the literature that provide significant opportunities for sustained interaction with experts in D&I (e.g., over a period of months or years), include the Training Institute for Dissemination and Implementation Research in Health (TIDIRH),[37,42,70] the Implementation Research Institute (IRI),[39,69,70] and the Mentored Training for Dissemination and Implementation Research in Cancer (MT-DIRC).[66] However, like many training initiatives, eligibility restrictions apply due to the scope of the training, trainers' capacity, and additional resources to deliver. For example, the IRI,[39,69,70] TIDIRH,[37,42] and MT-DIRC[38,66] were only open to early-career faculty. While TIDIRH and MT-DIRC are no longer active, IRI has recently been renewed, and other trainings have been developed. The challenge, however, is that these are in general trainings with emphasis on a specific topic (e.g., mental health, cancer), focused on research trainings, and very competitive. Currently, limited opportunities exist for the provision of ongoing support for those at any career stage[5] and for multidisciplinary researchers and practitioners. Equally, endeavors that focus more broadly on increasing organizational capacity in research universities (like that described in Reference 3) is lacking.[3]

Development of Core Competencies

Competency-based training helps shape the development of curriculum in D&I, enabling trainees' proficiency in meeting learning objectives (and, in turn, the effectiveness of the training) to be more readily assessed against standardize learning objectives.[87–89] For researchers, aiding understanding and assessment of effective approaches to translate evidence to the real world will be most relevant. For practitioners, understanding how to apply and adapt these approaches to achieve the best outcomes in different populations and contexts will be of more interest. While competency "lists" are increasingly developed and used for training related to research and practice,[90–92] the field of D&I is still very much learning about what it entails to be a D&I researcher and/or practitioner. While one could argue that there is tension about adding boundaries to define a D&I expert in a multidisciplinary field, experts in D&I capacity building have argued that more research is urgently needed on D&I competency development and assessment to ensure that trainees' needs are appropriately met.[71,80,88,93,94]

Efforts to generate and define core competencies for the D&I researcher (and practitioner) comprise various methods and have included card-sort techniques,[88] online surveys,[71] and scoping reviews.[95] In the most notable early attempt (in 2015),[88] a list of 43 D&I competencies were generated based on the research teams' experience with planning/delivering D&I training (e.g., the MT-DIRC[66] [see Case Study 30.2] and the TIDIRH)[37,42] and through consultation with colleagues (*N* = 16) and D&I researchers (*N* = 124). Using a card-sort technique, competencies were categorized into four broad domains: (1) background and rationale (e.g., identifying gaps in D&I research); (2) theory and approaches (e.g., identifying appropriate conceptual models); (3) design and analysis (e.g., describing core components of external validity) and (4) practice-based considerations (e.g., considering the perspectives of different stakeholders). Competencies were further split into experience levels ("beginner," "intermediate," "advanced," with most focused at the intermediate experiential level).[88]

A recent online survey asked a group of international multidisciplinary experts (N = 82) to name the competencies they considered most helpful for conducting D&I research and practice (the latter of which, with few exceptions, is a less-understood area).[71] Experts indicated whether they acquired the identified competencies through education, on-the-job training, self-study, or some other kind of training. Skills and knowledge relating to collaboration (e.g., networking and building relations) were considered most helpful for D&I practice, whereas (perhaps unsurprisingly) skills and knowledge relating to research (e.g., knowledge of study designs) were deemed most salient for researchers. Competencies relating to "practice" primarily were acquired through self-study or on the job, whereas research competencies were "learned" through professional education.[71]

Another study undertook a scoping review to establish competencies in knowledge translation (a related, interchangeable field to D&I).[95] Several health and interdisciplinary electronic databases were searched alongside the gray literature to produce 19 core competencies, categorized into three areas: (1) knowledge (e.g., understanding the context, "how things really work"); (2) skills (e.g., collaboration and teamwork, developing authentic and respectful working relationships); and (3) attitudes (e.g., confidence, belief in one's own abilities).[95] Initial and important steps have also been taken to develop competency lists and expectations for practitioners, with core competencies for the implementation specialist practice profile recently released by the National Implementation Research Network[96] and the "Core Competencies for Implementation Practice" report by the Center for Implementation Science, which identifies the many different roles and responsibilities implementation practitioners and intermediaries may take on so it is translatable to different initiatives and settings.[97]

Taken collectively, the evidence from the studies summarized above suggests that specific competences are required for researchers and practitioners if they are to work together in the most optimal ways.[71,88,95,96] Researchers need knowledge (and skills) to undertake methodologically robust and relevant implementation studies. Practitioners (i.e., those that "use" the research) need to be able to understand D&I methodology adequately enough to select D&I concepts of relevance and adapt these to address the specific practice problem in question. The degree of knowledge and skill of D&I competency may vary depending on the level of engagement with the D&I science[58]; however, rigorous testing of D&I competencies (like those described above) is required to assess their relevance to research and practice in different contexts, which competencies should be gained and how for the different levels of researcher and practitioner so that a benchmark for the standardization of training development and evaluation can be provided.[71,88,95,96]

TRAINING OPPORTUNITIES: AVAILABILITY AND ACCESSIBILITY

As the appetite for D&I training has grown and subsequently the interest in D&I research (and more recently practice), so has the need to examine the nature and range of training opportunities available.[5,7] Several publications provide more of a field-wide perspective on some of the training options to date, including both formal (i.e., training through established training initiatives) or more "informal" training (e.g., meetings to discuss D&I-related projects, training handbooks, or e-learning modules).[4,5,40,43,59,60,64,98–100]

However, while this research points toward the growing number of D&I training initiatives on offer, a notable deficit is evident: Current training options are not sufficient to fill the increasing demand to learn about D&I.[5] At present, only a limited number of universities offer structured D&I training programs, and while postdoctoral institutes have been set up to try to address some of the training gaps, these are heavily oversubscribed. For example, evaluations of the TIDIRH and IRI report acceptance rates of 13%[37] and 36%,[70] respectively. Equally, training initiatives may require travel for attendance, be held only once a year, and/or stipulate specific eligibility criteria (e.g., aimed at specific professions, qualifications, or levels of experience), meaning only a limited pool of individuals can apply.[5] As such, finding ways to speed up the pace of D&I training development and delivery has been highlighted as an international priority, with experts and organizations (e.g., the National Institutes of Health in the United States and the World Health Organization) concluding that we need widened access to training for all levels of D&I researchers (and practitioners).[6,101]

METHODOLOGICAL CHALLENGES

While training individuals (and teams) in D&I is integral to the process of building and sustaining the field, developing, implementing, and evaluating training is not without challenges.[3–5,44,59,61,102] Many obstacles are interrelated, further compounding complexities with building capacity. Here we discuss some of the key challenges, specifically in relation to the research areas described above.

Challenges Within the Field of "Needs Assessment"

Dissemination and implementation sit in no obvious disciplinary home,[3,37] holding relevance to academics and nonacademics from a wide range of backgrounds (e.g., social scientists, clinicians, economics, public health analysts, and patient representatives). These groups may have different training needs.[4,60,65,71] Researchers, for example, may be more interested in learning how you shift focus from the (more traditional) efficacy studies to those that are more generalizable (i.e., "effectiveness" and "pragmatic" trials). Conversely, practitioners may prioritize learning about the costs (in terms of time and money) attached to a specific intervention rather than the mechanics of the research methodology it is derived from. Equally, even those within the research field will have varying requirements based on their professional background. A research epidemiologist, for example, may want to know how an intervention focused on cardiovascular disease can improve the nature and scale of a stroke. Alternatively, a patient representative researcher may be most interested in the specifics of the language in which the intervention is communicated to the lay public in a way that they can understand and use.

While these differing perspectives are neither preventable nor unwanted, they present challenges to the development and delivery of training in terms of meeting individual needs.[103]

We illustrate this point by drawing from our own experience of running the Kings College London UK ISM[54] (see Case Study 30.1 for more information). A strong underlying aim of the ISM is its transdisciplinary and cross-professional approach. While we believe overall this is of benefit (given the importance of addressing healthcare problems from a variety of angles),[104] such diversity means the curriculum cannot be easily tailored to a specific discipline or context. Based on our evaluations of training over several years to date, some trainees (particularly those with less experience) reported this made it harder for them to assimilate taught concepts and methods in a way that made sense to their own research or practice setting. Equally, an intentional feature of the ISM is its dual focus on individuals newer to the field alongside early career and more established investigators; doing this, however, has both advantages and limitations for learning. Those with less experience can benefit greatly from learning from real examples from others on how D&I methods can be applied in practice. However, those with more experience need content tailored appropriately to them to avoid repetition in already learned concepts. As the ISM has grown (since its inception in 2014), the need to split specific sessions based on levels of expertise (e.g., in relation to training on theory and hybrid trials) has become more apparent (with wider literature in the field also supporting this view). However, when we integrated this thinking into our 2019 ISM through the inclusion of an advanced stream, we found it challenging knowing at what level to pitch the relevant ("advanced" vs. "beginner") content, and indeed feedback from delegates registering for the course suggested that some of them found it hard to judge whether they would consider themselves at an introductory or advanced level. While steps have been made to develop and categorize D&I competences based on expertise, these are yet to be tried and tested to produce a clear benchmark for training expectations. Some competences will be more basic (i.e., suitable for beginners) than others, hence knowing which these are would allow training initiatives to be pitched more suitably to delegates (and delegates would know where they stand in relation to competency mastery).

Challenges in Developing Competencies in D&I

The field of D&I, unlike more long-standing fields where individuals are overseen by professional bodies and regulators (e.g., in the United Kingdom, medics are overseen/regulated by the British Medical Association [https://www.bma.org.uk/) and General Medical Council [https://www.gmc-uk.org/], respectively), no such governance applies to D&I. Curricula (and related competencies) in D&I are therefore less obvious[71] and prescriptive, with the developers of the training making the decisions on what content should be covered and how it should be delivered and assessed. Given the multitude of methods one could draw on to teach, the field can appear somewhat overwhelming, with learners being introduced to a vast array of information[105] (e.g., on theories, frameworks,[106] and implementation strategies[107]) that can be hard to assimilate and digest in a way that individuals then feel able to apply to implementation research and practice. Equally, measures and methods in D&I are still developing[108] (and can be difficult to define),[64,109] so priorities for the content of training (and in turn the selection of relevant competencies) need to continually change to reflect these new insights. It can be difficult to unpick and agree on "who" should be taught "what."

Research that describes and/or evaluates established training initiatives can provide a useful starting point for testing different D&I competencies, outlining how training may be structured, in accordance with the current climate. However, while numerous examples of D&I training have been successfully launched (e.g., ISM,[37,54] IRI,[39,69,70] TIDIRH),[42] with evident similarities (e.g., covering content on theory, design, measurement), different topics are covered to varying degrees, and a consistent curriculum, focused on transdisciplinary competencies, has not been established.[88]

Given the multidisciplinary nature of D&I, many professions contribute to training development, with potentially differing perspectives not only on training needs but also their preferred language to communicate to their audience (for further discussion on debates in D&I terminology, see).[110–112] While such diversity reflects the field's evolution in different contexts and purposes, it potentially limits advances in training development and effective communication between disciplines. Advocating the adoption of a common set of terms attached to competencies would help to overcome some of these training issues. Steps to address this are evident in some areas already—for example, in relation to implementation outcomes[108] and implementation strategies,[107,113] both of which draw from clearly operationalized definitions and concepts that have transdisciplinary relevance.

Limited Availability and Access

Research indicates that the availability of training is not sufficient to cater for the growing workforce.[1,3–6,60] One approach to help address this issue is to develop training aimed at a large pool of individuals; but, while this has the advantage of greater efficiencies in scale, it can also present challenges. We illustrate this by drawing again from our own experience of delivering the ISM.

The ISM has grown considerably over the years.[54] It attracts an international range of expert faculty and delegates at a singular event, providing rich opportunities to network and learn from a wide pool of people. In the early years of delivery, when the ISM was smaller (i.e., approximately 40 delegates in attendance), delegates were able to benefit greatly from the wealth of experience of the faculty and could sign up for one-on-one time to gain feedback on their individual projects. It was also easier to split individuals into smaller group sessions, themed based on their interests and experience, providing an opportunity to discuss techniques and methods that could be used in specific contexts or projects of direct relevance to them. Over time, as demand for the ISM grew (and we increased the intake to cater for this), opportunities for personalized contextual feedback have become more difficult. This presents somewhat of a quandary: On the one hand we are trying to grow the ISM (to provide opportunity for a greater number of individuals to benefit), while also balancing this against meeting the individual needs of each trainee (which becomes harder as the number of trainees continues to rise).

Another issue is the need for ongoing support postcompletion of training (e.g., mentorship) to give trainees the knowledge and confidence to put what they have learned into action. To do this effectively, consistent involvement of experts in D&I is required.[3,64] For example, training initiatives (e.g., MT-DIRC)[66] report that senior-level faculty play an integral part in supporting trainees, with significant time spent on building infrastructure, providing technical support, and mentoring.[3]

However, aside from the mentorship embedded in these notable training initiatives, there are few established "experts" that can provide guidance to those newer to the field. Most universities encounter a deficit in academic leaders who can take on this role (with the availability of mentors in hospitals or health and social care settings even more problematic).[3,5] As funding in D&I becomes more available and more grants are subsequently awarded, the numbers of more mid- and early level investigators (employed to work on these grants) will increase, resulting in faculty leaders being even busier and less accessible.[3] The recently launched TRIPLE (Training in Implementation Practice Leadership)[48]is one example of a novel implementation leadership training initiative aimed at behavioral healthcare leaders (e.g., clinical supervisors) to develop and harness leadership skills and effective organizational change relating to evidence-based practice principles. More efforts like this to train leaders in D&I are urgently required.

When local D&I leadership is lacking, alternative approaches to providing support are required.[98] One example is an interactive web networking, developed based on feedback from trainees' experiences of the TIDIRH. This platform provides opportunities for discussion (e.g., on general issues related to the field), feedback (e.g., on research papers being written), and dissemination (e.g., to share lectures, funding opportunities[37]) but is open to TIDIRH trainees; thus, additional avenues for learning, open to a wider mass of individuals, are required.

Online D&I webinars (e.g., the Implementation Science Webinar Series)[114] and peer networks (e.g., the Society for Implementation Research Collaboration)[25] are examples of interactive forums providing an alternative avenue for learning. Alongside this (and when other options are lacking), individuals should be directed to the wealth of online tools and guides on implementation, research design, theory,[115] measurement,[116] implementation strategies,[117] and evaluation approaches,[118] as well as more general competencies on writing for publication and research funding.[57] While steps have been taken by individual organizations to develop lists of relevant D&I training guides and resources,[119–121] a more general repository covering all key resources is yet to be developed.

HEALTH EQUITY AND D&I TRAINING

Recently, there has been a paradigm shift in the field of D&I science to incorporate an explicit focus on enhancing health equity and reducing health disparities through equity-oriented D&I research, which occurs "when strong equity components—including explicit attention to the culture, history, values, assets, and needs of the community—are integrated into the principles, strategies, frameworks, and tools of implementation science."[122] Incorporating an equity lens in D&I training involves examining who is being trained and how the training is being delivered.[123] As the field grapples with issues of racism and colonialism in its knowledge production[124,125] in a field that tends to be highly centralized,[103] it will be important to critically examine who will be the next generation of leaders and mentors in the field of D&I.

Thinking about "who is being trained" and "how" these trainings will be delivered will affect the composition of the next generation of D&I scholars and the consequent knowledge production of the field. A challenge in achieving this goal lies in the very problem of equity: how to increase the reach of training programs and provide quality mentoring with limited funding. Freely available videos or modules can help increase reach,[101,126] but long-term solutions are needed. To be able to achieve this goal, we need to increase access to D&I trainings for all types of learners, especially scholars of color, scholars of varying levels of ability and socioeconomic status, and other scholars with lived experience of racism and discrimination. By increasing the diversity of implementation scholars and learning to collaborate and engage with our communities with reflexivity and examination of our positions of power and privilege[125] as we design and implement our interventions,[127] it is hoped we will avoid equity tourism.[128] In other words, as the field engages in conversations about equity,[129–131] we need to avoid the risk of implementation scientists without prior experience or commitment to health equity research parachuting into the equity field. Instead, it is only by critically thinking how to engage and train the next generation of D&I scholars that we will effectively promote health equity.

When thinking about equity in D&I training with an equity lens, therefore, there is a need to develop training with specific focus on equity-oriented D&I research,[71] rather than embedding one or two sections of equity or D&I as added components of current trainings. In doing so, focused training for equity D&I research could expand on going further than describing equity issues or health inequities and strengthen capacity through an increase in knowledge, skills, and reflection in "how to" address disparities (Baumann et al., under review).[132] Increasing the diversity of the leaders and engaging in collaboration with underrepresented scholars who have been doing equity work is of urgency. These include shifts in funding mechanisms to support recruitment, training, and retention of a diverse workforce (including those with lived experience with inequities). To be successful in this shift, however, D&I researchers need to reflect and examine how we recruit, train, and retain scientists of historically marginalized backgrounds to lead and collaborate on research and implementation. It is only by including a diverse pool of researchers, and by recognizing the long history and contribution of scholars of color in the health disparities research in the field of implementation science, that we will be able to advance the D&I field to promote equitable oriented research.

DIRECTIONS FOR THE FUTURE

The published evidence and the plethora of educational and training initiatives in the field of D&I that we have reviewed in this chapter support the view that the capacity development initiatives within D&I are several and continue to grow. The impetus for training and educational interventions, programs, and initiatives seems to be following the similarly expansive trajectory of the discipline: Having started as a small cross-cutting subspecialty, the D&I science has grown very rapidly, and demand for it among funders and clinical investigator and trial units has been growing steadily in the past 15 years. It appears that in our field growth of education goes hand in hand with growth in research and the need to achieve and demonstrate clinical and public health impacts and aims to support the delivery of high-quality research projects and programs. If this interpretation is correct (time will tell), then we anticipate the demand for capacity building and skills development to continue to grow in the coming years.

This is a pattern of, simultaneously, an opportunity and a significant challenge, which we feel the discipline needs to address systematically in the coming 5 years to 10 years. On the one hand, demand for D&I supports increased awareness of the need of implementation concepts, methods, and measures to complement clinical effectiveness studies and traditional change and project management approaches in practice. Increased awareness, on the other hand, is one of the levers for funders and health and social care organizations to invest in training and education programs for their staff and for universities and large academic health sciences centers to do the same for their students and clinicians. Some of the existing D&I training initiatives that we reviewed in this chapters will be well suited to cover such needs; however, current delivery models will always mean that access remains a problem, indeed one that will grow bigger as awareness and demand continue to increase. We would strongly advocate the development of e-learning and similar well-produced, educationally solid materials that can be scaled in an asynchronous manner, such that the global demand for D&I skills and competences can be addressed without always relying on the few available expert trainers and availability of funding to support training costs. The lessons we all had to learn by necessity during the last 2 years of the COVID-19 global pandemic have accelerated the view that virtual delivery is possible and can be time- and cost-effective for both trainers and trainees.

Further to expanded training and education provision through virtual means, we strongly advocate that D&I scientists and trainers reach out to education experts and learn from them. The medical and health sciences education communities have long established such relationships, such that the fields of medical and health sciences education are generating new evidence that has paved the way for competence-based (rather than time-based) clinical curricula, which at their best offer an individualized learning pace and experience, tailored ideally to individual learners. Not all medical and health science schools have achieved this, of course; however, educational expertise has steadily infused their curricula and training in the past two decades. Articulation of competences for implementation scientists, practitioners, and eventually educators is an important next frontier in our field: We need to understand competences not as long, unstructured checklists of "stuff to learn" but as frameworks and systems of knowledge that trainees can develop gradually. Mapping implementation research and practice activities onto such competences has already started; we recommend that such efforts be supported in the future, such that global curricula become available that are solidly based on needs assessments and systematically mapped onto curricula and delivered. We propose that this approach will generate coherence and a clear view of what makes a "proficient" implementation scientist or practitioner. We anticipate that a positive corollary of such systematization will be more clarity among non-expert colleagues regarding what implementation science and practice are about and reinforce the need for health and social care systems and funders to further invest in our discipline.

Further, systematization of competence frameworks and related curricula will also facilitate evaluative studies of D&I training and education interventions and programs, such that we begin to understand better how to optimally teach the requisite skills with good immediate and delayed retention and application to learners' practice. Importantly, the field now has several published educational courses and initiatives. Systematic mapping of the types of competences these instill and ongoing evaluation will assist those looking to develop/deliver training in D&I to understand what training approach, program, or initiative works for which learners in which context. Better understanding of the type of learning needs each available initiative addresses will allow our discipline to mix and match existing courses for the maximum educational effect. For example, a detailed masterclass-level course may be followed ideally by a course that offers asynchronous (postcourse) individualized mentoring to learners, such that they can design and implement their implementation projects successfully and reach the desired impact or outcomes. This would mean better use of the wide range of training opportunities currently available and maximal efficiency—and with virtual courses economies of scale can be achieved on a global scale as trainers and trainees are not restricted by geography or time. We expect that a "one-size-fits-all" approach to training content, delivery, or curriculum structure is unlikely to be adequate to meet either current or future needs; finding innovative and effective ways to tailor and combine should be technically feasible and facilitated by collaborative approaches to D&I education.

SUMMARY

In summary, while capacity building in D&I has seen considerable growth over the years (exemplified by the growing number of training opportunities available), we have discussed that the field still has much to learn. Equally, there appears to be a notable gap in the lack of training opportunities that would be accessible to all those interested in learning about D&I, particularly efforts to provide ongoing support to implementers, researchers, or educators in their workplace. Among the topics covered in this book, capacity building research is one of the least developed (and funded). Placing further emphasis on the research of training, and not just the development and delivery of training, will help pave the way for the improvement of existing training programs and the development of new ones. Efforts to further research what we should be teaching (i.e., competencies and further validation of these) and how we should be doing this for different types of learners could really maximize the "take-home" messages from training for learners. Ultimately, and arguably, this resultant newer and improved training could lead to a better understanding and application of core D&I concepts and methodologies in practice, which in turn would help to close the heavily cited "research-practice" gap that the field strives to close.

SUGGESTED READINGS AND RESOURCES

Readings

Brownson RC, Proctor EK, Luke DA, et al. Building capacity for dissemination and implementation research: one university's experience. *Implement Sci.* 2017;12(1):104.

This article presents and discusses a number of initiatives that have been implemented at Washington University St Louis that are focused on building D&I research capacity.

Chambers DA, Proctor EK, Brownson RC, Straus SE. Mapping training needs for dissemination and implementation research: lessons from a synthesis of existing D&I research training programs. *Transl Behav Med.* 2017;7(3):593–601.

Initiated from a 2013 NIH workshop, this article identifies training opportunities in D&I and maps them by different characteristics (e.g., career stage, format).

Davis R, D'Lima D. Building capacity in dissemination and implementation science: a systematic review of the academic literature on teaching and training initiatives. *Implement Sci.* 2020;15(1):97.

This systematic review identified D&I capacity-building initiatives that have been described and/or evaluated in the academic literature.

Luke DA, Baumann AA, Carothers BJ, Landsverk J, Proctor EK. Forging a link between mentoring and collaboration: a new training model for implementation science. *Implement Sci.* 2016;11(1):137. doi:10.1186/s13012-016-0499-y

This article presents evaluative findings of the value of mentoring over time through the National Institute of Mental Health (NIMH) supported by the Implementation Research Institute (IRI).

Selected Websites and Tools

European Implementation Collaborative. https://implementation.eu/training-and-education/

The European Implementation Collaborative has a curated list of education and training events and courses in the field of implementation research and practice, largely Europe-wide coverage.

Global Alliance for Chronic Disease. https://implementationscience-gacd.org/implementation-science2/toolkit/

Repository of useful tools and websites for implementation science research and practice including ongoing D&I projects, funding & collaboration opportunities, and other D&I-related activities.

Global Alliance for Chronic Disease. https://www.gacd.org/news/2021-03-15-launch-of-new-implementation-science-e-hub

The Global Alliance for Chronic Disease (GACD) provide an online learning hub providing knowledge and skill development in implementation research, particularly in relation to chronic and non-communicable diseases

National Implementation Research Network Active Implementation Hub. https://nirn.fpg.unc.edu/ai-hub

The National Implementation Research Network Active Implementation Hub provides free online learning to any audience interested in implementing and scaling up interventions.

Training Institute for Dissemination and Implementation Research in Cancer. https://cancercontrol.cancer.gov/is/training-education/training-in-cancer/TIDIRC-open-access

The Training Institute for Dissemination and Implementation Research in Cancer (TIDIRC) has open access training videos in implementation research.

UK Implementation Society. https://www.ukimplementation.org.uk/network-events-diary

The UK Implementation Society provides a curated list of events and training (and other implementation research- and practice-related resources), largely UK coverage.

UW Implementation Science Resource Hub. https://impsciuw.org/

The UW Implementation Science Resource Hub is a learning hub containing numerous resources to help you conduct implementation research.

REFERENCES

1. Norton WE, Lungeanu A, Chambers DA, Contractor N. Mapping the growing discipline of dissemination and implementation science in health. *Scientometrics.* Sep 2017;112(3):1367–1390. doi:10.1007/s11192-017-2455-2
2. Sales AE, Wilson PM, Wensing M, et al. Implementation science and implementation science communications: our aims, scope, and reporting expectations. *Implement Sci.* Aug 2019;14(1):77. doi:10.1186/s13012-019-0922-2
3. Brownson RC, Proctor EK, Luke DA, et al. Building capacity for dissemination and implementation research: one university's experience. *Implement Sci.* Aug 2017;12(1):104. doi:10.1186/s13012-017-0634-4
4. Chambers DA, Proctor EK, Brownson RC, Straus SE. Mapping training needs for dissemination and implementation research: lessons from a synthesis of existing D&I research training programs. *Transl Behav Med.* Sep 2017;7(3):593–601. doi:10.1007/s13142-016-0399-3
5. Davis R, D'Lima D. Building capacity in dissemination and implementation science: a systematic review of the academic literature on teaching and training initiatives. *Implement Sci.* Oct 2020;15(1):97. doi:10.1186/s13012-020-01051-6
6. Proctor E, Carpenter C, Brown CH, et al. Advancing the science of dissemination and implementation: three "6th NIH Meetings" on training, measures, and methods. *Implement Sci.* Aug 2015;10(1):A13. doi:10.1186/1748-5908-10-S1-A13
7. Straus SE, Sales A, Wensing M, Michie S, Kent B, Foy R. Education and training for implementation science: our interest in manuscripts describing education and training materials. *Implement Sci.* Sep 2015;10(1):136. doi:10.1186/s13012-015-0326-x
8. Bates I, Akoto AYO, Ansong D, et al. Evaluating health research capacity building: an evidence-based tool. *PLoS Med.* 2006;3(8):299. doi:10.1371/journal.pmed.0030299

9. Kislov R, Waterman H, Harvey G, Boaden R. Rethinking capacity building for knowledge mobilisation: developing multilevel capabilities in healthcare organisations. *Implement Sci.* Nov 2014;9(1):166. doi:10.1186/s13012-014-0166-0
10. Levine R, Russ-Eft D, Burling A, Stephens J, Downey J. Evaluating health services research capacity building programs: implications for health services and human resource development. *Eval Program Plann.* Apr 2013;37:1–11. doi:10.1016/j.evalprogplan.2012.12.002
11. Trostle J. Research capacity building in international health: definitions, evaluations and strategies for success. *Soc Sci Med.* Dec 1992;35(11):1321–1324. doi:10.1016/0277-9536(92)90035-o
12. Demakis JG, McQueen L, Kizer KW, Feussner JR. Quality Enhancement Research Initiative (QUERI): a collaboration between research and clinical practice. *Med Care.* Jun 2000;38(6)(suppl 1):17–25.
13. Kilbourne AM, Elwy AR, Sales AE, Atkins D. Accelerating research impact in a learning health care system: VA's Quality Enhancement Research Initiative in the Choice Act era. *Med Care.* Jul 2017;55 (7)(suppl 1):4–12. doi:10.1097/mlr.0000000000000683
14. Stetler CB, Mittman BS, Francis J. Overview of the VA Quality Enhancement Research Initiative (QUERI) and QUERI theme articles: QUERI Series. *Implement Sci.* Feb 2008;3:8. doi:10.1186/1748-5908-3-8
15. Dissemination and Implementation Seminar Series. Institute for Public Health. Washington University in St Louis. Accessed April 6, 2022. https://publichealth.wustl.edu/centers/dissemination-implementation/
16. Division of Cancer Control and Population Sciences. National Cancer Institute. Implementation Science Centers in Cancer Control (ISC3). Updated June 17, 2021. Accessed April 6, 2022. https://cancercontrol.cancer.gov/IS/initiatives/ISC3.html
17. Choosing Wisely Canada. Implementation and Research Network. Accessed April 6, 2022. https://choosingwiselycanada.org/implementation-research-network/
18. University of Newcastle. Priority Research Centre for Cancer Research, Innovation and Translation. Accessed April 6, 2022. https://www.newcastle.edu.au/research/centre/cancer
19. Kings College London. Centre for Implementation Science. Accessed April 6, 2022. https://www.kcl.ac.uk/research/cis
20. Global Alliance for Chronic Disease (GACD). World Health Organization Implementation Research Resources. Accessed April 6, 2022. https://implementationscience-gacd.org/who-ir/
21. Tinkle M, Kimball R, Haozous EA, Shuster G, Meize-Grochowski R. Dissemination and implementation research funded by the US National Institutes of Health, 2005–2012. *Nurs Res Pract.* 2013. doi:10.1155/2013/909606
22. National Implementation Research Network. Frank Porter Graham Child Development Institute. Home page. Accessed April 6, 2022. https://nirn.fpg.unc.edu/national-implementation-research-network
23. Washington University in St. Louis. Institute for Public Health. WUNDIR meetings. Accessed April 6, 2022. https://publichealth.wustl.edu/items/wundir/
24. UK Implementation Society. Home page. Accessed April 6, 2022. https://www.ukimplementation.org.uk/
25. Society for Implementation Research Collaboration. Home page. Accessed April 6, 2022. https://societyforimplementationresearchcollaboration.org/
26. Academy Health. 13th Annual Conference on the Science of Dissemination and Implementation in Health. Accessed April 6, 2022. https://academyhealth.org/events/2020-12/13th-annual-conference-science-dissemination-and-implementation-health
27. Global Implementation Conference. Home page. Accessed April 6, 2022. https://gic.globalimplementation.org/
28. King's College London. Implementation Science Masterclass. Accessed April 6, 2022. https://www.kcl.ac.uk/events/implementation-science-masterclass
29. Eccles MP, Mittman BS. Welcome to implementation science. *Implement Sci.* Feb 2006;1(1):1. doi:10.1186/1748-5908-1-1
30. BMC. *Implementation Science Communications.* Home page. Accessed April 6, 2022. https://implementationsciencecomms.biomedcentral.com/?gclid=EAIaIQobChMI7NyP7_fO9AIVc4BQBh1VngvLEAAYASAAEgJ9VvD_BwE
31. *Implementation Research and Practice.* Sage Publishing. Accessed April 6, 2022. https://us.sagepub.com/en-us/nam/implementation-research-and-practice/journal203691
32. *Implementation Science.* Frontiers in Health Services. Accessed April 6, 2022. https://www.frontiersin.org/journals/health-services/sections/implementation-science
33. Cochrane Qualitative and Implementation Methods Group. Home page. Accessed April 6, 2022. https://methods.cochrane.org/qi/welcome

34. Carlfjord S, Roback K, Nilsen P. Five years' experience of an annual course on implementation science: an evaluation among course participants. *Implement Sci*. Aug 2017;12(1):101. doi:10.1186/s13012-017-0618-4
35. Jones K, Armstrong R, Pettman T, Waters E. Knowledge translation for researchers: developing training to support public health researchers KTE efforts. *J Public Health*. 2015;37(2):364–366. doi:10.1093/pubmed/fdv076
36. Means AR, Phillips DE, Lurton G, et al. The role of implementation science training in global health: from the perspective of graduates of the field's first dedicated doctoral program. *Glob Health Action*. Dec 2016;9(1):31899. doi:10.3402/gha.v9.31899
37. Meissner HI, Glasgow RE, Vinson CA, et al. The US Training Institute for Dissemination and Implementation Research in Health. *Implement Sci*. Jan 24 2013;8:12. doi:10.1186/1748-5908-8-12
38. Padek M, Mir N, Jacob RR, et al. Training scholars in dissemination and implementation research for cancer prevention and control: a mentored approach. *Implement Sci*. Jan 2018;13(1):18. doi:10.1186/s13012-018-0711-3
39. Proctor EK, Landsverk J, Baumann AA, et al. The Implementation Research Institute: training mental health implementation researchers in the United States. *Implement Sci*. 2013;8(1):105. doi:10.1186/1748-5908-8-105
40. Ramaswamy R, Mosnier J, Reed K, Powell BJ, Schenck AP. Building capacity for public health 3.0: introducing implementation science into an MPH curriculum. *Implement Sci*. Feb 28 2019;14(1):18. doi:10.1186/s13012-019-0866-6
41. Ullrich C, Mahler C, Forstner J, Szecsenyi J, Wensing M. Teaching implementation science in a new master of science program in Germany: a survey of stakeholder expectations. *Implement Sci*. Apr 2017;12(1):55. doi:10.1186/s13012-017-0583-y
42. Vinson CA, Clyne M, Cardoza N, Emmons KM. Building capacity: a cross-sectional evaluation of the US Training Institute for Dissemination and Implementation Research in Health. *Implement Sci*. Nov 2019;14(1):97. doi:10.1186/s13012-019-0947-6
43. Albers B, Metz A, Burke K. Implementation support practitioners—a proposal for consolidating a diverse evidence base. *BMC Health Serv Res*. 2020;20(1):368. doi:10.1186/s12913-020-05145-1
44. Black AT, Steinberg M, Chisholm AE, et al. Building capacity for implementation—the KT challenge. *Implement Sci Commun*. Jul 2021;2(1):84. doi:10.1186/s43058-021-00186-x
45. Moore JE, Rashid S, Park JS, Khan S, Straus SE. Longitudinal evaluation of a course to build core competencies in implementation practice. *Implement Sci*. Aug 2018;13(1):106. doi:10.1186/s13012-018-0800-3
46. Center for Implementation. What we do. Accessed April 6, 2022. https://thecenterforimplementation.com/about-us
47. Metz A, Albers B, Burke K, et al. Implementation practice in human service systems: understanding the principles and competencies of professionals who support implementation. *Hum Serv Organ Manag Leadersh Gov*. May 2021;45(3):238–259. doi:10.1080/23303131.2021.1895401
48. Proctor E, Ramsey AT, Brown MT, Malone S, Hooley C, McKay V. Training in Implementation Practice Leadership (TRIPLE): evaluation of a novel practice change strategy in behavioral health organizations. *Implement Sci*. Jun 2019;14(1):66. doi:10.1186/s13012-019-0906-2
49. Provvidenza C, Townley A, Wincentak J, Peacocke S, Kingsnorth S. Building knowledge translation competency in a community-based hospital: a practice-informed curriculum for healthcare providers, researchers, and leadership. *Implement Sci*. Jul 2020;15(1):54. doi:10.1186/s13012-020-01013-y
50. Richter A, von Thiele Schwarz U, Lornudd C, Lundmark R, Mosson R, Hasson H. iLead—a transformational leadership intervention to train healthcare managers' implementation leadership. *Implement Sci*. Jul 2016;11(1):108. doi:10.1186/s13012-016-0475-6
51. Leppin AL, Baumann AA, Fernandez ME, et al. Teaching for implementation: a framework for building implementation research and practice capacity within the translational science workforce. *J Cli Transl Sci*. 2021;5(1):147. doi:10.1017/cts.2021.809
52. Boyce CA, Barfield W, Curry J, et al. Building the next generation of implementation science careers to advance health equity. *Ethn Dis*. 2019;29(suppl 1):77–82. doi:10.18865/ed.29.S1.77
53. Schmitt MH. Conceptualization: what is it and why is it important in the research process? *Oncol Nurs Forum*. Mar–Apr 1988;15(2):221–223.
54. Davis R, Mittman B, Boyton M, et al. Developing implementation research capacity: longitudinal evaluation of the King's College London Implementation Science Masterclass, 2014–2019. *Implement Sci Commun*. Sep 2020;1(1):74. doi:10.1186/s43058-020-00066-w
55. Baumann A, Brown M, Gerke D, et al. "Grant-writing bootcamp" and D&I toolkits: models for accelerating D&I research. In: *8th Annual Conference on the Science of Dissemination and*

Implementation; December 2015; Washington, DC.
56. Baumann AA, Morshed AB, Tabak RG, Proctor EK. Toolkits for dissemination and implementation research: preliminary development. *J Clin Transl Sci.* 2018;2(4):239–244. doi:10.1017/cts.2018.316
57. Proctor EK, Powell BJ, Baumann AA, Hamilton AM, Santens RL. Writing implementation research grant proposals: ten key ingredients. *Implement Sci.* Oct 2012;7(1):96. doi:10.1186/1748-5908-7-96
58. Tabak RG, Bauman AA, Holtrop JS. Roles dissemination and implementation scientists can play in supporting research teams. *Implement Sci Commun.* Jan 2021;2(1):9. doi:10.1186/s43058-020-00107-4
59. Chambers DA, Pintello D, Juliano-Bult D. Capacity-building and training opportunities for implementation science in mental health. *Psychiatry Res.* Jan 2020;283:112511. doi:10.1016/j.psychres.2019.112511
60. Proctor EK, Chambers DA. Training in dissemination and implementation research: a field-wide perspective. *Transl Behav Med.* Sep 2017;7(3):624–635. doi:10.1007/s13142-016-0406-8
61. Proctor EK, Landsverk J, Aarons G, Chambers D, Glisson C, Mittman B. Implementation research in mental health services: an emerging science with conceptual, methodological, and training challenges. *Adm Policy Ment Health.* Jan 2009;36(1):24–34. doi:10.1007/s10488-008-0197-4
62. Chambers D, Proctor EK. Advancing a comprehensive plan for dissemination and implementation research training 6th NIH Meeting on Dissemination and Implementation Research in Health: a working meeting on training. National Cancer Institute Division of Cancer Control & Population Science Implementation Science Webinar Series. January 28, 2014. Accessed April 6, 2022. Videocast available at: https://cancercontrol.cancer.gov/is/training-events/webinars/details/9
63. Brownson RC, Fielding JE, Green LW. Building capacity for evidence-based public health: reconciling the pulls of practice and the push of research. *Annu Rev Public Health.* Apr 2018;39:27–53. doi:10.1146/annurev-publhealth-040617-014746
64. Stamatakis KA, Norton WE, Stirman SW, Melvin C, Brownson RC. Developing the next generation of dissemination and implementation researchers: insights from initial trainees. *Implement Sci.* Mar 2013;8(1):29. doi:10.1186/1748-5908-8-29
65. Tabak RG, Padek MM, Kerner JF, et al. Dissemination and implementation science training needs: insights from practitioners and researchers. *Am J Prev Med.* Mar 2017;52(3)(suppl 3):322–329. doi:10.1016/j.amepre.2016.10.005
66. Brownson RC, Jacob RR, Carothers BJ, et al. Building the next generation of researchers: mentored training in dissemination and implementation science. *Acad Med.* Jan 2021;96(1):86–92. doi:10.1097/acm.0000000000003750
67. Jacob RR, Gacad A, Padek M, et al. Mentored training and its association with dissemination and implementation research output: a quasi-experimental evaluation. *Implement Sci.* May 2020;15(1):30. doi:10.1186/s13012-020-00994-0
68. Jacob RR, Gacad A, Pfund C, et al. The "secret sauce" for a mentored training program: qualitative perspectives of trainees in implementation research for cancer control. *BMC Med Educ.* Jul 2020;20(1):237. doi:10.1186/s12909-020-02153-x
69. Luke DA, Baumann AA, Carothers BJ, Landsverk J, Proctor EK. Forging a link between mentoring and collaboration: a new training model for implementation science. *Implement Sci.* Oct 2016;11(1):137. doi:10.1186/s13012-016-0499-y
70. Baumann AA, Carothers BJ, Landsverk J, et al. Evaluation of the Implementation Research Institute: trainees' publications and grant productivity. *Adm Policy Ment Health.* Mar 2020;47(2):254–264. doi:10.1007/s10488-019-00977-4
71. Schultes MT, Aijaz M, Klug J, Fixsen DL. Competences for implementation science: what trainees need to learn and where they learn it. *Adv Health Sci Educ Theory Pract.* Mar 2021;26(1):19–35. doi:10.1007/s10459-020-09969-8
72. Turner MW, Bogdewic S, Agha E, et al. Learning needs assessment for multi-stakeholder implementation science training in LMIC settings: findings and recommendations. *Implement Sci Commun.* Dec 2021;2(1):134. doi:10.1186/s43058-021-00238-2
73. Vroom EB, Albizu-Jacob A, Massey OT. Evaluating an implementation science training program: impact on professional research and practice. *Glob Implement Res Appl.* Sep 2021;1(3):147–159. doi:10.1007/s43477-021-00017-0
74. Friedman DB, Escoffery C, Noblet SB, Agnone CM, Flicker KJ. Building capacity in implementation science for cancer prevention and control through a Research Network scholars program. *J Cancer Educ.* 2022;37(6):1957–1966. doi:10.1007/s13187-021-02066-3
75. Gonzales R, Handley MA, Ackerman S, O'sullivan PS. A framework for training health professionals in implementation and dissemination science. *Acad Med.* 2012;87(3):271–278. doi:10.1097/ACM.0b013e3182449d33

76. Leung BM, Catallo C, Riediger ND, Cahill NE, Kastner M. The trainees' perspective on developing an end-of-grant knowledge translation plan. *Implement Sci.* Oct 14 2010;5:78. doi:10.1186/1748-5908-5-78
77. Norton WE. Advancing the science and practice of dissemination and implementation in health: a novel course for public health students and academic researchers. *Public Health Rep.* Nov–Dec 2014;129(6):536–542. doi:10.1177/003335491412900613
78. Osanjo GO, Oyugi JO, Kibwage IO, et al. Building capacity in implementation science research training at the University of Nairobi. *Implement Sci.* Mar 2016;11(1):30. doi:10.1186/s13012-016-0395-5
79. Park JS, Moore JE, Sayal R, et al. Evaluation of the "Foundations in Knowledge Translation" training initiative: preparing end users to practice KT. *Implement Sci.* Apr 2018;13(1):63. doi:10.1186/s13012-018-0755-4
80. Straus SE, Brouwers M, Johnson D, et al. Core competencies in the science and practice of knowledge translation: description of a Canadian strategic training initiative. *Implement Sci.* Dec 2011;6:127. doi:10.1186/1748-5908-6-127
81. Burton DL, Levin BL, Massey T, Baldwin J, Williamson H. Innovative graduate research education for advancement of implementation science in adolescent behavioral health. *J Behav Health Serv Res.* Apr 2016;43(2):172–186. doi:10.1007/s11414-015-9494-3
82. Wahabi HA, Al-Ansary LA. Innovative teaching methods for capacity building in knowledge translation. *BMC Med Educ.* Oct 2011;11(1):85. doi:10.1186/1472-6920-11-85
83. Gagliardi AR, Webster F, Perrier L, Bell M, Straus S. Exploring mentorship as a strategy to build capacity for knowledge translation research and practice: a scoping systematic review. *Implement Sci.* Sep 2014;9(1):122. doi:10.1186/s13012-014-0122-z
84. Allen TD, Eby LT, Poteet ML, Lentz E, Lima L. Career benefits associated with mentoring for proteges: a meta-analysis. *J Appl Psychol.* 2004;89(1):127–136. doi:10.1037/0021-9010.89.1.127
85. Burnham EL, Fleming M. Selection of research mentors for K-funded scholars. *Clin Transl Sci.* Apr 2011;4(2):87–92. doi:10.1111/j.1752-8062.2011.00273.x
86. Sambunjak D, Straus SE, Marusić A. Mentoring in academic medicine: a systematic review. *JAMA.* Sep 6 2006;296(9):1103–1115. doi:10.1001/jama.296.9.1103
87. Leung WC. Competency based medical training: review. *BMJ.* Sep 2002;325(7366):693–696.
88. Padek M, Colditz G, Dobbins M, et al. Developing educational competencies for dissemination and implementation research training programs: an exploratory analysis using card sorts. *Implement Sci.* Aug 2015;10(1):114. doi:10.1186/s13012-015-0304-3
89. Thacker SB, Brownson RC. Practicing epidemiology: how competent are we? *Public Health Rep.* Jan 2008;123(suppl 1):4–5. doi:10.1177/00333549081230S102
90. Campbell CR, Lomperis AM, Gillespie KN, Arrington B. Competency-based healthcare management education: the Saint Louis University experience. *J Health Adm Educ.* Spring 2006;23(2):135–168.
91. Gebbie K, Rosenstock L, Hernandez LM. *Who Will Keep the Public Healthy? Educating Public Health Professionals for the 21st Century.* Institute of Medicine; National Academies Press; 2003.
92. O'Donnell J. Competencies are all the rage in education. *J Can Educ.* 2004;19 2:74–75. doi:10.1207/s15430154jce1902_2
93. Alonge O, Rao A, Kalbarczyk A, et al. Developing a framework of core competencies in implementation research for low/middle-income countries. *BMJ Glob Health.* 2019;4(5):e001747. doi:10.1136/bmjgh-2019-001747
94. Shea CM, Young TL, Powell BJ, et al. Researcher readiness for participating in community-engaged dissemination and implementation research: a conceptual framework of core competencies. *Transl Behav Med.* Sep 2017;7(3):393–404. doi:10.1007/s13142-017-0486-0
95. Mallidou AA, Atherton P, Chan L, Frisch N, Glegg S, Scarrow G. Core knowledge translation competencies: a scoping review. *BMC Health Serv Res.* 2018;18(1):502. doi:10.1186/s12913-018-3314-4
96. Metz A, Louison L, Burke K, Albers B, Ward C. *Implementation Support Practitioner Profile—Guiding Principles and Core Competencies for Implementation Practice.* National Implementation Research Network, University of North Carolina at Chapel Hill; 2020.
97. Center for Implementation. Core competencies for implementation practice. Accessed April 6, 2022. https://thecenterforimplementation.com/core-competencies
98. Ford B, Rabin B, Morrato EH, Glasgow RE. Online resources for dissemination and implementation science: meeting demand and lessons learned. *J Clin Transl Sci.* 2018;2(5):259–266. doi:10.1017/cts.2018.337

99. Darnell D, Dorsey CN, Melvin A, Chi J, Lyon AR, Lewis CC. A content analysis of dissemination and implementation science resource initiatives: what types of resources do they offer to advance the field? *Implement Sci.* Nov 2017;12(1):137. doi:10.1186/s13012-017-0673-x
100. National Implementation Research Network. Active Implementation Hub. Accessed April 6, 2022. https://nirn.fpg.unc.edu/ai-hub
101. Hooley C, Baumann AA, Mutabazi V, et al. The TDR MOOC training in implementation research: evaluation of feasibility and lessons learned in Rwanda. *Pilot Feasibility Stud.* May 2020;6(1):66. doi:10.1186/s40814-020-00607-z
102. Ginossar T, Heckman CJ, Cragun D, et al. Bridging the chasm: challenges, opportunities, and resources for integrating a dissemination and implementation science curriculum into medical education. *J Med Educ Curric Dev.* 2018;5:2382120518761875. doi:10.1177/2382120518761875
103. Nooraie RY, Roman G, Fiscella K, McMahon JM, Orlando E, Bennett NM. A network analysis of dissemination and implementation research expertise across a university: central actors and expertise clusters. *J Clin Transl Sci.* 2022;6(1):e23. doi:10.1017/cts.2022.8
104. Dhand A, Luke DA, Carothers BJ, Evanoff BA. Academic cross-pollination: the role of disciplinary affiliation in research collaboration. *PLoS One.* 2016;11(1):e0145916. doi:10.1371/journal.pone.0145916
105. Curran GM. Implementation science made too simple: a teaching tool. *Implement Sci Commun.* Feb 2020;1(1):27. doi:10.1186/s43058-020-00001-z
106. Tabak RG, Khoong EC, Chambers DA, Brownson RC. Bridging research and practice: models for dissemination and implementation research. *Am J Prev Med.* Sep 2012;43(3):337–350. doi:10.1016/j.amepre.2012.05.024
107. Powell BJ, Waltz TJ, Chinman MJ, et al. A refined compilation of implementation strategies: results from the Expert Recommendations for Implementing Change (ERIC) project. *Implement Sci.* Feb 2015;10(1):21. doi:10.1186/s13012-015-0209-1
108. Proctor E, Silmere H, Raghavan R, et al. Outcomes for implementation research: conceptual distinctions, measurement challenges, and research agenda. *Adm Policy Ment Health.* 2011;38(2):65–76. doi:10.1007/s10488-010-0319-7
109. Chambers D. Preface. In: Brownson RC, Colditz GA, Proctor EK, ed. *Dissemination and Implementation Research in Health: Translating Science to Practice.* Oxford University Press; 2012:vii–x.
110. Colquhoun H, Leeman J, Michie S, et al. Towards a common terminology: a simplified framework of interventions to promote and integrate evidence into health practices, systems, and policies. *Implement Sci.* May 2014;9(1):781. doi:10.1186/1748-5908-9-51
111. McKibbon KA, Lokker C, Wilczynski NL, et al. A cross-sectional study of the number and frequency of terms used to refer to knowledge translation in a body of health literature in 2006: a Tower of Babel? *Implement Sci.* Feb 2010;5(1):16. doi:10.1186/1748-5908-5-16
112. Rapport F, Clay-Williams R, Churruca K, Shih P, Hogden A, Braithwaite J. The struggle of translating science into action: foundational concepts of implementation science. *J Eval Clin Pract.* Feb 2018;24(1):117–126. doi:10.1111/jep.12741
113. Waltz TJ, Powell BJ, Fernández ME, Abadie B, Damschroder LJ. Choosing implementation strategies to address contextual barriers: diversity in recommendations and future directions. *Implement Sci.* Apr 2019;14(1):42. doi:10.1186/s13012-019-0892-4
114. National Cancer Institute. Division of Cancer Control and Population Sciences. Implementation science webinars. Accessed April 6, 2022. https://cancercontrol.cancer.gov/is/training-events/webinars
115. Dissemination and Implementation Models in Health Research and Practice. Index. Accessed April 6, 2022. https://dissemination-implementation.org/tool/
116. National Cancer Institute. Division of Cancer Control and Population Sciences. Research Tools. Accessed April 6, 2022. https://cancercontrol.cancer.gov/is/tools/research-tools
117. Washington University in St Louis. Dissemination and Implementation Research. Toolkits. Accessed April 6, 2022. https://implementationresearch.wustl.edu/support-your-research/toolkits/
118. Mathematica Policy Research. PCORI dissemination and implementation toolkit. February 2015. Accessed April 6, 2022. http://www.pcori.org/sites/default/files/PCORI-DI-Toolkit-February-2015.pdf
119. Washington University in St Louis. Institute for Public Health. Resources for dissemination and implementation science. Accessed April 6, 2022. https://publichealth.wustl.edu/resources-dissemination-implementation/
120. NIH Fogarty International Center. Resources for implementation science researchers.

Accessed April 6, 2022. https://www.fic.nih.gov/About/center-global-health-studies/neuroscience-implementation-toolkit/Pages/resources.aspx

121. Global Alliance for Chronic Diseases (GACD). Implementation science. Accessed April 6, 2022. https://www.gacd.org/research/implementation-science
122. Baumann AA, Long PD. Equity in implementation science is long overdue. *Stanf Soc Innov Rev.* 2021;19(3):15–17. doi:10.48558/GG1H-A223
123. Brownson RC, Kumanyika SK, Kreuter MW, Haire-Joshu D. Implementation science should give higher priority to health equity. *Implement Sci.* Mar 2021;16(1):28. doi:10.1186/s13012-021-01097-0
124. Shelton RC, Adsul P, Oh A, Moise N, Griffith DM. Application of an antiracism lens in the field of implementation science (IS): recommendations for reframing implementation research with a focus on justice and racial equity. *Implement Res Pract.* Jan 2021;2. doi:10.1177/26334895211049482
125. Snell-Rood C, Jaramillo ET, Hamilton AB, Raskin SE, Nicosia FM, Willging C. Advancing health equity through a theoretically critical implementation science. *Transl Behav Med.* Aug 13. 2021;11(8):1617–1625. doi:10.1093/tbm/ibab008
126. Penkunas MJ, Chong SY, Rhule ELM, Berdou E, Allotey P. Designing the next generation of implementation research training for learners in low- and middle-income countries. *Glob Health.* Jun 2021;17(1):63. doi:10.1186/s12992-021-00714-3
127. Baumann AA, Cabassa LJ. Reframing implementation science to address inequities in healthcare delivery. *BMC Health Serv Res.* Mar 2020;20(1):190. doi:10.1186/s12913-020-4975-3
128. Lett E, Adekunle D, McMurray P, et al. Health equity tourism: ravaging the justice landscape. *J Med Syst.* Feb 2022;46(3):17. doi:10.1007/s10916-022-01803-5
129. Cabassa LJ, Baumann AA. A two-way street: bridging implementation science and cultural adaptations of mental health treatments. *Implement Sci.* Aug 2013;8(1):90. doi:10.1186/1748-5908-8-90
130. Shelton RC, Chambers DA, Glasgow RE. An extension of RE-AIM to enhance sustainability: addressing dynamic context and promoting health equity over time. perspective. *Front Public Health.* May 2020;8:article 134. doi:10.3389/fpubh.2020.00134
131. Woodward EN, Matthieu MM, Uchendu US, Rogal S, Kirchner JE. The health equity implementation framework: proposal and preliminary study of hepatitis C virus treatment. *Implement Sci.* Mar 2019;14(1):26. doi:10.1186/s13012-019-0861-y
132. Baumann AA, Woodward EN, Singh RS, Adsul P, Shelton RC. Assessing researchers' capabilities, opportunities, and motivation to conduct equity-oriented dissemination and implementation research: an exploratory cross-sectional study. *BMC Health Serv Res.* 2022;22:731.

INDEX

For the benefit of digital users, indexed terms that span two pages (e.g., 52–53) may, on occasion, appear on only one of those pages.

Tables, figures, and boxes are indicated by *t*, *f*, and *b* following the page number. Page ranges in bold indicate main discussions.